Orthopaedic Basic Science

Biology and Biomechanics of the Musculoskeletal System

2nd Edition

Orthopaedic Basic Science

Biology and Biomechanics of the Musculoskeletal System

2nd Edition

Edited by

Joseph A. Buckwalter, MD, MS

Professor and Chairman
Department of Orthopaedic Surgery
University of Iowa
Iowa City, Iowa

Thomas A. Einhorn, MD

Professor and Chairman
Department of Orthopaedic Surgery
Boston University School of Medicine
Boston, Massachusetts

Sheldon R. Simon, MD

Orthopaedic Department
Beth Israel Medical Center
New York, New York

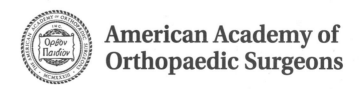

American Academy of
Orthopaedic Surgeons

Director, Department of Publications
Marilyn L. Fox, PhD

Senior Editor
Lisa Claxton Moore

Production Manager
Loraine Edwalds

Assistant Production Managers
David Stanley
Sophie Tosta

Production Assistants
Karen Danca
Geraldine Dubberke
Sharon O'Brien
Jana Ronayne
Vanessa Villarreal

Publications Secretary
Jackie Shadinger

Graphic Design Coordinator
Pamela Hutton Erickson

ORTHOPAEDIC BASIC SCIENCE: BIOLOGY AND BIOMECHANICS OF THE MUSCULOSKELETAL SYSTEM
American Academy of Orthopaedic Surgeons®

The material presented in *Orthopaedic Basic Science: Biology and Biomechanics of the Musculoskeletal System* has been made available by the American Academy of Orthopaedic Surgeons for educational purposes only. This material is not intended to present the only, or necessarily best, methods or procedures for the medical situations discussed, but rather is intended to represent an approach, view, statement, or opinion of the author(s) or producer(s), which may be helpful to others who face similar situations.

Some drugs or medical devices demonstrated in Academy courses or described in Academy print or electronic publications have not been cleared by the Food and Drug Administration (FDA) or have been cleared for specific uses only. The FDA has stated that it is the responsibility of the physician to determine the FDA clearance status of each drug or device he or she wishes to use in clinical practice.

At the time of this writing, bone screws placed posteriorly into vertebral elements have been cleared for use in this specific manner by the Food and Drug Administration (FDA) to provide immobilization and stabilization as an adjunct to fusion in the treatment of the following acute and chronic instability or deformities of the thoracic, lumbar and sacral spine: degenerative spondylolisthesis with objective evidence of neurological impairment; fracture; dislocation; scoliosis; kyphosis; spinal tumor and failed previous fusion (pseudoarthrosis). In addition, anterior vertebral body screws (cervical, thoracic, and lumbar) are Class II devices and can be used as labeled in vertebral bodies.

Furthermore, any statements about commercial products are solely the opinion(s) of the author(s) and do not represent an Academy endorsement or evaluation of these products. These statements may not be used in advertising or for any commercial purpose.

Second Edition

Copyright ©2000 by the American Academy of Orthopaedic Surgeons

ISBN: 0-89203-176-X (softcover)
         0-89203-177-8 (hardcover)

Library of Congress Cataloging-in-Publication Data

The histologic section on the cover is taken from a mouse tibia stained with trichrome, illustrating a bony fusion.
Courtesy of Jill A. Helms, DDS, PhD

Contributors

Hannu Alaranta, MD, PhD
Associate Professor, Head of the Rehabilitation Unit
The Invalid Foundation
Helsinki, Finland

Kai-Nan An, PhD
Director, Biomechanics Laboratory
Chair and Consultant, Division of Orthopedic Research
Professor of Bioengineering, Mayo Medical School
Mayo Clinic and Mayo Foundation
Rochester, Minnesota

Steven P. Arnoczky, DVM
Wade O. Brinker Endowed Professor
Director, Laboratory for Comparative Orthopaedic Research
College of Veterinary Medicine
Michigan State University
East Lansing, Michigan

Hannu T. Aro, MD
Professor of Surgery
Department of Surgery
University of Turku
Turku, Finland

Gerard A. Ateshian, PhD
Associate Professor of Mechanical Engineering
  and Biomedical Engineering
Department of Orthopaedic Surgery
Columbia University
New York, New York

Subhashis Banerjee, MD
Group Leader
Department of Pharmacology
BASF Bioresearch Corporation
Worcester, Massachusetts

Thomas M. Best, MD, PhD, FACSM
Assistant Professor of Family Medicine
  and Orthopaedic Surgery
University of Wisconsin Medical School
Madison, Wisconsin

Scott D. Boden, MD
Associate Professor of Orthopaedics
Director, The Emory Spine Center
Emory University School of Medicine
Atlanta, Georgia

Sue C. Bodine, PhD
Director, Muscle Research
Regeneron Pharmaceuticals
Tarrytown, New York

Earl Bogoch, MD, FRCSC
Associate Professor of Surgery
University of Toronto
Toronto, Ontario, Canada

Adele Boskey, PhD
Director of Research
Professor of Biochemistry
Hospital for Special Surgery
New York, New York

Mathias P. G. Bostrom, MD
Assistant Attending Orthopaedic Surgeon
Department of Orthopaedics/Research Division
Hospital for Special Surgery
New York, New York

Joseph A. Buckwalter, MD, MS
Professor and Chairman
Department of Orthopaedic Surgery
University of Iowa
Iowa City, Iowa

Edmund Y.S. Chao, PhD
Professor, Vice Chairman for Research
Department of Orthopaedic Surgery
Johns Hopkins University
Baltimore, Maryland

Denis R. Clohisy, MD
Associate Professor
Department of Orthopaedic Surgery
  and Cancer Center
University of Minnesota
Minneapolis, Minnesota

Andrew J. Cosgarea, MD
Assistant Professor, Orthopaedic Surgery
Assistant Director, Sports Medicine
Department of Orthopaedic Surgery
Johns Hopkins University
Baltimore, MD

William R. Creevy, MD
Assistant Professor and Vice Chairman
Department of Orthopaedic Surgery
Boston University School of Medicine
Boston, Massachusetts

Susan M. Day, MD
Attending Orthopaedic Surgeon
Grand Rapids Orthopaedic Surgery Residency
Grand Rapids, Michigan

John A. DiBattista, PhD
Associate Professor
University of Montréal
Hopital Notre-Dame du C.H.U.M.
Montréal, Québec, Canada

Frederick R. Dietz, MD
Professor of Orthopaedic Surgery
Department of Orthopaedic Surgery
University of Iowa
Iowa City, Iowa

Thomas A. Einhorn, MD
Professor and Chairman
Department of Orthopaedic Surgery
Boston University School of Medicine
Boston, Massachusetts

C. H. Evans, PhD, DSc
Professor
Orthopaedic Surgery
Center for Molecular Orthopaedics
Harvard Medical School
Boston, Massachusetts

David R. Eyre, PhD
Professor
Department of Orthopaedics
University of Washington
Seattle, Washington

Paul D. Fey, PhD
Assistant Professor
Medicine and Pathology and Microbiology
Department of Internal Medicine
University of Nebraska Medical School
Omaha, Nebraska

Gary S. Firestein, MD
Professor of Medicine
Chief, Division of Rheumatology, Allergy and Immunology
Department of Medicine
University of California, San Diego School of Medicine
La Jolla, California

Richard A. Fischer, MD
Department of Orthopaedic Surgery
Diagnostic Clinic
Clearwater, Florida

Evan L. Flatow, MD
Chief of Shoulder Surgery
Department of Orthopaedics
Mount Sinai Medical Center
New York, New York

Cyril B. Frank, MD, FRCSC
McMaig Professor in Joint Injury and
  Arthritis Research
Professor of Surgery
Chief, Division of Orthopaedics
University of Calgary and Calgary Regional
  Health Authority
Calgary, Alberta, Canada

Joel L. Frazier, MD
Assistant Clinical Professor of Surgery
Department of Orthopaedics
College of Medicine
The Ohio State University
Columbus, Ohio

William E. Garrett, Jr, MD, PhD
Associate Professor of Orthopaedic Surgery
  and Cell Biology
Duke University Medical Center
Durham, North Carolina

Kevin L. Garvin, MD
Professor of Orthopaedic Surgery
Department of Orthopaedic Surgery
University of Nebraska Medical Center
Omaha, Nebraska

Harry K. Genant, MD
Professor of Radiology, Medicine, Epidemiology
  and Orthopaedic Surgery
Department of Radiology
University of California
San Francisco, California

Steven Goldstein, PhD
Professor of Surgery
Director of Orthopaedic Research
University of Michigan Medical School
Ann Arbor, Michigan

Stuart B. Goodman, MD, PhD
Associate Professor and Head
Division of Orthopaedic Surgery
Stanford University School of Medicine
Stanford, California

Nadim J. Hallab, PhD
Assistant Professor
Department of Orthopaedic Surgery
Rush-Presbyterian-St. Luke's Medical Center
Chicago, Illinois

Joseph P. Iannotti, MD, PhD
Associate Professor, Orthopaedic Surgery
University of Pennsylvania School of Medicine
Philadelphia, Pennsylvania

Joshua J. Jacobs, MD
Crown Family Professor
Director, Section of Biomaterials
Department of Orthopaedic Surgery
Rush-Presbyterian-St. Luke's Medical Center
Chicago, Illinois

Frederick S. Kaplan, MD
Chief of the Division of Metabolic Bone Diseases
University of Pennsylvania School of Medicine
Philadelphia, Pennsylvania

David R. Karp, MD, PhD
Associate Professor of Internal Medicine
Simmons Arthritis Research Center
The University of Texas Southwestern Medical Center
Dallas, Texas

Jonathan J. Kaufman, PhD
Assistant Professor
Department of Orthopaedics
The Mount Sinai Medical Center
New York, New York

Christopher Keading, MD
Assistant Professor
The Ohio State University
Columbus, Ohio

Janet Kuhn, PhD
Assistant Professor of Surgery
University of Michigan Medical School
Ann Arbor, Michigan

Stephen L. Li, PhD
Senior Scientist
Biomechanics and Biomolecular Design
Hospital for Special Surgery
New York, New York

Richard L. Lieber, PhD
Professor, Department of Orthopaedics
  and Bioengineering
University of California, San Diego
San Diego, California

Louis Lipiello, MD
Professor and Director, Orthopaedic Research
University of Nebraska Medical Center
Omaha, Nebraska

Glen A. Livesay, PhD
Assistant Professor
Department of Biomedical Engineering
Tulane University
New Orleans, Louisiana

James V. Luck, Jr, MD
Professor
Department of Orthopaedic Surgery
UCLA Orthopaedic Hospital
University of California at Los Angeles
Los Angeles, California

C. Benjamin Ma, MD
Orthopaedic Resident
Musculoskeletal Research Center
Department of Orthopaedic Surgery
University of Pittsburgh
Pittsburgh, Pennsylvania

Cahir A. McDevitt, PhD
Staff Scientist
Department of Biomedical Engineering
Lerner Research Institute
Cleveland Clinic Foundation
Cleveland, Ohio

Henry J. Mankin, MD
Edith M. Ashley Professor of Orthopaedic Surgery
Harvard Medical School
Boston, Massachusetts

Carol D. Morris, MD, MS
Fellow, Orthopaedic Oncology
Department of Orthopaedic Surgery
Memorial Sloan-Kettering Cancer Center
New York, New York

John S. Mort, PhD
Associate Professor
Department of Surgery
McGill University
Montréal, Québec, Canada

Van C. Mow, PhD
Stanley Dicker Professor of Biomedical Engineering
  and Orthopaedic Bioengineering
Department of Orthopaedic Surgery
Columbia University
New York, New York

Michael Muha, MD
Hand Surgery Fellow
Department of Orthopaedics
The Ohio State University
Columbus, Ohio

Jeffrey C. Murray, MD
Professor of Pediatrics
University of Iowa
Iowa City, Iowa

Barry S. Myers, MD, PhD
Associate Professor
Department of Biomedical Engineering
Department of Biological Anthropology and Anatomy
Duke University
Durham, North Carolina

Elizabeth R. Myers, PhD
Associate Scientist
Biomechanics and Biomaterials
The Hospital for Special Surgery
New York, New York

Regis J. O'Keefe, MD
Associate Professor of Orthopaedics
Department of Orthopaedics
University of Rochester School of Medicine
Rochester, New York

Nancy Oppenheimer-Marks, PhD
Associate Professor
Department of Internal Medicine
University of Texas Southwestern Medical School
Dallas, Texas

Robert F. Ostrum, MD
Clinical Associate Professor of Orthopaedics
Ohio State University
Columbus, Ohio

Jacquelin Perry, MD, DSc (Hon)
Medical Consultant, Pathokinesiology Service
Professor Emeritus of Orthopaedics
Rancho Los Amigos National Rehabilitation Center
Downey, California

Charles G. Peterfy, MD, PhD
Assistant Clinical Professor
Department of Radiology
University of California at San Francisco
San Francisco, California

A. Robin Poole, PhD, DSc
Director, Joint Diseases Laboratory
Shriners Hospitals for Children
Montréal, Québec, Canada

Malcolm Pope, PhD, DMSc
McClure Professor of Orthopaedic Research
Department of Orthopaedics and Rehabilitation
University of Vermont
Burlington, Vermont

Peter Quesada, PhD
Assistant Professor, Orthopaedics
 and Biomedical Engineering
The Ohio State University
Columbus, Ohio

Bruce Rapuano, PhD
Assistant Scientist
Hospital for Special Surgery
New York, New York

Anthony Ratcliffe, PhD
Associate Professor
Department of Orthopaedic Surgery
Columbia University
New York, New York

Anneliese D. Recklies, PhD
Assistant Professor
Department of Surgery
McGill University
Montréal, Québec, Canada

Paul R. Reynolds, PhD
Associate Professor
Department of Orthopaedics
University of Rochester School of Medicine
 and Dentistry
Rochester, New York

Timothy P. L. Roberts, PhD
Assistant Professor of Radiology
Department of Radiology
University of California, San Francisco
San Francisco, California

Randy N. Rosier, MD, PhD
Professor of Orthopaedics, Oncology,
 Biophysics and Biochemistry
The University of Rochester
Rochester, New York

Clinton T. Rubin, PhD
Professor and Director
Center for Biotechnology
State University of New York
Stony Brook, New York

Mark E. Rupp, MD
Associate Professor of Medicine
Department of Internal Medicine
University of Nebraska Medical Center
Omaha, Nebraska

William Z. Rymer, MD, PhD
Professor, Departments of Physical Medicine and
 Rehabilitation, Physiology and Biomedical Engineering
Northwestern University
Chicago, Illinois

Robert Schneider, MD
Attending Radiologist and Director of Nuclear Medicine
Hospital for Special Surgery
New York, New York

Sheldon R. Simon, MD
Orthopaedic Department
Beth Israel Medical Center
New York, New York

Sharon Stevenson, DVM, PhD
Executive Director
Advanced Tissue Sciences
San Diego, California

Dale R. Sumner, PhD
Professor and Chairman
Department of Anatomy
Rush Medical College
Rush-Presbyterian-St. Luke's Medical Center
Chicago, Illinois

Wim van den Berg, PhD
Professor of Exp Rheumatology
Department of Rheumatology
University of Nymegen
Nymegen, The Netherlands

Cornelis van Kuijk, MD, PhD
Academic Specialist–Radiologist
Director, Imaging Research Center
Department of Radiology
Academic Medical Center, University of Amsterdam
Amsterdam, The Netherlands

John Varga, MD
Professor of Medicine
Department of Rheumatology
University of Illinois
Chicago, Illinois

Jennifer S. Wayne, PhD
Associate Professor, Department of
  Biomedical Engineering
Director, Orthopaedic Research Laboratory
Virginia Commonwealth University
Richmond, Virginia

Mark Weidenbaum, MD
Associate Professor of Clinical Orthopedic Surgery
Department of Orthopedic Surgery
Columbia University
New York, New York

Savio L.-Y. Woo, PhD
Ferguson Professor and Director
Musculoskeletal Research Center
Department of Orthopaedic Surgery
University of Pittsburgh
Pittsburgh, Pennsylvania

Timothy M. Wright, PhD
Senior Scientist
Hospital for Special Surgery
New York, New York

David J. Zaleske, MD
Chief of Pediatric Orthopaedics
Massachusetts General Hospital
Boston, Massachusetts

Jennifer Zeminski, BS
Graduate Research Associate
Musculoskeletal Research Center
Department of Orthopaedic Surgery
University of Pittsburgh
Pittsburgh, Pennsylvania

Yiping Zhang, MD
Associate Professor
Department of Medicine and Surgery
McGill University
Montréal, Québec, Canada

Reviewers

James R. Andrews, MD
Clinical Professor of Orthopaedic Surgery
University of Alabama at Birmingham
Alabama Orthopaedics and Sports Medicine Center
Birmingham, Alabama

James Aronson, MD
Chief, Orthopaedic Surgery
Arkansas Children's Hospital
Department of Orthopaedic Surgery
Little Rock, Arkansas

R. Tracy Ballock, MD
Assistant Professor of Orthopaedics and Pediatrics
Department of Orthopaedics
Case Western Reserve University
Cleveland, Ohio

Scott D. Boden, MD
Associate Professor of Orthopaedics
Director, The Emory Spine Center
Department of Orthopaedic Surgery
Emory University School of Medicine
Atlanta, Georgia

Mark E. Bolander, MD
Professor of Surgery
Department of Orthopaedic Surgery
Mayo Clinic
Rochester, Minnesota

Mathias P. G. Bostrom, MD
Assistant Attending Orthopaedic Surgeon
Department of Orthopaedics/Research Division
Hospital for Special Surgery
New York, New York

Barbara D. Boyan, PhD
Professor and Director of Research
Department of Orthopaedics
University of Texas Health Science Center
 at San Antonio
San Antonio, Texas

Eric Brandser, MD
Associate Professor
Department of Radiology
University of Iowa College of Medicine
Iowa City, Iowa

John J. Callaghan, MD
Professor
Department of Orthopaedics
University of Iowa Hospitals and Clinics
Iowa City, Iowa

Gregory Carlson, MD
Assistant Professor
Chief of Spine Surgery
Department of Orthopaedic Surgery
University of California, Irvine
Orange, California

Edmund Y.S. Chao, PhD
Professor, Vice Chairman for Research
Department of Orthopaedic Surgery
Johns Hopkins University
Baltimore, Maryland

Charles R. Clark, MD
Professor of Orthopaedic Surgery
 and of Biomedical Engineering
Department of Orthopaedic Surgery
University of Iowa
Iowa City, Iowa

Denis R. Clohisy, MD
Associate Professor
Department of Orthopaedic Surgery
 and Cancer Center
University of Minnesota
Minneapolis, Minnesota

William G. Cole, MD, PhD
Professor of Surgery
Department of Orthopaedics
The Hospital for Sick Children
Toronto, Ontario, Canada

Ernest U. Conrad III, MD
Professor of Orthopaedics
Department of Orthopaedics
University of Washington
Seattle, Washington

John Louis Esterhai, Jr, MD
Associate Professor of Orthopaedic Surgery
Department of Orthopaedic Surgery
University of Pennsylvania Medical Center
Philadelphia, Pennsylvania

Robert H. Fitzgerald, Jr, MD
Magnuson Professor and Chair
Department of Orthopaedic Surgery
University of Pennsylvania
Philadelphia, Pennsylvania

Mark C. Gebhardt, MD
Frederick W. and Jane M. Ilfeld
  Associate Professor of Orthopaedic Surgery
Harvard Medical School
Orthopaedic Department
Children's Hospital, Massachusetts General Hospital
Boston, Massachusetts

Richard H. Gelberman, MD
Reynolds Professor and Chairman
Department of Orthopaedic Surgery
Washington University School of Medicine
St. Louis, Missouri

Ronald P. Grelsamer, MD
Chief, Hip and Knee Reconstruction
Maimonides Medical Center
New York, New York

Jo A. Hannafin, MD, PhD
Assistant Professor of Orthopaedic Surgery
Associate Scientist
Department of Sports Medicine and Shoulder Service
Hospital for Special Surgery
New York, New York

John McArthur Harris III, MD
Associate Professor of Orthopaedics
Orthopaedic Section, Surgical Service
Boston VAMC
Boston, Massachusetts

Joshua J. Jacobs, MD
Crown Family Professor
Director, Section of Biomaterials
Rush-Presbyterian-St. Luke's Medical Center
Chicago, Illinois

Joseph M. Lane, MD
Professor of Orthopaedic Surgery
Weill Medical College of Cornell University
Department of Orthopaedics
Hospital for Special Surgery
New York, New York

Jay Lieberman, MD
Associate Professor
Department of Orthopaedic Surgery
UCLA School of Medicine
Los Angeles, California

Alan S. Litsky, MD, ScD
Associate Professor of Orthopaedics
  and Biomedical Engineering
Ohio State University
Columbus, Ohio

Cahir A. McDevitt, PhD
Staff Scientist
Department of Biomedical Engineering
Lerner Research Institute, Cleveland Clinic Foundation
Cleveland, Ohio

Shawn W. O'Driscoll, PhD, MD, FRCS(C)
Professor of Orthopedic Surgery
Director, Cartilage and Connective Tissue Research Unit
Department of Orthopedic Surgery
Mayo Clinic
Rochester, Minnesota

Theodore R. Oegema Jr, PhD
Professor
Department of Orthopaedic Surgery
University of Minnesota
Minneapolis, Minnesota

Vincent D. Pellegrini Jr, MD
Michael and Myrtle Baker Professor and Chair
Department of Orthopaedics and Rehabilitation
Milton S. Hershey Medical Center
The Pennsylvania State University College of Medicine
Hershey, Pennsylvania

Jacquelin Perry, MD, DSc (Hon)
Medical Consultant, Pathokinesiology Service
Professor Emeritus of Orthopaedics
Rancho Los Amigos National Rehabilitation Center
Downey, California

Scott Alan Rodeo, MD
Assistant Attending Surgeon
Assistant Professor of Orthopaedic Surgery
Cornell University Medical College
Hospital for Special Surgery
New York, New York

Clinton T. Rubin, PhD
Professor and Director
Center for Biotechnology
State University of New York
Stony Brook, New York

Thomas J. Santner, PhD
Professor and Chair
Department of Statistics
Ohio State University
Columbus, Ohio

Robert Schenck, Jr, MD
Associate Professor
Department of Orthopaedic Surgery
University of Texas Health Science Center
 at San Antonio
San Antonio, Texas

Thomas P. Schmalzried, MD
Associate Director
The Joint Replacement Institute
Los Angeles, California

Michael A. Simon, MD
Professor and Chairman, Orthopaedic Surgery
Department of Orthopaedic Surgery
University of Chicago
Chicago, Illinois

Harry B. Skinner, MD, PhD
Professor and Chair
Department of Orthopaedic Surgery
University of California, Irvine
Orange, California

Robert Lane Smith, PhD
Professor, Research
Department of Functional Restoration/Orthopaedics
Stanford University School of Medicine
Stanford, California

Marc F. Swiontkowski, MD
Professor and Chair
Department of Orthopaedic Surgery
University of Minnesota
Minneapolis, Minnesota

Richard M. Terek, MD
Associate Professor
Department of Orthopaedic Surgery
Brown University
Providence, Rhode Island

Laura L. Tosi, MD
Associate Professor of Orthopaedics and Pediatrics
Department of Orthopaedics
George Washington University
Washington, DC

Andrew J. Weiland, MD
Professor of Orthopaedic Surgery
Department of Orthopaedics
Hospital for Special Surgery
New York, New York

James Weinstein, DO, MS
Professor, Surgery and Community and Family Medicine
Center for Evaluative Clinical Sciences,
 Dartmouth Medical School
Dartmouth College
Hanover, New Hampshire

Orthopaedic Basic Science

Biology and Biomechanics of the Musculoskeletal System

2nd Edition

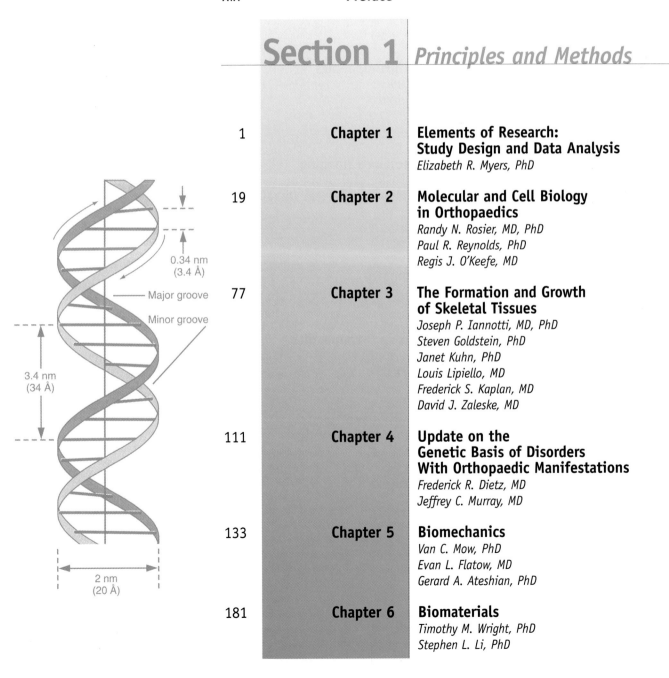

0.34 nm
(3.4 Å)

— Major groove

Minor groove

3.4 nm
(34 Å)

2 nm
(20 Å)

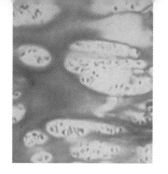

Section 1 Principles and Methods

Section 2 | Tissues and Pathophysiology

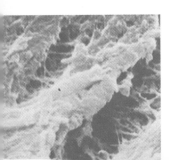
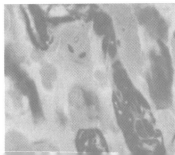

Section 2 *Tissues and Pathophysiology*

65°

70°

Section 2 | *Tissues and Pathophysiology*

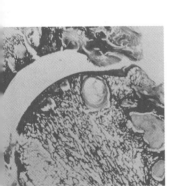

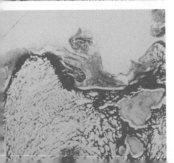

Preface

Optimal treatment of patients with diseases and injuries of the musculoskeletal system requires an in-depth understanding of the composition, structure, and function of the tissues that make up the musculoskeletal system and of how these tissues are integrated to form the organ system that provides the stability and mobility of the human body. Physicians and other health care personnel who treat patients with disorders of the musculoskeletal system need a comprehensive text that provides current information. This second edition of *Orthopaedic Basic Science: Biology and Biomechanics of the Musculoskeletal System* is an expanded and updated version of the previous text, *Orthopaedic Basic Science*, edited by Sheldon Simon. The goal of the editors and authors was to provide a useful, accessible synthesis of the basic science information needed for the care and treatment of patients with musculoskeletal disorders. In this text expert scientists and clinicians provide critical in-depth reviews of the structure and composition of the tissues that form the musculoskeletal system including bone, cartilage, tendon, ligament, muscle, and intervertebral disk. Other sections provide current reviews of essential information concerning the function of the musculoskeletal system and methods of evaluating and diagnosing disorders. Important new additions to the book include chapters on molecular and cell biology, genetic basis of disorders, pharmacology, MRI of the musculoskeletal system, bone densitometry, transplantation of musculoskeletal tissues, inflammation, neoplasia, and the intervertebral disk. Clinicians, scientists, and ancillary health personnel whose interests and efforts involve the musculoskeletal system will find this new edition a valuable resource for improving their understanding of the biology and biomechanics of the musculoskeletal system.

The editors and authors wish to express their appreciation to Marilyn L. Fox, PhD, Director of the Publications Department, Lisa Claxton Moore, Senior Editor, and Loraine Edwalds, Production Manager. Without their efforts it would not have been possible to complete the book and publish it in a timely fashion.

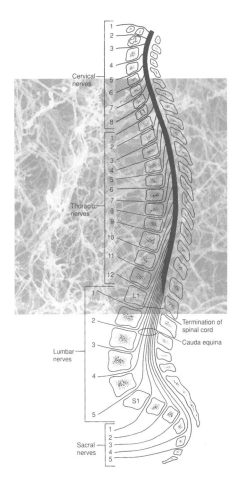

Joseph A. Buckwalter, MD, MS
Thomas A. Einhorn, MD
Sheldon R. Simon, MD

Section 1

Principles and Methods

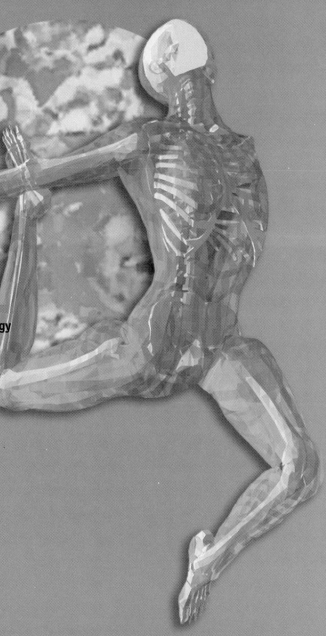

Chapter 1

Elements of Research: Study Design and Data Analysis

Elizabeth R. Myers, PhD

This chapter at a glance

This chapter describes the components of designing a study and the analytical approaches taken after data are collected, with the intent to provide an overview of analysis used in planning new research or in critically evaluating past and current studies.

Introduction

Many researchers have been faced with the problem of conducting a study and then not being able to reach a well-supported conclusion about the results. The reasons could range from not having enough subjects to performing an incorrect multivariate statistical analysis. When designing a study, steps should be taken to maximize the ability to reach conclusions and to infer from study findings the value of the work. This chapter first describes the components of designing a study followed by analytic approaches taken after data are collected. The intent is to provide an overview of analysis used in planning new research or in critically evaluating past and current studies.

Most orthopaedic research is probabilistic in nature, that is, the phenomena of interest occur with some random error. Each occurrence is not exactly the same as any other observation of the phenomenon. Probabilistic phenomena can be contrasted with deterministic problems, in which there is no allowance for error and each run gives the same value as the others. An example of a deterministic model is force = mass × acceleration, or Newton's Law. It is expected that an object of mass, under an acceleration, will generate force, with very little error in force for most practical purposes. The outcome is determined by the input values. There is little reason to apply statistical techniques of data analysis to deterministic problems because there is minimal variability associated with prediction of the results. However, in probabilistic research, analysis is required to determine if associations are likely caused by random error or are likely to be real. This aim is the basis behind most statistical analyses of research. This chapter deals with such techniques in orthopaedic research.

Such scientific studies can be broken down into 3 main components: a design phase, in which the scientist formulates a research question, chooses the subjects, determines the measurements, and plans the analysis; an implementation phase, during which the information is collected; and an analysis phase, in which descriptive summaries are generated and inferences are made based on the findings of the study. Overall goals of any scientific study are to be able to draw well-supported conclusions from the research and to convince others that the methods and interpretations are valid. To attain these goals, each component of research has specific aims. The aim of designing a study is to plan a convincing study and, when possible, to generalize the results to the world outside the study. The goal during implementation is to collect data while taking steps for quality control. The purpose of the analysis phase is to use appropriate statistical methods that estimate effects and assess the goodness of decision making.

Study Design

The point of designing a study in orthopaedic research before data collection is simple: to maximize the ability to draw valid and supported conclusions from findings in the study. In other words, the goal is to maximize both the internal and external validity of a study. Internal validity is the soundness of conclusions drawn within the study as based on the actual findings. External validity is the validity of inferences drawn from the study to the world outside the study. One recommended set of steps for designing a scientific study is shown in Outline 1. Maximizing the ability to generalize study results should be considered in all steps of study design. Reviewing the literature prior to beginning a study is essential; this information can impact proposed project design, analysis, and interpretation of results.

Research Question

The first step in planning a new study is to formulate a research question. Similarly, the first step in evaluating a completed study is to elucidate the research question. A research question is a statement of an unknown issue in science that the investigator wishes to address. Every study begins with a basic question or series of questions. Resolution of the research question is then considered by planning

---

Outline 1

Sequential Steps in Designing a Research Project

Research question:
Formulate the research question; review literature before proceeding

Study subjects:
Conceptualize the target populations
Plan the technique for obtaining the intended set of subjects from the populations
Establish a plan to minimize loss of actual subjects

Measurements:
Identify the properties of interest
Translate the properties of interest into intended variables of the study
Plan the actual measurements

Statistical analysis:
Formulate a working hypothesis based on the research question, subjects, and variables
Plan the statistical technique for testing the working hypothesis

Number of subjects:
Estimate the number of subjects or specimens

---

measurements or observations in subjects or specimens that represent appropriate characteristics in a population of interest. The research question should be new and important, but it must also be practical and workable. When stating the research question, the investigator should specify the unresolved issue, the properties of interest, and the general set of subjects or specimens. Some examples of research questions are: What is the prevalence of infection around a hip implant following joint replacement in patients with osteonecrosis? Does therapy that inhibits bone resorption result in a decrease in hip fractures in postmenopausal women? In the mature rabbit knee, does repaired cartilage have mechanical properties of normal cartilage in full-thickness cartilage defects?

During the formulation of the research question, it is important to decide whether to study the issue by observing events or by testing the effects of an active intervention or treatment (Fig. 1). If the investigator observes and measures uncontrolled events without altering them, then the study is considered nonexperimental or observational. However, if the investigator controls or manipulates events, then the study is considered an experiment. Observational studies can be further divided into descriptive studies, in which properties are described but relationships are not analyzed, versus analytic studies, in which relationships are analyzed. In analytic observational studies, the researcher must decide which properties are predictors and which are outcomes, although these designations are based on assumptions about cause and effect.

There are basic research questions that can be answered by either observational or experimental studies. For example, 2 possible studies could be designed and conducted to answer the question: Do high-impact forces during a fall contribute to hip fractures in elderly women? In the first study, the investigator decides to compute estimated impact forces by observing and gathering pertinent information about falls in female patients older than 65 years of age. The values for impact force are compared between a group with hip fractures and a group of control fallers without hip fractures. This is an analytic observational study in which the investigator does not impose controlled events on the subjects. In the second study, the investigator decides to study the effects of padding the trochanteric region in elderly female subjects. One group of patients wears an attenuating pad and a second group serves as controls with no padding, and the outcome of hip fracture is assessed. In this experiment, the investigator controls impact force with the trochanteric pad. There is no correct manner in which to conduct a study, and many issues enter into the decision of observational versus experimental investigations. Often a research question is first examined by an observational study to confirm significant associations between a predictor and an outcome, and then a more difficult interventional study is done to establish cause and effect. There are even some research questions that can only be studied by an observational approach.

Target Population and Study Subjects

The second step in designing a study or in evaluating an existing investigation is to delineate the target populations and the subjects or specimens to be assessed in the study. A population is the complete set of subjects or specimens of interest to the researcher with specified characteristics. In health research, these characteristics are defined typically by clinical and demographic traits. A sample is a subset that is selected from the population of interest. The units of study are the individual subjects or specimens that are assessed in a scientific investigation. In orthopaedic research, many clinical studies use individual humans as the units of study, but there are also musculoskeletal research projects that use organs, tissues, cells, specimens of synthetic material, or animals as the units of study. In the rest of this chapter, the terms subject and specimen will be used interchangeably to describe the unit of study.

The first consideration in choosing subjects for orthopaedic research is to envision the target populations. A population is defined by a set of clinical, demographic, geographic, and/or time-based selection criteria. An example of a target population is the set of adolescent females living in the United States with idiopathic scoliosis of a certain degree of deformity.

Next, a selection procedure is chosen to select a group of specimens from the population. In a few rare instances it is

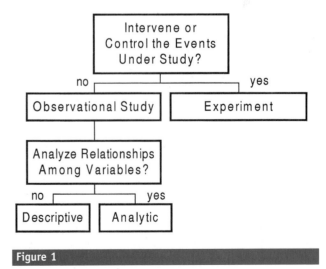

Figure 1

Comparison of observational versus experimental research studies.

possible to study the entire target population. However, the target population is often too large or unmanageable to study all members. In such cases, a procedure is required to select the subset of subjects that will make up the sample. External validity in choosing subjects is whether findings from the set of subjects can be generalized to a population of interest. External validity is of particular consideration in medical research using animals. Clearly, the animal subjects used in such a study are not a sample of the human target population. The process of generalizing, then, involves a judgment of what features in the animal study represent the human condition.

In clinical studies, there are several techniques for selecting the subjects. Random selection is marking every member of the population and then using a random technique for drawing a certain number of study units. Thus, random samples are those that each have an equal probability of being selected from the population. Selecting subjects randomly is a good method for obtaining a sample that will represent the underlying population, but it is often impractical to do in small, low-cost studies. Samples chosen by random selection are also called probability samples.

When it is not possible to draw a random sample, the subjects can be chosen by nonprobability methods. In consecutive selection, every available subject or specimen that meets the selection criteria is taken over a given time period or up to a certain number of units. As long as the time period is long enough to avoid seasonal effects, consecutive samples can work effectively. For example, all female patients between the ages of 12 and 18 years seen in a scoliosis clinic over 2 years from a given start date would make up a consecutive sample representing a population of adolescent girls with a certain degree of scoliosis in that geographic location.

There are many other selection techniques, including modifications of random sampling, and other nonprobability techniques such as selecting subjects based on convenience. Techniques that involve volunteers or convenience samples tend to be the least representative of the population. Findings from such a study can be distorted relative to phenomena in a population simply because the sample is nonrepresentative. Problems with such techniques include bias and confounding and can therefore yield limited conclusions.

During the design phase, it is important to establish strategies to retain as many subjects or specimens as possible within the intended set. If subjects or specimens are lost to measurements, then the internal validity of a study could suffer in that the actual subjects or specimens at the end of the study do not represent the intended set of subjects (bias). Minimizing such loss could require diverse approaches such as planning for effective recruitment and retention of human subjects or minimizing loss of specimens in cell culture. For example, an investigator is only able to contact and assess subjects who come into the scoliosis clinic during afternoons and, therefore, misses subjects participating in sports practice. The intended sample is meant to be a clinic-based consecutive sample, yet a group of important, active subjects is omitted. Strategies for encouraging participation in patient studies include making contact with every member of the intended sample and developing relationships between the study coordinator and subjects. Sometimes the best way to plan a study is to look at a previous study with successful recruitment strategies. For laboratory studies, strategies to reduce loss of specimens include providing training for technical personnel and establishing standard operating procedures for techniques.

Properties of Interest, Variables, and Measurements

A third step in the design phase of research is to identify the properties of interest, to define the intended variables, and to plan how the variables will be measured. The aim is to choose variables that represent the general properties of interest and to measure those variables with accuracy and precision. An example of a property of interest is infection around a hip implant, with the corresponding variable being the presence of bacteria after aspiration arthrogram, and the actual measurement being the reading of an investigator looking through a microscope at culture grown from the aspirate.

There are some basic concepts that must be understood to plan the variables effectively. The first is the idea of classifying the properties of interest into those that are predictive versus those that are responses or outcomes. The corresponding classification of the variables is into independent or dependent variables. Independent variables are those either controlled by the investigator in an experiment or chosen as predicting variables in an observational study. Independent variables are also known as factors, predictor variables, or effect variables. Dependent variables are the variables measured as outcome and are also called response or outcome variables.

The second concept is to determine the scale on which each variable is measured. Continuous variables take on values corresponding to points on a real number line. Discrete variables take on a finite number of values with quantified intervals. Categorical variables take on a finite number of values with qualitative intervals. The levels of a variable are the settings or possible values that the variable can take on; continuously scaled variables have an infinite number of possible levels, whereas discrete and categorical variables have a finite number of levels defined by the intervals. When levels are ordered in a categorical variable, it is called an ordinal variable. When there is no rank or order to the levels, the categorical variable is called nominal ("in name only"). Examples of each of these measurement scales are given in Table 1.

Considerations of validity should be made when planning

the variables and measurements. When picking variables to represent the properties of interest, the researcher should consider the external validity and make an informed judgment of how closely the variables represent the phenomena. For example, does the compressive failure load of a cadaveric spine specimen broken in the laboratory represent fracture risk in the elderly?

When designing the actual measurements, accuracy, the degree of agreement between the result of a measurement and the true value of the quantity measured, and precision, the degree of agreement of repeated measurements using the same protocol, are important to ensure that the values are valid internally. For instance, does the maximum axial force registered by a calibrated load cell during a compression test of an excised vertebra with end plates removed represent the failure load of the vertebra? Some strategies for increasing accuracy and precision include planning for calibration of the instruments, standard operating procedures, training time for the observer, automation of measurements, and use of objective measures if possible.

Testable Hypothesis

Once the research question is set, the subjects defined, and the variables identified, the fourth step is to take all that information, generate a working hypothesis, and plan the statistical approach. The working hypothesis is a formulation of the research question, and it includes a tentative statement that can be tested or investigated. The working hypothesis is a practical version of the research question. The immediate goal for stating this hypothesis is to set up a strategy for statistical analysis, and it is important to note

that this is done during the planning phase. The long-term goal is to be able to draw conclusions at the end of the study that answer the research question.

Research hypotheses involve an explanation of the phenomenon of interest and often provide explicit ideas about cause and effect. In an analytic study that will use statistical decision making, statistical hypotheses are also stated in addition to the research hypothesis.

Statistical hypotheses involve a concept called proof by contradiction. Both a null hypothesis and an alternate hypothesis are stated, and support for the research hypothesis is shown by rejecting or "nullifying" the null hypothesis. The null hypothesis (H_o) states that there is no association between predictor and outcome variables or that a treatment has no effect. The alternate hypothesis (H_a) states that there is an association between the variables or that the treatment has an effect. This alternate hypothesis is usually linked to the research hypothesis. By rejecting the null hypothesis, support is shown for the research hypothesis.

As an illustration of null and alternate hypotheses, the following research question should be considered: does therapy using dose A of Drug X increase bone density in the proximal femur of postmenopausal women in the United States? The specific research hypothesis is that hip bone mineral density measured by dual energy x-ray absorptiometry is changed by treatment with dose A of Drug X compared with placebo in a convenience sample of women aged 60 and older. The null hypothesis is that the mean bone mineral densities are equal between the treated and placebo groups, which are designated as group 1 and group 2:

$$H_o{:}(\mu_1 - \mu_2) = 0$$

and the alternate hypothesis is that the mean bone mineral densities are unequal;

$$H_a{:}(\mu_1 - \mu_2) \neq 0$$

where μ_1 = mean for group 1 treated with Drug X and μ_2 = mean for group 2 treated with placebo.

In studies of associations among variables, the statistical approach is determined primarily by the type and scale of the variables. This is why, in addition to considerations of validity, it is very important to plan the variables and to list the type and scale of each variable during the planning phase. If the researcher plans to use statistical significance testing, the choice of the statistical test is made during the design phase for several reasons: to assure that the working hypothesis is testable, to confirm that the capabilities for performing the analysis are available, and to determine the number of subjects or specimens.

The alternate hypothesis can be stated with or without a definite direction. A 1-sided or 1-tailed alternate hypothesis states that there is a specific direction to the association between variables or to the difference among groups. To

Table 1
Measurement Scales for Variables

Scale	Levels	Examples
Continuous	Infinite	Temperature
		Bone mineral density
		Fracture force
Discrete	Finite quantitative intervals	Temperature in intervals (30°, 35°, 40°)
		Number of alcoholic drinks per day
		Range of motion in intervals (10°, 20°, 30°)
Categorical	Finite qualitative intervals	
	Ordinal	Temperature (room, body)
		Pain (mild, moderate, severe)
	Nominal	Gender (male, female)
		Blood type
		Hip fracture (yes, no)

illustrate, a 1-sided hypothesis would state that there is a positive linear relationship between x and y or that group 1 has a greater mean value than group 2. A 2-sided or 2-tailed alternate hypothesis has no specific direction. One-sided tests should be planned when the scientist believes that medical or scientific meaning is only important in 1 direction. For example, a 1-sided hypothesis might be used in a study of compromised bone accumulation in girls wearing back braces for treatment of scoliosis. The hypothesis that brace treatment results in lower rates of bone accumulation may be of interest in musculoskeletal research, whereas the hypothesis that brace treatment results in greater bone accumulation than in unbraced subjects is not part of the research question and may not be of concern. When there is no clear, strong reason for directionality, it is recommended that the 2-sided approach be used.

It should be pointed out that confidence interval estimation is a strong alternative to statistical hypothesis testing that is gaining popularity in health research. The confidence interval is more informative than the significance test. A confidence interval is a bracket that has a certain level of confidence (often 95%) that the interval encloses a population parameter. Therefore, the confidence interval displays both the size of an effect and the variability of the estimate. Plans can be made during the design phase of a project to use interval estimation rather than or in addition to null hypothesis testing. Which method of analysis should be used? Both are used in basic and clinical orthopaedic science. A decision based on rejection of a null hypothesis is appropriate when the study is designed to make a choice between alternatives. The interpretation of the results is often clear and easy ("the difference in compressive strength between bone cement and the new polymer was significant"). In research areas such as epidemiology or orthopaedic treatment, however, confidence intervals are often preferred. Confidence interval estimation allows the clinical relevance of an effect to be evaluated because the magnitude and variability of the estimate are presented. Additional information and computational approaches for statistical decision making and confidence interval estimation are given in the section on data description and analysis.

Number of Subjects

A necessary step in designing any orthopaedic research project, before beginning the study, is to determine the number of subjects or specimens needed for an analytic study. There are very practical reasons for determining the number of subjects. The number of subjects impacts the feasibility, cost, ethical considerations, and the time scale of a project. If a large number of subjects is needed to ensure a certain probability of detecting an effect or a certain plausible range for a parameter, then it may not be feasible to perform the study at all.

What is involved in a determination of the number of subjects? It is necessary to know the statistical methods proposed for the study. Three other quantities are also needed: two originate from the probabilities the researcher is willing to accept in making a decision at the conclusion of the study and the third is based on the size of the impact that the predictor variables will have on the response. These 3 quantities are called the alpha level, the beta level, and the effect size; these terms are defined in the following paragraphs.

In statistical decision theory, 2 hypothetical states of reality are established. One is the null hypothesis (no association found) and the other is the alternate hypothesis (an association exists). After a study is implemented and results collected, a decision is made about whether there is sufficient evidence to reject the null hypothesis in favor of the alternate hypothesis. Thus, there are 4 possible outcomes after a study is completed (Table 2): the null hypothesis is rejected and in reality the alternate hypothesis is true (a correct and desirable decision); the null hypothesis is not rejected when in reality it is true (also a correct decision); the null hypothesis is rejected but in reality it is true (a type I error); and the null hypothesis is not rejected but in reality the alternate hypothesis is true (a type II error). Hopefully a correct decision will be made, but it is helpful to consider the probabilities of making the wrong decisions. Alpha is the probability of making the wrong decision when the null hypothesis is true (Table 2), that is, deciding that there is an association in the study when there is no association in the population. This type of decision is sometimes called a false positive, in that the result of the research study is positive (an association is found) but it is false. Alpha is then analogous to a false positive rate. Beta is the probability of making the wrong decision when the alternate hypothesis is actually true, that is, deciding that there is no association in the study when there is an association in the population. This decision can be thought of as a false negative; the study has a negative result (no association found) but that result is false. Beta is therefore analogous to a false negative rate. Scientific intuition should encourage the idea that alpha and beta (the false positive and false nega-

Table 2
Decisions in Analytic Studies

Statistical Decision in the Study	Reality	
	Null hypothesis is true	**Alternate hypothesis is true**
Do not reject null hypothesis	Correct $(1 - \alpha)^*$	Type II Error $(\beta)^*$
Reject null hypothesis	Type I Error $(\alpha)^*$	Correct $(1 - \beta)^*$

* Conditional probabilities of the decisions.

tive rates) should be set as low as possible to enhance the conclusions drawn at the end of a study. However, as described in the following sections, the number of subjects increases as the levels of alpha and beta are restricted, so a tradeoff is necessary in practice.

Power is the probability of rejecting the null hypothesis (in favor of the research hypothesis) in the study when the alternative is true in the population. This outcome often leads to support for the research hypothesis. Thus, it is important to have a study with high power.

Effect size is the magnitude of the effect of an independent variable on the dependent variable relative to the background variability or spread in the dependent variable. Consider the example of determining the impact of a categorical variable, drug treatment, with 2 levels (drug treatment can take on the value of "dose I" or "dose II") on a continuous response variable, bone mineral density (Fig. 2). For illustrative purposes, suppose that 2 separate studies are performed. The difference between doses I and II is the same for the data of study A and that of study B. However, the spread in the values for bone mineral density is much greater for the data of study B. For example, this greater spread could be caused by careless assessments in the second study resulting in more error in the determination of

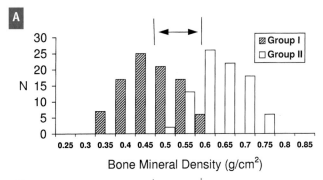

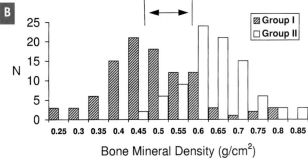

Figure 2

Example of how the effect size of a factor depends on both the magnitude of the effect and the spread in the data. Both parts of the figure show histograms of bone mineral density values in 2 groups. **A,** The difference in bone mineral density between Group I and Group II is large relative to the spread in values for bone mineral density. **B,** The difference between Groups I and II is the same as in study A, but the spread of data is much greater in both groups. Therefore, the effect size is smaller in study B compared with study A. More subjects would be required to detect the difference between groups in study B.

bone mineral density. The effect size would be smaller for the data of the second study compared with the first study. Furthermore, it would require more subjects to detect the difference for the second case at given levels of alpha and beta.

To determine the number of subjects needed for the study, the researcher first must decide on the maximum probability of making type I and type II errors. Ideally, alpha and beta should be set at small levels. Based on practical issues and tradition, alpha is often set at 0.05, but note that lower alpha levels should be used if it is critical to avoid false positives. Conversely, higher alpha levels could be used if avoiding false positives is not that important, such as for a therapy with clinically relevant potential benefits but with minimal side effects. Beta is often set at 0.05 to 0.2, which gives a power of 80% to 95%. These values for beta are also based on tradition and should be adjusted to suit a given study. Next the researcher estimates the effect size. This may seem like an example of the cart coming before the horse, but the estimate can be done based on pilot studies, values in the literature, or simply by making an educated guess at the size of the effect and the variability in the dependent variables. If an educated guess is used, it is helpful to estimate the number of subjects based on several reasonable values of the effect size.

It is worthwhile at this point to consider what strategies could enhance the probability of a successful outcome. There are 4 quantities involved: alpha, power (or beta), effect size, and number of subjects. Power is the probability of rejecting the null hypothesis when the alternative is true in the population (a successful positive outcome), so it is enlightening to consider the dependence of power on the other quantities. The relationships among power, effect size, and number of subjects are illustrated in Figures 3 and 4 for a Student's *t* test or comparison between 2 groups. The Student's *t* test is defined in the section on data analysis. Note that the power goes up as the number of subjects is increased for set values of alpha and effect size (Fig. 3). Thus, there is an obvious strategy that could be used to enhance the probability of a successful outcome: increase the number of subjects. When the total number of subjects is restricted, there are at least 2 other strategies that could help in certain designs. One is to amplify the "signal" of the information and the other is to reduce the "noise". Both of these act to increase the effect size, and the power of the study increases as the effect size goes up for set levels of alpha and number of subjects (Fig. 4). To increase the signal, a treatment or predictor variable can be planned that is thought to result in a large difference in the dependent variable. To reduce the noise of the study, precise assessments can be planned.

In summary, it is important to note that the components of a scientific study are sequential: a study must be planned and implemented before it is possible to make inferences based on the analysis. Steps in designing a study are straightforward: formulate a research question, pick the study subjects, determine the measurements, and plan the analytic approach and number of subjects. The benefits of giving consideration to the design of a study are also straightforward. Careful attention to the steps in study design can enhance the validity of conclusions after the study is completed.

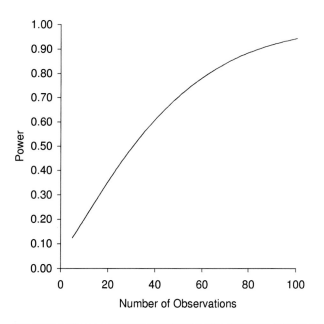

Figure 3

Relationship between power and number of observations for a comparison of 2 groups with a fixed effect size of 0.5 and a fixed type I error rate of 0.05. Power is related directly to number of observations or subjects.

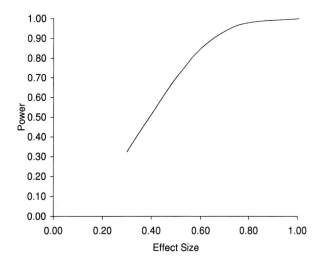

Figure 4

Relationship between power and effect size for a comparison of 2 groups with a fixed number of subjects (50) and a fixed type I error rate (0.05). The larger the effect size, the greater the power of a study for constant α and number of subjects.

Data Description and Analysis

Once the study is designed and implemented, the results need to be analyzed and inferences need to be made based on the study results. Just as there are practical steps in study design, there are also functional steps in analysis of results: screening data to maximize the quality, generating descriptive summaries of the data, checking assumptions, and performing analytic tests and calculating confidence intervals. These steps are shown in Outline 2.

Data Screening

Why screen the data? The main goal is to ensure an accurate data set. In the process, the researcher verifies that data are entered correctly, that each variable falls within a proper range, and that missing values are flagged.

Checks of data entry are perhaps the most tedious of the steps in the screening process but have been aided by the advent of computer programs for data entry. In the best of all worlds, a complete list of data is generated by the software program and checked on a cell-by-cell basis with the laboratory notebook or other original source of values. In addition, the investigator should check the following in the output: number of variables, number of observations, and format of each variable. Incorrect entries identified by this initial screening should be corrected.

Out-of-range values, or outliers, are observations that appear inconsistent with the remainder of the data set. Extreme values can be in a single variable only or in a combination of variables. Possible sources of extreme values include errors made in taking, recording, or entering data; cases that are not part of the population the investigator intended to represent; and values that are the result of extreme (but real) biologic variation. To detect outliers in a

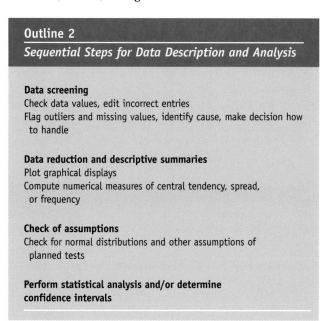

Outline 2

Sequential Steps for Data Description and Analysis

Data screening
Check data values, edit incorrect entries
Flag outliers and missing values, identify cause, make decision how to handle

Data reduction and descriptive summaries
Plot graphical displays
Compute numerical measures of central tendency, spread, or frequency

Check of assumptions
Check for normal distributions and other assumptions of planned tests

Perform statistical analysis and/or determine confidence intervals

single variable, the minimum and maximum values should be examined; to detect outliers in a combination of variables, more difficult multivariate procedures are needed.

What to do with outlying data depends on the source of the out-of-range value. If errors are made in data entry, the outlier is replaced with the correct value. If it is clear that the case is not from the target population, it is deleted from the data set. An example is the inadvertent inclusion of a young male cadaveric spine specimen with a fracture load of 10,000 N in a study of fracture in elderly female specimens only, with a range of fracture loads from 1,000 to 5,000 N.

If the outlier is suspected of being the result of extreme biologic variation, then the path to follow is not as clear. Most investigators simply live with the extreme value and accept any distortion caused by the outlier in the descriptive summaries and analysis. There are also mechanisms for handling outliers during analysis, such as techniques that adjust for skewed data. It should be noted that outliers may give insight into the phenomena under study and should therefore be examined carefully.

The approach to examining missing values is similar to that for out-of-range values. Sources of missing values include problems such as loss of specimens, poor patient recall, and equipment malfunction. Missing values should be detected and flagged in the data set. The cause should be determined if possible. The quantity and pattern of the missing information should be checked. Values that appear to be missing at random are much less of a problem in terms of distortion than values that are missing information in association with other variables in the study. For example, in a study of falls, impact location, and hip fracture, most of the subjects who cannot recall the location of impact during a fall are found to be in the fracture group. The subjects who readily identify the location of impact tend to be in the control group without fracture. Thus, there is an association between having a missing value for a key variable and fracture status. Consequently, deletion of these subjects could cause distortion of the sample.

The procedures for handling missing values should be done with care. Deletion of all data for a specimen or specimens with missing values is a possible alternative if there are only a few cases and they seem to be a random subset within the set. Similarly, the variable with missing values can be dropped from the data set, particularly if the missing values are concentrated within the variable and the variable is not crucial for answering the research question. Another common procedure is to impute the missing value based on nonmissing values for the variable or on relationships with other variables in the data set. A variable to be used in hypothesis testing with another variable should never be used to estimate missing values within this other variable.

Another approach sometimes used to handle missing information is to transform missing information into a new variable. This approach is taken when failure to have a value may itself be predictive of outcome. Such a tactic can yield interesting information about the phenomena under study but should be taken with caution. Typically, a dummy variable is created out of the variable with missing values. In the example used previously, the new variable would be labeled "ability to recall impact location" and would be coded as missing or complete. This new variable could then be used in the analysis. More complicated models can also be developed to describe the mechanism of missing data. For both outliers and missing values, the decision of how to handle the problem should be made before the data analysis.

Data Reduction and Descriptive Summaries

The second step in data description and analysis is to generate summaries of the data. How is a set of measurements described? The measurements could be presented in their entirety, but this would be of little help to the orthopaedic scientist in understanding the results. Instead, graphic displays are made or numeric measures are computed that represent the central tendency, the dispersion, or the frequency of the variables. There are many such methods for describing data sets; only a few methods used commonly in orthopaedic research are presented in this section.

Graphic methods for displaying distributions include frequency histograms and box plots. To form a frequency histogram, intervals are established from values of a variable and then the number of observations within each interval is determined. To form the histogram plot, the interval values of the variable are plotted on a horizontal axis and the vertical heights of bars are drawn proportional to the number of specimens within that interval. An example is shown in Figure 5 for fracture force from a study of cadaveric specimens from elderly female donors. The number of intervals is arbitrary but should be adjusted to the amount of data collected. Typically 5 to 20 intervals are used, with larger data sets requiring more intervals.

By examining the frequency histogram, the manner in which the measurements are distributed in the intervals is evident. In addition, the histogram can be used to determine what proportion of measurements have values greater or less than a certain value. For example, what fraction of spines broke at loads greater than 3,000 N? Based on Figure 5, six specimens out of 15 achieved fracture loads greater than 3,000 N, or 40%. Note that this is also the percent of the total area under the histogram. It is expected that the frequency histogram of a sample will provide information on the population frequency histogram, which is the histogram that would be generated if all values from the population were obtained.

A second method for graphic display of a set of measurements is the box plot. In contrast to the horizontal axis of a histogram, the distribution of a variable is displayed on a vertical scale in a box plot. First, a horizontal line is drawn at the midpoint of the measurements and then a box is constructed that divides the lower 25% of observations from the upper 75%. In addition, vertical lines mark the smallest and largest observations. Figure 6 is a box plot for the same data used to generate the histogram of Figure 5. If the actual data points are superimposed on the box plot, outlying values become readily apparent.

Numeric methods for describing data sets are intended to reduce the data to a limited set of numbers that conveys the

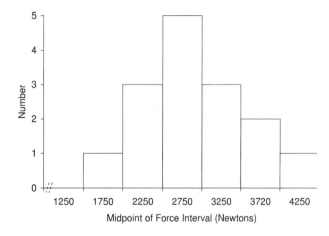

Figure 5

Example of a histogram. Data are plotted for the failure force in Newtons of 15 spine specimens. The horizontal axis depicts intervals of force values with interval widths of 500 N.

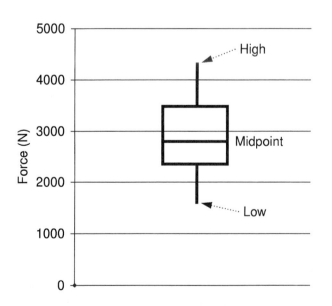

Figure 6

Example of a box plot. The same data as in Figure 5 are plotted in the box plot format. The vertical axis depicts force values on a continuous scale. The midpoint or median of the data array after ordering is plotted as a horizontal line. Then a box is drawn around the median line with the upper edge at the 75th percentile and the lower edge at the 25th percentile. The high and low values are also indicated by vertical lines.

distribution of the measurements. Scientists are often interested in numbers that describe the central tendency and the spread of observations within continuous and discrete variables. In certain cases, it is possible to summarize the entire set of measurements for a given continuous variable with two numbers, one that reflects the center and another that reflects the dispersion.

The sample mean is equal to the sum of a set of measurements divided by the number of observations:

$$Mean: \quad \bar{y} = \frac{\sum_{i=1}^{n} y_i}{n}$$

where y_i is the specific value of the variable y for the ith observation and n is the total number of observations. The sample mean can be used as a measure of central tendency for a continuous variable if the distribution is roughly bell-shaped (the histogram of Figure 5 is an example). The sample mean is used to estimate the population mean (μ), which is generally unknown. If the population distribution is bell-shaped, the population mean is the center of the distribution and the most probable value within the population.

Other measures of central tendency include the median and the mode. The median of a set of n measurements is the value that falls in the middle of the ordered measurements.

$$Median: \quad \frac{y_i + y_{i+1}}{2}, \, i = \frac{n}{2}, \, n \text{ even}$$

$$y_{i}, \, i = \frac{n+1}{2}, \, n \text{ odd}$$

The mode is the most frequently occurring measurement in a set of measurements and is often used with discrete and categoric data.

Measures of dispersion or spread in the data include the variance, standard deviation, range, and interquartile range. The sample variance (s^2) is:

$$s^2 = \frac{1}{n-1} \sum_{i=1}^{n} (y_i - \bar{y})^2$$

Note that y_i minus the mean is a measure of the deviation of that specific measurement from the mean. Thus, the variance reflects the average of the squares of the deviations of the measurements about their mean. When the variance is large, the data are more dispersed than when the number is small. The sample standard deviation (s) is the positive square root of the variance:

$$Sample \; standard \; deviation: \quad s = \sqrt{s^2}$$

The sample variance is an estimate of the population variance (σ^2), which, like the population mean, is generally unknown.

Other indicators of sample variability include measures such as the range, which is the difference between the largest and smallest value of y, and the interquartile range, which is the difference between the third quartile and the first quartile of a set of measurements. The first quartile is the value of y that separates the lower 25% from the upper 75% of values, and the third quartile is the value that separates the lower 75% from the upper 25%. Fifty percent of values fall within the interquartile range.

Several descriptors are used with nominal variables. A proportion is the number of measurements with a particular level of a nominal variable divided by the total number of measurements. For example, if 36 out of 50 patients with hip fracture are women, then the proportion of women is 36/50 or 0.72. A ratio is the number of measurements with a particular level of a nominal variable divided by the number of measurements without that value. The ratio of women with hip fracture to men with hip fracture is 36/14 or 2.6. A rate is a proportion determined over a period of time. A well known illustration of a rate in medicine is the incidence of a disease, which is the number of new cases of a disease divided by the total number of people at risk over a certain time period.

Checking Assumptions for Analytic Techniques

Parameters are numeric descriptive quantities that characterize the population, such as the population mean or standard deviation. Many analytic tests assume that the parameter being analyzed comes from a population with a certain frequency distribution called the normal probability distribution (Fig. 7). Therefore, before going on to the strategy for checking assumptions, it is necessary to review the concepts behind a normal distribution.

A large number of continuous variables in nature possess a frequency distribution with many values near the mean and progressively fewer values toward the extremes of the range. If the number of observations is large, the distribution is bell shaped and approximates a normal distribution. Examples include the height and weight of humans, bone mechanical properties, or bone density. In Figure 8, actual values for bone mineral density in a sample of 120 postmenopausal women are plotted in a frequency histogram. The cluster of values near the mean and the approximate bell shape can be seen.

The equation of the normal curve is given by the normal probability density function:

$$f(y) = \left(\frac{1}{\sigma\sqrt{2\Pi}}\right)e^{-[(y-\mu)^2/2\sigma^2]}$$

This is the equation of the bell-shaped curve illustrated in Figure 7 where μ is the population mean and σ is the standard deviation. Note that the area under the curve to the right of a given value of y represents the probability that y will be greater than or equal to the given value.

The normal score (z) gives the distance that y is from the mean in number of standard deviations:

$$z = \frac{y-\mu}{\sigma}$$

If z = 1, then the corresponding y is one standard deviation away from the mean. If z = 0, y is equal to the mean. The probability distribution for z is called the standard normal distribution (Fig. 9). The probability that z belongs to some interval is equal to the corresponding area under the standard normal curve, and the total area under the curve is equal to 1. To illustrate the use of the standardized normal curve, consider the following question: What is the value of z (call it z_0) such that 95% of z values fall within -z_0 and +z_0? Based on Figure 9, the area under the curve between z = 0

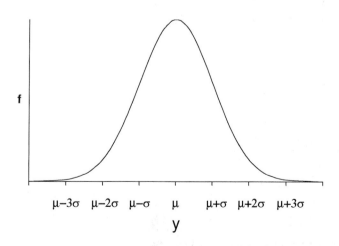

f

μ−3σ   μ−2σ   μ−σ   μ   μ+σ   μ+2σ   μ+3σ

y

Figure 7

Normal probability distribution. The horizontal axis depicts the variable y and the vertical axis is the value of the normal density at (f). The peak of the normal probability distribution corresponds to y = mean (μ).

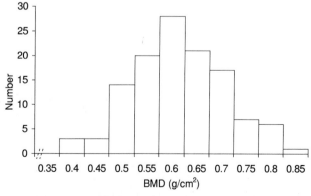

Figure 8

Histogram of bone mineral density in 120 postmenopausal women.

and 1.96 is 0.475 and, with symmetry, the area between z = -1.96 and +1.96 is 0.95. Therefore, z_0 = 1.96 and it can be seen that 95% of values fall within 1.96 or approximately 2 standard deviations of the mean.

Just as variables often have a bell-shaped distribution with many values near the mean and progressively fewer values near the extremes or tails, so do the means of a given variable from multiple random samples drawn from a population. In other words, if many samples are drawn randomly from a population, the means of these samples will form a normal distribution. Many of the means will be near the mean of the means but a few will be far away. Even if the underlying population is not normal, the distribution of the means will tend toward normality as the number of observations within each of the samples increases. This leads to the definition of the standard error of the mean, which should not be confused with the standard deviation. The sample standard error of the mean (SEM) is the square root of the sample variance of the distribution of means and is equal to the sample standard deviation divided by the square root of n:

$$SEM = \frac{s}{\sqrt{n}}$$

Note that the sample SEM is not a measure of the dispersion of a set of observations but a measure of the dispersion of the mean. Some call it an assessment of the precision of the estimate of the mean. It should not be used as an expression of the spread of a variable nor as an estimate of the population spread. SEM gives important information, however, when comparing means.

If an assumption for the analysis is that the observations have a normal distribution, then the sample distribution should be assessed before proceeding with analysis. A graphic display of the histogram should be checked for skewness and kurtosis. A skewed variable is one with the mean not in the center of the distribution. An example of a skewed distribution is shown in Figure 10 for the body mass index of 50 adolescent girls. Although many values tend to cluster near 18 to 20 kg/m², there are several subjects with quite high values for body mass index, resulting in positive skewness. A variable with kurtosis has either too many cases in the tails of the distribution or too few observations in the tails. There are also hypothesis tests for assessing departure from normality, such as the Shapiro-Wilk or W statistic and the Kolmogorow-Smirov test.

If there is departure from normality, there are nonparametric tests that do not rely on parameters such as the mean and standard deviation. There are also transformation functions that can be applied to variables to reduce skewness or kurtosis. This is often the reasoning behind logarithmic or square-root transformations of data in orthopaedic research. Taking the logarithm of y will sometimes pull in the tail of a skewed distribution. Note that transforming variables may make it difficult to describe and interpret results. For example, it is difficult to interpret the logarithm of body mass index.

The mean and standard deviation are appropriate measures of central tendency and dispersion only if the data have an approximate normal distribution. In situations with marked deviation from a normal distribution, the median and the range or interquartile range can be used as measures of central tendency and dispersion.

Other assumptions for analytic tests depend on the specific tests themselves. Some frequently required assumptions include independence of observations and equality of variances among groups. The researcher and critical

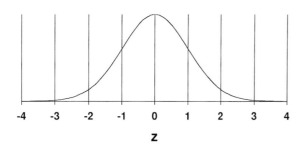

z	Area between 0 & z	Area to right of z
0	0	
1.645	0.45	0.05
1.96	0.4750	0.025
2	0.4772	0.0228
2.580	0.495	0.005
infinity	0.5	

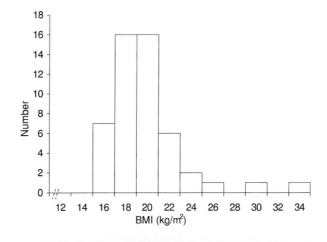

Figure 9

Standard normal distribution for the normal score (z). Area under the standard normal curve represents probability.

Figure 10

Histogram of the body mass index (BMI) of 50 adolescent female subjects.

reviewer should be aware that a given parameter estimate or hypothesis test may have underlying assumptions that should be checked.

Statistical Analysis

The culminating step to data description and analysis is to perform statistical analyses. The objective is to make inferences about a population based on information gathered in the sample of a research study. It is important to understand that parameters determined in a study (values such as the sample mean and standard deviation or the difference between 2 means) do not necessarily completely represent the values of the underlying population. Typically, studies are limited by factors such as small numbers of specimens or large biologic variability. Therefore, researchers are called upon to estimate population values and sometimes to make decisions concerning the value of a parameter.

Strategies to analyze results tend to fall into 2 categories: tests of hypotheses concerning values of parameters (statistical decision making; also called the significance test) and estimations of parameter values (point and interval estimates). Most everyone who has read scientific literature over the last century is familiar with the significance test. Some of the underlying ideas behind significance tests have been described in this chapter in the section on Study Design (see subsections Testable Hypothesis and Number of Subjects) and are covered in more depth in some of the suggested references. In many designs, a straw man (null hypothesis) is set up and an attempt is made to strike it down with the data of the study. The researcher and critical reviewer should keep in mind, however, that there are limitations to significance tests. Performing a significance test is a decision-making process. The significance test treats the acceptance or rejection of a hypothesis as a decision the researcher makes based on the data. As such, the test may only give a yes-no decision about a parameter. There is no sense of the size or strength of an effect or the nature of a relationship. An interval estimate, on the other hand, contains this important, additional information. Therefore, although reports of significant tests may be more familiar in orthopaedic publications, researchers should consider using confidence intervals to report results in the literature. Many experts have a strong preference for interval estimation over significance tests (see bibliography). Insomuch as both approaches are currently followed in orthopaedic science, techniques for performing significance tests and for determining point and interval estimates are described in the following sections.

A significance test involves a specific procedure that depends on the design of the study. Some of the frequently used parameters and the corresponding parametric significance tests are shown in Table 3. The anatomy of a statistical significance test is consistent among the many techniques (Outline 3). The basic question is whether an observed association in a sample could be the result of random error. Null and alternate hypotheses are stated and a single number called the test statistic is computed based on the sample information. If the magnitude of the test statistic is large enough, it is considered inconsistent with the truth of the null hypothesis and the null hypothesis is rejected. The p-value (p), also called the observed significance or associated probability, is the probability that the

Table 3
Techniques for Statistical Inference About Parameters

Parameter	Technique
Mean	One-sample t test
Difference between 2 means	Two-sample t test
Difference between paired means	Paired-difference t test
Difference between 2 variances	F test
Difference among > 2 means	Analysis of variance
Difference among > 2 means with trial factor	Repeated measures analysis of variance
Linear association between 2 variables	Correlation
Slope between 2 variables	Regression

Outline 3
Basic Setup for Statistical Significance Test

Null hypothesis (H_o):
No difference or no association

Alternate hypothesis (H_a):
Difference or an association specified by the investigator

Test statistic:
Function of the data and parameters that are known

Degrees of freedom:
Function of number of measurements

p-value:
Probability of obtaining a value of the test statistic at least as extreme as the value observed given that H_o is true; depends on magnitude of test statistic and degrees of freedom

Type I error rate (α):
Probability of erroneously rejecting H_o; set during design of study

Decision:
If $p \leq \alpha$, reject H_o

test statistic could be at least this extreme assuming the null hypothesis is true. The *p*-value is compared against the alpha level set during the design of the study. If the *p*-value is less than or equal to the alpha level, then the null hypothesis is rejected.

To illustrate the use of a significance test, consider the comparison of 2 means, which uses the test statistic called Student's t:

$$H_o: (\mu_1 - \mu_2) = D_o$$

$$H_a: (\mu_1 - \mu_2) \neq D_o$$

$$\text{Test Statistic: } t = \frac{(\bar{y}_1 - \bar{y}_2) - D_o}{S\sqrt{\frac{1}{n_1} + \frac{1}{n_2}}}$$

$$\text{Degrees of Freedom: } \nu = n_1 + n_2 - 2$$

Further details of the t test are given in Outline 4 and in the selected bibliography, but the basic idea behind a significance test can be understood by considering the test statistic. Note that the hypotheses are stated for the population parameters but that the test statistic is calculated from the sample data. The value of t will be large if the difference between the mean for sample 1 and the mean for sample 2 is large relative to the assumed difference, D_o. In most studies, the assumed difference is zero ($D_o = 0$). The value of t will also be large if the pooled standard deviation (s_p) is small. The statistic, therefore, captures important information about the comparison of 2 means. If the magnitude of t is very large, then it is plausible that the value is not the result of random error under the given condition (H_o) that there is no difference.

A case-control study of bone mineral density in hip fracture sufferers versus controls can be used as an example. The research question is whether bone mineral density is different in postmenopausal women with hip fracture than in controls without fracture. This question is translated into a 2-sided hypothesis test. Two samples are drawn in a consecutive fashion from a hospital orthopaedic floor: one group has hip fracture and the other has fallen without hip fracture. Bone mineral density is assessed in the proximal femur (Table 4), and the corresponding t value is:

$$t = \frac{0.64 g/cm^2 - 0.56 g/cm^2}{(0.12 g/cm^2)\sqrt{\frac{1}{10} + \frac{1}{12}}} = 1.56$$

For degrees of freedom equal to 20, the *p*-value (area under the t distribution to the right of t = 1.56 and to the left of t = -1.56) is *p* = 0.13. Thus, there is insufficient evidence to reject the null hypothesis or to support a conclusion of any difference between the means of the 2 populations.

A second analytic strategy is estimation of a population value based on data from the research study, including both point and interval estimates. A point estimate is a single number that estimates the parameter of interest. For instance, the difference between 2 sample means can serve as a point estimator of the difference between 2 population means. An interval estimate gives a plausible range for a parameter and, as such, contains very important information. To illustrate, the confidence interval of the difference between 2 means provides an assessment of the plausible range of the difference between 2 population means rather than just a point estimate. If this confidence interval overlaps zero, then it is plausible that the true values for the 2 means are not different. But if the range is large, then the plausible values for the difference cover broad ground.

The width of a confidence interval depends on the variability in the data, the number of subjects or specimens, and on a value called the confidence coefficient (1-α). The level of confidence is often expressed as a percentage: 100 (1-α). It is arbitrary but is often set at 90% or 95%. For a confidence level of 95%, the estimated interval would enclose the population parameter 95% of the time if repeated studies were performed.

The upper and lower bounds of a confidence interval are

Table 4

Example of Data for Comparison of Two Means: Femoral Bone Mineral Density (BMD) for Control and Hip Fracture Groups

Group	Mean BMD (g/cm²)	s (g/cm²)	n	95% confidence interval (g/cm²)
Control	0.64	0.13	10	0.55 - 0.73
Hip Fracture	0.56	0.11	12	0.49 - 0.63
Pooled		0.12		

Table 5

Nonparametric Counterparts for Some Common Parametric Tests

Parametric	Nonparametric
Student's t test	Mann-Whitney or Wilcoxon rank-sum
Paired difference t test	Wilcoxon signed rank
One-way analysis of variance	Kruskal-Wallis
Two-way analysis of variance	Friedman
Linear correlation	Kendall or Spearman rank correlation

Outline 4

Inference About Mean: One Sample t test

Null hypothesis (H_o):	$\mu = \mu_o$
Alternate hypothesis (H_a):	$\mu \neq \mu_o$ OR $\mu < \mu_o$ OR $\mu > \mu_o$ (specified by investigator)
Test statistic:	$t = \dfrac{\bar{y} - \mu_o}{s/\sqrt{n}}$
Degrees of freedom:	$\nu = n - 1$
p-value:	One-tailed: area under t_{n-1} distribution to the right of t if $H_a = \mu > \mu_o$ or to the left of t if $H_a = \mu < \mu_o$. Two-tailed: sum of areas under t_{n-1} distribution to the right of $\mid t \mid$ and to the left of $-\mid t \mid$
Decision:	If $p \leq \alpha$, reject H_o
Assumptions:	Random sample Sampled population has normal probability distribution with unknown mean μ and unknown variance
Confidence interval $100 \times (1 - \alpha)$:	$\bar{y} \pm \dfrac{t_{n-1,\alpha/2}s}{\sqrt{n}}$

calculated from formulas specific to the parameter of interest. For example, the confidence interval for the population mean is:

$$\bar{y} \pm \frac{t_{\alpha/2}s}{\sqrt{n}}$$

where $(1-\alpha)$ is the confidence coefficient. The 95% confidence intervals for the previous example of bone mineral density are given in Table 5. The plausible values for population mean bone density for hip fracture patients are between 0.49 and 0.63 g/cm^2.

Equations for the test statistics of a few of the most common parametric statistical tests are given in Outlines 4 through 6. In addition, the assumptions required for each test and the equations for computing the confidence interval of the parameter are also given. There are many other test statistics used to examine other null hypotheses, but the computations of these extensive tests are beyond the scope of this chapter. Several of the general statistics texts listed in the bibliography provide additional information.

When reporting results from significance tests, sometimes only the *p* value is given without also presenting additional information such as parameter estimates or confidence intervals. This omission is a common error in biomedical literature and should be avoided. An example is the following report: the drug raised the hip bone mineral density in postmenopausal women compared with placebo treatment ($p = 0.04$). Note that although the *p* value is given, indicating that there is an effect, there is no sense of the magnitude of the effect. An improved report is: the drug raised the hip bone mineral density in postmenopausal women by a mean of 0.06 g/cm^2 or 10% compared with placebo treatment ($p = 0.04$). The parameter in this case is the difference in bone mineral density between the two treatment groups. An even better account is to give the confidence interval for the difference.

Note that many parametric tests assume that the underlying population has a normal distribution (see Outlines 4 through 6). When sample size is large, many parametric tests are "robust" to deviations from the normal distribution. Robust means that the validity of the test is not seriously affected. When the assumption of normality is severely violated, however, nonparametric tests, which do not rely on an assumption of underlying normality, can be used. Many of the nonparametric tests use ranks rather than means and consequently do not rely on the shape of the distribution of the property being tested. Nonparametric counterparts to some common parametric tests are listed in Table 5. These tests are recommended for situations in which the investigator wishes to examine ranks or when the check of assumptions reveals severe violations.

Summary

There are many problems in research that can be improved by a sound understanding of study design and statistical analysis. Research is undoubtedly a creative process, but some practical skills will enhance the creativity. The approach and practical steps outlined in this chapter are idealized, but it is hoped that they will provide a rough framework for initiating new research studies or understanding current ones.

Outline 5
Inference About Difference Between 2 Means: Student's t Test

Null Hypothesis (H_o):	$\mu_1 - \mu_2 = D_o$
Alternate Hypothesis (H_a):	$(\mu_1 - \mu_2) \neq D_o$ or $(\mu_1 - \mu_2) > D_o$ or $(\mu_1 - \mu_2) < D_o$
Test Statistic:	$$t = \frac{(\bar{y}_1 - \bar{y}_2) - D_o}{S\sqrt{\frac{1}{n_1} + \frac{1}{n_2}}}$$ where $Sp^2 = \frac{(n_1 - 1)s_1^2 + (n_2 - 1)s_2^2}{n_1 + n_2 - 2}$
Degrees of Freedom:	$\nu = n_1 + n_2 - 2$
p-value:	One-tailed: area under t_ν distribution to the right of t if $H_a = (\mu_1 - \mu_2) > Do$ or to the left of t if $H_a = (\mu_1 - \mu_2) < Do$ Two-tailed: sum of areas under t_ν distribution to the right of $|t|$ and to the left of $-|t|$ (or 2x area to the right of $|t|$)
Decision:	If $p \leq \alpha$, reject H_o
Assumptions:	Random samples Sampled populations have normal probability distributions, population variances are equal, and samples are independent
Confidence Interval $100 \times (1-\alpha)$:	$(\bar{y}_1 - \bar{y}_2) \pm t_{\nu,\alpha/2} s \sqrt{\frac{1}{n_1} + \frac{1}{n_2}}$

Outline 6
Inference About Difference Between Paired Means: Paired Difference Test

Null Hypothesis (H_o):	$\delta = \delta_o$, where δ = mean of the differences
Alternate Hypothesis (H_a):	$\delta \neq \delta_o$, or $\delta < \delta_o$ or $\delta > \delta_o$
Test Statistic:	$$t = \frac{\bar{d} - d_o}{S_d / \sqrt{n}}$$ where d is the mean of the differences in the sample and s_d is the standard deviation of the differences
Degrees of Freedom:	$\nu = n-1$ where n = number of pairs
Associated probability (p):	One-tailed: area under t_{n-1} distribution to the right of t if $H_a = \delta > \delta_o$ or to the left of t if $H_a = \delta < \delta_o$ Two-tailed: sum of areas under t_{n-1} distribution to the right of $|t|$ and to the left of $-|t|$ (or 2x area to the right of $|t|$)
Decision:	If $p \leq \alpha$, reject H_o
Assumptions:	Random sample Sampled population has normal probability distribution
Confidence Interval $100 \times (1-\alpha)$:	$\bar{d} \pm \dfrac{t_{n-1,\alpha/2} s_d}{\sqrt{n}}$

Selected Bibliography

Study Design

Cohen J (ed): *Statistical Power Analysis for the Behavioral Sciences*, ed 2. Hillsdale, NJ, L Erlbaum Associates, 1988.

Hulley SB, Cummings SR, Browner WS (eds): *Designing Clinical Research: An Epidemiologic Approach*. Baltimore, MD, Williams & Wilkins, 1988.

Janssen HF: Experimental design and data evaluation in orthopaedic research. *J Orthop Res* 1986;4:504–509.

Lieber RL: Statistical significance and statistical power in hypothesis testing. *J Orthop Res* 1990;8:304–309.

Rothman KJ (ed): *Modern Epidemiology*. Boston, MA, Little, Brown & Co, 1986.

Winer BJ (ed): *Statistical Principles in Experimental Design*, ed 2. New York, NY, McGraw-Hill, 1971.

Analysis and Statistics

Dawson-Saunders B, Trapp RG (ed): *Basic and Clinical Biostatistics*. Norwalk, CT, Appleton & Lange, 1990.

Glantz SA (ed): *Primer of Biostatistics*, ed 3. New York, NY, McGraw-Hill, 1992.

Kleinbaum DG, Kupper LL, Muller KE (eds): *Applied Regression Analysis and Other Multivariable Methods*, ed 2. Boston, MA, PWS-Kent Publishing, 1988.

Lieber RL: Experimental design and statistical analysis, in Simon SR (ed): *Orthopaedic Basic Science*. Rosemont, IL, American Academy of Orthopaedic Surgeons, 1994, pp 623–665.

Mendenhall W (ed): *Introduction to Probability and Statistics*, ed 4. North Scituate, MA, Duxbury Press, 1975.

Munro BH, Page EB (eds): *Statistical Methods for Health Care Research,* ed 2. Philadelphia, PA, JB Lippincott, 1993.

Oakes MW (ed): *Statistical Inference.* Chestnut Hill, MA, Epidemiology Resources Inc, 1986.

Santner TJ: Fundamentals of statistics for orthopaedists: Part I. *J Bone Joint Surg* 1984;66A:468–471.

Santner TJ, Burstein AH: Fundamentals of statistics for orthopaedists: Part II. *J Bone Joint Surg* 1984;66A:794–799.

Santner TJ, Wypij D: Fundamentals of statistics for orthopaedists: Part III. *J Bone Joint Surg* 1984;66A:1309–1318.

Tabachnick BG, Fidell LS (eds): *Using Multivariate Statistics,* ed 2. New York, NY, Harper & Row, 1989.

Zar JH (ed): *Biostatistical Analysis,* ed 2. Englewood Cliffs, NJ, Prentice-Hall, 1984.

Special Topics

Browner WS, Newman TB: Are all significant P values created equal? The analogy between diagnostic tests and clinical research. *JAMA* 1987;257:2459–2463.

Cleveland WS (ed): *The Elements of Graphing Data,* rev ed. Murray Hill, NJ, AT&T Bell Laboratories, 1994.

DeMets DL: Statistics and ethics in medical research. *Science Eng Ethics* 1999;5:97–117.

Dorey FS, Nasser S, Amstutz H: The need for confidence intervals in the presentation of orthopaedic data. *J Bone Joint Surg* 1993;75A:1844–1852.

Friedman LM, Furberg C, DeMets DL (eds): *Fundamentals of Clinical Trials,* ed 2. Littleton, MA, PSG Publishing Company, 1985.

Glantz SA: Biostatistics: How to detect, correct, and prevent errors in the medical literature. *Circulation* 1980;61:1–7.

Lang TA, Secic M (eds): *How to Report Statistics in Medicine: Annotated Guidelines for Authors, Editors, and Reviewers.* Philadelphia, PA, American College of Physicians, 1997.

Mills JL: Data torturing. *N Engl J Med* 1993;329:1196–1199.

Vrbos LA, Lorenz MA, Peabody EH, McGregor M: Clinical methodologies and incidence of appropriate statistical testing in orthopaedic spine literature: Are statistics misleading? *Spine* 1993;18:1021–1029.

Chapter Outline

Chapter 2

Molecular and Cell Biology in Orthopaedics

Randy N. Rosier, MD, PhD

Paul R. Reynolds, PhD

Regis J. O'Keefe, MD

This chapter at a glance

This chapter presents the basic processes used to propagate and interpret genetic information, and the techniques of molecular biology that have made current understanding possible.

Introduction

The human body represents an exquisite integration of tissues and extracellular matrix. The tissues and matrix are comprised of and synthesized by hundreds of distinct cell types. The human body contains over 100 trillion cells, and each cell contains the same complement of hereditary information. Thus, individual cells must interpret their surroundings and specify which pieces of information to use at a particular time and place.

This chapter will present the basic processes used to propagate and interpret genetic information, and the techniques of molecular biology that have made current understanding possible, enabling the reader to better understand and appreciate the fundamentals of molecular biology and the potential applications of current knowledge.

Basics of Molecular Biology

Genetic information is contained within DNA molecules, which are polymers of deoxyribonucleotides. The central dogma of molecular biology holds that information in DNA is transmitted through RNA and converted into protein; that is, DNA serves as a template for RNA and RNA serves as a template for protein synthesis. All cellular activities are ultimately encoded in DNA, and the keys to understanding development, tissue homeostasis and repair, and disease are present within the DNA sequence. It is for this reason that enormous resources are now being directed toward the Human Genome Project, a federally funded program of the National Institutes of Health (NIH) and the Department of Energy, which is involved in determining the sequence of the entire human genome. This program began in 1993, and currently almost 200 Mb of the human genome have been sequenced. The most recent human genetic physical map now includes the locations of 30,000 genes, and may contain half of all human protein-coding genes. The timetable for completion of the human genome sequence has shortened because advances in technology have accelerated the pace of data acquisition, and may be as soon as the end of 2003. The genomes of *Escherichia coli* and yeast have been completely sequenced, and work is underway on *Drosophila melanogaster, Caenorhabditis elegans,* and mouse.

DNA serves as a template for synthesis of RNA in a process called transcription. There are 3 major forms of RNA: messenger (mRNA), ribosomal (rRNA), and transfer (tRNA); all are used in different aspects of protein synthesis in a process called translation. Proteins are polymers of amino acids that catalyze nearly all biologic reactions, and serve structural roles as well. The code for individual amino acids is contained in the DNA and RNA sequences as a series of triplets of the nucleotides, with different triplets or codons specifying particular amino acids to be added. The proteins produced are thus a function of the set of genes actively being transcribed, and in turn determine the behavior and

phenotypic expression of the cell. The transfer of information from nucleic acids to protein is unidirectional; information from proteins cannot generate nucleic acid sequences.

Gene expression determines cellular, and hence tissue, identity. Thus, processes of concern to the orthopaedist, such as skeletal formation, fracture repair, degeneration of cartilage, and prosthetic loosening can be traced to certain genes being transcribed or not transcribed in bone, cartilage, and certain hematopoietic cells. Molecular biology provides a set of sophisticated tools that facilitate understanding of the relationship between genotype (the complete genetic complement of an organism) and phenotype (the properties or qualities of an organism that result from expression of the genotype). In other words, it is becoming clear how similar genes determine segmentation of the body in both invertebrates and vertebrates, and how a bone cell is programmed to produce type I collagen, and a cartilage cell to produce type II collagen.

The insights into DNA and RNA function revealed by modern technology have revolutionized biomedical and biological sciences. Understanding the structure and function of genes has led to the identification of the causes of diseases. Recombinant DNA technology has led to novel diagnostic and therapeutic approaches and to production of recombinant proteins, and has paved the way for engineered tissues, genetically altered organisms, and gene therapies. For example, in orthopaedics, the bone morphogenetic proteins (BMPs) are in the vanguard of the application of molecular biology to clinical problems such as stimulation of fracture healing and regrowth of bone (to create a "living prosthesis"). The discovery, analysis, and production of BMPs for clinical trials would not have occurred without recombinant DNA technology.

DNA Structure

Plant heredity was first studied in the mid 19th century, and it was postulated that the presence of genes controlled the transmission of characteristics between generations. DNA was discovered in 1869, and the theory that heritable information was contained in DNA was initially formulated in 1894. Localization of DNA to the chromosomes was identified in the 1920s. However, proof of the concept that genetic information was contained in the DNA was not demonstrated until 1952, when it was shown that the genetic material within the bacteriophage consisted of DNA. The primary structure of the DNA molecule, with description of the double helical structure, was proposed in 1953. The pace of research and growth of knowledge of molecular biology has subsequently increased explosively since that time.

Genetic information is transported by DNA, which consists of 2 strands wound around one another in a double helix (Fig. 1). Each strand can serve as a template for synthesis of the other strand during semiconservative replication. A chromosome is a single DNA molecule that contains

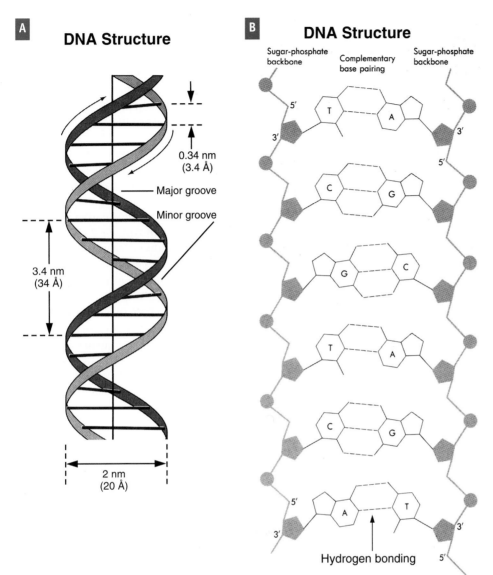

A   DNA Structure

0.34 nm
(3.4 Å)

Major groove

Minor groove

3.4 nm
(34 Å)

2 nm
(20 Å)

B   DNA Structure

Sugar-phosphate backbone

Complementary base pairing

Sugar-phosphate backbone

5′

3′

T — A

3′

5′

C — G

G — C

T — A

C — G

5′

3′

A — T

3′

5′

Hydrogen bonding

Figure 1

A, The double helical structure of DNA illustrated with hydrogen bonding between bases on the 2 strands represented as horizontal bars. The configuration results in a conformation with major and minor grooves. **B,** The hydrogen bonding between complementary base pairs is shown with the deoxyribose-phosphate backbone. (Reproduced with permission from Watson JD, Gilman M, Witkowski J, Zoller M: *Recombinant DNA,* ed 2. New York, NY, Scientific American Books, 1992.)

hereditary information and is transmitted from one generation to the next. *E. coli* has a single circular chromosome of 4 million deoxyribonucleic pairs (which are referred to as base pairs [bp]). Humans have 23 pairs of linear chromosomes that total 6 billion bp; the total DNA defines the human genome. Only certain segments of the DNA are transcribed, and these segments are called genes. In eukaryotes, each gene typically encodes a single protein.

The nucleotides, or individual building blocks, are comprised of a phosphate group, the carbon sugar 2′-deoxyribose, and 1 of the 4 bases guanine (G), adenine (A), cytosine (C), or thymine (T) (Fig. 2). The backbone of a single DNA strand is comprised of the phosphate and ribose groups, which connect the 5′ and 3′ carbon groups of the ribose; in the second strand the orientation of the 5′ and 3′ carbons is opposite to the first. The bases are attached to the ribose group and extend into the center of the helix in a plane perpendicular to the long axis of the helix. The elegant utility of the DNA molecule is derived from hydrogen bonds, the

weak chemical bonds that form between the purine (G,A) and pyrimidine (C,T) bases aligned in the center of the helix. Guanine forms 3 hydrogen bonds with cytosine, and adenine forms 2 bonds with thymine (Fig. 3). The sum of these weak bonds in a long double helix results in a stable structure at physiologic temperature, ionic strength, and pH. However, the bases can be separated sequentially with relatively small energy expenditure, "unzipping" the helix for replication, transcription, or repair. The complementary nature of the 2 strands of the DNA helix is the key to its capacity for self-replication. The 3 critical cellular functions of DNA are accurate self-replication during cellular division, transcription of mRNA, and the regulation of these processes.

Genomic DNA

The structure of DNA in eukaryotes differs from the structure found in prokaryotes. Unlike prokaryotic cells, eukaryotic cells possess a nucleus. Human chromosomes contain a total of 6 billion bp, which encode approximately 50,000 to 100,000 individual genes. The total DNA in a single cell would stretch for nearly 2 m if placed end to end; therefore, it is not surprising that several higher orders of folding are required for eukaryotic DNA to fit into a nucleus roughly 5 to 10 μm in diameter. The first order of packing in DNA is called the nucleosome, which is a unit of approximately 200 bp. Each nucleosome contains an octamer of histone proteins, 2 each of histone H2A, H2B, H3, and H4. The nucleosomal histones are small (molecular weight approximately 11,000 daltons), highly positively charged proteins; the high concentration of positive charge negates the repulsion that would occur with the packing of the phosphate groups. 146 bp DNA is wound around the histone octamer, with the remainder of the 200 bp forming a linker region to the next 146 bp nucleosomal unit. When these structures are spread out and examined by electron microscopy, they resemble beads on a string. A fifth histone protein, H1, is interposed between the nucleosomal units. The nucleosomes are coiled into units of 6 to form solenoidal structures referred to as 30-nm fibers (Fig. 4). The 30-nm fibers are looped out from attachments to a protein structure called the nuclear scaffold. Further packing of solenoidal segments occurs during chromosomal condensation at the time of cell repli-

cation. In all, the compaction of DNA is at least 4 orders of magnitude.

Only 5% to 10% of genomic DNA in the higher eukaryotes is transcribed. DNA of genes is organized into introns, or noncoding sequences, and exons, which contain the code for the RNA of the transcribed template that will be used to produce the proteins of the gene product. Some of the noncoding sequences contain promoter regions, regulatory elements, and enhancers. This portion of the genome accounts for approximately an additional 65% of the DNA. The average size of genes tends to increase with organism complexity, and ranges from 0.5 kb to over 100 kb in mammals. The majority of genes are single copies that occur within the genome as short segments (< 25 kb) of DNA, which are separated by repetitive DNA sequences. There are various types of repeated sequences that range from tens to hundreds of bp; the number of repeats can range into the thousands.

The 2 major types of repetitive DNA sequence are satellite DNA, which contains short, clustered tandem repeats, and interspersed DNA. The satellite DNA sequence constitutes

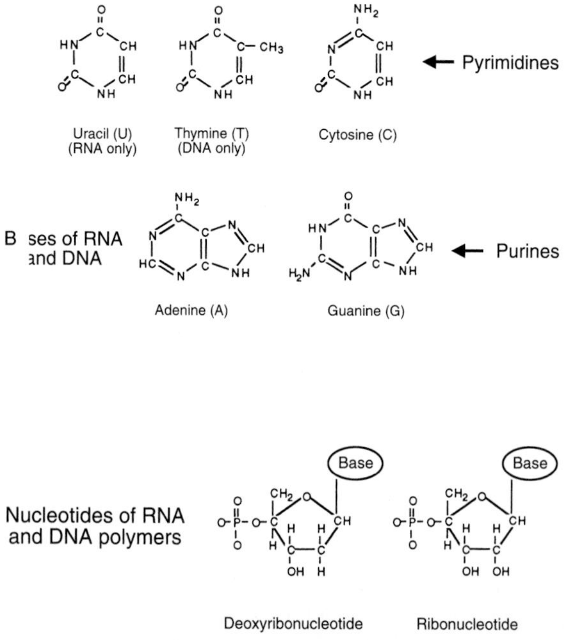

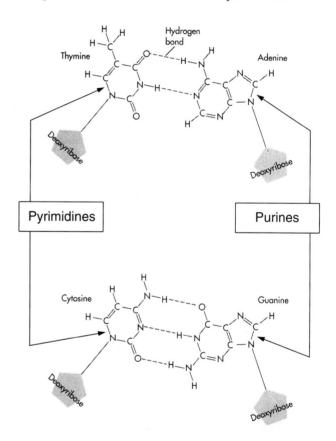

Figure 2

The bases comprising RNA and DNA. Uracil and thymine, respectively, are present in RNA and DNA only. The bases are covalently bound to the deoxyribose or ribose sugars as shown to constitute the nucleotides of DNA and RNA.

Figure 3

Specific base pairing and associated hydrogen bonding of purines and pyrimidines are shown. Note the stronger bonding between G and C pairs as opposed to the A and T pairs because of triple versus double hydrogen bonds. (Reproduced with permission from Watson JD, Gilman M, Witkowski J, Zoller M: *Recombinant DNA*, ed 2. New York, NY, Scientific American Books, 1992.)

about 10% of the genomic DNA, and tends to be concentrated in specific chromosomal regions such as the telomeres and centromeres. The ribosomal RNA genes are contained within regions of satellite DNA, and are clustered in locations on 5 different chromosomes and present in approximately 200 copies in the human genome. The remaining 15% of the genome is in the form of the interspersed repetitive DNA sequences, some of which represent evolutionary duplications with sequence similarities resulting in gene families. For example, the human *Alu* repeats are roughly 300 bp long and are repeated hundreds of thousands of times; therefore, *Alu* repeats comprise approximately 2% of the human genome. The function of these repeats is unknown, although aberrant recombination has been identified in a few genetic disorders, such as familial hypercholesterolemia. The location of the short tandem repeat satellites has been useful in providing a large number of markers dispersed along specific chromosomes used in mapping genes to specific locations.

DNA Replication

The nature of the 2 strands of DNA is the key to accurate duplication prior to cell division. DNA is replicated by a semiconservative process, meaning that each strand of DNA serves as a template for creation of a new strand. Replication usually starts at an origin and proceeds bidirectionally. Thus, after replication, there are 2 paired strands, each containing 1 original strand of DNA and 1 newly synthesized strand. DNA is replicated through the activity of DNA polymerases, which require a template and primer to synthesize the new strand, and a number of accessory proteins. The template is a strand of nucleotides that provide bases that will hydrogen bond to the bases on the strand being synthesized. The primer is a segment of newly synthesized DNA. The primer provides a 3′ hydroxyl (3′ OH) group to which the 5′ phosphate of the incoming nucleotide will be attached (Fig. 5). The incoming nucleotide is selected on the basis of its ability to hydrogen bond to the template base, so that G is always inserted across from C, A across from T, etc. The polymerization is said to proceed in a 5′ to 3′ direction, and may occur at a rate up to several thousand nucleotides per second. The accuracy, or fidelity, of replication is in the range of 1 mistake per million to 100 million nucleotides inserted. Fidelity is improved by a "proofreading" function built into certain polymerases that can sense the insertion of a mismatched base and replace it with the correct one. Overall fidelity of replication is also increased by enzymatic DNA repair systems that operate after replication. There are 5 identified mammalian DNA polymerase types. DNA polymerase a is involved in priming template strands for new synthesis; DNA polymerase b is the form involved in DNA synthesis; DNA polymerase g is involved in mitochondrial DNA replication; and polymerases e and d are involved in DNA repair.

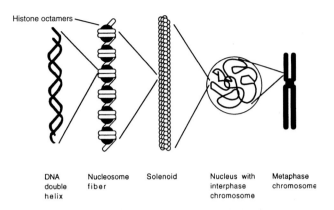

DNA double helix Nucleosome fiber Solenoid Nucleus with interphase chromosome Metaphase chromosome

Figure 4

Double helical DNA is further packed by wrapping around histone octamers, with 2 coils per octamer at 200 base-pairs intervals, and the histone/DNA complex is referred to as a nucleosome. The fibers of nucleosomes are further wound in groups of 6 into a solenoidal structure, which is further packed in the chromosomes. (Adapted with permission from Shore EM, Kaplan FS: Tutorial: Molecular biology for the clinician: Part I. General principles. *Clin Orthop* 1994;306:264–283.)

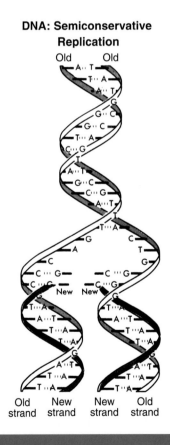

DNA: Semiconservative Replication

Old   Old

Old strand New strand New strand Old strand

Figure 5

DNA replication is semiconservative because 1 template strand is retained in the newly replicated double helix. (Reproduced with permission from Zubay GL, Parson WW, Vance DE (eds): *Principles of Biochemistry*. Dubuque, IA, Wm C. Brown, 1994, p 651.)

Retroviruses (RNA viruses) also have the ability to self-replicate after infection of cells, using a reverse transcriptase enzyme (RT), which is a DNA polymerase that converts the RNA of the virus into DNA, using the viral RNA as a template. RT initiates synthesis at the 3′ end of the viral RNA molecule, replicating in a 5′ to 3′ direction. RT also degrades the RNA portion of the RNA:DNA hybrid, then synthesizes the second DNA strand. The double-stranded DNA can randomly integrate into the host genome. The host cell machinery is then used to generate new retroviral genomes packaged into coat proteins.

T4 polymerase and the Klenow fragment of DNA polymerase I are general polymerases used for filling in sticky ends, for random priming (usually for labeling DNA with a radioactive or other detectable label to produce a probe), or for mutagenesis (changing 1 or more bases within a DNA sequence). These enzymes have a high degree of accuracy, or alternatively, a low base error rate. Sequenase (T7 polymerase) is an enzyme with a specialized function used in sequencing DNA by the dideoxy sequencing base termination method of Sanger (see below under DNA sequencing). This is also a highly accurate polymerase.

Cell Division

Mammalian cells all contain 2 sets of genetic material, or chromosomes, 1 set from each parent organism. Somatic mammalian cells therefore are referred to as having a diploid content of DNA. The gametes that fuse and combine genetic material during fertilization each contain half the genetic material of the offspring, and are referred to as haploid in DNA content. During cell division, the chromatin, that is, chromosomal DNA and associated proteins, changes from being dispersed throughout the nuclear matrix to a highly condensed form that can be seen microscopically. The individual chromosomes are replicated during the prophase period, and become aligned along the central axis of the cell during metaphase. The chromosome duplicates separate and move toward opposite poles of the cell during anaphase. At this point the cell has a tetraploid DNA content. During telophase, the segregated chromosomes reach the poles of the dividing cell and cytokinesis occurs, resulting in splitting of the cell into 2 diploid daughter cells.

The DNA content of the cell is thus an indicator of the phase of the cell cycle. This has been used as a means of assessing the proliferative proclivity of tumors using a technique called flow cytometry. The DNA of cells isolated from a tumor is labeled with a fluorescent compound (usually propidium iodide). The cells are then passed through an orifice where fluorescence induced by a laser is quantified by a detector. Cells with tetraploid DNA content demonstrate a twofold increase in fluorescence in comparison with diploid cells, and an increased tetraploid peak (poly-ploidy) indicates increased cellular proliferation. Both benign and malignant tumors can exhibit increased tetraploidy. Cells with an abnormally increased amount of DNA (but not a simple multiple of 2) are indicative of defective mitotic behavior and are referred to as aneuploid. This is always associated with malignancy, and histologically such cells appear to have enlarged, bizarre nuclei. Some correlations between biologic behavior and ploidy have been observed in musculoskeletal tumors, but in general ploidy has not proved to be an accurate predictor of behavior.

During cell division, an important activity resides in the telomeres, which seal and stabilize the ends of the chromosomes and contain large numbers of tandem repeat short sequences. The telomeric sequence can be extended during replication by an enzyme called telomerase. Inadequate replication of telomeric sequences by telomerase over successive mitoses may cause the telomeric shortening seen with aging of cells. The telomeric length may determine the possible number of cell divisions that can occur prior to cell senescence.

Defects in DNA and Its Replication

DNA replication, while remarkably accurate, is imperfect. There are separate mismatch systems that increase the overall fidelity of replication to an error rate of only 1 in 10^8 to 10^9, and occasionally result in errors that can disrupt function or expression of a particular gene. In addition, environmental agents, such as free radicals generated from chemical reactions or radiation, can result in alterations in the sequence of DNA that are not always repaired by the cell. These aberrations in DNA sequence are called mutations. The effects of mutations in DNA are highly variable, depending on the type and gene(s) involved, and can have no discernible effect on the cell or organism or, at the other extreme, be lethal.

Mutations can be broadly categorized as single bp changes, deletions or insertions, or rearrangements. Single bp changes can be silent if the codon changes to one that still codes for the same amino acid, or neutral if the codon changes the amino acid to a different one that is functionally equivalent. Change of a codon to an amino acid that is not functionally equivalent is called a missense mutation. An example of this type of mutation would be osteogenesis imperfecta, where a single glycine to cysteine mutation in the helical domain of the alpha 2 chain of type I collagen leads to an abnormal collagen and bone fragility. Deletions or insertions can result in a shift of the reading frame if such base changes do not occur in a multiple of 3. When a frame shift mutation occurs, the downstream coding sequence is functionally scrambled, and the altered protein may be nonfunctional or truncated.

Insertions or deletions in intronic locations can also markedly alter the involved gene product. Deletions or insertions of short repeated sequences in either intronic or coding sequences can also occur. Rearrangement types of mutations include inversions, where the orientation of a segment of DNA is reversed, or translocations, where a segment of DNA from one chromosome is transferred to another. An example of chromosomal translocation occurs in Ewing's sarcoma, where the translocation from chromosome 11 to chromosome 22 creates an abnormal transcription factor due to the fusion gene product between Fli-1 and EWS, resulting in malignant transformation of the cells containing the mutation.

Some benign mutations, introduced into the human genome many generations ago, are expressed in relatively large portions of the population. These changes are referred to as gene polymorphisms, or allelic variants. The susceptibility to some diseases may be related to certain polymorphic genes in a complex way. Examples include polymorphisms of the vitamin D and estrogen receptors, which may correlate with a predisposition to develop osteoporosis in some patients.

Somatic mutations occur in diploid cells, and can result in regional tissue abnormality or dysregulated cell growth. They cannot be passed on to the progeny of the affected individual. An example of a somatic mutation is monostotic fibrous dysplasia, which is caused by a mutation in a Ga_s protein in the involved tissue. Although a regional disturbance in the bone cells occurs as a result, the disease is not passed on to subsequent generations. A mutation within the DNA of a haploid germ cell (sperm or ovum) can be transmitted to progeny. Because there are 2 alleles (resulting from the maternal and paternal copies of every gene), whether a mutation is phenotypically expressed depends on the relative function of the 2 forms of the gene in the individual. In some cases, such as in hemophilias, a single functional copy is sufficient for a normal phenotype, and the mutated form will constitute a recessive trait. In other cases, such as in cleidocranial dysostosis or achondroplasia, a single dysfunctional copy causes an abnormal phenotype, and the abnormal gene will produce a dominant trait.

RNA Synthesis

RNA differs from DNA in 3 ways: (1) it has a hydroxyl group at the 2′ position in the ribose, rather than the hydrogen found in DNA (thus, the "deoxy" ribose in DNA); (2) the base uracil is used in place of thymine to hydrogen bond to adenine (Fig. 6); and (3) RNA is a single-stranded molecule, although intrastrand hydrogen bonds are an essential property of certain RNAs, enabling secondary structure.

Transcription is typically regulated by untranscribed DNA sequences proximal, or upstream, of the DNA template. These upstream sequences can specify the binding of spe-

cific proteins involved in or influencing transcription, and are generally referred to as promoter regions. Transcription of the different types of RNA is effected through several different forms of RNA polymerase, and involves the addition of single ribonucleotides to the growing RNA chain. In eukaryotes, RNA polymerase I transcribes the ribosomal RNAs, defined as class I genes based on their promoters, which are generally upstream of the encoded transcript and contain characteristic sets of short conserved sequences recognized by the polymerase and associated factors. RNA polymerase II generates the mRNA templates for protein production (class II genes), and the corresponding promoters of these genes have much greater diversity and complexity in upstream regulatory elements in the promoter regions. RNA polymerase III transcribes the class III genes, tRNAs and 5S rRNAs, which have promoters within the coding region and may also have downstream promoter regions.

As with replication, the nucleotide added during transcription is determined by the complementary base in the DNA: an adenine ribonucleotide is added to pair with a thymine deoxynucleotide in the template, and similarly, uracil (U), guanine, and cytosine nucleotides are added to

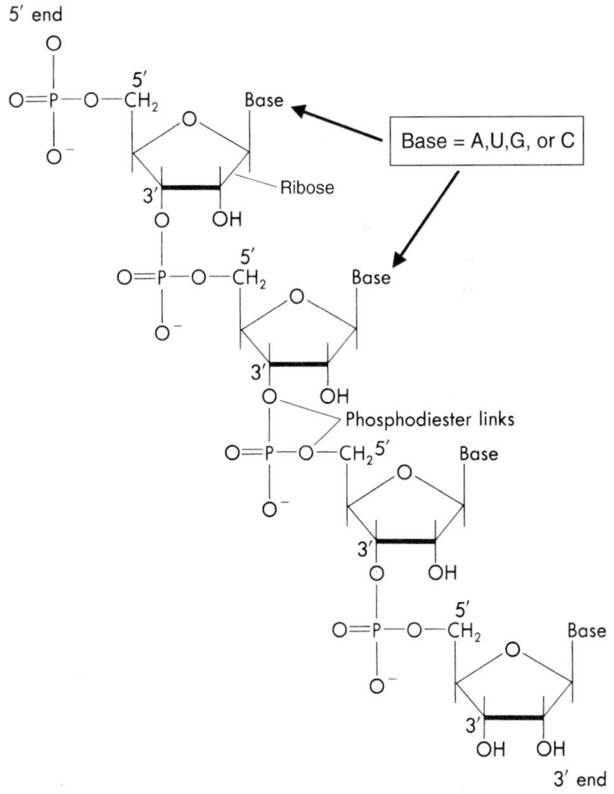

Figure 6

The structure of RNA resembles that of DNA, with ribose-phosphate linkages and purine or pyrimidine bases, although uracil replaces the thymine of DNA. As shown, the ribose in RNA contains a hydroxyl group not present in DNA.

pair with adenine, cytosine and guanine deoxynucleotides in the DNA, respectively. The RNA molecules are synthesized with a 5′ phosphate at the start, with subsequent 5′ phosphates on each nucleotide building block being added to the 3′ hydroxyl on the chain being synthesized. Thus, RNA polymerization is said to proceed in a 5′ to 3′ direction (Fig. 7), the same direction as DNA polymerase. However, unlike DNA polymerase, RNA polymerase does not require a primer to initiate synthesis, instead depending on short DNA sequences that serve as a collecting point for the RNA polymerase and its control proteins. To reiterate, the hydrogen bonding between the nucleotide pairs determines that transcribed RNA will be the complement of the template strand. As the strands are antiparallel, the synthesized strand is actually the reverse complement of the entire template.

Types of RNA and Roles in Protein Synthesis

Each type of RNA has a specific role in protein synthesis. rRNA is the most abundant type, accounting for over 90% of the total cellular RNA. It is contained within organized cytoplasmic structures called the ribosomes, which may migrate to the endoplasmic reticulum and dock there during synthesis, depending on the presence of a signal peptide as part of the protein being translated. The ribosomes function to allow translation of the mRNA into protein. At the site of protein synthesis, 2 multiprotein complexes assemble with rRNAs to form a large complex, the ribosome, that binds the mRNA strand and serves as a scaffolding to support assembly of the amino acid chain.

Ribosomes consist of 2 major subunit complexes, with rRNA constituting approximately 60% of the complex. The total mass of mammalian ribosomes is approximately 4×10^6 daltons, and the major subunits contain several rRNAs: the 60S subunit consists of 28S (4.7 kb), 5.8S (160 b), and 5S (120 b) rRNAs, while the 40S subunit contains 18S (1.9 kb) rRNA. The abundance of the 18S rRNA is approximately twice that of the 28S component. The ribosome binds to the translation start recognition site of the mRNA and initiates protein synthesis. Multiple ribosomal units (polyribosomes) will simultaneously move in a 5′ to 3′ direction along the mRNA template, producing individual nascent polypeptides.

The transport and polymerization of the specific amino acids, translation, is mediated through the tRNA, which is specific for each amino acid. tRNA is the molecule that interprets the code on the mRNA and delivers the appropriate amino acid to the elongating peptide chain. tRNA is structured through specific intrastrand bonds into a cloverleaf-like configuration. As the term "translation" implies, the information on the mRNA is in a genetic code. Each amino acid is encoded by a 3-nucleotide sequence on the DNA and mRNA referred to as a codon. Given that there are 4 bases, there are 64 different groups of 3 distinct sequences. The genetic code is degenerate: many amino acids are encoded by more than 1 codon; for example, glycine is encoded by GGA, GGC, GGG, and GGU. The tRNAs have anticodons that hydrogen bond to the complementary trinucleotide on the mRNA, thus decoding the information.

Each tRNA carries a specific amino acid at its 3′ end, and because of the architecture of the ribosome and the structure of the tRNA, the amino acid is placed in position to be added to the nascent peptide. Note that the codons for glycine differ only by their third nucleotide (Table 1). Many tRNAs have a "wobble" position at the third nucleotide of their anticodon, such that only the first 2 nucleotides are sufficient to encode an amino acid. A methionine (AUG) codon, generally in a context of GCC(A/G)CCAUGG, functions as the translation start signal, and defines the beginning of the amino acid sequence synthesis of the encoded protein. The ribosomal machinery recognizes the translation start site and binds to this region, allowing protein synthesis to begin. A specific initiator tRNA, which contains the AUG anticodon and carries a methionine initiates synthesis, and the mRNA template determines the subsequent sequence of tRNA binding and peptide amino acid elongation. Translation starts with the amino terminus of the protein and amino acids are added on the carboxyl end until the peptide is completed; therefore, the flow of amino acid sequence information for protein from N-terminus to C-terminus is from 5′ to 3′ mRNA sequence. Three codons stop translation: UGA, UAA, and UAG.

Bacterial mRNAs may be polycistronic, meaning that a single transcript has multiple start and stop codons with intervening untranslated intercistronic sequences. Thus, the single transcript can produce several proteins when translated. Eukaryotic mRNAs, however, are generally monocistronic, with each transcript encoding a single protein. The events constituting the function of RNA in transcription and translation of the genetic code into protein production are summarized in Figure 7.

RNA Splicing

The transcribed regions of genes, or exons, contain the coding sequence for the mRNA. Creation of a functional mRNA template requires splicing together the exons during transcription, a phenomenon that occurs in the nucleus. Because of the localization of the transcriptional apparatus and chromosomes within the nuclear envelope, translation does not occur concomitantly in eukaryotes the way it does in bacteria. This allows for posttranscriptional processing of the mRNA, another potential point of regulation of gene transcription in higher organisms. The average sizes of eukaryotic exons are 100 to 200 bp, while the intronic segments are generally much longer, and can range up to 20 kb. Some types of introns contain ribozyme type catalytic activity, and splice themselves out during transcription. Others require extraneous catalytic activity to accomplish

Table 1

The Genetic Dictionary from DNA to RNA to Amino Acids

Codon*	Amino Acid	Codon	Amino Acid	Codon	Amino Acid	Codon	Amino Acid
AAG	Lysine	CAG	Glutamine	GAG	Glutamate	TAG	STOP
(UUC)	LYS, (K)	(CAG)	GLU, (Q)	(GAG)	GLU, (E)	(UAG)	
AAA		CAA		GAA		TAA	
(AAA)		(CAA)		(GAA)		(UAA)	
AAC	Asparagine	CAC	Histidine	GAC	Aspartate	TAC	Tyrosine
(AAC)	Asn, (N)	(CAC)	His, (H)	(GAC)	Asp, (D)	(UAC)	Tyr, (Y)
AAT		CAT		GAT		TAT	
(AAU)		(CAU)		(GAU)		(UAU)	
ACG	Threonine	CCG	Proline	GCG	Alanine	TCG	Serine
(ACG)	Thr, (T)	(CCG)	Pro, (P)	(GCG)	Ala, (A)	(UCG)	Ser, (S)
ACA		CCA		GCA		TCA	
(ACA)		(CCA)		(GCA)		(UCA)	
ACC		CCC		GCC		TCC	
(ACC)		(CCC)		(GCC)		(UCC)	
ACT		CCT		GCT		TCT	
(ACU)		(CCU)		(GCU)		(UCU)	
AGG	Arginine	CGG	Arginine	GGG	Glycine	TGG	Tryptophan
(AGG)	Arg, (R)	(CGG)	Arg, (R)	(GGG)	Gly, (G)	(UGG)	Trp, (W)
AGA		CGA		GGA		TGA	STOP
(AGA)		(CGA)		(GGA)		(UGA)	
AGC	Serine	CGC		GGC		TGC	Cysteine
(AGC)	Ser, (S)	(CGC)		(GGC)		(UGC)	Cys, (C)
AGT		CGT		GGT		TGT	
(AGU)		(CGU)		(GGU)		(UGU)	
ATG	Methionine	CTG	Leucine	GTG	Valine	TTG	Leucine
(AUG)	Met, (M)	(CUG)	Leu, (L)	(GUG)	Val, (V)	(UUG)	Leu, (L)
ATA	Isoleucine	CTA		GTA		TTA	
(AUA)	Ile, (I)	(CUA)		(GUA)		(UUA)	
ATC		CTC		GTC		TTC	Phenylalanine
(AUC)		(CUC)		(GUC)		(UUC)	Phe, (F)
ATT		CTT		GTT		TTT	
(AUU)		(CUU)		(GUU)		(UUU)	

* RNA codons are shown in parentheses.

the splicing, and use protein/RNA complexes to achieve this. Exon/intron boundaries are defined by consensus sequences, GT at the 5′ end (GU in the RNA), and AG at the 3′ end of the intron, which also define the directionality of the splice site. Splice sites are not specific to either particular genes or cell types. The protein/RNA complexes that mediate splicing consist of large particles containing multiple proteins and short nuclear RNA (snRNA), and are referred to as the spliceosomes. This structure cleaves the intron/exon boundary at the 5′ end, loops the RNA of the intronic sequence toward the 3′ end in a "lariat" formation,

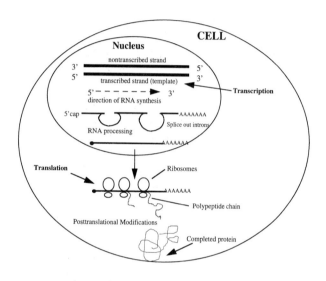

Figure 7

The general flow of genetic information from DNA to RNA to protein. See text for details.

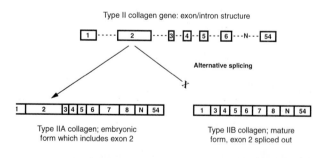

Figure 8

A good example of the alternative splicing process in skeletal tissues is presented here with the type II collagen gene, which exists in 2 tissue-specific alternative splice forms. The full-length protein includes exon 2, is expressed in embryonic tissues and precartilage, and is referred to as type IIA. In mature cartilage, a second splice variant which lacks exon 2 is produced.

cleaves the 3′ boundary, and then splices the exons together. This process is complex but occurs rapidly during transcription, with splicing of the 5′ introns occurring during transcription of the 3′ end of the mRNA. Many genes have alternative splicing pathways, where the arrangement of exons varies, so that differing protein products can be produced from a single gene. Inclusion or exclusion of specific exons during splicing determines the final form of the transcript and its protein product. Alternative splicing can occur in a tissue- or cell-specific manner during transcription of gene products, and it is increasingly recognized that alternatively spliced forms, or alternative transcripts, exist for a large number of genes. An important example in skeletal tissues is type II collagen, which exists in a type IIA (full length sequence) form that is expressed in embryonic cartilage and recapitulated during some injury and repair processes such as fracture healing, and type IIB, the mature form seen in adult cartilage tissues and in which exon 2 is spliced out (Fig. 8). Another example is *Bcl-2*, which is involved in the control of apoptosis, or programmed cell death. Alternative splicing results in the production of a long form ($Bcl-x_l$) and a short form ($Bcl-x_s$), which have opposing effects. $Bcl-x_l$ stimulates apoptosis while $Bcl-x_s$ prevents it. Increasing numbers of genes exhibiting this phenomenon of functionally significant alternative splice forms are being identified. The mechanisms regulating the selection of the alternative splicing pathways have not yet been elucidated.

Posttranslational RNA Processing

The mRNA ferries the code for a protein's amino acid sequence from the DNA in the nucleus (the gene) to the site of protein synthesis in the cytoplasm. Each gene usually has at least 1 mRNA, but there are many genes that produce more than 1 mRNA. Eukaryotic mRNA is polyadenylated on the 3′ end by a poly(A) polymerase in the nucleus prior to transport to the cytoplasm. The polyadenylation and cleavage signal is contained within a consensus sequence, AAUAAA, and is recognized by an endonuclease that cleaves the mRNA 20 nucleotides 3′ of the consensus sequence. Subsequently the poly(A) polymerase adds from 20 to 250 nucleotides of poly(A) to the 3′ end of each mRNA.

In addition, after mRNA transcription is complete, the 5′ end is modified with a guanine cap, which is added to the original RNA molecule by a nuclear guanylyl transferase enzyme. The guanine is inserted in a reverse orientation (5′-5′ bond) to the rest of the nucleotides in the mRNA, and is methylated. The guanine cap may enhance stability, maintain orientation of the transcript, and provide a recognition domain for the ribosome, which is thought to scan from the 5′ end to locate the binding domain of the translation start site. The mRNA usually contains untranslated sequences at the 3′ and 5′ ends of the coding sequence. The 3′ untranslated regions have been implicated in the control of mRNA stability, and can contain sequences that either enhance or decrease mRNA degradation rates via interaction with specific binding proteins and ribonucleases.

Catalytic RNA

Another type of RNA is the ribozyme, a segment of RNA that actually has DNA or RNA cutting enzymatic activity. Examples of this catalytic activity include some intronic sequences that can splice themselves out of the final transcript; such activity is a property of the secondary structure of the encoded RNA. In other cases ribozymes can modify transcribed sequences or cleave double-stranded DNA. Finally, RNA can also constitute a genome for certain organisms, called retroviruses. These viruses use a reverse transcriptase enzyme coded for in their genomic RNA and carried as the translated protein in the viral particle. This allows transcription of the viral genomic RNA into DNA in the cell immediately after infection into a double-stranded DNA representation of the viral genome. This is integrated into host DNA and through transcription produces single-stranded RNA replicates of the viral genome.

Posttranslational Protein Modification

Following protein synthesis by the ribosomes and tRNAs, the proteins undergo further posttranslational processing or modifications. Proper protein folding is essential for function, and generally occurs concomitant with synthesis. A class of proteins called chaperones is important in assuring proper conformation of many proteins, including collagens. Chaperones are ubiquitous and constitutively expressed proteins that bind reversibly to unfolded regions of nascent polypeptides and control folding to ensure proper functional conformation. Chaperones are also involved in intracellular protein transport, but their mechanisms of action are not well understood. Most proteins undergo specific proteolytic cleavages to achieve their final form. Some proteins can be targeted for specific organellar locations, such as the mitochondria or endoplasmic reticulum, or for secretion. This information is encoded in amino acid sequences in the N-terminal end (leader sequences) of the protein, which are usually cleaved when the protein is in the appropriate destination. In addition, appropriate glycosylation, cross-linking, and sulfhydryl bonds are essential for function of many mammalian proteins. Glycosylations generally occur in the endoplasmic reticulum and Golgi apparatus. A number of important skeletal growth factors, such as transforming growth factors-β (TGFs-β) and BMPs, exist as sulfhydryl bonded dimeric molecules.

A powerful result of knowing the genetic code is that the primary structure, the amino acid sequence, of a protein (the gene product) can be predicted by analysis of the DNA sequence. Thus, a gene product can be classified into a certain group of proteins based on homology to that group.

Analysis of so many varieties of proteins has facilitated the identification of the probable function of almost all cloned genes. This avoids the necessity of purifying the protein and running extensive tests to assay for a biochemical activity, and, if assays for activity are required, a predicted activity allows the biochemist to narrow the search. Because the functional (enzymatic, binding) domains of many proteins are similar, creating protein families, many new genes with known activity have been discovered from randomly cloned DNA fragments called expressed sequence tags.

Control of Gene Expression

The level of expression of certain gene products will determine cellular phenotype. There are an estimated 100,000 genes in the human genome, and approximately 5,000 genes are expressed in a single cell. Thus, control of gene expression is imperative. There are 6 potential control points for gene regulation: initiation of transcription; posttranscriptional processing of the mRNA; mRNA degradation; efficiency of translation; posttranslation processing; and protein degradation. The most significant among these control mechanisms is initiation of transcription. This is the most sensible of the control points because the cell does not waste energy synthesizing a useless RNA. Also, multiple genes may be required simultaneously, and a common control mechanism allows for coordinate expression at the appropriate time and place. Although initiation of transcription is the major control point for the expression of many genes, this form of control does not exclude others from providing a cell with the ability to fine-tune the expression of a particular gene.

Control of transcription is significantly different in prokaryotes and eukaryotes. RNA polymerase is a complex of 5 proteins in *E. coli*, and approximately 12 in eukaryotes. The RNA polymerase is directed to start RNA synthesis by interacting with other proteins, several in *E. coli*, and several dozen in eukaryotes. These proteins first bind to specific sequences in the upstream (promoter) region (Fig. 9), then with RNA polymerase to signal that transcription should begin. In *E. coli* the promoter region is usually within a few hundred nucleotides of the initiation site, and is mainly limited to two 6-base consensus sequences, 10 ("-10 box") and 35 ("-35 box") bases upstream of the transcription initiation site. In eukaryotes there is a proximal promoter region with 1,000 bp, and additional regulatory elements that can be tens of kb upstream or downstream. These distant regulatory elements are called enhancers, and elements that negatively affect transcription have recently been described as silencers.

There are several general terms that describe certain types of control. Usually genes that are expressed in every cell are termed housekeeping genes, and their expression is termed constitutive. Genes that are not normally on, but increase

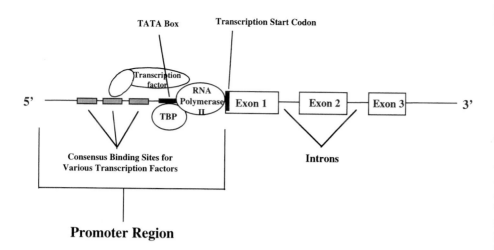

Promoter Region

Figure 9

The general scheme for promoter regulation of genes involves a sequence at the 5' end that contains specific binding sequences (consensus sequences) for portions of the transcriptional machinery and regulatory proteins such as transcription factors. The TATA binding protein (TBP) binds to the TATA box and associates with several proteins and the RNA polymerase. The transcriptional activity is regulated either positively or negatively by other transcription factors that bind to the consensus sequences and then associated with the transcription complex. Regulatory elements in intronic sequences or at distant sites, including the 3' flanking region of the gene, can also occur in some instances.

in response to an external signal or condition are inducible. Genes whose expression decreases in response to a signal are termed repressible. Activators are proteins that bind to DNA and facilitate transcription of a gene, in a process referred to as positive regulation. Repressors are proteins that bind to DNA and block transcription, and this process is referred to as negative regulation.

DNA sequences that bind proteins that regulate transcription are known as *cis* elements; the proteins that bind to the *cis* elements and influence transcription (and are products of other genes) are called *trans* acting factors. The affinity of binding of a protein to a DNA sequence usually extends over a region of 5 to 7 bp, and is strongly influenced by the exact sequence. Consensus sequences are those that bind a given regulatory protein with the highest affinity, although less tight association occurs with increasing mismatch of the consensus sequence from the ideal. Optimal matching of DNA binding sequences to regulatory factors enhances their binding by 10^6- to 10^7-fold. Promoter regions contain activation domains where specific regulatory proteins can bind, and then interact with the transcription complex to enhance the rate of transcription. Similarly, repressor elements bind proteins that either interfere with binding of one of the proteins of the transcriptional complex or the polymerase, or decrease the efficiency of the transcriptional complex in some manner through protein-protein interactions. Regulatory elements such as enhancers can be physically removed from the proximal promoter region by many kb of DNA, yet influence transcription of the noncontiguous transcribed gene. This is thought to occur through secondary structure of the DNA with loops that bring the enhancer element and its interacting regulatory protein into contact with the transcriptional complex (Fig. 10).

The RNA polymerase binds to the consensus binding site at -35, and unwinds the double-stranded DNA as it moves to the -10 binding site, creating a transcription bubble of single-stranded DNA approximately 17 bases in length that will accommodate the transcription complex and allow transcription of the exposed portion of the template DNA. In the promoters of most eukaryotic class II genes, there is a consensus sequence known as a TATAAA (usually called a TATA box), analogous to the *E. coli* -10 site, and generally located 25 to 30 bp upstream from the transcription start site. A binding protein (TATA binding protein, TBP, or transcription factor IID, TFIID) attaches here as the initial part of the transcription complex. Associated general transcription factor proteins TFIIA and TFIIB then bind to the promoter, followed by RNA polymerase II, as well as several other factors, including TFIIE and TAFs (TBP associated factors). This transcriptional complex then allows initiation of mRNA transcription, and represents the basal transcriptional apparatus (Fig. 11). Other sequences that can func-

Interaction of remote enhancer regions with transcription complex

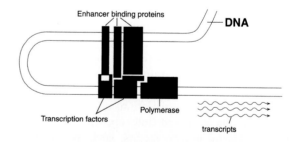

Figure 10

Possible mechanism by which remote upstream regulatory enhancer elements may influence the transcriptional complex. Looping of the DNA may bring sets of transcription factors into proximity to allow influence on the polymerase activity. (Reproduced with permission from Zubay JL, Parson WW, Vance DE (eds): *Principles of Biochemistry*. Dubuque, IA, WCB/McGraw-Hill, 1994, p 802.)

tion to control transcription in the proximal promoter include the CCAAT box (5'-GCCAAT-3') and the GC box (5'-GGGCGG-3'), which bind proteins Sp1 and C/EBP.

The regulatory proteins that interact with the promoter *cis* elements are loosely termed transcription factors. Several general classes of these proteins exist, all of which contain both DNA binding domains and protein-protein interaction domains through which they influence the transcriptional complex. The first type is the helix-turn-helix form. These are common in prokaryotes, and consist of 20 amino acid segments with 2 α helices of 7 to 9 amino acids separated by a β turn. The second type is the zinc finger transcription factor. These proteins contain groups of 4 cysteine or histidine residues that coordinate a zinc ion. Some regulatory proteins have multiple zinc finger regions, allowing multiple DNA interaction domains and thereby increasing specificity. Steroid receptors such as the vitamin D receptor, thyroid hormone receptor, and retinoid receptors contain a common central domain that binds DNA through 2 zinc finger regions. Homeodomain transcription factors are related to helix-turn-helix factors, and contain 3 α helices, one of which is the DNA recognition domain. These proteins are involved in patterning during early development, and are absent in prokaryotes.

Another class of factors important in development is the basic helix-loop-helix proteins (bHLH). These proteins have a basic DNA binding region, and are active as dimers. Myo D, which controls muscle differentiation, is an example of a bHLH factor. The last category of transcription factors, the leucine zipper, contains a helical domain with an exposed series of leucines that interact with similar leucines on a dimerization partner. Leucine zipper transcription factors can be heterodimeric or homodimeric. Transcription factor types are summarized in Figure 12. AP1 is an important transcription factor in many musculoskeletal tissues and processes, and consists of dimers of the Fos and Jun family members. AP1 activity is frequently associated with early response gene activation in signaling and control of cell proliferation. Some transcription factors, such as AP1, can be activated by phosphorylation. Note that the transcription factors are essentially instruments by which the cell turns genes off or on in response to various stimuli. These stimuli, such as growth factors or mechanical stress, set off a series of signals from the plasma membrane to the cytoplasm. The last members of these signaling pathways are transcription factors.

The state of activation of genes is related to the physical configuration of the genetic DNA in the chromosome. The extremely compact form of DNA in the nuclear chromatin and its association with histone complexes in the nucleosomes makes the majority of genetic DNA inaccessible for initiation of transcription. Thus, DNA may be present in open (accessible) or closed (inaccessible) configurations. An open chromatin configuration is sometimes found on flanking DNA sequences such as the locus control region (LCR) of the beta globin gene. Alterations of the LCR lead to closed chromatin pattern and are associated with the disease β-thalassemia.

DNA can also be methylated, which appears to maintain it in an inactive configuration. The best example of this is the X chromosome, a copy of which is inactivated in each cell. The inactivated X chromosome is heavily methylated and is not transcribed. Also, the methylation of histone proteins on lysine, arginine, and histidine residues, or acetylation of lysine residues can influence histone association with DNA and its accessibility for transcription or replication. Histones are also phosphorylated on serine and histidine residues. Phosphorylation of the H1 histone may be involved in mitotic condensation of chromatin. RNA polymerase is thought to displace histone octamers during transcription.

Transcription factor expression has tissue-specific consequences; tissue-specific transcription factors such as *Cbfa1*, which is also found in cartilage and has relatively restricted expression to osteoblastic cells, have recently been identi-

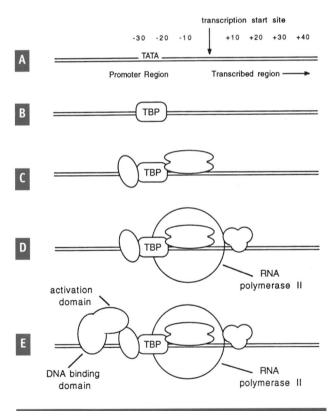

Figure 11

The transcriptional complex is assembled sequentially (**A**), with the initial event being binding of the TATA binding protein (TBP; also called transcription factor IID [TFIID]) to the TATA box (**B**). Subsequently TFIIA and TFIIB associate with TBP (**C**), followed by binding of RNA polymerase II (**D**). Finally, regulatory transcriptional factors that control the rate of transcription associate with consensus sequences in the promoter region and the transcriptional complex of proteins (**E**). (Reproduced with permission from Shore EM, Kaplan FS: Tutorial: Molecular biology for the clinician: Part I. General principles. *Clin Orthop* 1994;306:264–283.)

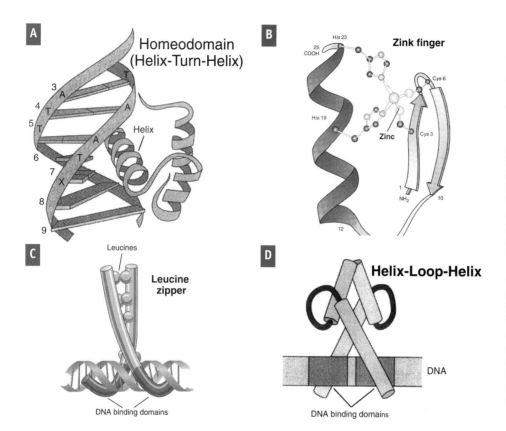

Figure 12

A, The general structure of the homeodomain subtype of helix-turn-helix transcription factors includes 3 helical domains, 1 of which interacts with the major groove of DNA to regulate gene expression. (Adapted with permission from Gilbert SF: *Developmental Biology*, ed 4. Sunderland, MA, Sinauer Associates, 1994, p 558.). **B,** Zinc finger proteins contain a zinc ion bound by coordinating histidine/cysteine pairs. (Figures B and C are adapted with permission from Zubay JL, Parson WW, Vance DE (eds): *Principles of Biochemistry*. Dubuque, IA, WCB/McGraw-Hill, 1994, p 815–816.). **C,** Leucine zipper transcription factors consist of homodimers or heterodimers that have leucine interaction domains (the "zipper") and DNA binding domains. **D,** Helix-loop-helix transcription factors are active only as homodimers. (Adapted with persion from Alberts B, Bray D, Lewis J, Raff M, Roberts K, Watson JD: *Molecular Biology of the Cell*. New York, NY, Garland Publishing, 1994, p 414.)

fied. Deletion of this gene in mouse models results in a perinatal lethal phenotype that fails to develop mineralized bones, and failure of expression of a number of other osteoblast genes that appear to be under its control. Mutations in *Cbfa1* have been associated with the cleidocranial dysostosis. An osteoblastic transcriptional coactivator protein, NAC, has also been identified. Expression of myoD in fibroblasts can transform the cells into myoblasts. Overexpression of c-fos in transgenic mice results in development of chondrosarcomas, and c-fos overexpression is observed in fibrous dysplasia, although the underlying mutation in this disorder is within a g protein, a membrane-associated protein which associates with signal-transducing receptors, and not c-fos itself.

Homeotic Genes and Development

Homeotic genes represent a widely used motif in transcription factors. These genes were first discovered through the study of mutant *Drosophila melanogaster* (the fruit fly), which has been an invaluable model for the study of development in complex multicellular organisms. The mutant flies had body segments that had acquired the identity of the neighboring segment. For example, flies mutated in *Ultrabithorax* had 2 sets of wings because the first abdominal segment developed into a structure resembling the third thoracic segment. In other words, the function of the homeotic gene *Ultrabithorax* is to confer identity to cells along the anteroposterior (head-to-tail) axis. In *Drosophila*

there are 8 homeotic genes in a single split cluster, named *HomC*, on chromosome 3 (Fig. 13). In a unique arrangement, the expression of each homeotic gene in *HomC* is sequential, and the timing of expression is aligned along development of the anteroposterior axis. Thus, the first homeotic gene in the cluster is highly expressed in the segments that become the head, followed by sequential expression of the rest of the genes in the thoracic and then abdominal segments. The expression of the last homeotic gene is highest in the distal abdominal segments.

Each homeotic gene product contains a highly conserved domain of 60 amino acids that bind to DNA. The DNA binding domain is referred to as the homeodomain, and the coding sequence in DNA for the homeodomain is called a homeobox. The primary sequence of the homeodomain is rich in the positively charged amino acids lysine and arginine. The structure of the homeodomain is distantly related to the helix-turn-helix domains of prokaryotic regulatory proteins; however, unlike prokaryotic helix-turn-helix proteins, homeodomain proteins bind singly and asymmetrically. The homeodomain forms 3 α-helices, one of which contacts the DNA recognition sequence in the major groove, and a nonhelical N-terminal portion of the homeodomain contacts the DNA in the minor groove. However, other regions of homeodomain proteins and protein-protein interactions are also critical for accurate function of these transcription factors.

Mammals possess 4 gene clusters similar to *Homc. Hoxa, Hoxb, Hoxc* and *Hoxd* are found on chromosomes 7, 17, 12,

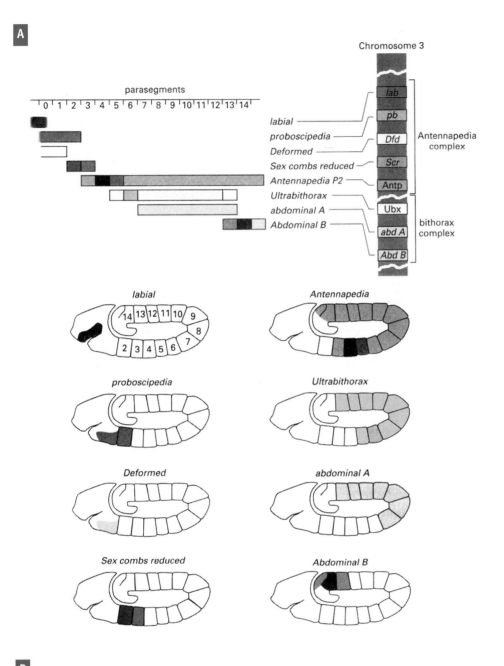

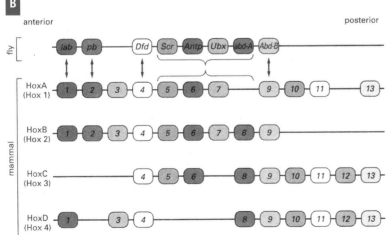

Figure 13

A, Homeobox genes that regulate patterning of body development are activated sequentially in a linear arrangement on the chromosome, reflecting the linear arrangement of the body parts whose development they control. **B,** Homeotic genes and their arrangement are highly conserved across species. (Reproduced with permission from Alberts B, Bray D, Lewis J, Raff M, Roberts K, Watson JD: *Molecular Biology of the Cell,* ed 3. New York, NY, Garland Publishing, 1994, pp 1095, 1104.)

and 2, respectively (Fig. 13). Each cluster has 9 to 11 genes, totaling 39 *Hox* genes for all 4 clusters, and each gene at a particular position number (such as position *Hoxa1, Hoxb1,* and *Hoxd1*) are called paralogs. As in *Drosophila*, the expression of each gene in the cluster is sequential, and peaks in neighboring segments of both the axial and appendicular skeleton and other tissues. Studies with genetically engineered mice that either overexpress or have deletions of various *Hox* genes have demonstrated that there is some overlap in activity of paralogous genes. In other words, a single *Hox* gene is not solely responsible for development of a single segment, as is found in *Drosophila*. Thus, loss of function of a single *Hox* gene in mammals does not typically result in homeotic transformation of neighboring segments.

Families that have defects in distal skeletal elements have recently been characterized as possessing mutations in either the *Hoxa13* or *Hoxd13* genes. Human synpolydactyly is a semidominant condition that results from a mutation in the Hoxd13 protein. Three separate families have been identified with insertion of different numbers of alanines in a polyalanine tract in the N-terminal of the Hoxd13 protein. The alanine tract is not in the homeodomain, and the altered polyalanine domain does not appear to block DNA binding. Instead, the increased numbers of polyalanines are believed to affect the interaction of the Hoxd13 protein with other transcription factors. Human hand-foot-genital syndrome is an autosomal dominant condition caused by a mutation in the homeodomain of *Hoxa13*. This defect affects the first digits in hands and feet, and results in alteration of a number of structures in the genital system. Therefore, *Hox* genes are critical for proper development of all tissues.

Finally, it should be noted that the homeodomain is not restricted to gene products from the clustered *Hox* genes. There are an estimated 300 homeodomain proteins encoded in the human genome, and a number of human defects have been assigned to mutations in these homeodomain proteins. Thus, the use of this particular DNA binding domain has been widespread throughout evolution.

Tools and Techniques of Molecular Biology

Recombinant technology refers to the manipulation of segments of DNA and/or RNA, such that genetic material is recombined with other portions of genetic material, usually in plasmid and bacterial systems. This allows production of specific desired sequences of DNA, RNA, or amino acids. A recombinant protein is one in which the genetic sequence coding for the desired protein amino acid sequence is introduced into the genome of an organism or cell. The transcriptional and translational machinery of the organism or cell is then used to produce the protein, which can be extracted and purified for its intended uses. Numer-

ous proteins for therapeutic use, including human growth hormone, insulin, erythropoietin, and clotting factors, are currently produced using recombinant technology, and the list of engineered recombinant materials is growing explosively. Recombinant DNA technology also has applications in diagnosis of disease and identification of genetic abnormalities that cause inherited disorders.

The molecular biologist has a basic set of tools (contained in tiny test tubes) that allow these same actions with DNA (recombining DNA). The ability to manipulate DNA depends on simple tools analogous to the cut, paste, and copy functions on the computer. The overall process of molecular cloning involves isolating a specific segment of DNA, and generating many identical copies of that specific DNA sequence. This is accomplished by cutting the DNA fragment of interest, called the target sequence, from adjoining DNA sequences using bacterial enzymes, called restriction endonucleases, which cut double-stranded DNA at specific sites based on the DNA sequence. An isolated fragment of DNA cannot replicate itself, and has to be incorporated into a form of DNA (vector) with replicative capability. Plasmids, a type of commonly used vector, consist of a simple circular double-stranded DNA genome that replicates by infecting bacteria, using the transcriptional machinery of the bacteria to make copies of the plasmid DNA. Bacteriophages, another type of commonly used but more complex vector, are functionally viruses that infect bacteria, and can multiply using the bacterial transcriptional and translational apparatus. The DNA target sequence is inserted into the vector DNA at specific cloning sites (regions of sequence with known specific restriction sites) by cutting the vector with restriction enzymes to produce complementary base pairing to the ends of the DNA target sequence. This is "pasted," or ligated, into the vector DNA using an enzyme called a ligase. When bacteria are induced to internalize the vector, the DNA target sequence is copied by the replication mechanisms along with the vector DNA, and the DNA molecules thus produced are referred to as recombinant DNA, because the target sequence has been recombined with the vector DNA.

Internalization of a plasmid in the bacteria is facilitated by altering chemical conditions and is referred to as bacterial transformation. Bacteriophage introduction into bacteria is referred to as bacterial transfection. Multiple copies of the vector containing the target sequence are produced by internal replication, and the target sequence DNA can be isolated from the bacterial and vector DNA by using restriction enzymes to excise it. Bacteria that contain the vector can be separated from those that do not by using antibiotics in the bacterial culture medium and incorporation of a resistance gene to the antibiotic within the vector DNA. The antibiotic is lethal to any bacteria that have not been transformed by the vector. Figure 14 summarizes the process of molecular cloning of recombinant DNA, and a detailed discussion of the process follows.

Cutting, Pasting, and Moving DNA

Restriction Endonucleases

Restriction digestion refers to cutting DNA into specific fragments using restriction enzymes. The genome of *E. coli* is 4 million bp, the genome of a human is 6 billion bp. In practice, such large pieces of DNA cannot be easily analyzed or manipulated. The discovery of restriction endonucleases (also called restriction enzymes) and their subsequent use enabled researchers to cut DNA into manageable pieces. These restriction enzymes are usually found in bacteria and act to guard against the invasion and expression of foreign DNA. A restriction enzyme cuts double-stranded DNA at a site of specific DNA sequence (usually 4 to 8 nucleotides in length) that is recognized by that particular enzyme. For example, *E. coli* makes an enzyme EcoRI, which cuts DNA at a specific sequence:

5'-NNNNNNGAATTCNNNNNNN-3'   EcoRI   5'-NNNNNNG-3'   5'- AATTCNNNNNN-3'

3'-MMMMMMCTTAAGMMMMMMM-5' ———→ 3'-MMMMMMCTTAA-5'   3'-   GMMMMMM-5'

N = any base; M = the complement to base (if N = A, M = T)

EcoRI cuts at the 6-base recognition site 5'-GAATTC-3'. This sequence is identical on both strands, and is referred to as a palindrome. Many restriction enzymes, particularly those that are used most frequently in the laboratory, cut at palindromic sequences. Given this activity in a cell, how does the bacteria recognize which DNA is foreign and which DNA is its own? In bacteria, restriction enzymes are paired with site-specific methylases, which modify a single base within the same recognition site by adding a methyl group ($-CH_3$). The EcoRI methylase modifies the first adenine in the GAATTC sequence. This methylation blocks the activity of the EcoRI restriction enzymes, and prevents cutting of the bacteria's own DNA.

Hundreds of restriction enzymes have been identified, and 50 to 70 have practical uses. In addition to the enzymes that cut at a 6-base recognition sequence (on the average, every 4,096 [4^6] base pairs), there are many that cut at 4 bp sites (every 1,012 bases) and 8 bp sites (every 16,384 bases). An unknown piece of DNA being analyzed is routinely cut with a panel of "6-base cutters." The data gleaned from such an experiment allows ordering of the various restriction sites along the piece of DNA to create a restriction map for the DNA segment under study. These sites can then be used to subdivide the fragment into specific pieces and to clone these smaller fragments to facilitate further analysis. Note that restriction enzymes can leave either 5' extensions (unmatched bases, called cohesive, or sticky ends), 3' extensions, or blunt ends after cutting. Restriction enzymes are named according to designations of the bacteria from which they were derived, generally with a letter abbreviation and sometimes a numeral. Table 2 shows some commonly used restriction enzymes and the recognition and cut sites.

DNA Ligation

In manipulating DNA, the ability to paste a DNA fragment into another or connect 2 fragments of DNA is as important a tool as restriction digestion, and is in effect the reverse of restriction. This process is called DNA ligation, and is accomplished by enzymes called ligases, which complete covalent phosphate bonds between adjacent nucleotides that have hydrogen-bonded complementary sequences.

Cloning a DNA Fragment

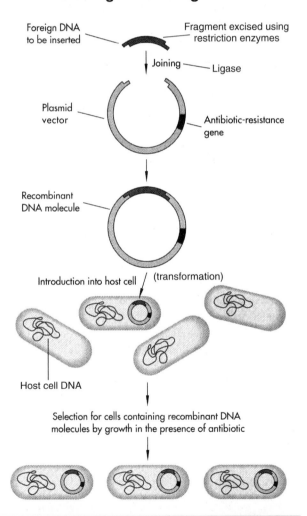

Figure 14

The general sequence of events for cloning a specific fragment of DNA using a plasmid vector. (Reproduced with permission from Watson JD, Gilman M, Witkowski J, Zoller M (eds): *Recombinant DNA,* ed 2. New York, NY, WH Freeman & Co, 1992, p 74.)

For instance, in the EcoRI example above, 2 DNA fragments cut with this enzyme will have cohesive complementary ends because of the palindromic nature of the restriction cut. Under proper conditions, hydrogen bonding of the complementary sequences can occur, linking the 2 ends of the different pieces of DNA together. Ligase enzymes can then complete the connection by making the appropriate 3′ to 5′ bonds in the same strands.

Restriction Mapping

After a DNA fragment is cut with restriction enzymes, the fragment(s) can be analyzed by agarose gel electrophoresis

Table 2
Common Restriction Enzymes

Restriction Enzyme	Sequence Recognition Site and Cut
Taql	5′ T C G A 3′ 3′ A G C T 5′
EcoRI	5′ G A A T T C 3′ 3′ C T T A A G 5′
Pstl	5′ C T G C A G 3′ 3′ G A C G T C 5′
Notl	5′ G C G G C C G C 3′ 3′ C G C C G G C G 5′
Smal	5′ C C C G G G 3′ 3′ G G G C C C 5′
Hindlll	5′ A A G C T T 3′ 3′ T T C G A A 5′
Pvul	5′ C G A T C G 3′ 3′ G C T A G C 5′

to determine molecular weight, which functionally is the same as the fragment length. Agarose, an extract of seaweed, is mixed with electrophoresis buffer and water, melted at 95° to 100°C, cooled, and then poured into a mold, forming a slab approximately 1/4″ thick. A comb is placed in one end of the gel mold, creating slots in the solidifying agarose. After the gel has set, the comb is removed, the gel is submerged in electrophoresis buffer, and the restriction digested DNA is then loaded into the slots, with molecular weight sizing standards loaded in a separate slot. As the DNA fragments are highly negatively charged because of the phosphate groups, the DNA fragments migrate toward the positive pole of the electrophoresis apparatus (Fig. 15). The agarose gel acts like a sieve, retarding larger molecular weight (longer) DNA fragments. Agarose gels usually contain ethidium bromide (EtBr), a dye that intercalates between the bases inside the helix. After the gel has been run, an ultraviolet (UV) light is used to cause the EtBr to fluoresce, identifying the location, and by comparison with the standards, the size, of the DNA fragments.

To create a restriction map of a DNA fragment of unknown sequence, the DNA is digested with several different restriction enzymes, and the digestions from different enzymes (or combinations) are electrophoresed in parallel lanes on an agarose gel. The restriction fragment patterns are used to assemble a map of the locations of the restriction sites in the DNA fragments relative to one another. An example of a restriction map is shown in Figure 16.

A restriction map of a DNA fragment is only the beginning of the analysis and use of the fragment. The DNA is usually subjected to sequence analysis, and may be used to express a protein. In order to use the DNA in this way, it is cloned into a vector, usually a plasmid. Cloning involves taking a DNA fragment and placing it into a compatible restriction site in the plasmid. The reason for this is again a practical one. To study a DNA fragment of interest, a certain amount of this fragment is needed, and so bacterial plasmids are

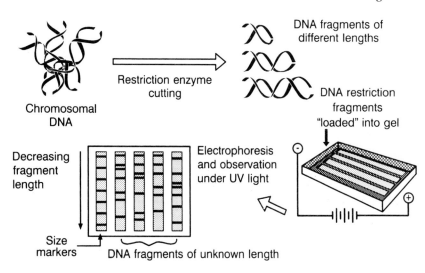

Figure 15

Agarose gel electrophoresis of DNA involves placing DNA fragment in wells at the top of an agarose gel suspended in a buffer; an electric voltage is applied. The highly negatively-charged DNA migrates toward the positive electrode, and the rate of migration is determined by the size of the fragment. Ethidium bromide binding to DNA can be visualized under ultraviolet light.

employed to supply the researcher with sufficient amounts of DNA, because they can replicate the target sequence in bacteria (usually *E. coli*).

Vectors for DNA Manipulation

Plasmids are extrachromosomal DNA, that is, not part of the circular *E. coli* chromosome. They are not subject to the same regulation on DNA synthesis as genomic DNA, and will continue to be replicated after the bacteria have stopped dividing. Thus, while any single *E. coli* will have 1 chromosome, it may contain over 50 copies of a plasmid. Plasmids are usually between 2.5 and 10 kb, and all contain 2 required sequences: an origin of replication, so that the

replication machinery can recognize the plasmid DNA, and a selectable marker, usually antibiotic resistance, so that only those cells harboring the plasmid survive. All plasmids of practical use contain multiple restriction sites grouped at a single location (called the multiple cloning site) in the plasmid, allowing for cloning of restriction fragments with a wide variety of ends (see example below). Insert sizes for plasmids and similar vectors called phagemids are generally less than 10 kb. Plasmids are introduced into bacteria by rendering the bacteria permeable (bacterial transformation). The plasmids then reproduce within the bacterial cells, and as the bacteria themselves replicate, the daughter plasmids are passed on along with the bacterial chromosome. The bacterial suspension is then plated in the presence of an antibiotic to kill all but the transformants, which survive because of the antibiotic resistance gene incorporated within the plasmid. The agar plates then develop individual colonies derived from single transformed bacteria as they continue to replicate. The colonies can be physically removed from the agar plate, regrown, and analyzed to confirm the presence of the plasmid and insert sequences.

For larger-sized DNA inserts, bacteriophage λ are often used, because these λ phage can accommodate inserts over 20 kb in size. λ phage DNA is double-stranded, can exist in either linear or circular forms, and is packaged in a protein coat. Phage particles containing the protein coat are infectious to bacteria, inserting their linearized DNA into the host organism, where the phage DNA circularizes and replicates. The packaged phage particles within the host bacteria eventually cause the bacteria to lyse and release the contained infective particles. These particles infect adjacent bacteria and repeat the process, resulting in areas of lysis on a "lawn" of uninfected bacteria on the surface of an agar plate. The phage can be recovered from the lytic areas on the plate and used for analysis or for reinfecting bacteria.

Cosmids are hybrid vectors between λ phage and plasmids, which accommodate inserts up to 45 kb in size. Cosmid DNA is packaged into phage particles but replicates within the bacteria like plasmids. Very large inserts can be cloned using yeast artificial chromosomes (YACs), which are engineered chromosomes containing cloning sites, selectable markers, and telomeric and centromeric regions that allow chromosomal segregation for proper replication during yeast cell replication. These vectors can handle inserts from 100 to 1,500 kb in size. They are used for chromosomal gene mapping studies because larger regions can be studied. YACs also allow study of some of the larger mammalian genes, which can exceed 100 kb in size.

Shorter restriction fragments can be introduced into plasmids using restriction digestion of the vector to produce a suitable end matching that of the fragment, and then using ligation to incorporate the fragment into the genome of the vector. Figure 17 demonstrates the process of cloning a restriction fragment. The *E. coli* strains used in the laboratory have been genetically altered to prevent human patho-

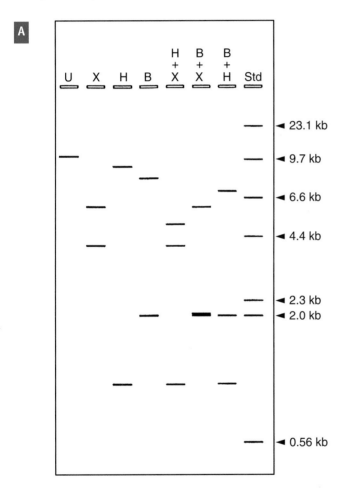

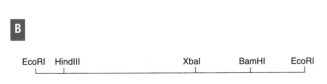

Figure 16

A, Analysis of DNA restriction fragments by agarose gel electrophoresis. **B,** Restriction map for the 10 kb fragment in **A.** X = XbaI, H = HindIII, B = BamHI, U = Undigested fragment, Std = Standards.

genicity, which also eliminates the risk of recombinant DNA being passed to humans working with these organisms.

Because bacteria contain ribosomes and can produce protein as well as transcribe RNA, a cloned DNA fragment can be used to produce the protein coded for by the DNA sequence as well as produce the DNA. Assuming the DNA sequence of interest is not a bacterial gene, expression of the gene product in the bacteria is known as heterologous expression. Protein extracts from transformed bacteria will contain the protein coded for by the DNA fragment cloned into the vector. Of course, the vector construction is critical; the introduced fragment must have an appropriate reading frame and, depending on the insertion site for the ligation, some of the plasmid DNA sequence will usually be included in the transcript, resulting in translation of additional amino acids not included in the ligated coding sequence. The resulting protein expressed in the bacteria is referred to as a fusion protein because it usually contains the segment of protein coded for by the cloned DNA fragment in addition to some amino acids derived from the upstream vector sequence. One problem in the heterologous production of mammalian recombinant proteins is that bacteria lack mammalian posttranslational processing mechanisms. Often, glycosylation and proper folding are blocked, making the recombinant protein nonfunctional. However, some fusion proteins may be functional, and this technique is also useful for producing proteins for use as antigens in the production of antibodies.

In vitro mutagenesis is a technique that takes advantage of the properties of the DNA-manipulating enzymes to alter sequences specifically in cloned DNA fragments. This allows specific mutations to be created to analyze effects on gene function. These techniques are facilitated by automated DNA synthesizers, which can readily and inexpensively produce specific DNA oligonucleotide sequences.

DNA Libraries

Genomic Libraries

A library, as the name implies, consists of a large collection of various cloned DNA fragments. Creation of a library is generally one of the first steps in isolating and cloning a specific gene or portion of a gene. The general approach is to extract DNA from cells or tissues, and then create a digestion with restriction enzymes, reducing the DNA to many small fragments that can be cloned into vectors. A genomic library involves digestion of genomic DNA extracted from cells of a particular species, which is then restriction digested and cloned into a vector with appropriate cloning sites. Bacteriophages, rather than plasmids, are usually used as vectors. The restriction fragments are ligated into the vector, and the recombinant bacteriophage DNA is then used to produce infectious phage particles. The phage contain-

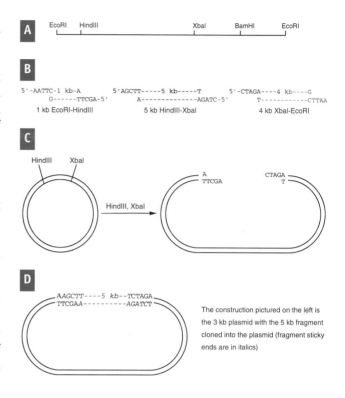

Figure 17

Cloning of DNA restriction fragments. **A,** Starting fragment. **B,** After digestion with the enzymes Hind III and XbaI. **C,** 3-kb plasmid with a multiple cloning site that contains Hind III and XbaI and cut with each of these enzymes. **D,** The 3-kb plasmid with the 5-kb fragment cloned into the plasmid (fragment sticky ends are in italics).

ing various inserts constitute the library of DNA restriction fragments. The phage replicates and lyses the bacteria, releasing progeny that infect adjacent bacteria, and a lytic plaque develops on a lawn of bacteria in culture. Such a plaque can be removed from culture and subcloned, and ideally will contain a single phage colony. Single clones containing a gene or part of a gene can be obtained in this manner. If plasmids are used as the cloning vector, the mix of plasmids carrying the various DNA inserts is used to transform bacteria after ligation of the restriction fragments. This results in replication of the plasmids and the bacteria containing them, effectively amplifying the amounts of individual genomic fragments in the library. The bacteria are adequately diluted and plated, so that colonies will develop containing individual clones with specific genomic fragments, and individual colonies are again subcloned as necessary to obtain single clones.

Complementary DNA Libraries

Because all somatic cells carry the same complement of genomic DNA, a genomic library is species-specific, but not tissue- or cell-specific. Libraries can also be created from mRNA isolated from cells, in which case only the expressed transcripts are incorporated into the library. This is accomplished by first converting the isolated mRNA into complementary DNA (cDNA). Libraries constructed from cDNA are specific for the cell or tissue type from which they are derived. Genomic libraries are useful for study of promoter and other regulatory elements that are not contained in the mRNA transcripts, and theoretically contain relatively equal representation of all single copy class II genes. cDNA libraries contain the representations of only the genes being actively expressed in the specific tissue, and will contain larger numbers of clones representing more abundant mRNA transcripts. In addition, the cDNA library is focused on a small fraction of the genome, because intronic sequences and genes not actively being transcribed are excluded.

To create cDNA, 3 processes are necessary: extraction of RNA from cells or tissues; purification of the total cellular RNA to obtain only the mRNA; and conversion of mRNA to cDNA using a reverse transcriptase enzyme. RNases are ubiquitous in the environment, and RNA is much more easily degraded and less stable than DNA. Consequently, strict attention to use of RNase-free glassware and reagents is essential to isolation of intact cellular RNA. RNA can be isolated by various methods, generally involving some variation on phenol/guanidinium isothiocyanate extractions and purifications by centrifugations and ethanol precipitations. The best way to handle tissue from human or animal samples being used for mRNA production is to place it in an RNase extraction solution in the operating room, or to freeze it in liquid nitrogen and then subsequently grind it to a powder and/or homogenize it within the RNA extraction solution with a sonicator called a polytron. These procedures prevent RNA degradation. Another common problem with RNA extraction can be contamination of the extracted RNA with DNA. The likelihood of contamination can be lessened by treatment of RNA preparations with DNase prior to reverse transcription procedures.

mRNA can be purified from total RNA to eliminate the more abundant rRNAs by recognizing that nearly all translated eukaryotic messages are polyadenylated at the 3′ end. The function of this poly(A) tail is uncertain, but it is of great practical use for isolating mRNA (also called poly(A)+ RNA). Short oligonucleotides containing only deoxythymidine residues [oligo(dT)] are attached to cellulose beads and placed in a small column. Under appropriate conditions to allow hydrogen bonding between the poly(dT) column and the poly(A) tails of the mRNAs, a solution containing total cellular RNA is poured through the poly(dT) column. The nonpolyadenylated RNA passes through the column, while the polyadenylated mRNA is retained on the column. Subsequently the mRNA is eluted by using a low salt buffer that disrupts the hydrogen bonding between the poly (dT) and the poly(A), and the poly(A)+ RNA is recovered in the eluting solution. mRNA yield from total RNA is usually only 1% to 3%.

Conversion of the mRNA to a complementary DNA sequence is accomplished using reverse transcriptase, an enzyme derived from retroviruses that function as primer-dependent DNA polymerase using an RNA template. Retroviruses use this enzyme to convert their genome (which is RNA) into DNA within the cell to allow subsequent replication using the cell's DNA transcriptional machinery and RNA polymerase to generate RNA copies of the virus. Like RNA polymerases, reverse transcriptase requires a primer to hybridize to the RNA template to permit transcription. In converting mRNA to cDNA, priming can be accomplished by either of 2 methods. The first uses the poly(A) tail and adds synthetic oligo(dT) as a primer to provide the 3′ OH group from which nucleic acid synthesis can extend. Alternatively, random synthetic short oligonucleotide primers can be used. The reverse transcriptase and primers are added to the solution of poly(A)+ RNA, and DNA synthesis occurs, generating a strand of cDNA for each mRNA transcript. Most manipulations of DNA require the DNA to be double-stranded; therefore, the mRNA must be removed (usually enzymatically, by addition of RNase), and then DNA polymerase and added deoxynucleotides are used to synthesize the strand complementary to the cDNA.

After the cDNA has been generated, the procedure for producing the cDNA library is similar to that described previously for genomic libraries. The cDNA is ligated into a cloning vector, creating a library of vectors containing cDNA representations of all of the expressed transcripts. Because most cDNAs are only a few kb long, the cloning vector can be either a plasmid or bacteriophage. The plasmids are used to transform bacteria, replicating the plasmids. The transformants can be plated at low density, and individual clones can be obtained using the antibiotic resistance selection procedure to select only bacteria containing the plasmid as previously described.

Another type of library is an expression library. In this case, the cDNA transformants heterologously produce the proteins encoded by the cDNA, and colonies containing a desired sequence can be selected either by protein-protein interactions using a labeled protein as a probe (in searching for ligands or binding proteins for the gene product, for example), or by using an antibody to a protein whose gene is being cloned.

Analysis of DNA and RNA With Hybridization Techniques

The property of hydrogen bonding of complementary bp allows use of a labeled segment of RNA or DNA to function as a probe, enabling detection of complementary sequences of either RNA or DNA. This process of hybridization technically refers to hybrids of DNA and RNA that form through hydrogen bonding of complementary bases. However, the term is more broadly applied to complementary binding strands of RNA or DNA as well. Hybridization, or efficient binding of complementary sequences, is affected by chemical conditions, including salt concentration, temperature, and presence of specific chemical constituents such as formamide that influence the hydrogen bonds. Higher temperatures and lower salt concentrations tend to dissociate hydrogen bonds and cause hybrids to separate, or denature. The optimal temperature for hybridization is a function of the type of polymers involved (RNA versus DNA), and is also dependent on the percentage of pyrimidine versus purine bases, because of the tighter binding of the triple hydrogen bonds of GC pairs as compared to the double hydrogen bonds of AT or AU pairs.

Nucleic Acid Probes

Any DNA or RNA sequence that contains some type of label to allow its detection is called a probe. The most common label is incorporation of radioactivity, often ^{32}P-labeled nucleotides. Other types of labels include fluorescently tagged nucleotides, or nucleotides with covalently bound organic molecules such as digoxigenin or biotin, which can be detected with specific antibodies. Incorporation of any of these labels into a fragment of RNA or DNA enables it to be used to identify the presence of complementary nucleic acid.

The 3 basic methods for labeling probes are nick translation, random priming, and end labeling. Nick translation is performed by treating double-stranded DNA with DNase I, an endonuclease that makes single-stranded nicks in the DNA, breaking the phosphodiester bond between 2 adjacent nucleotides. The exposed 3'-OH site at the nick serves as a primer site for DNA polymerase, which can then synthesize DNA extending 5' to 3' and degrading the unlabeled portion of the strand as it proceeds. The nick "translates" along the strand. The reaction mixture contains radiolabeled deoxynucleotide triphosphates, which are incorporated into the newly synthesized DNA and label the probe. In the random priming method, the double-stranded DNA is first denatured to separate it into single-stranded DNA. Next, random short synthetic oligonucleotide primers are added with labeled deoxynucleotide triphosphates and DNA polymerase, resulting in synthesis of complementary DNA at random sites along both strands wherever the primers bind. DNA molecules can also be labeled by end-labeling techniques. Use of a polynucleotide kinase adds a labeled phosphate to the 5' DNA end. Alternatively, enzymes called terminal transferases, which add a series of a single labeled nucleotides up to hundreds of bases in length to the end of the probe DNA, can be used.

One problem with double-stranded DNA probes is that the complementary strands compete with each other as well as with the target sequence. Single-stranded probes lack this disadvantage. Single-stranded probes can be generated by cloning the target DNA into a vector that enables an RNA polymerase to synthesize the probe from the template DNA in the presence of added labeled nucleotides. An RNA probe synthesized in this manner is called a riboprobe. Directional polymerases are available, which enable synthesis of either the sense or antisense strand, depending on the polymerase used.

Library Screening

The fact that a labeled DNA or RNA probe can be hybridized with complementary sequences to identify the presence of the target RNA or DNA sequence has numerous applications. One application is identification of clones that contain specific DNA sequences in a library of many sequences as discussed previously. Clonal plaques of phage or colonies of plasmid-transformed bacteria can be screened with the labeled probe complementary to the target DNA sequence, which is termed plaque or colony hybridization. Plaques or bacterial colonies can be lifted from an agar plate by placing a nitrocellulose or nylon filter disk on the surface of the culture. The filter is marked with reference marks that align with marks on the culture plate for orientation. Some of the phage or bacterial colonies will adhere to the filter when it is lifted off. The DNA is denatured and fixed to the filter. The filter is then incubated with a radioactively labeled probe complementary to the target sequence, allowing hybridization of the probe with the DNA from the phage or plasmids expressing the target DNA. The filter is washed to remove nonspecifically bound and excess labeled probe, using a series of washes with an increasing tendency to break hydrogen bonds, or denature weak interactions. This tendency is called stringency, and is accomplished with conditions of increasing temperature, or decreasing salt or formamide concentrations in the medium. High stringency conditions allow only the tightest hybrid bonds to remain intact, thus selecting for exact matches of the complementary sequence to the probe. If one were trying to clone a homologous gene from a different species that may not have the same sequence, lower stringency conditions may allow hybridization of a sequence with some degree of mismatched base pairing to identify a clone in the library for the homolog. After washing the filter, it is dried and placed on x-ray film, where hybridizing clones will result in dark spots on the film secondary to the binding of the radioactive probe. These regions can be mapped to their location on the original agar plate, and the corresponding plaques or colonies (clones) can be removed, recultured, and studied further (Fig. 18).

Southern Blotting

Another use for labeled probes is to identify specific DNA fragments separated by agarose gel electrophoresis using the Southern blot procedure. After restriction digestion, DNA fragments are separated as previously described for restriction mapping using agarose gel electrophoresis, including running 1 lane of labeled DNA molecular weight standards of known size. The double-stranded fragments are denatured after separation by size according to electrophoretic mobility by treatment with a strong base. Next, the gel is placed against a piece of nitrocellulose or nylon, and the single-stranded DNA fragments are transferred to the membrane by blotting and capillary action, preserving the relative positions of the DNA fragments as they are arranged on the gel (Fig. 19). This concentrates the DNA in a single plane and immobilizes it on the filter membrane. The filter is then hybridized with a labeled probe complementary to the target sequence, as described for library screening. After appropriate washes to remove excess probe, the filter is dried and analyzed by autoradiography. Regions of target sequence show up as dark bands on the film. The relative intensity of the band is proportional to the amount of complementary sequence present, and the length of the fragment can be ascertained by comparison with the molecular weight standards on the blot. Southern blotting is frequently used to determine presence of a gene in clinical specimens and can be useful for the diagnosis of genetic disorders.

Northern Blotting

Northern blots are used to identify and quantitate the presence of specific RNA species, usually mRNA (Fig. 19). mRNA is isolated from cells or tissues as described above, and may or may not be further purified with a poly(dT) column, depending on the abundance of the target transcript.

For rare transcripts, use of poly(A)+ RNA may be necessary to concentrate the transcript so it can be detected. As with Southern blots, the mRNA is subjected to agarose gel electrophoresis, and the shorter average length of mRNA transcripts obviates the need for restriction digestion.

After the mRNAs have been separated electrophoretically by size, the gel is blotted onto a filter membrane. The blot is hybridized with labeled cDNA probe or riboprobe complementary to the target sequence, and autoradiographed after appropriate washing. The intensity of the hybridizing bands on the autoradiograph indicates the presence and amount of target mRNA, and its molecular weight helps to confirm its identity. The amount of exposure on the film is proportional to the amount of mRNA, and can be digitized and quantitated by computer-assisted image analysis. Synthetic labeled oligonucleotides can also be used as probes, as can complementary riboprobes. Nonradioactive probes can also be used, in which case the blot is incubated with the appropriate chemical substrate or antibody after hybridization to develop a color reaction at the location of the mRNA/probe hybrid. The loading of RNA on the gel can vary considerably from lane to lane, and with Northern blots it is always important to include loading controls to allow normalization of the signal and correct measurement of the relative mRNA level. A number of genes, including GAPDH and actin, are constitutively expressed in most cells and are not regulated. These are known as housekeeping genes, and by hybridizing the Northern blot with a second probe for the housekeeping genes, mRNA (assuming the

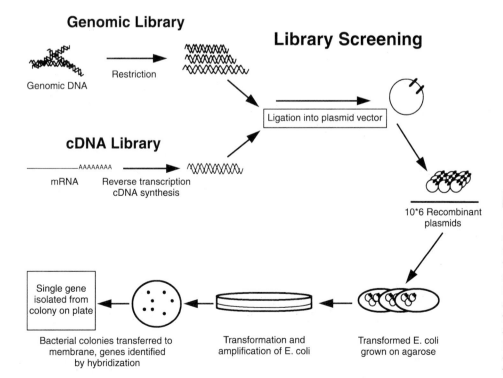

Genomic Library

Genomic DNA → Restriction →

Library Screening

cDNA Library

mRNA → Reverse transcription cDNA synthesis →

Ligation into plasmid vector

10*6 Recombinant plasmids

Single gene isolated from colony on plate

Bacterial colonies transferred to membrane, genes identified by hybridization

Transformation and amplification of E. coli

Transformed E. coli grown on agarose

Figure 18

Library screening involves restriction digestion of genomic DNA or cDNA, followed by ligation of the restriction fragments into plasmids. The plasmids are used to transform bacteria. Dilutions of the bacterial suspension are plated, and single colonies transferred to nitrocellulose membranes and hybridized with appropriate probe for gene of interest. Positive clones are then selected and grown in culture to produce the DNA fragment of interest.

molecular weight is different from the target mRNA) can allow normalization for loading. A second common method for normalizing Northern blot loading is ethidium bromide staining and UV photography of the gel prior to blotting (if total cellular RNA and not poly(A)+ RNA has been used). The highly abundant 18S and 28S rRNA bands are readily visible due to EtBr fluorescence, and the intensity of the bands can be digitally quantified by image analysis and used to normalize for lane loading differences in quantitating the mRNA signal. Figure 20 shows an example of a Northern blot.

RNase Protection Assay

This method is much more sensitive than the Northern blot and is used to detect mRNA transcripts present at very low levels. The basis of the technique is that RNA/RNA hybrids are only protected from RNase digestion when there is exact base complementary matching. Complementary radiolabeled riboprobes are used and hybridized in solution with the target sequence mRNA. The hybridization mixture is then digested with a mixture of RNases, and any single-stranded RNA (which is not protected) is degraded by the RNase. The mixture is then subjected to agarose gel electrophoresis and filter blotting as described. The labeled undigested riboprobes can be detected by autoradiography. This technique cannot determine the molecular weight or length of the mRNA, however, because of digestion of the unhybridized portions of the message.

DNA Sequencing

A simple restriction analysis of cloned inserts usually does not provide sufficient information about a gene. For exam-

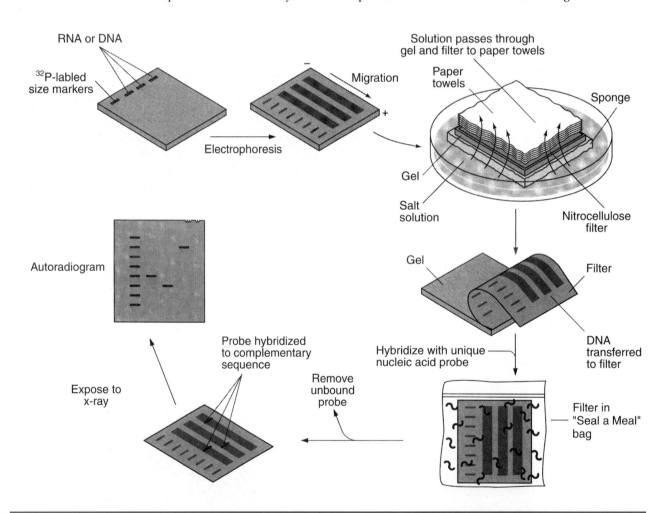

Figure 19

Northern blot analysis involves DNA electrophoresis as described to separate RNA species according to size. Following this the agarose gel is placed against a nitrocellulose filter in salt solution, with paper towels applied to the nitrocellulose. This results in diffusion of the RNA onto the nitrocellulose due to capillary action, where it is retained. The filter is then incubated with an appropriate probe complementary to the sequence of interest, and then washed to remove excess probe. After drying the filter is placed next to x-ray film and areas of radioactivity from bound probe expose the film resulting in bands of intensity that correspond to the mRNA of interest. (Reproduced with permission from Watson JD, Gilman M, Witkowski J, Zoller M (eds): *Recombinant DNA,* ed 2. New York, NY, WH Freeman & Co, 1992, p 129.)

ple, assume that the restriction fragment contains an entire gene. Sequencing will reveal the amino acid sequence of the protein (which frequently will suggest a function for the protein) and which parts of the fragment are likely to regulate gene expression, be transcribed into RNA, and be translated into protein (the coding sequence, or open reading frame). Several methods have been developed for determining the nucleotide sequence of DNA fragments. Obviously this has great importance in identifying genes, confirming sequences in cloned genes, and predicting protein products of genes. The most commonly used technique for sequencing DNA is the Sanger method of dideoxy chain termination. The DNA to be sequenced is used as a template for DNA polymerase I to synthesize a complementary strand. The technique makes use of the fact that the dideoxynucleotides do not have the 3'-OH group available for linking the next nucleotide, so chain termination occurs when a dideoxynucleotide is added by the polymerase. Because single-stranded DNA must be used as the template, the DNA must be denatured, or a single-stranded sequence of the target DNA must be generated by cloning the DNA into a bacteriophage

such as M13 or a phagemid, and using specific polymerases to synthesize the single DNA strand. An oligonucleotide primer is used to prime the DNA synthesis and must be complementary to either a portion of the target sequence or an adjacent known vector sequence if none of the target sequence is known. DNA is then synthesized from the template in 4 separate reactions, each containing all 4 nucleotide triphosphates (A,C,G,T), and one each of a dideoxynucleotide (a,c,g,t). Each reaction will generate a series of DNA fragments whose lengths change incrementally by the distance to the next dideoxynucleotide in the sequence (Fig. 21). The reaction mixtures also contain ^{35}S- or ^{32}P- labeled nucleotides so that the synthesized DNA incorporates a label to enable its detection. The reaction mixtures are subjected to high-resolution polyacrylamide gel electrophoresis, blotting, and autoradiography, producing 4 parallel lanes of bands corresponding to the fragment lengths. The sequence (which is complementary to the original target sequence) is read 3' to 5' from the shortest fragment to the longest (Fig. 18). Automated versions of the sequencing have been developed to permit computerized determination of the sequence. One modification involves use of fluorescently labeled dideoxynucleotides, which eliminates the need for radioisotopes. Because the 4 dideoxy bases can be labeled with different fluorescent tags, a single reaction mixture can be run. After DNA synthesis, the mixture is electrophoresed in a single lane, and a computerized fluorescent scanner scans the lane, in which the 4 different absorbances of the fluorescent tags will be interpreted as different bases.

Polymerase Chain Reaction

The polymerase chain reaction (PCR) was the third major technical advance in molecular biology, following the cloning and sequencing of DNA. PCR is a method of enzymatically amplifying a sequence of DNA to levels greater than 10^6, which permits acquisition of specific fragments of DNA in sufficient quantity for further use and analysis. With an estimated 100,000 genes in the human genome, and a total size of 6 billion bp, the ability to generate short fragments without conventional screening procedures has revolutionized molecular biology. PCR was developed in 1988, and is based on temperature-dependent hybridization of primers to a DNA template, polymerization, followed by denaturation of the double-stranded DNA synthesized, and a new round of polymerization. This results in a geometric amplification of the target DNA.

PCR is made practical by Taq polymerase, a thermostable enyme obtained originally from heat-resistant bacteria that inhabit thermal vents. A number of similar heat-stable polymerases have subsequently been developed with improved properties. Thermostable DNA polymerase is used for PCR, which uses thermal cycling to amplify DNA sequences. A DNA template with 2 primers (generally 15 to 30 bases)

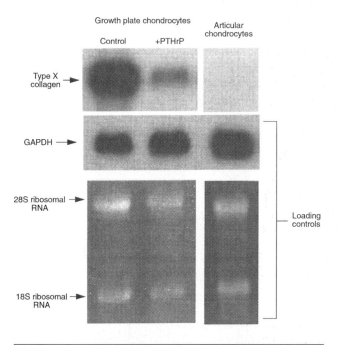

Figure 20

Results of a Northern blot performed to analyze type X collagen expression in chondrocytes. The intensity of the dark spot on the autoradiograph for the type X collagen and the housekeeping gene, GAPDH, corresponds to the amount of RNA loaded on the gel. Thus, the GAPDH is used to assure normalization of the total RNA under study in the different lanes. The type X collagen band is intense in the control and suppressed by parathyroid hormone related protein (PTHrP) treatment, indicating regulation of steady state mRNA levels by PTHrP. In contrast, articular chondrocytes, which do not make type X collagen, demonstrate no band for this mRNA. The 28S and 18S ribosomal bands of the total RNA extracts photographed under ultraviolet light before blotting the gel can also be used as loading controls to assure equal amounts of total RNA being analyzed in each lane.

complementary to sequence flanking the target sequence to be amplified is incubated with nucleotides and the Taq polymerase. At a low temperature (usually 50° to 60°C), the primers anneal (hybridize) to the template, the optimum annealing temperature being determined by the sequences. Then the mixture is heated to the optimum temperature for the polymerase (usually 72°C) and the polymerase fills in the template, starting from the primer, to produce a double-stranded DNA. The mixture is then heated to 92° to 94°C to denature the double-stranded DNA that has been produced, resulting in 2 complementary template strands. The thermal cycle is then repeated, resulting in a geometric amplification of the original template sequence (Fig. 22).

The products of the PCR reaction can be visualized by agarose gel electrophoresis and EtBr/UV photography. For low levels of DNA, labeled nucleotides can be included in the PCR reaction mix, and the gel can be blotted and autoradiographed to increase detection sensitivity. Molecular weight standards allow determination of the length of the amplified fragment to confirm its identity. The fragment can also be excised from the gel and reamplified to be cloned in a vector for further manipulation, or for sequencing. The primers used for PCR can be designed to incorporate restriction sites to facilitate cloning of the amplified fragments into a suitable vector. Also, the accuracy and specificity of PCR amplification can be improved by the use of nested primers, a second set of specific primers internally located on the target sequence to the first set of primers. After initial amplification with the first set of primers, further amplification is carried out using the second internal set of primers.

Evaluating Levels of Gene Expression With PCR

Reverse transcription PCR (RT-PCR) refers to amplification starting from RNA rather than DNA. The first step of the procedure involves use of reverse transcriptase to produce cDNA from the original RNA template. RT-PCR is most commonly used to amplify an mRNA sequence, and can be used to detect and quantitate expression of very low level mRNA messages. Relative levels of cDNA can be estimated from band intensity on the PCR gel, but minute variations in amounts of template DNA, temperature in different reaction tubes, and other variables can also greatly amplify these artifactual errors during the PCR reaction.

DNA amplification by PCR becomes nonlinear at higher numbers of cycles (> 20 to 25 amplification cycles, depending on the amount of template and reaction conditions). Theoretically, comparisons of PCR reaction product amounts on the linear part of the curve (that is, at lower numbers of amplification cycles) will be quantitatively related to the amount of original starting material template in each reaction tube. However, because of the abovementioned experimental variables, quantitative comparisons are not very accurate. These comparisons may be important in studies of gene regulation, which use PCR to amplify cDNA from mRNAs of interest. Several quantitative methods have been developed to improve the accuracy of comparisons with PCR. Quantitative PCR, of which one form is competitive PCR, uses known amounts of a mimic sequence (an arbitrary sequence similar in length to that of

Single strand DNA to be sequenced.

Four sequencing reactions. Each includes primer, DNA polymerase, nucleotides (A,C,G,T) and 1 of 4 dideoxynucleotides (a,c,g,t)

The sequencing reaction synthesized DNA fragments of different lengths, each synthesis terminated by the incorporation of a dideoxynucleotide (a,c,g,t).

The products of each sequencing reaction are separated by gel electrophoresis.

"Reading" the gel from the smallest fragment to the largest gives the complementary DNA sequence.

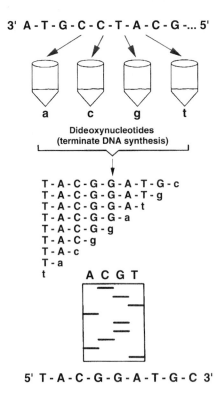

Figure 21

The Sanger method of sequencing involves use of dideoxynucleotides, which, when added to a DNA sequence by DNA polymerase, preclude further addition of nucleotides. By using 4 separate reactions with a different dideoxynucleotide in each, a series of fragments is generated that differ in length by the number of bases to the next like nucleotide. After high-resolution gel electrophoresis of the 4 reactions run in parallel (an appropriate label having been incorporated in the reactions), the sequence can be read by position of the bands on the gel from the shortest to the longest fragment.

the target sequence). Reaction tubes are prepared containing a series of dilutions (known concentrations) of the mimic sequence, and dilutions of the template sequence. The series of tubes is set up so that those containing the most dilute known concentrations of the mimic DNA contain the highest concentration of the unknown, and vice versa. Primers complementary to the 3′ and 5′ end of the mimic sequence as well as the primers complementary to the target sequence are added to all the reaction mixtures with the polymerase. The principle is that the template and mimic sequences will be identically amplified during PCR cycles. Therefore, when the PCR reaction products are run on a gel, 2 bands (the mimic and target sequence) will be present in each lane in relative proportion to the amount of starting material. By comparing the relative intensities of the 2 bands, the actual amount of the starting template can be estimated from the lane in which the 2 bands are of approximately equal intensity. A variation of this technique uses nucleotides with a fluorescent tag that does not fluoresce until the tag is released from the nucleotide at the time the tagged nucleotide is added to the DNA strand by the polymerase. Thus, the amount of fluorescence in the medium is proportional to the amount of DNA synthesized. This allows quantitation of PCR reaction products during the reaction by computerized monitoring of the fluorescence signals in multiple parallel reaction mixtures simultaneously, and is also accurately quantifiable using standards. An example of use of PCR is shown in Figure 23.

PCR-Based Cloning

An important use of PCR is in cloning new genes. For instance, if a portion of a protein sequence can be determined by amino acid analysis, PCR can be used to clone the gene. From the amino acid sequence, "degenerate" primers can be synthesized (that is, using all possible combinations at each position that could encode the given amino acid) that span a segment of the protein amino acid sequence. Genomic DNA or cDNA from the target species or tissue is then amplified by PCR using the degenerate primer mix, and the target DNA sequence will be selectively amplified by the primers with the correct matching complementary base sequences. This fragment can be radiolabeled during synthesis, or cloned into a vector and subsequently labeled, to be used as a probe to screen the appropriate genomic or cDNA library. Thus, clones containing all or a portion of the gene or its mRNA can be isolated and manipulated or further characterized.

Another use of PCR cloning is to generate a cloned gene homologous to a known gene that may be used to identify gene family members or homologs in other species. Primers are synthesized complementary to conserved regions of the gene (regions that are identical or similar across other known species or family member homologs), and usually represent functionally important domains of the encoded protein. The primers are then used to amplify the target sequence from DNA or cDNA using PCR, the amplified fragments then being gel purified, reamplified, and cloned into a vector to generate a labeled probe to screen the appropriate library and isolate the cloned gene homolog.

Taq polymerase is limited to less than 1 kb sequences, but newer enzymes can be used for so-called long PCR, which can amplify templates thousands of kb in length. Also, some of the newer DNA polymerases developed for PCR have proofreading and correction functions that correct PCR errors during polymerization, enhancing the accuracy of the amplified products. Variations on the PCR procedure include RACE (rapid amplification of cDNA ends), which makes use of the polyadenylated tail on all translated mRNAs to obtain further segments of DNA sequence beyond an available template sequence, and PCR differential display, which is used to compare a random set of genes expressed in 2-cell or tissue populations.

PCR has rapidly found innumerable applications in biology and medicine. Clinically, the use of PCR to amplify segments of genes to identify mutations that cause disease is a

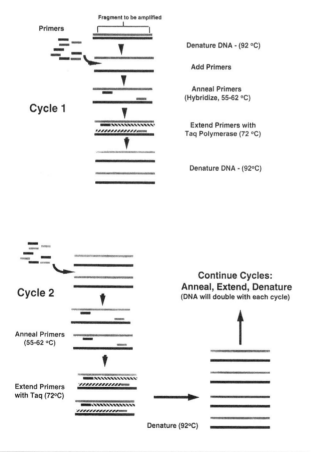

Figure 22

Double-stranded DNA is denatured by heating, and then primers complementary to the 5′ and 3′ ends of the target sequence are allowed to hybridize. Heating to optimum temperature for Taq polymerase synthesizes 2 new complementary strands. This cycle is repeated by thermal cycling, resulting in a doubling of the DNA with each cycle.

far more efficient method than creating a genomic library from an individual's DNA and screening it with specific probes to find abnormal genes. Amplification of DNA from minute clinical specimens is also possible, and has been applied in detecting bacterial genes to diagnose osteomyelitis or viral genes to diagnose acquired immunodeficiency syndrome as an extremely sensitive assay method. PCR is also widely used in forensic medicine to amplify human DNA from trace specimens. A number of genetic markers can be compared with an extremely high level of specificity in determining whether a trace tissue specimen is derived from a particular individual.

Analysis of Differential Gene Expression

As stated in the introduction, the genes expressed within a cell determine its identity and function. Many genes are expressed in all cell types; these genes encode proteins that are involved with intermediary metabolism, such as the enzymes involved in the use of glucose for energy. In contrast, there is a set of genes that will be specific to one or just a few cell types, such as the expression of urea cycle genes in the liver, the expression of neurotransmitter receptors in the brain, or the expression of type X collagen in the hypertrophic zone of the growth plate. Thus, the usefulness of methods to identify specifically expressed genes is evident. A variety of methods have been developed, with most of the

recently developed techniques employing PCR. Examples include 3 types: "classic" subtractive hybridization, which does not use PCR; differential display, which does; and subtractive suppression hybridization, which uses both a subtraction procedure and PCR.

The first method developed to evaluate differential gene expression between 2 cell populations or tissues was subtractive hybridization. This technique involves extraction of mRNA from both cell populations, and then reverse transcribing the mRNA from one population to form single stranded cDNA. The cDNA is separated from the RNA, and then hybridized with the mRNA from the second cell population. The DNA/RNA hybrids and unhybridized RNA are removed, leaving only single stranded cDNAs that did not hybridize, thus representing genes expressed in the first cell population that are not expressed in the second. The single stranded cDNA is converted to double-stranded DNA with a polymerase. These DNA fragments can be cloned into a vector, creating a library of the differentially expressed genes, or labeled and used as probes to screen an existing cDNA library.

The technique of differential display was first described in 1992, and uses PCR with short primers to randomly amplify cDNAs from different cell types. In its original formulation, the method makes use of the fact that all mRNAs are polyadenylated. Thus, oligonucleotides of deoxythymidine (oligo dT) are synthesized of the form $T_{11}MN$, where M is

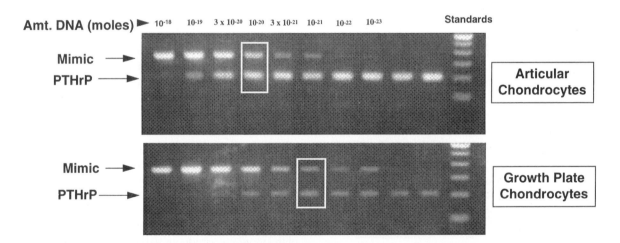

Competitive PCR

Figure 23

This example of competitive polymerase chain reaction (PCR) demonstrates differential expression of a very low level mRNA not detectable by Northern blot in articular and growth plate chondrocytes. A series of PCRs are run using dilutions of a known quantity of mimic sequence that incorporates complementary primer sites at the 3' and 5' ends to the primers to be used for amplification of the sequence under study (in this case, parathyroid hormone related protein [PTHrP]). Similar dilutions of the cDNA to be quantified are added to the reaction tubes in the reverse order, so that the tube with the highest amount of mimic sequence contains the lowest amount of unknown. After running the PCR reaction, the DNA samples are run on an agarose gel with ethidium bromide staining and photographed under ultraviolet light. Where the intensity of the bands is equal, the concentrations of the 2 DNA templates should be equal. Here, growth plate chondrocytes are shown to express PTHrP at mRNA levels approximately 1 order of magnitude lower than the articular chondrocytes.

A,G, or C, and N is A, G, C, or T. These are used as primers for cDNA synthesis from polyA⁺ mRNA templates using mRNA isolated from the cell populations to be compared. This set of random primers would theoretically represent 1/12 of all possible mRNAs, given the 12 possible combinations of M and N. PCR is then carried out using the oligo dT primers and a second set of completely random primers, usually 10 bases in length, with radiolabeled bases in the reaction mixture. The radiolabeled cDNAs generated from 2 or more cell populations are then separated in parallel lanes by gel electrophoresis and displayed by autoradiography. Comparison of band intensities in adjacent lanes indicates roughly the difference in gene expression between the cells or tissues being compared. Differentially expressed genes are documented by excising the band from the corresponding gel, and then reamplifying and cloning the resulting DNA fragment. The cloned fragment can be sequenced to determine its identity or any homologies, and used to produce a labeled cDNA probe to confirm differential expression in the cell populations by Northern analysis or RNase protection assay. An example of differential display is shown in Figure 24, which compares gene expression in articular and growth plate chondrocytes (AC and GPC). Bands marked with arrows represent cDNAs, which are differentially expressed in the 2 populations.

Differential display offers several advantages compared to subtractive hybridization. First, 2 or more cell types can be analyzed simultaneously, and genes either over- or underexpressed in one population as compared to another can be identified. Thus, in the chondrocyte example, both GPC and AC cDNAs could be identified. Second, differential display is less laborious and technically demanding, so that identification of potentially specific cDNAs is much more rapid than with subtractive hybridization. There are also a few drawbacks. This technique is more likely to identify the most abundant specific cDNAs, such as type X or alkaline phosphatase in GPC. There have also been problems with a high percentage of false positive results. Finally, the oligo-dT priming and short fragments result in cDNAs that are usually in the 3' untranslated portion of the cDNA. These regions are rarely conserved, so additional cloning is necessary to obtain coding sequences. Coding sequences are usually conserved, and may suggest a function for the gene product based on homology with other sequences in the national data banks.

Other Methods

Newer methods of screening thousands of genes simultaneously for differential expression have been developed. One method is known as suppressive subtractive hybridization, which is a variation on subtractive hybridization that normalizes abundant and rare cDNAs. The second new approach makes use of a device called a DNA microchip, a silicon or glass chip on which are immobilized tens of thousands of either synthetic oligonucleotides or DNA fragments of known sequences in a specific geometric array using the microscopic lithographic techniques of computer chip technology. The RNA, DNA, or cDNA to be analyzed is fluorescently labeled and hybridized with the chip array. A computerized laser scanner can determine the presence of hybrids at the sites of binding to the DNA array of known sequences. Simultaneous comparison of 2 or more populations, such as cDNA from a diseased versus normal tissue or cell type, can be readily accomplished by using different fluorescent labels to tag the cDNA from different sources. The DNA arrays can be made using particular sequences relevant to a specific disease state or gene category, and current examples include arrays specific for human immunodeficiency virus (HIV) genome mutations, cytochrome p450 (genes involved in drug metabolism), and p53, a tumor suppressor whose mutations are associated with many cancers. Microchips that can enable arrays of synthetic peptides to be screened to identify interaction domains of either DNA or other proteins using this technology have also been created. This technology is still in its infancy, but has enormous promise to accelerate the pace of information regarding differential gene expression in normal and diseased cells and tissues.

In Situ Hybridization

Gene expression can also be analyzed in intact sections of tissue, or in situ, which provides many insights not possible from analysis of tissue extracts of RNA. This is in part because most tissues contain multiple cell types; the cell type that is actually expressing the gene can be confirmed only by localizing a given mRNA or DNA sequence of interest to a specific cell. The basic technique involves preparation of tissue sections or cells on glass microscope slides, which are generally treated with a fixative to immobilize the RNA and DNA in the cells by causing crosslinking to proteins. Decalcification with an acidic solution or a calcium chelating solution (EDTA) is usually necessary to enable cutting of the bone-containing sections. The cells are then permeabilized by removing the lipids of the membranes with detergent or organic solvents to allow the probe to access the immobilized RNA or DNA. Probes can be either cDNAs, riboprobes, or synthetic oligonucleotides, and can be labeled with radioactive nucleotide incorporation (usually ³⁵S or ³²P) during synthesis, or with fluorescently tagged nucleotides or those tagged with immunodetectable organic molecules such as biotin or digoxigenin, as previously discussed.

After hybridization with the probe and increasing stringency washes to remove unbound probe, the slide is processed for detection of the probe signal. For radioactively labeled probes, the slide is coated with a photographic emulsion material, and areas of radioactivity will fix silver grains in the emulsion, leaving dark spots where the target sequence is found. For fluorescently tagged probes, the slide is viewed under a fluorescence microscope and the probe can be visualized directly. For immunodetectable tags, an antibody to the tag is incubated on the slide to allow binding to the probe, and then a chemical reaction produces a colored insoluble product using an enzyme conjugated to the antibody or to a secondary antibody. Areas of color on the slide indicate the location of the target sequence.

In situ hybridization can provide detailed information about the localization of gene expression in tissues and cells. Although short oligonucleotide probes can be useful, specificity is generally improved with longer probes, which are also somewhat more sensitive for detecting low level messages. Cocktails of probes to different parts of the mRNA can increase sensitivity. Riboprobes have generally better signal-to-noise ratios because of the higher stability of RNA/RNA hybrids compared with DNA/RNA hybrids. Controls are critical to correct interpretation of in situ hybridization because of the possibility of background nonspecific binding. Comparison of sections hybridized with sense and antisense probes is one way to assure specificity. Tissue sections may also contain elements that serve as informative internal controls, such as the presence of specific cells known to express or not express the target sequence. An example of in situ hybridization is demonstrated in Figure 25. Recently, in situ PCR techniques have been developed, in which PCR is performed on sections of suitably fixed and permeabilized tissues or cells using specific primers and labeled nucleotides in the reaction mixture, enabling in situ detection of very low level messages.

Methods of Protein Detection

Western Blotting

The Western blot is a method of detecting proteins that is analogous to Northern blots for mRNA detection. A solubilized protein extract from tissue or cells of interest is separated by sodium dodecyl sulfate polyacrylamide gel electrophoresis (SDS/PAGE), in which the SDS binds to the proteins, providing a negative charge to facilitate migration of the proteins toward the positive electrode during electrophoresis. The proteins are separated according to electrophoretic mobility, which is a function of molecular weight, conformation, and charge. As with Northern and Southern blots, the proteins on the gel are blotted onto nitrocellulose filters by electroblotting rather than capillary action (which uses an electrical current to cause the proteins to migrate onto the filter) where they are immobilized. The blot is first incubated with a mixture of proteins to saturate nonspecific binding sites, and then incubated with a specific antibody generated to recognize the protein of interest. After washing to remove unbound antibody, a secondary antibody to the antibody (from an animal of a different species, for example, goat anti-rabbit) is applied and

detected by any of a number of detection systems such as those described above for in situ hybridization. The secondary antibody may have a conjugated enzyme that mediates a chemical reaction to deposit a colored product, a radioactive or chemiluminescent tag that will expose an applied x-ray film, or a fluorescent tag that can be detected. Molecular weight standards are run in one lane next to the protein extracts so the molecular weight of the band that is detected is known.

Immunohistochemistry

Immunohistochemistry is similar to in situ hybridization, but uses specific antibodies to proteins of interest to localize protein expression in the cells or tissue. The tissue must be preserved in a manner that does not cause loss of antigenicity of the proteins, and different target proteins may require very different fixation and processing to enable detection. As with Western blots, tissue sections are incubated first with a blocking agent such as serum proteins to block nonspecific binding sites. Then the primary antibody is incubated with the sections, and any excess removed by

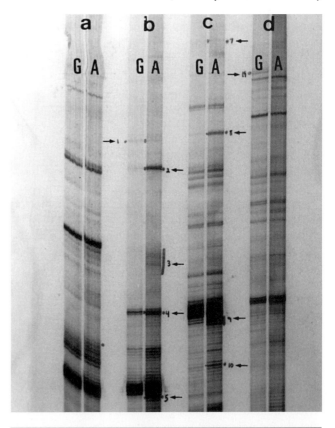

Figure 24

Differential display of polymerase chain reaction products from growth plate (G) and articular (A) chondrocytes. The bands that are expressed differentially in 1 cell type or the other are marked with arrows. The bands of interest are excised from the gel, amplified, cloned, and sequenced. Northern analysis is then used to confirm the differential expression in the 2 cell types.

washing. A secondary antibody tagged with one of a number of detectable labels is then applied and allowed to bind to the first antibody. The detection of the secondary antibody usually involves a chemical reaction to generate a colored product and is mediated by an enzyme bound to the secondary antibody. A common approach uses a biotinylated secondary antibody, which binds streptavidin, a protein with a high affinity and specificity for binding biotin. The streptavidin is conjugated to an enzyme, horseradish peroxidase, which generates a red- or brown-colored insoluble reaction product at the sites of antibody binding by conversion of a substrate (3-amino-9-ethylcarbazole) incubated with the section. An example of immunohistochemistry using the streptavidin/peroxidase technique is shown in Figure 26.

Another common method uses a secondary antibody conjugated to an alkaline phosphatase enzyme. When an appropriate substrate is added, the alkaline phosphatase converts it to an insoluble blue dye deposited at the site of the antibody localization. Alternatively, the secondary antibody can be tagged with a fluorescent label allowing it to be visualized on the tissue section with fluorescence microscopy. The advantage of the enzymatic detection methods is the amplification of the signal that occurs because of progressive deposition of reaction product by continued enzymatic reaction, creating many molecules of signal for a single molecule of antibody.

Some basic principles of immunohistochemistry include the need for appropriate positive and negative controls, the selection of the type of antibody as well as the detection system, and appropriate procedures to minimize background. In addition, the tissue fixation is critical to preserve antigenicity, and fixation requirements vary depending on the antigen and antibodies used. Polyclonal antibodies can be raised against either a fusion protein or synthetic peptide. A fusion protein is generated by inserting the DNA sequence of the protein of interest into a plasmid vector, which is then used to infect bacteria (usually *E. coli*), and the recombinant protein generally consists of the desired sequence with some additional adjoining sequences from the vector. This material is purified from bacterial extracts, and then used to inject animals to produce antisera. The antisera are generally purified using the fusion protein linked to an affinity column to select antibodies specific to epitopes of the desired sequence, or short sequences of amino acids that antibodies recognize.

Affinity-purified antibodies contain a complex mixture of antibodies to different regions or epitopes of the immunizing antigen, and thus tend to have better sensitivity than monoclonal antibodies. Monoclonal antibodies are produced by selecting clonal cell lines from hybridoma cells, which are clonal murine antibody-producing lymphocytes fused with human myeloma plasma cells so that each clone produces only a single specific antibody to a given epitope of the target protein or peptide. The advantage of the monoclonal antibodies is that a continuous supply of the identical antibody is produced from the immortalized hybridoma cell line, and the selection of a single antibody ensures a higher level of specificity. However, decreased sensitivity is usually the trade-off.

All antibodies, whether produced in a laboratory or obtained commercially, need to be titrated for sensitivity on a positive control tissue in the immunohistochemistry laboratory. The tissue is to be used to optimize the titer used under specific conditions. In addition, Western blots can be used from extracts of the tissues or cells to be tested as a control for specificity (that is, the molecular weight of the detected band[s] is appropriate to the target protein). An immunoabsorption control is also a strong confirmation of specificity of the immunostaining. In this procedure, differing titers of the purified antigen are mixed with the primary antibodies at the time of the incubation with the tissue, and will bind to the antibodies in solution or "absorb" the antibodies, so that the immunostaining signal in a positive control tissue disappears as the titer of antigen is increased.

Immunohistochemistry is now extensively used in the diagnosis of pathologic specimens such as tumors. Many specific antibodies are available that recognize markers of specific cell types. These include epithelial markers such as cytokeratin for diagnosis of carcinomas, mesenchymal markers such as vimentin, which is useful in diagnosis of sarcoma, and neural and lymphocytic markers.

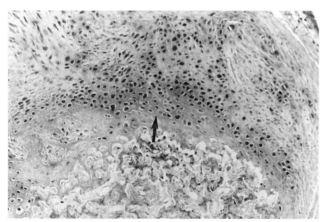

Figure 25

In situ hybridization is used to identify gene expression in fracture callus. The probe is a synthetic oligonucleotide cDNA to type IIA collagen, labeled with digoxigenin-d-UTP using a terminal transferase. An alkaline phosphatase-conjugated antidigoxigenin antibody generates a colored reaction product at sites of hybridization of the probe. Note the intense staining of the chondrocytes (*arrow*), as well as expression in the chondrocyte precursor proliferating mesenchymal cells adjacent to the cartilage.

Enzyme-Linked Immunosorbent Assay (ELISA)

ELISA is a commonly used method to detect and quantify specific proteins in solution. The assay relies on specific antibody binding to the protein of interest, followed by the use of an enzyme-linked secondary antibody, similar to the method for immunohistochemistry. The enzyme is usually a form of alkaline phosphatase, and incubation with an appropriate substrate will generate a soluble colored product that can be detected by measuring absorbance of the solution at an appropriate wavelength. In general, the method is performed by first immobilizing a specific antibody by binding it to a plastic well in a multiwell plate. The solution containing the protein of interest, for instance conditioned medium from a cell culture in which a secreted protein is to be measured, is incubated with the antibody and binds to it. A secondary antibody conjugated to the detection enzyme is subsequently incubated with the complex and, after washing away excess antibody, color reaction substrate is added. The absorbance is read by an automated plate reader after incubation to allow color development.

There are several variations on the technique, including binding the antigen to the plate first, or using 2 different antibodies (sandwich technique) and applying the second after the antigen is attached to the first antibody on the plate. The use of 2 different antibodies to the protein can enhance specificity. Standard reactions with known quantities of the protein are generally run parallel to allow quantitation of the samples. Like immunohistochemistry, ELISA does not have the specificity of Western blots, in which the molecular weight of the protein can be confirmed, but is an excellent technique for rapid and simple evaluation of large numbers of samples with a high level of sensitivity.

Analyzing Protein/DNA Interactions

The gel retardation technique, also known as gel mobility shift assay, is used to assess the interactions of proteins with specific DNA sequences, generally to identify proteins such as transcription factors that bind to portions of gene promoters. Nuclear extracts are prepared from cells to separate the nuclear proteins from the DNA. A segment of cloned double-stranded DNA containing a consensus binding sequence of interest is radiolabeled and mixed with the nuclear extract. Binding of the labeled DNA to specific interacting proteins will occur. The mixture is then subjected to polyacrylamide gel electrophoresis, and the migration of the DNA complexed to the protein is retarded as compared to unbound probe. The gel is blotted and autoradiographed, and the position of the bands corresponds to protein/DNA complexes.

Antibodies are available that recognize a number of different transcription factors. These antibodies can be added to the nuclear extract/DNA mixture prior to electrophoresis, and if a specific protein recognized by the antibody is present, the protein/DNA complex will be "supershifted," or further retarded in migration due to the additional protein of the antibody. Also, identity of a regulatory protein can sometimes be confirmed by adding unlabeled oligonu-

cleotide consensus sequence DNA to compete with the labeled probe for binding of the protein, thereby diminishing the band intensity.

A related approach called DNA footprinting is used to define the specific nucleotides that interact with areas of a binding protein. Labeled promoter DNA is mixed with nuclear proteins and then digested with DNase I prior to electrophoretic separation. The areas of the sequence that directly interact with the protein are protected from DNase degradation, and these fragments can be analyzed following electrophoresis to determine the exact portions of the sequence that interact with the binding protein.

Transfection

Transfection is a method of introducing a foreign DNA fragment into a cell or organism, as previously discussed with bacteriophage infection of bacteria. For some applications, such as the study of regulation of gene promoters, or production of functional mammalian recombinant proteins, transfection is ideally carried out with mammalian cells rather than bacteria. Unlike bacteria, in order for transfected DNA to be transcribed and ultimately translated, it must be transported into the nucleus. Extrachromosomal constructs can be transcribed and the mRNA translated. Such transfections are referred to as unstable or transient transfections, and are limited by the survival time of the foreign DNA, the extrachromosomal DNA being lost during cell division. If the DNA is integrated into the host genome by spontaneous recombination, stable transfected cell lines can be obtained, and the transfected DNA will continue to be expressed.

Transfection in mammalian cells is a relatively inefficient process, and selectable markers are usually included in the

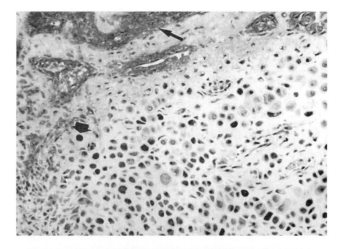

Figure 26

Immunohistochemistry of rat fracture callus using an antibody to osteocalcin with the immunoperoxidase technique demonstrates intense staining of the bone matrix (*thin arrow*), and staining of hypertrophic chondrocytes in the callus as well (*thick arrow*).

construct, such as a specific antibiotic-resistance conferring gene so that only those cells that successfully transfect and transcribe the introduced DNA will survive in the presence of the selection antibiotic. DNA can be introduced in the form of plasmids, or the cells can be infected with viral vectors containing the cloned target sequence. The most common viral vectors for transfection are retroviruses and adenoviruses. Introduction of plasmids can be accomplished by several techniques. The original technique used was calcium phosphate precipitation, which causes uptake of plasmid DNA into cells. Four techniques used recently include lipofection, which uses a compound such as lipofectamine to increase cell permeability to DNA; electroporation, which uses an electrical current to create holes in the plasma membrane of cells; microinjection, which directly injects the construct into a cell; and liposome delivery, which fuses liposomes containing the DNA with the plasma membrane to deliver the DNA into the cytoplasm.

Transfection vectors often incorporate a reporter gene, such as luciferase, beta galactosidase, or choramphenicol acetyltransferase, so that transcription of the sequence can be monitored by a chemical or chemiluminescent assay. The reporter can also be cotransfected as a separate construct to monitor transfection efficiency. Reporters are also useful in vectors containing a cloned promoter sequence. The activity of the reporter gene can be modulated transcriptionally by the promoter fragment, and specific segments of the promoter can be added or deleted and then transient transfection performed to determine the effect of specific regions and consensus binding sequences on the activity of the reporter gene. Promoter regions can be mapped and regulatory elements characterized in this manner.

Antisense Strategies

Antisense strategies involve introducing a complementary RNA (or a DNA sequence complementary to an mRNA of interest) into a cell. Theoretically, the antisense sequence will bind or hybridize to the mRNA of interest, preventing its translation. This method can be used to analyze the effect of shutting off a gene of interest. This can be accomplished by use of transfection techniques as discussed above, and has been used successfully in many cell systems to determine the effect of preventing or decreasing expression of a specific gene product.

Another method of preventing translation involves use of antisense synthetic thiolated base-containing oligonucleotide cDNAs, which are quite stable and not readily degraded intracellularly because of the synthetic thiolated base configuration. These cDNAs can enter cells spontaneously through endocytosis if the concentration is high enough (generally μM levels), or can be introduced through liposomes, electroporation, or lipofection. Use of antisense oligonucleotides has enabled demonstration that the differentiating effect of glucocorticoids on osteoblasts is mediated by BMP6; antisense oligonucleotides complementary to BMP6 mRNA prevented the effect. Some naturally-occurring antisense mRNAs have been identified, such as an antisense mRNA for fibroblast growth factor 2 (FGF2), but it is unknown if they have functional ability to inhibit translation or are involved in regulation in vivo.

Transgenics

The ability to transfect foreign DNA into mammalian cells eventually led to the introduction of genes into germ line cells and embryos. A transgenic animal is generated by introducing a cloned gene (called the *trans* gene) into a fertilized ovum by microinjection, or by transfection of embryonic stem cells in an embryo. If the gene integrates into the host genome, it may be expressed in the progeny after the altered ovum or embryo is implanted into a foster mother. Incorporation of the transgene into the haploid germ line cells of the reproductive system can enable stable transmission of the gene to further generations. The expression of the transgene can also be controlled using further modifications of the cloned gene. Overexpression can be obtained by using a constitutive promoter in the transgene, and controllable expression can be implemented by incorporating an inducible promoter. Some inducible promoters can be turned on by pharmacologic agents such as tetracyclines. Alternatively, tissue-specific expression of the transgene can be achieved by using a tissue-specific promoter in the transgene. For instance, a fragment of the type II collagen promoter can be incorporated into a transgene, and the transgenic mice that express the gene will only do so in areas of cartilage. This is particularly useful for studying genes that are ubiquitous regulators, such as transcription factors and signaling molecules, as diffuse expression in all tissues can be lethal. Transgenic techniques have been used to produce a number of useful altered agricultural plant products and animals. Recently, farm animals such as sheep and cattle have been cloned, by introducing somatic diploid DNA from an animal into a fertilized ovum from which the endogenous nuclear DNA has been removed by microscopic manipulation. The ovum is implanted and develops into a new copy, or clone, of the original animal. These experiments have proven that the entire genetic material to encode an organism is present within every somatic cell, and have raised some difficult ethical questions regarding manipulation of human embryos.

Deleting the function of a gene using transgenic techniques can also be accomplished, and is referred to as gene deletion or "knockout." Knockout mice are created through homologous recombination in embryonic stem cells. The stem cells are transfected with a defective (nonfunctional, or null mutation) gene targeted to the site of the endogenous gene. After a single copy of the gene is replaced with the mutated gene, those progeny with germ cell transmission of the defective gene copy are cross-bred to derive progeny that have both copies of the null mutation, effectively knocking out the expression of that gene in the animal. The phenotype of the animals can be studied to gain insights as to the function of the gene in the organism and its various tissues and organs. A huge number of transgenic and knockout mice have now been produced, and the technique is becoming quite common. Knockout mice have often been found to have either subtle or indiscernible phenotypic abnormalities, underscoring the crucial nature of homologous gene families in which one or more family members can sometimes substitute for the deleted gene. Mice are now being produced with several different genes deleted, to enable study of gene function with functional homologs.

Genetic Diseases

There are several thousand inherited diseases in humans, although the specific gene responsible has been identified and cloned in less than 100 of these disorders. Because gene mutations affecting the musculoskeletal system are less often lethal than many mutations in genes critical to other vital organ systems, inherited musculoskeletal disorders comprise a substantial proportion of the diseases in which the genetic cause has been identified. Many of the tools of molecular biology described above are being used to characterize the causes of inherited and some acquired disorders, to develop new diagnostic tests, and to develop therapies to treat these diseases. Genetic disease inheritance patterns usually are either dominant (mutation of one allele sufficient to cause expression of abnormal phenotype), recessive (mutation of both alleles, or homozygosity, necessary for expression of abnormal phenotype), autosomal (location of the gene on a chromosome other than the sex-defining X and Y chromosomes), or sex-linked (location of the gene on the X or Y chromosome). The trait determined by the abnormal gene can also display incomplete penetrance, indicating that other genes may influence expression of the mutant gene in complex and not readily predictable ways. Many diseases also appear to have complex inheritance patterns indicative of a polygenic etiology, where a single gene mutation may only contribute to a susceptibility to the disease.

Some of the major discoveries of genetic diseases relate to skeletal gene mutations. Osteogenesis imperfecta, characterized by bone fragility and fractures, has been found to be caused by a variety of mutations in both the COLIA1 and COLIA2 genes. The more severe forms are usually caused by point mutations within the helical domains of the collagen molecule that disrupt helix formation and result in abnormal fibril formation with impaired mechanical strength. Osteogenesis imperfecta is now known to be a heterogeneous group of mutations, and nearly every family analyzed has been found to have a different type I collagen mutation. Type II collagen mutations have been identified in some forms of familial osteoarthritis, Stickler syndrome (ophthalmoarthropathy), and hypochondrogenesis. The mutation responsible for the most common skeletal dysplasia, achondroplasia, has recently been identified as a point mutation in the FGF receptor 3 gene, which results in constitutive activation of the receptor (the receptor is permanently in the "on" position, signaling the chondrocytes in the absence of ligand binding). The mutation in this disorder is the same in nearly all families studied. The FGF receptors have also been associated with several other chondrodysplasias. Marfan's syndrome results from mutation of a gene called fibrillin, which encodes a fibrillar protein present in many connective tissues. The list of identified mutations is growing rapidly, and Table 3 presents a summary of some musculoskeletal disorders for which the genetic defect has been identified. A useful source for further information on inherited skeletal disorders is the Online Mendelian Inheritance in Man database available through the National Library of Medicine on the Internet (http//www.ncbi.nlm.nih.gov).

Linkage Analysis

Many genes are polymorphic, meaning that several forms of the gene, with some sequence alterations, exist as allelic variations in the normal population. When an individual's DNA is subjected to restriction digestion, a series of DNA fragments of varying lengths results, dependent on the location of restriction sites in the genomic DNA. Restriction map construction was explained previously, and is used to identify the relative positions of a number of different restriction sites in a segment of DNA. If a mutation in a gene alters one of the restriction sites, the DNA pattern of the digested fragments will differ. This is known as restriction fragment length polymorphism (RFLP). Restriction fragments can be identified and their length determined by agarose gel electrophoresis and Southern blotting using labeled probes. A large number of polymorphous markers have been mapped to specific chromosomal locations throughout the human genome. An example of RFLP analysis is shown in Figure 27 in the context of linkage analysis, showing association of the RFLP with the individuals exhibiting the disease phenotype.

A mutated gene can change position to the homologous chromosome of a chromosome pair by cross-overs, which occur by spontaneous recombination during meiosis when chromosome pairs segregate before cell division. Other genes or DNA sequences, including polymorphic sequences, near the mutated gene can be moved with it, and the closer the physical proximity of a DNA sequence is to the mutated gene, the greater the likelihood that it will segregate with the mutation during recombination events. The phenomenon of cosegregation during chromosomal recombinations is called linkage; a genetic sequence near a gene of interest may be linked to it and thus will display a similar inheritance pattern of expression. Two genes located on different chromosomes cannot be linked because cross-overs do not occur between nonhomologous chromosomes normally. Therefore, the likelihood of specific alleles on different chromosomes being coinherited is random, or 50%. The same is true for 2 genes located far apart on the same chromosome, because segregation of genes during recombination events requires physical proximity. The farther the physical separation of 2 genes on the same chromosome, the less likely they will move together, or exhibit linkage, with a lower limit of 59% probability, which is a random association.

Linkage analysis is a very powerful tool for identifying the specific physical chromosomal location of a disease-causing gene. By analyzing genomic DNA from a large family or group of families with an inherited disease, a statistical association of specific markers with the disease can be calculated, called the logarithm of the odds (LOD) score. This value determines the degree of likelihood that a marker is linked to a disease gene. If a polymorphic marker associates, or is linked, to the disease phenotype, the location of the mutated gene can be identified within a certain region of a specific chromosome. Demonstration of linkage of a disease to a polymorphic marker by RFLP analysis is shown in Figure 27.

Limitations of linkage analysis include the need for large kindreds to identify linkages, and the fact that even with the large number of mapped markers in the genome, the location of the gene is still narrowed down to only a region of the chomosome, and the distance between markers can be 10^5 to 10^6 bp of DNA sequence. Thus, identifying the specific disease-causing gene linked with the markers may still pose a challenging task unless a likely candidate gene is known to lie within the identified region. Cloning a gene using linkage analysis to progressively narrow the location is known as positional cloning, and has been successfully used to identify a number of musculoskeletal genetic mutations such as Stickler syndrome (type II collagen gene mutation) and X-linked hypophosphatemic rickets (PEX gene mutation).

More numerous than RFLP markers are variable number short tandem repeats of DNA sequences scattered throughout the genome, and microsatellite markers, which are short tandem repeat polymorphic markers. These markers have been cataloged and can be rapidly characterized in genomic DNA specimens using PCR with primers flanking the markers, allowing rapid identification of specific polymorphisms. The variation in length of the amplified PCR products corresponding to the polymorphism is detected on electrophoretic gels. Another PCR-based approach to localizing mutations is single-stranded conformational polymorphism. Single-stranded DNA in solution develops intrastrand hydrogen bonds, which cause a particular secondary structure or conformation. DNA fragments the same length but different in conformation will migrate dif-

ferently during gel electrophoresis. Therefore, PCR can be used to amplify specific marker regions of DNA, and the PCR fragment containing a mutation will migrate differently when the strands are denatured from the complementary strand containing the normal allele (Fig. 28).

Gene Therapy

Applying the tools of molecular biology not only provides a means to identify the genetic abnormalities that cause dis-

Table 3	
Musculoskeletal Disorders and Their Genetic Defects	
Musculoskeletal Genetic Disorder	**Genetic Mutation***
Achondroplasia	FGF receptor 3
Osteogenesis imperfecta	Type I collagen
Pseudoachondroplasia	Cartilage oligomeric matrix protein (COMP)
Marfan's syndrome	Fibrillin
Spondyloepiphyseal dysplasia	Type II collagen
Multiple epiphyseal dysplasia	COMP or type IX collagen (COL9A2)
Thanatophoric dysplasia	FGF receptor 3
Diatrophic dysplasia	Sulfate transporter
Duchenne muscular dystrophy	Dystrophin
X-linked hypophosphatemic rickets	PEX (a cellular endopeptidase)
Osteopetrosis	Carbonic anhydrase type II; proton pump—(humans) c-src, MCSF, beta3 integrin— (mouse models)
Fibrous dysplasia	$G_{s\alpha}$ (receptor-coupled signaling protein)
Schmid metaphyseal dysplasia	Type X collagen
Jansen metaphyseal chondrodysplasia	PTH/PTHrP receptor
Multiple hereditary exostoses	EXT1, EXT2 genes
Hypochondroplasia	FGF receptor 3

*   FGF = fibroblast growth factor; COMP = cartilage oligomeric matrix protein; MCSF = macrophage-colony stimulating factor; PTH = parathyroid hormone; PTHrP = parathyroid hormone related protein.

ease, but offers technical possibilities such as introducing normal genes to correct defects. The generation of transgenic animals has dramatically demonstrated the possibility of altering genes in a complex organism. Introduction of a specific gene product can also be used to treat acquired diseases and allow local biologic manipulation of the disease process. Gene therapy is already becoming a reality in experimental treatment of human diseases. Several methods of gene therapy have been developed. Viral vectors, such as adenovirus or adeno-associated virus, can be used,

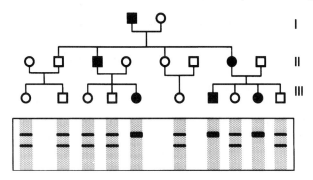

Figure 27

Linkage analysis correlates a genetic trait or disease with restriction fragment polymorphisms in the DNA of the affected and unaffected members of a kindred. In this example the polymorphism demonstrated by the single band is highly associated with the individuals expressing the genetic disease (the dark circles or squares), and therefore demonstrates linkage to the disease. This generally means that the gene represented by the restriction fragment polymorphism is physically located on the chromosome near the gene causing the disease, or it can be the causative gene itself.

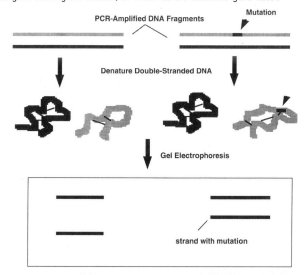

Figure 28

Single-stranded conformational polymorphism is a polymerase chain reaction (PCR)-based method allowing rapid screening of genes for mutations. When DNA is denatured, the single strands develop specific secondary structures or shapes due to intrastrand hydrogen bonds that depend on the sequence of the DNA. A mutation can change the conformation of the strand containing it, and the different conformations will migrate differently during gel electrophoresis. Thus, the conformational change allows identification of the presence of a mutation in the DNA fragment.

into which the appropriate gene and promoter have been cloned. The virus will infect cells with which it comes in contact, and the gene and its encoded protein product can be expressed. The virus can be introduced directly into the host, or can be used to transfect host cells ex vivo and then the transfected cells can be introduced into the host. The disadvantage of the ex vivo approach is that it takes more time, but the method retains better control of exactly which cells are infected. Recent studies suggest that the infected cells stay localized to the injection site, and may gradually disappear over a few weeks. Loss of expression over time is a problem with all gene therapy modalities when applied to problems of a chronic nature or to genetic disorders. Transfection of stem cells, so that a renewal source of genetically altered cells can be reimplanted, is one approach under study. This method has been used successfully with BMP2 in bone marrow stromal cells to induce bone formation in vivo. Also, enhancement of spinal fusion has been demonstrated by implantation of marrow cells transfected with a bone formation stimulating gene called LIM mineralization protein-1.

An alternative method for gene therapy involves direct introduction of DNA, such as a plasmid containing the desired construct, into the desired site. The uptake of plasmid into host cells is inefficient, but may be enhanced by immobilizing the DNA in a matrix such as a collagen framework (referred to as a gene-activated matrix). This method has been used successfully experimentally in animals to deliver stimulatory molecules in long bone critical-sized defect models, which will not heal spontaneously. As with viral vectors, the plasmid-containing cells remain localized to the application site and disappear gradually over time. Techniques are also being developed to use constructs that contain inducible promoters, so that the foreign gene can be turned on and off, such as with pharmacologic agents. Finally, future viral constructs may incorporate DNA sequences that allow inducible cell apoptosis, so that transfected cells can be eliminated in the host at will. Preliminary clinical trials of gene therapy have been carried out using plasmid DNA containing endothelial growth factor sequences to treat ischemic vascular disease, and a cytokine-inactivating protein gene has been introduced by intra-articular injection to treat rheumatoid arthritis in humans. Many other applications of gene therapy are under development.

Cell Biology of the Musculoskeletal System

The Cell Cycle and Its Regulation

Cell division is a complex, tightly regulated process, and the techniques of molecular biology have enhanced the understanding of the cell cycle and its control. Derangements of cell division are a central theme in the development of neoplasia, underscoring the clinical importance of this process. Cells are constantly bombarded with a myriad of signals from external stimuli, including hormones, growth factors, cytokines, mechanical perturbations, interactions with other cells and cellular matrix components, and from environmental influences such as temperature, pH, and ionic and osmotic influences. These signals result in activation of numerous interacting signal transduction pathways within the cell, which ultimately must be integrated and converted into activation of appropriate gene expression patterns to respond to the net sum of the various stimuli. Many of the signals influence different aspects of the regulation of cell proliferation and differentiation, and act at specific checkpoints in the cell cycle to stimulate or inhibit cell division.

The cell cycle is divided into 4 active phases and one inactive phase (Fig. 29). The resting phase, referred to as G_0, represents the time spent by a cell prior to preparation for active division, and is a state outside the cell cycle. When a signal causes a cell to reenter the cell cycle, the entry phase is called G_1 (G = growth). This phase lasts 6 to 12 hours, and the cell is involved in active RNA and protein synthesis during this time. The cell then enters the S (S = synthesis) phase, where DNA is replicated until the diploid cell doubles its DNA content by duplicating of all chromosomal material to become tetraploid. S phase usually lasts 6 to 8 hours, and its end is signified by completion of DNA replication. The nucleus increases in size significantly during S phase, and its protein content increases in conjunction with the increase in DNA content. Cells in S phase can be identified by exposing the cell to a labeled base, such as radioactive thymidine or a synthetic thymidine analog called bromodeoxyuridine (BrdU). The labeled base will be incorporated into the newly synthesized DNA, providing a means of identifying the cells in S phase. Radioactivity of the incorporated label can be measured by extracting the DNA from the cells, or by autoradiography of the cells in situ. Similarly, BrdU can be detected immunohistochemically with an antibody to this synthetic base.

G_2 phase represents the preparations for mitosis, lasts 3 to 4 hours, and is characterized by continued increase in RNA and protein synthesis without further DNA synthesis. The conclusion of G_2 is signaled by the onset of M phase (mitosis), during which the replicate chromosomes segregate under control of the mitotic spindle, an apparatus that forms from cytoskeletal microtubules at the onset of mitosis. The cell divides, signifying the conclusion of M phase, and the process of mitosis is relatively rapid. Almost all cells follow this pattern of cell division, although rapidly dividing cells in early embryogenesis may alternate S phase and M phase without growing in between. Following division the cell may then enter G_0 or proceed into G_1 to begin another cycle of division.

There are 2 major decision points in the cell cycle that determine whether a cell proceeds: the first is in G_1, when a commitment to chromosome replication occurs; the second is at the end of G_2, when commitment to mitotic division must be made. In most mammalian cells, the dominant controls of cell cycle progression occur in G_1. The proportion of cells in different phases of the cell cycle can be determined by DNA content, using flow cytometry as previously described. An increased proportion of cells with greater than diploid amounts of DNA, the G_2/M phase fraction, is indicative of a higher proliferative rate. Cell populations in which a high proportion are in the G_0 state will have few cells with greater than diploid amounts of DNA.

There are 2 key families of proteins that control the cell cycle: cyclins and cyclin-dependent kinases (cdk). The cdk are serine/threonine kinases that phosphorylate target regulatory proteins involved in cell cycle control. Cyclins are activator proteins that bind to cdk and control their kinase activity. The cyclic assembly, activation, and disassembly of cyclin cdk complexes are critical events driving the cell cycle. There are currently 7 families of cyclins that have been identified: A, B, C, D, E, F, and G; 10 cdk genes are known. Specific cyclin family members bind to specific cdk and regulate their kinase activity. The catalytic activity of the cdk is also controlled by specific phosphorylations. Pro-

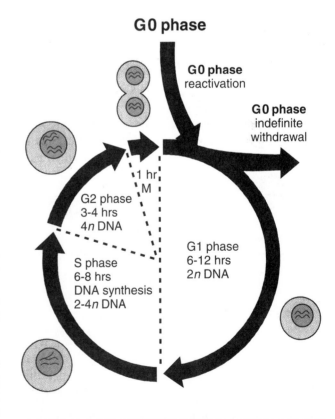

G0 phase

G0 phase
reactivation

G0 phase
indefinite
withdrawal

1 hr
M

G2 phase
3-4 hrs
4n DNA

G1 phase
6-12 hrs
2n DNA

S phase
6-8 hrs
DNA synthesis
2-4n DNA

Figure 29

The phases and approximate durations of the cell cycle. (Reproduced with permission from Lewin B: *Genes VI*. New York, NY, Oxford University Press, 1997, p 1089.)

teins such as p53 and Rb modulate cell cycle events involving cyclin activities, and mutations in these genes are important causes of loss of cell cycle control in cancers. The cdk/cyclin regulations of the cell cycle are summarized in Figure 30. For further details, see Chapter 16.

Cell Signaling

In differentiated cells, such as those that compose the musculoskeletal system, only a small subset of the total number of genes are actively transcribed. This transcriptional specificity determines the identity of the cell and influences the composition of the tissue, as well as tissue homeostasis and repair. The rate of transcription of the pool of potentially expressed genes can vary in musculoskeletal and other tissues and is responsive to a number of external influences. Cells integrate these influences, including mechanical forces, interactions with extracellular matrices, contact with other cells, and growth factor binding, into a coordinate series of intracellular signaling events that converge on the nucleus and regulate the synthesis of specific genes, many of which are central to control of proliferation and differentiation (Fig. 31).

Transcription factors are commonly directed to their cognate promoter binding sites as the terminal event in a signaling cascade that occurs in response to an external cellular signal. This process is referred to as signal transduction. The different transcription factors are each responsive to unique signaling pathways and have different modes of activation. Signal transduction frequently depends on successive phosphorylations and dephosphorylations of the participatory proteins. Phosphorylation is effected by enzymes known as kinases, and dephosphorylation is effected by phosphatases. The major classes of kinases are serine/threonine kinases or tyrosine kinases based on the

phosphorylated residue in the protein; there are corresponding phosphatases. The kinases and phosphatases currently identified number well into the hundreds, emphasizing the broad use of this mechanism for altering protein activity.

The response of cells to parathyroid hormone (PTH) and parathyroid hormone-related protein (PTHrP) illustrates how a single peptide can generate a cascade of signals. The pathway begins with binding of PTH or PTHrP to a receptor in the plasma membrane. The binding results in a conformational change in the receptor, which is transmitted to an associated protein trimer known as a G protein (G due to the binding of GTP by the α subunit). The α, β, and γ subunits of the G protein dissociate in response to ligand binding. The α subunit then interacts with adenylate cyclase, an integral plasma membrane enzyme. The interaction with G_a stimulates adenylate cyclase to convert ATP to cyclic adenosine 3'-5' monophosphate (cAMP). cAMP subsequently binds to protein kinase A (PKA), which is a tetramer of 2 regulatory (R) and 2 catalytic (C) subunits. The catalytic subunits are freed by the binding of cAMP to the R subunits. The C subunit translocates to the nucleus, where they phosphorylate cAMP response element binding protein (CREB) at a specific serine (Ser 133). While CREB binds to DNA in the absence of Ser[133] phosphorylation, activation of transcription by CREB is dependent on this event. Phosphorylated CREB is able to interact with other proteins (KBP/P300) to stimulate transcription (Fig. 32).

PTHrP binding to its receptor also activates another signaling pathway. A second type of G protein that is associated with the PTHrP receptor activates protein lipase C. The lipase cleaves phosphatidyl inositol-4,5-bisphosphate into inositol 1,4,5 triphosphate (IP_3) and diacylglycerol. The IP_3 is a soluble molecule that diffuses through the cytoplasm and binds to a receptor in the endoplasmic reticulum membrane. The IP_3 receptor is a calcium chan-

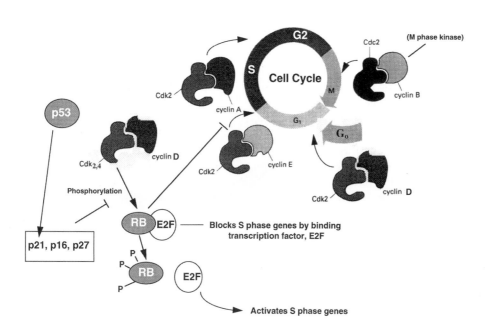

Figure 30

Cyclins and their associated kinases are involved in checkpoint control of the cell cycle. Cyclin B associates with the kinase Cdc2 and is critical to initiation of mitosis. Cyclin D associates with Cdk2 or Cdk4, and allows entry from G_0 into G_1. In addition, cyclin D/Cdk2,4 complexes phosphorylate RB, which releases E2F allowing transcription of S phase genes and therefore the transition from G_1 to S phase. Cyclin E/Cdk2 also acts to allow cell cycle progression into S phase, and cyclin A/cdk association is necessary for progression from S phase to G_2. *p53*, a tumor suppressor gene, induces transcription of *p21*, which is one of the inhibitors of the cyclin D/cdk mediated phosphorylation of RB that controls the G1/S phase transition.

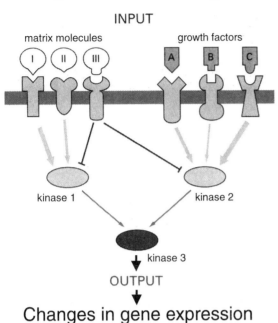

Integration of cellular signals

INPUT

matrix molecules   growth factors

kinase 1   kinase 2

kinase 3

OUTPUT

Changes in gene expression

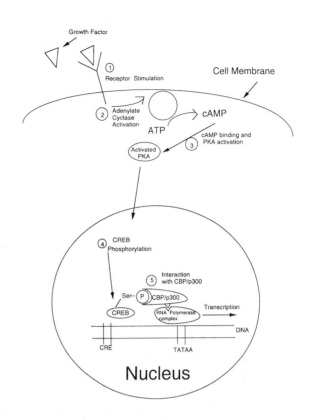

Nucleus

Figure 31

Cells ultimately must integrate signals from multiple pathways and stimuli into net changes in gene expression. Matrix/cell interactions cause kinase signals through integrins and other receptors, as does stimulation of multiple cell surface receptors by various growth factors or hormones. These signals have varying positive and negative influences on tissue-specific gene expression controlling proliferation and differentiated function, which integrate through kinase signaling pathways into a net resultant effect on the cell's behavior. (Reproduced with permission from Alberts B, Bray D, Lewis J, Raff M, Roberts K, Watson JD: *Molecular Biology of the Cell*, ed 3. New York, NY, Garland Publishing, 1994, p 781.)

Figure 32

A common example of a signal transduction pathway is the cyclic AMP (cAMP)/protein kinase A pathway, which is used by many receptors in skeletal tissues, including the parathyroid hormone related protein receptor. A surface receptor binds a specific ligand (1), which results in adenylate cyclase activation (2). This in turn causes cAMP production, which binds to protein kinase A (PKA), activating this enzyme (3). The activated PKA translocates to the nucleus, where it phosphorylates a cAMP response element binding protein (CREB protein) (4), which binds to a consensus sequence in the promoter of a gene and through the serine residue phosphorylated by PKA interacts with a protein called CREB binding protein (CBP), or p300 (5). The p300 then interacts with the transcription complex to regulate its activity, and thus the level of expression of the gene.

nel that opens in response to IP$_3$, transiently elevating cytosolic calcium levels from approximately 10^{-8} M to 10^{-6} M. Calcium itself is a powerful intracellular signal. Among the responders to elevated calcium is protein kinase C (PKC), which also requires diacylglycerol as a cofactor. PKC is a membrane-bound serine/threonine protein kinase. In contrast to PKA, it does not diffuse to different cellular compartments. Instead, the proteins phosphorylated by PKC are the first step in a series of phosphorylations that ultimately affect the activity of a subset of transcription factors.

A slightly different mechanism of a signal transduction pathway is found for the transcription factor nuclear factor kappa B (NFκB), which amplifies the inflammatory response and is responsive to tumor necrosis factor –2 (TNF) receptor activities. NFκB is normally found in the cytoplasm bound to IκB (inhibitor of kappa B). Upon binding ligand to the TNF receptor, a series of kinases are activated, which culminate in the phosphorylation of IκB at multiple sites. Following phosphorylation, IκB is bound to ubiquitin, a 76-amino acid protein that is used to "tag" proteins, usually for proteolysis. This IκB is targeted to the 26S proteosome, a large cylindrical protein complex that attaches to proteins bound to ubiquitin and proteolyzes them as the proteins are drawn through its "barrel." The released NFκB translates to the nucleus where it binds to its recognition sequences in the promoters of a variety of genes. NFκB is a widely used transcription factor with proven activities in apoptosis and limb development, in addition to its role in the inflammatory response.

Steroid receptors, another prevalent pathway, combine both receptor and signal transduction activities. There are a variety of these receptor types, which bind lipid soluble substrates such as vitamins A and D, thyroid hormone, and steroid hormones such as estrogen and glucocorticoids. Following ligand binding in the cytosol, the receptor-hormone complex translocates to the nucleus and binds to target DNA sequences. Many of these steroid hormones bind to DNA by virtue of a zinc finger DNA binding motif. The transcriptional regulating activity then influences the expression of specific genes.

These are but a few examples of many types of intracellular signaling pathways. All cells contain a large number of different signal transduction pathways that interact in extremely complex ways. Ultimately, the cell must integrate all of these various signals to enable meaningful responses to stimuli in its environment.

Apoptosis

Apoptosis is the phenomenon of programmed cell death, which is important in many physiologic and pathologic processes. There are a number of parallel signal pathways through which different stimuli can trigger apoptosis, and a common final pathway that actually mediates the disassembly of the cellular organellar and nuclear apparatus. Apoptosis is the normal differentiation pathway termination for certain cells, such as growth plate chondrocytes and osteoclasts. The balance of a number of competing regulatory proteins determines if a cell enters the apoptotic pathway. Cell necrosis that results from a chemical toxin causes the cells to swell and burst, spilling their intracellular contents, and is quite different from the controlled process of apoptosis. Cell necrosis can induce an inflammatory response to the cellular debris, whereas with apoptosis the systematically degraded components rapidly disappear without inducing inflammation. Apoptosis was initially characterized by its particular microscopic features, which include condensation and shrinkage of the nucleus, vacuolization of the cytoplasm, and fragmentation of the nuclear material. The cellular debris created as the cell disintegrates is rapidly and efficiently engulfed by macrophages or neighboring cells and degraded. Apoptosis can be induced by a number of different stimuli, including specific receptor/ligand interactions, chemical agents such as chemotherapy, glucocorticoid receptor stimulation, radiation, or hypoxia. Derangements of normal apoptotic pathways can enhance oncogenic potential in cells.

Apart from histologic determination, apoptosis can be identified by several methods. A defining terminal event in apoptosis is the fragmentation of the DNA, which is cleaved in internucleosomal intervals by a DNase called caspase activated DNase (CAD). Caspases are a family of 10 cysteine proteases that are the effectors of the apoptotic cascade. When activated, caspases cleave an inhibitor of the CAD, initiating DNase activity. Other targets of caspase proteolytic activity are members of a family of apoptosis-preventing proteins called Bcl2s and some of the proteins involved in cytoskeletal maintenance, gelsolin and focal adhesion

kinase (FAK). Gesolin, a protein involved in actin turnover, becomes activated and degrades actin filaments, and FAK function is disrupted.

The activation of CAD generates a series of DNA fragments varying in length by the approximately 200 bp between nucleosomes. Consequently, upon gel electrophoresis of DNA extracted from cells undergoing apoptosis, a ladder pattern of DNA fragments is characteristically obtained. Another method of detecting DNA fragmentation is referred to as the terminal uridine nicked end labeling (TUNEL) assay. The exposed nicked ends of DNA are labeled by incubation with a terminal transferase, which adds a tail of tagged nucleotides such as digoxigenin-deoxyuridine wherever a DNA end is exposed. This can be detected with an enzyme-conjugated antibody to the label using a simple immunohistochemical method. Other labeling methods as previously discussed are also possible. The TUNEL method can be used for identification of apoptotic nuclei in a tissue section or cultured cells.

Receptor-mediated apoptosis results from interaction of a ligand with one of a family of transmembrane receptors containing a cytoplasmic death domain. The 2 most studied family members are the Fas receptor (also called Apo1, or CD95), and the tumor necrosis factor receptor 1 (TNFR1). Binding of the Fas receptor by ligand causes the intracellular death domain to bind a protein called FADD, which activates caspase 8, leading directly to apoptosis. TNFR1 activation can trigger both proapoptotic and antiapoptotic signals. A similar death domain can bind either FADD or a kinase called RIP. Proteins that interact with RIP can then trigger activation of a transcription factor, NFκB, by catalyzing its release from its binding protein IκB, or stimulate a Jun kinase pathway that phosphorylates Jun, both of which inhibit apoptosis. On the other hand, the binding of FADD activates caspase 8 and promotes apoptosis directly as with CD95 activation. Other members of this receptor family have been identified, as have decoy receptors, which bind the ligands but lack death domains.

The Bcl-2 family of proteins consists of a group of 15 pro- and antiapoptotic molecules that can form heterodimers. Bcl-2 and antiapoptotic homologs such as Bcl-x_L are localized to intracellular membranes such as the endoplasmic reticulum, nuclear membrane, and particularly the outer membrane of mitochondria. Bcl-2 proteins may function as membrane channels, based on protein structure homologies. Bcl-2 bound to the mitochondrial membrane without a dimerization partner binds an adaptor protein called Apaf-1. Upon dimerization with a pro-apoptotic homolog, such as Bik, Bax, or Bad, two significant events are thought to take place: the Apaf-1 is released into the cytosol, and a permeability transition occurs in the outer membrane of the mitochondria that allows the release of soluble cytochrome c from the space between the inner and outer mitochondrial membranes. The Apaf-1 binds to procaspase 9, and cytochrome c in turn binds Apaf-1, catalyzing cleavage of the propeptide and activation of caspase 9. Caspase 9 can then carry out the apoptosis program. Increasing the expression of Bcl-2 decreases the ability of cells to undergo apoptosis, and increasing proapoptotic expression of Bax or other homologs enhances apoptosis. Bcl-2 also has an independent function that appears to inhibit entry into the cell cycle. Phosphorylations and other interactions also modulate the activities of these apoptosis gate-controllers. For instance, Raf, a kinase in the Ras signal pathway, phosphorylates Bad, which prevents its dimerization with Bcl-2. Similarly, phosphorylations of Bcl-2 have been shown to inhibit its antiapoptotic activity. However, the key point is that it is the overall balance between Bcl-2-like and Bax-like proteins that open or shut the pathway to caspase 9 activation. Figure 33 summarizes the major relationships of the apoptotic pathways.

Growth Factors

Local proteins secreted by many cell types that bind to specific receptors and mediate signaling events that modulate cell proliferation and differentiation are called growth factors. Cytokines are similar receptor-activating local protein factors, and in fact the distinction is somewhat artificial. However, historically cytokines are secreted factors initially characterized in cells of the hematopoietic and immune systems. Essentially all musculoskeletal tissues produce and respond to growth factors, and these proteins are involved in injury, disease, and repair processes as well as normal growth and development. Growth factors are also beginning to find clinical therapeutic applications. Growth factors are a part of the normal processes that regulate the cell cycle. Mutations in growth factors or growth factor receptors can be associated with derangements of cell growth in the case of cancers, or can result in skeletal malformations. Most growth factors are mitogenic, or stimulate cell proliferation. These proteins are secreted by a cell and activate cell surface receptors either on the same cell (autocrine stimulation) or on nearby cells (paracrine stimulation). The activity of some growth factors is regulated extracellularly by specific binding proteins that may either prevent interaction with the receptors, or in some cases be necessary to present the growth factor to the receptor. Growth factors have been named after their apparent functions or tissue of origin.

Epidermal growth factor (EGF) stimulates a broad range of cell types to undergo proliferation. EGF acts on bone and cartilage cells, but does not at present appear to be one of the more important regulators of skeletal tissues. Mutations of the EGF receptor that result in its activation have been associated with squamous cell carcinomas. Platelet-derived growth factor (PDGF) has mitogenic effects on a wide range of cell types, and is present in high concentrations in platelets and vascular endothelial cells. PDGF is a dimeric molecule, and 2 isoforms, A and B, exist and can form

either homodimers or heterodimers. PDGF overproduction has been associated with some tumors, and the proto-oncogene name for PDGF is c-sis. PDGF is released in large amounts by platelets at sites of injury, and may play an important role in initiating proliferation of reparative cell populations. PDGF has been shown to stimulate tendon healing, and also has stimulatory effects on chondrocyte and osteoblastic proliferation.

TGF-β is a ubiquitous family of structurally related dimeric growth factors. There are 4 primary mammalian forms of TGF-β and subfamilies including activins, gdf's and the BMPs. TGF-β1-4 have been identified in cartilage and bone, and have pleiotropic effects on these tissues. In general, TGF-βs stimulate proliferation of cells of mesenchymal origin, although in epithelial cells these proteins inhibit proliferation. TGF-βs are secreted in a latent propeptide form that requires enzymatic cleavage for activation. Activation can also be achieved by acid pH or heat. A binding protein secreted in many tissues that produce TGF-βs sequesters the proteins and prevents receptor activation. TGF-βs are dimeric, disulfide-bonded molecules.

Three receptors have been identified, type I (MW 50 to 60 kD), type II (MW 75 to 80 kD), and type III (MW 200 kD). The type III receptor is a cell surface proteoglycan with high affinity binding and is not a true receptor. Biologic effects are mediated through the type I and II receptors, which function as heterodimeric serine/threonine kinases. All forms of TGF-β bind to these receptors, but generally TGF-β2 has lower affinity than TGF-β1 and TGF-β3 for the type I and II receptors. The type II receptor has lower affinity for the TGF-β isoforms than the type I receptor. The type I, II, and III receptors have all been identified in cartilage, although changes in expression of these receptors during maturation have only been partially characterized to date. Progressive expression of the type II receptor (which may inhibit proliferation) occurs with chondrocyte maturation, and may be responsible for a decreasing mitogenic stimulation as the cells begin to hypertrophy.

Heterodimeric receptor-TGF-β complexes initiate signaling via receptor autophosphorylation, and subsequent signaling events involve a family of proteins activated downstream of the receptor called SMADs that are translocated to the nucleus following activation and regulate gene transcription (Fig. 34). However, the downstream signaling pathways responsible for initiating changes in gene transcription in response to TGF-β receptor activation are not fully understood. In articular chondrocytes, TGF-β stimulates proteoglycan synthesis and may reverse effects of other cytokines such as interleukin-1 (IL-1), which stimulate matrix degradation, but it is not mitogenic in chondrocytes that have not entered the pathway of endochondral ossification. In bone, TGF-βs stimulate osteoblast proliferation as well as matrix synthesis. TGF-β is stored in bone matrix in a latent form. During bone resorption, TGF-β is released from the bone matrix, and the acidic pH would

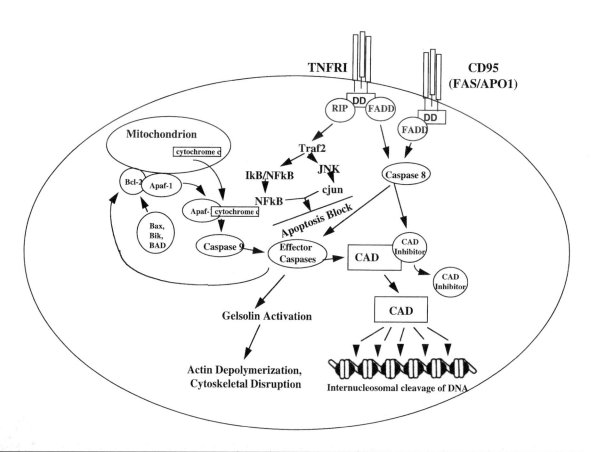

Figure 33

Regulation of apoptosis occurs through complex intersecting pathways. Ligand mediated activation of the process can occur through receptors such as tumor necrosis factor receptor 1 (TNFR1) or CD95. Upon ligand binding, the "death domains" of the receptors and kinases called FADD interact, resulting in activation of caspase 8. Caspase 8 results in activation of other effector caspases, such as caspase 3, and dissociation of the CAD (caspase-activated DNAse) from its inhibitor, resulting in internucleosomal cleavage of DNA. The effector caspases also activate gelsolin, disrupting the cytoskeleton. The TNF receptor can also exhibit anti-apoptotic effects in some cells through activation of a kinase called RIP, which activates a signaling protein (Traf2) resulting in both release of NFκB from its binding protein IκB and phorphorylation of c-jun by its kinase (JNK). These transcription factors can then block apoptosis. Other signals, including toxins, can cause apoptosis through activation of the caspase 9 pathway. In this pathway, Bcl-2 functions as an apoptotic inhibitor by binding of Apaf-1. Dimerization with proapoptotic proteins such as Bax, Bik, Bid, or Bad results in release of Apaf-1 and a permeability transition in the mitochondrial outer membrane, which releases cytochrome c. Cytochrome c binds Apaf-1 and activates caspase 9, which in turn activates effector caspases such as caspase 3, thus triggering apoptosis. The relative levels and states of phorphorylation of Bcl-2 and Bax family members control the levels of Apaf-1/caspase 9 activity. The expression of the *bcl-2/Bax* families of anti- and proapoptosic control genes and their phosphorylation is in turn regulated by numerous signaling pathways.

activate the protein. Therefore, TGF-β has been proposed as one of the molecules that may regulate osteoblast/osteoclast interactions in the local coupling of bone formation and resorption. It has been used to stimulate cartilage repair, and has shown modest effects in stimulation of fracture healing.

BMPs are a 15-member subfamily of the TGF-β superfamily of growth factors. BMPs are involved in regulation of growth and development. BMPs are dimeric disulfide bonded proteins, but are not secreted as latent polypeptides and consequently do not require proteolysis for activation. However, binding proteins such as noggin and chordin associate with BMPs extracellularly and inhibit their interaction with receptors, providing another level of cellular control over BMP activity. Most of the BMPs share

the ability to induce differentiation of cartilage and bone through the endochondral calcification pathway when implanted in an ectopic site. BMP1 is a metalloprotease that functions as a C-propeptidase for collagen types I, II, and III. BMP2 is an osteoinductive factor, and induces chondrogenic differentiation of mesenchymal cells. BMPs 5, 6, and 7 are closely related, and are also effective osteoinductive agents. BMPs 6 and 7 are located in hypertrophic cartilage, and promote cartilage maturation and commitment to the endochondral calcification pathway.

BMPs have also been identified in nerve tissue, and mutations causing overexpression of BMP4 in inflammatory cells are responsible for fibrodysplasia ossificans progressiva, a disease characterized by massive spontaneous heterotopic bone formation. BMP expression is also critical to induction of apoptosis in the interdigital web spaces to form the digits during embryonic development. Three BMP receptors have been identified that are similar to the TGF-β receptors. There are 2 type I receptors, A and B, and 1 type II receptor. The receptors dimerize upon binding the ligand, and the receptor autophosphorylates and then phorphorylates members of the SMAD family of signaling proteins, which dimerize and are transported to the nucleus where they in some way mediate changes in gene transcription (Fig. 34).

BMPs, in particular BMP2 and BMP7 (also known as osteogenic protein 1, or OP1), are being used in experimental clinical settings to induce bone regeneration. The typical delivery system for these growth factors is incorporation into a collagen sponge or collagen gel, which is implanted in the prospective site for bone induction. Efficacy in stimulation of critical defect and nonunion models in animals is abundant, although data from human trials have been published only for native and not recombinant molecules. Two human clinical trials for nonunions have been published, one using human native BMP with a bone matrix-derived substrate, and a second using a bovine BMP/plaster of Paris delivery. In both trials, 16 of 17 patients were healed using this treatment. One remaining question is why huge doses

(microgram to milligram range) of recombinant BMP are needed in defect models as opposed to native material. Heterodimers of different BMPs have recently been shown to have greater efficacy than the currently produced heterodimers, and this is an area of current research, although no heterodimeric factors have yet been produced for testing in clinical trials.

Delivery of BMPs using gene therapy approaches has successfully been demonstrated in animal models with either direct introduction of the plasmid in a collagen matrix formulated to enhance cellular uptake of the DNA, or introduction of transfected cells. Clinical trials involving spine fusion (in conjunction with titanium cages), osteonecrosis of the hip, and fracture healing are in progress. Trials suggesting efficacy in restoration of alveolar bone loss in periodontal disease have also been reported and further studies are ongoing. Reported preliminary human results with spinal fusion appear promising.

BMP6 is regulated in developing cartilage and in the growth plate cartilage by other locally produced growth factors, PTHrP, and a developmental patterning gene called indian hedgehog (*IHH*), in a paracrine fashion. Unlike PTH, PTHrP is a locally acting factor rather than a systemic hormone. It was initially identified in malignant tumors that overproduce it, causing hypercalcemia. PTH and PTHrP share a common receptor, the PTH/PTHrP receptor, in most tissues, although a second receptor has been identified that selectively binds PTH. The N-terminal sequence of PTH and PTHrP are similar, and constitute the binding domain for the receptor. The PTH/PTHrP receptor activates multiple signals upon binding ligand through g proteins that interact with the receptor. These include cAMP stimulation of protein kinase A and activation of phospholipase C with secondary production of inositol triphosphate, which causes a transient rise in cytosolic calcium levels and activation of the protein kinase C pathway. The protein kinases phosphorylate intracellular signaling molecules and alter gene transcription. Two of the important transcription factors activated by PTH/PTHrP receptor activation are CREB and AP1. The effect of PTHrP on chondrocytes is to stimulate proliferation and suppress genes associated with maturation such as alkaline phosphatase, *BMP6, IHH*, and type X collagen. PTH/PTHrP receptor expression is found in growth plate, but not articular or epiphyseal cartilage, and PTHrP produced in the epiphysis is thought to act on receptors in the growth plate chondrocytes in a paracrine fashion, stimulating proliferation and preventing premature hypertrophy, in part by suppression of *BMP6* expression. PTHrP expression is in turn stimulated by *IHH*, which is expressed in the growth plate chondrocytes. *IHH* induces PTHrP expression through a receptor-mediated mechanism via receptors called *patched* and *gli* in adjacent perichondrium and possibly the epiphysis, and PTHrP reciprocally inhibits IHH in a paracrine feedback loop. The balance between these factors controls the rate of chondrocyte pro-

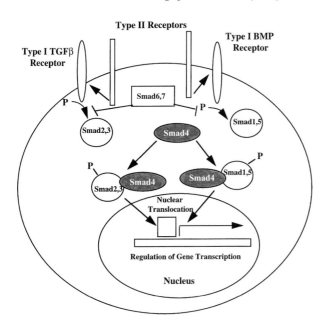

Figure 34

The TGF-β and BMP family members utilize the SMAD signaling pathways. When the appropriate ligand associates with the type I receptor, the type II receptor binds to and phosphorylates the type I receptor. This in turn results in phosphorlylation of the signaling proteins called SMADs. SMAD 2 or 3 can be phosphorylated by the TGF-β type I receptor, and SMAD 1 or 5 by the BMP type I receptor. Upon phosphorylation, the SMADs associate with another protein called SMAD4, resulting in translocation to the nucleus, where this complex associates with promoter elements and alters gene transcription. Other inhibitory SMADs (6 and 7) function to block the phosphorylation and can thus prevent signal transduction by the receptors.

liferation and maturation. The paracrine relationships between the growth plate and articular/epiphyseal cartilage during development are depicted in Figure 35. The critical nature of PTHrP and its receptor and *IHH* has been demonstrated in knockout mouse models. Deletion of the *PTHrP* gene results in a perinatal lethal dwarfed phenotype, with severe derangements of cartilage maturation typified by decreased proliferation and premature onset of hypertrophy in the growth plates. A similar result occurs with deletion of the PTH/PTHrP receptor. Deletion of *IHH* also results in severe disruption of the growth plate, along with a failure of mineralized bone formation even in areas of osteoblastic bone formation. The significance of *IHH* in developmental regulation of osteoblast function is not yet understood.

Insulin-like growth factors (IGFs) are also important in the regulation of many skeletal tissue types. IGF-I, also called somatomedin C, is produced in the liver and also in skeletal tissues in response to activation of cell surface receptors for growth hormone. Locally produced IGF-I in the growth plate has been shown to stimulate proliferation of chondrocytes, and probably contributes significantly to the stimulation of long bone growth by growth hormone. Growth hormone has also been demonstrated to stimulate expression of FGF-2 in cartilage. IGF-I stimulates proteoglycan synthesis as well as cell proliferation. IGF-II is expressed in bone, and can activate the IGF-II receptor, which is identical with the cation-independent mannose-6-phosphate receptor. IGF-II stimulates proliferation and matrix synthesis by osteoblasts. Cells that secrete IGFs also secrete binding proteins (BP) that control the activity of IGFs. Six IGF binding proteins have been identified, and most of the binding proteins inhibit IGF function, although IGFBP5 actually enhances the effect of IGFs on bone cells.

FGFs are a family of 11 growth factors, with FGF-1 and -2 the most abundant. FGFs are found in cartilage matrix and in bone. They stimulate proliferation of both cell types, and 4 different FGF receptors have been identified. FGF inhibits proliferation in vivo in the growth plate or in organ cultures, although in monolayer cultures of chondrocytes FGF is stimulatory. Mutations of the FGF receptors have been implicated in a number of human chondrodysplasias, including identification of an activating mutation of FGFR3 as the cause of achondroplasia. FGFs are also angiogenic, stimulating growth of vasculature. The angiogenic properties of FGF-2 have been used experimentally to revascularize infarcted areas of myocardium by implantation of the growth factor at the time of coronary bypass surgery. FGFs are tightly bound by many extracellular matrix molecules, including heparin-like carbohydrates and proteoglycans. The FGF receptors function as tyrosine kinases, triggering intracellular signaling pathways. FGFs can have synergistic effects on the stimulation of chondrocyte proliferation with IGF-I and TGF-β. FGFs have been used to stimulate tendon, ligament, and cartilage repair, but do not have major effects on fracture repair.

Vascular endothelial growth factor (VEGF) is another angiogenic growth factor found in endothelial cells. This growth factor stimulates endothelial cell proliferation in vitro; in vivo, it markedly stimulates formation of new vasculature. VEGF has been identified in the lower hypertrophic zone of the growth plate, where it may play a role in stimulating endothelial ingrowth into the calcified cartilage, triggering its conversion to bone. VEGF has also been localized to the tissue within the distraction gap during distraction osteogenesis lengthening of long bones. In fact, with each microdistraction caused by lengthening the fixation device there is a wave of VEGF expression. The histology of the distraction gap tissue demonstrates a highly vascularized fibrous interzone that develops abundant osteoblastic activity and bone formation along the developing vessels. This tissue supports the central role of VEGF in driving the vascularization necessary to support osteoblastic bone formation. VEGF does not appear to be highly expressed in normal bone, but is involved in angiogenesis in malignant tumors. VEGF has been used in experimental clinical trials of gene therapy for vascular ischemic disease and myocardial infarction. In one clinical trial, intra-arterial injection of naked plasmid DNA encoding VEGF resulted in dramatic clinical improvement in lower limb ischemia, and promising results in myocardial revascularization have been reported in animal models.

Cytokines

Cytokines are a diverse group of soluble peptide signaling molecules and more than 100 such molecules have been identified. Although cytokines are widely known for their role in inflammation, they also affect mechanisms such as tissue homeostasis and repair. Cytokines are produced by a variety of cells, but are sometimes referred to as lymphokines or monokines to denote a relative specificity of production by either activated lymphocytes or monocytes. The term chemokine is sometimes used to designate cytokines with chemoattractant activity for fibroblasts or leukocytes. Cytokines are typically produced locally and act in a paracrine or autocrine manner. However, cytokines can also have systemic effects ranging from an infection-mediated febrile response to the cachexia of malignancy. Elevated systemic cytokine levels have been associated with hypercalcemia of malignancy secondary to increased osteoclastic bone resorption.

Cytokines act on specific cell membrane-associated receptors and have pleiotropic effects on a variety of target cells. One of the most important effects of these molecules is their role in immunomodulation. Activation of monocytes/macrophages by phagocytosis or stimulation with bacterial lipopolysaccharide results in the synthesis of several important proinflammatory cytokines, including IL-1, IL-6, and TNF-α. These molecules increase vascular permeability, attract additional mononuclear cells to the site of

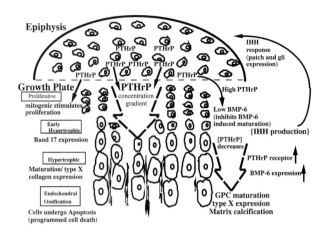

Figure 35

The paracrine regulatory loop of parathyroid hormone related protein (PTHrP) and Indian hedgehog (IHH) in developing cartilage is illustrated. IHH is produced in the growth plate in response to expression of BMP-6 in the early hypertrophic chondrocytes. IHH in turn signals to cells in the perichondrium and possibly, the epiphysis, through a receptor called patched and its intracellular signaling molecule called gli to stimulate PTHrP expression. PTHrP in the epiphysis then in turn inhibits expression of BMP-6 and IHH in the growth plate cells, suppressing hypertrophy and maturation in a feedback loop. The balance between PTHrP and BMP-6/IHH expression controls the rate of chondrocyte proliferation and maturation. (Reproduced with permission from Rosier RN, O'Keefe RJ, Reynolds PR, Hicks DG, Puzas JE: Expression and function of TGF-β and PTHrP in the growth plate, in Buckwalter JA, Ehrlich MG, Sandell LJ, Trippel SB (eds): *Skeletal Growth and Development*. Rosemont, IL, American Academy of Orthopaedic Surgeons, 1998, pp 285–300.)

inflammation, lead to the proliferation and differentiation of lymphocytes, and stimulate additional proinflammatory cytokine release. Thus, these molecules enhance and amplify the inflammatory response. Although important for the control of infection, the response results in tissue catabolism if left unchecked.

Regulation of the inflammatory response is probably provided in part by one or more anti-inflammatory cytokines, such as IL-4 or IL-10. IL-4 is made predominantly by lymphocytes, and IL-10 is produced by both monocytes and lymphocytes. Both peptides act via specific cell membrane receptors and decrease the expression and secretion of the proinflammatory cytokines in activated monoculear cells. IL-10 also decreases monocyte expression of HLA-DR. Because it is involved in antigen presentation to CD4+ lymphocytes, HLA-DR is essential for the immunologic activity of macrophages. Thus, IL-10 also indirectly downregulates the cell-mediated immune response. There is evidence to suggest that downregulation of IL-10 may play an important role in the pathogenesis and progression of some human inflammatory diseases, a concept supported by the limited life span of transgenic mice lacking the expression of IL-10. These animals die prematurely because they develop chronic inflammatory disease. Similarly, experi-

mental studies show the ability of exogenously administered IL-4 to control inflammatory arthritis in animal models. Thus, normal tissue homeostasis may depend on a balance between proinflammatory and anti-inflammatory cytokines.

Cytokines have a major role in both the health and disease of the musculoskeletal system. Inflammatory arthritis is associated with high levels of cytokine release, including the proinflammatory cytokines. These cytokines lead to tissue catabolism through both direct and indirect mechanisms. The proinflammatory cytokines stimulate matrix metalloproteinase (MMP) activity in synovial lining cells and incite the development of a proliferative, erosive pannus that invades and destroys the cartilage surface. However, the proinflammatory cytokines also have a wide range of direct effects on chondrocyte metabolism. Cytokine-stimulated articular chondrocytes secrete MMPs, which lead to cartilage degradation and production of aggrecanase, resulting in the breakdown of proteoglycans. In addition, proinflammatory cytokine-stimulated articular chondrocytes have diminished collagen and proteoglycan synthesis and secretion, furthering the catabolic effect of these agents.

Several human trials have recently been conducted, demonstrating that strategies aimed at blocking the proinflammatory cytokines can improve the clinical course of inflammatory arthritis. Administration of IL-1 receptor antagonist, a naturally-occurring soluble IL-1 blocking protein that binds and sequesters IL-1, resulted in improvements in clinical parameters and in radiographic evidence of joint damage over a 6-month period of investigation. Human gene therapy trials using vectors expressing IL-1 receptor antagonist are currently underway with promising early results. Recently, the Food and Drug Administration approved the use of a recombinantly produced soluble fusion protein containing TNF-α type I receptor binding sequences for use in rheumatoid arthritis. Injection of the fusion protein, which sequesters TNF-α, has resulted in marked and continuous improvement in the majority of patients with arthritis unresponsive to traditional therapies.

The proinflammatory cytokines IL-1, IL-6, and TNF-α are also important regulators of bone resorption. These cytokines stimulate osteoclast recruitment from undifferentiated cells in the granulocyte/macrophage lineage and mature osteoclast function. Thus, these cytokines have been implicated in the increase in bone resorption observed in a number of pathologic inflammatory conditions, including infection, periprosthetic osteolysis and loosening, and inflammatory arthritis. Recently, tumor-associated bone loss has been shown to be mediated by osteoclasts in response to cytokine production by tumor cells. Proinflammatory cytokine synthesis has been demonstrated in benign tumors such as pigmented villonodular synovitis, in primary bone tumors such as Ewing's sarcoma, and in the majority of metastatic tumors involving bone.

Animal studies have suggested that the increase in bone resorption that occurs during estrogen deficiency is related to increased levels of IL-6 secretion in marrow stromal cells, an effect that is blocked by the exogenous administration of estrogens. Thus, there is likely a role for these proteins in postmenopausal osteoporosis. Osteoclasts also synthesize IL-1, IL-6, and TNF-α, and may stimulate further bone resorption through an autocrine mechanism in conditions where there are excess numbers of osteoclasts, such as giant cell tumor of bone.

In addition to their responsiveness to cytokines, cells of the musculoskeletal system also secrete cytokines. Osteoblasts synthesize and secrete IL-6 in response to PTH as well as following stimulation with prostaglandins. Because PTH does not have direct effects on osteoclasts, the well known bone resorptive effects of PTH are probably mediated in part through the synthesis of IL-6 by osteoblasts. In addition to its effects on osteoblasts, IL-6 has been shown to stimulate both the differentiation and proliferation of osteoblasts and is a putative stimulator of bone formation. Thus, IL-6 demonstrates the pleiotropic effects that are characteristic of the cytokines.

Prostaglandins

Prostaglandins are lipid-derived signaling molecules that are important mediators of the inflammatory response. Prostaglandins are comprised of 20 carbon molecules that contain a 5-carbon ring. Arachidonic acid is the precursor of prostaglandins and other eicosanoids (molecules containing 20 carbon atoms), including leukotrienes and thromboxanes. Prostaglandins are the products of the cyclooxygenase pathway of arachidonic acid metabolism, and signal by binding to specific membrane receptors and different members of the prostaglandin family of molecules, stimulating various signaling pathways.

Cyclooxygenase is a membrane-associated enzyme and 2 isoforms have been identified and are referred to as cyclooxygenase 1 (COX-1) and cyclooxygenase 2 (COX-2). These isoforms have markedly different physiologic roles. COX-1 is constitutively expressed and is important in the normal physiology of a number of tissues. In the gastrointestinal system COX-1 is highly expressed in the stomach and provides a protective effect against the development of peptic ulcer disease. COX-1 is also involved in normal kidney physiology. In contrast, COX-2 is the inducible form of the enzyme, and is expressed primarily in the setting of inflammation. Nonsteroidal anti-inflammatory drugs (NSAIDs) inhibit COX activity and decrease the pain and edema associated with tissue injury and inflammation. Although these effects are associated with inhibition of COX-2, the deleterious effects of NSAIDs are associated with inhibition of COX-1. Recently, a class of drugs with selective inhibition of COX-2 has been developed. These new pharmacologic agents have the potential to inhibit the inflammatory effects of prostaglandins with a much lower risk of gastric and renal injury.

Cell-Matrix Interactions

The matrix is a key factor in influencing gene expression in skeletal tissues and allowing the cells to receive signals from the environment. This is particularly important in the musculoskeletal system because of the load-bearing functions of the tissues, which require responsiveness and adaptability to mechanical forces. Matrix proteins interact with cell surface receptors in a manner similar to growth factors, and this array of stimuli is transduced by intracellular signaling pathways that integrate them to cause activation of genes that control the cell cycle and the expression of proteins that define differentiated functions of the cell (Fig. 31).

Some interactions of the cell with surrounding matrix are mediated through the cytoskeleton. Cytoskeletal proteins are essential for several cellular functions, including mitosis, cell motility, and intracellular movement and organization of organelles. The cytoskeleton is composed of 3 major types of filaments made by reversible polymerization of specific proteins: actin filaments (actin polymer), microtubules (tubulin polymer), and intermediate filaments (polymers of vimentin or lamin). Cell surface movements are controlled by interactions of the actin molecules with myosins in the cytoplasm, enabling contractility and cell movement. Actin fiber formation is regulated by the Rho family of G proteins. Actin filaments are flexible, whereas microtubules are more rigid structures. Microtubules polymerize and depolymerize continuously in the cell, and mediate organelle transport and subcellular organization. Microtubules are critical in organizing the events of cell division, and radiate outward through the cell from origin sites within the centrosome, a structure adjacent to the nucleus. Proteins called kinesins and dyneins are cytoplasmic ATP-dependent motors that move in opposite directions along microtubules, carrying bound proteins or vesicles. The cytoplasmic intermediate filaments are thought to function within the cell to resist deformation to external mechanical stress, and have greater strength than actin and tubulin (Fig. 36). Numerous cytoplasmic proteins associate with the cytoskeletal proteins and control their structure, contractility, and stability.

One common mechanism linking cells to matrix is the integrin family of cell surface receptors that interact with specific matrix proteins. Integrins consist of transmembrane heterodimeric signaling molecules expressed on the cell surface, which can interact with matrix proteins containing a specific sequence of amino acids (arginine-glycine-aspartate, or RGD). Many extracellular matrix proteins, including collagens, contain RGD sequences enabling interaction with integrin receptors. The dimers consist of α and β subunits that associate in specific combinations in different cell types. All mesenchymal cells express specific subsets of integrin receptors on the cell surface. Over 20 heterodimers have been identified between 9 types of β subunits and 14 types of α subunits. In addition to the numerous isoforms of the 2 integrin subunits, some isoforms have a number of alternatively spliced forms of the protein, further increasing the diversity of this receptor family. The different heterodimers possess differing and sometimes overlapping specificity for particular matrix RGD-containing proteins.

Integrin receptors have relatively lower affinities for their ligands than growth factor and hormone receptors, and are 10 to 100 times more abundant on cell surfaces. The β subunit contains a binding domain that interacts with the cytoskeletal proteins talin and α-actinin, and upon ligand binding causes formation of linkages to the actin cytoskeleton. These areas of focal receptor/cytoskeletal contact can activate kinases such as the focal adhesion kinase or the tyrosine kinase product of the src gene. This in turn leads to a signal cascade that can result in changes in gene expression. Because cells are attached to their matrix by the integrins, perturbations of the mechanical environment couple to effects on the cytoskeleton and associated kinases, providing one mechanism whereby cells can respond with changes in gene expression to changes in mechanical loading.

Another class of adhesion molecules include the hyaluronan receptor family, which recognizes carbohydrates related to hyaluronate. This is also known as the CD44 receptor group, and consists of a number of isoforms. CD44 has been implicated in the attachment of tumor cells to matrix in target tissues during metastasis. Like other cell surface receptors, CD44 can activate intracellular processes. Some types of cell surface receptors, such as cadherins and receptors with some homology to immunoglobulins, known as CAMs (cell-cell adhesion molecules), mediate cell-cell contact events rather than cell-matrix interactions. Activation of cadherins results in binding of these receptors to cytoplasmic proteins called catenins, which interact with the actin cytoskeleton analogous to the manner in which talin and α-actinin link integrin activation to actin. Cadherins and CAMs are homophilic receptors, that is, they bind to a like receptor on a different cell to mediate signaling events. Alterations in cadherin expression can change chondrocyte differentiation pathways in embryogenesis, indicating that gene expression depends on cell-cell interactions as well as cell-matrix interactions.

Most cells possess stretch-activated ion channels in the plasma membrane, which provide another means of cellular response to mechanical stimuli. These channels control influx of K^+ or Ca^{++}, two cations that the cell actively maintains at low intracellular levels through the actions of the plasma membrane-based, energy-dependent pumps. When the matrix adjacent to an attached cell is mechanically deformed, transient elevations of cations can occur through the action of the stretch-activated channels. These cations can influence other signaling pathways within the cell, thus enabling mechanical input to influence the cell's transcrip-

tional machinery. Stretch-activated channels have been demonstrated in fibroblasts, osteoblasts, and chondrocytes.

A family of matrix-cell binding proteins called annexins has features of both a matrix receptor and an ion channel. Annexins are ubiquitous extracellular proteins that associate with the plasma membrane under certain conditions. Annexins II, V, and VI bind to collagen and to the plasma membrane, providing another mechanism for cell-matrix attachment. In addition, some annexins function as calcium channels in the plasma membrane. In chondrocytes, annexins V and VI may function as calcium channels that are activated by binding of type II and type X collagen. The phospholipid composition of the plasma membrane influences annexin association with the membrane, with acidic phospholipids enhancing membrane binding. Annexin V binding is enhanced by changes in the phospholipids of the plasma membrane that occur as part of the cascade of events in programmed cell death, or apoptosis, and binding of this annexin has been used as a marker for apoptosis. Annexins provide another connection between the matrix and intracellular signaling pathways.

Bone remodeling provides an excellent prototypical example of matrix control of cell behavior and communication, and integration of multiple signal inputs by cell-

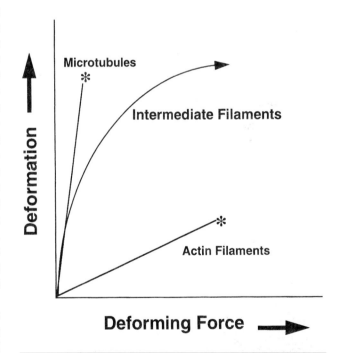

Figure 36

Mechanical properties of different cytoskeletal elements subjected to shear force. Microtubules readily deform with minimal force, while actin filaments are much more rigid, tolerating greater force with less deformation. The intermediate filaments such as vimentin are easily deformed, but withstand large forces without rupture. (Adapted with permission from Janmey P, Euteneuer V, Troub P, Schliwa M: Viscoelastic properties of vimentin compared with other filamentous biopolymer networks. *J Cell Biol* 1991;113:155–160.)

matrix interactions. Osteoblasts secrete the matrix of bone, incorporating growth factors that can be released and activated upon matrix resorption. Osteoblasts provide the initial signals for bone resorption by osteoclasts, responding to stimuli such as PTH with production of collagenase, which appears to clear an area for osteoclast attachment, as well as producing cytokines that stimulate osteoclast formation and activation. The osteoclast begins resorbing bone, organizing its functional apparatus in response to integrin signals upon contact with the bone matrix. The osteoclast releases and activates growth factors from the bone matrix as it resorbs bone, which in turn stimulate osteoblast progenitors nearby to differentiate. In addition, the osteoclast deposits signals on the resorption surface prior to moving on or undergoing apoptosis. These signals attract osteoblasts and stimulate matrix deposition at the previously resorbed surface, replacing the bone matrix. This functional cooperation of osteoblasts and osteoclasts, coupled by the matrix, is modulated by systemic hormonal controls such as PTH and vitamin D, which regulate systemic calcium metabolism. However, the remodeling process is also under local control through mechanical signal transduction through the bone matrix to the osteoblasts and/or osteoclasts, allowing the bone to remodel according to local mechanical stress. Finally, pathologic processes such as inflammation or tumors can produce local cytokines which alter the balance between formation and resorption, leading to pathologic loss of bone matrix.

Cellular Phenotypic Expression

The genotype of an organism or a cell refers to the genes present in its genome. However, in any somatic cell, only a fraction of the genes are expressed. The phenotype of a cell is defined by the array of genes that are expressed and their relative levels of expression. When the phenotype of a cell is characterized, the focus is usually on the genes expressed that are unique or relatively unique to that cell type, because there are thousands of genes that all cells express in common. Differentiation of cells refers to acquisition of a specific profile of gene expression that sets the cell apart from other types of cells, and determines its structure and function. In general, cell proliferation and differentiation tend to be inversely regulated. Proliferation of normal cells is prevented by cell-cell contacts, a phenomenon known as contact inhibition. When cells are plated at low densities in culture, there is no contact inhibition and they tend to enter the cell cycle and proliferate. During active proliferation, the expression of tissue-specific proteins by the cells diminishes. When confluency is attained, contact inhibition triggers mechanisms that inhibit the cell cycle, and cells tend to differentiate, expressing specific characteristics of the

tissue from which they were derived. This paradigm has been well demonstrated in a skeletally relevant tissue using osteoblasts in culture. When initially plated in culture, osteoblasts proliferate and exhibit minimal expression of proteins associated with normal osteoblasts in vivo. In the presence of appropriate differentiation-stimulating agents, the cells progressively express proteins characteristic of differentiation at confluency, such as alkaline phosphatase, osteocalcin, and osteopontin, and ultimately produce a mineralized osteoid matrix (Fig. 37).

The cells of most skeletal tissues, including muscle, tendon, ligament, connective tissue, bone, and cartilage, are derived from multipotent cells called mesenchymal stem cells (MSCs). MSCs give rise to the development of all the skeletal elements during development, and remain present in low numbers in sites such as periosteum and bone marrow throughout life. It is these cells that can differentiate into bone, cartilage, and fibrous tissue following a fracture and generate a reparative callus. Mesenchymal stem cells can be isolated from bone marrow, and under the correct culture conditions can be induced to differentiate into lipoblasts, myoblasts, fibroblasts, osteoblasts, or chondrocytes. Most likely they can also be induced to form tenocytes or fibrochondrocytes, although this has not yet been demonstrated specifically. The number of MSCs declines with age, as does their responsiveness to growth factors; hence, ability to regenerate various mesenchymal tissues declines as a function of aging. Use of MSCs for regenerating bone and repairing osteochondral defects is well underway, and feasibility has been demonstrated in several animal models. Several markers putatively specific for MSCs have been reported, such as STRO1, but further work needs to be done to fully characterize these markers.

Osteoblast Phenotype

There are a number of phenotypic parameters that characterize the osteoblast. Osteoblasts produce and secrete structural proteins (such as collagen) and regulatory proteins (such as growth factors). The study of osteoblasts has been facilitated by development of methods to isolate them from intact bone tissue, usually by collagenase digestion of calvarial or long bone specimens from rats or mice, or from trabecular bone specimens in humans. The cells can be grown in culture, and a number of transformed osteoblastic cell lines have been developed from mouse, human, and rat bone cells derived from tumors or immortalized by viral transformations. Commonly used cell lines include ROS17.28 (rat), UMR106 (rat), SAOS2 (human), MG63 (human), and MC3T3 (murine). The abundant extracellular matrix that osteoblasts produce is called osteoid and, when mineralized with crystalline hydroxyapatite, becomes bone. The major matrix protein synthesized by osteoblastic cells, which comprises more than 90% of the organic matrix of bone, is type I collagen. Type I collagen is synthesized and secreted as a triple helix with two α1 and one α2 chains (genes designated COLIA1 and COLIA2). The amino terminal and carboxyterminal propeptides are cleaved extracellularly, and the collagen molecules spontaneously self-assemble into collagen microfibrils and fibrils, with a quarter-staggered arrangement of the individual molecules. The C-propeptide is cleaved by proteolytic activity of BMP1, a member of the bone morphogenetic protein family that lacks osteoinductive capacity but has some homology to the other members. The C-propeptide and N-propeptide fragments can be detected in serum, and are indicative of bone formation rates.

Bone matrix also contains small amounts of type III and type V collagens. The collagen fibrils are laid down parallel to the surface of the osteoblast, and spontaneously nucleate hydroxyapatite crystals that initially form preferentially in the "hole zones" between the quarter-staggered collagen

molecules. With a periodicity related to the bone formation rate, the orientation of the fibrils changes 90° to the preceding layer, resulting in a layered structure similar to plywood that maximizes the tensile strength of the material. The mechanism that controls this ordered orientation of the matrix is unknown. Normal bone formation in this layered arrangement is referred to as lamellar bone, and is an important feature that distinguishes normal bone from bone formed by tumors or in injury and repair processes.

The carboxyglutamic acid-containing glycoprotein osteocalcin and 2 other glycoproteins, osteopontin and osteonectin, are the next most abundant extracellular matrix protein constituents produced by osteoblasts. Osteonectin may function to enhance binding of hydroxyapatite crystals to the collagen matrix as mineralization proceeds. Osteocalcin is thought to play a role in recruiting osteoclasts to bone surfaces for bone resorption, and the

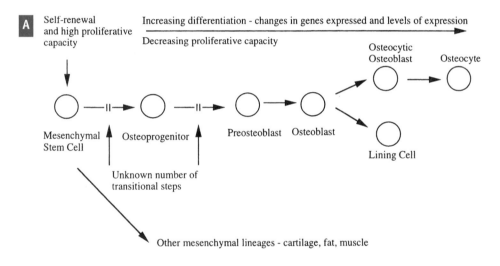

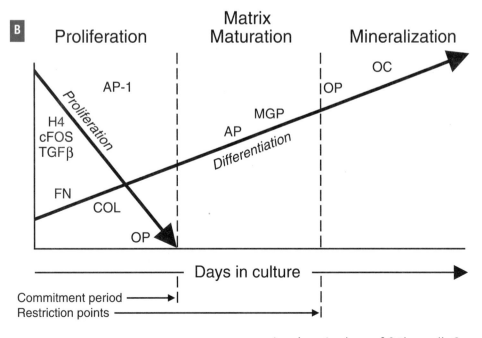

Figure 37

A, The pathways of bone cell progenitor differentiation from mesenchymal stem cell to osteoblast and osteocyte (Reproduced with permission from Aubin JE, Kahn A: The osteoblast lineage: Embryologic origins and differentiation sequence, in Favus MJ (ed): *Primer on the Metabolic Bone Diseases and Disorders of Mineral Metabolism,* ed 3. Philadelphia, PA, Lippincott-Raven, 1996, p 36.). **B,** Reciprocal relationship between genes associated with proliferation and differentiation in an osteoblast culture model. During early culture, genes associated with proliferation such as histone H4, c-fos, TGF-β and AP-1 activity are downregulated, while matrix genes such as fibronectin (FN) and type I collagen (COL) begin to increase. This continues through matrix maturation, when proliferation ceases and onset of expression of alkaline phosphatase (AP) and matrix glutamic acid containing protein (MGP) begins. During the final phases of differentiation, the matrix mineralizes, and osteopontin (OP) and osteocalcin (OC) are expressed. (Reproduced with permission from Lian JB, Stein GS: Development of the osteoblast phenotype: Molecular mechanisms mediating osteoblast growth and differentiation. *Iowa Orthop J* 1995;15: 118–140.)

function of osteopontin is unclear. Bone matrix also contains a sialoprotein and small amounts of several other glycoproteins and phosphoproteins of uncertain function. The extracellular matrix structural proteins are 1 set of phenotypic parameters that define the osteoblast. During osteoblast differentiation, there are a number of shifts in protein synthesis: from type III and type I collagen to type I collagen; from low to high levels of alkaline phosphatase; from versican to fibronectin expression, and from expression of an attachment protein called thrombospondin to expression of the bone glycoproteins osteonectin, osteocalcin, osteopontin, and sialoprotein.

Bone matrix contains a number of regulatory proteins deposited by osteoblasts as well. These include growth factors such as TGF-β, IGF-I and IGF-II, FGFs, PDGFs, and BMPs. Although present quantitatively in minute amounts, these proteins are extremely important in regulating bone remodeling and in conferring osteoinductive capacity on bone, which enables bone grafting and transplantation.

As part of their pheonotype, osteoblasts also express many genes that are not incorporated into the bone matrix. For instance, bone-specific alkaline phosphatase is an enzyme probably involved in mineralization of osteoid. Osteoblasts express PTH/PTHrP receptor, and exhibit intracellular signaling responses to PTH or PTHrP. Osteoblasts also express the vitamin D receptor and consequently vitamin D responsiveness. Some osteoblastic-specific transcription factors, Cbfa1 and a transcriptional co-activator called αNAC, have also recently been identified. Glucocorticoids have complex effects on bone, stimulating differentiation of preosteoblasts in culture through a BMP6-mediated pathway, while inhibiting bone cell proliferation and decreasing bone formation, resorption, and net mass when given systemically in vivo.

Osteocytes are fully differentiated osteoblasts that become encased in the secreted matrix. Because osteocytes are completely embedded in bone, their culture and study has been difficult, and less is known about their phenotype and function. Osteocytes have numerous long cell processes that extend throughout the bone matrix and are in contact with the cell processes of other osteocytes. The channels in the matrix through which these numerous connecting cell processes extend are called canaliculi. Recently it has been demonstrated that osteocytes express cell-cell channels called connexins, through which small molecules such as second messengers can pass. This implies that the networks of osteocytes are in communication with one another. It is also known that bone exhibits piezoelectric properties under mechanical loading because of its anisotropic nature, that is, bone develops surface electrical charges that are asymmetrically distributed when it is mechanically loaded. One putative function of osteocyte-osteocyte communication within the larger organization of bone as a tissue may be in sensing and modulating signals that control osteoblastic and osteoclastic activity, enabling the observed ability of bone to increase its mass in areas that are loaded and decrease mass in response to unloading. Osteocytes also express osteocalcin and fibronectin, although the role of these proteins in osteocyte function is unknown.

Chondrocyte Phenotype

Like osteoblasts, chondrocytes arise from undifferentiated mesenchymal stem cells. As chondrocytes differentiate, they also express a pattern of specific genes that define their function. Chondrocytes are characterized, like osteoblasts, by production of an abundant extracellular matrix. Chondrocytes undergo differentiation along 2 major distinct pathways: one in which the cells undergo maturation, hypertrophy, and matrix calcification (the endochondral calcification pathway), and one in which the cells are relatively quiescent, carrying out load-bearing and structural functions (the nonendochondral calcification pathway) (Fig. 38). Induction of chondrocyte differentiation from mesenchymal stem cell precursors occurs during embryogenesis, and also in injury and repair such as in fracture callus. The nonendochondral calcification pathway can be activated in quiescent chondrocytes as demonstrated by the onset of maturation and calcification in the deep layers of the articular cartilage during cartilage degeneration. Growth plate chondrocytes generate bone growth through proliferation and hypertrophy during maturation along the endochondral calcification pathway.

Chondrocytes can be isolated from cartilage by digestion of the tissue with collagenase or combinations of collagenase, hyaluronidase, and trypsin, and the cells can be grown and studied in culture. Chondrocytes in monolayer culture tend to dedifferentiate, and lose expression of type II collagen and other phenotypic markers such as proteoglycan synthesis. Instead, they take on a more fibroblastic phenotype and express type I collagen. When cultured in a suspension culture or in a 3-dimensional gel made of collagen, agar, or alginate, the cells will maintain a chondrocytic phenotype, emphasizing the importance of cell-matrix interactions in controlling gene expression.

The predominant matrix protein in cartilage is type II collagen, which is comprised of a single type chain forming a triple helix. Like type I collagen, type II collagen is secreted as triple helical proprotein that is cleaved extracellularly (gene designated as COLIIA1). The C-propeptide of type II collagen may also be cleaved by BMP1, which is constitutively expressed in cartilage. Type II collagen exists in 2 alternatively spliced forms, as previously mentioned. The embryonic form, type IIA, differs from the more mature IIB form by inclusion of exon 2 (Fig. 8). This exon is part of the processed portion of the mRNA and therefore does not alter the fibrillar structure of the collagen molecule. The other major organic component of the matrix is proteoglycan, which includes several proteins containing covalently bound glycosaminoglycan side chains. The major proteoglycan is aggrecan, which consists of a protein core and chondroitin sulfate and keratan sulfate side chains. The proteoglycans confer many of the unique mechanical properties on cartilage, including its ability to absorb repetitive compressive mechanical loads without damage. Aggrecan molecules form noncovalently bound aggregates with hyaluronic acid and a link glycoprotein. In addition, cartilage contains small proteoglycans such as decorin and biglycan. A series of minor collagens also associated with the chondrocyte phenotype includes type VI, IX, X, and XI collagens. Type VI collagen is a pericellular matrix protein, and type IX is a collagen molecule with a proteoglycan moiety. Type IX collagen molecules coat the outer surface of type II collagen fibrils and interact with the matrix proteoglycan via their own proteoglycan moieties. This is thought to serve to interconnect the collagen and proteoglycan matrix. Type XI collagen is localized within the type II fibrils, and may regulate fibril diameter.

Several chondrocyte phenotypic markers are specific to the differentiation pathway of the chondrocyte. For instance, type X collagen is only expressed by hypertrophic chondrocytes, and is a highly specific marker for this phenotype. In addition, these cells express high levels of alkaline phosphatase, in contrast to minimal expression in chondrocytes not committed to maturation. Chondrocytes committed to the endochondral calcification pathway also express several growth factors, including BMP-6 and BMP-7, that promote maturation. Differential expression of these genes in articular and growth plate chondrocytes demonstrates the critical role that regulatory gene products can play as determinants of phenotypes.

Osteoclast Phenotype

The osteoclast, the cell responsible for carrying out bone resorption, is extremely specialized, with an array of proteins responsible for resorbing calcified matrix. Osteoclasts are derived from monocytic precursors, and share some of the characteristics of monocytes and macrophages. Osteoclasts are multinucleated, and arise through a syncytium of several precursor cells under the influence of specific growth factors in the bone marrow. Functional osteoclasts have been isolated from animal and human models using several techniques. One of the earliest methods of obtaining sufficient numbers of osteoclasts for study was to rinse the marrow cavity of long bones of egg-laying chickens on low calcium diets. Later, cells with osteoclast-like characteristics were isolated from human giant cell tumors. Functional osteoclasts can also be generated from the marrow of long bones of neonatal rats or mice, and cultured on wafers of cortical bone in the presence of vitamin D and PTH. This procedure, although using a polymorphous cell population, readily enables the study of osteoclasts in vitro.

Osteoclasts attach to bone surfaces through a specific cell attachment receptor called an integrin. The osteoclast inte-

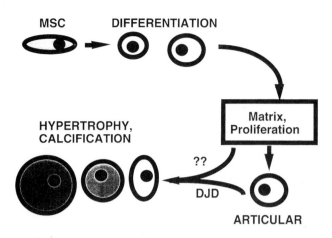

Figure 38

Under proper circumstances, mesenchymal stem cells (MSC) undergo differentiation to prechondroblast and chondroblast, associated with expression of chondrocyte specific genes such as type II and type IX collagen, and aggrecan. The cartilaginous matrix thus produced defines the phenotype. Chondrocytes can then differentiate along 2 pathways: the first is toward articular chondrocyte phenotype, in which the cells are not actively dividing although they are metabolically active in maintenance and turnover of the matrix; the second pathway is endochondral maturation, which results in hypertrophy, expression of type X collagen, and mineralization as a precursor to bone formation. The pathway of maturation may be activated during osteoarthritis, as evidenced by chondrocyte cloning (proliferation), hypertrophy, and type X collagen expression. DJD = degenerative joint disease.

grin receptor is also known as $\alpha_v\beta_3$, or the vitronectin receptor. A number of bone matrix proteins, including collagen, fibronectin, and osteopontin, contain the attachment RGD sequences. After attaching to a bone surface, the integrins activate focal adhesion kinases that in turn induce intracellular signals, including activation of c-src, a regulatory kinase that contributes to the induction of polarization of the osteoclast. An extensive series of microscopic invaginations of the plasma membrane surface against the bone matrix surface forms, called the ruffled border, which serves to markedly increase the surface area of membrane next to the bone. A plasma membrane proton pump moves to the ruffled border and pumps protons from the cytosol into the space between the osteoclast and the bone (Fig. 39). This acidifies the bone surface, resulting in dissolution of the hydroxyapatite mineral phase of the bone.

Lysosomes move to the ruffled border and discharge their contents of lysosomal enzymes into the resorption region. These include acid-activated hydrolases such as cathepsins, which degrade the collagen in the matrix. Osteoclasts also express a MMP (gelatinase B, or MMP9), although its function is unknown. An isoform of carbonic anhydrase (CAII) is expressed and generates intracellular protons for the acidification process. Osteoclasts also express a specific phosphatase called tartrate-resistant acid phosphatase (TRAP), but its function is unknown. TRAP and other glycosylated lysosomal enzymes are deposited on the resorption surface and remain there after the osteoclast has moved away. It is possible that these residues are important in attracting osteoblasts to the resorption sites. Many of these enzymes contain glycosylations that can bind to receptors such as the IFG-II/mannose-6-phosphate receptor. This receptor is expressed in osteoblasts, and when stimulated causes anabolic effects and matrix synthesis. Theoretically, the residue of glycosylated enzymes on the resorption surface may function to target osteoblasts to this location and initiate bone formation, thus representing part of the site-directing coupling mechanism between bone formation and resorption.

Osteoclasts contain a calcium receptor that may be involved in the induction of movement of the pseudopodia of the motile osteoclasts, which creep along the bone surface as they excavate the matrix. When the pseudopodia arise from the bone surface and move to reattach, the accumulated high concentration of inorganic ions such as calcium and phosphate resulting from the resorption of bone matrix is discharged into the extracellular space. Some of the matrix and mineral may be removed by endocytosis and transported across the osteoclast, but this is controversial. Osteoclasts have a finite lifetime, and are active in bone resorption for an estimated 10 to 14 days, after which they undergo apoptosis.

Several key hormones and local factors control osteoclast function. Systemically, PTH stimulates bone resorption. However, only osteoblasts express the PTH receptor. Therefore, the stimulation of resorption is by PTH mediated through signals from the osteoblast. One of these signals may be IL-6, a stimulator of osteoclast formation and resorption. TNF-α is an extremely potent stimulator of osteoclast progenitor proliferation, fusion, and activation of osteoclastic bone resorption, as is IL-1. TNF, IL-1, and IL-6 are produced in many inflammatory processes, and are known as proinflammatory cytokines. These factors are critical to many important clinical disorders, and have been implicated in pathologic bone resorption in metastatic and primary bone tumors, infection, prosthetic loosening, nonunion of fractures, osteoporosis, and periarticular bone loss in inflammatory arthropathies. Figure 40 summarizes the interactions of osteoblasts and osteoclasts in coupling bone formation and resorption during remodeling.

A new receptor similar to the TNF receptor, called RANK (receptor activator of nuclear factor kappa B), has recently been identified. This receptor is expressed during osteoclast development, and its ligand is similar to TNF and is called RANK ligand (RANKL, also known as osteoprotegerin ligand). RANKL is produced by osteoblasts as well as other cell types such as tumor cells. RANKL/osteoprotegerin ligand signals through the RANK receptor to induce osteoclast gene expression in precursor cells, and also activates bone resorptive functions in mature osteoclasts. RANKL may be one of the signals that allows osteoblast or tumor cell-mediated stimulation of bone resorption. A soluble binding protein for RANKL has also been identified, called osteoprotegerin. Binding of RANKL by osteoprotegerin prevents its interaction with the RANK receptor and therefore osteoprotegerin inhibits bone resorption.

Fibroblastic Phenotype

The hallmarks of the fibroblastic phenotype are synthesis of types I and III collagen, and a spindle cell shape with cell processes. There are relatively few specific markers for the fibroblastic phenotype, and it appears in some ways to be a default differentiation pathway for mesenchymal cells. Fibroblastic cells express fibronectin, and can differentiate along some specialized pathways in generating cells of tendon and ligament. Ligaments and tendons contain primarily type I collagen, as well as type XII, which coats the type I fibrils and is analogous to type IX collagen in cartilage in that it contains a proteoglycan-like moiety that is thought to interact with the proteoglycans within the matrix. Tendon and ligament contain only small proteoglycans, biglycan and decorin, rather than aggrecan. During compression, tendon can develop a more fibrocartilaginous phenotype, with expression of aggrecan, particularly when tendons are under chronic compressive force, such as in the posterior tibial tendon. Other important components of tendon and ligament are tenascin and elastin.

Two new BMPs, BMP-12 and BMP-13, which are homolo-

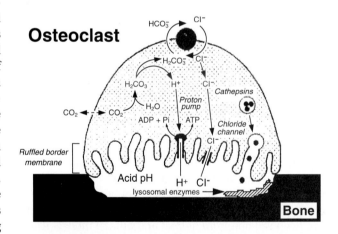

Figure 39

The osteoclast is an extraordinarily complex and functionally specific cell type. The cell attaches to bone through the vitronectin receptor, resulting in a series of intracellular activation steps that cause formation of the microvillous ruffled border and increase dramatically the amount of cell surface adjacent to the bone. The cell polarizes, with migration of the proton pump to the ruffled border and consequent acidification of the space between the cell and the bone, causing dissolution of mineral. Carbonic anhydrase II expression generates protons for this activity. Lysosomal enzymes, including cathepsins, are secreted by exocytosis into the region and degrade collagen and other proteins. Some of these lysosomal proteins are retained on the bone surface after the osteoclast undergoes apoptosis, possibly defining sites for subsequent osteoblastic bone formation.

gous to previously identified murine growth and differentiation factors (gdf7 and gdf6, respectively), have recently been identified through molecular cloning techniques. When implanted ectopically, instead of inducing bone production like the other BMPs, these molecules induce the formation of an organized fibrous tissue resembling tendon or ligament. This tissue also expresses tenascin, small proteoglycans, and elastin. Thus, these BMPs may play a role in regulating tendon and ligament morphogenesis. Embryologic studies have identified expression of these molecules during formation of the joint capsule, tendinous attachments to bone, and ligament sites. In addition, a recent study has shown stimulation of patellar tendon healing in an animal model by implantation of BMP-12. Growth factors such as bFGF, PDGF, and TGF-β have also been demonstrated in animal models to enhance the healing of ligaments and tendons.

Tendon and ligament cells also respond to mechanical stress, and this controls reorganization of the matrix during healing, to decrease the excessive amount of type III collagen expressed early in healing in favor of increased expression of type I and to allow realignment of the fibrils with the direction of mechanical force, which increases the strength of the structure. The realignment is thought to occur through matrix remodeling, but little is known about this process. The strength and rate of remodeling of healing tendons or ligaments is enhanced by application of mechanical tensile force, as long as it is not excessive (which will lead to laxity). In addition, crosslinking of collagen increases with progressive healing, as does the fibril diameter, and both factors enhance the mechanical structure of the healing tissue.

Cellular Biology of Neoplasia

The regulatory genes involved in control of cell proliferation offer numerous points of potential disruption because of mutations, which can result in loss of growth control, or neoplasia. Genes whose function becomes disrupted leading to malignant transformation of the cell are known as oncogenes. A large number of genes have been identified in which mutations are associated with specific types of cancer. Oncogenes are classified as either proto-oncogenes or antioncogenes. Proto-oncogenes are mutations in genes that stimulate cell proliferation, and are dominant mutations, because mutation in a single allele of the gene can lead to loss of growth control. Proto-oncogenes, the normal counterparts of mutated genes in cancers, were initially identified from viruses that induced malignant transformations in cells or caused tumors in animals. Some viruses can incorporate an oncogene through recombinant events, and overexpression of this gene in association with viral infection of a cell can cause uncontrolled cell proliferation, or neoplastic transformation. These oncogenes were later identified as normal growth regulators in cells, hence the

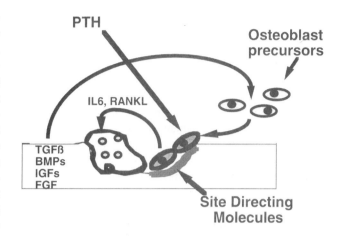

PTH

Osteoblast precursors

IL6, RANKL

TGFß
BMPs
IGFs
FGF

Site Directing
Molecules

Figure 40

Osteoblasts and osteoclasts communicate in a process known as coupling of bone formation and resorption. Upon resorption of bone by osteoclasts, bone matrix growth factors such as transforming growth factor-β (TGF-β) and bone morphogenic proteins (BMPs) are released and activated. These anabolic factors may stimulate osteoblastic precursors to differentiate into osteoblasts and begin bone formation. The carbohydrates of the glycosylated lysosomal enzymes deposited on the resorption surface by the osteoclasts may induce osteoblast attachment and matrix synthesis through cell surface receptors such as the mannose-6-phosphate/IGFII receptor, thus site-directing the replacement of the resorbed bone. The overall process is controlled by systemic hormones such as parathyroid hormone (PTH), which activates receptors on the osteoblast, triggering collagenase expression and release of osteoclast stimulating molecules such as interleukin-6 (IL-6), and the recently identified tumor necrosis factor-like molecule called osteoprotegerin ligand or RANKL. These effector molecules in turn stimulate osteoclast differentiation and function.

term proto-oncogene. Some proto-oncogenes associated with human cancers include *erbB1* (squamous cell carcinoma), *c-myc* (Burkitt's lymphoma), *brca1* and *brca2* (breast cancer), *L-myc* (lung carcinoma), *bcl-2* (follicular lymphoma), *ras* (lung carcinoma), *c-fos* (osteosarcoma, chondrosarcoma), and *c-src* (colon cancer).

Antioncogenes are also known as tumor suppressor genes, such as the *RB* and *p53* genes previously mentioned. These genes normally function to prevent cell proliferation, and when mutated in a way that interferes with their suppressive ability, permit excessive cell division. Antioncogenes are also known as recessive oncogenes, because it is an absence of their function that leads to malignancy. Some tumor suppressor gene mutations and associated cancers include *RB* (retinoblastoma, breast cancer, lung carcinoma, osteosarcoma), *APC* (colonic carcinoma in familial polyposis), *p53* (diverse mutations associated with 50% of cancers; colon carcinoma, osteosarcoma, breast and others), *NF* (neurofibromatosis), and *WT* (Wilms' tumor). For further detail on oncogenes in musculoskeletal tumors, see Chapter 16.

A new group of genes associated with tumor formation are the *EXT* genes, named for their association with hereditary multiple exostoses. Three *EXT* genes have been cloned (*EXT*1, 2, and 3) with 3 different chromosomal locations, and mutations in these genes are associated with multiple exotoses as well as with chondrosarcomas. The function of the *EXT* genes is not yet known, but they are hypothesized to be tumor suppressor genes, and are related to a group of *Drosophila* genes with a regulatory role in development.

Because of the redundancy of the growth regulatory proteins, frequently more than 1 gene must be altered in order for a cell to become malignant, particularly in the case of antioncogenes. The need for multiple "hits" to express a fully malignant phenotype is well accepted. In some cases, such as the *RB* gene, a germline mutation that confers a susceptibility does not lead to a malignancy until a second somatic mutation occurs affecting the other *RB* allele. Rare instances exist where a malignant tumor spontaneously regresses or disappears, and this is theorized to result from a further somatic mutation that interferes with cell proliferation or induces apoptosis. An example is occasional change of a neuroblastoma to a benign ganglioneuroma.

Another class of genetic abnormalities which can cause neoplasia are chromosomal translocations. These are somatic cell defects that occur during mitosis with recombinations of nonhomologous portions of chromosomes. Ewing's sarcoma is one of the best examples of a malignancy resulting from a chromosomal translocation. In 95% of Ewing's sarcoma (as well as in the closely related peripheral neuroectodermal tumor), there is a translocation between chromosomes 11 and 22, designated t(11;22), (q24;q12). It happens that the translocation results in joining 2 genes together, creating a fusion protein. The fused genes are the *EWS* gene and a member of the ETS transcription factor family called *Fli-1*. It is presumed that resulting dysregulation of the *Fli*-1 gene contributes to the malignant cell phenotype. For further information on chromosomal abnormalities, see Chapter 16.

Another important gene family that is a strong determinant of responsiveness to chemotherapy in musculoskeletal malignancies is the multidrug resistance (MDR) genes. Chemotherapeutic agents interfere with various aspects of cell proliferation, including DNA synthesis and protein synthesis. Many cells are able to detoxify the cells of foreign chemicals by actively pumping them out of the cell. MDR1 (the best characterized gene, also known as p-glycoprotein) is one such mechanism, which is a transmembrane ATPase that pumps a wide range of weakly charged organic compounds from the cytoplasm to the extracellular fluid. Multidrug resistance related protein is a related gene. Chemotherapeutic agents such as doxorubicin are efficiently extruded from cells expressing MDR1. A significant percentage of osteosarcomas express MDR1, and several studies have demonstrated an inverse correlation between gene expression and the responsiveness of the tumor, judged by the amount of necrosis following neoadjuvant chemotherapy. In some cancers, including lymphomas and sarcomas, attempts have been made to use pharmacologic agents to block MDR1 function in order to increase the efficacy of chemotherapy. However, drug toxicity to normal tissues is also enhanced, and results of this approach have been limited. Chondrosarcomas have recently been shown to constitutively express MDR1, with a tendency for increased levels of expression in higher grade tumors. This may explain the lack of sensitivity of chondrosarcomas to chemotherapy.

Metastasis

The hallmark of malignancy, in addition to the loss of growth control, is the ability cancer cells acquire to migrate to other organs, or metastasize. Metastasis is an extremely complex process, requiring a series of coordinated cellular events and unique behaviors. The steps in the process include: (1) cell motility; (2) invasion of normal tissue matrices; (3) transgression of endothelial basement membranes, or intravasation; (4) attachment to endothelium at remote site; (5) transgression of endothelial basement membrane in organ of implantation, or extravasation; (6) invasion of local host organ; (7) colony establishment and proliferation in new environment; (8) induction of local angiogenesis to support tumor growth; (9) possible repetition of the cycle of metastasis from the new site.

In addition to all of the required steps, there is a site selectivity that may depend on many host factors. For instance, sarcomas almost always metastasize to the lungs as the most common initial site. Clinical patterns of metastatic disease are common and are specific to different tumor types. Certain carcinomas such as those of the breast, prostate, and lung have a strong predilection for bone as a metastatic site, and specific locations show an order of preference: axial skeleton, proximal appendicular skeleton, and distal appendicular skeleton.

Metastasis is still presumed to operate on the seed and soil concept. Both the tumor and the host tissue express factors that facilitate the metastatic localization. Local growth factors and cytokines may play a key role in this site selection.

Metastasis also requires a number of cellular properties, which include (1) expression of degradative enzymes such as MMPs; (2) extracellular matrix receptors such as integrins or CD44; (3) cytoskeletal elements, which facilitate motility; (4) expression of angiogenic molecules such as FGFs or VEGFs; (5) systems to activate MMPs, including other proteases and urokinase-like plasminogen activator (UPA); and, for metastasis to bone, (6) cytokines to stimulate osteoclastic bone resorption. Figure 41 summarizes the events in metastasis.

MMPs are important in normal matrix remodeling as well as in pathologic conditions such as metastasis, where they allow passage through basement membranes and invasion in tissues. These zinc-dependent enzymes exhibit varying substrate specificity for extracellular matrix components, are secreted as latent propeptides requiring proteolytic cleavage for activation, and can activate one another in a cascade fashion. The family of MMPs and their substrates is shown in Table 4. Endogenous tissue inhibitors of MMPs (TIMPS) are secreted by all cells which produce MMPs. The net protein degrading activity present in a tissue, and in cancers the invasive and metastatic potential, depends on the balance between TIMPs and MMPs. Other types of protease inhibitors such as the serine protease inhibitors called serpins, may also play a role in determining the overall proteolytic capacity of tumor cells. Expression of MMP-1, -2, -3, -9, and -13 has been correlated with metastatic potential of diverse types of cancers, and are now increasingly recognized prognostic markers.

UPA is a serine protease that is capable of activating plasminogen to plasmin, which in turn activates a number of MMPs. The efficacy of UPA in inducing local matrix degradation may be enhanced by its binding to the plasma membrane by a specific receptor (UPAR). Recently UPA/UPAR and MMP-9 (gelatinase B) have been demonstrated to be critical, and possibly universal, elements in the process of intravasation, or the initial entry of tumor cells into vessels through their basement membranes.

Cytokines may also play an important role in metastasis, particularly in metastasis to bone. The expression of bone resorptive cytokines, including TNF, IL-1, and IL-6, may be essential to stimulate osteoclastic bone resorption, facilitating tumor cell attachment and local growth. Expression of these cytokines also enhances MMP expression by tumor and stromal cells, increasing metastatic capability. For further detail on aspects of metastasis, see Chapter 16.

Immunobiology

The immune system provides defense against foreign pathogens and is dependent upon an exquisitely regulated interaction between several different cell types. At the apex of the immune response is the antigen-presenting cell. Antigen-presenting cells phagocytose and present exogenous antigens to CD4 T lymphocyte cells. Following phagocytosis, antigens are processed in the cell within the lysosomal compartment. The processing includes proteolysis, and 10 to 18 amino acid fragments are noncovalently complexed with the type II major histocompatibility complex (MHC) molecule, HLA-DR, and transported to the plasma membrane. In contrast with type I MHC molecules, which are expressed on all cells, type II MHC molecules are expressed only on phagocytic antigen-processing cells. T lymphocytes possessing the CD4 receptor (T-helper cells) are able to interact with MHC type II expressing cells.

The immune response is dependent on the activation of CD4 cells. CD4 cells determine whether the antigen is "self," in which case there is no activation, or "non-self," which results in initiation of the immune response. The CD4 cells make this determination through a CD3 cell surface receptor complex which is also referred to as the T cell antigen receptor (TCR). The TCR contains disulfide linked alpha and beta chains, which are derived from genes that undergo combinatorial joining of variable regions; ie, generating numerous forms of alternatively spliced transcripts. In this

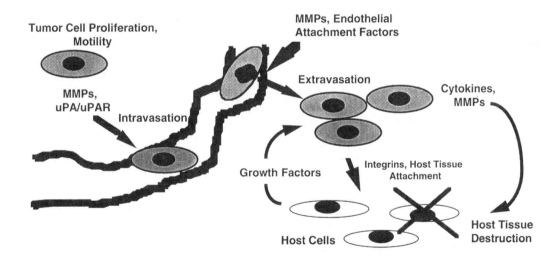

Figure 41

The process of metastasis involves a complex series of events. Tumor cells proliferate at the primary site and exhibit motility, allowing them to invade tissues and vascular or lymphatic channels. Matrix metalloproteinase (MMP)-9 and the UPA/UPAR receptor expression are essential to vascular invasion, possibly concentrating proteolytic activity at the invading leading edge of the cell along the vessel basement membrane. After intravasation, the cells attach to endothelium at a remote organ site via attachment factors, and extravasate utilizing MMP proteolytic activity again. The cells may attach to the host tissue through integrins, CD44, or other cell/matrix receptors, and then proliferate at the host site, elaborating MMPs which contribute to host tissue matrix destruction, and cytokines that can induce these and other degradative enzymes in the tumor and host cells. The host tissues in turn may produce growth factors which further stimulate the tumor cell growth.

process, which is also used to generate the diversity of immunoglobulins, variable regions are randomly mixed to create an unlimited number of binding sites with different specificities. As with B cells, which produce immunoglobulins, each CD4 cell produces a single CD3 receptor complex. The diversity of the immune system is derived from the large number of CD4 cells, each with a unique binding specificity.

Upon recognizing an antigen, the CD3 receptor complex initiates a signal transduction pathway that results in the synthesis and secretion of IL-2. IL-2 leads to clonal expansion of the CD4 cells and results in stimulation of CD8 lymphocytes (cytotoxic T cells). Stimulated CD8 cells also undergo clonal expansion and develop cytotoxic activity. Although B lymphocytes have the capacity to respond to exogenous antigens directly and undergo clonal expansion with antigen binding, this process is markedly enhanced by IL-2 and results in both clonal proliferation and differentiation into immunoglobulin-producing plasma cells. Thus, activation of CD4 lymphocytes is the critical event in immune activation. Depletion of CD4 cells occurs in HIV infections and is associated with increased rates of oportunistic infection.

Cytotoxic T cells, through expression of the CD8 receptor, recognize type I MHC molecules rather than the type II MHC molecules. Type I MHC molecules are less complex and have less antigen-binding specificity than type II MHC molecules. Class I MHC molecules are composed of an alpha chain encoded by genes at the A, B, and C loci of the HLA complex on chromosome 6. The alpha chains are polymorphic (with variable sequences) and are noncovalently associated with a small protein called β2-microglobulin. β2 microglobulin is probably associated with the transport of small endogenously produced peptide fragments (8 to 10 amino acids) to the cell surface where they become associated with the polymorphic regions of the α chain of the type I MHC molecule. This complex can subsequently interact with the CD3 antigen receptor complex (TCR) on cytotoxic T-cells. When activated CD8 cells recognize foreign antigens, the cytotoxic response is initiated. Thus, a cell infected with a viral particle would present viral antigens to CD8 cells through type I MHC molecules and the cytotoxic response would be initiated. MHC I molecules present endogenous antigens while MHC II molecules present exogenous antigens. The immune responses are summarized in Figure 42.

Inflammatory processes can occur in the absence of immunologic activation. An example of this is the inflam-

Table 4

Matrix Metalloproteinase Family Members and Substrates

MMP	Name	Substrates
MMP1	Interstitial collagenase	collagens I, II, III, VII, VIII, X, proteoglycan
MMP2	Gelatinase A	collagens I, IV, V, VII, X, XI, elastin
MMP3	Stromelysin	proteoglycans, fibronectin, laminin, collagen IV, V, IX, X, elastin, procollagen
MMP7	Matrilysin (PUMP1)	fibronectin, laminin, collagen IV, gelatin
MMP8	Neutrophil collagenase	collagen I, II, III, VII, VIII, X, proteoglycans
MMP9	Gelatinase B	collagen IV, V, elastin, proteoglycans
MMP10	Stromelysin 2	same as stromelysin 1
MMP11	Stromelysin 3	serpin
MMP12	Elastase	elastin
MMP13	Collagenase 3	fibrillar collagens
MMP14	MT-MMP	progelatinase A
MMP15	MT2-MMP	unknown
MMP16	MT3-MMP	progelatinase A
MMP17	MT4-MMP	unknown
MMP18*		unknown

*   Has not yet been given another name; only recently discovered

matory reaction that occurs in association with aseptic implant loosening. Although phagocytosis of particulate material by macrophages results in the secretion of proinflammatory cytokines such as TNF-α, IL-1, and IL-6 with subsequent tissue fibrosis, inflammation, and bone resorption, there is no evidence demonstrating immune activation during this process. In contrast, autoimmune disorders such as rheumatoid arthritis are associated with loss of self-tolerance and immune activation in response to the host's own proteins. The specific cause of autoimmune disease is unknown, but is multifactorial and probably includes a complex interplay of genetic susceptiblity, infectious agents, and environmental factors.

Rejection of allograft tissues is understandable considering the cellular immune response mediated by type I MHC molecules. Allogeneic tissues present "non-self" antigens to CD8 lymphocytes. CD8 cell activation is enhanced by CD4 activation by antigen-presenting cells that scavenge shed MHC I and MHC II molecules from the allogeneic tissue. Thus, live, vascularized allograft organs typically require the delivery of immunomodulatory agents to prevent rejection. In contrast, the implantation of allogeneic tissue with minimal cellular content (freeze-dried allograft bone) is not associated with inflammation or rejection. The importance of the immune response to fresh or fresh-frozen allografts, which are poorly revascularized and potentially have living cells only in avascular articular cartilage, is not clear. However, it is likely that the success of allograft implants is caused in part by subtle differences in the immune response to the implanted bone.

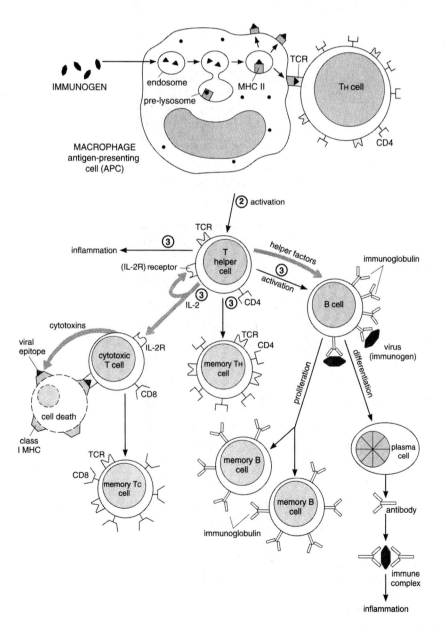

Figure 42

Immune response stimulation involves internalization of an antigen by macrophages, which is is then bound to a receptor, MHC II, and expressed on the cell surface. The CD4-expressing helper T cells are activated by receptor interaction with the antigen (2) if it is recognized as foreign. The activated CD4 cell elaborates factors which stimulate B cells to express antibody, and also inflammatory cytokines. B cells can differentiate into antibody-producing plasma cells, or remain as memory cells. Similarly, the sensitized T-cells can expand by proliferation and mediate cytotoxicity, or be retained as memory cells. (Reproduced with permission from Stites DP, Terr AI, Parslow TG: *Medical Immunology*, ed 8. Norwalk, CT, Appleton & Lange, 1994, pp 43–44.)

Selected Bibliography

Basics of Molecular Biology

Gilbert SF (ed): *Developmental Biology*, ed 4. Sunderland, MA, Sinauer Associates, 1994.

Lehninger AL, Nelson DL, Cox MM (eds): *Principles of Biochemistry*, ed 2. New York, NY, Worth Publishers, 1993.

Lewin B: *Genes VI*. Oxford, England, Oxford University Press, 1997.

Shore EM, Kaplan FS: Tutorial: Molecular biology for the clinician: Part I. General principles. *Clin Orthop* 1995;306:264–283.

Shore EM, Kaplan FS: Tutorial: Molecular biology for the clinician: Part II. Tools of molecular biology. *Clin Orthop* 1995; 320:247–278.

Zubay GL, Parson WW, Vance DE (eds): *Principles of Biochemistry*. Dubuque, IA, WCB/McGraw-Hill, 1994.

Tools and Techniques of Molecular Biology

Hicks DG, Stroyer BF, Teot LA, O'Keefe RJ: In situ hybridization in skeletal tissues utilizing non-radioactive probes. *J Histotechnol* 1997; 20:215–224.

Innis MA, Gelfand DH, Sninsky JJ (eds): *PCR Strategies*. San Diego, CA, Academic Press, 1995.

Liang P, Pardee AB: Differential display of eukaryotic messenger RNA by means of the polymerase chain reaction. *Science* 1992;257: 967–971.

Mullis KB, Ferre F, Gibbs RA (eds): *The Polymerase Chain Reaction*. Cambridge, MA, Birkhäuser Boston, 1994.

Service RF: Microchip arrays put DNA on the spot. *Science* 1998;282: 396–399.

Watson JD, Gilman M, Witkowski J, Zoller M: *Recombinant DNA*, ed 2. New York, NY, Scientific American Books, 1992.

Cell Biology

Alberts B, Bray D, Lewis J, Raff M, Roberts K, Watson JD: *Molecular Biology of the Cell*, ed 3. New York, NY, Garland Publishing, 1994.

Ashkenazi A, Dixit VM: Death receptors: Signaling and modulation. *Science* 1998;281:1305–1308.

Bilezikian JP, Raisz LG, Rodan GA (eds): *Principles of Bone Biology*. San Diego, CA, Academic Press, 1996.

Buckwalter JA, Ehrlich MG, Sandell LJ, Trippel SB (eds): *Skeletal Growth and Development: Clinical Issues and Basic Science Advances*. Rosemont, IL, American Academy of Orthopaedic Surgeons, 1998.

Evan G, Littlewood T: A matter of life and cell death. *Science* 1998; 281:1317–1322.

Favus MJ, Christakos S (eds): *Primer on the Metabolic Bone Diseases and Disorders of Mineral Metabolism*, ed 3. Philadelphia, PA, Lippincott-Raven, 1996.

Hunter T: Oncoprotein networks. *Cell* 1997;88:333–346.

Jacobson MD, Weil M, Raff MC: Programmed cell death in animal development. *Cell* 1997;88:347–354.

Levine AJ: The cellular gatekeeper for growth and division. *Cell* 1997; 88:323–331.

Lukashev ME, Werb Z: ECM signalling: Orchestrating cell behaviour and misbehaviour. *Trends Cell Biol* 1998;8:437–441.

Schenk PW, Snaar-Jagalska BE: Signal perception and transduction: The role of protein kinases. *Biochim Biophs Acta* 1999;1449:1–24.

Stites DP, Terr AI, Parslow TG (eds): *Medical Immunology*, ed 8. Norwalk, CT, Appleton & Lange, 1994.

Thomson AW (ed): *The Cytokine Handbook*, ed 3. San Diego, CA, Academic Press, 1998.

Thornberry NA, Lazebnik Y: Caspases: Enemies within. *Science* 1998; 281:1312–1316.

Chapter 3

The Formation and Growth of Skeletal Tissues

Joseph P. Iannotti, MD, PhD

Steven Goldstein, PhD

Janet Kuhn, PhD

Louis Lipiello, MD

Frederick S. Kaplan, MD

David J. Zaleske, MD

This chapter at a glance

This chapter reviews the current knowledge about the formation,
growth, remodeling, and maturation of skeletal tissues in health and
disease, with emphasis on the basic science of the growth plate and
endochondral ossification.

Introduction

As advances in molecular genetics and molecular biology elucidate the mechanisms underlying morphogenesis and cytodifferentiation, a fundamental understanding of cartilage and bone formation is also evolving. Bone formation and skeletal growth constitute an intricate program of molecular, biochemical, and cellular processes. These processes occur as an entire program in the embryo, constituting cytodifferentiation and morphogenesis of the musculoskeletal system, and are modulated somewhat during fetal development to produce fetal growth. Fetal growth, in turn, is transformed into the postnatal growth of the immature skeleton, with similar primordial events recapitulated in remodeling and fracture healing.

This chapter will review current knowledge about the formation, growth, remodeling, and maturation of skeletal tissues in health and disease, with emphasis on the basic science of the growth plate and endochondral ossification.

Hyaline cartilage is a heterogeneous tissue with 2 distinct types: articular cartilage and growth plate cartilage. This distinction may be made at several levels including nutritional supply, cellular subpopulation characteristics, molecular and biochemical markers, and terminal differentiation under normal conditions.

The bony skeleton is formed along 2 pathways: intramembranous and endochondral bone formation. Although the distinction between the pathways can readily be seen at the level of light microscopy, the bone ultimately formed has been regarded as the same tissue. Intramembranous bone formation occurs at the periosteal surfaces of all bones and in parts of the pelvis, scapula, clavicles, and skull, when osteoblasts form a calcified osteoid matrix within a collagenous framework; this process begins with the differentiation of primitive mesenchymal cells. Endochondral bone formation occurs at the growth plates and within fracture callus when osteoblasts form osteoid on a cartilaginous framework. The growth plates are formed within a cartilaginous mass of mesenchymal cells during embryonic and fetal development. The elucidation of fundamental molecular pathways in bone differentiation provides an increasingly robust understanding of mechanistic switches underlying these pathways.

Cartilage and Bone Development

Three lineages of vertebrate development have been described over the course of centuries. The craniofacial skeleton is derived from the neural crest and brachial arches. It is largely intramembranous bone; however, the base of the skull is endochondral. The axial skeleton is derived from the sclerotome of the somites. The appendicular skeleton is derived from the lateral plate mesoderm that contributes to the formation of the limb buds. The axial and appendicular skeletons are largely endochondral. Limb development is a particularly good model system for studying endochondral bone formation at several levels.

Aristotle noted that the embryogenesis of the chick could be observed by removing part of the shell. Darwin compared the similarity in limb development among different species. The chick limb has been used for experimental embryonic surgery with tissue ablations and transplantations that produce various dysmorphologies such as failure of formation of parts and duplication of parts. From these experiments, mechanisms underlying morphogenesis were formulated. The Saunders-Zwilling hypothesis, that pattern results from an interaction between the ectoderm and mesoderm of a limb bud, provides a basis for understanding vertebrate limb development at the tissue level and for reinterpretation at the molecular level.

The vertebrate limb begins as an outpouching from the lateral body wall of surface ectoderm and underlying mesoderm. Molecular information obtained from organisms even earlier in the phylogenetic tree indicate that the basic developmental mechanisms are widely conserved throughout phylogeny. Data obtained from a variety of organisms have direct relevance to humans. In humans, limb development begins at 4 weeks of gestation and limb morphogenesis is completed at 8 weeks (Fig. 1). The Saunders-Zwilling hypothesis, using the chick as a model, combines experimental data along the 3 cardinal axes of the limb bud as it is first forming. A genetic and epigenetic network is established along these axes. Outgrowth along the proximodistal (PD) axis is governed by the interaction between a thickening of the ectoderm at the distal end of the limb bud, the apical ectodermal ridge (AER), and the underlying mesoderm secretes an apical ectodermal maintenance factor. The underlying mesoderm adjacent to the AER is maintained in an undifferentiated, rapidly proliferating state. From this region, termed the progress zone, mesenchymal condensations are sculpted by a combination of different factors operating locally and diffusing through the limb bud across various gradients. These mesenchymal condensations are the first recognizable precursors of skeletal elements or anlagen (Fig. 2).

The formation of limb buds and the function of the AER have been studied at the molecular level. Fibroblast growth factors (FGF-1, FGF-2, and FGF-4) can induce ectopic limb buds on the flanks of chick embryos. In a mouse limb bud culture system, FGF-4 was shown to replicate the PD axis outgrowth shown to reside in the AER in tissue level experiments. The bone morphogenetic proteins (BMPs) also are part of the signaling mechanism at the progress zone. BMP-2 inhibits the outgrowth, and BMP signaling is required for cell death to separate the digits during embryonic formation.

Homeobox genes were originally described in *Drosophila* as the genes controlling body segment morphogenesis. The

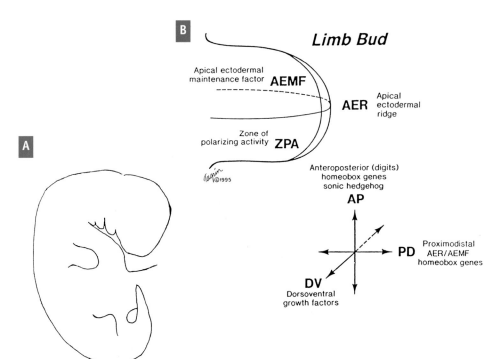

genes have subsequently been demonstrated to be highly conserved phylogenetically and to serve roles in vertebrate development analogous to their roles in *Drosophila.* The products of these genes are transcription factors, which contain a highly conserved 60-amino-acid sequence, or homeobox, that binds to DNA and regulates its transcription. These genes are organized along the genome in clusters. Their geographic location along the genome correlates directly with the sequence of their expression during embryogenesis. Homeobox genes located at the 3′ end of a cluster are expressed earlier in time and more anteriorly on the body during embryogenesis. Their expression antedates mesenchymal condensations that are the first recognizable precursors or anlagen of skeletal structures. Nomenclature for homeobox genes has been standardized to reflect their relationships throughout the vertebrates and to earlier ancestors. The abbreviation *hox* (*HOX* in humans) is reserved for those homeobox genes occurring in clusters related to the *Drosophila antennapedia* and *bithorax* complexes.

The formation of digits is specified along the anteroposterior (AP) axis of the limb bud. From earlier experiments in tissue ablation and transplantation in the chick, a zone of tissue at the posterior border of the limb bud, the zone of polarizing activity (ZPA), was crucial in ordering the number and type of digits. When the ZPA was transplanted anteriorly, extra digit duplications were produced. More recently, at the molecular level, a vertebrate gene *Sonic hedgehog* (*Shh*), related to the *Drosophila* gene *Hedgehog,* was demonstrated to mediate the activity of the polarizing zone. The *HoxD* genes (*HOXD* in humans) correlate with the specification of the digits along the AP axis. A developmental cascade initiated by *Shh* and retinoic acid activates the

sequential expression of the *HoxD.* The mechanism of gene action is not yet known, but the activity of the homeobox genes correlates with the mass of mesenchymal cells programmed to condense for the sheketal elements of the digits and their subsequent growth.

Along the dorsoventral axis of the limb bud, ectodermal and mesodermal interactions again specify the induction of another homeobox gene by the secreted protein WNT7a. Pattern of the limb and its skeletal elements is the epiphenomenon that results from a specific pattern of gene interactions mediated by transcription factors for downstream genes, signaling molecules, receptors, local growth factors, and both receptive and responsive cells. Mesenchymal condensations are the tissue-level manifestation of this molecular and cellular information network. It might be anticipated that such a complicated system could be disturbed by very slight changes upstream in the information cascade that could have increasing repercussions downstream. Conversely, information and network redundancy could repair or bypass a change that might be predicted to have otherwise major morphogenetic consequences. These theoretical predictions about mechanisms in morphogenesis have been experimentally confirmed with knockout mice. Such phenomena are also apparent in naturally occurring mutations in clinical practice, which will be discussed.

During the sixth week of human embryonic development, the mesenchymal condensations chondrify; that is, the mesenchymal cells of the anlagen differentiate into chondrocytes. Initially these chondrocytes are all the small, round cell phenotype. During the seventh embryonic week, at the central region of the cartilaginous anlagen, the chondrocytes become hypertrophic and local matrix begins to calcify. Simultaneously, a periosteal sleeve of bone forms circumferentially around the midshaft of each cartilage anlage; by direct ossification of a collagenous matrix, intramembranous bone formation occurs. At the end of the eighth week, capillary buds extending through the peripheral sleeve of bone invade the central portion of the hypertrophied and calcified cartilaginous anlage, expanding the primary center of ossification formed by replacement of the cartilage by endochondral ossification (Fig. 3). Vascular invasion into the cartilaginous anlagen occurs first at the humeri but in rapid succession, primary centers of ossification form throughout the skeleton. The formation of the primary center of ossification of the humerus establishes the transition from the embryonic period to the fetal period. The vascular invasion brings to the cartilaginous anlagen the blood-borne precursors that differentiate into osteoblasts and osteoclasts. The lineage of bone cells is often debated, but it is clear that the marrow/hematogenous component is crucial. The

osteoblasts produce an osteoid matrix on the surfaces of the calcified cartilaginous bars and form the primary trabeculae of the endochondral (or enchondral) bone. The osteoclasts remove the primary trabecular bone to form a medullary canal. From the process of advancing endochondral bone formation and trailing osteoclastic resorption, the primary center is enlarged. The cartilaginous regions at either end of the primary center of ossification become the growth regions, growing away from the advancing ossification fronts at either end.

The cytodifferentiation within these growth regions becomes characteristic of growth plates or physes, which subsequently will be described in detail (Fig. 3). Interstitial division within the cartilaginous growth plates is precisely met by appositional deposition or growth of bone at the metaphyseal side. The continual recapitulation of this process initially occurring at the central region of the original cartilaginous anlage produces the growth of each

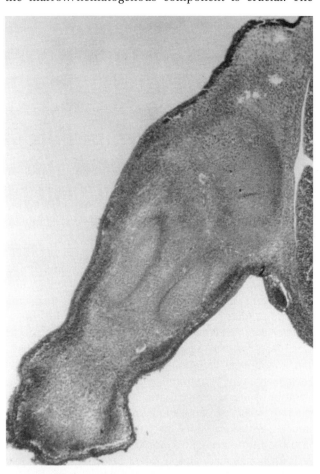

Figure 2

Hindlimb from a 13-day mouse embryo. Mesenchymal condensations are forming the anlagen or first recognizable precursors of skeletal elements. (Hematoxylin and eosin, × 40.) (Reproduced with permission from Zaleske DJ: Development of components of the skeletal system (bone, cartilage, synovial joints, growth plate), in Dee R, Hurst LC, Gruber MA, Kottmeier SA (eds): *Principles of Orthopaedic Practice*, ed 2. New York, NY, McGraw Hill, 1997, p 5.)

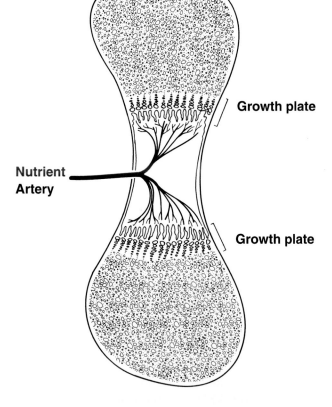

Figure 3

Development of a typical long bone. Formation of the growth plate and secondary centers of ossification. (Reproduced with permission from Brighton CT: The growth plate. *Orthop Clin North Am* 1984;15:571.)

individual bone as an organ and the collective growth of all the bones produces skeletal growth at the organismic level. This process continues until closure or obliteration of the growth cartilage with bone at skeletal maturity.

At the time of morphogenesis, the mesenchymal condensations are recognizable as discrete yet contiguous masses of cells. At the time of chondrogenesis the interzone regions between adjacent anlagen begin to break down in the process of joint cavitation (segmentation or cleft formation). Nomenclature may be used by different authors in different ways; the cartilaginous terminus may be called the chondroepiphysis. At specific times in the development of each long bone (usually postnatally, the sole exception being the distal femoral secondary center, which develops at 36 weeks of gestation), a secondary center forms (or multiple secondary centers form and eventually coalesce) within the chondroepiphysis of each bone. The development of the secondary center of ossification or bony epiphysis and its initially spherical enlargement within the chondroepiphysis provide centripetal growth to accompany the longitudinal growth of the plate. The contacts between adjacent chondroepiphyses at their articular surfaces constitute the articular cartilage of diarthrodial joints of the body (Fig. 4). The proliferating cartilage populations within the chondroepiphysis have many of the characteristics of the longitudinal growth plate and can be the characteristic site of pathophysiologic markers of genetic, mechanical, or hormonal clinical conditions.

As the secondary center of ossification enlarges within the

chondroepiphysis, it flattens on the surface adjacent to the longitudinal growth plate and becomes more hemispherical. For a long bone, the rate of interstitial cartilage division within the longitudinal growth plate is much greater than the rate of division within the chondroepiphyseal cartilage directing the growth of the secondary center of ossification. The relative rates of division lead to the final contour of each joint and the overall body proportions. The small or round bones also have proliferating cartilage but this remains as a roughly spherical growth plate.

Structure, Function, and Biochemistry of the Normal Growth Plate With Selected Examples of Pathophysiology

Overview

The process of endochondral bone formation, which occurs in all growth plates, is unique to the immature skeleton. This process comprises a series of events that occur on a daily basis in a well-defined sequence.

The function of the growth plate is related to its structure as an organ, which depends on the integrated function of 3 distinct tissue types. The growth plate is composed of a cartilaginous component that has 3 histologically distinct zones: reserve, proliferative, and hypertrophic; surrounded by a fibrous component; and bounded by a bony metaphyseal component. Each component has a unique structure, biochemistry, and function; together, these result in longitudinal and latitudinal growth and remodeling of the developing skeleton (Fig. 5). The vascular supply of the growth plate results in unique biochemical properties and is integral to normal function.

Vascular Supply to the Growth Plate

There are 3 major vascular supplies to the growth plate (Fig. 4). The epiphyseal artery enters the secondary center of ossification. The terminal branches of this artery pass through the reserve zone cartilage of the upper growth plate, terminate at the uppermost cell of the proliferative zone, and supply oxygen and nutrients to the proliferative zone chondrocytes. These vessels do not penetrate into the proliferative or hypertrophic zones. The main nutrient artery of the long bone enters at approximately the mid diaphysis, then bifurcates, sending an arterial branch within the medullary canal toward each metaphysis. The terminal branches in each metaphysis adjacent to the hypertrophic zone of the growth plate constitute the metaphyseal blood supply. Its capillary loops end at the last cartilaginous transverse septum of the bone-cartilage interface of the growth plate. These vessels turn back on themselves to

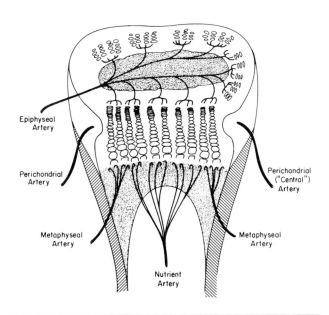

Figure 4

Structure and blood supply of a typical growth plate. (Reproduced with permission from Brighton CT: Structure and function of the growth plate. *Clin Orthop* 1978;136:24.)

form a venous return. This is an area of venous stasis and low blood flow; the vessels do not penetrate the hypertrophic zone of the growth plate. The structure of this vascular supply results in an avascular lower proliferative and hypertrophic zone, which is a major factor influencing growth plate chondrocyte physiology. The periphery of the growth plate is supplied by metaphyseal arteries with periosteal arteries providing a collateral supply. A perichondral artery supplies the perichondral ring of LaCroix.

Reserve Zone

The reserve zone, located just adjacent to the secondary center of ossification, is histologically characterized by a sparse distribution of single or paired round cells in an abundant matrix. These cells contain a well-developed endoplasmic reticulum characteristic of active protein synthesis. However, cellular proliferation in the reserve zone is sporadic. The reserve zone chondrocytes have the lowest intracellular and ionized calcium content, and they do not contribute to longitudinal growth.

The collagen content (type II collagen) is highest in the matrix of the reserve zone, and the collagen fibers are in an irregular pattern. There are a large number of matrix vesicles in the reserve zone matrix, but they do not participate directly in mineralization. The matrix proteoglycans are in an aggregated form, which is inhibitory to matrix mineralization. Although vascular channels pass through the reserve zone, they do not supply it with oxygen, and as a result the oxygen tension is low (20.5 ± 2.1 mm Hg).

The role of the reserve zone in growth plate function is not

clear. These data indicate that the reserve zone chondrocytes have the capacity to produce a cartilaginous matrix, but remain relatively inactive in cell or matrix turnover. The reserve zone does not actively participate in longitudinal growth through cell proliferation, matrix synthesis, or calcification. Although most growth plate abnormalities impact the reserve zone secondarily, no known disease state originates primarily from cytopathology unique to this zone alone.

Proliferative Zone

The proliferative zone is characterized histologically by longitudinal columns of flattened cells. The cytoplasm of these cells contains glycogen stores and an abundance of endoplasmic reticulum, suggesting a rich source of nutrients for aerobic glycolysis and a high capacity for protein synthesis. Of the 3 zones, this zone has the highest rate of proteoglycan synthesis and turnover. The total intracellular calcium content is approximately equal to that of the reserve zone, but the ionized calcium concentration is significantly greater in the proliferative zone, suggesting that the proliferative zone chondrocyte is not actively accumulating calcium for matrix mineralization.

The uppermost cell in each column is the progenitor cell for longitudinal growth of the cell column. This cell is not derived from the reserve zone cells. Longitudinal growth in the growth plate is equal to the number of cell divisions multiplied by the maximum height of the last hypertrophic zone cell. In addition, total longitudinal growth for the life span of the growth plate depends on the total number of progenitor cell divisions of each daughter cell derived from each progenitor cell division. The rate of cell division is influenced by hormonal and mechanical factors; the differential growth by growth plates at different anatomic locations is a function of multiple parameters including the size of the cellular population originally recruited to the proliferative zone as well as the chondrocyte kinetics.

The distribution of collagen fibrils and matrix vesicles in the matrix of the proliferative zone is nonuniform. The highest volume fraction and number of matrix vesicles is in the interterritorial matrix of the lower proliferative and upper hypertrophic zones. These matrix vesicles participate in matrix mineralization in the lower hypertrophic zone. The proteoglycans of the proliferative zone are in an aggregated form and, in this zone, they inhibit matrix mineralization. The oxygen tension is higher in the proliferative zone than in any other zone (57 ± 5.8 mm Hg). This high oxygen tension appears to be secondary to the rich vascular supply of the proliferative zone. The presence of rich glycogen stores and a high oxygen tension supports aerobic metabolism in the proliferative zone chondrocyte.

The functions of the proliferative zone—matrix production and cellular division—together contribute to longitudinal growth. All disease states that affect matrix will

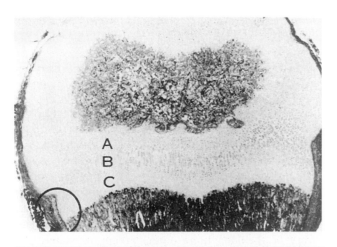

Figure 5

Zonal structure, function, and physiology of the growth plate. A = reserve zone; B = proliferative zone; C = hypertrophic zone; the black ring encircles the ossification groove and the perichondrial ring (hematoxylin-eosin, × 500). (Reproduced with permission from Brighton CT: Clinical problems in epiphyseal plate growth and development. *American Academy of Orthopaedic Surgeons Instructional Course Lectures XXIII*. St Louis, MO, CV Mosby, 1974, pp 105–122.)

also have an impact on this zone. Achondroplasia is the prototypical example of a condition whose origin is in the chondrocytes of the proliferative zone. The molecular basis for this is an abnormality in fibroblast growth factor receptor-3. Unlike the molecular heterogeneity that underlies osteogenesis imperfecta, the molecular basis for achondroplasia is remarkably homogeneous; most cases result from a single amino acid substitution in the receptor.

Hypertrophic Zone

The hypertrophic zone is characterized by cells that are 5 to 10 times the size of the proliferative zone cells. In early electron microscopy studies in which aqueous fixation techniques were used, the lowest cells of the hypertrophic zone were found to be fragmented and nonviable. Results of more recent morphologic studies, in which anhydrous fixation techniques were used, suggest that all of the hypertrophic zone cells maintain cellular morphology compatible with active synthetic cellular functions. Data from many biochemical studies support the active role of hypertrophic zone chondrocytes in synthesis of novel matrix proteins. Although hypertrophic zone chondrocytes are metabolically active, the data do not suggest or support the concept that the hypertrophic zone cell survives the process of vascular invasion or transforms to another cell type in the metaphysis. The ultimate fate of the hypertrophic zone cell is cell death.

Biochemical analysis shows that the hypertrophic zone cells are metabolically active. Of the 3 zones, the hypertrophic has the highest content of glycolytic enzymes. Hypertrophic zone chondrocytes synthesize alkaline phosphatase, neutral proteases, and type X collagen, thereby participating in matrix mineralization.

The hypertrophic zone is avascular and, as a result, the oxygen tension is quite low (29.3 ± 2.4 mm Hg). In the normally mineralized hypertrophic zone the diffusion coefficient is very high, resulting in a high barrier to the diffusion of oxygen and nutrients from the metaphysis.

In most normal cells, glucose is converted to pyruvate (through glycolysis), which is subsequently converted to glycerol-3-phosphate mediated by cytoplasmic glycerol phosphate dehydrogenase. The glycerol-3-phosphate so formed can readily enter the mitochondria (glycerol phosphate shuttle) and efficiently serve as a fuel for further generation of adenosine triphosphate (ATP) by the Krebs or tricarboxylic acid cycle. Chondrocytes from all zones of the growth plate lack glycerol phosphate dehydrogenase and are therefore incapable of forming glycerol-3-phosphate. Pyruvate can enter the mitochondria but does so less efficiently than glycerol-3-phosphate. In the proliferative and upper hypertrophic zones, mitochondria are generating ATP; however, lactate accumulates in the presence of ample oxygen tension while electron transport and the Krebs cycle continue in the mitochondria. Oxygen tension decreases along the hypertrophic zone. Energy production occurs by anaerobic glycolysis of the glycogen stored in the proliferative zone. Mitochondria can either form ATP or store calcium but not both. In the upper hypertrophic zone there is a switch from ATP production to calcium storage. In this region, the energy derived from electron transport is used primarily in the accumulation, storage, and release of calcium rather than for ATP production. The upper hypertrophic zone chondrocytes contain the largest amount of total cellular calcium and the greatest labile pool of stored calcium in their mitochondria. This zone also has the highest concentration of cytosolic ionized calcium.

In the lower hypertrophic zone, glycogen is completely consumed. Both ATP production and calcium storage by the mitochondria require energy. Following exhaustion of the glycogen energy supply, the mitochondria in the chondrocytes of the lower hypertrophic zone release calcium. One of the primary functions of the hypertrophic zone is to prepare the matrix for calcification and then to calcify it. The region of the hypertrophic zone adjacent to the metaphysis where matrix mineralization occurs is sometimes distinguished as a subzone, the zone of provisional calcification. The zone of provisional calcification is critical to normal function of the growth plate. Dysfunction of these cells results in specific pathologic changes of the entire growth plate.

The regulation of conversion from the small cell chondrocyte phenotype to the hypertrophic phenotype with the associated extracellular matrix changes is therefore an important control mechanism in the growth plate. A negative feedback loop governing this conversion has been demonstrated during limb development by the gene *Shh*. A related gene, *Indian hedgehog* (*Ihh*), is expressed in the prehypertrophic chondrocytes of the cartilaginous anlagen. *Ihh* indirectly slows the rate at which chondrocytes differentiate into the hypertrophic phenotype. *Ihh* signals the perichondrium to release another signaling molecule, parathyroid hormone-related protein (PTHrP). The receptor for PTHrP also responds to parthyroid hormone (PTH). This PTH/PTHrP receptor is present in several tissues including bone, kidney, and proliferating chondrocytes. PTHrP completes the negative feedback loop by direct action on the chondrocyte to slow the conversion from proliferating to hypertrophic chondrocytes. This *Ihh*-PTHrP negative feedback loop represents an example of autocrine/paracrine control; signaling molecules are produced and act on the same cell or on cells close to their site of production. A mutation in the PTHrP receptor that results in a constitutively active state is the molecular basis for Jansen chondrometaphyseal dysplasia. Jansen dysplasia has a radiographic similarity to rickets with widening of the hypertrophic zone. Because this abnormal receptor is also the shared receptor for PTH, hypercalcemia and hypophosphatemia with normal levels of PTH also occur in Jansen dysplasia.

Cartilage Matrix Turnover

Various genetic, humoral, and mechanical factors stimulate macromolecule and matrix vesicle biosynthesis in the growth plate. These factors are discussed later in this chapter. Several enzymes, along with tissue enzyme inhibitors and activators that regulate matrix degradation, are synthesized by the chondrocyte. The degradative enzymes found in the growth plate include a class of metalloproteinases that depend on zinc and calcium for enzyme activity. The enzymes found in the growth plate are collagenase, gelatinase, and stromelysin. The growth plate chondrocytes produce these enzymes in a latent (inactive) form, but the enzymes can be activated by interleukin-1 and plasmin. When activated, these enzymes, singularly or in combination, can degrade both the collagenous and proteoglycan components of the matrix. Their activity also is regulated by a locally produced tissue inhibitor, tissue inhibitor of metalloproteinase (TIMP), which can bind irreversibly to these enzymes to make them inactive. The presence and amount of metalloproteinases and their inhibitor (TIMP) vary among different zones of the growth plate. In addition, the factors produced in 1 zone can act at more distant sites within the growth plate. Thus, the activation of the enzymes is differentially regulated by interleukin-1 and TIMP. The coordinated effects of these factors within the growth plate, therefore, are complex and, at this point, remain incompletely elucidated.

The Metaphysis

The metaphysis functions in the removal of the mineralized cartilaginous matrix of the hypertrophic zone, the formation of bone, and the histologic remodeling of the cancellous trabeculae. It is characterized by anaerobic metabolism, vascular stasis, and low oxygen tension (19.8 ± 3.2 mm Hg). The vascular stasis and low oxygen tension result from the arteriovenous loops at the cartilage-bone junction and low blood flow. The metaphysis begins distal to the last intact transverse septum of each cartilaginous cell column of the hypertrophic zone (Fig. 4). The unmineralized last transverse septum is removed by lysosomal enzymes, the cartilaginous lacunae are invaded by endothelial and perivascular cells, and the hypertrophic zone cell is removed.

The factors that induce vascular invasion of the last hypertrophic zone cell are still being explained. The classic explanation of histologic data suggested that mineralization of the cartilage matrix is a prerequisite step in vascular invasion. The extremely orderly histologic progression from small cell chondrocyte to hypertrophic chondrocyte maintained in columnar array in the growth plate is the tissue level manifestation of genetic and epigenetic events mediated through transcription factors, messengers, receptors, and ultimately, cell biology.

After the last transverse septum is removed, osteoblasts from the metaphysis line the calcified longitudinal bars of cartilage. Between the capillaries and the osteoblasts lie polymorphic osteoprogenitor cells. The osteoblasts produce a bone matrix on the calcified cartilage bars. This area of sparse bone formed on a central core of calcified cartilage is termed the primary trabecular bone or primary spongiosa. The osteoblasts progressively lay down bone on the cartilage template and more distally in the metaphysis. The initial woven bone and cartilage bars of the primary trabeculae are resorbed by osteoclasts and are replaced by lamellar bone to produce the secondary trabecular bone or secondary spongiosa in a process termed histologic or internal remodeling.

The remodeling process at the metaphyseal-diaphyseal junction requires the synchronized functions of osteoclastic bone resorption and osteoblastic new bone formation. This process of external or anatomic remodeling occurs around the periphery and subperiosteal regions of the metaphysis, and results in narrowing of the diameter of the metaphysis to meet the diaphysis of the bone; the process is called funnelization. In the process of anatomic remodeling, osteoclasts remove bone from the periphery of the metaphysis, and new bone is formed at the endosteal surfaces.

The Fibrous Structure

Surrounding the periphery of the growth plate are a wedge-shaped groove of cells, the ossification groove of Ranvier, and a ring of fibrous tissue, the perichondrial ring of LaCroix (Figs. 4 and 5). The cells in the groove of Ranvier are active in cell division and contribute to an increase in the diameter, or latitudinal growth, of the physis. Three cell types constitute the groove of Ranvier. An osteoblast-type cell forms the bony portion of the perichondrial ring at the metaphysis; a chondrocyte-type cell contributes to latitudinal growth, and a fibroblast-type cell covers the groove and anchors it to the perichondrium above the growth plate. The structure of the perichondrial ring of LaCroix varies greatly among species, among different growth plates in the same species, or with age of the animal. The basic structure is a fibrous collagenous network that is continuous with the fibrous portion of the groove of Ranvier and the periosteum of the metaphysis. The perichondrial ring functions as a strong mechanical support at the bone-cartilage junction of the growth plate.

Growth Plate Mineralization

The mineralization of growth plate cartilage is unique and significantly different from the mineralization of bone (osteoid). The difference is based on the unique handling of intracellular calcium stores by the growth plate chondrocytes, the hypoxic environment, which results from the unique blood supply of the growth plate, its unique energy metabolism, the presence of matrix vesicles as the initial vehicle of mineralization, and the coordinated functions of several unique matrix macromolecules.

The many factors that play a role in growth plate mineralization (Fig. 6) may be divided into 4 major groups: intracellular calcium homeostasis, microenvironmental factors, the systemic hormonal milieu, and the extracellular matrix vesicles and macromolecules. The growth plate chondrocyte plays a central role in the process of matrix mineralization through intracellular calcium transport; the synthesis, secretion, and postsecretion modification of the matrix macromolecules that participate in mineralization; the ability to respond to systemic and microenvironmental factors; and the biogenesis of matrix vesicles.

Intracellular calcium apparently plays a significant role in

matrix calcification. In fact, the growth plate chondrocyte mitochondria seem to be specifically adapted for calcium transport. Electron-dense granules of calcium phosphate appear in hypertrophic zone mitochondria. Localization of mitochondrial calcium shows accumulation in the upper two thirds of the hypertrophic zone and depletion in the lowest chondrocytes. The loss of mitochondrial calcium in the lower hypertrophic zone is associated with matrix vesicle hydroxyapatite crystal nucleation (Fig. 7). These data suggest a transfer of intracellular calcium to extracellular sites during the process of hydroxyapatite crystal formation.

In isolated growth plate chondrocytes and mitochondria, there is a metabolic specialization for calcium transport. In comparison with nonmineralizing cells, the chondrocyte mitochondria have a greater capacity for calcium accumu-

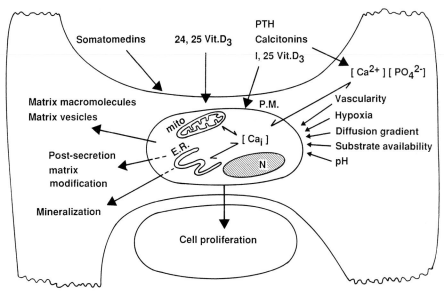

Figure 6

The factors influencing growth plate chondrocyte function and matrix mineralization. (Reproduced with permission from Iannotti JP: Growth plate physiology and pathology. *Orthop Clin North Am* 1990;21:1–17.)

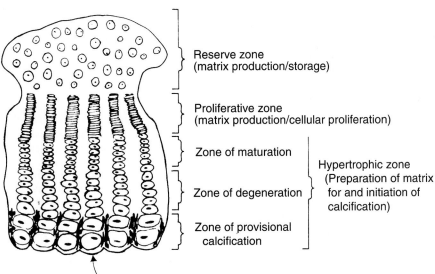

Figure 7

Zonal structure, function, and intracellular calcium transfer in the growth plate. (Reproduced with permission from Brighton CT: Structure and function of the growth plate. *Clin Orthop* 1978;136:24.)

lation and a greater ability to maintain these stores in a labile form for calcium release. In cells where the endogenous calcium stores are low, the endoplasmic reticulum is the major intracellular regulator of cytosolic (cytoplasmic) ionized calcium concentration. This is the situation in all nonmineralizing cells as well as in the reserve and proliferative zone chondrocytes. As the hypertrophic zone chondrocytes accumulate calcium, the capacity of the endoplasmic reticulum to accumulate calcium is saturated, and the mitochondria become the major source of calcium accumulation and regulation. Under high calcium-loading conditions, the mitochondria buffer the cytosolic ionized calcium concentration at an increased level. This ionized calcium pool is a major regulator of cellular metabolic function, and changes in the labile calcium pool have a profound effect on cellular functions. The high concentration of intracellular ionized calcium in the hypertrophic zone chondrocytes is correlated with matrix vesicle secretion from the plasma membrane of the isolated growth plate chondrocytes.

In summary, within the proliferative zone the oxygen tension and glycogen stores stay high, the cells have a low ionized and total calcium content, and the mitochondria are primarily involved in ATP production. The cells are actively involved in division and matrix production. In the hypertrophic zone the oxygen tension and nutrients are low, the mitochondria are initially active in calcium accumulation, and the cells secrete matrix vesicles. In the lower hypertrophic zone, mitochondrial calcium is released and matrix mineralization occurs (Fig. 8). The factors that initiate mitochondrial calcium accumulation and induce calcium release are poorly understood at this time.

Several other factors within the matrix affect mineraliza-

tion. Histochemical stains of the growth plate indicate that the hypertrophic zone matrix contains disaggregated proteoglycan. Electron microscopy reveals that the length of the proteoglycan aggregates and the number of subunits of the aggregate decrease from the reserve zone through the hypertrophic zone (Fig. 9). It is suggested that in vivo the disaggregated form of proteoglycan participates in matrix mineralization by binding and localizing calcium to the matrix. The disaggregation of proteoglycan in vivo results from enzymatic degradation by lysozyme or neutral protease. In vitro, aggregated proteoglycan inhibits calcium phosphate crystal formation. This inhibitory capacity is reduced by the treatment of the aggregates with physeal enzymes that digest the aggregates.

Although the major collagen in the hypertrophic zone is type II, the terminal hypertrophic chondrocytes also produce and secrete type X collagen into the matrix. The abrupt appearance of this unique collagen heralds the onset of endochondral ossification. Mutations in type X collagen are the molecular basis for the Schmid-type chondrometaphyseal dysplasia. Abnormalities in type II collagen underlie a variety of conditions currently described. These include achondrogenesis II/hypochondrogenesis, some types of spondyloepiphyseal dysplasia, Kniest dysplasia, and some forms of Stickler syndrome. Ascorbate (vitamin C) may play a role in mineralization by stimulating matrix vesicle formation and type X collagen synthesis. (For more information on collagen types refer to Chapters 17 and 18.)

The initial nucleation site for matrix calcification is controversial, although most data would support the primary role of the matrix vesicle in this process. Matrix vesicles are 100- to 150-µm trilamellar membrane structures produced

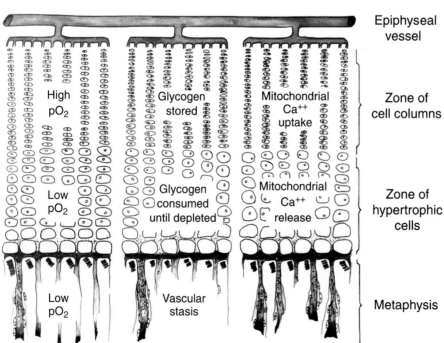

High pO₂

Low pO₂

Low pO₂

Glycogen stored

Glycogen consumed until depleted

Vascular stasis

Mitochondrial Ca⁺⁺ uptake

Mitochondrial Ca⁺⁺ release

Epiphyseal vessel

Zone of cell columns

Zone of hypertrophic cells

Metaphysis

Figure 8

Metabolic events in the growth plate. The growth plate showing the relative oxygen tensions in the various zones in the left-hand column, the change in glycogen storage and utilization in the center column, and the role of mitochondria in the right-hand column. (Reproduced with permission from Brighton CT, Hunt RM: The role of mitochondria in growth plate calcification as demonstrated in a rachitic model. *J Bone Joint Surg* 1978;60A:630–639.)

by the chondrocyte plasma membrane; they are rich in alkaline phosphatase and neutral proteases. Alkaline phosphatase may participate in mineralization by hydrolysis of pyrophosphate, a mineralization inhibitor. Hydrolysis of pyrophosphate, ATP, and other phosphodiesterases results in a local increase in phosphate. The neutral proteases of the matrix vesicles help degrade aggregated proteoglycans, producing disaggregated proteoglycans, which promote mineralization. The matrix vesicles can actively accumulate calcium by energy-dependent transport and are rich in calcium-binding phospholipids. The accumulation of calcium in the vesicle and the local increase in phosphate contribute to a local increase in the calcium phosphate product and thereby promote mineralization.

Other proposed sites of initial mineralization are associated with proteoglycans and a calcium-binding protein, chondrocalcin (C-propeptide of type II collagen). Chondrocalcin has been shown to be associated with the initial site of calcification, and is produced by the hypertrophic zone chondrocyte in response to stimulation by the vitamin D metabolite, 24,25-dihydroxy vitamin D. The precise relationship among these factors, mineralization, and matrix vesicles is not clear. The initial form of mineral deposition is also not clearly established although it has been studied extensively.

Effect of Hormones and Growth Factors on the Growth Plate

Overview

Many hormones, vitamins, and growth factors affect the growth plate by influencing chondrocyte proliferation,

maturation, macromolecule synthesis, intracellular calcium homeostasis, or matrix mineralization. Research in this area of growth plate physiology recently has led to new information and development of many new concepts. Although many more factors influencing the growth plate have been defined, the integrated view of all of these factors in the overall function of the growth plate is presently incomplete. Some of the factors (systemic hormones, vitamins, and growth factors) are produced at a site distant from the growth plate and, therefore, act on the chondrocytes through a classic endocrine mechanism. Other factors are both produced by and act within the growth plate and, therefore, function as paracrine or autocrine factors. Paracrine factors are produced by a particular cell within a tissue and affect a different cell in that tissue. Autocrine factors are produced by and affect the same cell in the tissue. Many of these factors that have a role in fetal and postnatal regulation of chondrocyte function were also an integral part of the histogenesis of cartilaginous anlagen during embryogenesis.

In the different zones of the growth plate, cells are distinguished by their involvement in the processes of division, maturation, and hypertrophy. Therefore, some factors have a specific effect on a particular zone (Table 1). In addition, the sensitivity of each zone of the growth plate to hormone stimulation can vary with the age of the animal. Some hormone effects may qualitatively or quantitatively depend on the species. To make matters even more complex, a combination of factors, acting in concert, influence the function of individual cells. Available evidence strongly suggests that each growth plate zone may be specifically targeted by 1 or more agents to mediate the cytologic characteristics unique to that zone (Fig. 8). This differential hormonal or growth factor sensitivity provides for a continuum of maturational events culminating in the accretion of bone tissue at the metaphyseal side of the growth plate. The total accretion over time is manifested as skeletal growth at the organismic level.

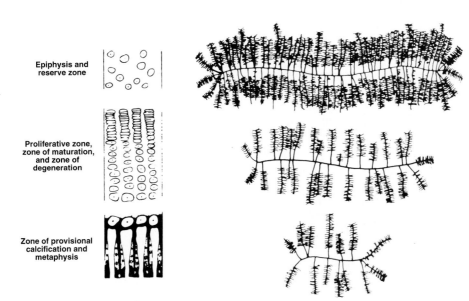

Epiphysis and reserve zone

Proliferative zone, zone of maturation, and zone of degeneration

Zone of provisional calcification and metaphysis

Figure 9

Scaled diagram showing the average relative size and form of aggregates from the three different regions of the growth plate. Aggregates from the epiphysis and reserve zone are not only larger, but also they have much closer spacing between subunits. (Reproduced with permission from Buckwalter JA: Proteoglycan structure in calcifying cartilage. *Clin Orthop* 1983;172:207–232.)

Table 1

Effect of Hormones and Growth Factors on the Growth Plate

Hormone/ Factor	Systemic/Local Derivation	Biologic Effect				Zone Primarily Affected
		Proliferation	Macromolecule Biosynthesis	Maturation Degradation	Matrix Calcification	
Thyroxine	Systemic (thyroid)	+ (T_3 with IGF-I)	0	+ (T_3 alone)	0	Proliferative zone and upper hypertrophic zone
Parathyroid	Systemic (parathyroid)	+	++ (proteoglycan)	0	0	Entire growth plate
Calcitonin	Systemic (thyroid)	0	0	+	+	Hypertrophic zone and metaphysis
Excess cortico-steroids	System (adrenals)	—	—	—	0	Entire growth plate
Growth hormone	Systemic (pituitary)	+ (through IGF-I locally)	+ (slight)	0	0	Proliferative zone
Somatomedins	Systemic Local paracrine (liver, chondrocytes)	+	+ (slight)	0	0	Proliferative zone
Insulin	Systemic (pancreas)	+ (through IGF-I receptor)	0	0	0	Proliferative zone
1,25 $(OH)_2D_3$	Systemic (liver, kidney)	0	0	+ (indirect effect serum [Ca] × [PQ])		Hypertrophic zone
24,25 $(OH)_2D_3$	Systemic (liver, kidney)	+	+ (collagen II)	0	0	Proliferative zone and hypertrophic zone
Vitamin A	Systemic (diet)	0	0	–	0	Hypertrophic zone
Vitamin C	Systemic (diet)	0	+ (collagen)	0	+ (matrix vesicles)	Proliferative zone and hypertrophic zone
EGF	Local paracrine (encothelial cells)	+	– (collagen)	0	0	Metaphysis
FGF	Local paracrine (encothelial cells)	+	0	0	0	Proliferative zone
PDGF	Local paracrine (platelets)	+	+ (noncollagenous proteins)	0	0	Proliferative zone
TGF-β	Local paracrine (platelets, chondrocytes)	±	±	0	0	Proliferative zone and hypertrophic zone
BDGF	Local paracrine (bone matrix)	0	+ (collagen)	0	0	Upper hypertrophic zone
IL-1	Local paracrine (inflammatory cells, synoviocytes)	0	–	++ activates tissue metalloproteinases	0	Entire growth plate
Prostaglandin	Local autocrine	±	+ (proteoglycan) – (collagen and alkaline phos-phatase)	0	Bone resorption osteoclasts	Hypertrophic zone and metaphysis

Effects are (+) increase stimulation; (0) no known effect; (–) inhibitory; (±) depending on the local hormonal milieu. Hormones/factors are epidermal growth factor (EGF); fibroblast growth factor (FGF); platelet-derived growth factor (PDGF); transforming growth factor-beta (TGF-β); bone-derived growth factor (BDGF); interleukin-1 (IL-1), insulin-like growth factor-I (IGF-I).

Systemic Hormones and Vitamins

Thyroxine

The thyroid hormones thyroxine (T_4) and 3,5,3´ triiodothyronine (T_3) are peptide hormones produced by the thyroid gland and transported to the target site on server proteins. T_4 is the primary secretory product of the thyroid, and 80% of T_3 is formed from deiodination of T_4 in the liver and kidney. Although there is less T_3 in the circulation, it has 3 to 4 times greater biologic activity than T_4. The thyroid hormones act on the proliferative and upper hypertrophic zone chondrocytes through a systemic endocrine mechanism (Fig. 10).

T_4 is essential for cartilage growth; it increases DNA synthesis in cells from the proliferative zone. T_4 has a second and independent effect on cell maturation, increasing glycosaminoglycan and collagen synthesis and alkaline phosphatase activity. Its effect on cartilage growth is mediated by a synergy between thyroxine and insulin-like growth factor/somatomedin-C (IGF-I/SM-C). For example, anti-IGF-I antibodies inhibit cartilage growth stimulation by T_3 but do not inhibit chondrocyte maturation as monitored by alkaline phosphatase activity. Administration of T_4 alone to thyroidectomized and parathyroidectomized animals results in hypertrophic chondrocyte maturation, but little growth; administration of growth hormone alone does not affect maturation, but generates normal cellular proliferation. Both agents together restore growth and maturation. T_3 does not stimulate IGF-I synthesis by chondrocytes; it simply enhances the growth effects of IGF-I. Excess T_4 results in protein catabolism, and a deficiency results in growth retardation, cretinism, and abnormal degradation of mucopolysaccharides.

Parathyroid Hormone

PTH, an 84-amino-acid protein produced by the parathyroids, acts primarily on the proliferative and upper hypertrophic zone chondrocytes (Fig. 10). Although PTH is found primarily bound to cells in the hypertrophic zone, it has the same qualitative effect on cells from different zones. This hormone has a direct mitogenic effect on epiphyseal chondrocytes and stimulates proteoglycan synthesis. Its effect on proteoglycan synthesis is mediated by an increase in the intracellular ionized calcium concentration and stimulation of protein kinase C. PTH has a synergistic effect that enhances the mitogenic effect of local growth factors.

Parathyroid Hormone-Related Protein

This protein was originally described in patients with humoral hypercalcemia of malignancy with normal levels of PTH. PTHrP shares significant amino acid sequence homology with PTH. Eight of the first 13 amino acids in PTH and PTHrP are identical. Moreover, the amino terminal portions of both PTH and PTHrP have nearly identical actions; both PTH and PTHrP share a common receptor. PTHrP is present in many tissues but apparently is not released into the circulation. Thus, although PTH has an endocrine function, PTHrP is a cytokine with autocrine or paracrine action. The common PTH-PTHrP receptor may be especially important in cartilage and bone. Its role in regulating the rate of conversion of small cell chondrocyte to hypertrophic phenotype via the *Ihh* loop has already

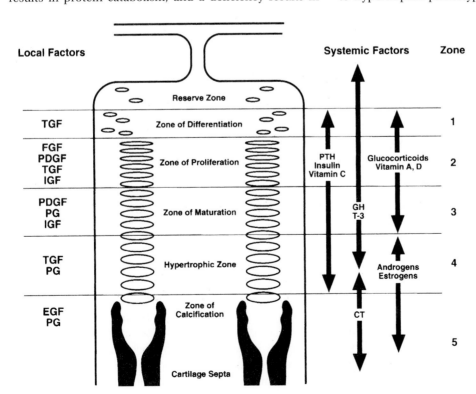

Figure 10

Schematic representation of the growth plate demonstrating the proposed site of action of local and systemic hormones, growth factors, and vitamins.

been described under the zones of the growth plate. An abnormal, persistently active PTH-PTHrP receptor as the molecular basis for Jansen metaphyseal chondrodysplasia has also been discussed under that topic.

Calcitonin

Calcitonin, a peptide hormone produced by the parafollicular cells of the thyroid, acts primarily in the lower hypertrophic zone (Fig. 10). It has been documented to accelerate growth plate calcification and cellular maturation.

Glucocorticoids

Adrenal corticoids (glucocorticoids), 4-ring steroid hormones produced by the adrenal cortex, primarily affect the zones of cellular differentiation and proliferation. Supraphysiologic amounts of glucocorticoids adversely affect growth and regeneration of epiphyseal cartilage, resulting in growth retardation. Excessive amounts of glucocorticoid from either endogenous or exogenous sources inhibit both the mitotic and the synthetic activity of chondrocytes. This catabolic effect of glucocorticoids has been documented at high concentrations where the growth rate of long bones is inversely correlated with hormone concentration. This metabolic suppression is attributed to a depression of glycolysis and a reduction of energy stores. The primary influence of glucocorticoids is a decrease in proliferation of chondroprogenitor cells in the zone of differentiation. An adverse effect of corticosteroids, apparent in the growth apparatus of young growing animals, is suppression of longitudinal growth and skeletal maturity.

Sex Steroids

Androgens (C_{19} steroids) function primarily in the lower portion of the growth plate to stimulate mineralization. Androgens are considered to be anabolic factors, and they stimulate proteoglycan synthesis in epiphyseal chondrocytes in vitro. This effect is age-dependent insofar as animals do not respond after reaching skeletal maturity. The anabolic effect of androgens is also manifested as an increased deposition of glycogen and lipids in cells and an increase in proteoglycans in cartilage matrix. Supraphysiologic doses of androgens depress growth and accelerate growth plate closure. According to results of recent studies, testosterone and dihydrotestosterone can stimulate DNA synthesis in chondrocytes of male growth plate tissue, whereas only dihydrotestosterone is active in female tissue. In both tissues, receptors were found only for the dihydrotestosterone metabolite, suggesting that this is the primary active androgen metabolite.

Estrogens (C_{18} steroids) decrease tibial length by specific inhibition of metaphyseal bone resorption, and thus, endochondral growth, increasing the thickness of the growth plate. It has been suggested that the acceleration of cell hypertrophy induced by estrogens may be interference in proteoglycan processing for extracellular transport.

Growth Hormone

Growth hormone (GH) is a peptide hormone produced by the pituitary. GH and its mediators, the somatomedins, act throughout the growth plate and primarily affect cellular proliferation. Hypophysectomy results in delayed or reduced osteogenesis, a decrease in mineralization, reduction in cartilage differentiation, and cessation of growth. GH is essential for growth plate function, but its mechanism of action remains unclear. The effects of GH are mediated by the production of a group of peptide factors termed somatomedins or, in current terminology, IGF. It is uncertain whether the effects of GH are indirect and result from the production of serum-derived IGF by the liver or whether there is a direct GH effect to induce chondrocytes to produce IGF locally (paracrine or autocrine effect). Earlier work suggested that GH effects were indirect, and were mediated only by the GH-dependent serum IGF. However, when GH binds to epiphyseal chondrocytes there is a local synthesis of IGF. Hence, the direct effect of GH creates target cells in which IGF-I induces a selective multiplication (clonal expansion) of differentiated cells.

Receptors for 2 members of the somatomedin family, IGF-I (somatomedin C or SM-C) and IGF-II (multiplication stimulatory activity), have been found in the growth plate. A complex pattern of graded specificity of receptors for each exists; cells in the zone of differentiation bind IGF-I, but the greatest binding is in the proliferative zone. GH regulates both the number of cells containing IGF receptors and the local synthesis of IGF-I by the chondrocytes in all zones of the growth plate. A "functional heterogeneity" exists in chondrocytes in the proliferative and hypertrophic zones, in that the cellular response to IGF-I declines with maturation and hypertrophy of the cells. IGF-II appears to be a more potent clonal growth effector during fetal life, and IGF-I has a greater effect during postnatal life. The structure and function of these factors are described in the chapter about articular cartilage.

Insulin

Patients with juvenile diabetes may exhibit a decrease in growth despite elevated levels of GH and normal IGF-I and IGF-II levels. It has been suggested that there is a decrease in a circulating growth plate factor, which contributes to growth retardation. Insulin can cross-react with IGF-I receptors and, therefore, may have some minor anabolic or permissive effect at physiologic insulin levels.

Vitamin D Metabolites

The active metabolites of vitamin D are the 1,25 and 24,25 dihydroxylated forms of vitamin D_3, both of which are produced by the liver and kidney. Vitamin D deficiency results in an elongation of the cell columns of the growth plate. This effect is considered to be secondary to a vitamin D-induced decrease in systemic calcium and phosphorus and the subsequent inhibition of mineralization. A direct mitogenic effect of vitamin D has been reported with 24,25-dihydroxy vitamin D ($24,25(OH)_2 D_3$), but not with $1,25(OH)_2 D_3$. The 24,25 $(OH)_2 D_3$ metabolite significantly increases DNA synthesis as well as inhibiting chondrocyte proteoglycan synthesis. The 1,25 $(OH)_2 D_3$ inhibits the proteoglycan synthetic response to local growth factors. The vitamin D metabolites are bound to cells in all growth plate zones except the hypertrophic zone. The highest levels are found in the zone of proliferation. Vitamin D excess is associated with atrophic changes mediated by an effect on the normal differentiation pattern. The pathologic effects of vitamin D excess and deficiency are discussed later in this chapter.

Vitamin A

The carotenes are essential for epiphyseal cartilage cell metabolism. A deficiency state results in impairment of cell maturation phenomena of the growth apparatus. This deficiency culminates in suppression of growth and in abnormal bone shape. Excessive vitamin A leads to bone weakness resulting from increases in lysosomal body membrane fragility.

Vitamin C

Ascorbic acid primarily influences the growth apparatus by virtue of its requirement as a cofactor in the enzymatic synthesis of collagen. Ascorbate has been shown to stimulate matrix mineralization in cultures of growth plate chondrocytes, through its stimulation of matrix vesicle formation and the synthesis of alkaline phosphatase and types II and X collagen.

Growth Factors

The growth factors or cytokines are generally regulatory peptides that are synthesized and exert their effects locally. They initiate their actions by binding to receptors on the surface membrane of the target cells. Thus, both the presence of the factor and a cell competent to respond are necessary to initiate a response. Moreover, the controlled conditions of an in vitro assay are not designed to replicate the extremely complex situation in vivo where a cell population is exposed to multiple endocrine as well as autocrine/paracrine molecules simultaneously. As has been described in the section covering development, the growth factors, which generally were described in postnatal regulatory roles, are intimately involved in the histogenesis of the tissues of the musculoskeletal system. With these complexities in mind, it is worthwhile to consider some general effects of the growth factors.

Epidermal growth factor (EGF) is generally found at high levels in platelets and glandular tissue. It also has an effect on the growth plate. It is found in endothelial lining cells in the growth plate, lying between invading capillaries and calcifying cartilage septa. EGF induces cell replication and inhibits collagen synthesis and alkaline phosphatase activity in calvarial cultures. Platelet-derived growth factor is generally a potent mitogen for cells of connective tissue origin. Its activation during injury such as fracture is an important initiator of the inflammatory and cellular response that leads to healing and bone formation.

FGF is a family of polypeptides derived from multiple areas, including endothelial cells. It will be recalled that in limb development FGF mediated the outgrowth of the limb bud along its longitudinal axis. FGF also upregulates chondrocyte replication as well as promotes neovascularization, both crucial functions in growth plate physiology. Basic fibroblast growth factor (bFGF) and IGF-I appear to interact to regulate growth. A more immature chondrocyte phenotype is apparently supported by bFGF, whereas IGF-I has a general anabolic role throughout the growth plate.

The transforming growth factor-β (TGF-β) superfamily includes a variety of growth factors including the bone morphogenetic proteins. TGF-β generally upregulates bone and cartilage components such as collagens and proteoglycans. Release of TGF-β is stimulated by PTH, but the overall effect of TGF-β appears to depend on constituent growth factors in the cell. Therefore, its effects may be stimulatory or inhibitory depending on the hormonal environment when TGF-β is introduced to the chondrocytes. TGF-β is a potent inhibitor of IL-1 and downregulates metalloproteinases by this inhibition.

Prostaglandins

These ubiquitous biologically active agents are present in nanomolar levels in growth plate cells and affect cellular processes by altering intracellular cyclic adenosine monophosphate levels. An acceleration in DNA synthesis has been observed in epiphyseal chondrocytes, as well as inhibition of alkaline phosphatase activity and collagen synthesis and stimulation of proteoglycan synthesis. Different types of prostaglandins are elaborated during different phases of endochondral ossification. Some evidence indicates that, at elevated levels, these factors delay proliferation and maturation of cells and inhibit bone elongation and cell production rate.

Biomechanics of the Growth Plate

Overview

As the weakest structure in the ends of the long bones of the immature skeleton, the growth plate is a common site for injury. Given that the growth plate is solely responsible for the longitudinal growth of the skeleton, the importance of understanding both the characteristics and consequences of growth plate injuries is clear. All injury is associated with failure, whether physiologic failure of systems or processes or mechanical failure of tissues. Mechanical disruption of the growth plate can lead to physiologic failure; appropriate treatment depends on comprehension of the mechanical properties of the growth plate, of the mechanical conditions that cause injury, and of the ultimate effect on growth.

When an injury will ultimately produce angular and/or longitudinal growth disturbance, intervention is indicated in various ways to avert, minimize, or correct the problem. The biomechanical properties of the growth plate need to be considered at each point in the treatment protocol.

The Mechanical Properties of Growth Plate Cartilage

Compared to the investigations into the mechanical properties of bone, tendon, ligament, and even articular cartilage, the investigations into the mechanical properties of physeal cartilage have been less numerous, at least until recently. The Hueter-Volkmann law for the growth plates has been more of a clinical observation than a quantitative description. This law is somewhat the inverse of Wolf's law for osseous tissue remodeling. The Hueter-Volkmann law notes that increasing compression across a growth plate leads to decreasing growth. Characterization of the many properties of the growth plate is essential for understanding the physis as an organ of growth and as a structural element within the immature musculoskeletal system.

The equilibrium compressive modulus (see section on the biphasic nature of articular cartilage) has been measured from cartilaginous tissues seemingly similar to the growth plate. Equilibrium moduli for articular, chondroepiphyseal, and reserve zone cartilage have been reported to be between 0.4 and 1.5 MPa, 0.7 MPa, and about 0.35 MPa, respectively. In recent studies, values for the equilibrium compressive moduli of bovine growth plate and rabbit growth plate have been found to be approximately 0.17 to 0.9 MPa and 0.044 MPa, respectively. Presently, no data exist to describe the failure, tensile, or shear properties of growth plate cartilage.

Although differences in mechanical test parameters, anatomic position, age, or species of test specimens may account for some of the large variation in modulus values, the intimate relationship between morphology and mechanical properties, or structure and function, must certainly play a significant role. Although the basic building blocks of cartilage, namely chondrocytes and matrix, appear common to articular, chondroepiphyseal, and physeal cartilages, specific cell and molecular types, amounts, and arrangement do vary among these cartilages and with developmental age. The relationship between growth plate morphology and tensile failure has been investigated using the proximal tibiae of growing rats. The weakest region within the growth plate was found to be the hypertrophic zone, in which the matrix volume is low and the cellular volume is high. At the onset of sexual maturation in the rat, the hypertrophic zone of the growth plate increases in width, and the tensile strength decreases. Cleavage through the hypertrophic zone at failure is consistent with the dependence of mechanical properties on regional morphology.

It should be appreciated that the clinical situation is considerably more complex. The status of the perichondrial ring of LaCroix, the anatomic relationship of ligaments, the nonplanar geometries of specific growth plates, and the application of combinations of compression, tension, and shear often lead to mechanical failure with significant undulations within or change in direction across the zones of the growth plate. Clinical growth plate fracture classification needs to accommodate these issues.

Factors Affecting Growth Plate Fracture and Failure Strength

Growth plate injuries occur when the mechanical demands placed on a bone exceed the mechanical strength of the epiphysis-growth plate-metaphysis complex. Two of the factors that determine the incidence of injury are the ability of the growth plate to resist failure (that is, the mechanical properties of the growth plate as discussed above), and the forces applied to the bone or the stresses induced in the growth plate. The characteristics of the fracture have great clinical significance for treatment options and predicted outcomes. The Salter-Harris classification system for growth plate injuries was proposed in an effort to relate the mechanisms, characteristics, and prognoses of these fractures.

As originally proposed, Salter-Harris type I injuries involve complete separation of the epiphysis from the metaphysis with no associated bone fracture, and are produced by shear or tensile forces (Fig. 11, A). This type of injury is most common in early childhood, when the growth plate is relatively thick. The fracture line propagates principally through the lower hypertrophic zone, leaving the reserve and proliferative zones attached to the epiphysis. In this situation, the cells responsible for interstitial growth within the physis and the epiphyseal vessels supplying these cells are left largely undisturbed. The prognosis for type I injuries for normal growth generally is quite good. (There are always clinical exceptions. For example, type I injuries with displacement of the distal femoral growth plate carry a more guarded prognosis. This growth plate is large and nonplanar. In displacing, the proliferative zone may also be injured. For a different reason, displaced type I injuries of the proximal femur carry an extremely guarded prognosis. Here epiphyseal vessels must travel along the femoral neck where they are vulnerable to direct disruption, leading to osteonecrosis of the entire chondroepiphysis.)

A type II injury (Fig. 11, B) is also thought to be produced by shear or tensile forces and is the most common injury. It consists of fracture along the growth plate with an attached metaphyseal bone fragment. The anatomic position of the metaphyseal fragment depends on load direction. With a bending or angulation force, the metaphyseal fragment is normally located on the compressive or concave side, whereas periosteum is torn on the tensile or convex side. The reserve and proliferative zones remain with the epiphysis, the circulation is usually preserved, and again, as a generalization, the prognosis for continued growth is excellent.

The type III injury (Fig. 11, *C*) is intra-articular and attributed to shear forces at the joint. The fracture passes from the joint surface to the growth plate and out toward the periphery along the lower hypertrophic zone. Accurate realignment is required for displaced fractures to restore the joint surface. This also implies reapproximation of the physis. As long as the epiphyseal blood supply is left intact, prognosis is good.

The type IV fracture (Fig. 11, *D* and *E*) is similar to the type III; however, the fracture crosses the growth plate and propagates across the metaphysis. If there is displacement, reduction must be performed accurately to minimize the formation of a physeal bar or bone bridge and subsequent growth arrest.

A type V injury (Fig. 11, *F* and *G*) results from a large compressive force that leads to necrosis of the proliferative zone. The occurrence of type V injuries as "pure" or isolated compressions as depicted in the figure have been questioned; they are certainly uncommon. However, this demonstrates another difference among tissue failure as defined in the laboratory, as illustrated by a medical artist, and as encountered in clinical practice. When a type I or II fracture displaces as the result of a high-energy accident such as vehicular trauma, the impaction of the growth plate against the metaphysis very well may also cause a secondary violent compression and terminal cellular damage within the growth plate. Therefore, the following caveat is worthwhile to remember.

Although the Salter-Harris classification is useful clinically, caution always needs to be exercised in conveying prognosis. It is important to reiterate that growth plate fractures are complex. Accurate assessment of the detailed histologic pattern of fracture is important because the location of damage determines the fate of proliferative cell activity and the status of the epiphyseal blood supply, and thus future growth. Although a consistent plane of separation through the hypertrophic zone has been seen in several experiments, other studies have revealed a more variable histologic pattern of fracture. It has been demonstrated that transphyseal fractures of the lower extremities of rats and rabbits did not exclusively produce damage to the hypertrophic zone. Although the greater proportion of each fracture involved the hypertrophic zone, damage was also noted in the proliferative and reserve zones. Only 15% of rat proximal tibiae tested in a separate study failed uniformly at the level of the growth plate-metaphysis junction, whereas 85% of the specimens displayed crack propagation through the upper proliferative and reserve zones.

The type of load applied to a bone also affects the fracture pattern. It has been shown that tensile forces applied to the rat proximal tibiae produce separation through the reserve

zone, whereas shear forces produce fractures through both the proliferative and hypertrophic zones. Even with the application of the same type of load, both the gross fracture pattern and the histologic fracture pattern (zones involved) can vary depending on the load direction.

As alluded to previously, unlike controlled laboratory tests, clinical fractures occur under multiaxial loading conditions, and failure is ultimately determined by the internally induced stresses in the bone and growth plate. These stresses must be distinguished from the externally applied load type. An externally applied compressive, tensile, or shear load cannot be expected to have the same effect on bones of different geometry and growth plate curvature, because these loads, singly or in combination, induce a complex 3-dimensional stress state within the structures. Any of these loading modes can induce all types of stresses (compressive, tensile, and shear) throughout the entire growth plate (Fig. 12) and, therefore, cause variable fracture patterns. In short, it is difficult to correlate fracture patterns to externally applied loads without consideration of other

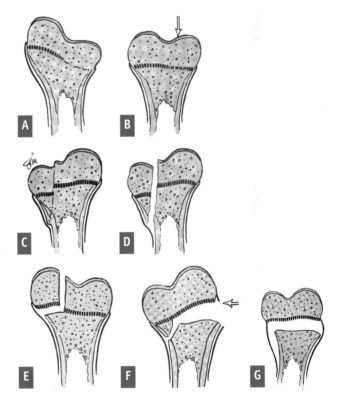

Figure 11

A, Type I epiphyseal plate injury: Separation of the epiphysis. **B,** Type II epiphyseal plate injury: Fracture-separation of the epiphysis. **C,** Type III epiphyseal plate injury: Fracture of part of the epiphysis. **D,** Type IV epiphyseal plate injury: Fracture of the epiphysis and epiphyseal plate. **E,** Bone union and premature closure. **F,** Type V epiphyseal plate injury: Crushing of the epiphyseal plate. **G,** Premature closure. (Reproduced with permission from Salter RB, Harris WR: Injury involving the epiphyseal plate. *J Bone Joint Surg* 1963;45A:587–622.)

factors, including regional geometry and local material (tissue) properties.

The majority of studies on the biomechanics of growth plate injuries have been conducted on a macrostructural whole bone level, in which the observed fracture or failure properties reflect the combined effects of the bone geometry and size, the growth plate topology, and the bone and growth plate cartilage mechanical properties. Experiments on isolated specimens of growth plate cartilage control for differences in the geometric and structural variables and reveal a relationship between mechanical stress and fracture pattern for growth plate cartilage alone. Isolated rectangular specimens of bone-growth plate-bone from the bovine femur and tibia have been tested, and the correlation between stress and histologic fracture pattern reported (Fig. 13). Tensile stresses cause the greatest damage in the upper proliferative zone. Shear stresses induce failure between the proliferative zone and the hypertrophic zone. Such damage may be deleterious to the activity of the dividing cells of the growth plate and can affect future growth. Under compressive stress, damage is found primarily in the metaphyseal trabeculae. This finding needs to be interpreted with the clinical observation previously discussed, namely "pure" type V injuries are uncommon. However, cellular damage from compression could occur in association with other types of fracture pattern and/or could occur without a change in conventional radiography or histology.

New clinical imaging modalities, specifically magnetic resonance, may become important as early warning systems of cellular jeopardy. Once this could be demonstrated reliably, treatment protocols to avert growth disturbance could be logically assessed.

Morphology

The growth plate adapts its form to follow the contours of principal tensile stresses. These contours allow the growth plate to be subjected mostly to compressive stress. The avoidance of shear stresses provides an optimal geometry for strength of the mechanical interface.

The gross morphology of the distal femoral bovine physis was studied and found to exhibit 3-dimensional undulations. The primary contours correspond to the 4 ridges and valleys. The distance between the apices is about 50 mm, and the amplitude is 10 mm. The secondary contours are a finer pattern of undulations within the primary contours, with a spatial periodicity of 5 mm and amplitude of 1 mm. The tertiary contours have an even smaller spatial periodicity (0.5 mm) and amplitude (0.1 mm). The primary and secondary contours are the same on the epiphyseal and metaphyseal sides of the physes. The tertiary contours, however, are unrelated on either side and appear to reflect the randomness of physeal growth. Radiographically a layer of dense trabecular bone is adjacent to and parallel to the primary contour of the growth plate on the metaphyseal side (Fig. 14).

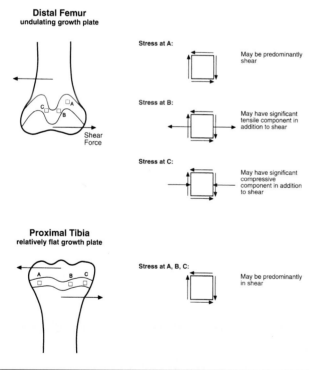

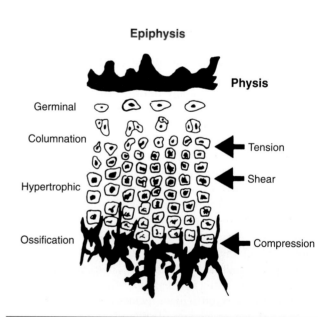

Figure 12

If the type of externally applied force is differentiated from the internally induced stresses, it can be better understood why different failure patterns can easily result when the same type of force is applied to different bones and growth plates.

Figure 13

The histologic zone of failure varies with the type of load applied to the specimens. (Reproduced with permission from Moen CT, Pelker RR: Biomechanical and histological correlations in growth plate failure. *J Pediatr Orthop* 1984;4:180–184.)

The Effect of Age on Failure Strength and Fracture Patterns

Mechanical tests on human cadaveric femoral heads of various ages (from younger than 13 months to older than 15 years) have shown that the shear strength of the capital femoral epiphysis increases with age. This increase in strength can be attributed both to the increasing overall size of the femoral head and to the developmental changes to the growth plate topology (Fig. 15). With increasing age, the growth plate becomes thinner and exhibits an increased number of mamillary processes and curves, thereby creating an undulating surface that imparts an increased resistance to shear. This finding has been reported consistently regardless of the type of applied force (shear or tension), the type of bone, or the species.

Experimental data have also been presented to support the fact that age or stage of skeletal development influences the growth plate fracture pattern. Under controlled shear tests on human and rabbit proximal femurs, it has been shown that the transphyseal fracture (type I) occurs most frequently in the very young as proposed by Salter and Harris; however, it may not pass exclusively through the lower hypertrophic zone. In older bones, fractures tend to pass through both the growth plate and the metaphysis or epiphysis (types II–IV).

The Effect of Surrounding Structures on Failure Strength

The growth plate is surrounded circumferentially by the perichondral region, which is composed of a dense cell layer, a loosely packed cell layer, an overlying fibrous tissue, and in some cases, an inner bony ring. The strongly oriented collagen fibers of the perichondral region are firmly anchored to the epiphysis and metaphysis, immediately adjacent to the growth plate. These characteristics of location and microstructure suggest a function of mechanical support, in which the perichondral region serves as a limiting membrane, providing lateral constraint to the growth plate cartilage. The perichondral region is included in Ogden's classification scheme for growth plate and epiphyseal injuries; an Ogden type VI injury describes the potential for osseous bridge formation and angular deformity as a result of damage to these peripheral structures.

In tension and shear tests on the proximal tibiae of rats, an intact periosteum/perichondral region has been shown to increase the failure strength significantly. It has also been demonstrated, using human cadaveric femoral heads, that an intact perichondral region can improve shear strength.

As a result of continued skeletal growth, generally the relative contribution of the perichondral region to the strength of the growth plate region diminishes. As the absolute and relative thickness and size of perichondral region decreases, the topologic and histomorphometric characteristics of the growth plate begin to account for a larger part of the biomechanical properties of the region. Yet the coordination of this load sharing has clinical significance. Slipped capital femoral epiphysis (idiopathic) is an entity that generally occurs during the growth spurt. Many

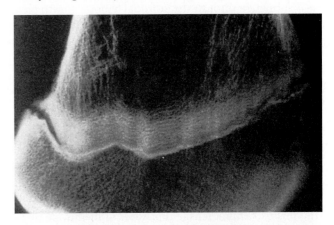

Figure 14

Radiograph of plate and trabecular bone structure in parasagittal section. (Reproduced with permission from Cohen B, Chorney GS, Phillips DP, et al: The microstructural tensile properties and biochemical composition of the bovine distal femoral growth plate. *J Orthop Res* 1992;10:263–275.)

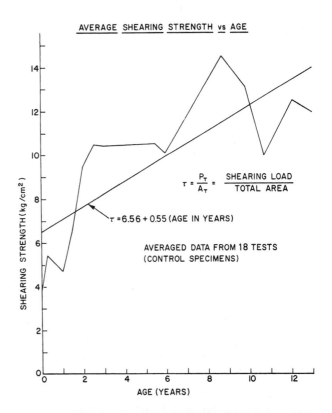

Figure 15

Shear stress (τ) for 18 control specimens versus age. The straight line represents a least-squares fit of the data. (Reproduced with permission from Chung SM, Batterman SC, Brighton CT, et al: Shear strength of the human capital epiphyseal plate. *J Bone Joint Surg* 1976;58A:94–103.)

mechanical factors, including body habitus, femoral neck-shaft angle (changing from relatively valgus to varus), and femoral torsion, are changing at this time as well as the diminished contribution of the perichondral region to strength. For some adolescents, this entity can cause a plastic deformation through the proximal femoral growth plate (clinical correlate, "chronic or stable slip") or failure (clinical correlate, "acute or unstable slip") that needs to be addressed surgically. In addition to idiopathic slipped capital femoral epiphysis, slips are known to occur with increasing incidence in endocrine conditions. In particular, in renal failure with associated hyperparathyroidism that weakens the attachment of the perichondral ring to the metaphysis, displacment of growth plates is common, not only at the proximal femur but at other locations as well.

Tensile and Compressive Properties

The microstructural tensile properties of the bovine distal femoral growth plate have been determined by controlled uniaxial tension tests. The tensile properties obtained from the stress-strain curves of such tests are shown in Table 2. The ultimate strain at failure (average 13.8%) has been noted to be fairly uniform throughout the growth plate. However, a significant difference has been noted among the anatomic sites for ultimate stress and tangent modulus. The anterior region of the growth plate seems stronger and stiffer than other sites. The growth plate is also stronger and stiffer at the periphery than in the interior. These findings correlate with biochemical studies showing that the collagen content is also highest in the anterior regions.

Compression studies on uniform cylindric specimens also have been performed on distal femoral growth plate specimens. The boundary conditions during fluid flow through the bony interfaces on either side of the growth plate are unknown; therefore, no assumptions on the boundary conditions have been made. Three models representing the different possibilities of boundary conditions have been used to analyze the experimental data: (1) both sides are completely permeable; (2) the metaphyseal side is free draining and the epiphyseal side is impermeable; and (3) both sides are impermeable.

The compressive modulus (equilibrium stress/applied strain) of growth plate has been found to be higher for the interior sites (0.90 MPa) than for the periphery (0.71 MPa). This difference between the interior and the periphery has been found to be independent of the boundary conditions.

The Response of the Growth Plate to Mechanical Stimuli

It has long been recognized that mechanical forces can influence the shape and length of growing bones for a given organism within limits selected over time and established by the genetic and epigenetic program. Both in vitro and in vivo studies on developing tissue have confirmed that mechanical factors can influence bone development during the earliest stages of endochondral ossification. At the end of the embryonic and beginning of the fetal periods, primary ossification centers form and advance toward either end of the long bones until the proliferative cartilages that are the growth plates are reached. From that time until skeletal maturity, the advance of the primary center will be matched by growth away from the ossification front at the metaphysis.

An alternative way to regard this is that the physeal regions are providing the motive force for internal distraction osteogenesis. The interface between the metaphyseal ossification front and the adjacent proliferative cartilage or developing growth plate may, in part, be determined or modified by mechanical forces. Initially, these forces are the first muscle contractions and joint reactive forces of development, and eventually they are the forces of the postnatal environment in which the organism will have to compete. Secondary centers within the chondroepiphyses are generally an evolutionary advance of mammals supporting the relatively fragile chondroepiphysis. As the secondary centers of ossification grow, initially spherically to occupy a larger volume of the chondroepiphysis, they advance and flatten at the reserve zone of the physis, which then is a "plate" albeit with undulations. Generally in humans the appearance of secondary centers of ossification are postnatal events, the single exception being that of the distal femur, which appears at 36 weeks of gestation. In mammalian quadrupeds, secondary centers of ossification may appear in utero.

Experiments have suggested that growth plates develop in a way that reduces shear stress at the bone-growth plate interfaces. Such a condition is attained by a growth plate contour that runs perpendicular to lines of principal compression or tension. These same studies further implied that growth plates composed of hyaline cartilage are subjected predominantly to compressive stresses, whereas growth plates or portions of growth plates composed of fibrocartilage primarily experience tensile stresses. These latter growth regions have sometimes been termed traction apophyses. However, the concept of a traction apophysis as a different type of growth plate needs to be considered with caution. A clinical situation may illustrate the problem. The anterior extension of the proximal tibial growth plate of humans is exposed to considerable tension through the patellar tendon, which inserts on the tibial tubercle on the proximal side of the growth plate. Yet, this region is contiguous with the remainder of the proximal tibial growth plate, which would function in a more compressive environment.

The influence of mechanical factors is exhibited throughout development and growth of the immature skeleton. The secondary centers of ossification are an excellent example. Finite element modeling techniques have been used to

Table 2

Tensile Properties by Various Anatomic Groupings (mean ± SD)

Region	Ultimate Stress[a] (MPa)	Ultimate Strain[b]	Tangent Modulus[a]
Anterior (n = 20)	4.0 ± 0.97	0.137 ± 0.05	48.6 ± 25.1
Posterior/lateral (n = 30)	3.05 ± 0.80	0.123 ± 0.04	37.9 ± 16.7
Posterior/medial (n = 29)	2.30 ± 0.68	0.160 ± 0.06	23.5 ± 14.9
Center (n = 7)	2.16 ± 0.79	0.1117 ± 0.06	27.0 ± 11.8
Average	2.97 ± 0.80	0.138 ± 0.06	34.6 ± 17.7
Periphery (n = 30)	3.50 ± 1.06	0.132 ± 0.06	44.5 ± 26.1
Interior (n = 56)	2.68 ± 0.96	0.141 ± 0.06	29.3 ± 14.2

[a] Significantly different, $p < 0.01$

[b] Not significantly different, $p > 0.1$

(Reproduced with permission from Cohen B, Ghorney GS, Phillips DP, et al: The microstructural tensile properties and biochemical composition of the bovine distal femoral growth plate. *J Orthop Res* 1992;10:263–275.)

evaluate the stress patterns in immature human bones. Specific functions of the calculated stresses have been found to correlate with the propensity for cartilage to be replaced by bone. One hypothesis proposes that intermittent shear stresses tend to accelerate, and intermittent hydrostatic compressive stresses tend to inhibit endochondral ossification. This hypothesis was used along with a series of geometric and analytical assumptions to predict formation of the secondary ossification center. With further experimental verification, this theory has the potential to be a powerful tool. Although many clinical correlates could be drawn, the proximal femur in pediatric orthopaedics provides several examples. In developmental dysplasia of the hip, displacement of the proximal femur from the acetabulum will delay the appearance of the secondary center of ossification and alter its location within the chondroepiphysis. In neuromuscular problems, the lack of muscle balance around the hip and abnormal function of the joint lead to abnormal growth of both the proximal femur and the acetabulum and can eventuate in pathologic dislocation.

The concept that mechanical factors can influence growth plate behavior is embodied in the previously mentioned Hueter-Volkmann law. Although certainly an oversimplication, this law states that compression forces inhibit growth, and tensile forces stimulate growth. Although some clinical treatments for bone deformities are predicated on it (the very name "orthopaedics" originates from the quest to form a straight child), this description of the interaction between mechanics and growth plate behavior lacks quantification.

No boundaries or ranges on the magnitudes of these forces have been identified, and because both compressive and tensile forces exist simultaneously within the skeleton, it is doubtful that all compressive forces inhibit growth and all tensile forces stimulate it.

Despite these shortcomings, experimental evidence for the general theme of the Hueter-Volkmann law is abundant. Many animal studies have been performed in which some alteration is made to the "normal" mechanical environment of a growing bone, and the resultant changes in bone growth measured. Metal staples applied asymmetrically across growth plates have been successfully used to treat angular deformities, especially valgus at the knees. Casting and bracing are time-honored methods of treating some problems in pediatric orthopaedics. Generally these are more helpful in treating deformations and averting secondary growth problems than in addressing malformations in which the growth problem has its origin in abnormalities of the genome and/or morphogenesis. Thus, a Pavlik harness generally works well in treating typical hip dysplasia, and casting generally is effective in treating positional clubfeet. Teratologic hip dislocations in association with syndromes and stiff congenital clubfeet are harder to address with external mechanical treatments and even prove challenging to correct with surgical realignments.

Periosteal/perichondral stripping has been used as a means of stimulating growth by releasing the presumptive compressive forces across the growth plate. In view of the complex relationship of this region to the normal physiology of the growth plate, the response to this intervention would be difficult to predict in theory. That has been the case in practice. External fixators have been applied across growth plates to apply tension and thereby stimulate growth. Chondrodiastasis is an example of such a procedure. Experimental and clinical results have been variable. The relationship between the ultimate number of divisions of chondrocytes of the proliferative zone (as opposed to the rate of divisions over a period of time) and all perturbations (physical force, endocrine/paracrine/autocrine factors, nutrition) has not been well defined. Therefore, at the present time, clinical practice for lengthening is largely being conducted as distraction osteogenesis.

An alternative principle has been proposed in which certain increases in both tension and compression can inhibit growth. This chondral modeling theory is described graphically by a chondral growth-force response curve (Fig. 16). It is an attractive theory because of its ability to describe many of the clinical findings noted. However, it also suffers from the same limitations that apply to the Hueter-Volkmann law.

The variability seen in outcomes from clinical attempts to alter growth and the lack of conclusive experimental data might be explained by a limited understanding of the mechanics that control the response. In vitro experiments on the effects of mechanical stress on the biosynthetic and mitotic activity of chondrocytes may aid in elucidating these mechanisms. Although no definitive conclusions have been reached, data from recent studies indicate that high static compressive stresses decrease the biosynthesis of extracellular macromolecules, whereas low intermittent compressive stresses increase matrix synthesis. Again, a clinical example may be illustrative of the difficulty of bridging the distance between the laboratory and the patient. The gold standard of demonstrating the efficacy of a clinical intervention is the prospective, double-blind, controlled study. Relative to the shape that the immature skeleton will ultimately achieve, clinical intervention with physical force such as a brace is difficult to apply in a way that demonstrates an incontrovertible difference. For example, bracing of various sorts has been used in an attempt to alter tibial torsion, yet the skeptic can easily question whether shape at maturity would have been the same whether or not the device had been used. This does not diminish in any way the need for scientific investigation into the role of physical force on the development and growth of the immature skeleton. It does emphasize the rigor that will be demanded in applying such information clinically with credibility.

In summary, both the function of the growth plate and its mechanical properties depend on a complex interaction between internal structure and external influences. Continuing research efforts are crucial for defining these mechanical properties, molecular biology, and their interaction in a manner that can be applied in clinical diagnosis and treatment.

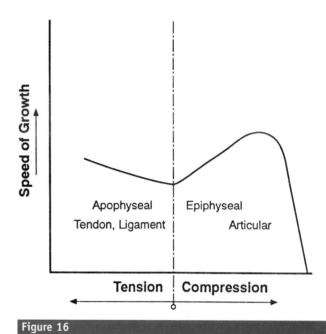

Figure 16

Growth response of cartilage types to physiologic loads. (Reproduced with permission from Frost HM: A chondral modeling theory. *Calcif Tissue Int* 1979;28:181–200.)

Pathologic States Primarily Affecting the Growth Plate

The primary function of the growth plate is longitudinal growth, which is accomplished through cellular proliferation and maturation, matrix production and mineralization, endochondral ossification, and resorption (remodeling). Several selected examples of pathophysiology were included in the section on structure and function as the prototypical examples of key disturbances in the program innate to abnormal development. The growth plate is also subject to environmental and nutritional disturbances as well as a broad spectrum of disturbances in cell biology, enzyme function, and structural molecules that will be subsumed under the category inheritable disorders.

Environmental Factors

Irradiation

Irradiation primarily affects longitudinal chondroblastic proliferation; it relatively spares latitudinal bone growth. Depending on dose, radiation can therefore result in shortened bones with relatively increased width. Such bones may radiographically resemble those seen in achondroplasia.

Bacterial Infection

The metaphyseal portion of the growth plate is affected by bacterial invasion. Bacteria lodge in the vascular sinusoids and soon produce one or more small abscesses. Explanations given for bacterial infection in the metaphysis include sluggish circulation, low oxygen tension, and deficiency of the reticuloendothelial system. Extension of the infection through the haversian canals results in osteomyelitis of cortical bone and subperiosteal abscess formation. In most long bones, the joint capsule and growth plate are strong barriers to bacterial extension. In the first year of life, cartilage canals may still persist across growth plates and serve as a conduit for extension. Further, in those joints in which the involved metaphysis is intracapsular, extension into the joint occurs once the bacteria have eroded outside the bony metaphysis. In the proximal femur, pyarthrosis often is associated with hematogenous osteomyelitis. This can result in proximal femoral osteonecrosis and chondronecrosis by compromise of the vascular supply and direct enzymatic digestion of the articular cartilage.

Although the cartilaginous portion of the growth plate is usually a barrier to bacterial infection, it is not impenetrable. Severe infection may result in local or total cessation of growth, even several years following the acute infection. Inhibited or angular growth usually results. Less commonly, there have been reports of stimulation of growth following infection.

Nutritional Disorders

Malnutrition or protracted illness, if severe enough, will result in depressed chondrogenesis and stunted growth. These disorders can also occur with growth plate injuries. Under such circumstances, metaphyseal bone formation continues until complete occlusion of the marrow space occurs at the cartilage-bone junction and a seal is formed.

When normal growth resumes, the growth plate moves away from the dense seal, which, by contrast with adjacent bone, is perceived on radiographs as a dense line. This is termed a Harris growth arrest or growth resumption line. Clinically this can be helpful in following growth after a growth plate injury. If the physis has uniformly resumed growth, it will move away from the line parallel to it. If, however, the physis has a terminally injured and nonfunctioning subpopulation in the center or at the periphery, the line will appear depressed centrally in the former case or tilted in the latter.

Rickets

Rickets results from several causes, including nutritional deficiency, malabsorption, and renal disease, that interfere with the normal processing of calcium, phosphorus, and vitamin D. The common end point disruption is failure to mineralize the matrix in the zone of provisional calcification. Histologically, the reserve and proliferative zones are normal, but the hypertrophic zone is greatly expanded. This can be noted on conventional radiographs as widening of the growth plates. Further findings are an absent zone of provisional calcification (normally denser than the metaphyseal bone as calcified cartilage has more calcium per unit volume than bone) and flaring of the metaphysis (Fig. 17, *A*). Cartilage bars persist into the metaphysis (Fig. 17, *B*). Osteoid remains unmineralized on these unmineralized cartilage bars and a primary spongiosa fails to form. In the rachitic growth plate, the hypertrophic chondrocyte mitochondria retain large amounts of calcium. These mitochondria do not discharge their calcium, and the surrounding matrix remains unmineralized until the metabolic problem causing the rickets is corrected. Because the matrix remains

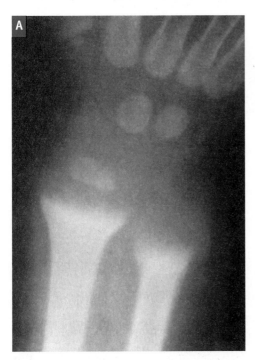

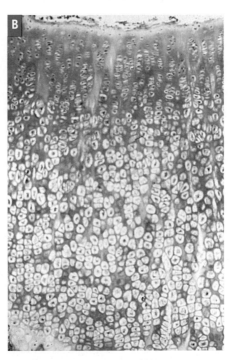

Figure 17

A, Radiographic features of rickets, distal radius, and ulna. Note the widened growth plates and flaring of the metaphyses. **B,** Histologic features of rickets. The zone of proliferation is largely unaffected, but the hypertrophic zone is markedly widened. (Photographs courtesy of Dr. Henry J. Mankin.)

unmineralized, nutrients can diffuse more readily than normal into the hypertrophic zone. This may explain the expansion of the hypertrophic zone. Further, the normal metaphyseal vascular invasion with aggressive capillary buds transgressing the last transverse septum also fails to occur in rickets (Fig. 18). It has been postulated that this cannot occur in mineral-deficient matrix. Also, vascular invasion may depend on the production of a chondrocyte-derived growth factor such as FGF and/or further angiogenic and angiotropic factors.

Scurvy

Scurvy is caused by vitamin C deficiency. Metabolically, vitamin C deficiency produces a decrease in chondroitin sulfate synthesis (enzymatic impairment of the conversion of glucose to galactosamine) and a deficiency in collagen synthesis (impaired hydroxylation of proline). The greatest deficiency in collagen synthesis is seen in the metaphysis. The microscopic appearance of the cartilaginous portion of the growth plate is normal, but that of the metaphysis is quite abnormal. The deficiency of type I collagen has its most disruptive impact where it is most in demand for the synthesis of new bone, namely the metaphysis. The calcified cartilage bars have a scant amount of osteoid, and they extend deep into the metaphysis. The accumulation of calcified cartilage at the zone of provisional calcification continues (unlike the situation in rickets). On radiographs, the calcium-rich zone of provisional calcification persists and, in contrast to the osteopenic metaphyseal bone, appears as a dense white line (line of Fraenkel). The bony trabeculae are sparse and thin. The osteopenia of the metaphysis on radiographs represents a true osteoporosis. The metaphyseal bone is weakened. Microfractures, hemorrhages,

debris, and fibrous tissue result. This region of detritus is called the zone of Trummerfeld. Collapse of the metaphysis along with continued latitudinal growth result in the formation of Pelkin's lateral spurs. Because of a marked change in the biomechanical properties of this region, growth plate displacement can occur.

Genetic Disorders

Defects in Matrix Synthesis: Chondrocytes

Because type II collagen and proteoglycans account for much of the matrix of cartilage, it would follow that disturbances in these structural molecules or in the enzymes that catalyze their metabolism would disturb their normal physiology. Such is indeed the case. Because of a great deal of work with clinical dysmorphology, discrete syndromes have been identified that were known to be abnormalities of cartilage. Kindreds of these syndromes can now be analyzed with the techniques of molecular biology. Molecular explanations for these syndromes are constantly being added to the literature.

All the cartilage matrix defects produce some degree of skeletal dysplasia with varying degrees of impact on articular and growth cartilage. Figure 19 categorizes the various abnormalities of the growth plate. Abnormalities in type II collagen underlie achondrogenesis II/hypochondrogenesis, some types of Stickler syndrome, some types of spondyloepiphyseal dysplasia, and Kniest dysplasia. Abnormalities in type IX collagen are found in some of the kindreds of Fairbanks multiple epiphyseal dysplasia. Mutations in type X collagen cause the Schmid-type chondroepiphyseal dysplasia. In a subset of Stickler syndrome distinct from that

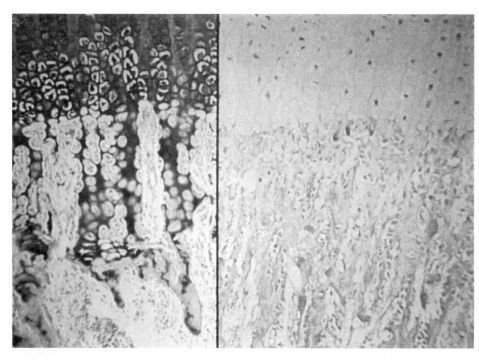

Figure 18

Vascular loops in rickets.

associated with the type II collagenopathy, a mutation has been described in type XI collagen.

The prototypical example of a defect of proteoglycan metabolism is diastrophic dwarfism. The mutation causing diastrophic dwarfism is in a sulfate transporter molecule, the diastrophic dysplasia sulfate transporter. Undersulfation of proteoglycans results. It will be remembered that proteoglycan size and hydration were critical to the function of the growth plate. This defect at the molecular level results in short stature and several deformities, in particular severe equinovarus feet, which is characteristic of this condition.

The 6 types of mucopolysaccharidosis result from systemic defects in enzymes that mediate proteoglycan metabolism. Lysosomal storage of undegraded glycosaminoglycans and large accumulations of these glycoproteins within the cell occur as a result (Table 3). As a group, the clinical presentation of the mucopolysaccharidoses is somewhat varied by the specific enzyme defect and glycoprotein accumulated. Each type of mucopolysaccharide has a varied toxic effect on the central nervous system, skeleton, ocular, or visceral organ systems (Table 3).

The general clinical characteristics of this group of diseases may not be specific for any type, but the pattern should suggest the presence of the disease. To variable degrees they share a spondyloepiphyseal dysplasia phenotype. All children have stunted growth and some degree of dysmorphic facies. Some have corneal clouding and mental retardation. Skull films may show thickening of the diploe and occasionally a "slipper-shaped" sella turcica. The chest radiographs may demonstrate paddle-shaped ribs. The pelvis films frequently show coxa vara with variable degrees of femoral capital dysplasia. The long bones typically demonstrate diaphyseal shortening and widening. The metacarpals demonstrate a "pencil sharpened" proximal epiphysis. Madelung wrist deformity may be present.

The developmental abnormalities with failure to recruit and program mesenchyme appropriately might be includ-ed in this category. An abnormal branching pattern and growth pattern in the human hand localized to a homeobox gene (*HOXD13*) is an example of this type of developmental abnormality that impacts cartilaginous anlagen and subsequently the growth plates. Another developmental abnormality of the human hand that has now been mapped to the genome is a complex polysyndactyly that is not in the homeobox cluster. Therefore, the developmental cascade for cartilage morphogenesis described at the outset of this chapter still has many steps that remain to be elucidated.

Defects in Matrix Synthesis: Osteoblasts

Osteogenesis imperfecta is really a spectrum of entities, all of which share the common feature of osseous tissue with diminished strength to failure. In clinical parlance this is manifested as bone fragility or ease of fracture. Osteogenesis imperfecta, as clinical presentations, has been classified in several ways to split the spectrum into discrete entities. The spectrum ranges from skeletons so fragile that fractures occur in utero and death ensues in the perinatal period, to skeletons extremely fragile and dysmorphic but compatible with life, to skeletons relatively unaffected except for an increased number of fractures that seem to occur less with increasing age. The molecular bases for the clinical entities have proved even more heterogeneous. Although type I collagen is usually affected in some way, the specific molecular defects can include a wide range of abnormalities in primary sequence and diminished synthesis.

The histologic and radiographic features of the severe, nonlethal type of osteogenesis imperfecta are depicted in Figure 20. Endochondral bone formation in the metaphysis and intramembranous bone formation are severely affected. The cartilaginous part of the growth plate region is at least relatively spared. The mineralized osteoid is scant; the trabeculae are thin and few in number; the cortices are thin and osteoporotic. Osteogenesis imperfecta ranks at the top of the differential diagnosis for osteoporosis presenting in childhood. As in scurvy, there is a large synthetic demand

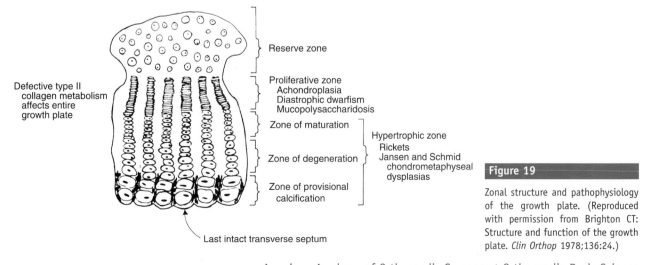

Defective type II collagen metabolism affects entire growth plate

Reserve zone

Proliferative zone
Achondroplasia
Diastrophic dwarfism
Mucopolysaccharidosis

Zone of maturation

Hypertrophic zone
Rickets
Jansen and Schmid
chondrometaphyseal
dysplasias

Zone of degeneration

Zone of provisional
calcification

Last intact transverse septum

Figure 19

Zonal structure and pathophysiology of the growth plate. (Reproduced with permission from Brighton CT: Structure and function of the growth plate. *Clin Orthop* 1978;136:24.)

for type I collagen in the metaphysis, but this cannot be met with a normal supply. Unlike scurvy, in which the metaphyseal region once had normal type I collagen, in osteogenesis imperfecta the collagen was never normal. Hence, the diaphysis is also abnormal. There is evidence of previous fractures and gross dysmorphology of all the bones. Fractures in osteogenesis imperfecta respond with the customary events of fracture healing, but the callus formed also has the abnormal collagen and thus the abnormal fragility.

The inferior mechanical properties of the osseous tissue in osteogenesis imperfecta are exposed most in those areas of the skeleton subject to the greatest force. Lower extremity long bones are particularly severely affected. (In the more mild forms of osteogenesis imperfecta, the frequent fractures usually have had a greater incidence in the long bones of the lower extremities.)

In analogy to the developmental abnormalities with failure to recruit and program mesenchyme appropriately to

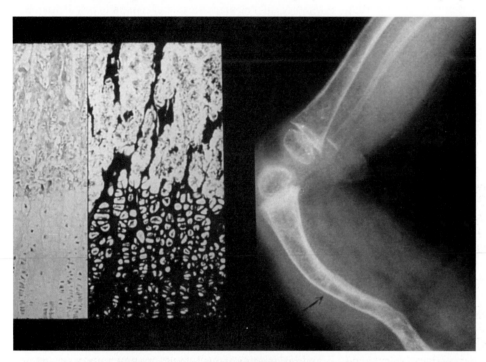

Figure 20

Histologic and radiographic features of osteogenesis imperfecta.

Table 3

Toxic Effects of Mucopolysaccharidoses

Syndrome	Skeletal Dysplasia	Mental Retardation	Corneal Clouding	Deafness	Inheritance	Glycoproteins Accumulated	Enzyme Defect
Hurlers (MPS-1H)	++	++	++	+	Autosomal recessive	Chondroitin sulfate B	α-L-iduronidase
Hunters (MPS-II)	+	+	–	++	Sex-linked recessive	Chondroitin sulfate B + heparitin sulfate	Sulfoiduronate sulfatase
Sanfilippo (MPS-III)	+–	++	–	+	Autosomal recessive	Heparitin sulfate	4 types–each a different enzyme
Morquio (MPS-OV)	++	–	+	+	Autosomal recessive	Keratan sulfate	Glucosamine-6 sulfatase
Scheie (MPS IS)	+	–	+	+	Autosomal recessive	Chondroitin sulfate B	α-L-iduronidase
Maroteaux-Lamy (MPS-VI)	++	–	+	+	Autosomal recessive	Dermatan sulfate	Arylsulfatase β

the cartilaginous sequence, a recent study has described the abnormality in the differentiation from a pluripotent mesenchymal cell to an osteoblast. Cleidocranial dysplasia results from a mutation in the transcription factor CBFA1. Again this leads to the issue of intramembranous and endochondral bone. Although the transcription factor CBFA1 has a clear role in osteoblast differentiation for intramembranous bone, it also seems to have an effect on the osseous lineage as it becomes involved in endochondral bone formation. This transcription factor may be involved in the *Ihh*-PTHrP signaling loop that was described in regulating the differentiation of chondrocytes from small to hypertrophic cell phenotype. If that is the case, then a very attractive candidate for coordinating the linkage between the cartilaginous elements of the growth plate and the osseous elements of the metaphysis has begun to be elucidated.

Defects in Calcification

Hypophosphatasia is an inherited autosomal recessive defect in alkaline phosphatase, an enzyme that degrades phosphate esters in cartilage and bone (for example, ATP and pyrophosphate). These phosphate esters inhibit cartilage calcification as was discussed in the section on zones of the growth plate and the role of matrix vesicles in mineralization. In hypophosphatasia, the serum calcium/phosphate product is normal, but the matrix does not calcify. The hypertrophic zone widens, and the osteoid formed on the cartilage bars does not mineralize. The histologic and radiographic findings in hypophosphatasia and rickets are very similar. The growth plate is widened because of an increase in the hypertrophic zone, but the proliferative and reserve zones are normal. The hypertrophic zone cells per-

sist into the metaphysis. The zone of provisional calcification and the primary spongiosa do not form. This failure occurs because of a slightly different abnormality from nutritional rickets, but the effect on histogenesis is similar, following a common pathway. Radiographically, the growth plate is widened, and there is flaring of the metaphysis. The end result is inhibition of growth.

Hypophosphatemic familial rickets (vitamin D-resistant rickets) results in the typical skeletal changes seen in vitamin D-deficient rickets, again by a different molecular mechanism that disrupts a common pathway. This disorder is a sex-linked dominant, characterized by low calcium and phosphorus, a high alkaline phosphatase activity, and abnormal conversion of vitamin D to its active metabolites.

Defects in Cell Proliferation

Achondroplasia was mentioned under the structure of the growth plate as the prime example of a defect in proliferation. It has been apparent for some time that achondroplasia is a defect in endochondral bone growth. Abnormalities were sought in various biochemical pathways but were never found. The molecular basis has now been established as abnormality in FGF-3. Unlike the molecular heterogeneity underlying osteogenesis imperfecta, most of the cases of achondroplasia occur because of a mutation in a single base pair resulting in a single amino acid substitution in the receptor. Interestingly, subsequent knockout studies of the FGF-3 receptors in mice indicate that the absence of the receptor results in longer bones. Hence, the mutation underlying clinical achondroplasia is a positive mutation, exerting a tighter brake on proliferation, not a negative mutation that would presumably fail to give a needed mito-

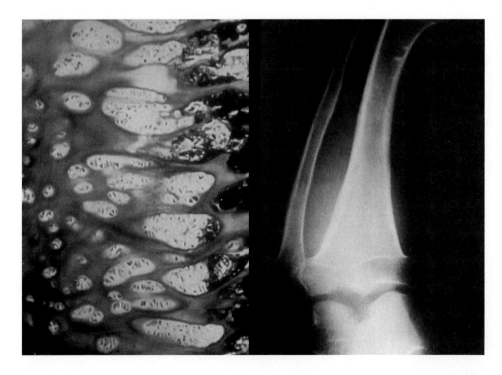

Figure 21

Histologic and radiographic features of achondroplasia.

genic stimulus. It is another indication that the coordination of the cartilaginous and osseous elements that result in normal growth are under very sophisticated control.

The typical radiographic and histologic characteristics of achondroplasia are depicted in Figure 21. The growth plates that would be most active in longitudinal endochondral growth are the most severely affected. The cell columns are very short, and the hypertrophic zone is narrow. The metaphysis reveals diminished calcified cores of cartilage and scanty new bone formation. Periosteal (intramembranous) bone formation is unaffected and latitudinal growth continues. This makes the metaphyses relatively wide.

An uncoupling of longitudinal and latitudinal growth can be seen in other conditions. This uncoupling can produce some phenotypic similarity among conditions caused by different mechanisms. Radiation was noted to inhibit longitudinal growth preferentially. Metatropic dwarfism also uncouples these separable pathways of bone growth.

Defects in Bone Remodeling

Osteopetrosis is characterized by abnormal internal or histologic remodeling. The typical radiographic and histologic characteristics are depicted in Figure 22. Osteopetrosis is also termed marble bone disease or Albers-Schönberg disease. It occurs in 2 forms: an autosomal recessive malignant form, which usually results in intrauterine death, and a relatively benign autosomal dominant form. In this disorder, there is an abnormality of osteoclast function and a defect in resorption of the primary spongiosa. The disease is characterized histologically by persistence of calcified cartilage bars in the diaphysis of the bone, and absence of a medullary cavity and marrow space. The interior of the bone is filled with chondro-osseous tissue. Radiographically, osteopetrosis is characterized by uniform opacity of the bones with no discernible internal architecture. In some less severely affected individuals, transverse radiodense banding may be seen in the metaphysis. Calcified cartilage has a higher mineral content per unit volume than bone, hence the radiographic appearance. The mechanical properties of calcified cartilage are inferior to those of bone; therefore, fractures occur. Healing ensues, but time to healing may be prolonged. The defect in osteoclast function appears to be caused by a defect in osteoclastic differentiation. This defect can be overcome with bone marrow transplantation which, if successful, reverses the histologic, radiographic, and clinical signs of the disease.

Osteochondromas (exostosis, multiple exostoses, diaphyseal aclasis) result from a defect in the perichondrial ring of LaCroix and the groove of Ranvier. In this disorder, chondrocytes from the cartilaginous region of the growth plate are displaced roughly orthogonal to the axis of growth. These cells continue to behave with the proliferative capacity of physeal chondrocytes. They form a cartilaginous cap that is in essence a heterotopic growth plate that forms bone at its base. While the skeleton is growing, the osteochondroma continues to grow and may become quite large. A solitary lesion overwhelmingly remains benign. In multiple familial exostoses, many of the lesions may form and grow. Presumably because sufficient proliferative cartilage is displaced from its normal alignment along the longitudinal axis, angular deformity can occur. Neoplastic degeneration can occur in this condition. Lesions in the axial skeleton are of particular concern.

Pyle disease or familial metaphyseal dysplasia is failure of

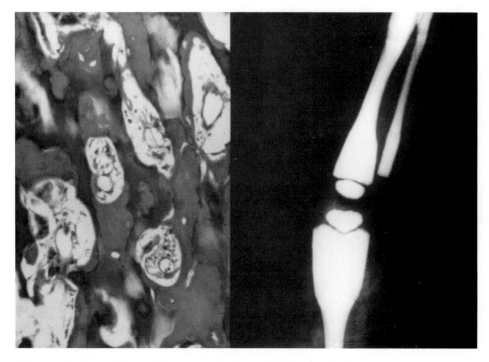

Orthopaedic Basic Science | American Academy of Orthopaedic Surgeons

Figure 22

Histologic and radiographic features of osteopetrosis.

external remodeling in the distal end of the metaphysis. The major clinical manifestation is genu varum. Histologically, the fiber bone of the secondary spongiosa is not resorbed or remodeled to lamellar bone until far down in the diaphysis.

Summary

The formation and growth of skeletal tissues are being explained at the molecular level. Embryology is a program with genes, messengers, receptors and cells precisely distributed during morphogenesis, and the cells acquiring or expressing specific characteristics with differentiation. The program is awe-inspiring in its complexity and fidelity. Yet examples of pathologic states of the growth plates exist at nearly every part of the program. These pathologic states not only can be correlated with molecular events but also help further elucidate the embryologic program itself. For those patients with problems of the growth plates, the challenge for physicians is to correct the specific defect. For all, the challenge is to employ embryologic processes for the repair of damaged or absent tissues.

Selected Bibliography

Introduction and Bone Development

Boskey AL: Current concepts of the physiology and biochemistry of calcification. *Clin Orthop* 1981;157:225–257.

Einhorn TA: The cell and molecular biology of fracture healing. *Clin Orthop* 1998:355(suppl):S7–S21.

Erlebacher A, Filvaroff EH, Gitelman SE, Derynck R: Toward a molecular understanding of skeletal development. *Cell* 1995;80:371–378.

Glowacki J: Editorial: The early revascularization of membranous bone. *Plast Reconstr Surg* 1985;76:515–516.

Heinegard D, Oldberg A: Structure and biology of cartilage and bone matrix noncollagenous macromolecules. *FASEB J* 1989;3:2042–2051.

Hinchliffe JR, Johnson DR (eds): *The Development of the Vertebrate Limb: An Approach Through Experiment, Genetics, and Evolution.* Oxford, England, Clarendon Press, 1980.

Hunter GK: Role of proteoglycan in the provisional calcification of cartilage: A review and reinterpretation. *Clin Orthop* 1991;262:256–280.

Iannotti JP: Growth plate physiology and pathology. *Orthop Clin North Am* 1990;21:1–17.

Muragaki Y, Mundlos S, Upton J, Olsen BR: Altered growth and branching patterns in synpolydactyly caused by mutations in HOXD13. *Science* 1996;272:548–551.

Poole AR, Matsui Y, Hinek A, Lee ER: Cartilage macromolecules and the calcification of cartilage matrix. *Anat Rec* 1989;224:167–179.

Riddle RD, Johnson RL, Laufer E, Tabin C: Sonic hedgehog mediates the polarizing activity of the ZPA. *Cell* 1993;75:1401–1416.

Riddle RD, Ensini M, Nelson C, Tsuchida T, Jessell TM, Tabin C: Induction of LIM homeobox gene Lmx1 by WNT7a establishes dorsoventral pattern in the vertebrate limb. *Cell* 1995;83:631–640.

Rodan GA, Harada S: The missing bone. *Cell* 1997;89:677–680.

Scott MP: Vertebrate homeobox gene nomenclature. *Cell* 1992;71:551–553.

Sledge CB, Zaleske DJ: Developmental anatomy of joints, in Resnick D, Niwayama G, (eds) *Diagnosis of Bone and Joint Disorders,* ed 2. Philadelphia, PA, WB Saunders, 1988, vol 2, pp 604–624.

Trippel SB: Basic science of the growth plate. *Curr Opin Orthop* 1990;1:279–288.

Structure, Function, and Biochemistry of the Normal Growth Plate

Zaleske DJ: Cartilage and bone development, in Cannon WD Jr (ed): *Instructional Course Lectures 47.* Rosemont, IL, American Academy of Orthopaedic Surgeons, 1998, pp 461–468.

Brighton CT: Longitudinal bone growth: The growth plate and its dysfunctions, in Griffin PP (ed): *Instructional Course Lectures XXXVI.* Park Ridge, IL, American Academy of Orthopaedic Surgeons, 1987, pp 3–25.

Brown CC, Hembry RM, Reynolds JJ: Immunolocalization of metalloproteinases and their inhibitor in the rabbit growth plate. *J Bone Joint Surg* 1989;71A:580–593.

Hunziker EB, Schenk RK, Cruz-Orive LM: Quantitation of chondrocyte performance in growth-plate cartilage during longitudinal bone growth. *J Bone Joint Surg* 1987;69A:162–173.

Lanske B, Karaplis AC, Lee K, et al: PTH/PTHrP receptor in early development and Indian hedgehog-regulated bone growth. *Science* 1996;273:663–666.

Le Merrer M, Rousseau F, Legeai-Mallet L, et al: A gene for achondroplasia-hypochondroplasia maps to chromosome 4p. *Nat Genet* 1994;6:318–321.

Rimoin DL: Molecular defects in the chondrodysplasias. *Am J Med Genet* 1996;63:106–110.

Schipani E, Kruse K, Juppner H: A constitutively active mutant PTH-PTHrP receptor in Jansen-type metaphyseal chondrodysplasia. *Science* 1995;268:98–100.

Shapiro F, Holtrop ME, Glimcher MJ: Organization and cellular biology of the perichondrial ossification groove of Ranvier: A morphological study in rabbits. *J Bone Joint Surg* 1977;59A:703–723.

Shiang R, Thompson LM, Zhu Y-Z, et al: Mutations in the transmembrane domain of FGFR3 cause the most common genetic form of dwarfism, achondroplasia. *Cell* 1994;78:335–342.

Vortkamp A, Lee K, Lanske B, Segre GV, Kronenberg HM, Tabin CJ: Regulation of rate of cartilage differentiation by Indian hedgehog and PTH-related protein. *Science* 1996;273:613–622.

Warman ML, Abbott M, Apte SS, et al: A type X collagen mutation causes Schmid metaphyseal chondrodysplasia. *Nat Genet* 1993;5: 79–82.

Wilsman NJ, Farnum CE, Leiferman EM, Fry M, Barreto C: Differential growth by growth plates as a function of multiple parameters of chondrocytic kinetics. *J Orthop Res* 1996;14:927–936.

Growth Plate Mineralization

Boskey AL, Maresca M, Armstrong AL, Ehrlich MG: Treatment of proteoglycan aggregates with physeal enzymes reduces their ability to inhibit hydroxyapatite proliferation in a gelatin gel. *J Orthop Res* 1992;10:313–319.

Brighton CT, Hunt RM: Mitochondrial calcium and its role in calcification: Histochemical localization of calcium in electron micrographs of the epiphyseal growth plate with K-pyroantimonate. *Clin Orthop* 1974;100:406–416.

Buckwalter JA: Proteoglycan structure in calcifying cartilage. *Clin Orthop* 1983;172:207–232.

Buckwalter JA, Glimcher MJ, Cooper RR, Recker R: Bone biology: Part I: Structure, blood supply, cells, matrix, and mineralization. *J Bone Joint Surg* 1995;77A:1256–1275.

Poole AR, Pidoux I, Reiner A, Choi H, Rosenberg LC: Association of an extracellular protein (chondrocalcin) with the calcification of cartilage in endochondral bone formation. *J Cell Biol* 1984;98:54–65.

Effect of Hormones and Growth Factors on the Growth Plate

Atkin I, Pita JC, Ornoy A, Agundez A, Castiglione G, Howell DS: Effects of vitamin D metabolites on healing of low phosphate, vitamin D-deficient induced rickets in rats. *Bone* 1985;6:113–123.

Balogh K Jr, Kunin AS: The effect of cortisone on the metabolism of epiphyseal cartilage: A histochemical study. *Clin Orthop* 1971;80: 208–215.

Barling PM, Bibby NJ: Study of the localization of [3H]-bovine parathyroid hormone in bone by light microscope autoradiography. *Calcif Tissue Int* 1985;37:441–446.

Bauer GC, Carlson A, Linquist B: Evaluation of accretion, resorption and exchange reactions in the skeleton. *Kungl Fysiogr Sallsakp Lund Forhandl* 1955;25:1–16.

Burch WM, Corda G: Calcitonin stimulates maturation of mammalian growth plate cartilage. *Endocrinology* 1985;116:1724–1728.

Burch WM, Van Wyk JJ: Triiodothyronine stimulates cartilage growth and maturation by different mechanisms. *Am J Physiol* 1987;252: E176–E182.

Canalis E: Effect of growth factors on bone cell replication and differentiation. *Clin Orthop* 1985;193:246–263.

Canalis E, McCarthy T, Centrella M: Growth factors and the regulation of bone remodeling. *J Clin Invest* 1988;81:277–281.

Carrascosa A, Audi L, Ferrandez MA, Ballabriga A: Biological effects of androgens and identification of specific dihydrotestosterone-binding sites in cultured human fetal epiphyseal chondrocytes. *J Clin Endocrinol Metab* 1990;70:134–140.

Chandrasekhar S, Harvey AK: Transforming growth factor-beta is a potent inhibitor of IL-1 induced protease activity and cartilage proteoglycan degradation. *Biochem Biophys Res Commun* 1988;157: 1352–1359.

Corvol MT, Carrascosa A, Tsagris L, Blanchard O, Rappaport R: Evidence for a direct in vitro action of sex steroids on rabbit cartilage cells during skeletal growth: Influence of age and sex. *Endocrinology* 1987;120:1422–1429.

Dearden LC, Mosier HD Jr, Brundage M, Thai C, Jansons R: The effects of different steroids on costal and epiphyseal cartilage of fetal and adult rats. *Cell Tissue Res* 1986;246:401–412.

Dorfman A, Schiller S: Effects of hormones on the metabolism of acid mucopolysaccharides of connective tissue. *Recent Prog Horm Res* 1958;14:427–456.

Fahmy A, Talley P, Frazier HM, Hillman JW: Ultrastructural effects of estrogen on epiphyseal cartilage. *Calcif Tissue Res* 1971;7:139–149.

Fine N, Binderman I, Somjen D, Earon y, Edelstein S, Weisman Y: Autoradiographic localization of 24R,25-dihydroxyvitamin D 3 in epiphyseal cartilage. *Bone* 1985;6:99–104.

Goldstein S, Unterman TG, Phillips LS: Nutrition and somatomedin: XV. Growth plate, growth factor and biologically active somatomedins in rats with streptozotocin-induced diabetes. *Ann Nutr Metab* 1987;31:367–377.

Iannotti JP, Brighton CT, Iannotti V, Ohishi T: Mechanism of action of parathyroid hormone-induced proteoglycan synthesis in the growth plate chondrocyte. *J Orthop Res* 1990;8:136–145.

Isaksson O, Binder C, Hall K, Hokfelt B (eds): *Growth Hormone: Basic and Clinical Aspects*. Amsterdam, The Netherlands, Excerpta Medica, 1987.

Jingushi S, Scully SP, Joyce ME, Sugioka Y, Bolander ME: Transforming growth factor-(1 and fibroblast growth factors in rat growth plate. *J Orthop Res* 1995;13:761–768.

Kapur SP, Reddi AH: Influence of testosterone and dihydrotestosterone on bone-matrix induced endochondral bone formation. *Calcif Tissue Int* 1989;44:108–113.

Loder RT, Wittenberg B, DeSilva G: Slipped capital femoral epiphysis associated with endocrine disorders. *J Pediatr Orthop* 1995;15:349–356.

Maor G, Silbermann M: In vitro effects of glucocorticoid hormones on the synthesis of DNA in cartilage of neonatal mice. *FEBS Lett* 1981;129:256–260.

Martineau-Doize B, Lai WH, Warshawsky H, Gergeron JJ: In vivo demonstration of cell types in bone that harbor epidermal growth factor receptors. *Endocrinology* 1988;123:841–858.

Nilsson A, Isgaard J, Lindahl A, Dahlstrom A, Skottner A, Isaksson OG: Regulation by growth hormone of number of chondrocytes containing IGF-I in rat growth plate. *Science* 1986;233:571–574.

Ogden JA, Southwick WO: Endocrine dysfunction and slipped capital femoral epiphysis. *Yale J Biol Med* 1977;50:1–16.

O'Keefe RJ, Crabb ID, Puzas JE, Rosier RN: Effects of transforming growth factor-(1 and fibroblast growth factor on DNA synthesis in growth plate chondrocytes are enhanced by insulin-like growth factor-I. *J Orthop Res* 1994;12:299–310.

O'Keefe RJ, Crabb ID, Puzas JE, Rosier RN: The influence of prostaglandins on DNA and matrix synthesis by growth plate chondrocytes. *Trans Orthop Res Soc* 1989;14:535.

O'Keefe RJ, Puzas JE, Brand JS, Rosier RN: Effects of transforming growth factor-beta on matrix synthesis by chick growth plate chondrocytes. *Endocrinology* 1988;122:2953–2961.

Preece MA: The effect of administered corticosteroids on the growth of children. *Postgrad Med J* 1976;52:625–630.

Ray RD, Asling CW, Walker DG, Simpson ME, Li CH, Evans HM: Growth and differentiation of the skeleton in thyroidectomized-hypophysectomized rats treated with thyroxin, growth hormone, and the combination. *J Bone Joint Surg* 1954;36A:94–103.

Salmon WD Jr, Daughaday WH: A hormonally controlled serum factor which stimulates sulfate incorporation by cartilage in vitro. *J Lab Clin Med* 1957;49:825–836.

Simon MR, Cooke PS: Cellular heterogeneity and insulin-like growth factor I immunoreactivity among epiphysial growth plate chondrocytes in the pig. *Acta Anat (Basel)* 1988;133:66–69.

Sporn MB, Roberts AB (eds): *Handbook of Experimental Pharmacology: Peptide Growth Factors and Their Receptors, Parts I and II.* Berlin, Germany, Springer-Verlag, vol 95, 1990.

Tapp E: The effects of hormones on bone in growing rats. *J Bone Joint Surg* 1966;48B:526–531.

Trippel SB, Chernausek SD, Van Wyk JJ, Moses AC, Mankin HJ: Demonstration of type I and type II somatomedin receptors on bovine growth plate chondrocytes. *J Orthop Res* 1988;6:817–826.

Trippel SB, Wroblewski J, Makower AM, Whelan MC, Schoenfeld D, Doctrow SR: Regulation of growth-plate chondrocytes by insulin-like growth-factor I and basic fibroblast growth factor. *J Bone Joint Surg* 1993;75A:177–189.

Ueno K, Haba T, Woodbury D, Price P, Anderson R, Jee WS: The effects of prostaglandin E2 in rapidly growing rats: Depressed longitudinal and radial growth and increased metaphyseal hard tissue mass. *Bone* 1985;6:79–86.

Uhthoff HK, Wiley JJ (eds): *Behavior of the Growth Plate.* New York, NY, Raven Press, 1988.

Vetter U, Zapf J, Heit W, et al: Human fetal and adult chondrocytes: Effect of insulin-like growth factors I and II, insulin, and growth hormone on clonal growth. *J Clin Invest* 1986;77:1903–1908.

Weintroub S, Wahl LM, Feuerstein N, Winter CC, Reddi AH: Changes in tissue concentration of prostaglandins during endochondral bone differentiation. *Biochem Biophys Res Commun* 1983;117:746–750.

Wu LN, Sauer GR, Genge BR, Wuthier RE: Induction of mineral deposition by primary cultures of chicken growth plate chondrocytes in ascorbate-containing media: Evidence of an association between matrix vesicles and collagen. *J Biol Chem* 1989;264:21346–21355.

The Mechanical Properties of the Growth Plate and Its Response to Mechanical Stimuli

Amamilo SC, Bader DL, Houghton GR: The periosteum in growth plate failure. *Clin Orthop* 1985;194:293–305.

Arkin AM, Katz JF: The effects of pressure on epiphyseal growth: The mechanism of plasticity of growing bone. *J Bone Joint Surg* 1956;38A:1056–1076.

Blount WP, Clarke GR: Control of bone growth by epiphyseal stapling: A preliminary report. *J Bone Joint Surg* 1949;31A:464–478.

Bonnel F, Peruchon E, Baldet P, Dimeglio A, Rabischong P: Effects of compression on growth plates in the rabbit. *Acta Orthop Scand* 1983;54:730–733.

Brashear HR Jr: Epiphyseal fractures: A microscopic study of the healing process in rats. *J Bone Joint Surg* 1959;41A:1055–1064.

Bright RW, Elmore SM: Physical properties of epiphyseal plate cartilage. *Surg Forum* 1968;19:463–464.

Bright RW, Burstein AH, Elmore SM: Epiphyseal-plate cartilage: A biomechanical and histological analysis of failure modes. *J Bone Joint Surg* 1974;56A:688–703.

Brown TD, Singerman RJ: Experimental determination of the linear biphasic constitutive coefficients of human fetal proximal femoral chondroepiphysis. *J Biomech* 1986;19:597–605.

Carter DR: Mechanical loading history and skeletal biology. *J Biomech* 1987;20:1095–1109.

Carter DR, Orr TE, Fyhrie DP, Schurman DJ: Influences of mechanical stress on prenatal and postnatal skeletal development. *Clin Orthop* 1987;219:237–250.

Carter DR, Wong M: Mechanical stresses and endochondral ossification in the chondroepiphysis. *J Orthop Res* 1988;6:148–154.

Chung SM, Batterman SC, Brighton CT: Shear strength of the human femoral capital epiphyseal plate. *J Bone Joint Surg* 1976;58A:94–103.

Cohen B, Chorney GS, Phillips DP, et al: The microstructural tensile properties and biochemical composition of the bovine distal femoral growth plate. *J Orthop Res* 1992;10:263–275.

Elmer EB, Ehrlich MG, Zaleske DJ, Polsky C, Mankin HJ: Chondrodiatasis in rabbits: A study of the effect of transphyseal bone lengthening on cell division, synthetic function, and microcirculation in the growth plate. *J Pediatr Orthop* 1992;12:181–190.

Frost HM: A chondral modeling theory. *Calcif Tissue Int* 1979;28:181–200.

Glucksmann A: The role of mechanical stresses in bone formation in vitro. *J Anat* 1942;76:231–239.

Glücksmann A: Studies on bone mechanics in vitro: II. The role of tension and pressure in chondrogenesis. *Anat Rec* 1939;73:39–55.

Gray ML, Pizzanelli AM, Grodzinsky AJ, Lee RC: Mechanical and physiochemical determinants of the chondrocyte biosynthetic response. *J Orthop Res* 1988;6:777–792.

Gray ML, Pizzanelli AM, Lee RC, Grodzinsky AJ, Swann DA: Kinetics of the chondrocyte biosynthetic response to compressive load and release. *Biochim Biophys Acta* 1989;991:415–425.

Greco F, de Palma L, Specchia N, Mannarini M: Growth-plate cartilage metabolic response to mechanical stress. *J Pediatr Orthop* 1989;9:520–524.

Haas SL: Retardation of bone growth by a wire loop. *J Bone Joint Surg* 1945;27:25–36.

Haas SL: The localization of the growing point in the epiphyseal cartilage plate of bones. *Am J Orthop Surg* 1973;15:563–586.

Hall BK: In vitro studies on the mechanical evocation of adventitious cartilage in the chick. *J Exp Zool* 1968;168:283–305.

Hall BK: Immobilization and cartilage transformation into bone in the embryonic chick. *Anat Rec* 1972;173:391–403.

Houghton GR, Rooker GD: The role of the periosteum in the growth of long bones: An experimental study in the rabbit. *J Bone Joint Surg* 1979;61B:218–220.

Jaramillo D, Laor T, Zaleske DJ: Indirect trauma to the growth plate: Results of MR imaging after epiphyseal and metaphyseal injury in rabbits. *Radiology* 1993;187:171–178.

Jenkins DH, Cheng DH, Hodgson AR: Stimulation of bone growth by periosteal stripping: A clinical study. *J Bone Joint Surg* 1975;57B:482–484.

Jones IL, Klamfeldt A, Sandstrom T: The effect of continuous mechanical pressure upon the turnover of articular cartilage proteoglycans in vitro. *Clin Orthop* 1982;165:283–289.

Klein-Nulend J, Veldhuijzen JP, Burger EH: Increased calcification of growth plate cartilage as a result of compressive force in vitro. *Arthritis Rheum* 1986;29:1002–1009.

Lee KE, Pelker RR, Rudicel SA, Ogden JA, Panjabi MM: Histologic patterns of capital femoral growth plate fracture in the rabbit: The effect of shear direction. *J Pediatr Orthop* 1985;5:32–39.

Mankin KP, Zaleske DJ: Response of physeal cartilage to low-level compression and tension in organ culture. *J Pediatr Orthop* 1998;18:145–148.

Moen CT, Pelker RR: Biomechanical and histological correlations in growth plate failure. *J Pediatr Orthop* 1984;4:180–184.

Morscher E: Strength and morphology of growth cartilage under hormonal influence of puberty: Animal experiments and clinical study on the etiology of local growth disorders during puberty. *Reconstr Surg Traumatol* 1968;10:3–104.

Morscher E, Desaulles PA, Schenk R: Experimental studies on tensile strength and morphology of the epiphyseal cartilage at puberty. *Ann Paediatr (Basel)* 1965;205:112–130.

Mow VC, Proctor CS, Kelly MA: Biomechanics of articular cartilage, in Nordin M, Frankel VH, (eds): *Basic Biomechanics of the Musculoskeletal System*, ed 2. Philadelphia, PA, Lea & Febiger, 1989, pp 31–58.

Ogden JA: Injury to the growth mechanisms of the immature skeleton. *Skeletal Radiol* 1981;6:237–253.

Porter RW: The effect of tension across a growing epiphysis. *J Bone Joint Surg* 1978;60B:252–255.

Rudicel S, Pelker RR, Lee KE, Ogden JA, Panjabi MM: Shear fractures through the capital femoral physis of the skeletally immature rabbit. *J Pediatr Orthop* 1985;5:27–31.

Ryoppy S, Karaharju EO: Alteration of epiphyseal growth by an experimentally produced angular deformity. *Acta Orthop Scand* 1974;45:490–498.

Sah RY, Kim YJ, Doong JY, Grodzinsky AJ, Plaas AH, Sandy JD: Biosynthetic response of cartilage explants to dynamic compression. *J Orthop Res* 1989;7:619–636.

Salter RB, Harris WR: Injuries involving the epiphyseal plate. *J Bone Joint Surg* 1963;45A:587–622.

Siffert RS: The effect of staples and longitudinal wires on epiphyseal growth: An experimental study. *J Bone Joint Surg* 1956;38A:1077–1088.

Simon MR, Holmes KR: The effects of simulated increases in body weight on the developing rat tibia: A histologic study. *Acta Anat (Basel)* 1985;122:105–109.

Smith WS, Cunningham JB: The effect of alternating distracting forces on the epiphyseal plates of calves: A preliminary report. *Clin Orthop* 1957;10:125–130.

Smith JW: The relationship of epiphysial plates to stress in some bones of the lower limb. *J Anat* 1962;96:58–78.

Smith JW: The structure and stress relations of fibrous epiphysial plates. *J Anat* 1962;96:209–225.

Van Kampen GP, Veldhuijzen JP, Kuijer R, van de Stadt RJ, Schipper CA: Cartilage response to mechanical force in high-density chondrocyte cultures. *Arthritis Rheum* 1985;28:419–424.

Warrell E, Taylor JF: The role of periosteal tension in the growth of long bones. *J Anat* 1979;128:179–184.

Pathologic States Primarily Affecting the Growth Plate

Boden SD, Kaplan FS, Fallon MD, et al. Metatropic dwarfism: Uncoupling of endochondral and perichondral growth. *J Bone Joint Surg* 1987;69A:174–184.

Briggs MD, Choi H, Warman ML, et al: Genetic mapping of a locus for multiple epiphyseal dysplasia (EDM2) to a region of chromosome 1 containing a type IX collagen gene. *Am J Hum Genet* 1994;55:678–684.

Cole WG: Etiology and pathogenesis of heritable connective tissue diseases. *J Pediatr Orthop* 1993;13:392–403.

Hastbacka J, de la Chapelle A, Mahtani MM, et al: The diastrophic dysplasia gene encodes a novel sulfate transporter: Positional cloning by fine-structure linkage disequilibrium mapping. *Cell* 1994;78:1073–1087.

Maynard JA, Ippolito EG, Ponseti IV, Mickelson MR: Histochemistry and ultrastructure of the growth plate in achondroplasia. *J Bone Joint Surg* 1981;63A:969–979.

Mundlos S, Otto F, Mundlos C et al: Mutations involving the transcription factor CBFA1 cause cleidocranial dysplasia. *Cell* 1997;89:773–779.

Neufeld EF, Muenzer J: The mucopolysaccharidoses, in Scriver CR, Beaudet AL, Sly WS, Valle D (eds): *The Metabolic and Molecular Bases of Inherited Disease*, ed 7. New York, NY, McGraw-Hill, 1995, vol 2, pp 2465–2494.

Rimoin DL, Cohn DH, Eyre D: Clinical-molecular correlations in the skeletal dysplasias. *Pediatr Radiol* 1994;24:425–426.

Shapiro F: Osteopetrosis: Current clinical considerations. *Clin Orthop* 1993;294:34–44.

Shapiro F, Simon S, Glimcher MJ: Hereditary multiple exostoses: Anthropometric, roentgenographic, and clinical aspects. *J Bone Joint Surg* 1979;61A:815–824.

Spranger J: Pattern recognition in bone dysplasias, in Papadatos CJ, Bartsocas CS (eds): *Endocrine Genetics and Genetics of Growth*. New York, NY, Alan R. Liss, 1985, pp 315–342.

Spranger J, Winterpacht A, Zabel B: The type II collagenopathies: A spectrum of chondrodysplasias. *Eur J Pediatr* 1994;153:56–65.

Stanescu V, Stanescu R, Maroteaux P: Pathogenic mechanisms in osteochondrodysplasias. *J Bone Joint Surg* 1984;66A:817–836.

Tsukurov O, Boehmer A, Flynn J, et al: A complex bilateral polysyndactyly disease locus maps to chromosome 7q36. *Nat Genet* 1994;6:282–286.

Zaleske DJ: Metabolic and endocrine abnormalities, in Morrissy RT, Weinstein SL (eds): *Lovell and Winter's Pediatric Orthopaedics*, ed 4. Philadelphia, PA, Lippincott-Raven, 1996, pp 137–201.

Chapter 4

Update on the Genetic Basis of Disorders With Orthopaedic Manifestations

Frederick R. Dietz, MD

Jeffrey C. Murray, MD

This chapter at a glance

This chapter summarizes current genetic information about disorders with orthopaedic manifestations.

Introduction

New technology in molecular biology and quantitative analysis has led to an explosion in the knowledge and understanding of inherited diseases. Efforts to map the entire human genome are ahead of schedule. Gene therapy is being investigated for a host of diseases ranging from cystic fibrosis to cancer. Presymptomatic diagnosis is possible for people at risk for some diseases with delayed onset, such as Huntington's disease, Alzheimer's disease, and familial breast cancer.

Molecular advances in the 1980s made it feasible to sequence the 3 billion nucleotides of DNA that make up the human genome. International efforts, called the Human Genome Project, initiated under the auspices of the Human Gene Mapping Conferences, were formalized through the Human Genome Organization (HUGO). In the United States, the efforts have been jointly funded and coordinated by the National Institutes of Health and the Department of Energy since 1990, although private organizations also play a prominent role. In addition to the support for scientific inquiry, the National Institutes of Health and the Department of Energy allocate approximately 5% of their funding for study of the ethical, legal, and social issues relating to the human genome project.

During the first 5 years of funding, significant progress was made toward the development of high-resolution genetic maps, improvements in analytic strategies, and tremendous increases in the numbers of available polymorphic markers, physical mapping reagents, and genes. Genetic mapping provides a rough approximation of the location of a gene to a region on one of the 23 pairs of chromosomes. The next phase, physical mapping, identifies the gene exactly and gives its DNA sequence and structure. Presently genetic maps composed of markers that are easy to use, inexpensive, and efficient (ie, polymerase chain reaction [PCR]-based) make the mapping of genes in a few years practical by even modest-sized investigative groups. This is in contrast with the hundreds of person-years required in earlier successful searches, such as finding the causative gene for cystic fibrosis. Similarly, advances in analysis allow the practical study of even complex disorders such as clubfoot or scoliosis. Tremendous strides in physical maps mean that once a gene is localized by genetic mapping the gene itself may be identified more quickly. There is now an emphasis on finding and mapping all of the approximately 80,000 human genes, along with mouse homologs. The effort to complete the full human DNA sequence is well advanced and is targeted for completion in a rough draft form by 2001. In the last 5 years alone, the numbers of polymorphisms has increased from 2,000 to 15,000; the number of mapped genes from 1,500 to over 30,000; and the amount of DNA sequenced in humans from 5 million to over 200 million base pairs.

Disease-causing genes have been identified or localized for many conditions, including skeletal dysplasia (achondroplasia, pseudoachondroplasia, spondyloepiphyseal dysplasia, multiple epiphyseal dysplasia, diastrophic dysplasia, metaphyseal chondrodysplasia, precocious osteoarthritis); connective tissue disorders (Marfan syndrome, Ehlers-Danlos disease); metabolic diseases (hypophosphatemic rickets, osteoporosis, osteopetrosis); muscular dystrophies (Duchenne and Becker, facioscapulohumeral dystrophy, limb girdle dystrophy, myotonic dystrophy); peripheral neuropathies (Charcot-Marie-Tooth); and syndromes with orthopaedic manifestations (Apert syndrome, McCune-Albright polyostotic fibrous dysplasia, distal arthrogryposis). The mechanisms by which mutations in the disease-causing genes result in the disease phenotype are being actively investigated. These investigations are producing new information concerning the biology of normal and abnormal growth and development and tissue function at the molecular level.

Gene mapping and identification is only the initial step in understanding the complex biologic interactions that must be defined to make use of this information in a therapeutic way. After a disease gene is identified, cell biologists, embryologists, biochemists, clinicians, anatomists, physiologists, and others must work together to make sense of these preliminary data in a way that will benefit patients and their families.

It is important for the orthopaedic surgeon to be aware of the genetic cause of a disease in order to make appropriate referrals for genetic counseling, and to make specific diagnoses based on genotype as well as phenotype so that the prognosis for many disorders can be refined. Awareness of investigations in progress will allow more collaboration with researchers. A single patient with a rare translocation or deletion can provide the key for identifying a disease-causing gene, as occurred in the search for the gene causing Duchenne muscular dystrophy. Knowledge of primarily orthopaedic disorders can aid in the search for their causes. Accuracy in diagnosis in the patients studied is vital in the common approaches used for isolating disease-causing genes. Assigning the correct diagnosis is not always straightforward. Identification of an idiopathic clubfoot is more readily done by an orthopaedist than a pediatrician or geneticist. Including the wrong diseases in a genetic analysis (misascertainment) can delay diagnosis or mislead the investigator. Furthermore, knowledge of the pathology of orthopaedic disorders can help in the selection of appropriate candidate genes for investigation.

The approach most commonly used to find a new gene is positional cloning (previously called reverse genetics). This is done by finding an allele of a polymorphic marker of known location that is inherited with the disease in a family more commonly than would occur by chance. This statistical inference suggests that the disease gene is near the polymorphic marker. The marker and the disease are said to be linked. Sets of highly polymorphic markers are available that allow rapid screening of the entire genome in disorders with mendelian inheritance for which large families are available to establish linkage.

After the approximate chromosomal location is found by linkage, genes in this region are physically isolated. When a biologically plausible gene is shown to be mutated in patients with the disease, and no mutations are found in unaffected individuals it is probable that this is the causative gene. If confirmed, the possibility exists for diagnostic testing of individuals based on analysis of their DNA or the protein product of the gene.

Other approaches to identifying disease-causing genes exist. The candidate gene approach may prove more valuable than positional cloning in orthopaedic disorders with complex inheritance patterns. Families with many affected members, a necessary factor for standard linkage analysis, are rare in disorders with complex inheritance. The candidate gene approach uses an understanding of the biology of the disorder to suggest genes that may be involved in pathogenesis. Polymorphisms in the candidate genes are directly investigated by a variety of statistical techniques (ie, association studies and affected pedigree member analysis) to determine if a specific allele of the candidate gene is inherited by people affected by the disorder more commonly than would occur by chance.

Population-based association analysis is a case-control method using only the biologically affected persons in a family. It relies on a nonrandom similarity in polymorphisms present in the candidate gene when compared to an ethnically similar but unrelated control population. In other words, the frequency of a particular polymorphism at a candidate gene is compared between affected people and unrelated controls. The best known and documented associations are between the HLA blood antigens and insulin-dependent diabetes mellitus, multiple sclerosis, duodenal ulcers, and Graves' disease. A potentially major problem with the population-based association study is the choice of an appropriate control group. Ethnic differences between families with affected members and the controls (population stratification) may result in false positive or false negative associations. One solution is the use of parental alleles at the marker locus of interest that are transmitted to the affected children as "case" alleles and the parental alleles that are not transmitted to the affected children as the "control" alleles. By using these haplotype relative risk and related methods, problems with a noncomparable control population are avoided.

Affected-sib-pair analysis is a widely used and powerful technique for linkage analysis. The method is based on a comparison of the observed and expected distributions of the number of alleles shared by affected siblings. A great increase in the observed allele sharing among affected relatives over that expected of a particular marker is evidence of linkage. This is an optimal method for establishing lineage in disorders of complex inheritance, such as clubfoot, for which large pedigrees with multiple affected members are rarely available to perform standard linkage analysis.

New, efficient methods that combine elements of different analytic techniques offer promise for increasing the pace of disease-causing gene identification. For example, an analytic strategy called shared segment analysis has been used successfully to localize a susceptibility locus in nonsyndromic atrioventricular canal defects, Hirschsprung's disease, hereditary ataxia, and recurrent intrahepatic cholestasis.

The strategy is based on the fact that if a necessary (but not sufficient) locus exists for the occurrence of a disorder of complex inheritance, affected individuals should share alleles in a segment of the genome containing the locus. Genotyping DNA from a few distantly related affected individuals with densely spaced short tandem repeat polymorphisms will give numerous alleles for which the affected individuals are identical by state. By examining the haplotypes of markers in these regions, the markers for which the affected individuals are identical by descent can be determined. Clusters of contiguous alleles that are shared by the affected individuals are then sought, which further reduces the number of candidate regions. Genotyping with additional markers between and flanking the shared contiguous markers establishes a suspected susceptibility locus.

This chapter will summarize current genetic information about disorders with orthopaedic manifestations. For many of the listed disorders the specific gene is not known; only an approximate location has been found. Between the time of submission and publication of this chapter, additional disorders will be localized or the specific gene identified. There are numerous on-line services that allow access to public information and services relevant to genetics, ranging from the clinically oriented to ones specific for the molecular biology of particular organisms such as the fruit fly or yeast. One database that contains a wealth of clinical data on specific syndromes of all types is Online Mendelian Inheritance in Man (OMIM), which provides profiles of specific disorders with clinical and gene mapping data, and an extensive list of references. It can be searched using key words. It is found on the World Wide Web at: http://www3.ncbi.nlm.nih.gov/omim/

A second resource is a GeneTests database of laboratories doing research and/or clinical testing for specific disorders. GeneTests can provide contacts if a physician is interested in testing a particular family or learning if any groups are doing research on a rare disorder. It can be accessed at: http://healthlinks.washington.edu/helix

Skeletal Dysplasias

Fibroblast Growth Factor Receptor 3 Disorders

Achondroplasia, the most common form of dwarfism, is an autosomal dominant disorder. The majority of affected individuals represent new mutations. In a study that attempted to ascertain all dwarfs in the state of Victoria, Australia, only 2 of 60 achondroplasts had a positive family history. In another study, there were 31 familial cases of achondroplasia out of 148 achondroplasts attending regional and national meetings of the Little People of America. People with achondroplasia often have varus deformity of the legs and are at risk for atlantoaxial instability and spinal stenosis. The cause of achondroplasia is a point mutation in the gene coding for fibroblast growth factor receptor 3 (FGFR3). This mutation is almost always (~98%) at the same nucleotide (number 1138) and causes a single amino acid change (arginine to glycine) in the transmembrane portion of this cell surface receptor. This receptor is expressed in all prebone cartilage as well as diffusely in the central nervous system. The remarkable homogeneity of the phenotype in achondroplasia results from the remarkable homogeneity of the mutation in this disorder. No other autosomal dominant disorder whose gene defect is known has such a homogeneous mutation. In fact, this is the most mutable single nucleotide known in the entire human genome.

The function of FGFR3 has been studied in mice by disrupting the normal gene. Mice deficient in FGFR3 have elongated vertebral columns and long bone because of accelerated and prolonged growth compared to normal mice. Malfunction of the FGFR3 causes inhibition of chondrocyte proliferation in the proliferative zone of the physis. Thus, FGFR3 seems to regulate bone growth by limiting endochondral ossification. A possible explanation for the dwarfing phenotype in humans with an abnormal gene for FGFR3 is that the human mutation results in a receptor that is active even without the binding of a fibroblast growth factor ligand to the receptor. The receptor function in limiting endochondral ossification is overactive (called a gain of function mutation).

Hypochondroplasia is similar to achondroplasia, except for milder dwarfing and normal skulls and facies in affected persons. Associated problems, such as spinal stenosis and severe genu varum, are less common in hypochondroplasia. Most people with this disorder who have been studied have a mutation of the FGFR3 gene, as do those with achondroplasia. The mutation in hypochondroplasia affects the tyrosine kinase domain instead of the transmembrane domain of FGFR3 found in achondroplasia.

Thanatophoric dysplasia, the most common neonatal lethal skeletal dysplasia, is also caused by a mutation of the FGFR3 gene. This association was suggested by a phenotypic similarity between thanatophoric dysplasia and homozygous achondroplasia.

Although most syndromes with craniosynostosis are caused by a mutation in FGFR1 or FGFR2, a new craniosynostosis syndrome has been identified with a mutation of FGFR3. This syndrome has been defined in 61 individuals from 20 unrelated families, all of whom have a single amino acid substitution. All affected individuals have coronal synostosis. Variable features include abnormalities of the hands and feet, including syndactyly, brachydactyly, thimble-like middle phalanges, cone epiphyses, and carpal and tarsal fusions. A small number of individuals have delayed development and/or sensorineural hearing loss. Affected individuals have normal stature, which differentiates this disorder from other known FGFR3 disorders. Interestingly, the mutation occurs between the second and third immunoglobulin-like domains of the FGFR3 protein, which is analogous to the location of mutations in FGFR1 and FGFR2, which cause Pfeiffer and Apert syndromes.

Cartilage Oligomeric Protein Disorders

Pseudoachondroplasia is one of the more common skeletal dysplasias and is characterized by disproportionate short-limbed dwarfism and ligamentous laxity. Pseudoachondroplasia is not clinically apparent at birth, although platyspondyly is evident on radiographs. Growth retardation becomes apparent between 1 and 3 years of age. The disproportionate limb shortness increases with growth. The hands and feet are short and broad. The facies are normal but tend to resemble those of other pseudoachondroplasia patients.

Electron microscopy demonstrates dilated rough endoplasmic reticulum containing material that shows a laminar structure in epiphyseal and physeal chondrocytes. Immunostaining suggests that this material includes proteoglycan link protein and aggrecan. Accumulation of structurally abnormal cartilage oligometric matrix protein (COMP) is also likely. The cause of this disorder, however, is a mutation in the calmodulin-like calcium binding region of the gene coding for COMP. The mutations causing pseudoachondroplasia are deletions or alterations causing important changes in protein structure. This protein is present at high levels in the territorial matrix of cartilage. The mechanism by which this defective gene causes pseudoachondroplasia is speculative. It may be the result of a disruption of calcium-dependent proteoglycan binding by COMP, which might result in proteoglycan accumulation in chondrocytes, giving the typical endoplasmic reticulum findings. Although most cases of pseudoachondroplasia are new mutations, it is a dominant disorder caused by the pentameric structure of COMP. Only 3% of COMP molecules would have 5 normal subunits. This results, therefore, in a "dominant negative" effect on COMP function.

Whether inadequate COMP reaches the extraterritorial matrix or adequate amounts of defective COMP are present in the extraterritorial matrix is unknown.

Multiple epiphyseal dysplasia denotes a group of disorders with dysplasia of the epiphyses of the tubular bones and normal or near-normal vertebrae. Dwarfing is mild and presentation varies from childhood (a waddling gait and difficulties with running or stair climbing) to adulthood (premature osteoarthritis). Pain, limp, or decreased range of motion in the weightbearing joints are symptoms that prompt evaluation.

Several disorders with different causes are subsumed under the multiple epiphyseal dysplasia (MED) label. One such disorder (MED 1) that shows dilated rough endoplasmic reticulum with lamellar inclusions (similar to those seen in pseudoachondroplasia) has a known cause; it is a mutation in the gene coding for COMP. The mutations occur in the calmodulin-like domain as in pseudoachondroplasia, but appear to cause a more subtle structural alteration in the protein. Presumably, different sorts of mutations in the COMP gene result in the differing phenotypes of MED 1 and pseudoachondroplasia.

A second form of multiple epiphyseal dysplasia (MED 2) is caused by a mutation in the gene coding for the alpha-2 polypeptide chain of collagen type IX. Collagen IX is located on the surface of collagen II fibrils. Because defects in collagen IX cause early, noninflammatory articular cartilage degeneration in both humans and mice, it is hypothesized that collagen IX is essential in the long-term integrity of articular cartilage. Families with the MED phenotype that are not linked to the genes coding for COMP or collagen IX have been identified.

Type II Collagen Disorders

Collagen type II is the major structural component of cartilage. The structural characteristics of collagen II are affected by water content, proteoglycans, and collagens IX and XI (which bind to the surface of collagen II) as well as other matrix components. Different mutations of collagen II cause chondrodysplasias of varying severity. Single codon mutations causing a substitution of glycine in the triple helix cause 50% of reported mutations. Glycine, the smallest amino acid, is normally present as every third amino acid in the restricted space at the center of the collagen II triple helix. Substitution by bulkier amino acids disrupts the integrity of the collagen fibril. The perinatally lethal collagen II disorders usually have such a substitution of glycine. Other mutations are caused by duplications, deletions, insertions, or premature stop codons that often cause a quantitative defect of collagen II, rather than a severe, structural defect.

The collagen II disorders (also called type II collagenopathies or the spondyloepiphyseal dysplasia family of osteochondrodysplasias) are named descriptively based on phenotypic or radiographic features. Some are commonly referred to by eponym. Increased understanding of the cause of these disorders will lead to improved classification in the near future. Families of chondrodysplasias are being defined because the members all have the same known or presumed abnormal gene. The collagen II family denotes a group of allelic chondrodysplasias that are caused by different mutations in the gene coding for type II collagen. The most severe disorders in this family are the perinatally lethal achondrogenesis type II and hypochondrogenesis.

Spondyloepiphyseal dysplasia congenita, Kniest type spondyloepiphyseal dysplasia, Stickler syndrome (hereditary arthro-ophthalmopathy), and precocious osteoarthropathy are progressively milder disorders. Spondyloepiphyseal dysplasia congenita is characterized by disproportionate short trunk dwarfing. Most of these clinically heterogeneous disorders are evident at birth and are termed congenita. The facies show mild midface flattening. The neck is short and the chest is barrel-shaped. There is usually a thoracolumbar kyphosis with excessive lordosis in walking-age children. Rhizomelic shortening of the limbs is present, with fairly normal appearance of the hands and feet. The vertebral bodies are ovoid in the newborn and become markedly flattened with irregular end plates during childhood. The iliac bones are short and square. The tubular bones are short with mild metaphyseal irregularity. The epiphyses show delayed ossification and are usually fragmented in appearance. These changes are most pronounced in the capital femoral epiphyses. The features of spondyloepiphyseal dysplasia become more apparent with growth. Biochemical investigations of individuals with spondyloepiphyseal dysplasia congenita have shown abnormal α1(II) chains that form triple helical fibrils but make structurally abnormal collagen II. This results in a moderately severe phenotype.

Kniest type spondyloepiphyseal dysplasia is characterized by short stature, disproportionate short trunk, kyphoscoliosis, enlarged and stiff joints, cleft palate, hearing loss, and a flat nasal bridge. Multiple mutations have been identified that cause the Kniest phenotype. Disrupted triple helix formation, abnormal fibril formation, and significant errors in α1(II) chain formation have been found.

Stickler syndrome (hereditary arthro-ophthalmopathy) is an autosomal dominant disorder with myopia, vitreoretinal degeneration, retinal detachment, and premature osteoarthritis. Approximately two thirds of families with this phenotype have a mutation of the collagen II gene.

Stickler syndrome without eye involvement is caused by a gene coding for type XI collagen. This collagen is a minor fibrillar collagen that is important in determining collagen II fiber diameter and orientation. Refined classification based on the gene mutation will enhance diagnostic and prognostic accuracy in individuals with Stickler syndrome.

Osteoarthritis

That osteoarthritis (OA) runs in some families has been long recognized. That some people will never develop OA, barring trauma or infection, is also clear. The age of onset of nontraumatic osteoarthritis varies greatly. OA has been considered a multifactorial disorder; that is, a combination of genetic predisposition and unknown environmental factors has been thought to be the cause. A prospective epidemiologic study of patients undergoing total joint replacement of the hip or knee assessed the heritability of primary OA by comparing siblings of the probands with the probands' spouses. The siblings were at significantly higher risk of having OA than were spouses with a heritability estimate of 27% in this population. Stronger evidence comes from a study of 500 female twins aged 45 to 70 years. Radiographically proven OA was twice as common in the 130 sets of monozygotic twins than in the 120 sets of dizygotic twins. The genetic contribution to the liability to develop OA was estimated to be 35% to 65% in this study.

One reason that disorders with nonmendelian inheritance patterns may be categorized as multifactorial is the mixing of several different disorders, with different causes and different inheritance patterns. It is important to be as specific about the phenotype that causes inclusion in a group as possible. Although all end-stage arthritic joints look alike, perhaps people who develop arthritis in the second to fifth decades of life have a different cause than do people developing arthritic joints in their seventh and eighth decades. This appears to be true in OA.

Familial, generalized precocious OA has been associated with a mutation in the gene coding for collagen II in several large families. Furthermore, a small percentage of primary OA results from a rare allele coding for type II collagen that causes reduced gene expression. Premature OA accompanied by chondrocalcinosis has been localized to chromosome 8. Although specific genetic causes have been identified for only a tiny proportion of OA, discovery of involved genes will provide diagnostic, prognostic, and therapeutic insights. Much of what is now considered primary OA may have a detectable genetic cause or predisposition.

The X-linked form of spondyloepiphyseal dysplasia tarda has been localized to band p22, but the gene has not been identified. This rare disorder is seen in patients with disproportionate short stature who are between 5 and 10 years of age and causes severe degenerative changes of the spine and hips in midlife.

Diastrophic Dysplasia Transporter Disorders

Diastrophic dysplasia is a well characterized skeletal dysplasia featuring short limbs, short stature, kyphoscoliosis, generalized joint dysplasia with limitation of finger flexion, hitchhiker thumbs, and foot deformities ranging from the more common valgus of the hindfoot and adductus of the forefoot to clubfeet. The joint abnormalities in this disorder result in painful OA at an early age. The patients, who are of normal intelligence, are severely handicapped by their joint abnormalities. Although there is an increased mortality in infancy, life span after that time is not markedly decreased. Diastrophic dysplasia is caused by a mutation in a gene coding for a sulfate transporter protein located on chromosome 5. The sulfate transporter function of the gene product was suggested by protein sequence analysis showing an amino acid sequence similarity to known sulfate transporter proteins and was supported by greatly diminished sulfate uptake in skin fibroblasts from a patient with diastrophic dysplasia. This gene has been named diastrophic dysplasia sulfate transporter (*DTDST*).

In normal cartilage, proper sulfation of proteoglycans is necessary for them to be sufficiently negatively charged to function properly. There is evidence that the sulfation of proteoglycans is sensitive to both extracellular and intracellular sulfate concentrations. A defect in the sulfate transporter protein could easily explain the defective cartilage in this disorder. The gene responsible for the synthesis of this protein is expressed in virtually all cell types. The reason that its effects are most pronounced in cartilage-producing cells may simply be because of the greater requirement for sulfate for proteoglycan synthesis in cartilage than in other tissues. Specifically, a defect in sulfate transport across the cell membrane results in inadequate intracellular sulfate and undersulfation of proteoglycans.

Mutations of the *DTDST* have also been found to cause the neonatally lethal achondrogenesis type IB and atelosteogenesis type II. The most severe cases of diastrophic dysplasia overlap phenotypically and by mutation analysis with atelosteogenesis type II. The severity of these 3 autosomal recessive chondrodyplasias correlates well with the severity of dysfunction of *DTDST* protein that is predicted by mutation analysis.

Schmid Metaphyseal Chondrodysplasia

This autosomal dominant disorder is characterized by short stature, bowed legs, coxa vara, and a waddling gait. The metaphyses of the long bones are flared and the physes are wide and irregular. The defective gene codes for an abnormal type X collagen. Normal type X collagen is a short-chain collagen that is present predominantly in the hypertrophic zone of the physis and is thought to be important in endochondral ossification. Type X collagen exists as a homotrimer (3 identical chains linked together) in the pericellular matrix of hypertrophic chondrocytes. The mutations in this disease occur in the carboxy-terminal, noncollagenous domain of the protein and may limit the ability of the collagen to form trimers. Type X collagen appears to play a role in organizing matrix components of cartilage. Its absence results in alteration of the supporting properties of the physis as well as mild decrease in trabecular bone formation and mild disorganization of mineralization.

Jansen Metaphyseal Chondrodysplasia

Jansen metaphyseal chondrodysplasia is a rare autosomal dominant disorder characterized at birth by severe limb shortening with a prominent forehead and micrognathia. The tubular bones are short and the metaphyses are markedly flared with irregular ossification.

A patient with Jansen metaphyseal chondrodysplasia has been shown to have a mutation in the gene coding for parathyroid hormone-parathyroid hormone-related peptide (PTH-PTHrP) receptor. This explains the hypercalcemia and hypophosphatemia often associated with Jansen syndrome. Furthermore, this receptor is expressed in the growth plate and animal models suggest that parathyroid-related protein is important in bone elongation and ossification.

Craniosynostoses

Several disorders with premature fusion of the cranial suture and variable anomalies of the hands and feet are caused by mutation of the gene *FGFR2*. Apert's syndrome, Jackson-Weiss syndrome, Crouzon's disease, and most Pfeiffer's syndromes are autosomal dominant disorders caused by *FGFR2* mutations. Of these disorders, Apert's syndrome has the most extensive syndactyly of the fingers and toes. Specific mutations within the *FGFR2* gene have been correlated with different phenotypes between diseases and for different phenotypes within diseases, such as the severity of syndactyly and cleft palate in Apert's syndrome. Interestingly, new mutations in 57 Apert's syndrome families were all found to be of paternal origin, which explains the paternal age effect for new mutations causing Apert's syndrome.

Boston-type craniosynostosis has been shown to be caused by mutations in the *MSX2* gene—a DNA transcription factor called a homeobox gene.

Cleidocranial Dysplasia

Cleidocranial dyplasia (cleidocranial dysostosis syndrome) is a generalized skeletal dysplasia whose most prominent features include hypoplasia or aplasia of the clavicles, persistently open skull sutures with a bulging calvarium, midface hypoplasia, wide symphysis pubis, mild to moderate short stature, short middle phalanx of the little finger, dental anomalies, and often vertebral malformation. The disorder was linked to 6p21 and the region refined until an area with 3 known genes was identified. One of these genes, *cbfa1*, was a particularly attractive candidate because of its homology to the 'runt' family of genes in mice, which are

bone-specific nuclear-matrix-binding transcription factors. *cbfa1* was shown to cause cleidocranial dysplasia by mutation analysis. *cbfa1* encodes a protein that binds to an element in the promoter of the gene for osteocalcin and acts as an osteoblast-specific transcription factor and a regulator of osteoblast differentiation. Mice with homozygous mutation of *cbfa1* die at birth and completely lack skeletal ossification. Both intramembranous and endochondral ossification were absent, suggesting that *cbfa1* is essential for osteogenesis.

Metabolic Bone Diseases

Osteoporosis

Osteoporosis is a major individual and public health problem. Femoral neck fracture resulting from senile osteoporosis continues to result in a high rate of mortality. Peak bone mass is a major determinant of the occurrence of osteoporosis. Multiple nongenetic factors are important in determining peak bone mass, including exercise, drug use, alcohol intake, nutrition (including calcium intake), and smoking. A study of Caucasians of Anglo-Irish background living in Australia showed that the genetic contribution to peak bone mass can be explained by differing alleles for the gene coding for the receptor for 1,25 dihydroxyvitamin D. Other studies have not found an association between vitamin D receptor genotype and osteoporosis, or have found a minor effect that is overwhelmed by other variables, such as obesity. Another study found a correlation between bone mineral density and vitamin D receptor genotype in nonobese, postmenopausal women, but not in obese, postmenopausal women. Twin studies comparing bone mineral density and vitamin D receptor genotype found that dizygotic twins sharing the same vitamin D receptor genotype are similar to monozygotic twins and different from dizygotic twins not sharing the same vitamin D receptor genotype, with respect to bone mineral density.

Although a genetic influence seems likely, there are methodologic issues that make all associations reported to date tentative. It must be established that the alleles associated with low bone mass are the proximate cause and not merely a chance association with some other process that actually results in low bone mass. If different alleles coding for this vitamin D receptor (or different alleles in other genes affecting bone turnover such as the gene coding for transforming growth factor beta 1) result in clinically important differences in peak bone mass, specific allele identification could be used clinically to identify a population at particular risk early in life. This population could be targeted for aggressive prophylactic treatment and education before bone mass falls below the critical level necessary to avoid osteoporotic fractures.

Hypophosphatemic Rickets

The most common cause of vitamin D-resistant rickets is X-linked hypophosphatemic rickets. This disorder causes short stature, lower extremity deformities, and bone pain. A decrease in proximal tubular resorption of phosphate causing hypophosphatemia causes the disorder. Recent evidence indicates that an intrinsic renal defect is not responsible for this disorder but rather a humeral factor is produced that actively induces phosphate wasting. This situation has been shown by performing transplant experiments in an analogous disorder in mice. Normal kidneys transplanted into mice with X-linked hypophosphatemia waste phosphate, whereas kidneys from phosphate-wasting mice function normally in normal mice. Furthermore, the gene in humans that codes for the sodium phosphate transport protein is on chromosome 5, whereas X-linked hypophosphatemic rickets has been linked to an area of the X chromosome (the X P 22.1 region).

A gene called *PEX* (phosphate regulating gene with homologies to endopeptidases, on the X chromosome) was identified by linkage studies and confirmed by mutation analysis to cause hypophosphatemic rickets. Not all families studied have shown mutations in this gene. The gene has not been completely characterized so mutations in some families may have been missed. But, it is likely that more than 1 loci is responsible for this disease. *PEX* is similar to a class of endopeptidases that function to activate or inactivate hormones. The tissue of origin of *PEX* and its possible target hormone have not been identified.

Identification of the abnormal gene and its protein that results in phosphate wasting holds promise for developing specific therapies to counteract this humeral protein and ameliorate the effects of this disorder. Current treatments with phosphate and active vitamin D metabolites are only partially effective in avoiding short stature, deformity, and bone pain.

Connective Tissue Disorders

Type 1 and 2 Fibrillinopathies

Marfan syndrome is an autosomal dominant disorder affecting 1 in 10,000 to 20,000 people. The expression of the disorder is variable within and among different families. Several named variants with phenotype similarity are listed above. Typical Marfan syndrome features include dolichostenomelia (long, thin limbs), pectus excavatum or carinatum, scoliosis, high and narrow palate, ectopia lentis, myopia, dilatation of the ascending aorta, aortic dissection, and dural ectasia. Because of the wide distribution of affected tissues, a connective tissue defect was suspected for decades.

In 1991 the defective gene causing Marfan syndrome, located on chromosome 15, was found to encode for fibrillin (*FBN1*). Fibrillin is a large glycoprotein that is a structural component of elastin-containing microfibrils and is present in many tissues. The gene defect usually results in decreased amounts of fibrillin and, presumably, a structurally weakened elastin. The gene mutations occur throughout this large gene and are usually unique to the affected individual. Clear genotype/phenotype correlations are not apparent except for a clustering of mutations causing the severe, neonatal forms in a specific region of the gene. The entire gene has been sequenced and gene-based diagnosis is now possible through research laboratories.

A second, distinct, fibrillin protein is coded for by a gene on chromosome 5 (*FBN2*). A mutation in the fibrillin gene causes congenital contractural arachnodactyly, an autosomal dominant disorder that has the same skeletal features as Marfan syndrome, but joints are contracted instead of loose.

Osteogenesis Imperfecta

With rare exceptions, osteogenesis imperfecta is an autosomal dominant disorder caused by a mutation in either of the 2 chains that form type I collagen. Two copies of the $\alpha 1$ chain (coded for on chromosome 17) and 1 copy of the $\alpha 2$ chain (coded for on chromosome 7) form a triple helix approximately 1,000 amino acids long with repeated triplets of glycine-X-Y. Three triple helices wind around each other to form a superhelix. Type I collagen is the predominant structural protein in bone and connective tissue. Clinically, osteogenesis imperfecta is classified as type I, mild; type II, perinatally lethal; type III, progressively deforming; and type IV, moderately severe (between types I and III in severity).

Most type I disease is caused by mutations that reduce the amount of type I collagen in the collagen fibrils. The mutated messenger RNA is rapidly degraded and does not, therefore, result in the formation of structurally abnormal collagen. In types II, III, and IV disease, the majority of mutations are point mutations that cause substitutions of the repeated glycine amino acids. Severe phenotypes result from the incorporation of structurally abnormal chains into the type I collagen fibrils. Similar to the situation with achondroplasia and Apert's syndrome, many cases of the severe forms of osteogenesis imperfecta (types II and III) result from new, dominantly acting mutations often arising in the paternal germ line. In rare cases, clinically unaffected parents may be germline mosaics for a predisposing mutation so that the risk of a subsequent affected child is greater (1% to 5%) than the new mutation rate alone.

Two approaches to gene therapy are being actively explored in cell culture and/or animal models. Bone marrow transplantation holds some promise for increasing the amount of normal collagen I. Antisense gene therapy seeks to form complementary molecules that will bind with the mutated RNA, thus stopping expression of the abnormal chain. This would result in a diminished amount of collagen I and transformation of severe phenotypes into the type I, mild phenotype.

Ehlers-Danlos Syndromes

Ehlers-Danlos syndromes (EDS) are a heterogeneous group of disorders characterized by laxity and weakness of the dermis, ligaments, and blood vessels. Nine clinical and genetic subtypes have been described and all, whose etiology is known, are caused by mutations in fibrillar collagen genes or genes for enzymes that modify the fibrillar collagens.

EDS I is an autosomal dominant condition characterized by lax joints, hyperextensible skin, and wide, atrophic scars. EDS II is a milder form with the same clinical problems. Both disorders result from mutation of the gene coding for collagen V. Collagen V is coexpressed with collagen I in many tissues and is important for proper formation of collagen I fibrils.

EDS IV is a clinically heterogeneous subtype but is characterized by the tendency for rupture of large- and medium-sized arteries. Fatal ruptures often occur in the second or third decade of life. The etiology of EDS IV is a mutation in the gene coding for a chain of collagen III that interrupts the helical structure of this fibular collagen. Collagen III constitutes 50% of the collagen in blood vessel walls (the majority of the remaining collagen is type I) and 15% of the collagen in skin.

EDS VII A and B are caused by mutations in the structural gene coding for collagen I, whereas EDS VI and VIIC have mutations in genes coding for enzymes involved in collagen I synthesis.

Neuromuscular Disorders

Duchenne and Becker Muscular Dystrophies

The dystrophinopathies, Duchenne and Becker muscular dystrophies, have traditionally been considered 2 different diseases. When the gene, dystrophin, was cloned in 1987, it became clear that these diseases represent different phenotypes resulting from different mutations in a single gene.

The more severe form, Duchenne muscular dystrophy, presents in early childhood with proximal muscle weakness and calf hypertrophy. In affected boys there is mild delay in attaining motor milestones. Toe walking may be an early manifestation of the disease. The course is one of steadily worsening weakness.

The milder dystrophinopathies vary in clinical phenotype. Affected males who present in childhood with proxi-

mal weakness, calf hypertrophy, and very high creatine kinase values, but follow a more indolent course than the Duchenne muscular dystrophy patients, are given the diagnosis of Becker muscular dystrophy. Dystrophinopathies may be indistinguishable from limb girdle dystrophy. Seven of 41 patients (17%) in one series with the clinical diagnosis of limb girdle dystrophy had dystrophin mutations. Carrier females may be symptomatic on the basis of skewed X-inactivation. They usually present with limb girdle weakness and an elevated creatine kinase. Cardiomyopathy can be clinically significant and, rarely, is the primary manifestation of dystrophinopathy.

Dystrophin is an intracellular protein that is associated with 2 transmembrane complexes—the dystroglycan complex and the sarcoglycan complex. Loss of dystrophin leads to loss of all components of these complexes. The dystrophin gene is the largest human gene identified to date. This makes it a very large target for new mutations, and one third of dystrophinopathy cases are new mutations. In 55% to 70% of cases, a deletion or duplication can be identified by DNA testing (based on a review of all reported series up to 1993). In these cases a muscle biopsy is not necessary to make the diagnosis, though sometimes it will be done to allow more accurate predictions about the clinical course. (Duchenne muscular dystrophy has absent dystrophin in muscle, and the milder phenotypes have decreased or abnormal dystrophin.)

Because there is no effective treatment for the dystrophinopathies, there is great interest in the possibility of introducing a functional dystrophin gene into the muscle fibers, and thus curing the disease (gene therapy). There are many problems to be overcome before this is a viable treatment option; among these are identifying an appropriate vector for the new gene, overcoming host immune response to the vector or the expressed new protein, targeting muscle, and regulating the expression of the gene. These problems are the focus of active research. Most of the hurdles to be overcome before gene therapy is clinically useful are not specific to a missing protein, such as dystrophin. If the problems are solved for 1 type of muscular dystrophy, it is likely that the protocol will be adapted relatively quickly for other muscular dystrophies with similar pathogenesis.

Autosomal Recessive Limb Girdle Dystrophies

The autosomal recessive limb girdle dystrophies are progressive muscular dystrophies that predominantly affect the pelvic and shoulder girdle musculature. The severity ranges from forms manifesting weakness in the first decade of life and having rapid progression (called Duchenne-like muscular dystrophy) to forms with late onset and slow progression.

Seven genetic loci have been identified in families with this phenotype. Four loci code for proteins that are part of the sarcoglycan complex. The sarcoglycan complex and the dystroglycan complex are part of the dystrophin-glycoprotein complex that spans the muscle membrane from the cytoskeleton to the basal lamina. One hypothesis is that the dystrophin-glycoprotein complex functions to stabilize the sarcolemma, thereby protecting the muscle fiber from damage caused by repeated contractions. The genes for 2 forms of this disorder have not been identified, and 1 form is caused by a mutation in the gene coding for calpain-3, a proteolytic enzyme.

Hereditary Spastic Paraplegias

The hereditary spastic paraplegias (familial spastic paraparesis, Strümpell-Lorrain syndrome) are characterized by progressive spasticity of the legs. Symptoms usually manifest in the second to fourth decade with a slow and steady worsening gait. These disorders have been classified by mode of inheritance and whether the lower extremity spasticity is the only finding (uncomplicated) or whether other neurologic problems, such as optic neuropathy, dementia, ataxia, mental retardation, or deafness are present (complicated). Inheritance may be autosomal dominant, autosomal recessive, or X-linked.

Autosomal dominant forms have been linked to loci on chromosomes 2p, 14q, and 15q; an autosomal recessive form has been linked to 8q; and X-linked, to Xq28 and Xq22. Other loci for each disorder are suggested by families that do not link to the known loci. The Xq22 gene codes for a proteolipoprotein. The gene and gene product are not known for the remaining loci. The clinical phenotype is similar among families with mutations at the same loci.

Hereditary Motor Sensory Neuropathies (Charcot-Marie-Tooth Disease)

Charcot-Marie-Tooth disease has been subdivided on clinical grounds into type I and type II disease. More recently these were subsumed in the classification of hereditary motor sensory neuropathies in which Charcot-Marie-Tooth disease type I became hereditary motor sensory neuropathy I, and Charcot-Marie-Tooth type II became hereditary motor sensory neuropathy II. Hereditary motor sensory neuropathy I is autosomal dominant and the most common inherited neuromuscular disorder. It is characterized by progressive distal muscle wasting and weakness, areflexia, and foot deformities, most commonly cavovarus feet. Nerve conduction velocities show severe slowing and nerve pathology reveals simultaneous demyelination and remyelination. This disorder has variable expression but usually begins in childhood. Patients with foot deformities usually present to the orthopaedic surgeon in late childhood or early adolescence.

Seven different gene loci have been identified for the hereditary motor sensory neuropathy phenotype. Mutations in at least 3 loci (chromosomes 17, 1, and X) result in autosomal dominant hereditary motor sensory neuropathy type I. The most common cause is a duplication of 17p11.2-p12 (called hereditary motor sensory neuropathy IA). This duplication leads to trisomy for the peripheral myelin protein 22 (*PMP22*) gene. It is rare for patients with point mutations in this gene to have also had the hereditary motor sensory neuropathy type I phenotype, providing strong evidence for the primary role of *PMP22* in disease causation. Although *PMP22* is expressed in myelinating Schwann cells, its function is unknown and a wide range of disease severity occurs with very similar mutations of this gene. Interestingly, a chromosome 17 deletion reciprocal to the hereditary motor sensory neuropathy IA duplication causes hereditary neuropathy with a propensity for pressure palsies, another autosomal dominant neuropathy.

A second hereditary motor sensory neuropathy I locus, found on chromosome 1 (hereditary motor sensory neuropathy IB), codes for the protein myelin Po, and is the rarest locus identified thus far. A third locus (hereditary motor sensory neuropathy IC) has not yet been mapped. Another hereditary neuropathy with severe slowing of nerve conduction velocities is autosomal recessive. This phenotype has been localized to regions on both chromosome 5 and 8 in different families. In addition to these autosomal loci, there are 3 X-linked loci. The gene mutated in one of these is connexon 32; the gene product has not been identified for the other two. The phenotype associated with connexon 32 mutations is X-linked dominant, and families with these mutations cannot be reliably distinguished from families with the autosomal dominant forms on a clinical basis.

Hereditary motor sensory neuropathy II, the axonal form, doesn't map to any of the above locations, confirming that this is a distinct disease at both the clinical and molecular levels. Three loci (1p36, 3q13-q22, 7p14) have been identified so far.

It is difficult to determine accurate population-based frequencies for the various genetic loci associated with the hereditary motor and sensory neuropathy phenotype. The University of Iowa is a referral center for the genetic analysis of patients with hereditary neuropathy. Of 95 families studied, 77 families have the hereditary motor and sensory neuropathy type I phenotype. Of these 77 families, 54 show linkage to chromosome 17, and 50 have duplication of the *PMP22* gene. One family maps to the chromosome 1 locus, and 20 families have an X-linked dominant disorder (15 of these have demonstrated connexon 32 mutations). Eighteen of the 95 families have a hereditary motor and sensory neuropathy type II phenotype (axonal neuropathy). The final 2 families are X-linked recessive by pedigree analysis. This is not a population-based study, and the referral pattern may alter the frequencies slightly; however, it is like other studies in demonstrating that the great majority of families with hereditary motor and sensory neuropathy type I have chromosome 17 mutations. Mutations in *PMP22* or connexon 32 can be identified in peripheral blood by commercial laboratories. Thus, in the Iowa series, for 65/77 type I patients (84%), a specific diagnosis could be made through DNA analysis, allowing accurate genetic counseling and presymptomatic diagnosis.

Spinal Muscular Atrophy

Spinal muscular atrophy (SMA) has been classified into 3 clinical forms. (1) Werdnig-Hoffmann disease is characterized by generalized muscle weakness and hypotonia at birth and early death. (2) The intermediate type of spinal muscular atrophy afflicts patients who have normal motor milestones initially, but never gain the ability to walk. (3) Kugelberg-Welander syndrome is the mildest type; patients have muscle weakness that becomes evident after the age of 2. All 3 types of SMA are characterized by anterior horn cell degeneration and result in limb and trunk paralysis with muscle atrophy. Patients' major orthopaedic problems are scoliosis and hip instability. It has long been recognized that there is a continuum from the most severe early forms through the milder, later onset disease. This clinical impression has been borne out by the mapping of all forms of SMA to one small region of chromosome 5. Several genes have been identified in this region, including the survival motor neuron (*SMN*) gene, the neuronal apoptosis inhibitory protein, and the *p44* gene. This is a very complex and unstable segment of the genome. Two copies of the *SMN* gene with very minor differences are present in this region; one centromeric and the other telomeric to each other. More than 90% of SMA patients have deletions (or conversion of the telomeric *SMN* to the centromeric *SMN* type) in a specific portion (exons 7 and 8) of the telomeric *SMN* gene. SMA types II and III appear to have a conversion of the telomeric *SMN* to the centromeric *SMN* gene and have more copies of the centromeric *SMN* gene than exist in type I disease. The telomeric *SMN* gene encodes the fully functional protein, whereas the centromeric *SMN* gene encodes a transcript lacking exon 7.

The neuronal apoptosis inhibitory protein may provide an additional explanation for the variations in genotype/phenotype correlation. The neuronal apoptosis inhibitory protein gene functions to inhibit motor neuron programmed cell death. Programmed cell death is a normal occurrence in the development of the nervous system. Failure to inhibit cell death at the appropriate time could be part of the explanation for the anterior horn cell loss seen in SMA. In a group of patients with the most severe type of SMA, a high percentage of deletions in this gene was found. However, deletion of this gene may simply be coincidentally associated with more disease because of a more severe interruption in the *SMN* gene function.

Trinucleotide Repeat Disorders

Repeated sequences of nucleotides occur throughout the human genome and are the basis for inherited polymorphisms that have allowed the dramatic increase in identification of disease-causing genes in the last decade. Expansion of certain trinucleotide repeats causes 11 known neurologic disorders. These disorders are myotonic dystrophy, Friedreich's ataxia, fragile X syndrome, X-linked spinal and bulbar muscular atrophy, Huntington's disease, spinocerebellar ataxia type 1, spinocerebellar ataxia type 2, spinocerebellar ataxia type 6, spinocerebellar ataxia type 7, spinocerebellar ataxia type 3 (Machado-Joseph disease), and dentatorubral-pallidoluysian atrophy. The repeated sequences are unstable and change size in successive generations, usually becoming longer. Myotonic dystrophy and fragile X syndrome contain repeat sequences that are not within the protein coding region and, probably, cause disease by altering gene expression rather than by altering the protein product. Expansion of trinucleotide repeats (CAG repeats) in the coding region cause Huntington's disease, spinal and bulbar muscular atrophy, spinocerebellar ataxia type 1 and 6, dentatorubral-pallidoluysian atrophy, and Machado-Joseph disease. The CAG repeat results in polyglutamine amino acid sequences, and evidence suggests these polyglutamine regions are specifically neurotoxic by themselves. Friedreich's ataxia is caused by a repeat expansion in introns. The location of the repeats in the remaining diseases has not been identified. Myotonic dystrophy and Friedrich's ataxia will be discussed in more detail later in this chapter.

The trinucleotide repeat expansion provides a molecular basis for "anticipation," a phenomenon recognized by astute clinical geneticists, but discounted by colleagues in part because it failed to conform to classical mendelian genetics. Anticipation, in genetic parlance, is the worsening of the clinical phenotype (earlier onset, more severe disease) in succeeding generations. It is now clear that the trinucleotide repeats tend to lengthen in succeeding generations and the severity of the disease correlates, although not perfectly, with the length of the repeat segment.

Not all trinucleotide repeat disorders cause neurologic diseases. In fact, grouping of trinucleotide repeat disorders is somewhat artificial in that the gene involved and the nature of the trinucleotide repeat are often more important in determining the disease characteristics than the fact that a trinucleotide repeat, per se, is the type of mutation. For example, synpolydactyly is an inherited disorder that affects the hands and/or feet with various combinations of syndactyly and polydactyly. It is caused by a trinucleotide repeat resulting in an expansion of a polyalanine stretch in the amino terminal region of *HOXD13*. Increasing size of the polyalanine repeat regions may correlate with increasing numbers of involved limbs, from monomelic through tetramelic involvement.

Myotonic Dystrophy

Myotonic dystrophy is an autosomal dominant, multisystem disease that has marked clinical variability with an incidence of 1 per 8,000. The most severely affected patients are infants with congenital myotonic dystrophy. These children have severe hypotonia and weakness and often require ventilatory support and nasogastric feedings. Clubfeet and dislocated hips are common. These children are almost always born to myotonic mothers rather than affected fathers. If they survive the neonatal period, these children show improvement in strength, but have persistent motor disability. In addition, they are uniformly mentally retarded. At the other extreme, the only manifestation of myotonic dystrophy in the most mildly affected individuals may be cataracts.

After the neonatal period, the disease presents with mild muscle weakness and myotonia exacerbated by cold. Wasting of the temporalis muscles contributes to the typical phenotype of long narrow faces with bitemporal narrowing. Cardiac conduction defects are common, and may necessitate a pacemaker. Diabetes mellitus, male pattern baldness, infertility, and mental retardation are also manifestations of myotonic dystrophy.

The abnormal gene, myotonin, is a protein kinase. The substrate for the kinase and the pathophysiology of the disease remain unknown. The protein location has been shown by immunoelectron microscopy to be membrane bound in the terminal cisternae of the sarcoplasmic reticulum, mainly in the I-band. The mutation is an expansion of a trinucleotide repeat in the 3´ untranslated region of the gene. The normal gene has 5 to 30 copies of this CTG repeat. This is expanded in myotonic dystrophy patients, reaching thousands of copies. The congenitally affected infants have the largest expansions, on average, and the mildest phenotypes are associated with the smallest expansions into the disease-associated range.

Friedreich's Ataxia

Friedreich's ataxia is the most common early onset hereditary ataxia and occurs in approximately 2 to 4 per 100,000 in ethnically European populations. It is an autosomal recessive disorder characterized by progressive ataxia beginning before age 25 years. Muscle weakness, cardiomyopathy, and diabetes mellitus are frequent accompanying conditions. Scoliosis and pes cavus are common orthopaedic manifestations that often require treatment. The cause of Friedreich's ataxia is a mutation of the gene X25, which codes for protein named frataxin. The function of frataxin is as yet

unknown. Earlier age of onset and more frequent occurrence of associated problems such as diabetes and cardiomyopathy are associated with larger repeat expansions.

Miscellaneous Syndromes and Disorders

Hereditary Multiple Exostosis

This autosomal dominant disorder is viewed as a single clinical phenotype, but has localized to 3 different chromosomal locations: chromosome 8q24.1 (*EXT1*), chromosome 11p11-p13 (*EXT2*), and chromosome 19p (*EXT3*). The *EXT1* and *EXT2* genes have been cloned and are hypothesized to be a new family of tumor suppressor genes. The main evidence for this is that mutations of both alleles of the *EXT* genes have been identified in chondrosarcomas arising from both sporadic and hereditary exostoses. The *EXT1* gene has been shown to be expressed in many tissues, but the only known effect is on growing bones.

A current hypothesis is that exostosis formation fits the "2-hit" model of tumorigenesis. Both alleles must be mutated for an exostosis to form. This explains why hereditary exostoses occur at a younger age and in more sites than sporadic exostoses. That is, individuals who inherit an abnormal allele need a cartilage cell to undergo a mutation of only the second allele to form an exostosis; whereas sporadic exostoses require new mutations of both alleles in a cell. Presumably, malignant degeneration occurs when an additional mutation happens to another tumor suppressor gene or proto-oncogene.

Neurofibromatosis

Neurofibromatosis is one of the most common single gene disorders with an incidence of 1 in 3,000. It is autosomal dominant, with a nearly complete penetrance. Half of reported cases are new mutations.

There are 2 forms of neurofibromatosis. NF-1 has an incidence of 1 in 3,500 live births. The clinical features of NF-1 include café-au-lait spots, neurofibromas, dysostosis, congential pseudarthrosis of the tibia, and scoliosis. The gene responsible codes for a protein named neurofibromin. Neurofibromin is believed to be a tumor suppresser gene that normally functions to control cell growth and differentiation. Neurofibromas occur if the unaffected allele coding for neurofibromin (that is, the allele not carrying the mutation causing NF-1) undergoes a somatic mutation. This "2-hit" hypothesis of neurofibroma causation is supported by mutation analysis of neurofibromas from a large number of individuals in different families.

NF-2, with a gene location on chromosome 22, is far less

common, with a prevalence of 1 in 50,000 births. NF-2 is associated with a high prevalence of acoustic neuromas and rarely has orthopaedic complications. The mutant gene codes for merlin or schwannomin, which is a protein that links the cytoskeleton to the plasma membrane. This gene also appears to be a tumor suppressor gene, and the severity of the disorder correlates with how severe a truncation of the protein is caused by the specific mutation.

McCune-Albright Syndrome/Monostotic Fibrous Dysplasia

McCune-Albright syndrome is sporadic and is characterized by polyostotic fibrous dysplasia, sexual precocity, hyperplastic endocrine disorders, and café-au-lait spots. A mutation of the gene for the alpha subunit of stimulatory guanine-nucleotide-binding protein (Gs), a protein that stimulates cyclic adenosine monophosphate (cAMP) formation, has been found in patients affected with this disorder. The mutation seems to result in an inappropriate stimulation of adenyl cyclase. There is strong evidence that the mutation of this gene is a somatic rather than a germline mutation—meaning that the mutation occurred after fertilization in some subsequent cell division. The variation in the distribution of the abnormality in individuals can be explained by the tissues that have the mutated gene as opposed to the normal gene. In all patients studied so far, the abnormal gene was found in fibrous dysplasia material.

Abnormal tissues in this disease have been found by in situ hybridization to have increased expression of the c-*fos* proto-oncogene. Transgenic mice that overexpress the c-*fos* proto-oncogene have bone marrow fibrosis, increased formation of woven bone, and disordered bone remodeling. The abnormal stimulatory guanine-nucleotide-binding protein may create the abnormal cells by increasing the level of cAMP in affected tissues and, thereby, increasing the expression of the c-*fos* proto-oncogene, which is responsive to increased levels of cAMP.

Mutations in this gene have also been found, as well in patients with monostotic fibrous dysplasia. It seems likely that different mutations within this gene might result in lesser or greater involvement of bones and other tissues. Both monostotic and polyostotic fibrous dysplasia lesions show an increase in cell proliferation with a diminished synthesis of osteocalcin suggesting a reduction in cell differation as the cause of the lesions.

Paget Disease

Paget disease is an extremely common disorder of bone remodeling, with an incidence of approximately 3.3% of people older than 40 years. Paget disease has long been known to have a strong familiarity, with more than 40% of affected people having a first-degree relative with the disease. Because paramyxovirus-like nuclear inclusions have been found in osteoclasts, a viral etiology has been suggested as the cause. In a single large family, in which Paget disease had an autosomal dominant segregation pattern, Paget disease was found to be strongly linked to a region on chromosome 18, REF K. The authors surmise that a gene mutation might either confer a susceptibility to viral infection or be involved directly in osteoclast function. The authors searched this region of the genome because of the histologic similarity of Paget disease to an extremely rare disorder—familial expansile osteolysis—which had previously been linked to the same region of chromosome 18.

Polydactyly

Polydactyly, whether isolated or associated with other anomalies, is usually an inherited condition. Given the complex interactions that occur in limb pattern specification, it is not surprising that a number of causes of this condition are being found.

Grieg cephalopolysyndactyly is an autosomal dominant disorder characterized by postaxial polysyndactyly of the hands and preaxial polysyndactyly of the feet and dysmorphic facies. A DNA binding transcription factor, GLI 3, is the cause of this disorder. Its expression is restricted to the interdigital mesenchyme and joint-forming regions of the digits. A mouse mutant with a defect in the homologous gene has ectopic expression of both sonic hedgehog and FGF-4 in the anterior limb bud.

Another mutation causing human polydactyly is in the *Hox D* cluster of homeobox genes that has been implicated in digit specification. Synpolydactyly is caused by a mutation of *Hox D-13*.

Disorders of Complex Inheritance

Most orthopaedic disorders are not strictly mendelian in their inheritance. Disorders with complex inheritance are more interesting to most orthopaedists because they comprise many idiopathic disorders. These disorders are usually more common than mendelian disorder; for example, Wynne-Davies found that idiopathic clubfoot occurred in 163 of 131,452 live births in Devonshire, England (1.24 per 1,000 live births); Rogala and associates found idiopathic scoliosis of greater than 10° by the Cobb angle method in 2% of 26,947 screened children in the at risk age group; and Lawrence and associates report a 0.9% prevalence of rheumatoid arthritis in 6,672 noninstitutionalized civilians in the United States who were evaluated by clinical examination, radiographs of the hands and feet, and serum assays for rheumatoid factor and the bentonite flocculation test. The risk of near relatives being affected by the disorder is much less than with mendelian disorders.

Three explanations for such data exist: (1) there is a non-genetic cause, such as an environmental factor; (2) there is a polygenic cause with the genes not acting in a strictly additive fashion (otherwise it would look dominant); or (3) there is a major gene effect responsible for a weak predisposition in most people or a strong predisposition in a subset of people with a disease phenotype. Various combinations of these possibilities can blur their borders.

Complex Segregation Analysis

A sophisticated way of distinguishing between the possible causes of disorders with mild to moderate familial aggregation is by complex segregation analysis. Segregation analysis per se generally refers to assessing whether a trait segregates in a mendelian fashion. Complex segregation analysis refers to sophisticated mathematical analyses of pedigrees that can simultaneously look for apparent genetic and nongenetic components of the segregation of a trait or disease within families. Nongenetic components include environmental effects such as diet, geographic location, socioeconomic status, birth order, maternal age at pregnancy, and exposure to a common virus. Complex segregation analysis was developed in the 1970s by Elston and Howard. It requires the power of computers to assess the likelihood of various models accurately representing the cause of familial clustering of traits or disorders because the pedigree data usually includes hundreds of families, with several generations in each family.

This technique has advanced understanding of how traits cluster in families for specific disorders. In general, there are 4 types of models of inheritance tested by genetic epidemiologists. (1) Oligogenic or major gene models posit a single locus or a few loci that account for inheritance completely (mendelian inheritance is subsumed in this category). (2) Polygenic models presuppose many contributing factors that are separately indistinguishable. However, cumulatively their effects are transmissible and model multifactorial inheritance. Major gene effects are not detectable. (3) Nontransmitted models describe disorders that cluster in families but are not transmitted between generations in a way that suggests genetic inheritance. These models suggest environmental causation. (4) Mixed models combine oligogenic and polygenic models. Major gene effects are detectable but other factors appear to be influencing disease expression. These other factors are assumed to be polygenes or environmental effects. Basically, disorders with a major gene effect can be identified without requiring that a major gene alone accounts for the occurrence of the disorder. This is an important factor for planning research strategies. If a single gene is found to account for a large proportion of clustering of a disorder in families, molecular genetic techniques to find this gene are appropriate. If nonhereditary explanations fit the data best, then epidemiologic studies are more likely to identify the cause of disorder clustering. This sort of analysis has been applied to diseases of special interest to orthopaedists in all branches of medicine. Rheumatoid arthritis and idiopathic clubfoot are examples of diseases of special interest to orthopaedists that were studied with complex segregation analysis.

Lynn and associates evaluated the families of 247 consecutive patients presenting for treatment of rheumatoid arthritis. After eliminating families in which there was misdiagnosis of affected relatives or inability to ascertain affection status, the authors analyzed first-degree relatives from 30 families with more than 1 affected member and 135 families with only 1 affected member. They compared the fit of the data to a major gene model with those of multifactorial transmission and environmental transmission.

The best explanation of the pedigree data was a highly penetrant recessive gene with a prevalence in the population of 0.005. Not all pedigrees supported this result. The pedigrees that supported this result most strongly were families with an excess of affected males and a young age at onset of the disease. This information makes a molecular genetic search for a causative gene reasonable. The families with many males and early age of onset are the best families to use in the search for a causative gene.

Rebbeck and associates used the regressive logistic model of complex segregation analysis in a study of families with idiopathic clubfoot. This technique can evaluate disorders with a large number of genes and environmental factors contributing to statistical dependence among relatives without presupposing any genetic model. The technique lets all variables vary to fit the pedigree data in the best possible way. Models of major gene effect, multifactorial effect, and environmental effect are then compared to the best fit of the data.

Pedigrees from 143 consecutive idiopathic clubfoot probands were used for this study. This study strongly rejected the multifactorial and environmental models. A single major gene effect with an additional effect (polygenes or environmental factors) shared among siblings gave the best fit of the data. This result is supported by 2 other studies that came to the same conclusion using different models for complex segregation analysis of clubfoot.

Complex segregation analysis is a useful tool as a first step in investigating the etiology of disorders with nonmendelian clustering within families of the disorder. The results can aid the investigator in the effective allocation of resources in seeking causative factors.

The Orthopaedic Surgeon and the Geneticist at the End of the 20th Century

Genetic research will continue to alter the understanding and treatment of many disorders. Prenatal and presymptomatic diagnosis will become available for an increasing number of diseases. Gene therapy or gene product replacement will become available with the potential for ameliorating or eliminating the effects of abnormal genes. The orthopaedist must stay abreast of this knowledge to participate in advances in diagnosis and treatment, and to appropriately counsel his/her patients. Molecular genetics and biology will find inherited susceptibilities to diseases that are not mendelian in inheritance. Identifying subpopulations of patients within a single disease phenotype based on differing genetic backgrounds may allow improved treatment for individual patients. If its members are to remain orthopaedic physicians and not to become surgical technicians, the orthopaedic community must stay informed of and involved with the revolution in understanding the genetic and molecular bases of diseases.

It is probably prudent for the orthopaedic surgeon who takes care of patients with heritable disorders to consult regularly with a medical geneticist familiar with new developments in orthopedic genetics. The new information is accumulating too rapidly for most practicing orthopaedic surgeons to stay abreast of new developments. Patients, however, expect physicians to be at least as informed as they are, and rightly so. Educational lecture series in teaching institutions should include medical geneticists to relate new information concerning orthopaedic disorders. National educational meetings should include guest speakers with expertise in genetics to allow a broad dispersion of this new knowledge in the orthopaedic community.

A large family with an inherited disorder of unknown etiology should prompt a call or referral to a medical geneticist. He or she will be able to discover if active research into that disorder is occurring. If so, participation by said family in ongoing research may result in identification of the disease-causing gene.

A geneticist should be consulted before a diagnostic biopsy is performed, if any question exists about the availability of gene-based diagnosis. Most cases of Duchenne muscular dystrophy and Charcot-Marie-Tooth disease, for example, can be diagnosed by blood analysis, rather than muscle or nerve biopsy.

If the orthopaedic surgeon is unfamiliar with the empirical risk of recurrence of a disorder, a medical geneticist should be consulted. Idiopathic clubfoot is an example of a disorder in which the recurrence risk is often underestimated.

Patients with multisystem congenital anomalies should be referred to a geneticist to attempt to identify a unifying diagnosis. Also, families with diseases with mendelian inheritance should be offered referral for genetic counseling. The practicing orthopaedist does not have the time or teaching aids to adequately explain genetics to most families.

Selected Bibliography

Ahmad NN, McDonald-McGinn DM, Dixon P, Zackai EH, Tasman WS: PCR assay confirms diagnosis in syndrome with variably expressed phenotype: Mutation detection in Stickler syndrome. *J Med Genet* 1996;33:678–681.

Alman BA, Greel DA, Wolfe HJ: Activating mutations of Gs protein in monostotic fibrous lesions of bone. *J Orthop Res* 1996;14:311–315.

Anderson IJ, Goldberg RB, Marion RW, Upholt WB, Tsipouras P: Spondyloepiphyseal dysplasia congenita: Genetic linkage to type II collagen (COL2A1). *Am J Hum Genet* 1990;46:896–901.

Arikawa E, Hoffman EP, Kaido M, Nonaka I, Sugita H, Arahata K: The frequency of patients with dystrophin abnormalities in a limb-girdle patient population. *Neurology* 1991;41:1491–1496.

Baldwin CT, Farrer LA, Adair R, Dharmavaram R, Jimenez S, Anderson L: Linkage of early-onset osteoarthritis and chondrocalcinosis to human chromosome 8q. *Am J Hum Genet* 1995;56:692–697.

Bellus GA, McIntosh I, Smith EA, et al: A recurrent mutation in the tyrosine kinase domain of fibroblast growth factor receptor 3 causes hypochondroplasia. *Nat Genet* 1995;10:357–359.

Bleasel JF, Holderbaum D, Mallock V, Haqqi TM, Williams HJ, Moskowitz RW: Hereditary osteoarthritis with mild spondyloepiphyseal dysplasia: Are there "hot spots" on COL2A1? *J Rheumatol* 1996;23:1594–1598.

Bogaert R, Wilkin D, Wilcox WR, et al: Expression, in cartilage, of a 7-amino-acid deletion in type II collagen from two unrelated individuals with Kniest dysplasia. *Am J Hum Genet* 1994;55:1128–1136.

Briggs MD, Choi H, Warman ML, et al: Genetic mapping of a locus for multiple epiphyseal dysplasia (EDM2) to a region of chromosome I containing a type IX collagen gene. *Am J Hum Genet* 1994;55:678–684.

Briggs MD, Hoffman SM, King LM, et al: Pseudoachondroplasia and multiple epiphyseal dysplasia due to mutations in the cartilage oligomeric matrix protein gene. *Nat Genet* 1995;10:330–336.

Campbell L, Potter A, Ignatius J, Dubowitz V, Davies K: Genomic variation and gene conversion in spinal muscular atrophy: Implications for disease process and clinical phenotype. *Am J Hum Genet* 1997;61: 40–50.

Campuzano V, Montermini L, Molto MD, et al: Friedreich's ataxia: Autosomal recessive disease caused by an intronic GAA triplet repeat expansion. *Science* 1996;271:1423–1427.

Candeliere GA, Glorieux FH, Prud'homme J, St-Arnaud R: Increased expression of the c-fos proto-oncogene in bone from patients with fibrous dysplasia. *N Engl J Med* 1995;332:1546–1551.

Chance PF, Matsunami N, Lensch W, Smith B, Bird TD: Analysis of the DNA duplication 17p11.2 in Charcot-Marie-Tooth neuropathy type 1 pedigrees: Additional evidence for a third autosomal CMT1 locus. *Neurology* 1992;42:2037–2041.

Chen L, Yang W, Cole WG: Alternative splicing of exon 12 of the COL2A1 gene interrupts the triple helix of type-II collagen in the Kniest form of spondyloepiphyseal dysplasia. *J Orthop Res* 1996;14: 712–721.

Chitnavis J, Sinsheimer JS, Clipsham K, et al: Genetic influences in end-stage osteoarthritis: Sibling risks of hip and knee replacement for idiopathic osteoarthritis. *J Bone Joint Surg* 1997;79B:660–664.

Chong SS, McCall AE, Cota J, et al: Gametic and somatic tissue-specific heterogeneity of the expanded SCA1 CAG repeat in spinocerebellar ataxia type 1. *Nat Genet* 1995;10:344–350.

Clerk A, Rodillo E, Heckmatt JZ, Dubowitz V, Strong PN, Sewry CA: Characterisation of dystrophin in carriers of Duchenne muscular dystrophy. *J Neurol Sci* 1991;102:197–205.

Cobben JM, van der Steege G, Grootscholten P, de Visser M, Scheffer H, Buys CH: Deletions of the survival motor neuron gene in unaffected siblings of patients with spinal muscular atrophy. *Am J Hum Genet* 1995;57:805–808.

Cohn DH, Briggs MD, King LM, et al: Mutations in the cartilage oligomeric matrix protein (COMP) gene in pseudoachondroplasia and multiple epiphyseal dysplasia. *Ann N Y Acad Sci* 1996;785:188–194.

Collins FS, Ponder BA, Seizinger BR, Epstein CJ: The von Recklinghausen neurofibromatosis region on chromosome 17: Genetic and physical maps come into focus. *Am J Hum Genet* 1989;44:1–5.

Collod-Béroud G, Béroud C, Adès L, et al: Marfan database (second edition): Software and database for the analysis of mutations in the human FBN1 gene. *Nucleic Acids Res* 1997;25:147–150.

Cook A, Raskind W, Blanton SH, et al: Genetic heterogeneity in families with hereditary multiple exostoses. *Am J Hum Genet* 1993;53:71–79.

Defesche JC, Hoogendijk JE, de Visser M, de Visser O, Bolhuis PA: Genetic linkage of hereditary motor and sensory neuropathy type 1 (Charcot-Marie-Tooth disease) to markers of chromosomes 1 and 17. *Neurology* 1990;40:1450–1453.

Deng C, Wynshaw-Boris A, Zhou F, Kuo A, Leder P: Fibroblast growth factor receptor 3 is a negative regulator of bone growth. *Cell* 1996;84: 911–921.

De Paepe A, Nuytinck L, Hausser I, Anton-Lamprecht I, Naeyaert JM: Mutations in the COL5A1 gene are causal in the Ehlers-Danlos syndromes I and II. *Am J Hum Genet* 1997;60:547–554.

Dharmavaram RM, Elberson MA, Peng M, Kirson LA, Kelley TE, Jimenez SA: Identification of a mutation in type X collagen in a family with Schmid metaphyseal chondrodysplasia. *Hum Mol Genet* 1994;3:507–509.

Dietz HC, Cutting GR, Pyeritz RE, et al: Marfan syndrome caused by a recurrent de novo missense mutation in the fibrillin gene. *Nature* 1991;352:337–339.

Dietz HC, Pyeritz RE, Hall BD, et al: The Marfan syndrome locus: Confirmation of assignment to chromosome 15 and identification of tightly linked markers at 15q15-q21.3. *Genomics* 1991;9:355–361.

Donofrio PD, Challa VR, Hackshaw BT, Mills SA, Cordell AR: Cardiac transplantation in a patient with muscular dystrophy and cardiomyopathy. *Arch Neurol* 1989;46:705–707.

Dubé MP, Mlodzienski MA, Kibar Z, et al: Hereditary spastic paraplegia: LOD-score considerations for confirmation of linkage in a heterogeneous trait. *Am J Hum Genet* 1997;60:625–629.

Ducy P, Zhang R, Geoffroy V, Ridall AL, Karsenty G: Osf2/Cbfa1: A transcriptional activator of osteoblast differentiation. *Cell* 1997;89: 747–754.

Econs MJ, Rowe PS, Francis F, et al: Fine structure mapping of the human X-linked hypophosphatemic rickets gene locus. *J Clin Endocrinol Metab* 1994;79:1351–1354.

Eisman JA, Morrison NA, Kelly PJ, et al: Genetics of osteoporosis and vitamin D receptor alleles. *Calcif Tissue Int* 1995;56(suppl 1):S48–S49.

Fertala A, Ala-Kokko L, Wiaderkiewicz R, Prockop DJ: Collagen II containing a Cys substitution for Arg-α1-519: Homotrimeric monomers containing the mutation do not assemble into fibrils but alter the self-assembly of the normal protein. *J Biol Chem* 1997; 272:6457–6464.

Filla A, De Michele G, Cavalcanti F, et al: The relationship between trinucleotide (GAA) repeat length and clinical features in Friedreich ataxia. *Am J Hum Genet* 1996;59:554–560.

Fink JK, Heiman-Patterson T, Bird T, et al: Hereditary Spastic Paraplegic Working Group: Hereditary spastic paraplegia. Advances in genetic research. *Neurology* 1996;46:1507–1514.

Fu YH, Friedman DL, Richards S, et al: Decreased expression of myotonin-protein kinase messenger RNA and protein in adult form of myotonic dystrophy. *Science* 1993;260:235–238.

Gennarelli M, Novelli G, Andreasi Bassi F, et al: Prediction of myotonic dystrophy clinical severity based on the number of intragenic [CTG]n trinucleotide repeats. *Am J Med Genet* 1996;65:342–347.

Ghishan FK, Knobel S, Dasuki M, Butler M, Phillips J: Chromosomal localization of the human renal sodium phosphate transporter to chromosome 5: Implications for X-linked hypophosphatemia. *Pediatr Res* 1994;35: 510–513.

Giunti P, Sweeney MG, Spadaro M, et al: The trinucleotide repeat expansion on chromosome 6p (SCA1) in autosomal dominant cerebellar ataxias. *Brain* 1994;117:645–649.

Godfrey M, Olson S, Burgio RG, et al: Unilateral microfibrillar abnormalities in a case of asymmetric Marfan syndrome. *Am J Hum Genet* 1990; 46:661–671.

Griffiths LR, Zwi MB, McLeod JG, Nicholson GA: Chromosome 1 linkage studies in Charcot-Marie-Tooth neuropathy type 1. *Am J Hum Genet* 1988; 42:756–771.

Guyer MS, Collins FS: How is the Human Genome Project doing, and what have we learned so far? *Proc Natl Acad Sci USA* 1995;92: 10841–10848.

Hahnen E, Schönling J, Rudnik-Schöneborn S, Zerres K, Wirth B: Hybrid survival motor neuron genes in patients with autosomal recessive spinal muscular atrophy: New insights into molecular mechanisms responsible for the disease. *Am J Hum Genet* 1996;59: 1057–1065.

Hallam PJ, Harding AE, Berciano J, Barker DF, Malcolm S: Duplication of part of chromosome 17 is commonly associated with hereditary motor and sensory neuropathy type 1 (Charcot-Marie-Tooth disease type 1). *Ann Neurol* 1992;31:570–572.

Hamshere MG, Brook JD: Myotonic dystrophy, knockouts, warts and all. *Trends Genet* 1996;12:332–334.

Hanauer A, Chery M, Fujita R, Driesel AJ, Gilgenkrantz S, Mandel JL: The Friedreich ataxia gene is assigned to chromosome 9q13-q21 by mapping of tightly linked markers and shows linkage disequilibrium with D9S15. *Am J Hum Genet* 1990;46:133–137.

Harley HG, Brook JD, Rundle SA, et al: Expansion of an unstable DNA region and phenotypic variation in myotonic dystrophy. *Nature* 1992;355:545–546.

Harley HG, Rundle SA, MacMillan JC, et al: Size of the unstable CTG repeat sequence in relation to phenotype and parental transmission in myotonic dystrophy. *Am J Hum Genet* 1993;52:1164–1174.

Hästbacka J, de la Chapelle A, Mahtani MM, et al: The diastrophic dysplasia gene encodes a novel sulfate transporter: Positional cloning by fine-structure linkage disequilibrium mapping. *Cell* 1994; 78:1073–1087.

Hästbacka J, Superti-Furga A, Wilcox WR, Rimoin DL, Cohn DH, Lander ES: Atelosteogenesis type II is caused by mutations in the diastrophic dysplasia sulfate-transporter gene (DTDST): Evidence for a phenotypic series involving three chondrodysplasias. *Am J Hum Genet* 1996;58:255–262.

Hecht JT, Hogue D, Strong LC, Hansen MF, Blanton SH, Wagner M: Hereditary multiple exostosis and chondrosarcoma: Linkage to chromosome II and loss of heterozygosity for EXT-linked markers on chromosomes II and 8. *Am J Hum Genet* 1995;56:1125–1131.

Hecht JT, Hogue D, Wang Y, et al: Hereditary multiple exostoses (EXT): Mutational studies of familial EXT1 cases and EXT-associated malignancies. *Am J Hum Genet* 1997;60:80–86.

Hecht JT, Nelson LD, Crowder E, et al: Mutations in exon 17B of cartilage oligomeric matrix protein (COMP) cause pseudoachondroplasia. *Nat Genet* 1995;10:325–329.

Heuertz S, Smahi A, Wilkie AO, Le Merrer M, Maroteaux P, Hors-Cayla MC: Genetic mapping of Xp22.12-p22.31, with a refined localization for spondyloepiphyseal dysplasia (SEDL). *Hum Genet* 1995;96: 407–410.

Hewett D, Lynch J, Child A, Firth H, Sykes B: Differential allelic expression of a fibrillin gene (FBN1) in patients with Marfan syndrome. *Am J Hum Genet* 1994;55:447–452.

Hoffman EP: Genotype/phenotype correlations in Duchenne/Becker muscular dystrophy, in Partridge T (ed): *Molecular and Cell Biology of Muscular Dystrophy*. London, England, Chapman and Hall, 1993, pp 12–36.

Hoffman EP, Kunkel LM: Dystrophin abnormalities in Duchenne/Becker muscular dystrophy. *Neuron* 1989;2:1019–1029.

Holm IA, Huang X, Kunkel LM: Mutational analysis of the PEX gene in patients with x-linked hypophosphatemic rickets. *Am J Hum Genet* 1997;60:790–797.

Holmans P: Asymptotic properties of affected-sib-pair linkage analysis. *Am J Hum Genet* 1993;52:362–374.

Hoogendijk JE, Janssen EA, Gabreëls-Festen AA, et al: Allelic heterogeneity in hereditary motor and sensory neuropathy type 1a (Charcot-Marie-Tooth disease type 1a). *Neurology* 1993;43:1010–1015.

Horton WA: New insights into the chondrodysplasias. *Surg Rounds Orthop* 1990;4:24–30.

A gene (PEX) with homologies to endopeptidases is mutated in patients with X-linked hypophosphatemic rickets: The HYP Consortium. *Nat Genet* 1995;11:130–136.

Imbert G, Saudou F, Yvert G, et al: Cloning of the gene for spinocerebellar ataxia 2 reveals a locus with high sensitivity to expanded CAG/glutamine repeats. *Nat Genet* 1996;14:285–291.

Ionasescu VV: Charcot-Marie-Tooth neuropathies: From clinical description to molecular genetics. *Muscle Nerve* 1995;18:267–275.

Ionasescu V, Anderson R, Burns TL, Searby C, Ionasescu R, Ferrell R: Evidence for linkage of Charcot-Marie-Tooth neuropathy (CMT1) to apolipoprotein A2 (Apo-A2). *Am J Hum Genet* 1988;42:74–76.

Ionasescu VV, Ionasescu R, Searby C, Barker DF: Charcot-Marie-Tooth neuropathy type 1A with both duplication and non-duplication. *Hum Mol Genet* 1993;2:405–410.

Ionasescu V, Searby C, Sheffield VC, Roklina T, Nishimura D, Ionasescu R: Autosomal dominant Charcot-Marie-Tooth axonal neuropathy mapped on chromosome 7p (CMT2D). *Hum Mol Genet* 1996;5:1373–1375.

Ionasescu VV, Trofatter J, Haines JL, Summers AM, Ionasescu R, Searby C: Heterogeneity in X-linked recessive Charcot-Marie-Tooth neuropathy. *Am J Hum Genet* 1991;48:1075–1083.

Jacenko O, Olsen BR, Warman ML: Editorial: Of mice and men. Heritable skeletal disorders. *Am J Hum Genet* 1994;54:163–168.

Jodice C, Malaspina P, Persichetti F, et al: Effect of trinucleotide repeat length and parental sex on phenotypic variation in spinocerebellar ataxia I. *Am J Hum Genet* 1994;54:959–965.

Karpati G, Acsadi G: The potential for gene therapy in Duchenne muscular dystrophy and other genetic muscle diseases, *Muscle Nerve* 1993;16: 1141–1153.

Knapp M, Seuchter SA, Baur MP: The haplotype-relative-risk (HRR) method for analysis of association in nuclear families. *Am J Hum Genet* 1993;52:1085–1093.

Knowlton RG, Katzenstein PL, Moskowitz RW, et al: Genetic linkage of a polymorphism in the type 11 procollagen gene (COL2A1) to primary osteoarthritis associated with mild chondrodysplasia. *N Engl J Med* 1990; 322:526–530.

Koch MC, Grimm T, Harley HG, Harper PS: Genetic risks for children of women with myotonic dystrophy. *Am J Hum Genet* 1991;48:1084–1091.

Koenig M, Hoffman EP, Bertelson CJ, Monaco AP, Feener C, Kunkel LM: Complete cloning of the Duchenne muscular dystrophy (DMD) cDNA and preliminary genomic organization of the DMD gene in normal and affected individuals. *Cell* 1987;50:509–517.

Komori T, Yagi H, Nomura S, et al: Targeted disruption of Cbfa1 results in a complete lack of bone formation owing to maturational arrest of osteoblasts. *Cell* 1997;89:755–764.

Kwan KM, Pang MK, Zhou S, et al: Abnormal compartmentalization of cartilage matrix components in mice lacking collagen X: Implications for function. *J Cell Biol* 1997;136:459–471.

Lamont PJ, Davis MB, Wood NW: Identification and sizing of the GAA trinucleotide repeat expansion of Friedreich's ataxia in 56 patients: Clinical and genetic correlates. *Brain* 1997;120:673–680.

Lander ES, Schork NJ: Genetic dissection of complex traits. *Science* 1994;265:2037–2048.

Langdahl BL, Knudsen JY, Jensen HK, Gregersen N, Eriksen EF: A sequence variation: 713–8delC in the transforming growth factor-beta 1 gene has higher prevalence in osteoporotic women than in normal women and is associated with very low bone mass in osteoporotic women and increased bone turnover in both osteoporotic and normal women. *Bone* 1997; 20:289–294.

Lawrence RC, Hochberg MC, Kelsey JL, et al: Estimates of the prevalence of selected arthritic and musculoskeletal diseases in the United States. *J Rheumatol* 1989;16:427–441.

Lebo RV, Lynch ED, Bird TD, et al: Multicolor in situ hybridization and linkage analysis order Charcot-Marie-Tooth type 1 (CMT1A) gene-region markers. *Am J Hum Genet* 1992;50:42–55.

Lefebvre S, Bürglen L, Reboullet S, et al: Identification and characterization of a spinal muscular atrophy-determining gene. *Cell* 1995;80: 155–165.

LeGuern E, Guilbot A, Kessali M, et al: Homozygosity mapping of an autosomal recessive form of demyelinating Charcot-Marie-Tooth disease to chromosome 5q23-q33. *Hum Mol Genet* 1996;5:1685–1688.

Le Merrer M, Legeai-Mallet L, Jeannin PM, et al: A gene for hereditary multiple exostoses maps to chromosome 19p. *Hum Mol Genet* 1994;3:717–722.

Lindblad K, Savontaus ML, Stevanin G, et al: An expanded CAG repeat sequence in spinocerebellar ataxia type 7. *Genome Res* 1996;6:965–971.

Loprest LJ, Pericak-Vance MA, Stajich J, et al: Linkage studies in Charcot-Marie-Tooth disease type 2: Evidence that CMT types 1 and 2 are distinct genetic entities. *Neurology* 1992;42:597–601.

Loughlin J, Irven C, Athanasou N, Carr A, Sykes B: Differential allelic expression of the type 11 collagen gene (COL2A1) in osteoarthritic cartilage. *Am J Hum Genet* 1995;56:1186–1193.

Lynn AH, Kwoh CK, Venglish CM, Aston CE, Chakravarti A: Genetic epidemiology of rheumatoid arthritis. *Am J Hum Genet* 1995;57: 150–159.

Mackay K, Raghunath M, Superti-Furga A, Steinmann B, Dalgleish R: Ehlers-Danlos syndrome type IV caused by Gly400Glu, Gly595Cys and Gly1003Asp substitutions in collagen III: Clinical features, biochemical screening, and molecular confirmation. *Clin Genet* 1996;49:286–295.

MacKenzie JJ, Jacob P, Surh L, Besner A: Genetic heterogeneity in spinal muscular atrophy: A linkage analysis-based assessment. *Neurology* 1994;44:919–924.

MacKenzie JJ, Fitzpatrick J, Babyn P, et al: X linked spondyloepiphyseal dysplasia: A clinical, radiological, and molecular study of a large kindred. *J Med Genet* 1996;33:823–828.

Mahadevan MS, Amemiya C, Jansen G, et al: Structure and genomic sequence of the myotonic dystrophy (DM kinase) gene. *Hum Mol Genet* 1993;2:299–304.

Marie PJ, de Pollak C, Chanson P, Lomri A: Increased proliferation of osteoblastic cells expressing the activating Gs alpha mutation in monostotic and polyostotic fibrous dysplasia. *Am J Pathol* 1997;150: 1059–1069.

Marini JC, Gerber NL: Osteogenesis imperfecta: Rehabilitation and prospects for gene therapy. *JAMA* 1997;277:746–750.

McGrory J, Weksberg R, Thorner P, Cole WG: Abnormal extracellular matrix in Ehlers-Danlos syndrome type IV due to the substitution of glycine 934 by glutamic acid in the triple helical domain of type III collagen. *Clin Genet* 1996;50:442–445.

McIntosh I, Abbott MH, Warman ML, Olsen BR, Francomano CA: Additional mutations of type X collagen confirm COL10A1 as the Schmid metaphyseal chondrodysplasia locus. *Hum Mol Genet* 1994;3:303–307.

McKusick VA: The defect in Marfan syndrome. *Nature* 1991;352: 279–281.

Mirabella M, Servidei S, Manfredi G, et al: Cardiomyopathy may be the only clinical manifestation in female carriers of Duchenne muscular dystrophy. *Neurology* 1993;43:2342–2345.

Moloney DM, Slaney SF, Oldridge M, et al: Exclusive paternal origin of new mutations in Apert syndrome. *Nat Genet* 1996;13:48–53.

Monaco AP, Kunkel LM: Cloning of the Duchenne/Becker muscular dystrophy locus, in Harris H, Hirschhorn K (eds): *Advances in Human Genetics*. New York, NY, Plenum Press, 1988, vol 17, pp 61–98.

Monrós E, Moltó MD, Martínez F, et al: Phenotype correlation and intergenerational dynamics of the Friedreich ataxia GAA trinucleotide repeat. *Am J Hum Genet* 1997;61:101–110.

Moreira ES, Vainzof M, Marie SK, Sertié AL, Zatz M, Passos-Bueno MR: The seventh form of autosomal recessive limb-girdle muscular dystrophy is mapped to 17q11-12. *Am J Hum Genet* 1997;61:151–159.

Morrison NA, Qi JC, Tokita A, et al: Prediction of bone density from vitamin D receptor alleles. *Nature* 1994;367:284–287.

Muenke M, Gripp KW, McDonald-McGinn DM, et al: A unique point mutation in the fibroblast growth factor receptor 3 gene (FGFR3) defines a new craniosynostosis syndrome. *Am J Hum Genet* 1997;60:555–564.

Muenke M, Schell U: Fibroblast-growth-factor receptor mutations in human skeletal disorders. *Trends Genet* 1995;11:308–313.

Müller B, Melki J, Burlet P, Clerget-Darpoux F: Proximal spinal muscular atrophy (SMA) types II and III in the same sibship are not caused by different alleles at the SMA locus on 5q. *Am J Hum Genet* 1992;50:892–895.

Mundlos S, Otto F, Mundlos C, et al: Mutations involving the transcription factor CBFA1 cause cleidocranial dysplasia. *Cell* 1997;89:773–779.

Mundy GR: Osteoporosis: Boning up on genes. *Nature* 1994;367: 216–217.

Munsat TL, Skerry L, Korf B, et al: Phenotypic heterogeneity of spinal muscular atrophy mapping to chromosome 5q11.2-13.3 (SMA 5q). *Neurology* 1990;40:1831–1836.

Muragaki Y, Mariman EC, van Beersum SE, et al: A mutation in the gene encoding the alpha 2 chain of the fibril-associated collagen IX, COL9A2, causes multiple epiphyseal dysplasia (EDM2). *Nat Genet* 1996;12:103–105.

Muragaki Y, Mundlos S, Upton J, Olsen BR: Altered growth and branching patterns in synpolydactyly caused by mutations in HOXD13. *Science* 1996;272:548–551.

Murdoch JL, Walker BA, Hall JG, Abbey H, Smith KK, McKusick VA: Achondroplasia: A genetic and statistical survey. *Ann Hum Genet* 1970;33: 227–244.

Murray JC, Buetow KH, Weber JL, et al: A comprehensive human linkage map with centimorgan density: Cooperative Human Linkage Center (CHLC). *Science* 1994;265:2049–2054.

Murray LW, Bautista J, James PL, Rimoin DL: Type 11 collagen defects in the chondrodysplasias: I. Spondyloepiphyseal dysplasias. *Am J Hum Genet* 1989;45:5–15.

Nesbitt T, Coffman TM, Griffiths R, Drezner MK: Crosstransplantation of kidneys in normal and Hyp mice: Evidence that the Hyp mouse phenotype is unrelated to an intrinsic renal defect. *J Clin Invest* 1992;89:1453–1459.

Nicholls AC, De Paepe A, Narcisi P, et al: Linkage of a polymorphic marker for the type III collagen gene (COL3A1) to atypical autosomal dominant Ehlers-Danlos syndrome type IV in a large Belgian pedigree. *Hum Genet* 1988;78:276–281.

Oberklaid F, Danks DM, Jensen F, Stace L, Rosshandler S: Achondroplasia and hypochondroplasia: Comments on frequency, mutation rate, and radiological features in skull and spine. *J Med Genet* 1979;16:140–146.

Oldridge M, Lunt PW, Zackai EH, et al: Genotype-phenotype correlation for nucleotide substitutions in the IgII-IgIII linker of FGFR2. *Hum Mol Genet* 1997;6:137–143.

Palotie A, Vaisanen P, Ott J, et al: Predisposition to familial osteoarthrosis linked to type II collagen gene. *Lancet* 1989;l:924–927.

Park WJ, Theda C, Maestri NE, et al: Analysis of phenotypic features and FGFR2 mutations in Apert syndrome. *Am J Hum Genet* 1995;57: 321–328.

Paschalis EP, Jacenko O, Olsen B, Mendelsohn R, Boskey AL: Fourier transform infrared microspectroscopic analysis identifies alterations in mineral properties in bones from mice transgenic for type X collagen. *Bone* 1996;19:151–156.

Paulson HL, Fischbeck KH: Trinucleotide repeats in neurogenetic disorders. *Annu Rev Neurosci* 1996;19:79–107.

Peacock M: Vitamin D receptor gene alleles and osteoporosis: A contrasting view. *J Bone Miner Res* 1995;10:1294–1297.

Phillippe C, Porter DE, Emerton ME, Wells DE, Simpson AH, Monaco AP: Mutation screening of the EXT1 and EXT2 genes in patients with hereditary multiple exostoses. *Am J Hum Genet* 1997;61: 520–528.

Poole AR, Pidoux I, Reiner A, et al: Kniest dysplasia is characterized by an apparent abnormal processing of the C-propeptide of type II cartilage collagen resulting in imperfect fibril assembly. *J Clin Invest* 1988;81: 579–589.

Poole AR, Rosenberg L, Murray L, Rimoin D: Kniest dysplasia: A probable type II collagen defect. *Patho Immunopathol Res* 1988;7: 95–98.

Prior TW, Bartolo C, Pearl DK, et al: Spectrum of small mutations in the dystrophin coding region. *Am J Hum Genet* 1995;57:22–33.

Radhakrishna U, Blouin JL, Mehenni H, et al: Mapping one form of autosomal/dominant postaxial polydactyly type A to chromosome 7p15-q11.23 by linkage analysis. *Am J Hum Genet* 1997;60:597–604.

Rass-Rothschild A, Manouvrier S, Gonzales M, Farriaux JP, Lyonnet S, Munnich A: Refined mapping of a gene for split hand-split foot malformation (SHFM3) on chromosome 10q25. *J Med Genet* 1996;33: 996–1001.

Rebbeck TR, Dietz FR, Murray JC, Buetow KH: A single-gene explanation for the probability of having idiopathic talipes equinovarus. *Am J Hum Genet* 1993;53:1051–1063.

Rodrigues NR, Owen N, Talbot K, et al: Gene deletions in spinal muscular atrophy. *J Med Genet* 1996;33:93–96.

Rogala EJ, Drummonds DS, Gurr J: Scoliosis: Incidence and natural history. A prospective epidemiological study. *J Bone Joint Surg* 1978; 60A:173–176.

Rogers J, Mahaney MC, Beamer WG, Donahue LR, Rosen CJ: Beyond one gene-one disease: Alternative strategies for deciphering genetic determinants of osteoporosis. *Calcif Tissue Int* 1997;60:225–228.

Rossi A, van der Harten HJ, Beemer FA, et al: Phenotypic and genotypic overlap between atelosteogenesis type 2 and diastrophic dysplasia. *Hum Genet* 1996;98:657–661.

Roy N, Mahadevan MS, McLean M, et al: The gene for neuronal apoptosis inhibitory protein is partially deleted in individuals with spinal muscular atrophy. *Cell* 1995;80:167–178.

Ruttledge MH, Andermann AA, Phelan CM, et al: Type of mutation in the neurofibromatosis type 2 gene (NF2) frequently determines severity of disease. *Am J Hum Genet* 1996;59:331–342.

Schipani E, Kruse K, Juppner H: A constitutively active mutan PTH-PTHrP receptor in Jansen-type metaphyseal chondrodysplasia. *Science* 1995;268:98–100.

Serra E, Puig S, Otero D, et al: Confirmation of a double-hit model for the NF1 gene in benign neurofibromas. *Am J Hum Genet* 1997;61:512–519.

Sheffield VC, Pierpont ME, Nishimura D, et al: Identification of a complex congenital heart defect susceptibility locus by using DNA pooling and shared segment analysis. *Hum Mol Genet* 1997; 6:117–121.

Shenker A, Chanson P, Weinstein LS, et al: Osteoblastic cells derived from isolated lesions of fibrous dysplasia contain activating somatic mutations of the Gs alpha gene. *Hum Mol Genet* 1995;4:1675–1676.

Shenker A, Weinstein LS, Sweet DE, Spiegel AM: An activating Gs alpha mutation is present in fibrous dysplasia of bone in the McCune-Albright syndrome. *J Clin Endocrinol Metab* 1994;79: 750–755.

Sher C, Ramesar R, Martell R, Learmonth I, Tsipouras P, Beighton P: Mild spondyloepiphyseal dysplasia (Namaqualand type): Genetic linkage to the type II collagen gene (COL2A1). *Am J Hum Genet* 1991;48:518–524.

Sheth P, Abdelhak S, Bachelot MF, et al: Linkage analysis in spinal muscular atrophy, by six closely flanking markers on chromosome 5. *Am J Hum Genet* 1991;48:764–768.

Shiang R, Thompson LS, Zhu Y-Z, et al: Mutations in the transmembrane domain of FGFR3 cause the most common genetic form of dwarfism, achondroplasia. *Cell* 1994;78:335–342.

Shimokawa M, Ishiura S, Kameda N, et al: Novel isoform of myotonin protein kinase: Gene product of myotonin dystrophy is localized in the sarcoplasmic reticulum of skeletal muscle. *Am J Pathol* 1997;150:1285–1295.

Slaney SF, Oldridge M, Hurst JA, et al: Differential effects of FGFR2 mutations on syndactyly and cleft palate in Apert syndrome. *Am J Hum Genet* 1996;58:923–932.

Soares VM, Brzustowicz LM, Kleyn PW, et al: Refinement of the spinal muscular atrophy locus to the interval between D5S435 and MAP1B. *Genomics* 1993;15:365–371.

Spector TD, Cicuttini F, Baker J, Loughlin J, Hart D: Genetic influences on osteoarthritis in women: A twin study. *Br Med J* 1996;312: 940–943.

Steinmann B, Royce PM, Superti-Furga A: The Ehlers-Danlos syndrome, in Royce PM, Steinmann B (eds): *Connective Tissue and Its Heritable Disorders: Molecular, Genetic, and Medical Aspects*. New York, NY, Wiley-Liss, 1993, pp 351–407.

Stevanin G, Trottier Y, Cancel G, et al: Screening for proteins with polyglutamine expansions in autosomal dominant cerebellar ataxias. *Hum Mol Genet* 1996;5:1887–1892.

Superti-Furga A: A defect in the metabolic activation of sulfate in a patient with achondrogenesis type IB. *Am J Hum Genet* 1994;55: 1137–1145.

Tamai M, Yokouchi M, Komiya S, et al: Correlation between vitamin D receptor genotypes and bone mineral density in Japanese patients with osteoporosis. *Calcif Tissue Int* 1997;60:229–232.

Tavormina PL, Shiang R, Thompson LM, et al: Thanatophoric dysplasia (types I and II) caused by distinct mutations in fibroblast growth factor receptor 3. *Nat Genet* 1995;9:321–328.

Thomas PK, Marques W Jr, Davis MB, et al: The phenotypic manifestations of chromosome 17p11.2 duplication. *Brain* 1997;120: 465–478.

Thomson G, Bodmer W: HLA haplotype associations with disease. *Tissue Antigens* 1979;13:91–102.

Tiller GE, Polumbo PA, Weis M, et al: Dominant mutations in the type II collagen gene, COL2A1, produce spondyloepimetaphyseal dysplasia, Strudwick type. *Nat Genet* 1995;11:87–89.

Tiller GE, Rimoin DL, Murray LW, Cohn DH: Tandem duplication within a type II collagen gene (COL2A1) exon in an individual with spondyloepiphyseal dysplasia. *Proc Natl Acad Sci USA* 1990;87: 3889–3893.

Tiller GE, Weis MA, Polumbo PA, et al: An RNA-splicing mutation (G+5IVS20) in the type II collagen gene (COL2A1) in a family with spondyloepiphyseal dysplasia congenita. *Am J Hum Genet* 1995; 56:388–395.

Timchenko LT, Caskey CT: Trinucleotide repeat disorders in humans: Discussions of mechanisms and medical issues. *FASEB J* 1996;10: 1589–1597.

Tsipouras P, Del Mastro R, Sarfarazi M, et al: The International Marfan Syndrome Collaborative Study: Genetic linkage of the Marfan syndrome, ectopia lentis, and congenital contractural arachnodactyly to the fibrillin genes on chromosomes 15 and 5. *N Engl J Med* 1992;326:905–909.

Vainzof M, Passos-Bueno MR, Canovas M, et al: The sarcoglycan complex in the six autosomal recessive limb-girdle muscular dystrophies. *Hum Mol Genet* 1996;5:1963–1969.

Vandevyver C, Wylin T, Cassiman JJ, Raus J, Geusens P: Influence of the vitamin D receptor gene alleles on bone mineral density in postmenopausal and osteoporotic women. *J Bone Miner Res* 1997;12: 241–247.

Van Hul W, Bollerslev J, Gram J, et al: Localization of a gene for autosomal dominant osteopetrosis (Albers-Schonberg disease) to chromosome 1p21. *Am J Hum Genet* 1997;61:363–369.

Wang JH, Palmer RM, Chung CS: The role of major gene in clubfoot. *Am J Hum Genet* 1988;42:772–776.

Wenstrup RJ, Langland GT, Willing MC, D'Souza VN, Cole WG: A splice-junction mutation in the region of COL5A1 that codes for the carboxyl propeptide of pro(1(V) chains results in the gravis form of the Ehlers-Danlos syndrome (type 1). *Hum Mol Genet* 1996;5: 1733–1736.

Williams CJ, Jimenez SA: Heredity, genes and osteoarthritis. *Rheum Dis Clin North Am* 1993;19:523–543.

Willing MC, Deschenes SP, Slayton RL, Roberts EJ: Premature chain termination is a unifying mechanism for COL1A1 null alleles in osteogenesis imperfecta type 1 cell strains. *Am J Hum Genet* 1996;59:799–809.

Winterpacht A, Superti-Furga A, Schwarze U, et al: The deletion of six amino acids at the C-terminus of the α1(II) chain causes overmodification of type II and type XI collagen: Further evidence for the association between small deletions in COL2A1 and Kniest dysplasia. *J Med Genet* 1996;33:649–654.

Wu Y-Q, Heutink P, de Vries BB, et al: Assignment of a second locus for multiple exostoses to the pericentromeric region of chromosome 11. *Hum Mol Genet* 1994;3:167–171.

Wuyts W, Ramlakhan S, Van Hul W, et al: Refinement of the multiple exostoses locus (EXT2) to a 3-cM interval on chromosome 11. *Am J Hum Genet* 1995;57:382–387.

Wynne-Davies R: Family studies and the cause of congenital club foot: Talipes equinovarus, talipes calcaneo-valgus and metatarsus varus. *J Bone Joint Surg* 1964;46B:445–463.

Yang HY, Chung CS, Nemechek RW: A genetic analysis of clubfoot in Hawaii. *Genet Epidermiol* 1987;4:299–306.

Zhuchenko O, Bailey J, Bonnen P, et al: Autosomal dominant cerebellar ataxia (SCA6) associated with small polyglutamine expansions in the α1A-voltage-dependent calcium channel. *Nat Genet* 1997;15: 62–69.

Chapter Outline

Chapter 5

Biomechanics

Van C. Mow, PhD

Evan L. Flatow, MD

Gerard A. Ateshian, PhD

This chapter at a glance

This chapter provides a review of some fundamental principles of mechanics and demonstrates the use of these principles in some specific orthopaedic biomechanics problems.

Introduction

The musculoskeletal system, although complex, obeys the basic laws of mechanics. Biomechanics is the branch of science that deals with the effects of energy and forces on biologic systems. The study of biomechanics involves the application of Newton's laws of mechanics to models of biologic objects in order to describe their behavior and their functions. Orthopaedic biomechanics has focused on the effects—motions and deformation—of forces and moments acting on tissues such as bone, cartilage, growth plate, ligament, meniscus, synovial fluid, and tendon. The study of biomechanics has been important in the development and design of many of the joint replacement and fracture fixation devices commonly used in orthopaedic surgery today. Kinematics describes motions within the musculoskeletal system, such as those of diarthrodial joints (hip, knee, shoulder, etc), as well as locomotion and gait. Biotribology is the study of friction, lubrication, and wear resulting from the interaction of apposed articular surfaces in relative motion.

In addition to describing normal structure and function, clinical orthopaedic biomechanics seeks to examine specific pathologic conditions through the study of joint instability, gait pathologies, and fracture healing. Furthermore, surgical procedures designed to restore normal mechanics may be critically evaluated, using techniques such as force analysis of tendon transfer, kinematic studies of ligament repair, and finite element analysis of joint replacements.

This chapter provides a review of some fundamental principles of mechanics and demonstrates the use of these principles in some specific orthopaedic biomechanics problems. It includes definitions of forces and moments and examples of their calculation in specific cases (knee, hip, shoulder, spine, etc), as well as definitions of stresses and strains and examples of how these provide the intrinsic material properties of biologic materials. Furthermore, this chapter covers the friction, lubrication, and wear mechanisms existing in diarthrodial joints. Finally, some basic concepts of biomaterials and prosthesis design will be surveyed.

Skeletal Forces

Vectors and Forces

There are many types of physical quantities. Temperature, mass, volume, density, etc, are scalar physical quantities. Only one number is needed to quantify the magnitude of a scalar quantity. For example, temperature is quantified in degrees Celsius, mass in kilograms, volume in cubic meters, and density in kilograms/m³. Vectors are quantities that have direction and magnitude. Velocity, acceleration, force, and moment are all vectors. A vector is portrayed by an arrow; its direction is indicated by the direction of the arrow, and its magnitude is represented by the length of the arrow. For example, the velocity of a car going from east to west at 80 km/hr is defined by a vector; its direction is east to west and its magnitude is the speed 80 km/hr. Although body weight commonly is thought of as a magnitude, for example, 150 lb, it also has direction, which is down. Thus, the weight of a limb or body segment must always be portrayed by a vector in the direction of gravity (down), with its length defined relative to the weight of the limb applied at its center of gravity. The importance of direction is illustrated in Figure 1. When the arm is at the side of the body, the weight of the forearm will tend to extend the elbow; when the arm is elevated overhead, this weight will act to flex the elbow.

A force, in its most elementary definition, is a "push" or a "pull." For example, when the foot contacts the floor during standing, a force exists between the foot and the floor. The foot pushes on the floor and the floor pushes back, because

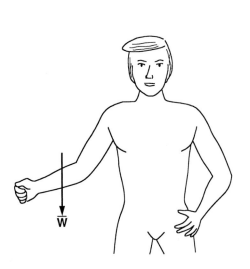
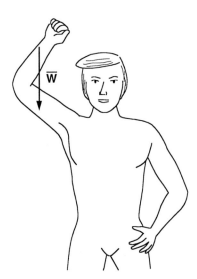

Figure 1

A force is a vector. The importance of direction is illustrated here.

according to Newton's third law, for every force (action) there is an equal and opposite force (reaction). Figure 2, *A*, illustrates an example of a force exerted on the foot. The unit most commonly used for force is the newton (N).

Two vector quantities, such as forces, may be added according to the parallelogram law of vector addition. This is done by using the 2 vectors as 2 sides of a parallelogram and then drawing a new arrow along the diagonal (Fig. 2, *B*). A vector is usually denoted by a boldface letter or a letter with an arrow, →, or bar, –, over it. Figure 3 shows that the force of the quadriceps F_Q, pulling the patella proximally, added to the force of the patellar tendon F_P, pulling it distally, results in a force R, which tends to compress the patella against the femur.

A bit of reflection will show that the parallelogram law also means that any vector may be broken down into component forces along any specified mutually perpendicular coordinate axes. The original vector F is the sum of its components along these axes:

$$F = F_x + F_y + F_z,$$

as shown in Figure 4. The magnitudes of F_x, F_y, F_z are denoted by $|F_x|$, $|F_y|$, $|F_z|$, or F_x, F_y, F_z, and they are known as the components of the vector F with respect to the xyz coordinate system.

The magnitude of the force F, denoted by $|F|$, is given by the Pythagorean theorem:

$$|F|^2 = |F_x|^2 + |F_y|^2 + |F_z|^2.$$

Figure 5 illustrates how the force of the deltoid F_D acting on the humerus may be broken down into a compressive force F_C acting perpendicularly ("normal") to the glenoid joint surface and a "shear" force F_S acting parallel (tangential) to the surface. This deltoid force also creates a moment (or rotation), which is defined next.

Moments

A force applied to an object may both push or pull and twist that object. That action of a force applied to an object, which tends to rotate the object about an axis, is called a moment. The force applied to the wrench handle in Figure 6 will generate a moment about the axis OO´ of the bolt. The magnitude of the moment about the axis OO´, M_o, caused by this force is equal to the magnitude of the force F multiplied by the perpendicular distance d from the axis

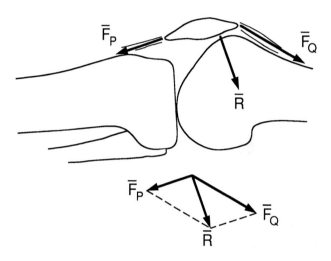

Figure 3

The force of the quadriceps F_Q added to the force of the patellar tendon F_P, in accordance with the parallelogram law, produces the resultant force R, which tends to compress the patella against the femur.

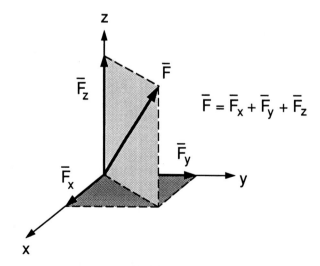

$$\bar{F} = \bar{F}_x + \bar{F}_y + \bar{F}_z$$

Figure 4

The parallelogram law of vector addition permits any vector to be resolved into its component vectors along any set of mutually orthogonal coordinate axes. This resolution is expressed by the equation $F = F_x + F_y + F_z$.

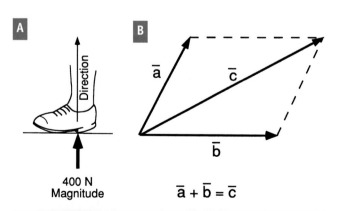

Figure 2

A, An example of the reaction force exerted on the foot by the floor. **B,** Two vector quantities are added according to the parallelogram law of vector addition; a and b are the sides of the parallelogram and c is the diagonal, which is known as the resultant vector.

OO´ of the bolt to the line of action A-A of the force; $M_o = F \times d = F \times l\sin\theta$. Clearly, M_o is also equal to $F\sin\theta \times l$, that is, to the component of F perpendicular to the wrench multiplied by the length of the wrench l. The distance d is often referred to as the moment arm. The units used for a moment are N·m. In the example shown in Figure 6, there is a 200 N force applied on the handle at a perpendicular distance of 25 cm from the bolt. The moment applied to the bolt is therefore 200 N × 25 cm or 50 N·m. The magnitude of a moment is a torque. Using the right hand rule, the direction of the moment is given by the thumb of the right hand when the fingers of the right hand are taken to be along the direction of rotation caused by the force. Note that a moment corresponds to a specific axis about which it turns. It does not matter whether any rotation ever occurs. Thus, it is possible to choose the most convenient axis for the problem at hand, and, indeed, any force will exert a moment around any point not located along its line of action.

When a moment is created by equal, noncolinear, parallel but oppositely directed forces F and -F, the moment created is called a couple. The simplest examples are the thumb and index fingers twisting off a bottle cap, or 2 hands turning a steering wheel. Figure 7, A, shows such a pair of forces in the xy plane. Obviously, the resultant force is zero. The magnitude of the couple is Fd, where d is the perpendicular distance between the 2 forces. Although the torque created by a single force is dependent on the location of the reference point O (Fig. 6), the torque of the couple is not. Thus, a couple is a free pure moment vector with no resultant force, and may be applied anywhere in the plane determined by the 2 vectors F and -F. The couple is a very important concept, because the effects of any force may be made equivalent to a couple and a force. This is shown in Figure 7, B, by a force F applied at a point A. The line of action of F closest to O is at A´; the distance d is the moment arm of F relative to point O. A pair of imaginary forces F and -F is added at the origin O. The original problem has not changed because these opposite forces cancel each other. The pair of forces composed of -F at O and the original force F at A is a couple. Its magnitude is Fd, and it is a free pure moment acting in the xy plane. The remaining force is the force F acting at O. Thus, the force F acting at A is equipollent to a force F acting at O and a couple. This important result is very useful in understanding the effects of muscle action around a joint.

Dynamics

An unopposed force acting on an object will accelerate the object; that is, it will change the velocity of the object. This is known as a nonequilibrium (dynamic) condition. It is important to note that, because velocity is a vector, a

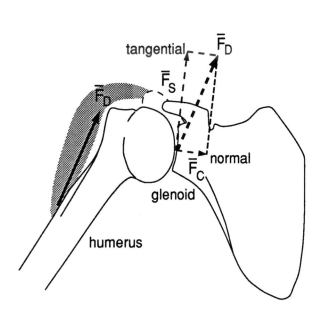

Figure 5

The force of the deltoid muscle F_D acting on the humerus may be resolved into a compressive force F_C, acting perpendicularly or normal to the glenoid joint surface, and a shear force F_S, acting parallel or tangential to the surface. F_D also creates a moment, which is not shown.

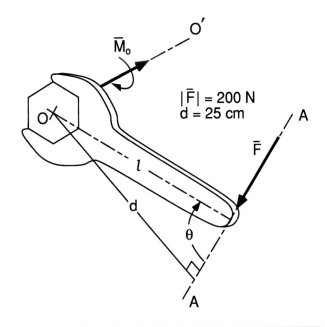

Figure 6

The magnitude of the moment about OO´, perpendicular to the face of the wrench, caused by the force F, parallel to the face of the wrench, is equal to the magnitude of the force multiplied by the perpendicular distance d from the axis OO´ to the line of action A-A of the force; $M_o = F \times d = F \times l\sin\theta$. The direction of the moment is given by the right hand rule.

change of velocity could mean a change of direction or of speed (magnitude) or of both. For example, a ball on the end of a string being twirled around at a constant speed moves in a circular path. Because its direction is constantly changing, there is an acceleration. In this case the tension (force) in the string produces a centripetal (toward the center) acceleration. If the string breaks, the ball will fly off in a straight line.

An acceleration produced by a force occurring along a straight line is called a linear acceleration. An acceleration produced by a torque occurs about an axis of rotation and is called an angular acceleration.

Figure 8 shows an example of linear deceleration. Here, the force of the floor is pushing up on the feet of a person who has just landed from a jump. This force is acting to decelerate, and eventually stop, the person's downward motion and, therefore, would be much greater than if the person were standing, when the force from the floor was balancing only body weight. The increase in force is proportional to the deceleration, which is, on average, equal to the change in speed divided by the time interval during which the change occurs. Thus, factors that lengthen this time interval, such as soft, compressible running-shoe heels or bending the knees, will diminish the decelerating force, that is, soften the impact.

Figure 9 shows an example of angular acceleration. The knee extensor force F_e generates a moment about the center of rotation O in the knee. The magnitude of the moment is given by $M_o = F_e \times d$. It provides an angular acceleration to the lower leg in rotation about the center of rotation of the knee O. The greater the magnitude of the force F_e, the greater the impact will be at the instant the foot strikes the football. The moment M_o can be changed in only 2 ways: (1) change d (for example, total knee replacement or tibial tubercle elevation); or (2) change the magnitude of F_e. The first option is surgical; the second option is exercise or physical therapy.

The knee extensor force F_e is equivalent to a force F_e acting at the center of the knee O, causing compression of the tibial plateau and femoral condyle surfaces, and a pure moment (couple) $M_o = F_e \times d$, rotating the lower leg about O. Thus, contrary to popular notions, during a "free" swing of the upper or lower extremity, compressive forces may be generated at the articulating surfaces when the muscles are active; the faster the swing, the larger the compressive force.

Most musculoskeletal movements are caused in this way. Limbs are rotated about joints as a result of the moments produced by the skeletal flexor and extensor muscles. Thus, it is apparent that the musculoskeletal system is essentially a collection of lever systems (shoulder, hip, knee, ankle, etc) linked together. The facts that the lever arms of muscles and tendons are generally very small and the moment arms of the extremities themselves are generally large result in a mechanical disadvantage that requires generation of large muscle forces to create moments large enough for movement.

Statics

Biomechanical Modeling Concepts

Biomechanics and, indeed, mechanics provide a means to study a problem through its representation by a physical model. Assumptions about the isolated unit must be made to construct the model. These assumptions deal with the geometry of the unit (size and shape) and the nature of the material(s) of which the unit is composed. Furthermore, assumptions must also be made about the nature of forces

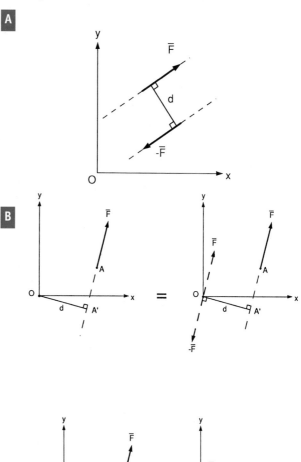

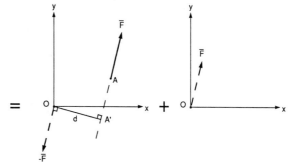

Figure 7

A, A couple is created by 2 equal, noncolinear, parallel but oppositely directed forces F and -F. The magnitude of the couple is Fd, where d is the perpendicular distance between the 2 forces. The resultant force of a couple is zero. **B,** A single force F applied at a point A acting along A-A', whose perpendicular distance to O is d, is equipollent to a force acting at O and a couple of magnitude Fd.

and moments acting on the surface of the object. These forces and moments move and deform the object. Clearly, the accuracy and acceptability of predictions based on the model depend on how well the model is constructed, especially on how closely it represents the actual unit with respect to the specific types of questions being pursued in the study. For example, modeling the action of a muscle on a bone as a single resultant force applied to the muscle's point of insertion may be reasonable if the aim of the study is to understand the muscle's moment about an adjacent joint, or to help predict the effect of a tendon transfer on

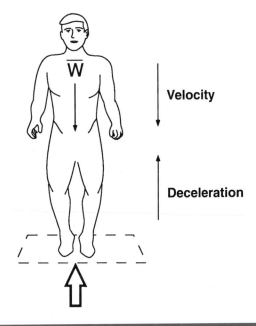

Orthopaedic Basic Science | American Academy of Orthopaedic Surgeons

gait. However, this model would be totally inadequate in a study aimed at understanding modes of tendon failure in tension, in which the precise geometry of the tendon and its insertion, the pattern of stress and strain within the tendon under load, and the material properties of the tendon are crucial to the problem.

A rigid body is an idealization of a real object; it assumes that the body is absolutely rigid so that it does not stretch, compress, or otherwise deform no matter how large are the forces and moments acting on it. This assumption, for example, usually is made in gait analysis models. Here, the model for the musculoskeletal system assumes bones to be absolutely rigid rods (stick figures) and joints to be rigid frictionless hinges. The important elements of rigid body mechanics are: (1) the magnitude and direction of forces and moments acting on the object; (2) the total mass of, and its distribution within, the object; and (3) the size and geometric form of the object.

Equilibrium

When the sum of all forces acting on an object is zero and the sum of all moments acting on an object also is zero, there will be no linear or angular acceleration; the object is said to be in equilibrium, at rest, or at constant velocity.

Large forces may be involved within a system at equilibrium, although the sum of all forces is zero when added together. For example, 2 evenly matched men playing tug-of-war will be at equilibrium so long as they pull equally hard on each end of the rope. Static analysis examines systems in equilibrium in this fashion. Although biologic systems are rarely in complete equilibrium, static analysis often is helpful in estimating skeletal forces.

Figure 10 illustrates the concept of both force and moment equilibrium. In this example, 2 children, one weighing 600 N and the other weighing 300 N, are sitting on

Figure 8

The reaction force provided by the floor pushing up on the feet of a person landing from a jump decelerates his/her downward motion.

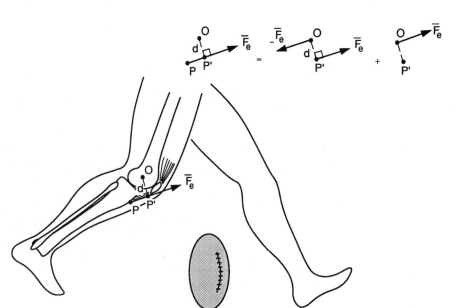

Figure 9

The knee extensor force F_e generates a moment about the center of rotation O in the knee. The magnitude of the moment is given by $M_o = F_e \times d$. Note that from the concept of the equipollent force systems, the knee extensor force F_e is equivalent to a force F_e acting at the center of the knee O, compressing the tibial plateau and femoral condyle surfaces together, and a pure moment $M_o = F_e \times d$, rotating the lower leg about O.

the seesaw. At equilibrium, the amount of force applied at the hinge support of the seesaw must equal the sum of the weight of the 2 children. Thus, the reaction force R at the hinge may be calculated by summing all the forces acting on the seesaw: -300 N (down) -600N (down) + R (up) = 0. Hence, the reaction force R at the hinge is a vector of magnitude 900 N pointing up.

For an object to be in equilibrium, the sum of all the moments must also equal zero. In this example, because the seesaw is not rotating, the net moment about the hinge supports must equal zero. Thus, for the sum of the moments about the hinge O to balance, the 300-N child must be sitting at a distance of 2 m to the right of the hinge to cancel the moment of the 600-N child sitting 1 m to the left of the hinge. The moment 300 N × 2 m clockwise must be equal to the moment 600 N × 1 m counterclockwise. The reaction force of 900 N at the hinge does not cause a moment about the hinge, because the moment arm of this force is zero. For many applications, a hinge is used because it cannot transmit a moment.

Thus, static equilibrium analysis examines a system at rest in which all the forces are balanced, allowing unknown forces, which must exist to balance the known forces, to be determined.

Problem: When an object is in static equilibrium, any point may be used to calculate the moment, and the sum of all these moments will still be zero. Demonstrate this principle by calculating the moments caused by the 2 children and the reaction force about A.

Free-Body Diagrams

The forces acting on any limb or body part may be identified by isolating that body part as a free body. For a portion of the body to be at equilibrium, the sum of all forces must be zero, and the sum of all moments must be zero. Because both forces and moments are vectors, they must sum to zero in each of 3 perpendicular directions. Thus, in 3 dimensions, there are a total of 6 equations of equilibrium, and a maximum of 6 unknowns may be solved.

Statically determinate problems are ones in which the number of unknown forces and moments is equal to the number of available equations. These equations may then be solved to determine the unknown forces. In statically indeterminate problems, the number of unknowns exceeds the number of equations available. Thus, there are not enough equations to solve for the unknowns, and if a solution for the unknowns is available, it will not be unique. To illustrate this point, consider the seesaw problem shown in Figure 10. Is it possible to determine the weights of 2 persons by seating them at known distances from the hinge at one side when the weight of the third person at the other side of the hinge is known, and that person's seating position relative to the hinge is specified so that the seesaw is balanced horizontally? The seesaw is similar to the old-fashioned, lever-arm balance scale used to determine weights. However, in this seesaw problem, there are 3 unknowns: the vertical reaction force at the hinge and the weights of the 2 persons, and there are only 2 equations: the vertical component of force and the moment about an axis perpendicular to the plane of the seesaw (the axis may be taken to be the hinge). Clearly, in this problem, no unique solution can be found, because an infinite variation of weights for the 2 individuals may be chosen to balance this seesaw. Unfortunately, in nearly every problem encountered in orthopaedic biomechanics, which involves the determination of muscle and joint forces, the situation is statically indeterminate because of the large number of muscles spanning the joint. This problem may be remedied by drastically simplifying the model, sometimes even in an unrealistic manner, so that an estimate of the important muscle or joint force may be obtained. Once again, of course, the reliability and accuracy of any model calcula-

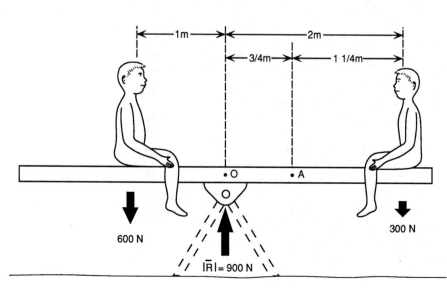

Figure 10

Force and moment balance must occur for motion equilibrium to exist. The reaction force at the hinge (900 N) may be determined by setting the sum of all vertical forces to zero. The sum of the moments must also equal zero so that the seesaw does not rotate.

tions depend on how realistic that model is in replicating the actual anatomic and physiologic circumstances.

A method frequently used in modeling is to assume that a muscle force exists only in tension; that is, to assume that muscles cannot exert compressive forces. Another commonly used method is to assume that the joint-reaction force only can be compressive; that is, tension force at the joint will cause the joint surfaces to lose contact. If the line of action of the muscle force is defined by assuming that it always acts along the center of the cross-sectional area of the muscle mass, the magnitude of the muscle force is the only remaining unknown. Another common simplifying assumption is to model a joint as a hinge (for example, the ankle), eliminating 2 of 3 possible axes of rotation and ignoring translations.

In this method of solving for the forces and moments around a joint at equilibrium, only the external forces and moments acting on the free body are considered. Internal forces within the free body cancel out. However, if care is taken in choosing the part to be modeled as a free body, it is possible to expose an internal force.

Forces on the Hip Joint

The free-body method of solution will be illustrated by calculating the abductor and joint-reaction forces at the hip. Figure 11, A, illustrates the case of a person standing on the right leg. In this free-body diagram, the body and the left leg have a weight of 5 W/6, where W is the total weight of the person. This weight must be supported and balanced by the force acting on the right acetabulum, joint-reaction force F_j, and by the action of the abductor muscles, F_{AB}. The moment equilibrium equation can be applied to determine the abductor force acting about the hip joint. The weight, 5 W/6, which tends to rotate the upper body about the center of the femoral head O, is counteracted by the pull of the abductor muscles on the pelvis. The hip joint is assumed to be frictionless so no reaction moment exists. Thus, for the body to be in equilibrium, the unknown counterclockwise moment (+) created by the abductor muscles must be balanced by the known clockwise moment (-) created by the gravitational forces of 5 W/6. In this model, the point of application and direction of the abductor force F_{AB} are assumed to be known from anatomic data; thus, only the magnitude of F_{AB} is unknown. Taking the moments about the center of the femoral head O, with b the distance from O to the line of action of the 5 W/6 weight and a the distance from O to the abductor muscle force F_{AB}, the magnitudes of the 2 moments are -(5 W/6) × (b) and (F_{AB}) × (a), respectively. For equilibrium, the sum of these 2 moments must equal zero. Thus, given a body weight W and a measured distance of a = 5 cm and b = 15 cm, the magnitude of the abductor muscle force F_{AB} will be 2.5 W (Fig. 11, A). The reaction force at the joint F_j does not create a moment about the joint center (center of rotation), similarly to the reaction force at the hinge in the seesaw.

The hip-joint-reaction force F_j can be calculated by applying the force equilibrium condition that the sum of all forces acting on the pelvis must equal zero. This calculation is made by using a force triangle, based on the parallelogram law of vector addition (Fig. 11, B). When only 3 forces are acting on a body in equilibrium, these forces must form a closed force triangle, because the 2 forces 5 W/6 and F_{AB} must add, by the parallelogram law, to equal the third unknown force F_j. Therefore, by simple geometric construction with the 2 known sides of the triangle, the gravitational force on the body, 5 W/6, and the abductor muscle force, 2.5 W, drawn to scale, the third side of the triangle also can be drawn to scale. The length of this third side is the magnitude of F_j and the direction of the arrow is the direction of the force F_j. In this simple example, the magnitude of the joint-reaction force F_j is calculated to be 3.3 W. Both the

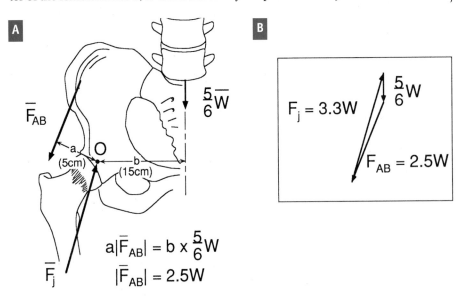

$$a|\overline{F}_{AB}| = b \times \frac{5}{6}W$$

$$|\overline{F}_{AB}| = 2.5W$$

Figure 11

A, A free-body diagram of the hip of a man standing on his right leg; the body and the left leg weighs 5 W/6, where W is the total weight of the person. The magnitude of the abductor muscle force F_{AB}, the direction of which is assumed known, may be determined by setting the sum of the moments about O equal to zero. B, A force triangle may be constructed to determine the joint-reaction force F_j.

muscle force and the joint-reaction force are considerably greater than the weight of the body and leg they are supporting because of the lever action of muscle forces around the hip joint.

Problem: During osteoarthritis of the hip, where the near frictionless cartilage has been totally worn away, frictional force of significant magnitude exists between the femoral head bone and the acetabular bone. This frictional force exerts a resisting moment so that the perfectly frictionless ball and socket joint is not a good modeling assumption. To account for this, suppose in a model for the osteoarthritic hip that friction between the 2 articulating surfaces can exert a resisting torque of 25 N·m. In this model, calculate the abductor reaction force required to maintain this osteoarthritic hip in equilibrium in the above example.

Forces on the Spine

The free-body diagram (model) shown in Figure 12 can be used to show how the musculoskeletal lever system can magnify the compressive force acting on the spine during an ordinary daily activity such as holding a weight W_1 with an outstretched hand. Calculation of the compressive force F_N in the spine begins with consideration of the moment equilibrium condition about the center of a vertebral body

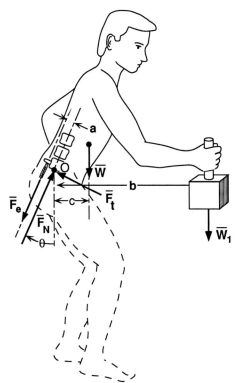

A free-body diagram of the spine. The normal compressive force F_N acting on the spine is 2,100 N even during an ordinary daily activity such as holding a 100-N weight by an outstretched hand (at 50 cm).

O. The moment that the weight W_1 creates about O is clockwise and is equal to $-(W_1) \times (b)$. Similarly, the moment of the upper body weight is $-(W) \times (c)$. The extensor muscle force F_e creates a counterclockwise moment about O given by $+ (F_e) \times (a)$. For equilibrium, these 3 moments must balance; therefore, $F_e = (W_1 b + Wc)/a$. For an upper body weight $W = 500$ N ($\frac{2}{3}$ of a body weight of 750 N), a held weight of $W_1 = 100$ N, and the distances a = 5 cm, b = 50 cm, and c = 8 cm, the magnitude of the extensor muscle force F_e required to hold this weight is calculated to be $(1,000 + 800)$ N. Note that the 100-N weight held at 50 cm produces a 1,000-N force in F_e while the 500-N upper body weight produces only 800 N in F_e.

For the portion of the upper body to be at equilibrium, the sum of the vertical components of all forces must add to zero: $F_N\cos\theta - F_e\cos\theta - W - W_1 + F_t\sin\theta = 0$. The sum of the horizontal components of all forces must also add to zero: $F_N\sin\theta - F_e\sin\theta - F_t\cos\theta = 0$. If $\theta = 60°$, then the 2 equations can be solved to give $F_t = (W + W_1)\sin60° = 520$ N and $F_N = F_e + (W + W_1)\cos60° = 2,100$ N. Hence, the component of the compressive force acting perpendicularly to the face of the vertebral body F_N is many times the weight supported. The major contribution to the compressive force on the vertebral body derives from the extensor muscle force (1,800 N), and the major component of that force (1,000 N) results from holding the relatively small force (100 N) at 50 cm in the outstretched hand. If the distance b is reduced by holding the weight W_1 closer to the body, the magnitude of the normal compressive force F_N acting on the vertebral body will be reduced dramatically. The contribution of body weight to the compressive force is usually much less than that of a weight held by an outstretched hand. This finding illustrates the large forces that may be generated in the spine from simple activities, causing fracture in some patients, especially those with osteoporosis.

Problem: Assuming everything else remains the same as in the example discussed above, describe how the compressive force on the lumbar intervertebral disks will vary going from L1 to L5.

Forces on the Shoulder

Figure 13 shows how the muscle and joint-reaction forces acting about the shoulder can be calculated when a weight is held at arm's length. In this problem, the free-body diagram consists of the extended arm with 3 forces acting on it: the weight W being held; the deltoid muscle force F_D; and the joint-reaction force F_J between the humeral head and the glenoid fossae. In this example, the weight of the arm (30 N) is neglected while determining only the extra deltoid muscle force and the glenohumeral joint force resulting from the held weight W (100 N). In this free-body diagram, 4 modeling assumptions for the unknown forces have been made: (1) a 2-dimensional (2-D) plane model is chosen; (2) the location of the deltoid force is at the centroid of the muscle (d = 5 cm from the center of the humeral head) and is given from anatomic data; (3) the deltoid force is tensile; and (4) the glenohumeral joint force is compressive. The held weight W is 100 N in the direction of gravity (down), and is located 60 cm from the center of the humeral head O. When the arm is in equilibrium, these 3 forces and their moments must sum to zero. Again, by taking the moments about O, the clockwise moment of the deltoid muscle force is $-(F_D) \times d$ and must balance the counterclockwise moment of the weight $+ (W) \times 60$; thus, $F_D = 1,200$ N. This equals about 1.5 times the average body weight of an adult; this is a result of lever action.

The joint-reaction force F_J can be found by using the force triangle concept shown in the lower right-hand side of the figure. By drawing the sides of the triangle proportional to the length of the forces, the joint-reaction force is found to be 1,150 N in the direction shown.

Problem: Find the total joint-reaction force F_J and the total deltoid muscle force F_D if the weight of the arm (30 N), located at the centroid of the arm 30 cm from O, is also included in the above problem.

Forces on the Knee Joint

If a person is slowly climbing steps, the inertial force (that is, force due to acceleration) on the leg may be neglected. Thus, the leg may be considered to be in static equilibrium (Fig. 14, *A*). The floor is pushing up on the foot with a force

equal to body weight; otherwise the body would be falling. This ground-reaction force passes 7.5 cm posterior to the center O of the knee joint, creating a counterclockwise flexion moment about the knee (Fig. 14, *B*). For the lower leg to be in equilibrium, 3 major forces must be acting: the ground-reaction force W; the tension on the patellar tendon F_P; and the compressive force on the tibial plateau of the knee joint F_J (Fig. 14, *C*). Here F_P is assumed to be acting at 2.5 cm from the center O of the knee (Fig. 14, *B*). To satisfy moment equilibrium about the center of the knee joint O, the flexion moment (counterclockwise) caused by the ground-reaction force $+ (W) \times (7.5)$ must equal the extension moment (clockwise) caused by the patellar tendon force $- (F_P) \times (2.5)$. Thus, the magnitude of the patellar tendon force F_P is 3 W, showing the lever action again. By using the force triangle, the joint-reaction force F_J is determined to be 3.5 W (Fig. 14, *D*). Thus, large forces can be created at the knee even during very slow stair-climbing and other ordinary activities.

Problem: Specifically identify the modeling assumptions used to arrive at the free-body diagram for the lower leg of the illustrative example discussed above.

Problem: If during a sudden application of stepping, the reaction force at the foot is 2 W, find F_P and F_J in this problem.

Forces on the Ankle

When a person does a bilateral toe raise, large forces may also be generated on the ankle. Half of the body weight

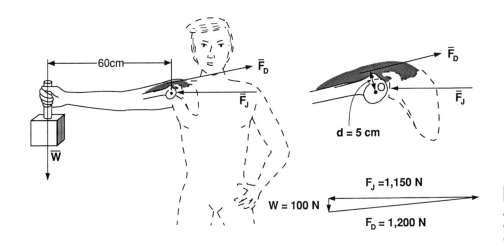

Figure 13

A man holds a weight W at a distance of 60 cm from the center of rotation of the humeral head. After determining the magnitude of the deltoid muscle force F_D (its direction is given) by summing the moments about O, F_J may be found from the force triangle.

(W/2) is supported by each foot. As illustrated in Figure 15, the ankle dorsiflexion moment (counterclockwise) created by the ground reaction is + (0.5 W) × 16 and is balanced by the plantarflexion moment (clockwise) created by the tension of the Achilles tendon, equal to - (F_A) × (4). The moment arms for both of these forces were obtained from radiographic measurement. For equilibrium, these 2 moments are equal; thus the force F_A in the Achilles tendon must be 2 W. If θ = 75°, then $F_t = F_A \cos 75° = 0.52$ W and $F_N = F_A \sin 75° + (W/2) = 2.43$ W. Therefore, the joint-reaction force is $(F^2_N + F^2_t)^{1/2} = 2.49$ W.

In all the examples discussed, the large forces at the joint surface F_J result from the lever action of the muscle forces required to balance the relatively low applied loads. If the applied loads are high, then the joint-reaction loads will be proportionally higher. For high-performance athletes, such as a baseball pitcher accelerating a baseball up to 150 km/hr during a pitch, or soccer players kicking the ball at 80 km/hr, very high muscle forces are required to accelerate

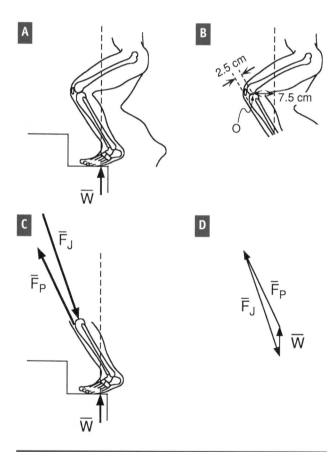

Figure 14

A, If during slow stair-climbing the inertial force on the leg may be neglected, then the ground-reaction force on the foot is W, the weight of the person. **B,** The knee is flexed so that the ground-reaction force passes 7.5 cm posterior to the center O of the knee joint. The patellar tendon force F_p acts 2.5 cm from O. **C,** The three major forces acting on the lower leg are the ground-reaction force W, the patellar tendon force F_P, and the compressive force on the tibial plateau of the knee joint F_J. **D,** Force triangle to determine the joint-reaction force F_J acting on the lower leg.

the limb and ball. These forces will produce a correspondingly higher joint-reaction force.

Kinematics

Kinematics is the study of the relationships between positions, velocities, and accelerations of rigid bodies, without concern for how the motions are caused (that is, without concern for forces and moments acting on the body). In other words, kinematics describes the geometry of motion.

Position Vectors

The position of an object at any time is always defined relative to a reference frame. In this chapter, the reference frame is assumed to be the x-y plane with origin O. The position of an object such as the femur (Fig. 16), which is assumed to be a rigid body in this discussion, may be defined by the points P and Q (in 3 dimensions, 3 points would have to be specified to fully define an object's position). These points are located in the x-y plane by the vectors R_P and R_Q. The vector locating the point P relative to Q, $R_{P/Q}$, is given by the parallelogram law of vector addition:

$$R_Q + R_{P/Q} = RP \text{ or } R_{P/Q} = R_P - R_Q.$$

Because P and Q are arbitrarily chosen on the femur, the definition of a rigid body is given by:

$$| R_{P/Q} | = \text{constant.}$$

This means that the distance between any pair of points on the femur remains constant. If it were to change, then internal deformation would be taking place, and the body would no longer be rigid.

In 3-D space, 6 coordinates are required to locate and orient the rigid body. These 6 coordinates may be defined as: (1) the 3 coordinates of a point such as Q; and (2) the 3 orientation angles of the body relative to an x,y,z reference frame. This corresponds to the intuitive notion that a rigid body may be translated in 3 perpendicular directions, and rotated about 3 axes. In Figure 17, the center of the humeral head is placed at the origin O defined by the 3 coordinates (0,0,0) in the x,y,z reference frame. The position of the humerus relative to the origin can be defined by the 3 angles θ,φ,ψ. The humerus may be translated anteroposterior (x-direction), superior-inferior (z-direction), or toward or away from the glenoid (joint compression or distraction; y-direction). Possible rotations of the humerus are abduction/adduction θ in a vertical plane, for example, the scapular plane; flexion/extension φ relative to the scapular plane, or axial rotation ψ around the longitudinal axis of the humerus. These 6 possible motions corresponding to the 6 coordinates are described as the 6 degrees of freedom of a rigid body. If a fixed fulcrum were implanted (for example, a constrained shoulder replacement), then translation would no longer be possible, and only 3 degrees of freedom, corresponding to rotation, would remain.

Velocity Vectors: Translation and Rotation

Velocity is defined as the change of position with respect to time. Because the position of any point P is defined by a vector, velocity is also a vector, having both magnitude (speed) and direction. Speed is measured in units of meters/second (m/s).

Translation occurs when all points on a body are moving in the same direction. If 2 points on the rigid body are moving in 2 different directions, then the body will be both translating and rotating. The rotation of an object is described by an angular velocity vector, usually denoted by ω. In general, the motion of any rigid body can be described in terms of a combination of a translation plus a rotation. The velocity of a point P on any rigid body is given by the velocity of any point Q, V_Q, plus the relative velocity of point P with respect to Q, $V_{P/Q}$ (Fig. 18, *A*). For rigid bodies, this relative velocity $V_{P/Q}$ is equal to the product $\omega \times R_{P/Q}$. This simple result means, for example, that if the motion of the center of a ball is known, as well as the way the ball is turning about the center, then the motion and position of the ball have been described fully.

Instant Center of Rotation

When a 2-D body is rotating without translation, for example, a rotating stationary bicycle gear, any marked point P on the body may be observed to move in a circle about a fixed point called the axis of rotation or center of rotation. When a rigid body is both rotating and translating, for example, the motion of the femur during gait, its motion at any instant of time can be described as rotation around a moving center of rotation (Fig. 18, *B*). The location of this point at any instant, termed the instant center of rotation (ICR), is determined by finding the point (ICR) which, at that instant, is not translating. Then by definition, at that instant, all points on the rigid body are rotating about the ICR. For practical purposes the ICR is determined by noting the paths traveled by 2 points, P and Q, on the object in a very short period of time to P´ and Q´. The paths PP´ and QQ´ will be perpendicular to lines connecting them to the ICR because they approximate, over short periods, tangents to the circles describing the rotation of the body around the ICR at that instant. Perpendicular bisectors to these 2 paths (Fig. 18, *B*) will intersect at the (approximate) center of rotation.

Problem: Suppose 2 radiographs of a patient's knee were taken at 2 slightly different flexion angles, say 30° and 35°. Describe how to find the ICR of the knee of this patient.

Screw Axis

In 3-D, instead of describing a body's motion with respect to an ICR, the concept of a screw (or helical) axis is used. Any rigid body's motion may be described, at any instant, as a combination of rotation about an axis and translation

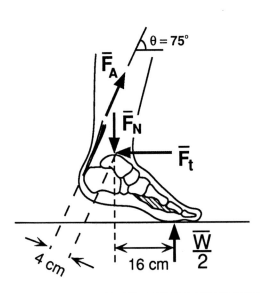

Free-body diagram of the ankle during dorsiflexion. The major forces acting on the foot are the Achilles tendon force F_A, the tangential F_t and the normal F_N components of the joint-reaction force, and the floor-foot reaction force W/2.

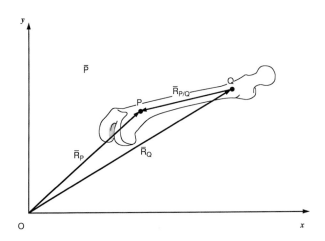

The position of the rigid body (femur) is defined by the 2 points P and Q located in the x-y plane by the 2 vectors R_P and R_Q. The vector locating the point P relative to Q, $R_{P/Q}$, is given by the parallelogram law of vector addition: $R_{P/Q} = R_P - R_Q$.

along (parallel to) that same axis. This axis does not have to be within the body. In fact, as the rotational component of the motion becomes smaller, the axis comes to be farther and farther away, approaching infinity for pure translation. At the other extreme, a ball-and-socket joint such as the hip will have more rotation than translation, and its screw axis will pass close to the geometric center of the femoral head. The screw axis description is often used for its elegance and an intuitive conceptualization of 3-D motion, but motions may be described in other ways. For example, because a rigid body's position may be specified by the location of a single point and the orientation of the body around it, any motion may be described as the translation of any given point (from its original to its final location) plus a rotation of the body around an axis passing through that point.

Relative Motion at the Articulating Surfaces of Diarthrodial Joints

Although in principle 2 objects may move relative to one another in any combination of rotation and translation, diarthrodial joint surfaces are constrained in their relative motion, by their surface geometry, the ligamentous restraints, and the action of muscles spanning the joint. In general, joint surface separation (or gapping) and impaction are small compared to overall joint motion.

When surfaces remain in contact in this fashion, they may move relative to each other in either sliding or rolling contact. In rolling contact (Fig. 19, A), the contacting points on the 2 surfaces have zero relative velocity, namely, no slip. In such a case, the rolling contact by an automobile tire would leave a clear impression of its treads. Because the point P on the wheel, which contacts the ground at any instant, is not moving, it is, by definition, the ICR for the wheel during rolling (Fig. 19, B), and the arrows define the actual velocities of points on the wheel. Rolling and sliding contact occur together (Fig. 19, C) when the relative velocity at the

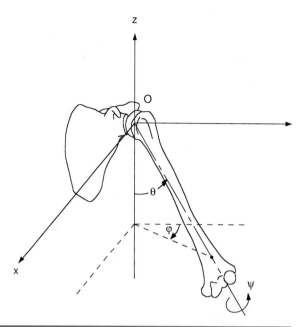

Figure 17

Illustration of the 6 degrees of freedom of a rigid body: the position of 1 point of the rigid body must be specified (for example, the 3 coordinates locating the humeral head); and the 3 angular orientations θ,ϕ,ψ are relative to a set of xyz coordinate axes.

contact point is not zero. The instant center will then lie between the geometric center and the contact point. Under these conditions, in the example of a tire, a skid mark would be left on the ground. In spinning motion (Fig. 19, D), the center of rotation will be the axis of the vehicle. This is the case if there is a total loss of traction between a tire and the ground, and the wheel is in pure rotation, with no forward translational motion of the vehicle. This situation often occurs with the tire spinning on icy pavement.

All diarthrodial joint motion consists of both rolling and sliding motion. In the hip and shoulder, sliding motion pre-

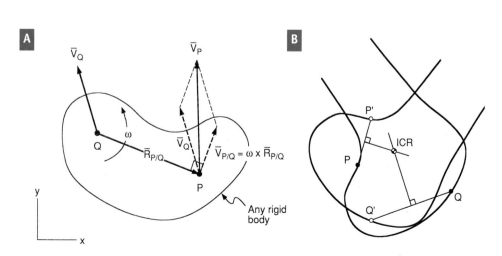

Figure 18

A, For rigid bodies, the velocity of point P, V_P, is equal to the sum of the velocity of point Q, V_Q, plus a relative velocity $V_{P/Q}$ of point P with respect to Q ($\omega \times R_{P/Q}$): $V_P = V_Q + V_{P/Q} = V_Q + \omega \times R_{P/Q}$. **B,** The instant center of rotation (ICR) may be found by drawing: (1) lines connecting 2 nearby successive positions P-P′ and Q-Q′ of 2 arbitrary points P and Q on the body; and (2) lines perpendicular to two lines P-P′ and Q-Q′ at their midpoints. The intersection of these 2 perpendicular bisectors locates the ICR. The reason why this construction works is that all points must rotate about the ICR.

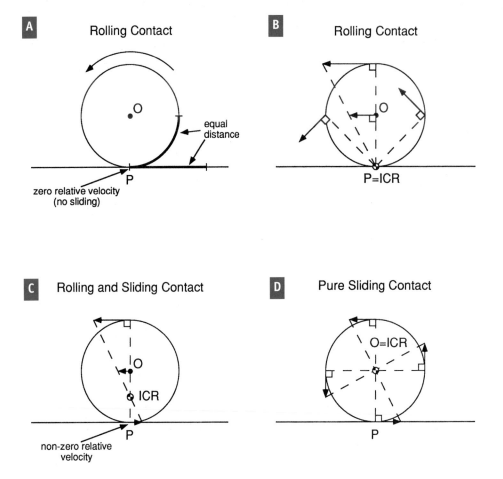

A, Rolling Contact

equal distance

O

P

zero relative velocity (no sliding)

B, Rolling Contact

P=ICR

Figure 19

A, Rolling contact occurs when the circumferential distance of the rolling object equals the distance traced along the plane. This can only occur when there is no sliding, that is, the relative velocity at the point of contact P is zero. **B,** For rolling contact, the point P of the wheel has zero velocity because it is in contact with the ground. Therefore, P is the instant center of rotation (ICR) of the wheel. This diagram shows the actual velocity of points along the wheel as it rolls along the ground. **C,** Sliding contact occurs when the relative velocity at the contact point is not zero. **D,** Pure sliding occurs when the wheel rotates about a stationary axis O. In this case, the car would have no forward motion.

C, Rolling and Sliding Contact

O
ICR
P

non-zero relative velocity

D, Pure Sliding Contact

O=ICR

P

dominates over rolling motion. In the knee, both rolling and sliding articulation occur simultaneously. These simple concepts affect the design of total joint prostheses. For example, some total knee replacements have been designed for implantation while preserving the posterior cruciate ligament, which appears to help maintain the normal kinematics of rolling and sliding in the knee. Other knee prostheses substitute for ligament control of kinematics by alterations in articular surface contour.

Three-Dimensional Modeling of the Patellofemoral Joint

Though the concepts of joint kinematics and static analysis are presented separately in the previous sections, they are intimately related when analyzing diarthrodial joints. The various examples of static analysis (Figs. 9, 11, 13, and 14) demonstrate that knowledge of the location of the joint center of rotation (the ICR, used in 2-D analyses) or axis of rotation (the screw axis, used in 3-D analyses) may be required in order to determine the moment arm of the muscles crossing the joint when no other information is available about the joint articular surface geometry. Indeed, there are various experimental techniques for measuring or estimating the muscle moment arm about the joint axis of

rotation, in vitro and in vivo. However, if the articular geometry is known, the joint kinematics and muscle moment arms may also be determined from analysis. Typically, because of the complexity of joint anatomy, these static analyses are most efficiently performed on computers, although they are based on the same vector equations of static equilibrium described in the previous sections.

The 3-D computer model of a knee patellofemoral joint shown in Figure 20 illustrates the capabilities and usefulness of static analyses for understanding the mechanics of complex joint structures. The geometry of the articular and bone surfaces employed in such a model can be measured accurately using various methods, including noninvasive methods such as computed tomography and magnetic resonance imaging. Similarly, the tendon and ligament insertions and the lines of action of the muscle forces can also be obtained from direct measurements. The magnitude of the muscle forces is prescribed in this analysis, and distributed according to the physiologic cross-sectional area of each muscle (in Fig. 20, the vastus lateralis and vastus medialis obliquus are modeled separately while the rectus femoris and vastus intermedius are bundled together). The choice of muscle force magnitudes at each flexion angle is based on the simulation of 3 activities: (1) squatting from a standing position to about 90° of knee flexion (closed-chain exercise); (2) extending the knee from 90° to 0° against a constant external moment from a seated position, simulating a typical open chain rehabilitation exercise; and (3) extending the knee from 90° to 0° with no external load or moment other than that caused by gravity (open-chain exercise). The tibiofemoral kinematics are determined from experimental measurements. The purpose of these analyses is to determine the range of contact forces, areas, and stresses that might develop at the articular surfaces of the patellofemoral joint for various activities; such results may be useful in the planning of rehabilitation exercises or conservative treatment for patients with patellofemoral joint disorders. Similar measures can be obtained from cadaver experiments, although it is often difficult to test multiple load configurations at several flexion angles on the same cadaver specimen. Therefore, computer analyses of this type are ideal for supplementing cadaver or in vivo studies and for the efficient and relatively inexpensive exploration of various hypotheses prior to initiating experiments.

According to the results of this computer analysis conducted on 5 models derived from distinct cadaver joints, the patellofemoral joint reaction force (PFJR) is seen to vary significantly depending on the type of exercise (Fig. 21). Because the leg extension requires the least amount of quadriceps force, it is not surprising that it produces the smallest amount of contact force at the joint. The squatting exercise is the most strenuous of the 3 simulated cases, causing contact forces as high as 4,000 N (4 to 5 times body weight) at 90°. The contact area size also varies significantly with flexion angle and activity (Fig. 22), ranging from 1 to 7 cm²; in comparison, the average articular surface area of

the patella is approximately 11 cm². Because the PFJR and contact area size both vary with flexion angle, the mean articular contact stress need not assume the same trend for the various activities; indeed, as observed in Figure 23, the average contact stress decreases moderately with increasing flexion angle for the leg extension, while it increases moderately with flexion angle during the constant-moment open-chain exercise. The squatting exercise causes the largest and most rapid increase in contact stress with increasing flexion angle, with contact stress values reaching as high as 6 MPa on average at 90°.

It is important to note that these computer analyses do not require knowledge of the muscle moment arms beforehand, because the kinematics of the patellofemoral joint is determined from the joint anatomy, which is faithfully reproduced in the model. In fact, it is possible to obtain the muscle moment arm from the results of the analysis, using an inductive approach. For example, a quantity of interest would be the moment arm of the patella tendon force about the tibiofemoral joint axis of rotation, because it would enter the calculation of the moment acting about the knee. The first step is to determine the screw axis for the tibiofemoral joint. As observed from Figure 24, the axis of rotation does not remain fixed as the knee flexion angle varies. Indeed, as the knee flexes the screw axis will sweep out a ruled surface in space, known as the axode. This fluctuation in the screw axis signifies that the knee is not truly a hinge joint, for which the axode would degenerate to a fixed line in space. Nevertheless, the knee is often approximated as a hinge joint, a simplification that may be acceptable for flexion angles between 45° and 90° where the moving screw axis remains very close to the line passing through the centers of curvature of the 2 posterior femoral condyles. Because the screw axis never lies near the articular surfaces

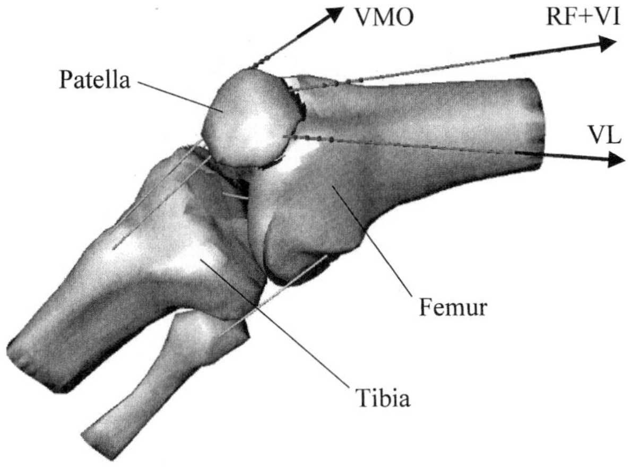

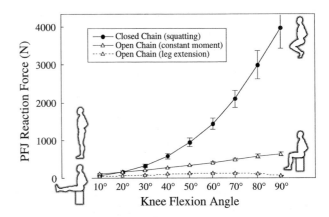

Figure 20

A 3-D multibody model of the patellofemoral joint can be constructed from accurate image data. This model includes a representation of the patellar, femoral, tibial, and fibular bones, the retropatellar and distal femoral articular surfaces, the patellar tendon, and the quadriceps forces. RF = rectus femoris; VI = vastus intermedius; VL = vastus lateralis; VMO = vastus medialis obliquus.

Figure 21

Patellofemoral joint (PFJ) reaction force (PFJR) as a function of knee flexion angle, for 3 typical exercises simulated on the multibody models of 5 joints: closed chain squatting, open chain exercise against a constant moment of 10 N·m about the knee, and open chain leg extension. Results are reported as mean values with standard deviation bars.

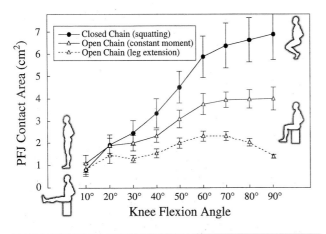

Figure 22

Patellofemoral joint (PFJ) articular contact area size for the 3 simulated exercises.

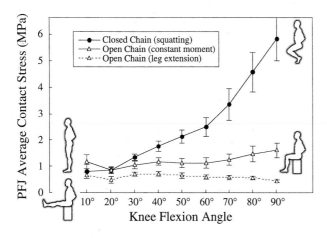

Figure 23

Patellofemoral joint average contact stress for the 3 simulated exercises.

of the tibiofemoral joint, it can be construed that the motion at the articular surfaces is not one of pure rolling, but a combination of rolling and sliding, in analogy to the ICR analysis of Fig. 19. Once the screw axis has been determined from the kinematic analysis, the moment arm of the patella tendon force about the screw axis can be calculated. As observed in Figure 25, this moment arm varies as a function of flexion angle; once again, however, the assumption of a constant moment arm over the range of 10° to 60° is not unreasonable when performing simplified 2-D analyses.

Mechanical Properties of Materials

Although modeling skeletal members as rigid bodies can be very useful in many orthopaedic applications, for example, gait analysis, the deformation experienced by the object is of major concern in many problems. Deformation must be

considered to understand how a bone may be fractured, how the anterior cruciate ligament may be torn or avulsed, or how the prosthetic femoral stem may be fatigued and fail. In these problems, the rigid body model is no longer appropriate. Understanding these problems requires analysis of the stresses and strains produced inside the body when forces and moments are applied onto the surface of the body.

Forces and moments (excluding electromagnetic effects) can be applied only to the external surface of a body, and stresses and strains inside the body can only be calculated, they can never be measured. However, strains on the surface may be measured experimentally. This distinction between the loading conditions on a body (forces and moments applied to a body) and the state of stress within a body is very important. For example, a frictionless joint surface can be loaded only in compression, but this loading will still produce shear and tensile stresses, as well as compressive stress inside the compressed articular cartilage.

All musculoskeletal tissues, for example, bone, cartilage, intervertebral disk, ligament, meniscus, and tendon, are deformable to some degree. Some are more deformable than others; cartilage is more deformable than bone. The degree of deformability depends on the intrinsic properties of the material of the object (for example, bone versus intervertebral disk) as well as its size and shape. When the

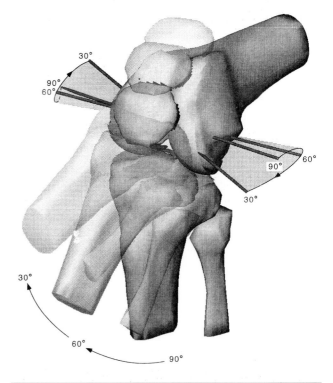

Figure 24

Screw axis for a typical knee joint during squatting. As the knee extends from 90° to 30°, the screw axis sweeps a surface in space called the "axode." At higher flexion angles, the screw axis passes very nearly through the centers of curvature of the posterior condyles.

deformational response of a material object depends on its size and shape, as well as its intrinsic properties, this response is called a structural property. For example, a 1.0-cm diameter rod would be structurally 4 times stiffer than a 0.5-cm diameter rod even if both were made of the same material, because the structural stiffness of each rod depends on its cross-sectional area $A = \pi r^2$.

Deformational properties of an object that do not depend on its size and shape are called intrinsic material properties. Load-deformation tests often are used to describe the structural response of a material object. For example, the structural response of the femur-prosthesis composite structure (Fig. 26, *A*), could be measured by loading the entire structure in a testing machine and measuring its bending behavior. To determine the intrinsic material properties of bone or steel, the effect of geometry must be eliminated. This may be done by making geometrically precise specimens for testing (Fig. 26, *B*), by dividing the load (force) by the object's cross-sectional area to determine stress, F/A, and by dividing the elongation by the original length to determine strain, $\Delta l/l_o$. For metals, the strain is usually very small and is measured in microstrain units. The stress-strain behavior of the object describes its intrinsic material response, and all physical quantities obtained from the stress-strain response are intrinsic material properties. In biomechanics, unfortunately, it is often difficult to obtain geometrically well defined specimens from which stress-strain tests may be performed.

Directional Properties

Isotropy
Isotropy is the property of a material such that its intrinsic material properties do not depend on the direction of loading. In general, the internal structure of such materials is very small and randomly dispersed. Metals, glasses, and plastics are isotropic materials. For isotropic elastic materials, there are only 2 material constants: Young's modulus E and Poisson's ratio υ. Once these 2 constants have been determined for an isotropic material, its elastic properties have been fully characterized.

Often, in the literature, other moduli are presented: shear modulus G, bulk compressive modulus k, aggregate modulus H_A, modulus of rigidity G or μ, Lamé coefficients λ, μ. All of these moduli are related to each other; once any two are known, the others may be calculated using very simple formulas. Investigators use different forms for these 2 isotropic coefficients because, in a particular experiment, a specific modulus may be the easiest to use and the most meaningful in terms of physical interpretation.

Anisotropy
Anisotropy is the property of a material such that its intrinsic material properties depend on the direction of loading. In general, the internal structures of such materials are large and observable, similar in size to the specimens, and arranged in an orderly manner. Wood, fiber-reinforced composite materials, and practically all materials of interest in the musculoskeletal system, such as articular cartilage, cancellous and cortical bone, intervertebral disk, ligament, meniscus, and tendon, are anisotropic. For such materials, more than 2 material constants are required, although the "apparent" Young's modulus E and Poisson's ratio υ still are used commonly to describe their stress-strain behavior. For example, the meniscus is highly anisotropic. Table 1 provides the tensile modulus of bovine meniscus for specimens taken parallel to the predominant collagen fiber direction and radial to the collagen fiber direction. Bone, ligament, and tendon are often considered to be transversely isotropic. Five constants are required to determine the elastic properties of this type of material. Articular cartilage and meniscus are considered to be orthotropic, and 9 constants are required to determine their elastic properties. Besides the isotropic coefficients, very little is known of the other coefficients for these materials.

Strain

Figure 27, *A*, shows how a rectangular block of material (solid lines) will deform when stretched by a force F_x in the x-direction. This deformation will be an elongation Δl in the x-direction and a contraction $-\Delta d$ in the y-direction. The original lengths of the sides are l_o and d_o. The lineal strain in the x-direction is defined by $\varepsilon_{xx} = \Delta l/l_o$.

The contraction in the y-direction is also a lineal strain, but it is caused by the force applied in the x-direction. In a similar manner, it is possible to define ε_{yy} and ε_{zz} caused by forces applied in the y- and z-directions, respectively. The Poisson's ratio, if only F_x is applied, is defined as the ratio:

$$\upsilon = -(\Delta d/d_o)/(\Delta l/l_o).$$

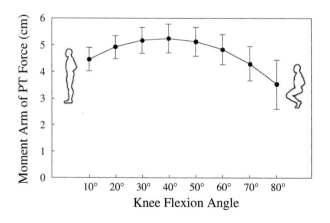

Figure 25

Moment arm of the patellar tendon (PT) force about the screw axis for knee flexion angles between 10° and 90°, for the closed-chain squatting exercise.

Table 1

Material Properties of Cartilage and Meniscus

	Bovine (‖)*	Tensile Modulus (MPa) Human (‖ Normal)	Human (‖ Fibrillated)
Cartilage			
Surface zone	42.2	10.1	8.5
Middle zone	13.0	5.9	8.4
Deep zone	2.6	4.5	4.0
Meniscus	198 (c)	93–160 (M)	
	4.6 (r)	159–294 (L)	

*   ‖ = parallel specimen; c = circumferential direction parallel to the collagen fibrillar network; r = radial direction perpendicular to the collagen fibrilar network; M = medial meniscus in the circumferential direction; and L = lateral meniscus in the circumferential direction

Because Δd and Δl are always in opposite directions, one being (+) and one being (-), the Poisson's ratio is always positive. The Poisson's ratio, which is an important intrinsic property of deformable materials, may be thought of as a measure of how much a material thins when it is stretched (as with a piece of taffy being pulled) and how much it bulges when compressed (as with a piece of clay or intervertebral disk being squeezed). Obviously, the Poisson's ratio may be defined in the y- and z-directions also. These 3 Poisson's ratios may or may not be equal depending on the microscopic structure of the material. Poisson's ratio is a measure of a material's compressibility. For isotropic materials, a Poisson's ratio of 0 indicates a highly compressible material, such as cork, a cylinder of which does not bulge sideways when compressed. A ratio of 0.5 indicates an incompressible material, such as natural rubber, a cylinder of which will bulge just enough to maintain a constant volume.

Figure 27, *B*, shows how a square block of material (solid lines) will deform when sheared by 2 pairs of forces **S** in the

x- and y-directions as shown. (For both force and moment equilibrium, the magnitude of forces in the x- and y-directions must be equal.) The deformation caused by these forces will be a change of the angle between the lines OA and OB, which were originally perpendicular. This change of angle is called the shear strain and is denoted by γ_{xy}. Obviously, if the square block of material is taken in the y-z plane or in the x-z plane, and sheared in a similar manner, then shear strains γ_{yz} and γ_{xz} will be created, respectively. For most hard materials, the shear strain is small.

In summary, the complete description of deformation in an object is given by the 3 lineal strain components, ε_{xx}, ε_{yy}, ε_{zz}, and the 3 shear strain components, γ_{xy}, γ_{yz}, γ_{xz}. These 6 components define the strain *tensor*, which is a mathematical construct that fully specifies the strain state at each point within deforming objects (for example, bone). The details of how tensors are manipulated are beyond the scope of this book, but it is important to understand that these 6 components completely define the state of strain. To actually analyze the strain, a coordinate system must be

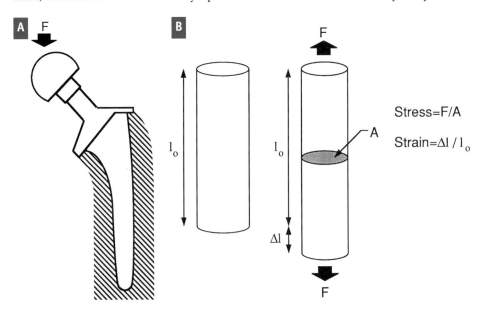

Stress=F/A

Strain=Δl / l$_{o}$

Figure 26

A, A femur-prosthesis composite structure is loaded for its structural response. The deformation of the structure depends on its geometry (size and shape) as well as the materials it is made of. **B,** To determine the intrinsic material properties, the stress-strain behavior of the material must be measured. Stress is defined as force/area F/A, and strain is defined as change of length/original length Δl/l$_{o}$.

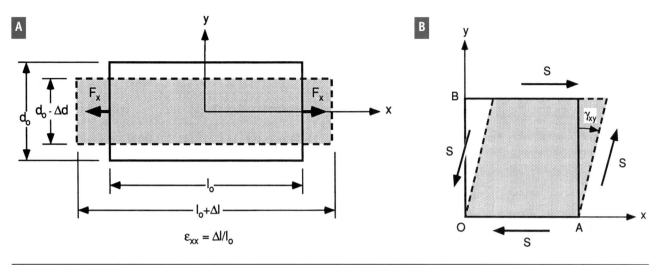

Figure 27

A, A rectangular block of material (solid lines) will deform when stretched by a force F_x in the x-direction. This deformation will be an elongation Δl in the x-direction. The lineal strain in the x-direction is defined by $\varepsilon_{xx} = \Delta l/l_0$. F_x causes a contraction $-\Delta d$ in the y-direction. **B,** A square block of material (solid lines) will deform when sheared by 2 pairs of forces S as shown. The deformation will be a change of angle between the lines OA and OB, denoted by γ_{xy}.

chosen. This is an extremely important concept. For example, in Figure 28, a strip is being loaded in uniaxial tension. The corners of a small block of material oriented parallel to the loading direction will all remain right angles, and no shear strain will be observed in this x-y orientation. If, on the other hand, the block is oriented at 45°, the angles at the corners will change, and shear strain will be observed. How is it that a test in uniaxial tension can cause shear? The force acting on each face of the block oriented at 45° in Figure 29, A, can be resolved into 2 components; one parallel and the other perpendicular (Fig. 29, B). The parallel components are shear stresses that will distort the square block of material. This simple example shows that the stress state is a sum of the normal stresses and shear stresses (Fig. 29, C). This notion is very counter-intuitive at first, and much confu-

sion will occur if the loading condition (tensile force F) is not carefully distinguished from the states of stress and of strain within the material. These stresses are complex and depend on the coordinate system chosen. As with strain, there are 6 components of stress; 3 normal stress components and 3 shear stress components. These components define the stress tensor.

Normal Stress and Shear Stress

Determination of forces acting on the femur in rigid body models has been discussed. Figure 30 shows how these externally applied forces on the femur (Fig. 30, A) will pro-

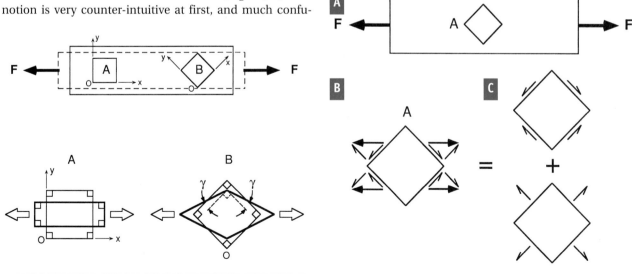

Figure 28

A strip loaded in uniaxial tension. No shear strain will be observed for block A but shear strain will be observed for block B.

Figure 29

A strip loaded in uniaxial tension (**A**); the stresses acting on block A (**B**) are equivalent to the normal stresses plus the shear stresses (**C**).

duce internal forces within the bone. Figure 30, *B (left)*, shows a thin section of the femur and a cube of the diaphyseal bone within the thin section. Only those forces acting on the top and bottom faces of this cube are shown in Figure 30, *B (right)*. The top and bottom faces of this cube are subjected to 2 types of forces: F_y, which is perpendicular (normal force), and S, which is parallel (shear force), to these faces (Fig. 30, *C*). The normal stress σ_{yy} is defined by F_y/A. This stress can be either compressive or tensile in nature. For the shear force S acting on this y-plane, there are 2 components: S_x and S_z. Thus, the components of the shear stress acting on the y-planes (top and bottom planes of the cube) are defined by

$$\tau_{xy} = S_x/A \text{ and } \tau_{zy} = S_z/A.$$

Similarly, it is possible to define σ_{xx}, τ_{yx}, τ_{zx} acting on the x-planes (left and right planes), and σ_{zz}, τ_{xz}, τ_{yz} acting on the z-planes (front and back planes). Because the moments must balance,

$$\tau_{xy} = \tau_{yx}, \tau_{zx} = \tau_{xz}, \text{ and } \tau_{yz} = \tau_{zy}$$

Thus, the 6 components of stress are the 3 normal stresses σ_{xx}, σ_{yy}, and σ_{zz} and the 3 shear stresses τ_{xy}, τ_{yz}, and τ_{xz} corresponding to the 6 components of strain.

Stress Analysis

These definitions can be used to analyze the state of stress in the simplest of all possible problems. Figure 31, *A*, shows a rectangular bar being stretched by a single tensile force F. By the definition of stress, to determine the state of stress at point P inside the bar (Fig. 31, *B*), the plane (the coordinate system) on which the stress will be defined must be identified. On the plane defined by $\theta = 0°$, the normal stress $\sigma_o = F/A_o$, and the shear stress $\tau_o = 0$. If the plane is at an angle $\theta \neq 0°$ from the horizontal (Fig. 31, *C*), the force F has 2 components with respect to this plane: a normal component given by $F\cos\theta$ and a shear component $F\sin\theta$. However, the area on which these normal and shear forces are acting is also different from the $\theta = 0°$ case. This area A_θ, by simple trigonometry, is equal to $A_o/\cos\theta$ (Fig. 31, *C*). Thus, the normal stress σ_θ acting on the θ-plane is given by $\sigma_\theta = (F\cos^2\theta)/A_o$ and the shear stress by $\tau_\theta = (F\sin2\theta)/2A_o$. The normal stress σ_θ goes from a maximum of F/A_o on the $\theta = 0°$ plane (Fig. 31, *B*) to zero on the $\theta = 90°$ plane. The shear stress τ_θ goes from zero on the $\theta = 0°$ plane to a maximum of $F/2A_o$ on the $\theta = 45°$ plane; beyond the 45° plane the shear stress decreases to zero at $\theta = 90°$. This analysis is also valid if F is taken to be compressive.

This stress analysis of the simplest possible problem indicates that, even for uniaxial tensile loading, shear stresses

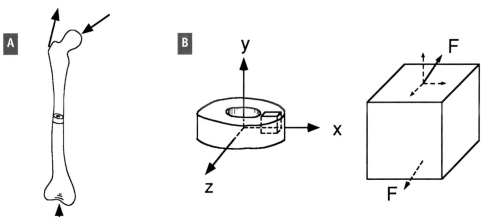

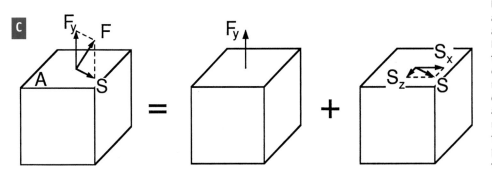

Figure 30

A, Externally applied forces on a femur will cause internal stresses to be developed. **B,** A thin section of the femur, and a cube of diaphyseal bone. Forces are shown acting on the top and bottom faces of a cube (y-plane). Similar forces also act on the left and right (x-plane), and front and back faces (z-plane) of the cube and have been omitted for clarity. **C,** Resolution of the force acting on the top face of the cube into a normal component Fy and a shear component S. The normal stress σ_{yy} is defined by F_y/A. The shear force S acting on this y-plane has 2 components: S_x and S_z. The components of the shear stress acting on the y-planes are defined by $\tau_{xy} = S_x/A$ and $\tau_{zy} = S_z/A$.

exist inside the object. Thus, material weak in shear will fail along the $\theta = 45°$ plane when subject to tension or compression. Concrete is such a material. When a concrete bar is overloaded in compression, its failure surface is oriented at 45° from the line of loading. Materials weak in tension, such as cast iron, will fail in a plane perpendicular to the line of loading. Once again, the distinction between loading condition and stress inside the object is crucial.

Figure 32, *A*, shows a square block of material being sheared by the forces S acting on each side of the element. Again, obviously, this system of forces is in equilibrium. A free-body diagram of the section of the square created by passing a plane through P along BPD shows that there must be a force F given by $\sqrt{2}$S (Fig. 32, *B*). This is from the Pythagorean theorem for right triangles. Using the definition $A = A_o/\cos\theta$ (Fig. 31, *C*), at 45° the tensile stress acting on the BPD plane is S/A_o. On this plane no shear stress exists, and this is the maximum tensile stress acting inside the square block under the pure shear condition. Similarly, it can be shown that the maximum compressive stress acts on the APC plane (Fig. 32, *C*). Thus, if a material such as bone, which is weak in tension, is sheared, it will fail along the 45° plane BPD. This is the basis for the often observed spiral fracture of the tibia from skiing injuries in which the tibia is torqued by the ski during a fall. The failure surface forms a spiral whose tangent is very close to 45° from the long axis of the tibia.

The results of these stress analyses are valid regardless of the nature of the material, for example, steel, titanium, bone, cartilage, etc. The results of these 2 stress analysis problems indicate that it is important to know the intrinsic properties of materials. Knowledge is required of materials'

intrinsic stiffness in tension, compression, and shear; their respective strengths; and for materials used in prostheses, their fatigue life.

Elastic Properties of Metals and Biologic Tissues

A linear elastic material has 3 fundamental stress-strain characteristics: (1) stress and strain are directly proportional to each other; (2) the strain is totally recovered when the stress is removed; and (3) the material is insensitive to the rate of loading. For a linear elastic material, the straight line OP shows the stress σ to be proportional to the strain ε (Hooke's law), that is,

$$F/A = E(\Delta l/l_o),$$

where F, A, Δl, and l_o are all measured quantities on precisely prepared specimens (Fig. 33). Young's modulus E, an important property of the material, is expressed in units of MPa or GPa. For elastic materials, if in an experiment the maximum load is below point P, Δl will vanish if the load is released.

The proportional limit P is the point beyond which stress is no longer proportional to the strain. The elastic limit (not shown) is the point beyond which further deformation is no longer purely elastic. These 2 limits are generally regarded to be the same. If the specimen is stretched beyond P, a small but permanent plastic deformation is created, that is, if the load F is released (shown by the down arrow), a small residual or permanent deformation remains (Fig. 33). This permanent deformation is caused by damage to the inter-

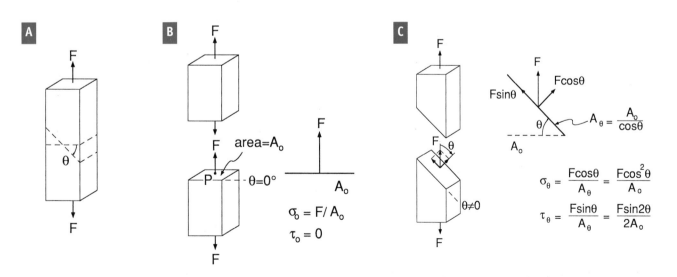

Figure 31

A, A rectangular bar being stretched by a single tensile force F. **B,** The normal stress F/A_o acting at point P on a plane defined by $\theta = 0°$. No shear stress exists on this plane. **C,** On an inclined plane ($\theta \neq 0°$) the force F has 2 components with respect to this plane: a normal component, $F\cos\theta$, and a shear component, $F\sin\theta$. The area A_θ on this inclined plane is $A_o/\cos\theta$. Thus, the normal stress σ_θ acting on the θ-plane is equal to $F\cos^2\theta/A_o$ and the shear stress τ_θ is equal to $(F\sin2\theta)/2A_o$.

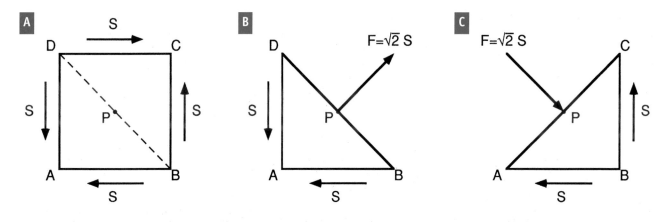

Figure 32

A, A square block of material being sheared by the forces S acting on each side of the element. **B,** A free-body diagram of a section of the square created by passing a plane through P along BPD. The force F, acting on the plane BPD, is equal to √2S. This is the maximum tensile stress created during pure shear and it always acts on a plane inclined at 45° with respect to the directions of shear. **C,** A free-body diagram of the section APC. This is the plane of maximum compressive stress created during pure shear. Its magnitude is the same as that for maximum tension.

nal microstructure of the specimen. The yield strength Y is the point at which a large plastic flow occurs, such that strain increases with little or no increase in stress. The ultimate tensile strength U (failure stress) is the point at which the specimen fails. The maximum stress that a material attains is known as its strength; this usually coincides with U. The strain at which failure occurs is known as the failure strain ε_f. Tables 1 to 3 provide some material constants for some common orthopaedic materials.

Toughness

Figure 33, shows the typical stress-strain behavior of solid materials such as steel, titanium, or bone and collagenous tissues. The energy a structure absorbs as it is deformed by an applied force is equal to the work done by that force. This energy is calculated as the magnitude of the force times the deformation produced and is equal to the area under the load-deformation curve. The energy required to bring the

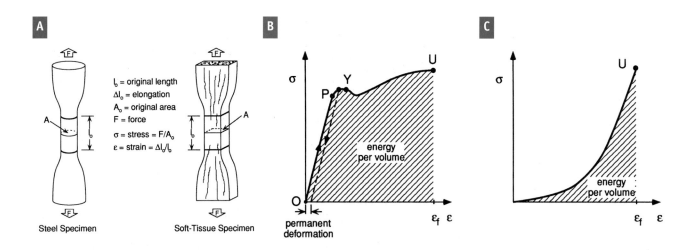

Figure 33

A, Two typical well prepared specimens for stress-strain testing. The circular cylindrical specimen is usually used for hard solid materials. The thin dumbbell strip is usually used for fibrous collagenous tissues. Dumbbell-shaped specimens are used to avoid gripping effects, and the middle section of the dumbbell is used for strain measurement. **B,** Typical stress-strain curve of a ductile metal or cortical bone: P is the proportional limit; Y is the yield strength; and U is the ultimate tensile strength. **C,** Typical stress-strain curve of collagenous tissues; U is the ultimate tensile strength.

structure to failure can thus be calculated. This concept is useful because many injuries may impart a specific energy to the body. For example, a fall from a height may turn the potential energy of the body weight at the original height into the energy of deformation of the lumbar spine or hip, causing fracture. To eliminate the effects of size, this energy is divided by the volume of the material being deformed. Because volume equals area × length:

energy/volume
= [force × deformation]/[area × length]
= [force/area] × [deformation/length]
= stress × strain
= area under the stress-strain curve

The amount of energy/volume a material can absorb before failure defines the intrinsic toughness of the material. For example, a brittle material often will fail at point P of the stress-strain curve. Such materials as ceramics and cast iron are brittle and are easily fractured. Although they are very stiff, these materials are not tough because they cannot absorb much energy. Ductile or annealed steel will fail only after significant amounts of stretching. These materials are intrinsically stiff and tough. Plastics and rubber are relatively soft (not stiff), but will stretch a great amount before failure. Thus, these materials are intrinsically soft and tough. This is the reason why rubber or similar substances are used for bumpers or tires. Collagenous tissues are soft and not particularly tough (Fig. 33); thus, these tissues fail easily.

Fatigue

Thus far material behavior has been discussed without considering the number of times the loading cycle is repeated. If subjected to large numbers of such cycles, most materials will fail at a stress lower than their ultimate tensile stress U, which is the stress at failure from only 1 cycle. The number of loading cycles required to cause failure is determined by performing a cyclic stress-strain experiment on the material. For such an experiment, the number of loading cycles required to cause specimen failure is plotted against the maximum stress level attained during the cyclic test. This is known as a σ-n curve (Fig. 34). As the magnitude of the stress decreases from the ultimate stress σ_{ult} (for 1 cycle), the number of cycles required to induce failure increases until a stress is reached for which failure will not occur, no matter how often the cycle is repeated. This is known as the endurance limit σ_E.

Viscoelasticity

Linear elasticity is an idealized model for real material stress-strain behavior. It is the basis for practically all structural analysis of buildings, bridges, airplanes, etc. Modern

orthopaedic prostheses are usually developed using finite element analysis with an elastic model for the bone, the prosthesis, and polymethylmethacrylate (PMMA).

As a reminder, linear elasticity has 3 fundamental stress-strain assumptions: (1) stress and strain are directly proportional to each other; (2) the strain is reversible when the stress is removed; and (3) the material is insensitive to the

Table 2

Material Properties of Commonly Encountered Prosthesis Materials

Material	Tensile Modulus E (GPa)	Ultimate Tensile Strength U (MPa)	Yield Strength Y (MPa)
Aluminum alloy	7.0	300	275
Alloy steel	20.6	600	540
Titanium	110.0	650	550
PMMA	2.07	30	

Table 3

Material Properties of Bone

	Tensile Modulus E	Shear Modulus G	Ultimate Tensile Strength U
Cortical bone	17 GPa	3.3 GPa	130 MPa
Trabecular bone	100 MPa	(NA)	50 MPa

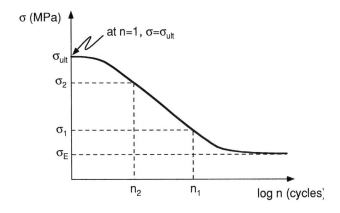

Cyclic fatigue failure will occur
at n_1 cycles of stress σ_1
<u>or</u> n_2 cycles of stress σ_2

Figure 34

The number of loading cycles n required to fail the specimen plotted against the maximum stress level σ attained during the cyclic test. This is known as a σ-n curve. The endurance limit σ_E is the stress below which cyclic fatigue of the material will not occur.

rate of loading. The proportionality relationship between stress and strain is given by $\sigma = E\varepsilon$. The definitions of σ and ε are used to obtain the relationship

$$F/A = E(\Delta l/l_0), \text{ or } F = k\Delta l$$

where $k = AE/lo$ is the structural stiffness of the material (in N/m), depending on the geometry of the object, A, l_0. This relationship between F and Δl is often written as $F = kx$ and the structure is designated by a spring (Fig. 35, *A*). Thus, for this linear, elastic spring, the F-x diagram (load-deformation) is a straight line, the slope of which defines the stiffness (Fig. 35, *B*). According to the elastic modeling assumptions stated, this straight line behavior does not change with time, nor does it depend on the rate of loading. In other words, as long as the deformation x (stretch) is maintained on the spring, a constant force is required to maintain the elongation, and vice versa.

This type of behavior often fails to occur, particularly in soft collagenous tissues. Articular cartilage, intervertebral disk, ligament, tendon, and even bone exhibit pronounced viscoelastic behavior, in which there is time-dependence. A syringe with a thin needle exhibits time-dependent behavior, because the faster the plunger is compressed the greater is the resistance generated.

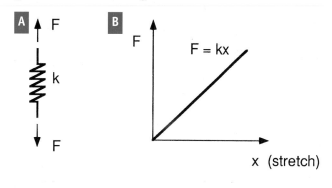

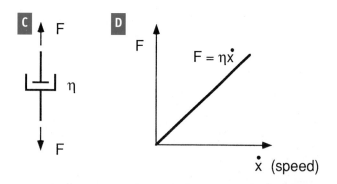

Figure 35

A linear elastic spring element (**A**) and its linear load-deformation (stretch) response (**B**). A linear viscous dashpot element (**C**) and its linear load-rate of deformation (speed) response (**D**).

These viscoelastic behaviors are the manifestations of the internal friction within the material, which may arise from many sources. To describe the viscoelastic behavior of materials, this friction is usually modeled by a linear viscous dashpot (Fig. 35, C) analogous to the linear elastic spring element already described. For the linear viscous dashpot, the relationship is

$$F = \eta \dot{x}$$

where force F is the applied force, x is the rate of deformation (speed) or flow, and (is the "structural" viscosity of the dashpot. Figure 35, *D*, shows the linear load-rate of deformation response of this dashpot. Implicit in this linear viscous dashpot model are the following: (1) if flow velocity is zero, no force exists (even if the element has been deformed); (2) if a force exists, flow will always occur; and (3) the force response increases with the speed of deformation. These response characteristics are those of a viscous fluid, and are fundamentally different from the response characteristics of a solid. Thus, any material model that includes a dashpot will have some of these basic flow characteristics.

For such materials, a constant force will produce creep, that is, the deformation will increase with time as long as the force is maintained on the material (like the motion of a bicycle pump plunger), until equilibrium is reached. Conversely, for viscoelastic materials, a constantly held deformation will cause stress relaxation to occur, that is, the force required to maintain the deformation will diminish with time until equilibrium is reached. For example, when a rubber ball is stepped on in a muddy field, the ball initially is elastically compressed by the force applied by the foot. Gradually, however, the ball sinks into the mud, and less and less force need be applied to keep the foot at a constant position. Figure 36 shows compressive creep and recovery and ramp loading and stress-relaxation behavior typical of hydrated soft collagenous tissues such as articular cartilage, intervertebral disk, and meniscus. All viscoelastic materials are sensitive to strain rate. Structures made of these viscoelastic materials (all diarthrodial joints and each spinal motion segment) will also exhibit creep and stress-relaxation behavior.

Viscoelastic materials are modeled by linking the elastic springs and viscous dashpots in series or parallel, or some other combination. Figure 37 illustrates 3 commonly used viscoelastic models: the Maxwell viscoelastic fluid where the spring and dashpot are linked in series (*A*); the Kelvin-Voigt solid where the spring and dashpot are linked in parallel (*B*); and the standard three-element solid (*C*).

When loaded, the Maxwell fluid will respond instantaneously (spring) and flow indefinitely (dashpot) by virtue of the serial arrangement. However, when loaded, the Kelvin-Voigt solid, by virtue of the parallel spring-dashpot arrangement, cannot respond instantaneously because this would require an infinite force on the dashpot, and it will not flow indefinitely because a force balance between the stretched spring and the load must exist at equilibrium. The creep and stress-relaxation of these idealized materials may be determined using engineering analysis. Figure 38 shows the creep and stress-relaxation response of 3 linear viscoelastic models. By comparing these responses with real creep and stress-relaxation responses, it is easy to see which is the most realistic model to use. Indeed, in principle, the number of springs and dashpots can always be increased in series or parallel ad infinitum to model the behavior of any real viscoelastic material. However, this usually is not done because of the complexity of the calculations involved.

Tensile Stress-Strain Behavior of Articular Cartilage and Meniscus

Because the composition of biologic materials often is complex (for example, collagen and proteoglycans of the extracellular matrices and water) and their structures are observable (for example, trabecular bone, ligament, and

tendons) their intrinsic properties are more complex. These properties often depend on the orientation of the specimen relative to, for example, the predominant directions of the collagen fibrous ultrastructure (anisotropic) and the location (inhomogeneous) from which the specimen is obtained. As examples, the swelling properties of the anulus fibrosus are not the same as those of the nucleus pulposus, and the tensile properties of the articular cartilage surface are very different from those of the deeper regions. In addition, in many hydrated soft materials (for example, articular cartilage, meniscus, and intervertebral disks), the movement of the interstitial fluid during deformation exerts the major force in governing their viscoelastic behaviors. The tensile properties of 2 important orthopaedic materials, articular cartilage and knee meniscus, will be presented in this section.

The anisotropic properties of these collagenous tissues are closely related to their composition and fibrillar structure. At the articular surface, collagen is arranged in a specific pattern, which depends on the joint. This may be illustrated by puncturing the surface with a round awl. The holes produced are not round, but rather oblong in shape, much like a split formed in lumber when punctured by a large nail. Figure 39 shows a split-line pattern on the surface of a human femoral condyle. This pattern is believed to reflect the predominant collagen fibril arrangement along the surface of the joint. Each joint surface, for example, femoral head, glenoid, humeral head, patella, etc., has specific characteristic split-line patterns. Each feature mentioned here has an influence on the properties of articular cartilage, and, thus, on its function in the joint. (See Chapters 17 and 18 for more details.)

Figure 40 is a schematic depiction of the collagen fibrillar structure of the meniscus. The articulating surfaces of meniscus are composed of fine collagen fibrils organized in a random fashion. These surface layers are approximately

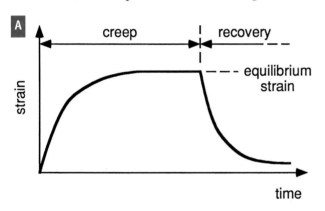

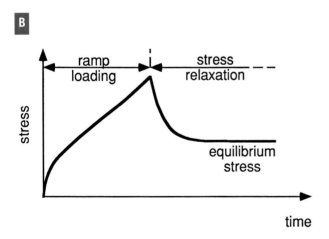

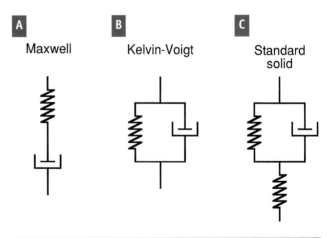

Figure 36

Typical compressive creep and recovery (**A**), and ramp loading and stress-relaxation behaviors (**B**) of hydrated soft collagenous tissues such as articular cartilage, intervertebral disk, and meniscus.

Figure 37

A, A Maxwell viscoelastic fluid with a spring and dashpot linked in series. **B**, A Kelvin-Voigt viscoelastic solid with a spring and dashpot linked in parallel. **C**, A standard 3-element viscoelastic solid.

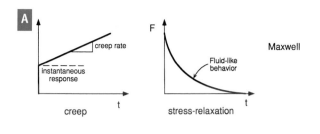

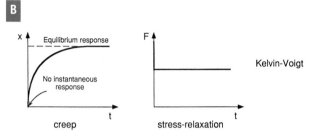

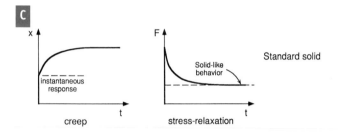

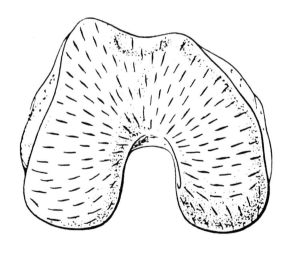

Figure 38

A, The creep and stress-relaxation response of a Maxwell viscoelastic fluid. **B,** The creep and stress-relaxation response of a Kelvin-Voigt viscoelastic solid. **C,** The creep and stress-relaxation response of a standard 3-element viscoelastic solid.

Figure 39

The split-line pattern on the surface of a human femoral condyle. This pattern is believed to reflect the predominant collagen fibril arrangement along the surface of the joint. (Reproduced with permission from Norden M, Frankel VH, Forseen, K: *Basic Biomechanics of the Musculoskeletal System.* Philadelphia, PA, Lea & Febiger, 1989, p 323.)

300 μm thick. In the deeper regions, very large collagen fiber bundles, visible to the naked eye, are found coursing around the circumferential direction. Occasionally, small radial fibers are seen randomly distributed around the circumference. These radial fibers are believed to function as ties that hold the large circumferential fiber bundles together.

Figure 33, *C*, illustrates a typical exponential tensile stress-strain curve for collagenous tissues such as articular cartilage and meniscus. The exponential shape means that the tangent to the stress-strain curve increases with increasing strain. Remember, for linearly elastic materials, the slope, that is, the Young's modulus, is a constant. The explanation for this increasing stiffness with strain may be found in the collagen ultrastructure. In these tissues, collagen is never laid down straight nor organized in a linear fashion. There is always slack or "crimp." Thus, as strain increases during a tensile test, more and more collagen fibers are straightened, and thus "recruited" to bear load. Usually, before the ultimate stress U is attained, there is a linear region in the stress-strain curve. It is believed that in this region all the available collagen fibers in the specimen are straight and have been recruited to bear load. Indeed, under the microscope, researchers have shown that the crimp pattern may be removed by stretching the collagenous tissue. (See Chapters 20 and 24 for more details.) This "recruitment model" for the tensile stress-strain behavior of collagenous tissues is also an idealization. The behavior of most tissues does not follow this neat pattern. Other organic matter such as proteoglycan and physical interactions between collagen and proteoglycan often play important roles in influencing the properties of tissues such as cartilage and meniscus. Swelling, which is an aspect of this, will be discussed below.

The anisotropic and inhomogeneous tensile properties of articular cartilage and meniscus are shown in Figure 41. For cartilage specimens taken parallel to the split-line pattern (Fig. 41, *A*) the surface zone is much stiffer than the middle and deep zone tissue. This situation is consistent with the layering morphology of the collagen network inhomogeneity. The tensile stiffness of specimens taken perpendicular to the split-line pattern is much less than that of specimens taken parallel to the split-line (Fig. 41, *A* and *B*). Again, this is consistent with overall understanding of the cartilage collagen network organization. Also, all of these stress-strain curves do not strictly follow the idealized exponential recruitment model. Figure 41, *C*, shows the tensile stress-strain behavior of meniscal specimens taken in the circumferential and radial directions. In the deep zone, circumferential specimens are much stiffer than the radial specimens. No statistically significant differences for the surface zone have been reported between these 2 directions. Figure 41 shows the dramatic anisotropic (circumferential versus radial) and inhomogeneous (surface versus deep) characteristics of meniscal tissue. These 2 tissues clearly illustrate the profound effect collagen structure has on their material properties.

Swelling Behavior of Articular Cartilage

An example of collagen-proteoglycan interaction may be seen from studies on the swelling properties of articular cartilage. In general, proteoglycan tends to produce swelling while collagen tends to limit swelling. Changes in proteoglycan content or damage to the collagen network will cause an increase in the tissue's water content. This is a very important area of investigation because in the earliest stages of osteoarthritis, articular cartilage swells because of a weakened collagen network.

Figure 42 shows the nature of cartilage swelling, which also is anisotropic and inhomogeneous. Figure 42, A, shows that increased NaCl concentration in solution around a cartilage specimen will produce greater contraction, and the relationship between NaCl concentration and contraction is linear. The slope of this linear relationship is known as the coefficient of chemical contraction. Because there is less collagen and more proteoglycan in the deeper zones than in the surface zone, contraction increases with depth: deep > middle > surface. Figure 42, B, shows that the contraction coefficient is anisotropic. Swelling is greatest in the thickness direction where there is a significant amount of crimping of the collagen fibers and least in the direction parallel to the split-lines (length direction) where the collagen fibers are likely to be straight.

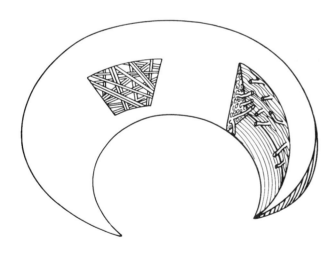

Figure 40

Schematic depiction of the collagen fibrillar structure of the meniscus. The articulating surfaces are composed of fine collagen fibrils and organized in a random fashion. In the deeper regions, very large collagen fiber bundles are found coursing around the circumferential direction. Small radial fibers are seen randomly distributed around the circumference serving to tie the large circumferential fiber bundles together. (Reproduced with permission from Fithian DC, Kelley MA, Mow VC: Material properties and structure function relationships in the meniscus. *Clin Orthop* 1990;252:19–31.)

Flow-Independent and Biphasic Flow-Dependent Viscoelastic Material Properties

The basic mechanisms responsible for the viscoelastic behavior of tissues are: (1) internal friction caused by sliding of one microstructural element past another (for example, collagen fibrils rubbing against collagen fibrils); and (2) viscous drag of interstitial fluid as it flows through the porous-permeable solid matrix (analogous to the resistance encountered when water is forced through coffee grounds in an espresso machine). Internal friction caused by interlamellar sliding within osteons has been reported as being responsible for the long-term creep behavior of bone. For ligaments and tendons under tensile loads, the major cause of internal friction arises from the "uncrimping" of the collagen fiber bundles as they slide through the thick viscous proteoglycan gel.

Viscous drag of interstitial fluid flow becomes the dominant cause of the viscoelastic response of articular cartilage, intervertebral disk, and meniscus, where the dominant mode of loading is compression. To account for this, these tissues have been modeled as biphasic materials. The solid phase is linearly elastic and porous (70% to 85% porosity). The fluid phase (mostly water) is incompressible. The solid matrix compresses elastically, thereby forcing out fluid, like water being squeezed out of a sponge. The frictional drag of this fluid is greater, the faster it is being forced (time-dependent). Obviously, if the cartilage is compressed very slowly the frictional drag will be negligible, and the cartilage will behave nearly elastically. Furthermore, the smaller the pores (lower permeability), the harder it is to force fluid through them; thus, the greater the drag. Because the pores are part of the solid matrix, compressive strain of the matrix makes the pores smaller, increasing the viscous drag. Thus the viscous behavior is both time- and strain-dependent. Finally, at equilibrium, when the fluid ceases to flow, all of the load is borne by the solid matrix at the same position on the stress-strain curve that it would have reached if it had been elastically compressed. (For details, see Chapters 17 and 18.)

Behavior of Simple Structures

Size and Shape of Geometric Forms

If an object is rectangular, its size may be described by the length of its sides, a,b,c,d. To characterize a sphere, it is necessary only to specify the radius r. How then is the size of a femur quantitatively defined? If shaft fracture from a bending load is of concern, shaft diameter and length are

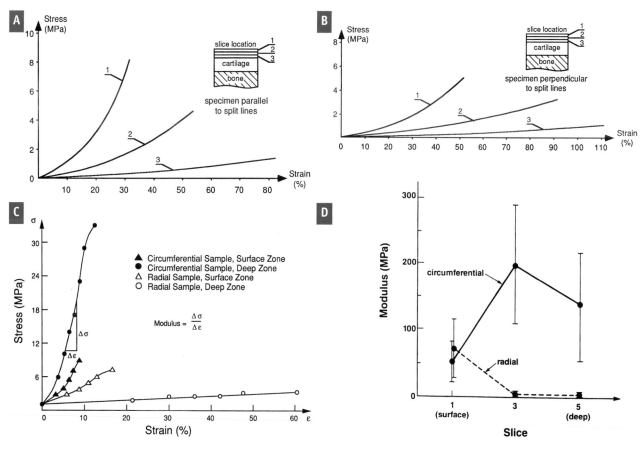

Figure 41

The anisotropic and inhomogeneous tensile properties of articular cartilage; specimens parallel to the split-line pattern (**A**) and specimens perpendicular to the split-line pattern (**B**). The surface zones are stiffer than the deep zones. **C,** Tensile stress-strain behavior of meniscal specimens taken in the circumferential and radial directions. In the deep zone, circumferential specimens are much stiffer than radial specimens. **D,** The anisotropic (circumferential versus radial) and inhomogeneous (surface versus deep) tensile properties of meniscal tissue. (**C** and **D** reproduced with permission from Proctor CS, Schmidt MB, Whipple RR, et al: Material properties of the normal medial bovine meniscus. *J Orthop Res* 1989;7:771–782.)

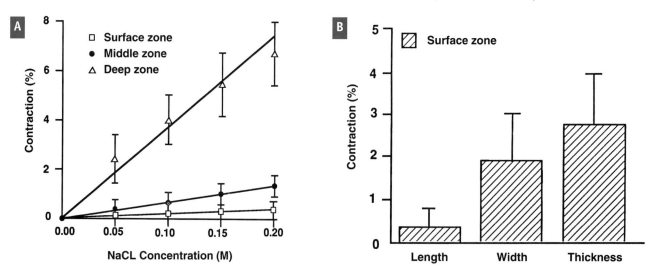

Figure 42

A, The inhomogeneous swelling properties of articular cartilage. With increased NaCl concentration, the cartilage specimen will contract. This swelling behavior increases with depth from the surface. **B,** The anisotropic swelling property of cartilage. The contraction coefficient is greatest in the thickness direction and least in the direction parallel to the split-lines (length). (Reproduced with permission from Myers ER, Lai WM, Mow VC: A continuum theory and an experiment for the ion-induced swelling behavior. *J Biomech Eng* 1984;106:151–158.)

important. If joint-reaction force is of concern, the trochanter-head distance (abductor moment arm) is crucial. If femoral neck fracture is of concern, the size of the femur from the femoral head to the distal medial condyle is less important than the length of the femoral neck. In general, it is important to remember that different geometric parameters are important in determining the structural response to different loading conditions. For an object of given shape and size, different orientations of the load with respect to the object will produce different responses. For example, it is far easier to bend a flat ruler perpendicular to its flat surface than along its edge. Thus, how tissue functions as a structure depends not only on its intrinsic material properties but also on its size and shape. This section covers the important geometric properties of objects, which influence the structural behavior of material objects.

Areas and Centroids

Recall that in describing the behavior of a bar of a material in tension, the important geometric quantities are A (cross-sectional area) and l_0 (the length along the direction of applied load). In many other problems, the "geometric center" of an area or a volume must be known. The geometric center is known as the centroid. For areas such as a circle or a rectangle, at least 2 lines of symmetry are obvious. Intuitively, the geometric center of these areas may be thought of as the intersection of these lines of symmetry. For volumes such as spheres and cubes, the geometric center may be thought of as the intersection of 3 planes of symmetry. How then is it possible to find the centroid of a more complex shaped object (triangle, trapezoid, etc) or an arbitrarily shaped object (femur, patella, etc) that does not have lines or planes of symmetry? This is done by defining the first moment of an area or volume.

Consider a very small bit of area ΔA (for example, ΔA = 0.005 mm²) located at a point x and y (3 cm and 4 cm) in the x-y plane. The first x-moment of this bit of area ΔA is defined to be x times ΔA (that is, 30 mm × 0.005 mm² = 0.15 mm³), and the first y-moment to be y times ΔA (that is, 40 mm × 0.005 mm² = 0.2 mm³). Note that for areas, the first x- and y-moments are also known as the first moments about the y and x axes, respectively. Now, any arbitrarily shaped area with a total area A (500 mm²) may be subdivided into tiny bits. In this example, the 500 mm² area could be divided into 100,000 equal bits of ΔA, and each ΔA in the x-y plane would have a contribution to the first x- and y-moments of area. The shape of the area comes into play in computation of the contribution of each ΔA to the first moment. The contribution of each ΔA would depend on where it is located relative to a set of reference axes x and y; the farther away from the axes, the greater would be the contribution to the first moment of area. The first x-moment of the area A is calculated by simply adding the contributions (that is, xΔA) of all the ΔAs. The first

y-moment may be similarly calculated. The x coordinate of the centroid (denoted by x_c) of any arbitrary area is defined by dividing the first x-moment of the area A by the total area A; y_c is similarly defined. If the object is a 3-D volume, then there are first x-, y-, and z-moments of volume with respect to the yz, xz, and xy planes, respectively.

Example: If the x-axis lies along the center line of a straight intermedullary rod with uniform circular cross section, and y and z axes are perpendicular to the rod and at the end of the rod, then the rod would have zero as the first y- and z-moments and a large first x-moment. In this case, the x axis is known as the centroidal axis.

It is important to remember that the first moment of area (or volume) is a measure of how far the centroid of the area (or center of the volume) is with respect to a coordinate system used to describe the area (or volume).

Physically, if the area A is a thin homogeneous steel plate weighing W (for example, 10 N), it is held in the x-y plane, and the z axis is the direction of gravity (down), then the first moments of area of the plate are proportional to the components of the moment vector exerted by the weight of the plate about the x and y axes; the proportionality constant being the specific weight of the steel plate (N/mm²). The centroid of the plate located at x_c, y_c is then defined as the point at which the weight W may be considered to be located. In other words, the moment components $M_x = y_c W$ and $M_y = x_c W$ are proportional to the first moments of area of the steel plate.

Problem: Explain why it is possible to balance this plate with one finger located at the centroid.

For each bit of the steel plate ΔA, gravity exerts a bit of force ΔW. The total weight W is the sum of all the ΔWs because all these gravitational forces are parallel. This simple example illustrates the general principle that any arbitrary distribution of parallel forces ΔWs all acting in one direction may be represented by an equipollent single force W acting at the centroid. This is a very fundamental result and it is commonly used in musculoskeletal biomechanics. Almost always, researchers will use the centroid of the physiologic cross-sectional area (commonly denoted as PCSA) of a muscle as the point through which the resultant muscle force acts. In ligament and tendon biomechanics studies, the resultant force also always is assumed to act through the centroid. The implication of this assumption is that the investigator has assumed that all the collagen fiber bundles in ligaments and tendons are parallel, are stretched by the same amount, and have the same material properties, so that the force per unit area is the same everywhere.

Problem: In light of what you know about the structure of the human anterior cruciate ligament, provide arguments for and against the assumption that the force carried by the ACL must pass through the centroid of the cross section.

For other loading states, different aspects of the geometry come into play. For example, in the case of bending of the long stem of a hip prosthesis, an entirely different aspect of structural geometry must be considered. To resist bending, the second moment of area or moment of inertia plays the dominant role. To define the second moment of area, consider again an area A in the x-y plane, in which A is subdivided into many tiny bits of ΔAs, and x and y specify the location of ΔA in the x-y plane. The second moment of area of A with respect to the x-axis (second y-moment) is the sum of the product of y^2 and ΔA over all subdivided areas; this is always denoted by the symbol I_{xx}. Similarly I_{yy} is the sum of the product of x^2 and ΔA over all the subdivided areas.

While the second moments of area I_{xx} or I_{yy} are important in resisting bending, the polar moment of inertia, usually denoted by I_p or I_{zz}, is fundamental in resisting torsion. The polar moment of inertia is also a second moment of area, but is given by the sum of the products $(x^2 + y^2)\Delta A = r^2\Delta A$ over all subdivided areas. More simply, the polar moment of inertia is given by the formula

$$I_p = I_{xx} + I_{yy}$$

Figure 43 provides the location of the centroid, x_c,y_c, of 3 common simple areas and the second moment of area about a set of x and y axes and the centroidal axes x_c and y_c.

Problem: For the rectangular area shown in Figure 43, describe how you would determine the second moment of area I_{xx} from $I_{x_c x_c}$ and knowledge of the position of the centroid C.

The concept of the second moments of area naturally arises when bending of beams and torsion of shafts are considered (for details, see sections below). In bending, the resistance to a bending moment is inversely proportional to the second moment of the cross-sectional area, say I_{yy}, and in torsion the resistance to a torque is inversely proportional to the polar moment of the cross-sectional area I_p.

To explain why a meter stick of length x = 1,000 mm, thickness y = 2 mm, and width z = 30 mm will appear very flexible in the thickness direction and very stiff in the width direction, consider a small area ΔA = 0.02 mm^2 in the cross section (y-z plane) of the meter stick. If, for example, in the thickness direction, the centroid of this ΔA is located at 0.25 mm below the surface (that is, y = 0.75 mm), then its second moment of area about the z axis I_{zz} will be $y^2\Delta A = (0.75$ mm$^2)0.02$ mm$^2 = 0.01125$ mm^4. Now, if in the width direction z, the centroid of this ΔA is also located at 0.25 mm below the surface (that is, z = 14.75 mm), then its second moment of area about the y axis I_{yy} will be $z^2\Delta A = (14.75$

mm$^2)0.02$ mm$^2 = 4.351$ mm^4. Thus, the same ΔA (0.02 mm^2) located at the same relative position will contribute 386.8 times more to the resistance of bending in the width direction when compared to that in the thickness direction.

There are 3 other second moments of area, I_{xy}, I_{yz}, I_{xz}. These are given by the sum of the products of xyΔA, yzΔA, and xzΔA, respectively, and are known as the products of inertia of the area A. They are a measure of the symmetry of an area with respect to the set of coordinates x,y,z used to describe that area. If x is an axis of symmetry for the area A, for every ΔA above the axis x there is an identical ΔA below x, that is, the locations of both ΔAs above and below the x-axis are identical. For example, in Figure 43, x_c is an axis of symmetry for the rectangle and the circle, but not for the triangle. If x is an axis of symmetry of A, then at each value of x, for each xyΔA there is a -xyΔA, and when xyΔA and -xyΔA are summed they must cancel each other. Thus, I_{xy} must be zero. A similar argument must hold if the y axis is an axis of symmetry. That is, if either x or y is an axis of symmetry, I_{xy} = 0. In general, even if there are no axes of symmetry, there exist at least 3 directions for which all 3 products of inertia, I_{xy}, I_{yz}, I_{xz}, will be zero.

For 3-D objects, there are 6 components of the second moment of area, I_{xx}, I_{yy}, I_{zz}, I_{xy}, I_{xz}, I_{yz}, that have the same mathematical properties as the stress tensor and the strain tensor, thus the identical tensorial analysis may be used to describe the second moments of area, otherwise known as the moment of inertia tensor.

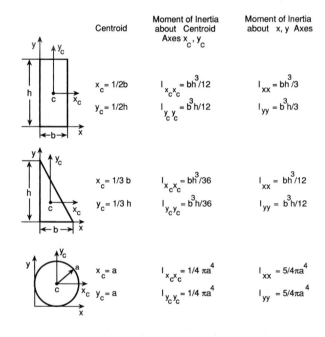

	Centroid	Moment of Inertia about Centroid Axes x_c, y_c	Moment of Inertia about x, y Axes
	$x_c = 1/2b$	$I_{x_c x_c} = bh^3/12$	$I_{xx} = bh^3/3$
	$y_c = 1/2h$	$I_{y_c y_c} = b^3h/12$	$I_{yy} = b^3h/3$
	$x_c = 1/3 b$	$I_{x_c x_c} = bh^3/36$	$I_{xx} = bh^3/12$
	$y_c = 1/3 h$	$I_{y_c y_c} = b^3h/36$	$I_{yy} = b^3h/12$
	$x_c = a$	$I_{x_c x_c} = 1/4\,\pi a^4$	$I_{xx} = 5/4\pi a^4$
	$y_c = a$	$I_{y_c y_c} = 1/4\,\pi a^4$	$I_{yy} = 5/4\pi a^4$

Figure 43

The centroid, and second moment of area (or moment of inertia) about the centroid axes x_c,y_c and the x,y axes of some common areas.

Problem: In Figure 43, x_c, y_c are axes of symmetry for the rectangle, therefore $I_{x_c y_c} = 0$. For another set of coordinate axes x', y' chosen to be rotated at an arbitrary angle θ with respect to the x_c, y_c axes, but sharing the same origin, is the product of inertia $I_{x'y'}$ with respect to $x'y'$ also zero? Yes or no, and explain why.

Uniaxial Tension and Compression of Bars

Structures are materials fashioned into specific sizes and shapes to serve a specific function. Thus, structures have dimensions and shapes. The simplest load-carrying structural element is a straight bar of cross-sectional area A and length l_0 that is loaded in a uniaxial manner, for example, the gauge section of a test specimen (Fig. 33). When a bar is loaded in uniaxial tension (or compression), the elongation Δl will be inversely proportional to the cross-sectional area A and stiffness of the material (Young's modulus E), and directly proportional to the load F and length l_0. Thus, Δl is given by the simple relation $\Delta l = Fl_0/AE$. Clearly, this gives Hooke's law $\varepsilon = \sigma/E$ where $\varepsilon = \Delta l/l_0$ and $\sigma = F/A$, as discussed in an earlier section. Again, for the bar, the structural stiffness is $k = AE/l_0$ and the intrinsic material modulus is E. The bar, as an example of a simple structure, clearly demonstrates the difference between structural response, which depends on the geometry of the structure, and material response, which depends only on the intrinsic properties of the material. For many linearly elastic materials, or even for materials that are not linearly elastic, the uniaxial test is universally used to determine the stiffness k or Young's modulus of the material.

Problem: The stress-strain behavior of soft biologic tissues such as the cruciate ligaments of the knee, glenohumeral ligaments, etc, usually looks like that shown in Figure 33, *C.* Describe how to determine the stiffness of such materials, using the simple linear relationship $\sigma = E\varepsilon$.

Torsion of Circular Shafts

A cylinder loaded in torsion is a common model used to help understand problems such as a tibia being twisted in a skiing accident, or a femoral intramedullary nail resisting torsion. Figure 44, *A,* shows a circular shaft of radius a and length l_0 subject to twisting couple M_t on either end; thus, both force and moment equilibrium conditions are satisfied. In this figure, x is the coordinate along the axis of the shaft through the center of the circular cross-sectional area, and y,z are axes perpendicular to the shaft. Under this torque, any line along the shaft AB will be twisted. This twist follows a helical path from the left face to the right face, assuming the left face is fixed. From theory of elasticity, the total angle of twist θ between the right face and the left face is given by $\theta = (M_t l_0/GI_p)$, where I_p is the polar moment of inertia (Fig. 44, *B*), and G is the linear elastic shear modulus. For a given applied torque, the angle of twist θ (the structural response) will depend directly on the length of the rod (the longer the rod the larger the angle) and inversely on its polar moment of inertia. Many geometric properties will affect the polar moment; for example, adding slots on the surface of an intramedullary nail will greatly reduce it. For a cylindrical rod, the polar moment will vary as the fourth power of the radius, so a rod or bone that is twice as thick has 16 times the torsional rigidity.

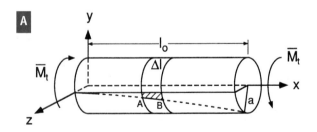

A

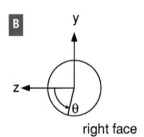

B

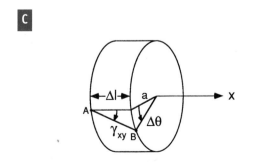

C

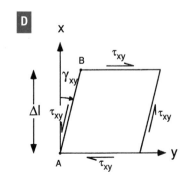

D

Figure 44

A, A circular shaft subject to twisting by a couple M_t at either end. **B,** The angle of twist θ between the right and left faces is given by $\theta = M_t l_0/GI_p$. **C,** The shear modulus G may be determined from the twist angle $\Delta\theta$ between 2 nearby surfaces separated by Δl: $G = (M_t\Delta l)/(\Delta\theta I_p)$. **D,** In the pure shear state, the shear stresses τ_{xy} act on each face.

To determine the shear modulus G of the material of the shaft, look at the twist angle $\Delta\theta$ between 2 nearby surfaces, separated by Δl (Fig. 44, C). Thus, in an experiment, if the twist angle $\Delta\theta$ and the geometry of the circular-cylindrical specimen, I_p, are prescribed, and the torque M_t response is measured, it is possible to calculate $G = (M_t \Delta l)/(\Delta\theta I_p)$. The shear modulus determined in this manner satisfies the shear component of Hooke's law $\tau_{xy} = G\gamma_{xy}$ in the same way the Young's modulus satisfies the lineal component of Hooke's law $\sigma_{xx} = E\varepsilon_{xx}$. For isotropic materials the only independent elastic coefficients are E,G; all other material coefficients may be derived from them. For example, the Poisson's ratio may be calculated from the simple relationship $\nu = (E - 2G)/2G$. Figure 44, D, shows how a square area is deformed when sheared. In the torsional configuration, the shear stresses τ_{xy} shown are acting on each face of a rectangular element; this is known as the pure shear state. A word of caution: There are no other easy test configurations for which a state of pure shear may be achieved. Often, for expediency, experimenters use a simple shear test, where the stresses τ_{xy} are applied to the top and bottom surfaces. Such a test clearly is not in rotational equilibrium; thus, other stresses (normal stresses) must be added at the top and bottom face to balance the torque. Because of this addition, results from simple shear tests are difficult to interpret.

Inside the circular cylindrical shaft, the magnitude of the shear stress τ increases linearly with the distance r from the center; this relationship is given by $\tau = M_t r/I_p$. This shear stress increases with the applied torque M_t and decreases inversely with Ip. If this shear stress were plotted along an arbitrary circle of radius r in the shaft, the shear τ would be tangent to that circle, (Fig. 45, A), and its magnitude would increase in the manner shown in Figure 45, B. The maximum shear stress would occur at the circumference of the cross-section.

For stress analysis, look at the specific case of a hollow circular shaft (tibia) with inner radius a and outer radius b (Fig. 46, A). As indicated in the preceding discussion, the square denoted by ABCD in the section Δl will be sheared as shown. The magnitude of the shear stress τ varies from a to b as shown in Figure 46, B. For the hollow tube, the polar moment of inertia I_p must be equal to I_p(outer cylinder) minus I_p(inner cylinder).

Problem: The average outer and inner diameters of the humerus for males are 2.45 cm and 0.97 cm, respectively, and for females they are 2.07 cm and 0.87 cm, respectively. For an applied torque of 5 N•m, calculate the maximum shear stress acting inside the humeral shaft. If the shear moduli of males and females are the same (800 MPa), and the length of the humeral shafts are 30 cm and 28 cm, respectively, calculate the angle of twist between the humeral head and the epicondylar axis of the elbow.

Figure 46, C, illustrates that plane BC in the deformed square ABCD is the plane on which the tensile stress inside the shaft is a maximum given by $\sigma_{max} = M_t b/I_p$. This maximum always occurs at the surface, and the plane is always oriented at 45° from the horizon. Figure 46, D, shows the orientation of a failure surface along the cylinder under pure shear for materials weak in tension. This forms a 45° spiral along the surface of the shaft. Clinically, this failure surface resembles that seen in a spiral fracture of the tibia in ski injuries resulting from torsion, because cortical bone is weak in tension.

Bending of Beams

A straight beam of cross-sectional area A and length l_o is subject to pure bending M_b on either end (Fig. 47, A). Again, x is the coordinate along the axis of the beam through the centroid C of the cross section; y and z are perpendicular to the beam axis as shown. For pure bending, any cross-sectional plane such as AA′ perpendicular to the centroidal axis remains a plane after bending (Fig. 47, B). Because of this, the normal stress σ_{xx} acting on the planes AA′ or BB′ must vary linearly from the plane containing the centroidal axis (known as the neutral plane) (Fig. 47, C). The stress is compressive from O to A′ and O to B′, and it is tensile from

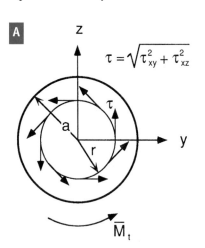

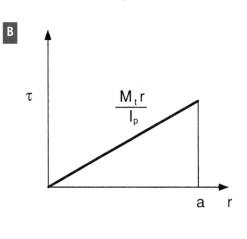

Orthopaedic Basic Science | American Academy of Orthopaedic Surgeons

Figure 45

Shear stress along an arbitrary circle in a shaft subject to torsion (**A**). The magnitude of the shear stress varies from 0 to $M_t a/I_p$ (**B**).

O to A and O to B. Maximum tension occurs along AB, and maximum compression occurs along A´B´. The normal stress along line OO is zero. Line OO is also known as the neutral axis. For a straight beam, the neutral axis and the centroidal axis are coincident. These axes are not coincident for curved beams. This difference is the origin of the often discussed tension-band concept in the orthopaedics literature.

As in torsion, the state of stress within the beam may also be calculated. In the bending configuration (Fig. 47), the normal stress σ_{xx} acting on any plane (for example, AA´) is given as $\sigma_{xx} = M_b z/I_{yy}$, which is known as the simple flexure formula in bending. Maximum compression occurs at $z = -h/2$ ($-M_b h/2I_{yy}$) and maximum tension occurs at $z = h/2$ ($M_b h/2I_{yy}$). Hooke's law $\sigma_{xx} = E\varepsilon_{xx}$ may be used to calculate the lineal strain ε_{xx} from the flexure formula, and the change of length Δl may be calculated from the relationship $\varepsilon_{xx} = \Delta l/l_o$.

The 3 formulas (bar, torsion, and bending) are very important, and they are the most frequently used formulas in structure mechanics. However, biologic structures such as bone are usually more complex geometrically; they are heterogeneous and anisotropic, and they are subjected to more complex forms of loading, which involve combinations of these pure forms. Thus, caution is always advised in interpreting data based on the 3 simple structure formulas.

Problem: For femoral cortical bone, the tensile strength is 60 MPa. If the femoral shaft is modeled as a straight, hollow, circular cylinder that is 42 cm long with inner and outer radii of 1.5 cm and 2.0 cm, respectively, and if a bending moment of 20 N•m is applied, calculate the maximum tensile stress. Will the femoral shaft fail?

Large tensile, compressive, and shear stresses exist inside the beam as a result of pure bending. From stress analysis, the plane of maximum shear stress occurs at 45° from the horizontal direction (Fig. 48). If, for example, a long bone such as the tibia is subject to large bending moments and begins to fail at the tension side, it also could induce failure in the shear mode as the tensile crack propagates into the bone. These 2 failure modes are responsible for the often observed butterfly fragment in bone fractures.

Problem: In finding the stress in the beam, the intrinsic material properties do not enter into consideration; for example, the stress in the beam would be the same if the meter stick were made of steel or wood. Does that mean any material may be used to construct a bridge, for example?

Combined Compression and Bending

So far, the behaviors that have been considered address only simple structures subjected to pure tension or compression, pure shear (or torsion), or pure bending. In this section, the case of combined compression and bending

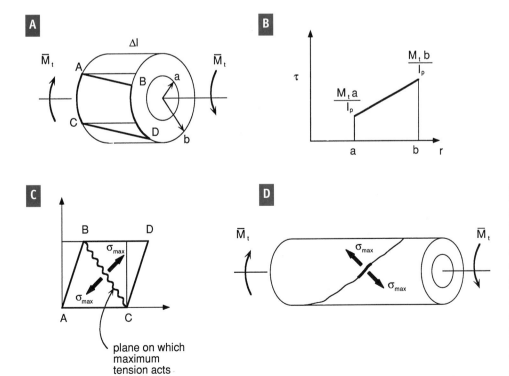

Figure 46

A, Stress analysis of a hollow circular shaft with inner radius a and outer radius b. The square denoted by ABCD in the section Δl is sheared as shown. **B,** The magnitude of the shear stress τ varies from a to b. **C,** The plane BC in the square ABCD is the plane on which the tensile stress inside the shaft is a maximum. This plane is oriented at 45° from the horizontal. **D,** The orientation of a tensile failure surface along the cylinder under pure shear for materials weak in tension.

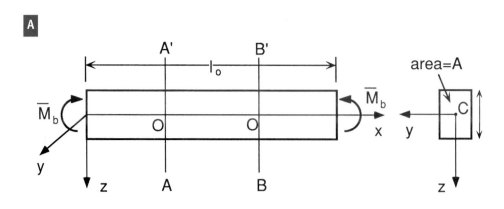

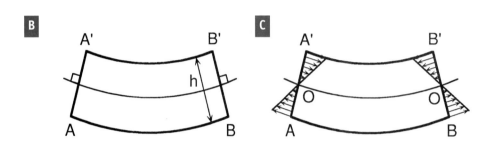

Figure 47

A, A straight beam of cross-sectional area A, length l_o, and centroid C subject to pure bending M_b on either end. **B,** Any straight plane such as AA′ perpendicular to the centroidal axis remains a plane after bending. **C,** The normal stress on the plane AA′ or BB′ varies linearly from the plane containing the centroidal axis 0-0.

will be considered as an illustration of how more complex loading conditions may be described. This model often has been applied to describe the state of stress within the femoral neck and fractures (Fig. 49).

The stress distribution in the femoral neck resulting from loading of the femoral head by the acetabulum can be described as follows. The resultant force produced by the acetabulum occurs at an angle to the transverse plane through the femoral neck. This situation cannot be analyzed by considering any one of the pure forms of loading alone. However, the state of stress may be determined by considering the components of the resultant force acting parallel to and perpendicular to this transverse plane (Fig. 49, *A*). The x axis is taken perpendicular to this plane and through the centroid of the cross-sectional area, and the y axis is taken parallel to this plane. The z axis is taken perpendicular to the x-y plane through the centroid of the cross-sectional area. Assume that F_R has no component in the z direction for this example. The resultant force may then be resolved into its x and y components F_x and F_y.

To see how these force components contribute multiple effects, first isolate the femoral neck, cut by the imaginary plane of interest as a free body (Fig. 49, *B*). If forces in the y direction are summed, a force F'_y, which is equal and opposite to F_y, must act at O to balance the force F_y. When forces are summed in the x direction, a force F'_x, equal and opposite to F_x, must act at O. This force results in a normal (compressive) stress $\sigma_{xx} = -F_x/A$, where A is the cross-sectional area of the cut surface (bar formula). Now summing moments about O, the force F_y produces a counterclockwise moment M equal to $+ (F_y) \times (d)$, which must be

balanced by a clockwise moment M′ on the right side of the section equal to $- (F_y) \times (d)$. The effect of these moments may be approximated by the pure bending case discussed above. It results in a stress σ_{xx}' on the cut surface equal to M_y/I_{zz}. The resultant stress across the cross-sectional area must then be the sum of σ_{xx}, produced by compression, and σ_{xx}', produced by bending, and is therefore equal to $(-F_x/A) + (M_y/I_{zz})$ (Fig. 49, *bottom*). There is also a shear component acting through the femoral neck as a result of F'_y at the section. This force produces a shear stress $\tau_{xy} = -F'_y/A$. As the resultant force F_R acting on the femoral head approaches the direction perpendicular to the axis of the femoral neck, large bending moments and shear forces will be developed, resulting in tensile stresses at the superior aspect of the femoral neck and a large shear stress across the neck.

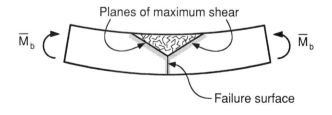

Planes of maximum shear

Failure surface

Figure 48

If a long bone subject to bending begins to crack at the side under tension, failure could be induced in the shear mode along the planes of maximum shear stress (45° from the horizontal direction) creating a butterfly fragment.

Problem: If the force F_R applied to the femoral head is 1,500 N at an angle of 45°, d = 4 cm, and the outer and inner diameters of the femoral neck cortex are assumed to be 3 cm and 2.5 cm, respectively, what is the maximum value of σ_{xx} on the cut surface? If the tensile strength of the cortical bone there is 100 MPa, will the femoral neck break?

Stress Concentration

These analyses compute average stresses over uniform geometries and loading conditions. In fact, structural imperfections, sudden changes in cross-sectional area, discontinuities, cracks, drill-holes, and other irregularities may concentrate stress locally, resulting in failure if the local material's ultimate strength is exceeded. The stress-concentration factor K_c is defined as the ratio of the maximum stress at the site of the discontinuity to the average stress in the region. This may be determined empirically, with a photoelastic method, or estimated by other techniques. Tables of stress-concentration factors for defects of known geometry are available. A more complete discussion of the stress-concentrating effects of cracks in cortical bone may be found in Chapter 14.

Finite Element Analysis

The discussions provided above are only for structures such as the bar, beam, and shaft under simple loading conditions such as uniaxial tension or compression, pure bending, and pure shear. For more complicated geometric forms and loading conditions, and for more complex materials, the state of stress inside the material becomes very complex. Thus, when the idealized assumptions are not met, the simple analyses cannot be used to assess the state of stress inside the body, or they must be used with great caution. For example, to treat the stress analysis problem of an actual femur with a femoral head prosthesis in place, the following must be known: (1) the actual loading conditions on the bone and the prosthesis; (2) the actual geometric form of the femur-prosthesis configuration; (3) the material properties of bone (inhomogeneous and anisotropic) and the prosthesis; and (4) the interface conditions between the bone and the prosthesis. Obviously, none of the required information is known precisely. First, better estimates of joint loadings may be obtained by increasing the sophistication of the statically indeterminate problems to solve for muscle and joint forces. Second, better geometric data may be obtained from mechanical sectioning or radiographic imaging procedures. Third, more tests may be

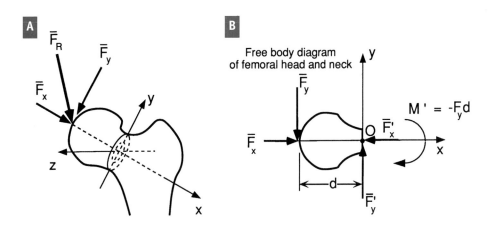

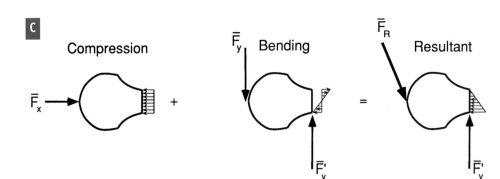

Figure 49

A, The force F_R acting on the femoral head may be resolved into components F_x and F_y. **B,** Free-body diagram of the femoral head. The effects of F_x and F_y are balanced at the right side by the moment M' and the forces F'_y and F'_x. **C,** The resultant effect of the compressive and bending loads on the femoral head.

made on the material properties of the femur. Finally, better educated guesses may be made on the mechanical interactions occurring at the prosthesis-bone interface. Suppose all this information is now available. Has the bone-prosthesis interface problem been solved? The answer is no. A detailed stress analysis must be performed of the bone-prosthesis problem by calculating the stresses and strains inside the bone, the PMMA, and the prosthesis. But the geometric form and other complexities prevent simple solutions from being obtained. This is where finite element analysis is used.

To solve a problem with complex geometric form and material property distributions, the finite element approach is to break the problem up into smaller "finite elements" with simple geometric form. Usually triangular or quadrilateral elements are used. A computer program is written to balance the forces and moments acting on each element, and match these forces and moments with those of its neighboring elements. For large structures with a large number of elements, the computer must solve thousands of algebraic equations to make sure all the forces are balanced in the interior of the body and at the surface where the forces are applied. Usually, in finite element analysis of linear elastic material structures, the principle of minimum energy is invoked, that is, the energy of deformation caused by the external loading is a minimum at equilibrium. While the finite element procedure is conceptually simple, the technical details for actual implementation of the computer programs are very complex. For most finite element analyses of bone and prostheses, linear elasticity is assumed as the model for their stress-strain behavior.

Biotribology of Diarthrodial Joints

Introduction

Diarthrodial joints have some common features. First, they are all enclosed by a strong fibrous capsule lined with the metabolically active synovium (Fig. 50, *A*). Second, the load-supporting bony ends of these joints are lined with a thin layer of articular cartilage (see Chapters 17 and 18 for more details). These linings form the joint cavity, which contains the synovial fluid (Fig. 50, *B*). The synovial fluid, articular cartilage, and supporting bone form the smooth, nearly frictionless bearing system of the body. For the human knee, the intra-articular fibrocartilaginous meniscus is also important for load bearing.

Although diarthrodial joints are subjected to an enormous range of loading conditions, the cartilage surfaces undergo little wear and tear under normal circumstances. For example, the human hip joint sustains a variety of loading conditions. Under relatively high speed motion, for example, during the swing phase of walking or running, low loads are sustained. However, during stance phase, especially at heel-strike, forces 5 to 10 times body weight across the hip and knee joints may be generated. Human diarthrodial joints must be capable of functioning effectively under these very high loads and stresses, and at generally very low operating speeds for 7 or 8 decades. This demands an efficient lubrication process to minimize friction and to pre-

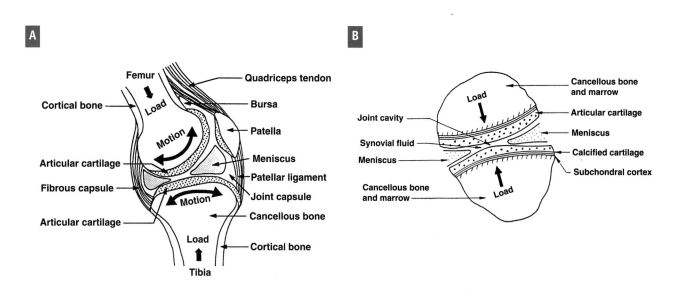

Figure 50

Schematic of a diarthrodial joint showing the strong fibrous capsule, articular cartilage (**A**), synovial fluid, and joint cavity (**B**).

vent wear of cartilage in the joint. Breakdown in cartilage by either biochemical or biomechanical means may lead to arthritis.

Tribology is defined as the science that deals with the friction, lubrication, and wear of interacting surfaces in relative motion. Biotribology, the branch of tribology that focuses on the understanding of the friction, lubrication, and wear phenomena found in diarthrodial joints, has been an intense area of investigation for over 50 years. Precise and meticulous measurements have been made on the frictional properties of joints and wear properties of cartilage. The biphasic nature of articular cartilage is important in these functional characteristics of diarthrodial joints.

Synovial Fluid

Synovial fluid is a clear, or sometimes slightly yellowish, highly viscous liquid secreted into the joint cavity by the synovium. Minute amounts of this fluid are contained in various human and animal joints. Approximately 1 to 5 ml of fluid is contained in a healthy human knee joint. Synovial fluid is a dialysate of blood plasma, without clotting factors, erythrocytes, or hemoglobin, but containing hyaluronate, an extended glycosaminoglycan and a lubricating glycoprotein that aids in friction reduction. A typical long-chain hyaluronate molecule has a molecular weight of 1 to 2 million daltons.

Newtonian and Nonnewtonian Fluids

Synovial fluid exhibits nonnewtonian flow properties, which include a shear thinning viscosity effect and viscoelastic effects. Newtonian viscosity of a fluid is defined by an equation very similar to the dashpot equation $F = \eta \dot{x}$ except it is now written for shear stress τ and shear-rate $D: \tau = M^D$. This equation is entirely analogous to Hooke's law for linearly elastic solids, that is, a newtonian fluid is a linearly viscous fluid. The viscosity μ is an intrinsic property of the fluid, whereas η is the structural viscosity or the damping coefficient of the dashpot, and they both represent resistance to flow. A newtonian fluid has no shear stiffness. For newtonian fluids such as air and water, the viscosity coefficient μ is a constant at a given temperature. For nonnewtonian fluids, the viscosity coefficient μ is not a constant; instead, it depends on the shear-rate D. Newtonian fluids are also purely dissipative materials (analogous to the dashpot). They cannot store energy, that is, there is no elastic spring element in the fluid. If the fluid contains a macromolecule in solution that is capable of forming networks, the energy of deformation may be stored by deforming the network. Such fluids are also known as viscoelastic fluids, and they may be modeled, for example, by the Maxwell model.

Figure 51 shows the shear-rate dependent viscosity η and shear stiffness (or modulus) G of synovial fluid. These char-

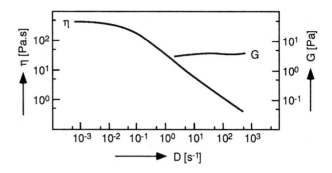

Figure 51

The shear-rate dependent viscosity η and the shear modulus G of normal synovial fluid: D = shear rate.

acteristics demonstrate that synovial fluid is a nonnewtonian fluid. In this figure, the viscosity of synovial fluid from normal knee joints decreases from 500 to 0.5 Pa as the shear rate increases from 0.001 to 1,000 s^{-1}. Normal synovial fluid also has significant shear stiffness (1 to 10 Pa), which remains relatively constant. The shear-rate dependent viscosity derives from the alignment of the long-chain hyaluronate molecules as the synovial fluid is sheared in the viscometer, and the shear stiffness derives from the entanglement of these long chain molecules forming elastic networks (springs) in the synovial fluid. The "stringiness" of synovial fluid is caused by the hyaluronate network in solution.

Synovial fluids from rheumatoid patients usually contain enzymatically degraded hyaluronate molecules. The viscosity of rheumatoid synovial fluid does not have these nonnewtonian flow properties; thus, researchers believe that rheumatoid synovial fluid is less effective as the lubricant in diarthrodial joints. Hyaluronates of synovial fluids from osteoarthritic joints (without inflammation) are not degraded. They maintain their nonnewtonian fluid properties.

Synovial fluid not only aids in lubrication, but also provides the necessary nutrients for cartilage. Furthermore, synovial fluid acts as a medium for osmosis between the joint and the blood supply, and as protection for cartilage against enzyme activity.

Anatomic Forms of Diarthrodial Joints

A major consideration in determining the frictional characteristics between two surfaces sliding over each other is the topography of the given surfaces. Changes in the anatomic form affect the way in which loads are transmitted across joints, altering the mode of lubrication in that joint and, thus, the physiologic state of cartilage.

Microscopically, articular surfaces are relatively rough compared to machined bearing surfaces (Table 4). In fact, the natural surfaces are much rougher than joint replacement prostheses. The mean of the surface roughness R_a for articular cartilage ranges from 1 to 6 µm, while the metal femoral head of a typical artificial hip has a value of approximately 0.025 µm, that is, the metal femoral head is much smoother. Topographic features on the joint surfaces are commonly described as follows: (1) primary anatomic contours; (2) secondary roughness less than 0.5 mm in diameter and less than 50 µm deep; (3) tertiary hollows on the order of 20 to 45 µm deep; and, (4) quaternary ridges 1 to 4 µm in diameter and 0.1 to 0.3 µm deep.

Scanning electron micrographs of arthritic cartilage usually depict a large degree of surface irregularity. Normal articular surface texture is shown in Figure 52, A, which depicts a tightly woven texture with fine pores. Degenerative tissues often exhibit tears (Fig. 52, B) and peeling (Fig. 52, C) on their surfaces. These surface irregularities have profound effects on the lubrication mechanism involved, and thus greatly affect the friction and the rate of degradation of the articular cartilage.

On the macroscopic level, the types of surface interactions occurring between different joints in the body vary greatly. For example, the hip joint is a deep congruent ball and socket joint; this differs greatly from the femoral condyles of the knee joint, which are bicondylar in nature, or from the saddle shape of the carpometacarpal joint of the thumb. Furthermore, these anatomic forms can vary with age and disease. The degree of matching between the various bones and articulating cartilage surfaces composing a joint is a major factor affecting the distribution of stresses in the cartilage and subchondral bone.

Motion and Forces on Diarthrodial Joints

In vivo experimental measurements on the relative motions between articulating surfaces of a joint, which correspond to daily activities, are limited. Most quantitative information is obtained from gait studies that do not provide the detailed information required for lubrication studies. However, simple calculations show that translational speeds between 2 articulating surfaces can range from approximately 0.06 m/s between the femoral head surface and the acetabulum surface during normal walking, to approximately 0.6 m/s between the humeral head surface and the glenoid surface of the shoulder when a baseball pitcher throws a fastball.

The loads transmitted across a joint may be carried by the opposing joint surfaces by means of cartilage to cartilage contact, through a fluid-film layer, or a mixture of both. As in joint motion, the load on the joint surface is dependent on the type of activity, that is, the loading sites change drastically as the articulating surfaces move relative to each other. During a normal walking cycle, the human hip, knee, and ankle joints can be subjected to loads on the order of 6 times body weight, with these peak loads occurring just

after heel-strike and just before toe-off. The average load on the joint is approximately 3 to 5 times body weight, which lasts as long as 60% of the walking cycle. During the swing phase of walking, only light loads are carried. During this phase, the articular surfaces move rapidly over each other. In addition, extremely high forces occur across the joints in the leg during jumping.

Friction

Basic Concepts

Friction is defined as the resistance to sliding motion between 2 bodies in contact. The first type of friction, called surface friction, comes either from adhesion of one surface to another caused by roughness on the 2 surfaces or from the viscosity of the sheared lubricant film between the 2 surfaces. In the case of "dry friction," that is, surface friction without a lubricant, the following laws have been defined by Amonton (1699) and Coulomb (1785): (1) frictional force F is directly proportional to the applied load W; (2) F is independent of the apparent area of contact; and (3) the kinetic F is independent of the sliding speed V. These laws help to define a coefficient of friction μ_f by the simple well-known equation $F = \mu_f W$.

The second type of friction, called bulk friction, occurs from the mechanisms for dissipation of internal energy within the material (viscoelasticity) or within the lubricant (viscosity). For cartilage, an internal friction is produced by the frictional drag caused when interstitial fluid flows through the porous-permeable solid matrix. Ploughing friction is a specific form of internal friction and may occur, for example, in diarthrodial joints when a load moves across a joint surface causing interstitial fluid flow. Experimentally, it is very difficult to distinguish the contributions of plough-

Table 4	
Typical Values of Mean Surface Roughness (R_a) for Various Surfaces	
Components	**R_a (µm)**
Plain bearings	
Bearing (bush or pad)	0.25 to 1.2
Journal or runner	0.12 to 0.5
Rolling bearings	
Tracks	0.2 to 0.3
Rolling element	0.05 to 0.12
Gears	0.25 to 1.0
Articular cartilage	1.0 to 6.0
Endoprostheses	
Metal (eg, femoral head)	0.025
Plastic (eg, acetabulum)	0.25 to 2.5

ing versus surface friction; however, recent theoretical calculations suggest that ploughing friction is negligible in articular cartilage.

Measurements of Coefficients of Friction

For friction between articular surfaces, μ_f has remarkably low values in comparison to other engineering materials (Tables 5 and 6). This friction coefficient μ_f for articular surfaces of joints has been measured in 2 ways. First, specially designed "arthrotripsometers" or pendulum devices have been used on intact joints. The second method involves sliding excised pieces of cartilage over another surface. The pendulum type experimental configuration uses a diarthrodial joint, usually the hip, as the fulcrum of a simple pendulum where one of the joint surfaces rocks freely over the other (Fig. 53, A). When the pendulum is set into motion, the frictional dissipation between the sliding surfaces and the dissipation within the bearing materials would eventually bring the motion to a stop (Fig. 53, B). The parameter α denotes the damping coefficient. This method provides a way to calculate the coefficient of friction. From these studies, the coefficient of friction of diarthrodial joints has been calculated to range from 0.003 to 0.06.

The second type of experimental configuration involves the sliding of small pieces of cartilage over another surface (Fig. 53, C). The advantage of this technique is that it offers greater control over the geometry of the test configuration, which may help in the interpretation of results. The coefficient of friction μ_f from this experiment may also be as low as 0.003 (Fig. 54). This interfacial friction has the following characteristics: (1) μ_f increased with time after application of the load; (2) μ_f increased with magnitude of the load; (3) μ_f was lower when synovial fluid instead of buffer saline was used as the lubricant; and (4) μ_f was very sensitive to small vertical oscillations of the annular plug of cartilage and actually decreased in magnitude under such motions. This last observation may be a result of the pressurization of interstitial fluid caused by the applied dynamic compressive load (see discussion below).

Table 5
Coefficients of Friction for Typical Materials

Material Combination	Coefficient of Friction
Gold on gold	2.8
Aluminum on aluminum	1.9
Silver on silver	1.5
Steel on steel	0.6–0.8
Brass on steel	0.35
Glass on glass	0.9
Wood on wood	0.25–0.5
Nylon on nylon	0.2
Graphite on steel	0.1
Ice on ice at 0°C	0.1

Table 6
Coefficients of Friction for Articular Cartilage in Synovial Joints

Joint Tested	Coefficient of Friction
Human knee	0.005–0.02
Porcine shoulder	0.020–0.35
Canine ankle	0.005–0.01
Human hip	0.010–0.04
Bovine shoulder	0.002–0.03

Role of Synovial Fluid

Many experiments have been performed in an attempt to assess the role of synovial fluid or its components in joint lubrication. This role has been difficult to quantify because it differs under varying circumstances and with different material properties of cartilage and synovial fluid. In general, synovial fluid affects joint lubrication in the following manner: (1) some of its constituents that adsorb to the cartilage surface may act as boundary lubricants (see below); (2) it reduces the cartilage-cartilage interface frictional

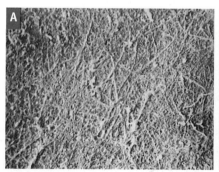
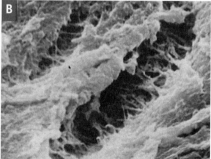
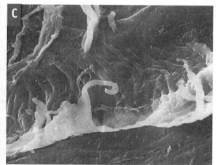

Figure 52

Normal articular surface texture depicting a tightly woven texture with fine pores (**A**). Degenerative tissue exhibiting tears (**B**) and peeling (**C**) on their surfaces.

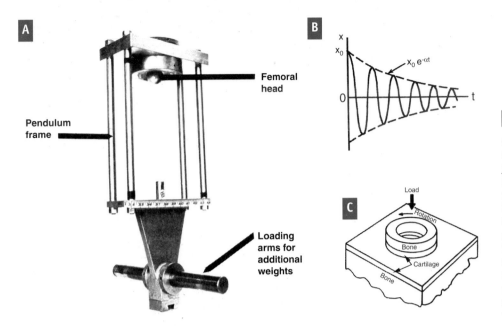

Figure 53

A, The pendulum type experimental configuration in which one of the joint surfaces (femoral head) rocks freely over the other (acetabulum, not shown). **B,** When the pendulum is set into motion, the frictional dissipation eventually brings the motion to a stop. The coefficient of friction may be calculated from the damping coefficient α. **C,** An experimental configuration in which small pieces of cartilage slide over another surface. This configuration is effective in preventing ploughing friction.

coefficient significantly at light loads (Fig. 54); (3) it reduces the cartilage-glass interface frictional coefficient from 0.02, when using buffered saline, to 0.01; (4) it reduces the cartilage-synovium friction from 0.4 to 0.2; and (5) at high loads, no additional benefit is seen with synovial fluid.

In summary, very low friction appears to exist within diarthrodial joints even after wiping away the synovial fluid. Dynamically applied loads, as is almost always the case physiologically, and oscillations or sliding tend to lower the coefficient of friction, and static loads act to increase frictional resistance.

Wear

Wear of bearings is a progressive loss of bearing substance from the material as a result of chemical or mechanical action. Chemical wear is usually a result of corrosion (see Chapter 6). The conventional types of mechanical wear are fatigue wear and interfacial wear. Fatigue wear is independent of the lubrication phenomena occurring at the surfaces of the bearing. It occurs because of the cyclic stresses and strains generated within the cartilage as a result of the application of repetitive loads caused by joint motion. A typical human joint has been estimated to experience 1 million cycles of loading in a year. These large cyclical stresses and strains may cause fatigue failure within the bulk material and may grow by an accumulation of microscopic damage within the material (Fig. 52, *A* and *C*). These internal failures within diseased tissues have been observed in the forms of collagen fiber buckling and loosening of the normally tight collagen network. Eventually, the internal failures can extend to the material surface, causing cracks and fissures. If the rate of damage exceeds that by which the cartilage cells may regenerate the tissue, an accumulation of fatigue microdamage will occur, which

may lead to bulk tissue failure. Thus, in vivo wear is a balance of mechanical attrition and biologic synthesis.

Interfacial wear occurs as a result of solid-solid contact at the surface of bearing materials. There are 2 basic types of interfacial wear. Adhesive wear, the most common, occurs when a junction is formed between the 2 opposing surfaces as they come into contact. If this junction is stronger than the cohesive strength of the individual bearing material surface, fragments of the weaker material may be torn off and adhere to the stronger material. Abrasive wear occurs when a soft material comes into contact with a significantly harder material. Under these circumstances, the

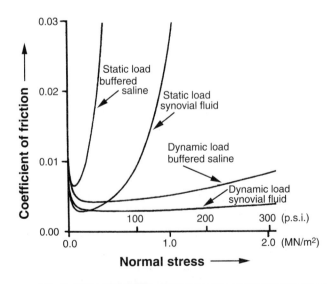

Figure 54

The coefficient of friction μ_f determined from sliding small pieces of cartilage over another surface under various lubrication and loading conditions.

microasperities of the harder material surface may cut into the softer counterpart, causing abrasive wear. This harder material may be either the opposing bearing surface or loose particles between the bearing surfaces. When loose particles between the surfaces cause abrasive wear, the process is termed 3-body wear. This type of wear occurs frequently in orthopaedics, for example, when PMMA cement particles are trapped in the joint space between an endoprosthesis and cartilage.

Wear is measured either as the mass of material removed from interacting surfaces per unit time, or as the volume lost. At present, wear measurement is mostly an empiric science. Therefore, it is difficult to predict either wear rates or their dependency on other physical parameters. Little or no quantitative information exists on wear mechanisms or wear rates for biologic materials. For hydrated tissues such as cartilage, it is very difficult to quantify either loss of mass or of volume as a result of the phenomenon of swelling. The only available data on cartilage wear were obtained from rubbing cartilage against stainless steel plates. Figure 55 shows the measured wear and wear rates for cartilage using collagen and hexosamine as markers at 2 compression levels.

In general, different types of wear produce different wear rates. Fatigue wear depends on the frequency and magnitude of the applied loads and on the intrinsic material properties of the bulk material. Interfacial wear depends on the roughness of the bearing surfaces, the true size of the contact area of the 2 surfaces, and the magnitude of the applied load. Some general rules on wear are: (1) wear rates increase with increasing applied normal load; (2) wear rates increase with increasing sliding contact area between the 2 opposing bearing surfaces; and, (3) the wear rate of the softer bearing surface is higher than that of the harder bearing surface.

The function of typical engineering bearings often is impaired if even a relatively small amount of the bearing volume is lost. Minute changes of bearing surface geometry can greatly affect the hydrodynamics of the thin lubricant film, usually no more than 25 µm thick, in the worn bearing. Despite its topographic roughness, an extremely low wear rate is seen for articular cartilage.

Repetitive joint motion and loading could cause cartilage fatigue damage and wear. Usually, normal chondrocyte activity and turnover are sufficient to maintain tissue homeostasis. Cartilage damage may be accelerated by blunt impact loading. As normal cartilage is compressed, redistribution of fluid within the tissue occurs, causing stress relaxation. Because fluid redistribution in the tissue is not possible during high speed impact loading, high pressures are built up within the tissue and high tensile stresses are built up near the articular surface.

Experiments have shown that a single impact on the patellofemoral joint can cause cartilage damage at the surface and shear fracture at the tidemark. Early accelerated biologic remodeling of patellar cartilage after impact in the region of the tidemark also has been observed. This impact-induced mechanical damage, followed by biologic remodeling, causes tidemark advancement and thinning of cartilage. The number of tidemarks has been found to increase with age. In general, cartilage thins dramatically during aging. Thus, these studies indicate that in vivo wear of articular cartilage is fundamentally different from wear of machine bearings. Biologic wear is caused by an imbalance of biologic turnover and mechanical attrition. (See Chapter 17 for a more detailed discussion on cartilage pathology.)

Diarthrodial Joint Lubrication

Many theories of lubrication have been proposed to explain the minimal friction and wear characteristics of cartilage found in diarthrodial joints. Basically, these various theories fall under the 2 fundamental modes of fluid film lubrication and boundary lubrication. Both modes of lubrication are believed to account for friction and wear of these joints under specific loading and motion conditions. Because today's technology is not able to detect the presence or absence of a fluid film between contacting articular surfaces, researchers have had to rely on theoretical models and predictions to help elucidate the lubrication mechanism of diarthrodial joints. For fluid film lubrication to exist, the minimum synovial fluid film thickness predicted from any of the various proposed theories must exceed the known average surface roughness of cartilage. If the predicted fluid film gap is too thin to produce fluid film lubrication at given loading and motion conditions, then boundary lubrication must be present. When both modes coexist, that is, when a synovial fluid film is still present

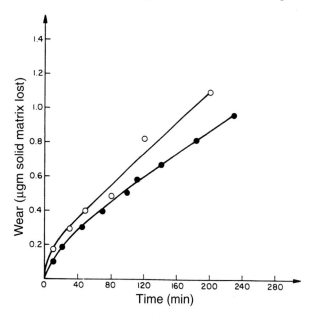

Figure 55

The measured wear and wear rates for cartilage at 2 compression levels: open circle, 4.62 MPa; closed circle, 1.66 MPa.

between the cartilage surfaces but surface asperities come into contact, this condition is known as mixed lubrication. Therefore, the fundamental questions are: Under what conditions is the synovial fluid film maintained? What substance provides the boundary lubrication in diarthrodial joints?

Fluid-Film Lubrication

Hydrodynamic Lubrication

To address the question of what conditions are required to maintain a fluid film in joints, many models have been suggested (Fig. 56). Hydrodynamic lubrication occurs when the speed of sliding and the viscosity of the lubricating fluid are sufficient to create a thin fluid film capable of supporting the applied load (Fig. 56, A). Because the bearing surfaces do not come into contact, there is virtually no wear under these conditions; hydrodynamic lubrication is known to occur in engineering bearings (for example, ball-bearings) under sufficiently high speeds and low loads. The essential assumptions of this model are: (1) the bearing surfaces are rigid and nonporous; (2) the surfaces form a wedge-shaped gap; (3) the lubricant viscosity is constant (newtonian); (4) the relative sliding speed is high; and (5) loads are light. In general, obviously, higher speeds and viscosities promote greater load-carrying capacities. This model is not a very good approximation of diarthrodial joints except, possibly, as might prevail during high-speed, nonaccelerating, rotatory motion of the femur during the swing phase of gait. However, if acceleration occurs, high compressive joint-reaction forces must exist. If the joint-reaction force exceeds the capacity of the lubricant film to support the load, the fluid film gap will close and boundary lubrication will occur.

Elastohydrodynamic Lubrication

The hydrodynamic lubrication model assumptions for cartilage are really far from reality. Improvement may be gained by considering the "elastic" deformation of the cartilage. In this model, cartilage surface deformation acts to: (1) spread the joint load over a larger surface area; (2) decrease the shear rate between the 2 surfaces; and, (3) by virtue of item (2) and the nonnewtonian behavior of synovial fluid, increase the synovial fluid viscosity. All these effects produce gains in the capacity of the fluid film to carry load as well as decreasing stresses within the cartilage. In engineering terminology, this lubrication mode, where both the viscous resistance of the lubricant and the elastic deformation of the bearing surfaces play a prominent role, is called elastohydrodynamic lubrication. For the hip and knee joints, film thickness has been estimated by this mechanism to range up to 1.0 µm under normal loads. This value is too small in comparison to cartilage surface roughness to support this mode of lubrication under all conditions of joint loading, although some researchers have

suggested that the surface roughness may decrease substantially under the high pressures prevailing in the fluid film (microelastohydrodynamic lubrication), which may make this mode of lubrication viable.

Squeeze-Film Lubrication

In squeeze-film lubrication, 2 bearing surfaces simply approach each other without relative sliding motion (Fig. 56, B). Because a viscous lubricant cannot instantaneously be squeezed out from the gap between 2 surfaces that are approaching each other, a pressure is built up as a result of the viscous resistance offered by the lubricant as it is being squeezed from the gap. The pressure field in the fluid film formed in this manner is capable of temporarily supporting large loads. Because the bearing surfaces are deformable layers of articular cartilage, the large pressure generated can cause localized depressions where the lubricant film can be trapped. Typically, with rigid bearings, a 20-µm thick film of fluid can resist several MPa of pressure for up to 1 or 2 seconds before the film becomes depleted. The nonnewtonian behavior of synovial fluid prolongs the squeeze-film time. Because of the intermittent motion of lower extremity diarthrodial joints, squeeze-film lubrication may operate in combination with hydrodynamic or elastohydrodynamic lubrication, for example, elastohydrodynamic lubrication during the swing phase of gait followed by squeeze-film action during heel strike. However, for periods of stationary loading of lower or upper extremity joints that exceed a few seconds, theoretical predictions suggest that

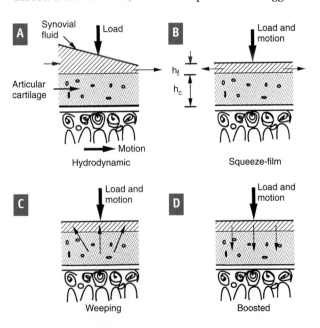

Figure 56

Models of fluid film lubrication: Hydrodynamic (**A**), squeeze-film (**B**), weeping (**C**), and boosted (**D**). (Reproduced with permission from Mow VC, Soslowsky LJ: Friction, lubrication and wear of diarthrodial joints, in Mow VC, Hayes WC (eds): *Basic Orthopaedic Biomechanics.* New York, Raven Press, 1991, pp 245–292.)

the fluid film gets depleted from the loaded regions between the articular surfaces.

For many years, researchers have debated whether the porous-hydrated nature of articular cartilage could promote better conditions for fluid film lubrication, for example, by exchanging water with the fluid film. Recent squeeze-film lubrication calculations, using the biphasic model for cartilage that accounts for the presence of its interstitial fluid (Fig. 57), suggest that the porous nature of cartilage does not provide a particular benefit to fluid-film lubrication, although other benefits may derive as described in the following sections.

Weeping Lubrication

In many engineering applications, hydrostatic lubrication is developed by providing an externally pressurized source of fluid to supply the lubricant film. Exotic applications such as large astronomic telescopes are floated on precisely ground smooth plates separated by a thin film of pressurized gas, and ordinary hydraulic lifts in many auto garages work on this principle. If the fluid in articular cartilage somehow could be imagined to flow out of the tissue, then a similar mechanism might occur in diarthrodial joints. In this proposed model, the fluid in cartilage is assumed to be "self-pressurized" and "wept" uniformly from the tissue into the joint space, serving as the lubricant in joints (Fig. 56, C). According to this weeping lubrication theory, lubricant fluid film between the 2 articulating surfaces is generated by the compression of articular cartilage during joint function.

Boosted Lubrication

Another model of lubrication for diarthrodial joints is known as boosted lubrication. In this model, as the articulating surfaces approach each other under squeeze-film action, the solvent component of synovial fluid, that is, water, passes into the articular cartilage over the entire load-support region during squeeze-film conditions, leaving behind a concentrated pool of hyaluronic acid-protein complex to lubricate the surfaces (Fig. 56, D). During squeeze-film lubrication, as the size of the gap between articulating surfaces decreases, the resistance of sideways efflux of the lubricant will eventually become greater than the resistance of flow into the articular cartilage (Fig. 56, B). Because the pores in normal articular cartilage (20 to 70 Å) are much smaller than the hyaluronate molecules (solution diameter range: $[1$ to $4] \times 10^3$ Å), the molecules cannot penetrate the cartilage surface and, thus, are left behind in the joint gap. In this manner the articulating surfaces act as filtration membranes through which only water and low molecular weight electrolytes and nutrients are capable of passing into cartilage. During this process, the hyaluronate concentration increases in the joint space, and synovial fluid viscosity is correspondingly increased; hence, the load-carrying capacity of this fluid is boosted.

Boundary Lubrication

Boundary lubrication occurs when the fluid film has been depleted and the contacting bearing surfaces are separated only by a boundary lubricant of molecular thickness, which prevents excessive bearing friction and wear. In articular cartilage, it has been proposed by some researchers that a monolayer of glycoprotein is adsorbed on each of the opposing articular surfaces. This hydrophobic monolayer functions like the pile of a carpet to provide a cushioning layer and protect the articular surface from abrasion (Fig. 58). Its thickness ranges from 10 to 1,000 Å, and it has the ability to carry weight and reduce friction. The glycoprotein that makes up this monolayer is called lubricin, and its molecular weight is approximately 2.5×10^2 kd. It is a single polypeptide chain with many oligosaccharides distributed along its length. Other researchers have suggested that the boundary lubricant is dipalmitoyl-phosphatidyl-choline, a phospholipid. Both of these boundary lubricants have been extracted from synovial fluid and have been shown to moderately decrease the friction coefficient when tested on various materials, including cartilage. However, there is some evidence that they are not as effective at high loads. In the joint under heavy loading, some combination of fluid-film lubrication and boundary lubrication may coexist (Fig. 59).

Interstitial Fluid Pressurization Flow and Diarthrodial Joint Lubrication

It is well known that the interstitial water of articular cartilage pressurizes substantially when the tissue is loaded; this phenomenon has been verified both theoretically and experimentally (Fig. 60). In fact, shortly after loading

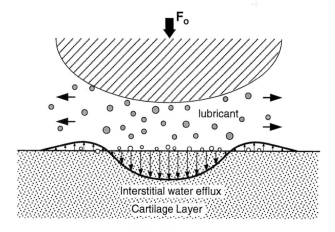

Figure 57

Under squeeze-film action, the lubricant squeezes out laterally away from the high-pressure region; as the gap between the approaching surfaces decreases and the resistance to sideways flow increases, a greater amount of lubricant will permeate into the cartilage layer in the central, high pressure region, while some fluid will exude from the cartilage at the periphery of the loaded region. (Reproduced with permission from Hou JS, Mow VC, Lai WM, Holmes MH: An analysis of the squeeze-film lubrication mechanism for articular cartilage. *J Biomech* 1992;25:247–259.)

(t < 300 s), of the total load acting across the articular surfaces of a joint, it is estimated that 90% to 95% is supported by the pressurized interstitial fluid when the cartilage surfaces are in direct (boundary) contact. This interstitial fluid load support is not unlike the mechanism by which a pressurized fluid film can support 100% of the applied load when fluid film lubrication prevails. Depending on the loading conditions, the interstitial fluid load support may vary with time, or with the magnitude of the applied load and sliding velocity of the articular surfaces. For healthy cartilage, however, even a stationary load may produce interstitial fluid load support in excess of 80% for 15 minutes or longer, and this pressurization will increase as soon as the cartilage surfaces begin to slide again. The reason that the fluid pressurization is so significant and lasts for so long is that the permeability of healthy cartilage is extremely low, which causes the fluid to flow very slowly away from the loaded region; this impediment to fluid flow contributes to the pressurization and delays its subsidence. This mechanism is also aided by the relatively low stiffness of cartilage, which causes the articular layers to deform significantly and conform together closely under normal loading; this conformity means that the size of the contact region is typically much greater than the thickness of the cartilage, forcing the fluid to flow a relatively long pathway to escape to the low-pressure regions outside of the contact area.

Some researchers have suggested that this interstitial fluid pressurization may contribute significantly to the reduction of the friction and wear between contacting articular surfaces when the fluid film has been depleted and boundary contact is taking place. Because the interstitial fluid may be supporting up to 95% of the total applied load, only the remaining 5% will be supported by the contacting collagen-proteoglycan matrix of the opposing surfaces. Thus, the friction coefficient of cartilage may be up to 20 times smaller (100% ÷ 5%) than if all the load were supported by the collagen-proteoglycan matrix, as would occur when the interstitial fluid pressure has completely subsided. Because

this mechanism is dependent on the amount of pressurization, it can explain the experimentally observed dependence of the cartilage friction coefficient on the duration of loading (Fig. 61); furthermore, because solid matrix-to-matrix loading is still present under this mechanism, the presence of a boundary lubricant adsorbed to the cartilage surface may further reduce the friction and wear in the joint. For example, if the friction coefficient of solid matrix-on-matrix is measured at 0.15 in the absence of interstitial fluid pressurization, the actual friction coefficient between the articular surfaces under physiologic loading, that is, in the presence of interstitial fluid pressurization, can be as low as 0.15 ÷ 20 = 0.007. If a boundary lubricant is present, this value may be reduced even further, for example, down to the lowest values listed in Table 6.

Summary of Joint Lubrication

There are 2 fundamental types of lubrication, fluid-film and boundary. Fluid-film lubrication can operate in many forms, such as hydrodynamic, elastohydrodynamic, or squeeze-film lubrication. The lubricant for fluid-film lubrication is synovial fluid. The nonnewtonian properties of synovial fluid, specifically its shear thinning effect, act to increase the load-carrying capacity, the area over which a load is spread, and the duration of the squeeze-film time. However, fluid-film lubrication cannot be sustained under all loading conditions of diarthrodial joints, particularly under high loads or when loading durations exceed a few seconds. Boundary lubrication involves a monolayer of lubricant molecules, which is adsorbed on each bearing surface. It is active when the surface roughnesses of the opposing articular surfaces come into contact, or when the fluid film is depleted under severe loading conditions. Pressurization of the cartilage interstitial fluid provides an interesting mode of mixed lubrication whereby the interstitial fluid supports most of the applied load (but not all of it, as would occur in fluid-film lubrication), while boundary lubrication occurs between the contacting collagen-pro-

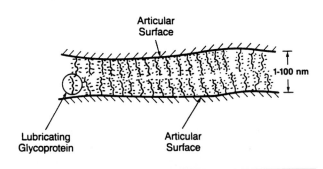

Figure 58

Boundary layer lubrication. A monolayer of glycoprotein provides a cushioning layer, protecting the articular surface from abrasion. (Reproduced with permission from Mow VC, Soslowsky LJ: Friction, lubrication and wear of diarthrodial joints, in Mow VC, Hayes WC (eds): *Basic Orthopaedic Biomechanics*. New York, Raven Press, 1991, pp 245–292.)

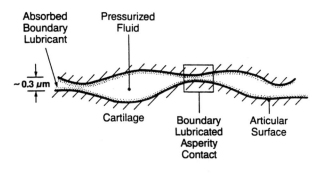

Figure 59

A combination of fluid-film lubrication and boundary lubrication. (Reproduced with permission from Mow VC, Soslowsky LJ: Friction, lubrication and wear of diarthrodial joints, in Mow VC, Hayes WC (eds): *Basic Orthopaedic Biomechanics*. New York, Raven Press, 1991, pp 245–292.)

teoglycan matrices that support the remainder of the load. This mixed lubrication mode can explain the low friction and wear of diarthrodial joints, as well as the observed dependence of the friction coefficient on the duration and magnitude of loading, as well as sliding velocity. The details of which specific lubrication mode predominates may depend on the specific joint in question and the particular type of loading applied. Under pathologic conditions, the lubrication mechanisms within a joint will be affected as the properties of the synovial fluid and/or the properties of the articular cartilage are altered as a result of degenerative changes.

Clinical Applications

Prosthetic Design Considerations: Shoulder

In this section, a clinical problem is discussed, using some of the basic biomechanics concepts presented. The design of a shoulder prosthesis must take into account a variety of factors peculiar to that joint. The glenohumeral joint functions in concert with the acromioclavicular, sternoclavicular, and scapulothoracic articulations during normal shoulder use. Thus, knowledge of shoulder anatomy and cartilage material properties is needed to define shoulder motion and articulation. The ligamentous stabilizers are

complex, and because of the unique anatomy of the coracohumeral and glenohumeral ligaments, stress is distributed among varying regions depending on arm elevation and rotation. The muscles, especially the rotator cuff, not only are important for dynamic stability, but their precise lever arms and lines of action are vital to generating the moments required to rotate the arm. Required knowledge includes the tensile properties of the glenohumeral ligament and lines of action of forces exerted by the shoulder muscle forces. Clearly, from this description, all the biomechanical concepts discussed must be brought to bear to understand shoulder biomechanics.

Constrained total shoulder replacements have had the same difficulties with loosening and mechanical failure as constrained replacements of other joints. The ideas of fatigue and failure stress within the bone and PMMA must be appreciated here. The initial appeal of the concept was the hope that the constrained articulation would provide stability to a joint whose small socket (glenoid) could not enclose the entire ball (humeral head). This articulation also was expected to assure a fulcrum for the deltoid in cases without a functioning rotator cuff. Joint-reaction loads and contact areas within the glenohumeral articulation must be determined by biomechanical investigations.

Figure 62, *A*, shows a 2-D model of a total shoulder replacement, which is assumed to be frictionless; the deltoid force and the rotator cuff force have been drawn. Both forces tend to abduct the humerus and, along with the weight of the arm, can be resolved into a resultant force acting at the center of the glenoid. This resultant force produces a uniform compressive loading pattern on the cement and bone. If the rotator cuff is torn or nonfunctional, the unopposed deltoid force will tend to act superiorly

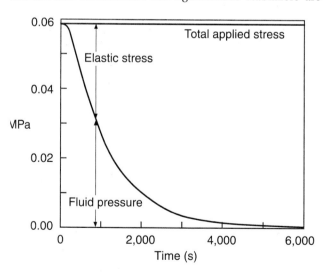

Figure 60

When a constant load is applied across the articular layers of a joint, the total applied stress at the articular surface consists of the elastic stress due to the deformation of the solid collagen-proteoglycan matrix, and the interstitial fluid pressure. The fluid pressure can support up to 100% of the total applied stress in the initial stages of loading, depending on the loading configuration, but will eventually subside to zero after 1 to 2 hours. (Adapted with permission from Wang LH, Soltz MA, Ateshian GA: Interstitial fluid pressurization regulates the frictional response of cartilage. *Trans Orthop Res Soc* 1997;22:83.)

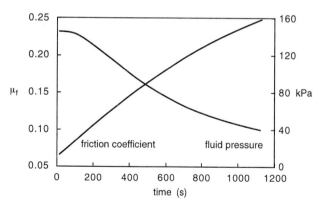

Figure 61

Experimental measurements and theoretical analyses confirm that the friction coefficient of cartilage achieves its lowest value when the cartilage interstitial fluid pressure is at its peak. As the fluid pressure subsides, the friction coefficient increases. Under physiologic loading conditions where the duration of sustained static loading rarely exceeds 1 minute, the interstitial fluid pressurization remains high, keeping the friction coefficient low. (Data taken from Soltz MA, Ateshian GA: Experimental verification of cartilage fluid pressurization in confined compression creep and stress relaxation. *Trans Orthop Res Soc* 1998;23:224.)

and eccentrically load the humerus, thus producing a tendency to subluxate the humeral component (Fig. 62, *B*). A rocking action would then be generated, causing the glenoid component to rotate against the restraining cement in the bone. This action has been clinically associated with glenoid component loosening.

Figure 63 shows the contact stresses on the surface of the humeral component. With the prosthetic surfaces assumed to be frictionless, only normal contact stresses may be developed. If the rotator cuff muscle force is present, the resultant force on the glenoid component may be centered to give a uniform contact stress pattern (Fig. 63, *A*). If the rotator cuff muscles are weak, a greater stress will be exerted on the "overhang" of the glenoid component (Fig. 63, *B*) used in some prostheses to "substitute" for the head-depressing effect of the rotator cuff. However, as shown in the figure, these forces have the same tendency to rock the glenoid as noted before. The risk of loosening rises as more constraint is added, because the moment arm will be increased.

It is often stated that the normal shoulder has a relatively flat glenoid articulating with a more curved humeral head, and, thus, that even a glenoid component of normal size adds constraint if it is manufactured to the same radius of curvature as the humeral component. However, recent precise quantitative assessments of glenohumeral articular geometry have shown that the normal humeral head and glenoid surfaces are conforming spheres within less than a millimeter difference. Impressions of glenoid shallowness probably resulted from its flatter appearance on radiographs that show only the subchondral bone, because cartilage thickness is greatest peripherally on the glenoid. Thus, the need to obtain precise anatomic information in prosthesis design is obvious.

Early experience with total shoulder replacement revealed an occasional fracture of a glenoid component at the junction of the fin and the socket. This fracture may have been caused in part by the stress concentration effect of a notch at that junction, which was eliminated on subsequent designs. Also, however, early techniques often built up areas of uneven glenoid wear with cement (Fig. 64). Given the different Young's moduli of bone and cement, a uniformly distributed load on the glenoid would nevertheless

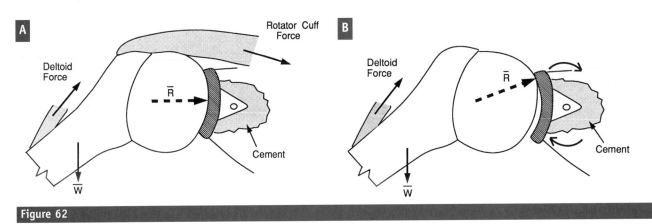

Figure 62

Model of a total shoulder replacement. **A,** With a functional rotator cuff, the resultant force is centered toward the glenoid, resulting in a uniform compression of the cement and bone. **B,** With a nonfunctional rotator cuff, the deltoid will eccentrically load the glenoid, causing it to rotate against the restraining cement in the bone.

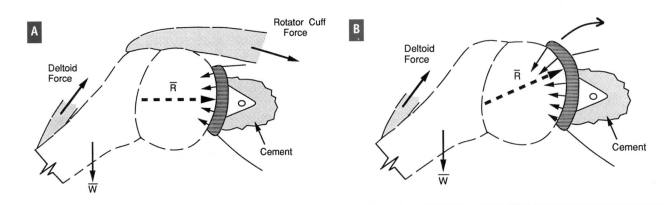

Figure 63

The contact stresses on the surface of the humeral component. **A,** The rotator cuff resists the superiorly directed force exerted by the deltoid. **B,** If the rotator cuff muscles are weak, stress will be exerted on the overhang of the glenoid component, which will tend to rock the glenoid.

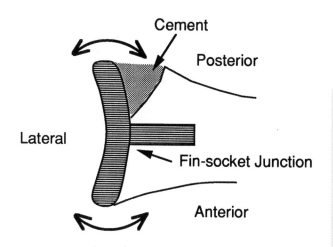

Figure 64

Area of glenoid wear built up with cement. The differences in the Young's moduli of bone and cement result in a different amount of displacement between the 2 sides, thus toggling and fatiguing the fin-socket junction.

result in a different displacement on the side of the cement buildup, thus toggling around and fatiguing the fin-socket junction. Therefore, the surgical technique was altered, either lowering the "high" side, bone grafting the "low" side, or altering the component version (or a combination) so that the glenoid component rests on bone evenly.

Metal backing of the glenoid component has been suggested to improve the evenness of stress transfer to bone according to finite element analysis, but clinical evidence of this is not yet available. Modular heads have been introduced to allow precise tensioning of the soft tissues and adjusting of muscle moment arms. Clearly, an understanding of the biomechanical principles presented in this chapter facilitates understanding of these considerations.

Conclusion

Although all material objects are subject to the laws of mechanics, the precise relation between form and function, so dear to the orthopaedist, may be, in practice, difficult to work out. This difficulty is caused by not only the technical and mathematic complexities involved, but also the variation in the anatomy and constitution of living tissues. Furthermore, living systems change rapidly, so that, for example, a bone undergoing stress remodeling may be difficult to subject to precise stress analysis.

Nevertheless, this chapter should enable the reader to: (1) work out forces and moments to estimate loads in clinical situations; (2) understand the assumptions that underlie biomechanical modeling; (3) understand the principles of deformation mechanics, especially the distinction between loading conditions and the states of stress and strain within the material; (4) understand the difference between a structural response and a material property; (5) be comfortable with kinematic analysis; and (6) have a general grasp of the frictional and wear properties of diarthrodial joints.

Selected Bibliography

Elementary Engineering Textbooks

Hibbeler RC: Engineering Mechanics: *Combined Statics and Dynamics*, ed 8. Upper Saddle River, NJ, Prentice Hall, 1998.

Lai WM, Rubin D, Krempl E: *Introduction to Continuum Mechanics.* Oxford, England, Pergamon Press, 1993.

Munson BR, Young DF, Okiishi T: *Fundamentals of Fluid Mechanics*, ed 3. New York, NY, John Wiley, 1997.

Riley WF, Sturges L, Morris D: *Mechanics of Materials*, ed 5. New York, NY, John Wiley, 1996.

Advanced Engineering Textbooks

Hertzberg RW (ed): *Deformation and Fracture Mechanics of Engineering Materials*, ed 3. New York, NY, John Wiley & Sons, 1989.

Johnson KL (ed): *Contact Mechanics.* Cambridge, England, Cambridge University Press, 1985.

Moore DF (ed): *Principles and Applications of Tribology.* Oxford, England, Pergamon Press, 1975.

Timoshenko SP, Goodier JN (eds): *Theory of Elasticity*, ed 3. New York, NY, McGraw Hill, 1969.

Yih CS: Fluid Mechanics: *A Concise Introduction to the Theory.* New York, NY, McGraw Hill, 1969.

General Biomechanics

Fung YC (ed): Biomechanics: *Mechanical Properties of Living Tissues.* New York, NY, Springer-Verlag, 1981.

Fung YC (ed): *Biomechanics: Motion, Flow, Stress, and Growth.* New York, NY, Springer-Verlag, 1990.

Skalak R, Chien S (eds): *Handbook of Bioengineering.* New York, NY, McGraw Hill, 1987.

Orthopaedic Biomechanics

Mow VC, Hayes WC (eds): *Basic Orthopaedic Biomechanics*, ed 2. New York Philadelphia, PA, Lippincott-Raven Press, 19971.

Mow VC, Ratcliffe A, Woo SL-Y (eds): *Biomechanics of Diarthrodial Joints.* New York, NY, Springer-Verlag, 1990.

Ozkaya N, Nordin M (eds): *Fundamentals of Biomechanics: Equilibrium, Motion, and Deformation.* New York, NY, Van Nostrand Reinhold, 1991.

Woo SL-Y, Buckwalter JA (eds): *Injury and Repair of the Musculoskeletal Soft Tissues.* Park Ridge, IL, American Academy of Orthopaedic Surgeons, 1988.

Articular Cartilage and Extracellular Matrices

Ateshian GA, Wang H, Lai WM: The role of interstitial fluid pressurization and surface porosities on the boundary friction of articular cartilage. *J Tribology* 1998;120:241–248.

Brandt KD (ed): *Cartilage Changes in Osteoarthritis.* Indianapolis, IN, University of Indiana Press, 1990.

Brandt KD, Doherty M, Lohmander LS (eds): *Osteoarthritis.* Oxford, England, Oxford University Press, 1998.

Comper WD (ed): *Extracellular Matrix, vol 1: Tissue Function,* and *vol 2: Molecular Components and Interactions.* Amsterdam, Netherlands, Harwood Academic Publishers, 1996.

Maroudas A, Kuettner K (eds): *Methods in Cartilage Research.* London, England, Academic Press, 1990.

Mow VC, Arnoczky SP, Jackson DW (eds): *Knee Meniscus: Basic and Clinical Foundations,* New York, NY, Raven Press, 1992.

Mow VC, Ratcliffe A (eds): *Structure and Function of Articular Cartilage.* Boca Raton, FL, CRC Press, 1993.

Mow VC, Ratcliffe A: Structure and function of articular cartilage and meniscus, in Mow VC, Hayes WC (eds): *Basic Orthopaedic Biomechanics,* ed 2. Philadelphia, PA, Lippincott-Raven, 1997, pp 113–177.

Bone

Cowin SC (ed): *Bone Mechanics.* Boca Raton, FL, CRC Press, 1989.

Ligaments

Daniel DM, Akeson WH, O'Connor JJ (eds): *Knee Ligaments: Structure, Function, Injury, and Repair.* New York, NY, Raven Press, 1990.

Woo SLY, Livesay GA, Runco TJ, Young EP (eds): Structure and function of tendons and ligaments, in Mow VC, Hayes WC (eds): *Basic Orthopaedic Biomechanics,* ed 2. Philadelphia, PA, Lippincott-Raven Press, 1997, pp 209–251.

Chapter 6

Biomaterials

Timothy M. Wright, PhD

Stephen Li, PhD

This chapter at a glance

This chapter discusses how a material's physical properties result from its chemical composition and structure, and fundamentals of mechanical performance in terms of the important material properties that determine the behavior of implant structures.

Introduction

The term biomaterials refers to synthetic and treated natural materials that are used to replace or augment tissue and organ function. Biomaterials must meet several criteria to perform successfully. They must be biocompatible, or able to function in vivo without eliciting an intolerable response in the body either locally or systemically; resistant to corrosion and degradation, meaning that the body environment must not adversely affect material performance; and possess adequate mechanical properties, an especially important criterion for those biomaterials used in devices intended to replace or reinforce load-bearing skeletal structures. In addition, orthopaedic biomaterials intended for total joint replacement must possess adequate wear resistance to maintain proper joint function and to minimize biocompatibility problems caused by biologic reactions to particulate debris. They must be capable of reproducible fabrication to the highest standards of quality control and, of course, at a reasonable cost.

Biomaterials that meet these criteria are fundamental to the practice of orthopaedic surgery. They have been used successfully to develop devices for internal fixation of fractures, osteotomies and arthrodeses, wound closure, soft-tissue reconstruction, and total joint arthroplasty that have advanced significantly the treatment of musculoskeletal diseases. But at the same time, limitations in biomaterial performance, failure of the implant designer to understand the limitations, or inappropriate application of the technology often are directly related to clinical failure.

Therefore, an understanding of the physical and chemical properties of orthopaedic biomaterials is an important consideration in selecting and using implant devices and in providing a realistic expectation of clinical performance. This chapter will discuss how a material's physical properties result from its chemical composition and structure, and fundamentals of mechanical performance in terms of the important material properties that determine the behavior of implant structures. Common metallic, polymeric, and ceramic orthopaedic biomaterials are described in terms of their molecular structures, microstructures, composition, and properties, and how their properties are influenced by processing and manufacturing variables is discussed as well.

Fundamentals of Mechanical Behavior

The choice of an appropriate device for an orthopaedic application requires the ability to predict the device's mechanical performance. For example, in choosing a femoral component for a total hip replacement, the surgeon must select a device with a functional life of sufficient length to meet the patient's expectations. Predicting a structure's mechanical performance depends on several factors: the forces to which it is subjected; the mechanical burdens that those forces place on the material from which it is fabricated; and the capability of the material to withstand those burdens over the structure's expected lifetime.

Stress Versus Strain
Elastic Behavior

A force acting on an object causes both an external effect (change in velocity) and an internal effect (deformation). The external effects can be considered under Newton's laws of motion to solve biomechanical problems in dynamic and static situations, such as determination of the forces and moments that act on skeletal joints (discussed in Chapter 5). From that discussion, it is clear that to maintain force equilibrium, an applied force that is causing the object to deform must be counteracted by an internal force of equal magnitude and opposite direction that is created within the structure itself. These internal forces arise from the resistance to deformation, no matter how small, that is produced in the material. The material's capability to withstand external forces can be described, therefore, in terms of the distribution of internal forces generated by the material (the stress) and the resulting deformation (the strain).

Consider, for example, a metallic bone plate manufactured from stainless steel and gripped at the ends (Fig. 1, A). An instrument called an extensometer is attached to the plate's surface and measures the change in distance between its 2 attachment points. A tensile load is applied through the grips, pulling at the ends of the plate. The external load is resisted by an internal load acting perpendicular to the cross section of the plate and evenly distributed over the plate's cross-sectional area. The resulting tensile stress within the bone plate has a magnitude equal to the applied load divided by the cross-sectional area. The tensile load causes the bone plate to elongate. The elongation can be described as tensile strain by normalizing the amount of elongation measured by the extensometer by the original distance between the attachment points when no load was applied.

If the applied load is plotted against the amount of elongation, the initial relationship is linear, so that load is proportional to elongation (Fig. 1, B). When the load reaches 500 N, the plate will have elongated 0.75 microns. Knowing the cross-sectional area of the plate (50 mm^2) and the original distance between the attachment points of the extensometer (15 mm), the force and elongation data can be converted to stress and strain, respectively, resulting in a stress versus strain curve. At 500 N, the stress and strain in the plate would be:

$$\text{Stress} = 500 \text{ N}/50 \text{ mm}^2 = 10 \text{ N/mm}^2 = 10 \times 10^6 \text{ N/m}^2 = 10 \text{ MPa}$$

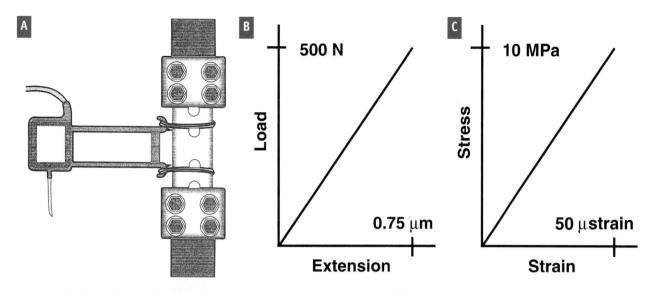

Figure 1

A, An extensometer, used to measure the change in distance between the two attachment points, has been fastened to the central portion of a bone plate prior to a tensile test of the plate. **B,** As tensile load is applied to the plate, the plate elongates. For a load of 500 N, the elongation measured by the extensometer is 0.75 microns. **C,** The load can be used, together with the cross-sectional area of the plate, to calculate the stress (stress = load/area), and the elongation can be used to determine the strain (change in distance divided by the original distance). The result is a stress versus strain curve for the material from which the plate is fabricated. (Reproduced with permission from Burstein AH, Wright TM: *Fundamentals of Orthopaedic Biomechanics.* Baltimore, MD, Williams & Wilkins, 1994.)

Strain = 0.75 microns/15 mm = 0.00075 mm/ 15 mm = 50×10^{-6} = 50 microstrain

Stress is represented in megapascals (pascal [Pa] is the unit of stress in the international system (SI) of units and the prefix mega- [M] represents a million). Strain is dimensionless, but is usually a quite small quantity and so is commonly expressed as microstrain (one-millionth).

The corresponding stress-strain curve, like the load-elongation curve, is a straight line (Fig. 1, *C*). If the 500 N load applied to the plate is removed, the stress and strain will return to zero (that is, the curve retraces itself back to the origin). Repeating the loading process up to 10 MPa reproduces the original curve. A stress versus strain curve that is fully reversible implies that the stainless steel in the plate is behaving elastically, so that after the load is released, there is no change in the plate's shape and no damage to the metal.

The ratio of stress to strain (that is, the slope of the stress versus strain curve) will be the same throughout this region of elastic behavior:

Stress/Strain = 10 MPa/50 microstrain = 10×10^{6} Pa/50×10^{-6} = 200 GPa

where the unit GPa (gigapascal) is equal to one billion (10^{9}) pascals. If many such experiments were conducted on different sizes and shapes of bone plates made from the same metal, the applied loads and the resulting elongations would change, but the relationship between the resulting stresses and strains would stay the same, so the stress-strain ratio would not change.

The ratio of stress to strain is, therefore, a material property of the stainless steel and not of the bone plate. The ratio is termed the modulus of elasticity, E:

E = stress/strain

The modulus of elasticity is constant for each material. Stainless steel, therefore, has an elastic modulus of 200 GPa.

Plastic Behavior

If tensile load is again applied to the bone plate and allowed to continually increase, the stress-strain curve will eventually become nonlinear. Removal of the load will reveal permanent elongation of the plate (permanent or "plastic" deformation of the stainless steel). The material has yielded its ability to behave elastically. As the load continues to increase, the bone plate (the stainless steel) eventually ruptures. The plastic portion of the stress-strain curve can be used to define important failure criteria for the stainless steel material. To impose sufficient stress on the stainless steel to cause it to yield, the material must undergo permanent structural change caused by some form of mechanical damage. In stainless steel, this form of damage occurs at an ultrastructural scale, involving the movements of imperfections through the crystalline structure of the metallic atoms. Although these individual damage mechanisms are invisible, the macroscopic result is the permanent deformation seen in the plate.

For materials like stainless steel that first exhibit elastic and then exhibit plastic behavior, there are 2 failure criteria that can be considered. The first is defined from the transition between elastic behavior and plastic behavior. The second is the point of rupture of the material. Some orthopaedic problems require knowledge of the onset of plastic behavior (the initiation of permanent deformation). For example, the determination of the maximum load that can be imposed on a hip nail-plate before it permanently deforms is important in defining the performance of the device in fracture fixation. Solutions to other problems, such as the joint reaction force needed to fracture a polymethylmethacrylate (PMMA) cement mantle around the femoral component of a total hip replacement, require knowledge of the rupture strength of the material.

These 2 failure criteria are usually described as stresses. The stress corresponding to the transition between elastic and plastic behavior in the stress-strain curve is called the yield stress. The maximum stress prior to rupture of the material is called the ultimate stress. For stainless steel, for example, the ultimate stress is considerably higher than the yield stress, while for cortical bone tissue the ultimate stress is closer in value to the yield stress (Fig. 2). The ultimate strain for stainless steel is several orders of magnitude higher than the yield strain. For bone tissue, the ultimate strain is only 3 or 4 times higher. Such distinctions are important when choosing materials for orthopaedic applications. If overloads producing rupture cannot be tolerated, such as in a fracture fixation application, a material such as stainless steel with a high value of ultimate strain must be chosen. The importance of ultimate strain has led to yet a third material property, ductility, defined as the strain at rupture (ultimate strain) in a material that undergoes plastic deformation.

Ductile Versus Brittle Behavior

Not all materials possess the capability of permanently deforming prior to fracture. For example, PMMA bone cement exhibits an elastic tensile stress-strain curve up to the point of rupture, in contrast to ultra-high molecular weight polyethylene (UHMWPE), which shows nonlinear, ductile stress-strain behavior in tension and compression (Fig. 3). Thus, PMMA does not exhibit plastic behavior and, therefore, has no yield stress. The stress at failure is the ultimate stress. Such materials are called brittle. Rupture of a brittle material produces a fracture pattern that allows reassembly of the broken fragments back into the original shape.

It is important to distinguish between brittle and ductile behavior. Both PMMA and rubber, for example, are brittle materials. Under tensile loading, both fail by brittle fracture, although rubber clearly suffers much greater elastic deformation. Thus, brittle failure is not defined from how high the material's elastic modulus happens to be or from how much deformation the material undergoes before frac-

ture. The same is true for a ductile material. Ductile materials can undergo very small strains prior to rupture. Bone tissue, for example, undergoes about the same strain as PMMA before rupture, although bone tissue is ductile (Fig.2) and PMMA is brittle (Fig. 3).

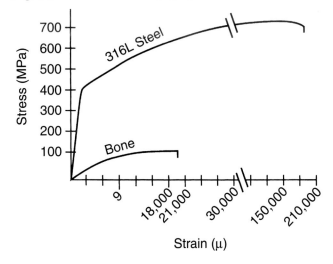

Figure 2

Stress versus strain curves for type 316L stainless steel and for cortical bone tissue show that both are ductile materials, though stainless steel has a much higher elastic modulus, yield stress, ultimate stress, and ductility. (Reproduced with permission from Burstein AH, Wright TM: *Fundamentals of Orthopaedic Biomechanics.* Baltimore, MD, Williams & Wilkins, 1994.)

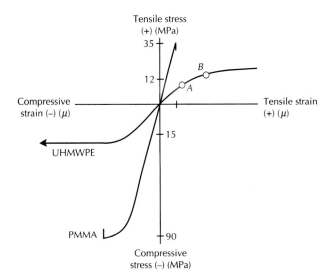

Figure 3

Stress versus strain curves in both tension and compression for ultra high molecular weight polyethylene and polymethylmethacrylate. If polyethylene is loaded to point A on the curve (within the elastic region), removal of the load will result in no permanent strain (i.e., both stress and strain will return to zero upon removal of the load). If, on the other hand, the material is loaded to point B on the curve (beyond the yield stress), removal of the load will result in recovery of elastic strain, but permanent strain will result (shown by the tick mark on the tensile strain axis). (Reproduced with permission from Burstein AH, Wright TM: *Fundamentals of Orthopaedic Biomechanics.* Baltimore, MD, Williams & Wilkins, 1994.)

Another way of contrasting brittle and ductile behavior is to consider toughness, the amount of energy that the material can withstand before rupture. Toughness is proportional to the area under the material's stress-strain curve. The stress reflects the load and the strain reflects the deformation, so the area under the stress-strain curve at any point reflects the amount of work (load moving through a distance) that was applied to the material to cause the deformation. A brittle material can be tough, even though it cannot plastically deform, because it has a high modulus and high strength. A ductile material can absorb large amounts of energy even if it is not very strong, provided it can undergo large amounts of plastic deformation before failing (Fig. 4).

Properties such as ductility, yield stress, and toughness can be significantly altered by mechanical or thermal treatments. One common method used to make stainless steel "stronger" is to cold work the material. The material is squeezed as rectangular plates between rollers or is drawn as cylindrical bars through a series of reduced diameter dies to reduce its cross-sectional size. Both methods are performed at temperatures well below the melting point of the steel (hence, the term "cold work"). The energy put into the material alters its microstructure and builds up permanent damage. The structural changes increase the yield stress and decrease the ductility (Fig. 5). The gains in yield stress can be quite impressive with only minor decreases in ductility, making the process useful for stainless steel in most orthopaedic applications.

Combined Stress States

The tensile test conducted on the bone plate proved instructive to describe the stress-strain behavior and to define important failure criteria for the material. However, orthopaedic devices such as bone plates and skeletal structures such as the femur rarely experience such simple loading regimens. As discussed in the chapter on biomechanics, these structures usually experience combinations of axial, bending, and torsional loads that result in complex distributions of stresses within the materials from which they are made. A bone plate, for example, often experiences a combination of axial compressive load and bending that causes both tensile and compressive stresses in the stainless steel. Similarly, the tibia experiences a large external torque that causes shear stresses in the cortical bone tissue when the leg is externally rotated in a violent fashion (for example, during a skiing accident). Even in the illustrative case of pure tensile loading on the bone plate, combinations of shear and tensile stress occur on every plane through the material other than the transverse plane.

In the more realistic loading situations encountered in the musculoskeletal system, it is often difficult to calculate the types, magnitudes, and distributions of stresses at any location within the material, especially in implant and skeletal

structures with complex shapes. Computer techniques, such as finite element modeling, are often employed to determine the stresses and to predict failure by comparing the predicted stresses to failure criteria for the material. It is important, therefore, to understand the material behavior under more than just tensile loading.

For example, in the case of the tibia resisting applied torque, shear stresses are created in the bone tissue as a means of generating an internal torque to oppose the externally applied torque. To examine the behavior of bone tissue under torsional load, tissue specimens can be tested under torsional load, and the shear stress can be plotted against the shear strain (analogous to plotting tensile stress versus tensile strain for the bone plate example). The resulting curve will exhibit a linear elastic region, the slope of which can be used to determine the shear modulus (analogous to the elastic modulus). Both yield stress and ultimate stress in shear can be determined from the curve and compared to the tensile (and compressive) yield and ultimate stresses. The data from these types of tests show that bone tissue is strongest in compression and relatively weak in tension and shear (Table 1). This data must be considered in predicting bone failure under combined load conditions in which tissue may undergo all 3 types of stress of different magnitudes at different locations throughout the bone.

Isotropic Versus Anisotropic Behavior

The test results described for the stainless steel bone plate are based on loading the plate along a direction corresponding to the long axis of a bone on which the plate might be attached for fracture fixation. If the plate were loaded in tension in another direction (for example, per-

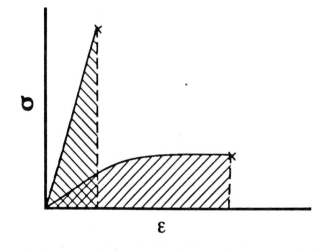

Figure 4

Toughness is the energy absorbed prior to failure, indicated by the area under the stress versus strain curve. These 2 materials are equally tough (the areas under the curve are the same), even though one is stiff and brittle, and the other is flexible and ductile.

pendicular to the longitudinal direction), the stress-strain curve measured for the stainless steel would be identical. Materials such as stainless steel that exhibit the same mechanical properties regardless of the direction of loading are said to be isotropic. Most common orthopaedic biomaterials (metals such as stainless steel and cobalt-chrome and titanium alloys), polymers (PMMA and UHMWPE), and ceramics (alumina and zirconia) are isotropic, so that defining their properties in 1 direction is sufficient to define their properties in all directions.

Many materials, however, possess different mechanical properties in different directions. This is true for materials such as biologic tissues (bone, cartilage, muscle, ligament, and tendon) and composites (fiberglass and carbon fiber-reinforced resins). Such materials are called anisotropic. Cortical bone tissue, for example, will exhibit very different stress-strain behavior if it is loaded in a direction corresponding to the long axis of the bone compared with a transverse direction (Fig. 6). When loaded transversely, the tissue is much weaker in terms of both yield and ultimate strength, is much less ductile, and has a much lower elastic modulus. Anisotropic behavior can often be predicted by considering the material's structure. Bone tissue at an ultra-

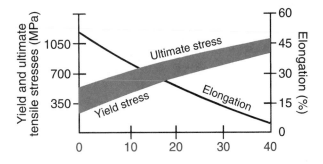

Figure 5

Metallic materials such as 316L stainless steel can be cold-worked to improve the yield and ultimate stress, though the ductility is decreased. Stainless steel in orthopaedic implants is often cold-worked about 30%. (Reproduced with permission from Burstein AH, Wright TM: *Fundamentals of Orthopaedic Biomechanics*. Baltimore, MD, Williams & Wilkins, 1994.)

Table 1
Strength of Femoral Cortical Bone*

Loading Mode	Ultimate Strength (MPa)
Longitudinal	
Tension	133
Compression	193
Shear	68
Transverse	
Tension	51
Compression	133

*   Data obtained from Reilly DT, Burstein AH: The elastic and ultimate
      properties of compact bone tissue. *J Biomech* 1975;8:393-405.

structural scale has both collagen fibrils and mineral crystals both aligned in a generally longitudinal direction in the cortices of the long bones of the skeleton. At a microstructural scale, the osteons are also generally aligned longitudinally, as are the cement lines between osteons. Given such an organization of the material's components, it is easy to understand why the tissue has its greatest strength in the longitudinal direction.

Man-made composite materials use the same approach to alter mechanical properties in preferred directions. This is most easily done by aligning strong fibers along preferred directions and then impregnating the fibers within a usually weaker matrix. The resulting material will display mechanical properties that depend on the properties of the fiber and the matrix, the relative amounts of fiber and matrix, the bonding between the fiber and matrix, and the geometry and orientation of the fibers. Such composite materials have been developed for artificial ligaments, for biodegradable fracture fixation devices, as scaffolds for tissue engineering applications, and even for total joint components, although none have gained widespread clinical use.

Perhaps the most common man-made composite material in orthopaedics is made right in the hospital: plaster casts. Plaster itself is brittle and relatively weak, particularly in tension. But impregnating the plaster around a stronger, more ductile gauze results in a laminated composite that has sufficient mechanical properties. Because of the weave of the gauze, the composite has the same mechanical properties in any direction within the plane of the gauze material, but different (and inferior) properties in other directions. Hence, the plaster cast material is anisotropic.

Plaster is formed by roasting crushed gypsum powder at 120° to 130°C to decrease the naturally occurring water content from about 21 wt% to 6 wt%. The powder is bonded to the gauze using either methylcellulose or polyvinyl acetate, with an added accelerator (such as potassium sulfate) often included to decrease setting time. When the plaster bandage is immersed in water, the calcium sulfate in the plaster material reacts with the water to form crystalline calcium sulfate dihydrate through an exothermic reaction. As the excess water slowly evaporates, the cast continues to solidify and the crystalline structure achieves its full mechanical properties.

Fiberglass casts substitute a polyurethane resin for the plaster and woven fibers for the gauze. A fabric carrier is used for structural integrity, and water is used to initiate the polymerization process. Although more expensive than plaster and more difficult to mold, fiberglass has advantages over plaster, including radiolucency, greater strength, lower weight, improved endurance, and water resistance.

Viscoelasticity

The tensile test of the bone plate (Fig. 1) could be performed at many different rates of loading. The rate was never specified in the previous discussion because for the case of stainless steel, the resulting stress-strain curve would be the same regardless of loading rate. This would be true for other metallic alloys and ceramics. However, for many other materials, loading rate will have a profound effect on the mechanical properties. When a material's properties are time-dependent, the material is said to be viscoelastic. For example, bone tissue is viscoelastic (Fig. 7). Specimens loaded at 3 different rates exhibit three different stress-strain curves, with elastic modulus, yield stress, and ultimate stress increasing, and strain rate and ductility decreasing as the rate increases.

The effect of loading rate must be considered, therefore, in predicting failure. A clinical example is failure of the anterior cruciate ligament (ACL). Ligament tissue exhibits less viscoelastic behavior than bone tissue. At low loading rates, the bone tissue is weaker than the ligament tissue. At high loading rates, the bone tissue is stronger than the ligament. This transition in strength can be used to explain the transition from bone avulsion to midsubstance ligament tears in ACL injuries as loading rate increases.

Viscoelastic materials often display hysteresis in their stress-strain curves. The loading and unloading curves do not overlap, forming a closed loop called a hysteresis loop (Fig. 8). The loop can be thought of as inefficiency in the process of storing and releasing energy as the material is loaded and unloaded. The loading curve represents the strain energy stored in the material during loading. This area exceeds the area under the unloading curve (that represents the release of strain energy during unloading). The difference (the area enclosed within the hysteresis loop)

represents the energy dissipated within the material, primarily by internal friction within the material. Polymers, for example, are often viscoelastic, with energy dissipated through friction between the polymer chains as the material is deformed. When cyclically loaded and unloaded, such viscoelastic materials actually generate heat as a result of the friction. Metallic materials, on the other hand, have crystalline, ordered material structures with few mechanisms for internal friction. Metallic materials, therefore, do not typically exhibit a hysteresis loop as part of their stress versus strain behavior.

Fatigue

The failure criteria defined thus far, namely yield and ultimate strength, are pertinent to questions concerning trauma or other situations involving maximum tolerable loads. These criteria were defined from a single, static application of load to the material. Most instances in orthopaedics, however, involve repeated, cyclic loads. For example, active total hip patients may take millions of steps each year, thus applying millions of cycles of load to their lower extremities. Such repeated loading and unloading can cause failure, even though each individually applied load creates stresses in the cement or in the metallic alloy of the stem that are below their ultimate strengths.

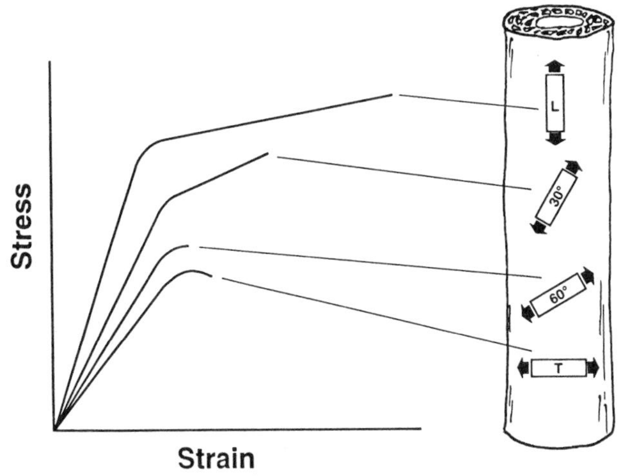

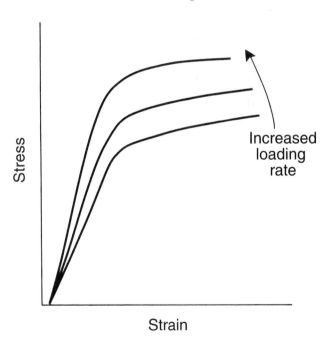

Figure 6

Cortical bone tissue is anisotropic. Specimens taken in different orientations within the cortex of a long bone and loaded in tension will exhibit very different stress-strain behavior. In general, the longitudinal direction exhibits a higher elastic modulus and greater strength, while the transverse direction exhibits the lowest elastic modulus and strength. (Adapted with permission from Nordin M, Frankel VH: *Basic Biomechanics of the Musculoskeletal System,* ed 2. Philadelphia, PA, Lea & Febiger, 1989.)

Figure 7

Cortical bone tissue is viscoelastic. Specimens of cortical bone loaded at 3 different rates will exhibit 3 different stress-strain curves, with both elastic modulus and strength increasing as rate increases. (Reproduced with permission from Burstein AH, Wright TM: *Fundamentals of Orthopaedic Biomechanics.* Baltimore, MD, Williams & Wilkins, 1994.)

Such failures are termed fatigue and are in fact the product of 2 separate events. The first is the accumulation of microstructural damage within the material with each loading cycle. The damage accumulates faster at higher intensities of cyclic loading. Eventually sufficient damage accumulates so that the material can no longer remain intact in the damaged region, and a crack is initiated. The second event is crack propagation, in which the crack continues to grow with each loading cycle until it reaches such a length that the remaining cross-section cannot sustain the next load cycle and the material breaks.

For a smooth metallic implant, a large portion of the fatigue life (typically the first 80%) is associated with damage accumulation and crack initiation. Subsequent crack propagation and final fracture requires far fewer loading cycles. Any factor that encourages crack initiation will have a disastrous effect on the fatigue life. For example, scratching or nicking the surface of a metallic orthopaedic device creates damage that under cyclic loading could quickly become a crack, thus greatly decreasing the fatigue life (the number of cycles to failure). Conversely, any factor that acts to arrest or slow crack propagation will increase fatigue life. Cracks growing through the matrix of a composite, when reaching stronger fibers within the matrix, will stop growing until enough damage accumulates to break the fibers.

Fatigue failure is the most common mode of failure in orthopaedic devices. Bone plates, femoral components from total hip replacements, tibial trays from total knee replacements, intramedullary nails, and other devices fabricated from metallic alloys can all suffer fatigue failure if loaded at sufficient magnitudes for a sufficient number of cycles. Even UHMWPE surfaces in total knee implants fail by fatigue-related wear mechanisms because of the cyclic nature of the loads applied.

There is a strong negative correlation between the intensity of loading and the number of loading cycles required for failure. This can be seen in a plot of applied cyclic stress versus number of cycles (Fig. 9). A smooth curve has been fit through data obtained from specimens that had been loaded to different stress levels and the number of cycles until failure recorded. Such plots are used to define the fatigue strength or endurance limit of the material, the stress at which the material can withstand 10 million cycles without experiencing fatigue failure. Given that patients can apply millions of cycles each year and that orthopaedic implants such as total joint components are intended to be permanent, it is obviously desirable to maintain the stresses induced in orthopaedic implants well below the endurance limit.

Metals

Metallic alloys have found widespread use in orthopaedic surgery. Alloys are metals composed of mixtures or solutions of metallic and nonmetallic elements. The combination of elements is used to impart the high strength, ductility, and elastic modulus, the corrosion resistance, and the biocompatibility required for load-bearing applications, such as fracture fixation devices and implant components for total joint arthroplasty. The 3 common alloys used in

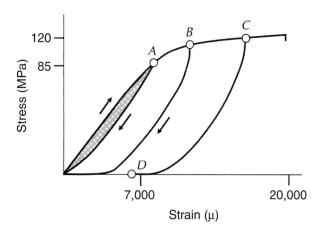

Figure 8

When a specimen of cortical bone is loaded to point A, and the load is then removed, the bone immediately returns to its original length, although not along the same path as the loading process. When the specimen is loaded to point B, and the load is released, the elongation does not immediately return to zero. It requires several seconds for the specimen to return. Loading to point C results in a change in length that is not reversible. (Reproduced with permission from Burstein AH, Wright TM: *Fundamentals of Orthopaedic Biomechanics*. Baltimore, MD, Williams & Wilkins, 1994.)

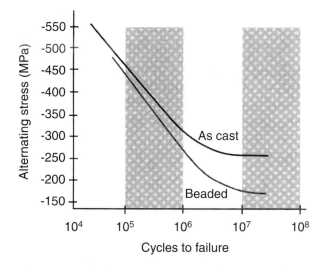

Figure 9

Cyclic stress amplitude is plotted against number of cycles to failure for a fatigue test of cast cobalt alloy and cobalt alloy with a sintered, beaded surface. The specimens in the test were exposed to reverse bending, subjecting the material to alternating compression and tension stresses. (Reproduced with permission from Burstein AH, Wright TM: *Fundamentals of Orthopaedic Biomechanics*. Baltimore, MD, Williams & Wilkins, 1994.)

orthopaedics are stainless steel, cobalt chromium alloy, and titanium alloy. None of these alloys were developed specifically for orthopaedic or biomedical applications. Instead, their proven strength and corrosion resistance in the aerospace, marine, and chemical industries have led them to be adopted for implant use. Their specific properties can be understood from their molecular structure, microstructures, and composition.

Metallic Bonding

The elements in a metallic alloy are held together by metallic bonds. These bonds are quite strong, accounting for the high strengths and high melting points of the alloys. Metallic bonds can best be described as crystalline arrays in which the nuclei of the atoms are closely packed in an orderly array that repeats in a 3-dimensional pattern. The valence electrons (the loosely bound electrons in the outer shells of the atoms) flow easily from adjoining atoms. Thus, the nuclei can be considered positive ions surrounded by a sea of negatively charged valence electrons. The ease with which valence electrons flow through the crystalline structure is responsible for the high electrical and thermal conductivities and the chemical reactivity of metals. The structure is on average neutrally charged because the positive ions are "glued" together by the negative charge that surrounds them.

The strength of the bond increases the more tightly packed the atoms become, leading to a lowest energy state where the atoms are as close together as possible (that is, until their inner electron orbits begin to overlap). There are 3 typical configurations in which the atoms pack together (Fig. 10), touching either 12 (in face-centered cubic and hexagonal arrays) or 8 (in a body-centered cubic array) neighboring atoms and filling about 70% to 75% of the possible volume. Metallic bonds are nondirectional in that atoms are free to associate in any direction with neighboring atoms. Atoms from the alloying elements can fill in gaps and crevices in the crystalline structure. The nondirectional nature of the bond allows for plastic deformation, as defects in the crystalline packing flow through the structure.

Metallic Microstructures

When atoms in a molten state are cooled to form a solid material, many small crystals of atoms nucleate and grow until they begin to impinge on one another. When all the molten liquid has solidified, the resulting solid is a polycrystalline array of individual crystals, typically of irregular shape and of a size visible in the light microscope or macroscopically. The microstructure can be revealed by polishing a flat surface of the metal, etching the surface with a mild corrosive to reveal the boundaries between the crystals (called the grain boundaries), and viewing the surface in a reflecting microscope under incident light (Fig. 11). Grain size is one of the most important microstructural features of metals and metallic alloys. The finer the grain size, the more homogeneous and isotropic the material will be, but more importantly, the greater its strength. This has proved to be an important consideration, for example, in cobalt-chromium femoral components for total hip replacement. Unacceptably large grain sizes have been shown to be responsible for insufficient fatigue strength in the alloy, resulting in clinical failures (Fig. 12).

In a pure metal, all of the grains have the same structure and thus differ only in the crystalline orientation of the atoms. The lack of directional bonding in metals, however, allows the introduction of other elements into the crystalline matrix. If the atomic sizes and the electronic structure of the 2 elements are similar, the elements can form a single-phase solid solution possessing a homogeneous microstructure, similar to the pure elemental case. For example, titanium in its commercially pure form (so-called

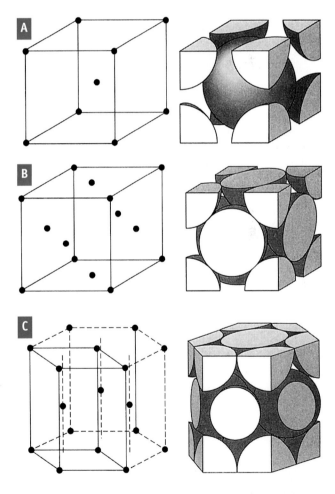

Figure 10

Common unit cell structures for crystalline arrangements of atoms can be body-centered cubic (**A**), face-centered cubic (**B**), or hexagonal close-packed (**C**). (Adapted with permission from Rolls KM, Courtney TH, Wulff J: *Introduction to Materials Science and Engineering*. New York, NY, John Wiley & Sons, 1976.)

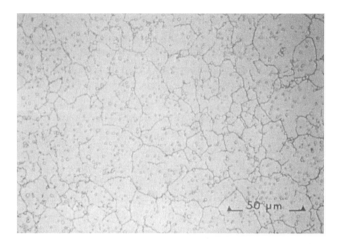

Figure 11

Microstructure of the American Society for Testing and Materials F75 cobalt alloy showing the polycrystalline nature and the intergranular matrix carbides. (Reproduced with permission from Ratner BD, Hoffman AS, Schoen FJ, Lemons JE (eds): *Biomaterials Science: An Introduction to Materials in Medicine.* San Diego, CA, Academic Press, 1996.)

CP-titanium) is a single-phase solid solution of oxygen in titanium. If the atoms possess dissimilar sizes and electronic structures, 2 or more phases can be formed. The solubility of the alloying element in the metallic alloy is limited, so as concentration continues to increase, a second phase begins to precipitate.

The grains of any single phase will have the same composition and crystalline structure, but will differ in composition and structure form grains of the other phases. Titanium alloy, for example, is a 2-phase solid solution: a body-centered cubic beta phase and a hexagonal close packed alpha phase. Similarly, chromium can substitute for iron in the face-centered cubic crystal structure of iron to form

stainless steel. As the chromium concentration is increased, a second phase that is rich in chromium precipitates. Carbon, an alloying element in all steels, will also form a second phase if concentrations are large enough. This second phase, however, weakens the steel, limits ductility, and decreases corrosion resistance, and thus carbon concentrations in stainless steel for orthopaedic applications are deliberately kept low.

Stainless Steel

The most common form of stainless steel used in orthopaedic applications is 316L, grade 2, designated by the American Society for Testing and Materials (ASTM) specification F138. The numeric designation "316" places the alloy within the so-called austenitic stainless steels; the "L" denotes low carbon concentration (typically below 0.03 wt%). As with all steels, 316L stainless steel is an alloy of iron and carbon. The other major alloying elements include chromium, nickel, and molybdenum, with minor amounts of manganese, phosphorous, sulfur, and silicon (Fig. 13). The alloying elements affect the microstructure and hence the mechanical and corrosion properties of the steel. Chromium in the microstructure forms a strongly adherent oxide (Cr_2O_3) on the surfaces of the metal that are exposed to the environment, thus providing corrosion resistance by forming a passive layer between the environment and the bulk material. Stainless steel devices are passivated by immersion in a strong nitric acid bath as part of the manufacturing process to assure the creation of the oxide layer.

The creation of a "passive" oxide layer limits the rate of electrochemical corrosion by about a thousand to a million times compared to the rate of corrosion in the absence of the oxide. Most of the metallic alloys are highly reactive

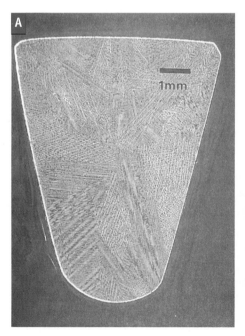

A

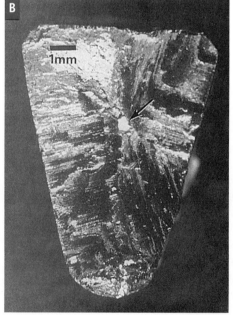

B

Figure 12

Etched cross-section of the femoral component of a total hip replacement fabricated from cast cobalt alloy showing dendritic structure and very large grain size (**A**). The fracture surface of the same component, which failed in vivo, including a large inclusion (arrow) that probably contributed to the failure (**B**). (Reproduced with permission from Ratner BD, Hoffman AS, Schoen FJ, Lemons JE (eds): *Biomaterials Science: An Introduction to Materials in Medicine.* San Diego, CA, Academic Press, 1996.)

with oxygen, so that the oxide layer forms naturally as the base metal is exposed to the atmosphere. Standardized methods (such as the nitric acid bath) are used to enhance the layer and ensure appropriate resistance to corrosion.

Though chromium provides the "stainless" quality to the steel, it also stabilizes the ferritic, body-centered cubic phase that is weaker than the face-centered cubic austenitic phase. Molybdenum, added to provide additional corrosion resistance, and silicon, added with manganese to aid in the manufacturing process, also stabilize the ferritic phase. To offset this tendency, nickel is added to stabilize the austenitic phase and thus assure an appropriately strong microstructure.

Carbon concentration must be kept low in 316L stainless steel to maintain corrosion resistance. At higher carbon concentrations, there is a tendency for the carbon to combine with the chromium to form a brittle carbide that robs the microstructure of much of the chromium and that tends to segregate to the grain boundaries, significantly weakening the material by making it prone to corrosion-related fracture. Such a condition, called sensitization, has been directly responsible for mechanical failures of orthopaedic implants made from stainless steels in which carbon content has been too high.

ASTM specifications for 316L stainless steel call for an austenitic microstructure free of carbides or inclusions that might remain from the steel-making process (and that can reduce corrosion resistance). The recommended grain size is small (about 100 microns in any dimension) to assure adequate strength for orthopaedic applications. Grain size

can be controlled by the solidification process and by post-solidification heat treatments and cold working of the material. Stainless steel is typically cold-worked by about 30% for orthopaedic applications. Mechanical properties of 316L stainless steel are provided in Table 2 in both the annealed (not cold-worked) and 30% cold-worked condition.

A potential disadvantage of stainless steel in implant applications is its susceptibility to crevice and stress corrosion. In any corrosion process, there are 2 reactions, an anodic reaction in which the metal is oxidized to its ionic form ($M \rightarrow M^{n+} + n$ electrons) and a cathodic reaction in which the electrons are consumed (in an aqueous solution with dissolved oxygen, $O_2 + 2H_2O + 4e \rightarrow 4OH^-$). These reactions could initially be progressing at an even rate over the surface of a stainless steel implant, such as a bone plate or a bone screw. But as the reactions progress in the crevice between the underside of the head of the screw and the countersunk area of the plate, the crevice becomes depleted of oxygen. The anodic reaction continues in the crevice while the remainder of the plate and screw undergo the cathodic reaction. The oxygen concentration is not readily replenished by the fluids outside of the crevice, though smaller chlorine ions flow into the crevice, drawn there by the metal ions being released by the anodic reaction. The crevice region decreases in pH, causing accelerated metal oxidation.

Stress corrosion cracking results when the combination of an applied stress and a corrosive environment lead to mechanical failure of the material, even though the environment or load in and of itself would be insufficient to

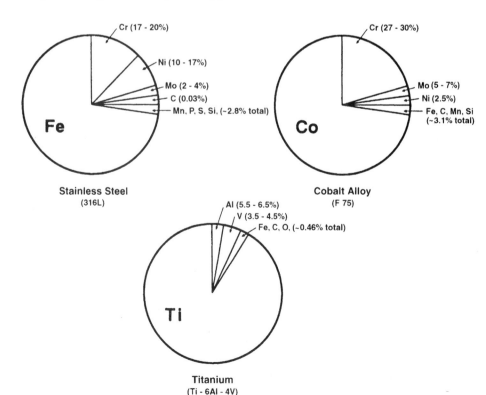

Stainless Steel
(316L)

Cr (17 - 20%)
Ni (10 - 17%)
Mo (2 - 4%)
C (0.03%)
Mn, P, S, Si, (~2.8% total)
Fe

Cobalt Alloy
(F 75)

Cr (27 - 30%)
Mo (5 - 7%)
Ni (2.5%)
Fe, C, Mn, Si (~3.1% total)
Co

Titanium
(Ti - 6Al - 4V)

Al (5.5 - 6.5%)
V (3.5 - 4.5%)
Fe, C, O, (~0.46% total)
Ti

Figure 13

The composition of the 3 common orthopaedic metallic alloys.

cause failure. Stress corrosion cracking has been shown to occur even under low levels of constant stress, such as might occur in an implant with residual stresses. Crack initiation is accelerated by the corrosion process, as is the subsequent crack growth that occurs under the applied stress.

Because of concerns about corrosion and subsequent long-term biocompatibility, stainless steel has been used primarily in fracture and spinal fixation applications. These applications often allow removal of the device or require strength only until healing occurs. Permanent implants, such as femoral components of the Charnley design of hip replacements, have also been made from stainless steel, demonstrating that stainless steel can be used safely even in these high-demand applications.

Cobalt-Chromium Alloys

Cobalt-chromium alloys include compositions intended to be manufactured by casting (ASTM F75 alloy) and by forging (ASTM F799 alloy), as well as alloy compositions that obtain excellent mechanical properties through cold working (ASTM F90 and F562). All of these alloys are primarily cobalt with significant amounts of chromium added for corrosion resistance. As with stainless steel, the chromium forms a strongly adherent oxide film that provides a passive layer shielding the bulk material from the environment. The F75 and F90 alloys contain about 60% cobalt with about 28% chromium (Fig. 13). The F799 and F562 alloys have less cobalt and chromium, and in their place have large amounts of other alloying elements (about 15% tungsten in F799 and about 35% Ni in the F562).

The alloys display a range of mechanical properties (Table 2) that can be understood from the processes and the resulting microstructures used to fabricate devices from the materials. The F75 alloy, for example, has commonly been used for investment (or so-called lost wax) casting. Wax molds of near-final dimensions of devices such as total hip femoral stems are coated with a ceramic slurry. The slurry is fired in a furnace (and the wax is lost as it melts away from the inside of the ceramic mold). Molten F75 alloy is poured or pressurized into the molds and allowed to solidify. The ceramic mold is broken away from the underlying metal part, which can then be finished into the final device.

Quality control can be a problem during the casting process. If solidification proceeds too slowly, grains have ample time to grow quite large, thus significantly diminishing the material's strength (Fig. 12). If solidification proceeds too quickly, air from inside the mold and gases that are released during the solidification process can become entrapped in the microstructure, causing undesirable stress concentrations that can cause premature failure. Finally, if cooling conditions are not ideal, carbides that naturally occur within the alloy's microstructure segregate to too great a degree, which can weaken the material, reduce ductility, and decrease corrosion resistance. To overcome these problems, the alloy can be fabricated by powder metallurgy. Fine powder of the alloy is compacted and sintered together to form a near net shape. The shape is then forged under pressure and heated into the final shape. The resulting microstructure has a smaller grain size and more evenly distributed carbides than the cast alloy, leading to improved properties (Table 2).

Table 2
Typical Mechanical Properties of Implant Metals

Material	ASTM Designation	Condition	Elastic Modulus (GPa)	Yield Strength (MPa)	Ultimate Strength (MPa)	Endurance Limit (MPa)
Stainless steels	F55, F56, F138, F139	Annealed	190	331	586	241–276
		30% Cold-worked	190	792	930	310–448
		Cold forged	190	1213	1351	820
Cobalt alloys	F75	As cast/annealed	210	448–517	655–889	207–310
		Hip*	253	841	1277	725–950
	F799	Hot forged	210	896–1200	1399–1586	600–896
	F90	Annealed	210	448–648		951–1220
		44% Cold-worked	210	1606	1896	586
	F562	Hot forged	232	965–1000	1206	500
		Cold-forged/aged	232	1500	1795	689–793
Titanium alloy	F67	30% Cold-worked	110	485	760	300
	F136	Forged annealed	116	896	965	620
		Forged/heat treated	116	1034	1103	620–689

*   HIP = hot isostatically pressed; ASTM = American Society for Testing and Materials. (Reproduced with permission from Ratner BD, Hoffman AS, Schoen FJ, Lemons JE (eds): *Biomaterials Science: An Introduction to Materials in Medicine*. San Diego, CA, Academic Press, 1996.)

F75 alloy is used to fabricate porous coatings for biologic fixation of orthopaedic implants. The resulting properties of the porous-coated device will depend on the microstructure of the substrate metal and the porous beads, as well as the thermal sintering process that is used to connect the two. Sintering involves very high temperatures (near the 1225°C melting temperature), which can significantly decrease the fatigue strength of the substrate material. Together with the stress concentrations caused at the attachment points with the porous coating, the result is a fatigue strength of only about 200 MPa, even after additional thermal treatments are used to restore some of the strength. This strength is well below that achieved for other cobalt alloys that are not porous-coated (Table 2).

The forging alloy, F799, possesses mechanical properties that are superior to that of the cast alloy (Table 2). Hot forging effectively reduces grain size, "heals" pores through the combination of pressure and heat, and breaks up the carbides into an even distribution. The thermomechanical forging operation also induces an additional microstructural phase that contributes to the improved properties.

The F90 and F562 alloys obtain substantial mechanical properties through more than 40% cold-working. The tungsten addition in F90 improves machinability and fabrication via cold-working. The cold working of F562 alloy provides additional energy for the transformation of some of the face-centered cubic phase into a hexagonal phase that emerges as fine platelets throughout the microstructure. The combination of a very fine grain size (the face-centered cubic grains are less than 0.1μ in any dimension) and the dispersed platelets impede plastic deformation, strengthening the material. In addition, the material can be thermally treated to precipitate a uniform distribution of very fine cobalt-molybdenum (Co_3Mo) precipitates that act to further strengthen the material. The result is among the strongest of the orthopaedic implant alloys (Table 2).

The ease of fabrication and the range of properties available for cobalt alloys make them ideal for a wide range of orthopaedic applications, including all metallic components of all joint replacements as well as fracture fixation devices. The chromium content of these alloys provide excellent corrosion resistance, with superior resistance to crevice corrosion than stainless steel. Long-term clinical use has proved that these alloys also have exceptional biocompatibility in bulk form.

Titanium and Titanium Alloys

Titanium and its alloys are of particular interest for biomedical applications because of their outstanding biocompatibility and corrosion resistance. Their corrosion resistance, provided by an adherent passive layer of titanium oxide (TiO_2), significantly exceeds that of stainless steel and the cobalt alloys. Uniform corrosion even in saline solutions is extremely limited, and resistance to pitting and intergranular and crevice corrosion is excellent. Experimental studies in animal models and long-term clinical use in humans confirm truly superior biocompatibility. Furthermore, the oxide surfaces of titanium and its alloys are well tolerated in contact with bone, becoming osseointegrated with little evidence of a fibrous layer between bone and implant.

CP-titanium (ASTM F67) is used more extensively in dental implants, but is used in orthopaedic surgery primarily in the form of wire mesh for porous coatings that is sintered onto titanium alloy joint replacement components. The properties of CP-titanium depend on the amount of oxygen contained in the metal. At small concentrations, increased oxygen content improves the mechanical properties. Grade IV CP-titanium, for example, with an oxygen concentration of 0.40 wt% has a yield strength of about 485 MPa, while grade I with an oxygen concentration of 0.18 wt% has a yield strength of only 170 MPa. The CP-titanium microstructure consists of grains of a single, hexagonal close-packed phase, and the material can be cold-worked. Additional strengthening of the microstructure comes from interstitial solid solution strengthening, in which atoms of oxygen, carbon, and particularly nitrogen harden the material by being encased in the interstices of the crystalline, hexagonal arrangement of titanium atoms.

The most common form of titanium used in orthopaedic applications is titanium-aluminum-vanadium alloy (ASTM F-136). The primary alloying elements, aluminum and vanadium, are limited to 5.5 wt% to 6.5 wt% and 3.5 wt% to 4.5 wt%, respectively (Fig. 13), so that the alloy is often called Ti-6Al-4V or simply Ti-6-4. Developed by the aerospace industry as a high strength-to-weight ratio material, the alloy is used in orthopaedic implants in the extra low interstitials form, in which the oxygen concentration is kept very low to avoid embrittlement and to maximize strength and ductility. The microstructure of Ti-6Al-4V contains 2-phase grains, the alpha phase being a hexagonal-close packed phase that is stabilized by the aluminum alloying element and the body-centered cubic beta phase stabilized by the vanadium. The distribution and amount of the phases dictate the material's properties and can be altered by prior thermal treatments. The alloy can also be mechanically worked to alter its properties. Typically, the microstructure is a fine-grained alpha phase with the beta phase present as isolated particles that precipitate at the grain boundaries; this microstructure possesses excellent fatigue resistance compared to other forms of titanium alloy microstructures.

The mechanical properties of Ti-6Al-4V are more than adequate for most orthopaedic applications (Table 2). The elastic modulus for the alloy is about half that of stainless steel and the cobalt alloys, making the alloy an ideal candidate for lowering the structural stiffness of a device without changing its shape. For example, the axial, bending, and torsional stiffnesses of a bone plate fabricated from titanium alloy will be half that of a bone plate of the same size and shape made from stainless steel or cobalt alloy. Thus, the severity of stress shielding when the plate is rigidly attached to the bone (so that the bone and the plate share load) would be less for the titanium alloy plate. This mechanical consideration has led to the use of titanium alloy in fracture and spinal fixation devices, including plates, nails, and screws. The same consideration has led to the use of titanium alloy in stems for total joint replacements.

A disadvantageous trait of titanium alloy is its notch sensitivity. A stress concentration, such as a notch or scratch, on the surface of a titanium alloy implant significantly reduces the fatigue life of the part. The same is true for the type of stress concentrations that occur when a porous coating is applied to the surface of a titanium alloy total joint component. The severe changes in geometry that result from the sharp angles that are created wherever the coating is sintered to the substrate act as points of stress concentration. Therefore, care must be taken in designing porous-coated total joint implants with titanium alloy.

Another disadvantage of titanium alloy is its lower hardness (in comparison, for example, to the cobalt alloys). An ambiguous term, hardness encompasses a number of mechanical properties, but mostly measures the material's resistance to elastic and plastic deformation. Several standard tests for measuring hardness exist, most involving the forced indentation of a fixed geometry indentor into the surface of a material. Hardness measurements are determined from the geometry of the resulting indentation (for example, the depth or the circumference). Hardness can be empirically related to other properties, such as yield strength, but in general it is most useful in terms of comparison between materials. Microhardness measurements, for example, in which a diamond-tipped, pyramid-shaped indentor is pressed into the surface under a 10-g load, show titanium alloy to be about 15% "softer" than cast cobalt alloy. The decreased hardness of titanium alloy that must be considered in total joint applications is due to its wear resistance. Clinical observations have demonstrated significant scratching and wear of total hip femoral heads made from titanium alloy. Measurements of the levels of titanium and aluminum in the tissues and fluids taken from the hip joint have confirmed the release of significant amounts of these elements from the femoral head. These observations suggest that titanium alloy that has not undergone additional surface processing (for example, ion implantation) should not be used as an articulating surface. Despite the long-term clinical evidence of the excellent biocompatibility of titanium alloy, the concern that the release of cytotoxic elements such as vanadium could cause local and systemic problems has led to the limited introduction of other titanium alloys in which the vanadium has been replaced by more inert elements such as niobium.

Beta titanium alloys have also been advocated for orthopaedic implants. These alloys have molybdenum con-

centrations greater than 10% to allow the beta phase to be stable at room temperature. Beta alloys can be processed to possess lower elastic modulus (by about 20%) and slightly better crevice corrosion resistance than Ti-6Al-4V, while maintaining other important mechanical properties at levels comparable or better than the conventional aluminum-vanadium alloy. Together with excellent formability, the beta alloys are candidates for a wide range of orthopaedic applications.

Polymers

This section begins with a definition and description of basic polymer science concepts generally applicable to all polymeric materials and concludes with a detailed look at bone cement, UHMWPE, and resorbable polymers, 3 specific families of polymers used extensively in orthopaedic applications.

Definition and Properties

Polymers are large molecules made from combinations of smaller molecules. These small molecules are called "mer" units from the Greek word "meros," which means part. For the purposes of this discussion, polymers will be limited to "organic" monomers, which are molecules based predominantly on carbon (C), hydrogen (H), oxygen (O), and nitrogen (N). The properties of a polymer are dictated by its chemical structure (the monomers used to make the polymer); physical structure (the manner in which the monomers are attached to each other); isomerism (the different possible orientation of certain atoms in some polymers); molecular weight (the number of monomers used to make the polymer); and crystallinity (the packing of the polymer chains into ordered atomic arrays).

Chemical Structure

Classes of polymer are determined by the presence of certain chemical combinations (moieties). A list of some common polymeric moieties and the classes of polymers they represent are provided in Table 3. Table 4 provides a list of specific polymers commonly found in medicine and in particular, orthopaedics, with their repeating structural units. Note that simple alterations to the chemistry of the monomers often yield dramatic differences in the final properties of the polymer.

Structural Isomers Copolymers are polymers that contain more than 1 type of monomer. For instance, bone cement, while predominantly PMMA, in some cases also contains a copolymer of methylmethacrylate and polystyrene or methylmethacrylate and methacrylic acid. In the case of copolymers, the distribution of the different monomers can also provide very different properties. For instance, for a copolymer made of 2 different monomers, A and B, the monomers may be randomly distributed (AABABB-

BABAAABB...), alternating (ABABAB..) or in blocks (AAABB-BAAABBBAAA...).

The manner by which each monomer is linked to the overall polymer structure can also provide different structural arrangements. Polymers may either be linear, branched, or cross-linked. Linear polymers have monomers that are linked end to end. Branched polymers have side chains attached to the main chain. The length of each branch, the number of branches, and the distribution of branches can all be used to alter the properties of the resulting polymer. Cross-linked polymers have polymeric chains that are bound to each other. These different structures are provided in Figure 14. These apparently subtle differences lead to very different polymer properties.

Geometric Isomers In addition to the different structural possibilities mentioned previously, there are additional variations that occur. Using polypropylene as an example, there are 3 possibilities for the placement of the pendant CH3 group in each monomer segment. They can all be on the same side of the backbone (isotactic), alternating sides with each monomer (syndiotactic), or they may be randomly placed (atactic). These 3 isomers are shown in Figure 15.

The most subtle of isomers is optical activity. This is a special case when a central carbon atom has 4 different atoms around it. In these cases, the central carbon is termed to be chiral or an optically active center. This type of isomerism may be especially important in determining the biologic activity and the physical properties. Figure 16 shows the 2 optical isomers of lactic acid, a monomer used in resorbable polymers. It is reminded that these structures are 3-dimensional in nature. This is represented in Figure 16 by the dashed lines, which indicate that the bond goes behind the plane of the paper and the filled triangle bonds indicate bonds that are above the plane of the paper. The 2 structures are not superimposable and thus are 2 different molecules, although they are chemically identical. These structures are also termed to be enantiomers. Enantiomers are characterized in the manner in which a sample will rotate plane, polarized light. If plane polarized light is exposed to an enantiomer, the sample will cause the plane of light to rotate to the left or right as it passes through the sample. If the light is rotated to the right, the enantiomer is termed the dextrorotatory or D form. If the light is rotated to the left, the enantiomer is termed the levorotatory or L form. It is this rotation of plane polarized light that gives rise to the description of enantiomers as optically active.

Molecular Weight

The molecular weight of a polymer is determined by the number of monomer units used to make up the polymer. Polyethylene is the simplest possible polymer. The number of ethylene units in a polymer chain determines the molecular weight of that chain. For instance, each ethylene monomer has a molecular weight of 28. A polymer made up of 1000 ethylene units has a molecular weight of 28,000. However, during the polymerization of ethylene, not all chains will be made of the exact same number of ethylene units so not all chains will have the same molecular weight. This results in a distribution of molecular weights.

There are several ways to characterize the molecular weight distribution. If a polymer sample has several different molecular weight fractions, then M_i is the mean molecular weight of fraction i, and x_i is the molar fraction of the sample that has molecular weight M_i. The number average molecular weight, M_n, is defined by the following equation.

$$M_n = \sum_{i=1}^{n} x_i M_i$$

In a similar manner, the weight average molecular weight, M_w, is defined as:

$$M_w = \sum_{i=1}^{n} W_i M_i$$

W_i is the weight fraction of molecules with molecular weight M_i. The different possible values for M_n and M_w are shown in Figure 17 for a polymer of typical molecular weight distribution. The polydispersity of a polymer is the ratio of M_w/M_n. Large values for polydispersity indicate that M_n and M_w are very different because the distribution of molecular weight is not a "normal" distribution. All other factors being equal, changes in molecular weight or polydispersity can significantly influence the stiffness, strength, toughness, and wear properties of a polymer. For example,

Linear

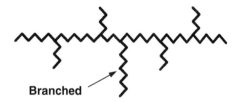

Branched

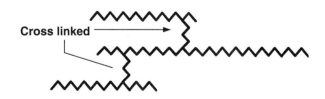

Cross linked

Figure 14

Polymer structures.

high density polyethylene is a polymer of ethylene that can have molecular weights of 50,000 to 200,000 (1800 to 7150 ethylene units). However, UHMWPE with a molecular weight > 2,000,000 (71,000 ethylene units) is also a polymer of ethylene but has very different properties than high density polyethylene.

Crystallinity

The crystallinity of the polymer should be considered as well. Some segments of the polymer chains can have a structural order, in addition to the factors previously discussed. Parts of the polymer that are random are the noncrystalline or amorphous sections of the polymer. The ordered areas are the crystalline areas. Virtually all polymers are semicrystalline in that only some areas of the structure are ordered. The degree of crystallinity can greatly influence the properties of the polymer. Crystalline regions can form lamallae as seen in Figure 18. The lamal-

Table 3

Classes of Polymers and Their Identifying Structural Units

Structural Unit	Polymer Class
$\begin{matrix} O \\ \| \| \\ -C-O- \end{matrix}$	Polyester
$\begin{matrix} O \\ \| \| \\ -C-NH- \end{matrix}$	Polyamide, nylon
$\begin{matrix} O \\ \| \| \\ -O-C-O- \end{matrix}$	Polycarbonate
$\begin{matrix} O \\ \| \| \\ -O-C-NH- \end{matrix}$	Polyurethane

Table 4

Polymers in Medicine and Orthopaedics

Repeating Unit	Name	End Use
$-CH_2-CH_2-$	Polyethylene	Joint replacements
$\begin{matrix} CH_3 \\ \| \\ -CH_2-CH_2- \end{matrix}$	Polypropylene	Ligament augmentation
$-CF_2-CF_2-$	Polytetrafluoroethylene	Early joint replacements
$-CH_2-CHCl-$	Polyvinyl chloride (PVC)	Surgical tubing, clips
$\begin{matrix} CH_3 \\ \| \\ -CH_2-C- \\ \| \\ C=O \\ \| \\ O-CH_3 \end{matrix}$	Polymethylmethacrylate	Bone cement
$\begin{matrix} H \\ \| \\ -CH_2-C- \\ \| \\ C=O \\ \| \\ O-CH_3 \end{matrix}$	Methacrylic acid	Bone cement copolymer
$\begin{matrix} -O-CH_2-C-O- \\ \| \| \\ O \end{matrix}$	Polyglycolic acid	Resorbable polymer
$\begin{matrix} -O-CH(CH_3)-C-O- \\ \| \| \\ O \end{matrix}$	Polylactic acid	
$-CH_2-O-$	Polyethylene oxide (polyacetal)	Early joint replacements, plastic trial inserts, surgical clips
$-CH(C_6H_6)-$	Polystyrene	Tissue culture plates, bone cement copolymer

lae size, orientation, and distribution affect polymer properties. This property is discussed in more detail in the section on UHMWPE.

A road map of the discussed polymer factors is provided in Figure 19. Depending on the application, any of these factors can be critical and may determine the success or failure of a particular material. All of these factors should be considered in testing, evaluating, or using a polymer in a medical device.

Mechanical Properties

The key physical properties of polymers are mechanical (modulus, yield strength, ultimate tensile strength, elongation to break), along with fracture, fatigue, and wear. The mechanical properties are determined with a standard dog

bone-shaped specimen as described in ASTM D638. As with the bone plate example (Fig. 1, C), strain is applied to the specimen and the resulting stress is recorded (Fig. 20). The modulus, yield point, ultimate tensile strength, and elongation to break are determined in the same fashion as described earlier in this chapter.

Figure 21, A shows a pliable polymer that can be strained to a large degree prior to breaking. This quality would be typical for a material such as UHMWPE. Figure 21, B shows a material much stiffer than UHMWPE, as indicated by the high initial slope of the line. The material in Figure 21, B is also more "brittle" in that it breaks at much lower strains that the material in Figure 21, A.

Glass Transition Temperature

Temperature can have a great effect on polymer properties. The critical temperature for a polymer is the glass transition temperature T_g. At temperatures below the T_g, a polymer is "glassy" in nature and is generally stiff, strong, and brittle. Above the T_g, the polymer properties are termed to be "leathery" in nature and are generally less rigid and tougher than values below the T_g. The T_g for UHMWPE is around -40°C, so for all medical applications, the properties of UHMWPE are "leathery" in nature. Below -40°C, UHMWPE becomes brittle and more stiff. In contrast, the desired properties of bone cement PMMA are that it be stiff, hard, and strong. The T_g for PMMA is >60°C and is thus used clinically below the T_g for bone cement.

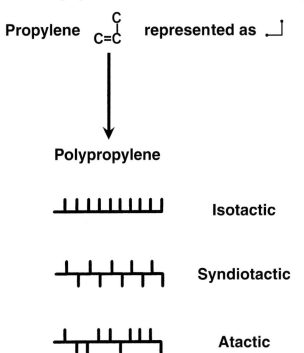

Figure 15

Polymer structural isomers.

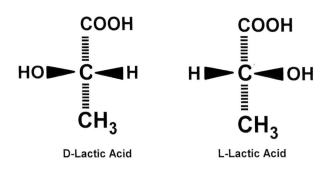

Figure 16

D- and L-forms of lactic acid.

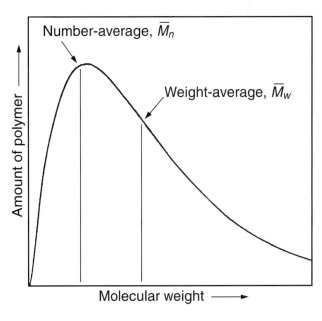

Figure 17

Molecular weight distribution showing average molecular weights, M_n and M_w.

Fatigue and Fracture Properties

The fracture properties of a polymer are determined by the energy or force required to break the polymer with a single loading. There are various methods in which these properties are determined. It is important to know that fracture properties cannot be accurately predicted from other physical properties and must be measured directly. The fracture properties may also be design- and environment-dependent.

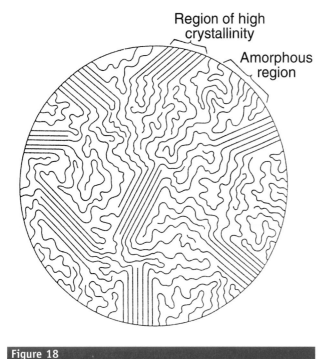

Figure 18

Crystalline lamellae and amorphous regions in semicrystalline polymer.

Fracture toughness of a polymer is a term that is much misused in the orthopaedic literature. The fracture toughness of a material is a measurement of its ability to withstand brittle fracture from a single applied load. There is a common desire to use the area under a stress/strain curve, such as in Figure 20, as the measure of the toughness of a material. However, in many instances, the polymer may elongate many times its original length prior to failure and it is difficult to call this brittle failure. In addition, the stress/strain curves are obtained only in tension and, as previously discussed, are sensitive to the rate of testing. For these reasons, the area under the stress curve is a poor predictor of polymer fracture.

Fracture mechanics is the study of the relationships between material properties, applied stresses, and brittle failure mechanisms. An inherent tenet of fracture mechanics is that there is always a flaw somewhere in the material. Criteria were developed to define the relationship between applied stresses and the size of the flaw as related to a brittle fracture process. This relationship provides information on fracturing a sample with a single load. This fact, and the geometry of the specimens clearly separates fracture testing from fatigue testing. The relationship is:

$$K_c = Y\sigma\sqrt{\pi a}$$

K_c is the fracture toughness of the material, σ is the applied stress, a is the size of the flaw, and Y is a factor that takes into account the geometry of the specimen. K_c is also a function of the thickness of the sample, as seen in Figure 22. Note that at some thicknesses, K_c is independent of the sample thickness. The value of K_c under these conditions is termed the plane strain fracture toughness, K_{1c}. This is the value of fracture toughness that is most often used because it represents the lowest toughness value for a material. In other words, if a device is designed not to fracture based on a K_{1c} value of

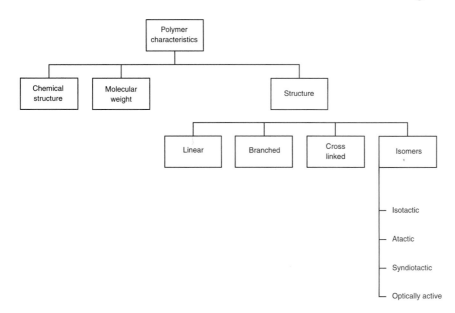

Figure 19

"Roadmap" of polymer characterization.

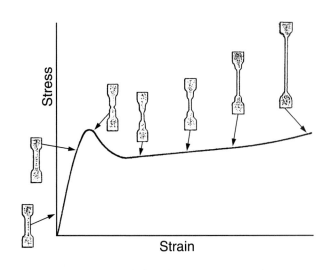

Figure 20

Stress versus strain curve. The drawings on the curve are a depiction of how the test sample is stretched during the test.

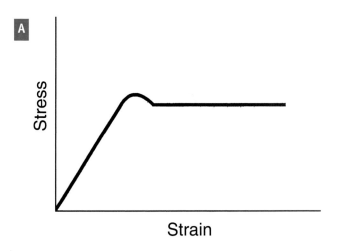

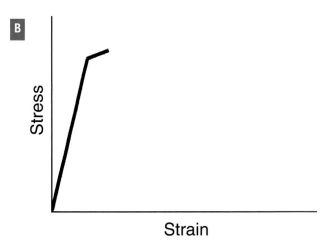

Figure 21

Example of stress/strain curves. **A,** Lower modulus, low elongation to break, pliable. **B,** Higher modulus, brittle, less pliable.

the structural material, then the device will not fracture regardless of the sample thickness. This relationship is powerful in that if the K_{1c} of a material and the size of the flaw in the material (a) are known, then the stress needed to cause a brittle fracture can be calculated. Some K_{1c} values for different materials are presented in Table 5.

The fatigue properties of a polymer indicate the ability of the material to withstand repetitive loads. In most cases, these tests are conducted by placing a razor notch in a sample and applying a predetermined number of loading cycles. At the end of the cycles, the razor notch, of length a, is measured to determined how much the crack grew. Additional loading cycles are then applied to the same sample until a relationship between the number of cycles (dn) and crack growth (da) can be determined. Like fracture properties, fatigue properties cannot be accurately predicted from other properties and values can be test- and environment-dependent. Each material must be evaluated in the manner that is best suited for its intended application. Figure 23 shows the da/dN curves for 2 different types of UHMWPE. Material B is more fatigue-resistant than material A; as for any given stress intensity, K, the crack growth (da) for material B is less than that of material A. This would suggest material A is the tougher, preferred material.

It is critical to note that other material properties such as elongation to break, yield, etc are not predictors of fatigue or fracture properties. In addition, it is possible to have 2 materials where A has a higher K_{1c} than B, but B may have more fatigue resistance. Additionally, the magnitude of the difference of K_{1c} values between samples is not an indication of the difference between fatigue values. For instance, it is common to have difference of a factor of 2 in K_{1c} between 2 different materials, but the difference in fatigue crack growth properties between the materials may be different by a factor of 100 or more. This apparent discrepancy is caused by the multiple modes of failure, such as creep, surface deformation around a crack, blunting of the crack during fatigue, and temperature effects, that can occur during a fatigue test. These different modes of failure and mechanisms are purposely avoided in K_{1c} determinations.

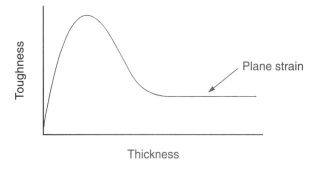

Figure 22

Effect of sample thickness and fracture toughness of the material (Kc).

Finally, it is important to note that there is no single fatigue or fracture test that will provide an adequate materials evaluation for all possible applications. For each application, the appropriate test must be determined as a function of the material properties, use conditions, loading, and known failure modes.

Polymers in Orthopaedics

Bone Cement

PMMA has been the polymer of choice since its introduction by Charnley in the 1970s. PMMA has several constituents in its actual formulation. The surgeon typically receives the bone cement kit in 2 parts: a liquid in a sealed glass ampule and a powder in a bag.

The liquid is predominantly methylmethacrylate monomer but also contains hydroquinone, a polymerization inhibitor, to insure that the liquid does not polymerize prematurely because of heat or light. The liquid also contains N, N, -dimethyl-p-toluidine, which helps to accelerate the polymerization and offset the effect of the hydroquinone once the reaction has begun.

The liquid does not polymerize until it comes into contact with the initiator, dibenzoyl peroxide, which is mixed in with the powder. There is a sufficient amount of the initiator in the powder to overcome the presence of the hydroquinone inhibitor in the liquid so that polymerization will begin. In addition to the initiator, the powder is composed mainly of PMMA or a blend of PMMA polymer with a copolymer of either PMMA and polystyrene or PMMA and methacrylic acid, depending on the grade and manufacturer of the cement. The copolymers are used to provide more toughness to the cement. Finally, there is a radiopaque material, either $BaSO_4$ or ZrO_2, which allows the cement to be visualized on radiographs. Compositions for several commonly used cements are presented in Table 6. Molecular weights of the different constituents are presented in Table 7.

Note that the polydispersity, M_w / M_n, of the polymers are high, indicating a broad range of molecular weights in both the powder as received and in the final mixed and set form.

There are 2 basic types of cement viscosity available: doughy (high viscosity) cement and injectable (low viscosity) cement. A doughy cement has a high viscosity almost from the instant of mixing and cannot be easily delivered with a mechanical device such as a cement gun. In contrast, the injectable cements have several minutes between the time of mixing and the time of hardening where viscosity is low enough so that the cement can be mixed with a vacuum mixer or centrifuge and delivered by a cement gun. The properties of the cement are dictated and controlled by varying the molecular weight and its distributions.

Once the polymerization process begins, the methylmethacrylate monomers are linked as the original carbon-to-carbon double bonds in methylmethacrylate are broken and new carbon-to-carbon single bonds are formed in the polymer chain. The heat given off during this process is 130 calories/g of methylmethacrylate monomer. The actual temperature rise, however, will be dictated by several factors including the actual amount of cement, heat transfer to surrounding areas, and the thickness of the cement. For instance, in the laboratory, a 3-mm thick section of cement around a femoral stem may provide a temperature rise to 60°C, while a 6-mm thick section may rise to over 100°C. These temperatures are high compared with the estimated 56°C that causes protein denaturation and the 47°C reported to cause bone necrosis. However, the actual in vitro bone cement temperatures have been reported to be as low as 40°C. This result and the general long-term success of cemented implants strongly indicate that thermal necrosis is not an important factor in the overall performance of the prosthesis.

Although there is still some discussion over the issue, it is common practice today to prepare the lower viscosity cements either using a vacuum mixing or centrifugation system to minimize the number of voids in the cement. It has been reported that the use of centrifugation or vacuum during mixing can reduce the porosity by greater than 50% over that of hand mixing. The mixing method exerts a definitive effect on the tensile properties and both vacuum

Table 5
Representative K_{1c} Values

Material	K_{1c} Mpam$^{1/2}$
Ti-6Al-4V	44–66
Nylon 6,6	3.5–4
Bone cement	1–2
Ultra High Molecular Weight Polyethylene	2–4

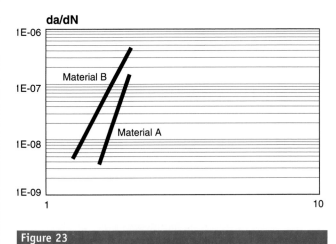

Figure 23

Crack growth/number of cycles versus change in stress intensity.

Table 6

Bone Cement Compositions

Component*		CMW-1	CMW-2	Palacos R	Simplex P	Zimmer Regular
Powder	Benzoyl Peroxide	2.6	2.2	.5–1.6	1.2	.75
	BaSO$_4$	9.1	10		10	10
	ZrO$_2$			14.9		
	PMMA	88.3	87.8		16.6	89.3
	PMMA/MA			83.5–84.7		
	PMMA/PS				82.3	
Liquid	MMA	98.7	98.1	97.9	97.5	97.3
	N,N' dimethyl toluidine	.4	1.0	2.1	2.5	2.7
	Hydroquinone (ppm)	15–20	15–20	64	75	75

* PMMA = polymethylmethacrylate; MMA = methylmethacrylate; MA = methacrylic acid; PS = polystyrene. All numeric values are expressed in wt%.

mixing and centrifugation lead to a mean 44% increase in ultimate tensile strength relative to hand-mixed cement. However, not all reports have duplicated these results and there are several instances where there is no apparent correlation between porosity and the mechanical properties. The differences in these results may lie in differences in cement, mixing technique, and testing method. Typical bone cement properties are provided in Table 8.

Differences in these values may be caused by differences in mixing methods (hand, vacuum, centrifuge), temperature (room temperature or 0°C), and postcuring times of samples before testing. The physical form of the cement may also be affected by these variables leading to different porosity levels and shrinkage of the cement.

Multiple investigations have examined the fracture toughness, K_c, for different cements. Different sample geometry and testing protocols prevent absolute comparisons between reported values. Toughness values, K_c, differ by a factor of 2.5. K_c values have been reported over a range of 1.03–1.55 MPam$^{1/2}$ for Simplex P; 1.18 to 1.41 MPam$^{1/2}$ for Zimmer Regular; and 1.96 to 2.32 MPam$^{1/2}$ for Palacos.

Bone cement properties may also be altered by the addition of antibiotics during the mixing process. The diffusion of the antibiotic to surrounding tissue is dictated by the chemistry and surface area of the cement as well as the manner in which the cement is prepared prior to delivery into the patient. For instance, all else being equal, the diffusion of gentamycin from Simplex or CMW cements has been reported to be much less than that from Palacos. Although there have been a few reports where the mechanical properties of the cement have been reduced with the addition of antibiotics, in general, therapeutic levels of antibiotics can be added to the cement without any measurable reduction of properties.

The performance of cement has been enhanced by improved protocols in cement handling, bone preparation, and cement delivery. The protocol improvements have been placed into 3 different generations. The protocols for

Table 7

Molecular Weight of Typical Bone Cement Mixture

	Monomer	Powder	After Curing
M_n	100	44,000	51,000
M_w	100	198,000	242,000

each generation of cement use are provided in Table 9. This table illustrates the importance of considering both materials and handling factors in the determination of the overall performance of a polymeric system.

Polymeric Bearing Materials

Since the advent of total hip replacements, relatively few polymeric materials have actually been used in total joint replacements. In 1936, Judet introduced PMMA as the first synthetic polymeric material used as a replacement for the femoral head. However, the press-fit acrylic devices became loose and were not extensively used.

Charnley originally chose polytetrafluoroethylene (PTFE) as a bearing material sometime between 1956 and 1958, based on its general chemical inertness and low coefficient of friction. The actual PTFE materials used were Fluon G1 and Fluon G2, products of Imperial Chemical Industries (not Teflon). There were also design issues surrounding these PTFE-based devices. PTFE was first used to make what is now termed a surface replacement prostheses. The femoral head was covered with a "cup" of PTFE and the acetabulum was lined with another layer of PTFE, making a PTFE against PTFE wear couple. A procedure that replaced the femoral head and neck with a metal femoral stem and metal 42-mm ball to articulate against the PTFE cup was developed next, followed by the introduction of the 22.225-mm metal femoral head and the use of acrylic bone cement for fixation of both the femoral stem and the acetabular cup. The wear of PTFE against a stainless steel head in this prosthesis provided 7 to 10 mm of linear wear in less than 3 years. These clinical failures were attributed to creep deformation of PTFE resins and their relatively poor abrasive wear characteristics.

The first hips using UHMWPE as a bearing surface were implanted in the early 1960s. The UHMWPE family remains the material of choice as the bearing surface in total joint replacements today. However, there were many efforts to test other polymers in the 1970s and 1980s in the hopes of finding a material with better wear properties or lower cost than UHMWPE. Very few of these materials, however, made it into actual clinical practice. Only PMMA, polyester, polyacetal, and carbon fiber-reinforced UHMWPE were used clinically to any significant extent.

As mentioned earlier, PMMA was used to fabricate the Judet hip prosthesis. The PMMA was cast and then shaped into a replacement for a femoral head. This device was used for a short period because of rapid wear of the PMMA, poor fixation, and generally poor results.

The 3 most notable efforts to use polymers other than UHMWPE involved the use of polyacetal (in the Christiansen hip), polyester and Poly II (a carbon fiber-reinforced UHMWPE used in acetabular cups), and tibial and patellar components in total knee replacements.

Polyacetal, sometimes called polymethylene oxide, had the potential advantages of higher yield strength, higher crystallinity, and ease of manufacturing in comparison to UHMWPE. It is important to note that this device was different from current hip prostheses in both design and materials. The 37-mm head in this device was mounted on a trunnion with an interposed polyacetal sleeve. This arrangement allowed the femoral ball to rotate relative to the stem. Polyacetal was also used to make the acetabular cup. This design provided 2 metal/polyacetal bearing surfaces. It is estimated that over 20,000 devices containing Delrin polyacetal were implanted from 1970 to 1986. The early results were sufficiently positive that in 1977 the FDA considered reclassifying the Christiansen hip from the most demanding class III regulatory category to the less demanding class II device category. However, by the mid to late 1980s, several groups reported significantly higher rates of revision of these devices and found that the wear was, in fact, over 7 times higher than for the Charnley prostheses. Polyacetal is still in orthopaedic use today, it is the common material used in the production of the colored trial components used to check the fit of the prosthesis during surgery.

Table 8
Range of Reported Bone Cement Mechanical Properties

Property	Range	% Variation
Tensile strength	23–45 MPa	89
Modulus	1.1–4.1 GPa	273
Elongation to break	.8–2.5%	213

Table 9
Generations of Bone Cement Application

First Generation	Second Generation	Third Generation
Hand mix with spatula	Hand mix with spatula and place into cement cartridge	Vacuum or centrifuge mixing
Leave cancellous bone	Remove cancellous bone near endosteal surface	Remove cancellous bone near endosteal surface
Vent femoral canal	Distal cement restrictor	Distal cement restrictor
Minimal canal preparation	Brush, pulsatile irrigation	Brush, pulsatile lavage
Irrigate and suction canal	Irrigate, pack and dry canal	Irrigate, pulsatile lavage, pack with adrenaline soak sponge, dry
Manual insertion at dough stage	Cement gun injection	Cement gun injection and pressurization
Manual position of stem to neutral	Manual position of stem	Distal and proximal centralizers
Femoral stem shapes with high stress transmission to interface	Improved stem shapes	Surface texturing and coating of femoral stem

Polyester was also used in another trunnion-bearing total hip prosthesis designed and implanted in the early 1970s. Polyester was apparently chosen for its ease of manufacture and its success in some industrial bearing applications. This device had stem and neck geometry similar to the Charnley except it had a 32-mm femoral ball made of polyester. Like the Christiansen hip, the femoral head was free to rotate on the femoral neck as well as the acetabular component. The polyester devices were soon abandoned because they showed progressive bone resorption in a 3- to 4-year time period.

Ultra High Molecular Weight Polyethylene

Polyethylene is, chemically, the simplest organic polymer possible. Depending on the conditions of polymerization, different types of polyethylene can be prepared as seen in Figure 24. The distinctions between the polyethylene types are due to molecular weight differences and the extent and type of branching (side chains to the backbone of the polymer) present. Each type of polyethylene has a very different set of properties and common uses. The material used in orthopaedics, UHMWPE, has often been incorrectly called high density polyethylene in the literature. Table 10 presents a comparison of properties of UHMWPE versus high density polyethylene. Note that differences in molecular weight are reflected in differences in density, impact strength, and abrasive wear. Although the difference in density values is only .007 to .02 g/cc, this is a meaningful difference for polyethylene materials. For comparison, low density polyethylene has density values that range from .925 to .935g/cc. UHMWPE has a density value closer to that of low density polyethylene than high density polyethylene. UHMWPE has a much higher molecular weight, significantly higher impact strength and toughness, and better abrasive wear characteristics than high density polyethylene.

Nomenclature Several different polyethylene resins and methods of tibial bearing manufacture have been used during the last 3 decades. These resins differ predominantly in the average molecular weight and the presence of the antioxidant calcium stearate. The names of the resins have also changed over the last 5 years, and it is becoming more difficult to identify the actual resin that is being used (Table 11).

Prior to 1998, Hoechst used a naming system that indicated the source of the powder, presence or absence of calcium stearate, and molecular weight. The first digit of the resin name was either a 1 or 4 depending if the material was synthesized in the Germany or Texas manufacturing facility, respectively. The second digit was either 0, indicating the absence of calcium stearate, or 1, indicating the addition of calcium stearate. The third digit was either 2 corresponding to a lower average molecular weight grade, or 5 corresponding to the higher molecular grade. However, since 1998, the first digit is 1 regardless of the origin of the powder.

Historically, RCH1000 was the name specifically used for compression molded 412GUR resin sheet made in Europe. RCH1000 was used extensively in Europe mostly for producing machined components such as the Charnley acetabular cup.

There are 3 different methods by which UHMWPE resin is formed into a device. The first method is to extrude the resin under heat and pressure to form a bar of UHMWPE and then machine the bar into the final form (ram extrusion). The second method is to compression mold the resin into a sheet of UHMWPE and then machine the component from the sheet. The third method is to directly mold the resin into the finished part (met-shape or direct molding). In the direct molding process, it is often common to machine the backs, or locking features, of the inserts, but the articular surfaces are not machined.

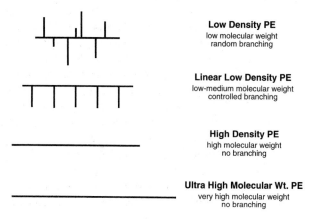

Low Density PE
low molecular weight
random branching

Linear Low Density PE
low-medium molecular weight
controlled branching

High Density PE
high molecular weight
no branching

Ultra High Molecular Wt. PE
very high molecular weight
no branching

Figure 24

Types of polyethylene (PE).

Table 10
High Density Polyethylene and UHMWPE* Properties

Property	High Density Polyethylene	UHMWPE	Units
Molecular weight	50,000–100,000	> 2,000,000	
Density	.952–.965	.930–.945	g/cc
Melting point	130–137	125–135	°C
Tensile yield	26.2–33.1	19.3–21	MPa
Tensile modulus	.9–1.6	.8–1.0	GPa
Elongation @ break	10–2200	200–350	%
Impact strength	.4–4.0	> 20, no break	ft-lb/in

* UHMWPE, Ultra high molecular weight polyethylene

Sterilization Since its commercial availability in the late 1960s, the dominant method for the sterilization of UHMWPE components has been gamma irradiation from a Co^{60} source. Although it has been known for some time that UHMWPE oxidizes after gamma sterilization, it wasn't until the connection between polyethylene debris and osteolysis was suggested in 1988 that oxidation effects on the performance of UHMWPE became a topic of major interest. Postirradiation oxidation of UHMWPE adversely affects the properties of UHMWPE as it increases the modulus, decreases the elongation to break, and decreases fracture toughness of the material. Oxidation is characterized by loss of molecular weight, an increase in the density and often, the introduction of oxygen-containing moieties into the polymer. The extent of oxidation is determined by the dose of irradiation received and the environment in which the irradiated component is subjected. Postirradiation aging "on the shelf" appears to be more extensive and chemically different from any oxidation that occurs in vivo.

In brief, oxidation is a process that causes chemical changes in the UHMWPE. The process is initiated by the gamma radiation used during sterilization. The gamma rays break either carbon-hydrogen (C-H) or carbon-carbon (C-C) bonds, which results in the formation of free radicals (atoms with an unpaired electron) that can then react further. These free radicals undergo one of three reaction pathways: (1) recombination, (2) chain scission, or (3) cross-linking. Each pathway has different consequences. Recombination simply reforms the bonds that were broken and provides no net change in chemistry.

In chain scission, a fragment of the polymer chain is removed from the original polymer chain. This process is driven by the presence of oxygen, which reacts readily with free radicals resulting in loss of molecular weight of the original polymer chain. The progressive loss of molecular weight in this manner results in a material that is more like high density polyethylene.

With cross-linking, 2 radicals from different polymer sections combine to form chemical bonds between 2 polymer chains. A cross-linked polymer may be harder and more abrasion-resistant than its non-cross-linked precursor. However, extremely high levels of cross-links may result in the material becoming extremely brittle.

Oxidation and Polyethylene Quality In addition to the chemical and physical property changes, oxidation has also been associated with the quality of the UHMWPE. There have been reports of "defects" found in UHMWPE devices. These "defects" are poorly consolidated particles of UHMWPE that can be seen in cross sections of aged implants as seen in Figure 25. In some extreme cases, the nonconsolidated particles are easily visible in the component by the unaided eye. Another feature found within postirradiation aged polyethylene components is a subsurface white band seen when components are divided into thin cross sections. These white bands are caused by the microtoming procedure and are typically 1 to 2 mm below the surface of the polyethylene and often closely follow the surface contours of the components (Fig. 26). The material in these white bands exhibits high density values and high levels of carbonyl-containing species, which is consistent with high oxidative damage. The high oxidative damage caused by postirradiation aging embrittles the polyethylene. The maximum oxidation generally occurs between .5 and 1.5 mm below the surface of the component. The white bands are formed during microtome sectioning because the material has oxidized to the point of embrittlement. The polyethylene then fractures as the sample is being cut.

The formation of nonconsolidated particles and white bands is a time-dependent process that occurs because UHMWPE continues to oxidize after gamma irradiation in air. These post-irradiation changes, as reflected by density measurements, continue to increase for as long as 13 years. At shelf life times of greater than 4 years post gamma sterilization, it is common for the polyethylene to have high oxidation levels, nonconsolidated particles, subsurface white bands and be embrittled. Figure 27 shows the increase in density, as a result of progressive oxidation, with postirradiation time for extruded 4150HP polyethylene gamma irradiated in air.

The level of degradation due to postirradiation may be altered in 2 ways. The first is to use a nonirradiation sterilization method such as ethylene oxide or gas plasma. These nonirradiation methods provide surface sterilization without forming the free radicals that lead to oxidative degradation. However, nonirradiation methods also do not provide any cross-linking of the polyethylene, which is known to reduce wear. The second method is to conduct the irradia-

Table 11
*Ultra High Molecular Weight Polyethylene Resin Designations**

Supplier	Name	Production Location	Calcium Stearate Added
Ticona	4150HP	USA	Yes
	4050HP	USA	No
	4120HP	USA	Yes
	4020HP	USA	No
	1150HP	Germany	Yes
	1050HP	Germany	No
	1120HP	Germany	Yes
	1020HP	Germany	No
Montel	1900	USA	Yes and no

*   Resins ending with "50" have average molecular weights of ~ 4-6 million

Resins ending with "20" have average molecular weights of ~ 2-4 million

For 1900, the presence of calcium stearate is not reflected in the resin name

tion in an environment with no oxygen present. This would include packaging the polyethylene in a vacuum or in an inert atmosphere such as nitrogen or argon. Irradiation in the absence of oxygen will minimize degradation and maximize cross-linking. To illustrate this, the hip simulation wear rates for cups sterilized by ethylene oxide, gamma irradiation in air, and gamma irradiation in a vacuum are 71, 51 and 35 mg/million cycles, respectively. This decreasing order of wear rates mirrors the increasing level of cross-linking.

Postirradiation aging continues due to the presence of free radicals. These radicals, however, may be quenched by treating the irradiated polyethylene with heat. For instance, melting the polyethylene for 5 hours after irradiation quenches the radicals to the point where subsequent shelf aging will no longer occur. However, as will be discussed below, these quenching treatments can also adversely affect mechanical properties.

Oxidation of UHMWPE may play an important role in surface damage of knees. There is a strong correlation between oxidation level in the polyethylene and tibial surface damage modes involving pitting and delamination. Minimizing oxidation may minimize these types of damage mechanisms, which can sometimes be catastrophic.

Crystallinity As discussed in an earlier section, the crystallinity of the polymer can significantly effect properties. Table 12 illustrates the effect of altering the crystallinity of one type UHMWPE resin from 50% to 68%. Table 12 provides some properties of the same UHMWPE material whose crystallinity has been altered by the use of pressure, temperature, and cooling rates to demonstrate the sole effect of crystallinity.

Cross-Linking Since the mid 1970s, it has been known that cross-linking UHMWPE can result in a very low wear rate. The current trend is to induce cross-linking by conducting the gamma sterilization in an oxygen-free environment (nitrogen, argon, or vacuum atmospheres). This reduces the wear rate of the resultant material. However, cross-linking also adversely affects fracture and fatigue properties so that in the final manufacturing process, there will be a balance between low wear and reduction of other physical proper-

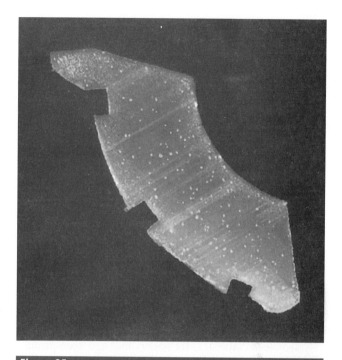

Figure 25

Nonconsolidated particles in cross-sectional view of postirradiation aged cup.

ties. In 1999, several companies have introduced a version of a cross-linked polyethylene with a density higher than that of commonly available materials. Although these materials are termed cross-linked polyethylene, these materials are different in the resins used, the manner in which the resin is formed into the device, and the irradiation and posttreatment conditions. The clinical consequences of these differences are not known.

In the past 3 years, there has been a renewed interest in the modification of existing UHMWPE materials by subjecting them to processes that involve either high doses of irradiation or chemical treatments. These processes modify the UHMWPE by forming "cross-links" within the polymer. This will be discussed in more detail in the following discussion. Cross-linking UHMWPE has been demonstrated to significantly lower hip simulator wear rates while adversely affecting other mechanical properties.

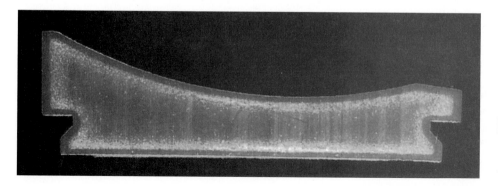

Figure 26

Subsurface white bands in cross-sectional view of post irradiation aged tibial insert.

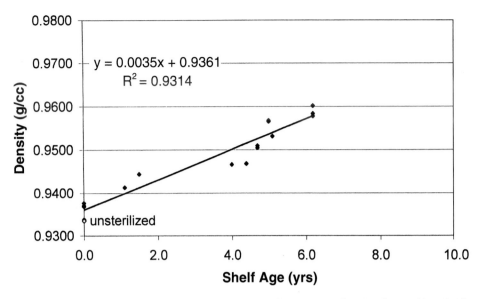

Figure 27

Oxidation rate for shelf aged extruded rod 4150.

Background: 1971–1996 The first clinical use of cross-linked UHMWPE was in 1971 when Oonishi implanted polyethylene acetabular components that had been irradiated with 100 Mrads of gamma irradiation. This dosage was determined by laboratory experiments where they studied the effect of gamma dosages on laboratory material property and wear tests. These laboratory wear rates were determined using a reciprocating "ball on flat" wear testing device. The metal ball had a diameter of 10 mm. A reciprocating stroke of 6 mm was applied at a frequency of 2 Hz and a load of 4.9 N. The test was conducted both dry and in water and terminated at 10,000 cycles. Under these conditions, it was found that the amount of polyethylene removed was a function of irradiation dose. Table 13 shows the volume loss as a function of irradiation dose. It can be seen that there was a large decrease in wear above 50 Mrads. There was an approximate 4-fold to 5-fold decrease in wear at 100 Mrads.

Additionally, they found the debris particles from the 200 Mrad treated samples to be smaller than those found in the nonirradiated control group. However, the collection of particles was not quantitative and it is not known what overall size distributions were present. However, it does raise the issue that although there is less debris from cross-linked UHMWPE, the size of the debris may be smaller and, in principle, may be more biologically active.

These cross-linked polymers were clinically used between 1971 and 1979. At that time, highly cross-linked polymers were part of a study where different stem designs and different metal materials were also being studied. In 1971, the SOM hip prosthesis, which was made from COP alloy (stainless steel with 20% Cobalt added) was developed. The femoral head was presumably made from this same alloy, but it is not explicitly identified in the literature. The polymeric cup was high density polyethylene (not UHMWPE) which had been gamma irradiated at 100 Mrads. A variation on this system was the Bioceram hip system which had an

alumina femoral head. All cups were cemented without metal shells. Table 14 provides a summary of the overall study.

The key findings are that there were much smaller differences between clinical wear rates of the high dose gamma irradiated cups and the control cups than found in the laboratory wear tests. In fact, the differences are not statistically significant between the 2 Bioceram groups in Table 14. Furthermore, the steady state wear rates of .072 and .076 mm/yr are not much lower than the .1 mm/yr wear rates for the best performing hip systems that do not use a cross-linked UHMWPE material. Oonishi recently reported that the wear rates were .06 mm/yr for his irradiated cups compared to .29 mm/yr on this same series. No explanation on the slight change in wear values was provided.

More recently, Wroblewski reported that, on average, cross-linked cups made with a different technology had

Table 12
*Effect of Crystallinity on Polyethylene Properties**

Property	UHMWPE Product Name			
	4150HP	Hylamer M	Hylamer	units
Crystallinity	50	57	68	%
Density	.934	.946	.955	g/cc
Melting point	135	147	149	°C
Modulus	1.0	2.0	2.5	GPa
Yield strength	23.3	26.5	28.6	MPa
Ultimate tensile strength	33.8	37.9	40.7	MPa

*   UHMWPE = Ultra high molecular weight polyethylene

clinically lower rates (.022 mm/yr) than the non-cross-linked cups (.07 mm/yr) in a very small series (19 cups). However, the method of cross-linking was not specifically provided and no information regarding the material was provided. It is generally believed that the material is a chemically cross-linked polyethylene with silanes used as the cross-linking moieties. Further, although the overall wear was low for the cross-linked cups, these cups demonstrated wear between .1 and .4 mm/yr during the first 1 to 2 years. After this time, they report no wear but the follow-up is not rigorous. It is difficult to provide any interpretation of this report without more details on the material and the longer term fate of these patients.

Current State of the Art In the mid 1990s, there was renewed interest in this technology and there are currently several methods that have been disclosed to cross-link UHMWPE to provide low wear rates. These methods are summarized in Table 15.

Characterizing Cross-Linked UHMWPE The extent of cross-linking is inferred through nondirect test methods such as extraction or polymer swell tests. The most common method of cross-link detection is through extraction tests. The principle in extraction test is that upon cross-linking, the amount of extractable material is reduced as the cross-links make it impossible for a molecule to be removed from the matrix. In cross-linking methods using more than 20 Mrads of irradiation, the amount of extractable material is zero.

Additional information can be obtained by determining the swell ratio of the material. This ratio provides the amount of a particular solvent that is "soluble" in the polymer at a given temperature. The more cross-links there are, the less solvent the material can absorb. Thus, as cross-linking goes up, the swell ratio goes down.

Wear The wear of cross-linked UHMWPE in both pin-on-disk and hip simulation tests can be significantly reduced from non-cross-linked material. The wear rate is dependent upon the level of cross-linking. When the irradiation does is greater than 20 Mrads, the hip simulator wear rate is immeasurable.

In addition to the early work of Oonishi, Grobbellar also used 15 Mrads of high density polyethylene and reduced the wear by 30% in a sand slurry abrasion test. Later, Rose found that cross-linking polyethylene by either molding high density polyethylene in the presence of peroxide or increasing the gamma irradiation dose from 2.5 to 5 Mrads, provided more wear resistant materials. It should also be noted that there are a few reports such as that of Streicher that showed that the wear resistance decreased after high dosage electron beam treatments up to 30 Mrads. This provides a good reminder that the method of testing can greatly influence the outcome of these wear tests and care should be taken to ensure that the evaluation tests are as representative as possible of the clinical situation.

It is interesting to note that Oonishi did not see the same magnitude of wear benefit in patients that he did in his laboratory wear tests. It is also important to point out in this light, that the current cross-linking methods may not have the same benefit as found in hip simulators. Oonishi's data only reports average wear rates and does not indicate standard deviations or if any of the cross-linked UHMWPE had higher wear rates than expected.

Table 13
Volume Loss as a Function of Irradiation Dose

Irradiation (Mrads)	Volume Loss Dry ($\times 10^{-3}$ mm^3)	Volume Loss Wet ($\times 10^{-3}$ mm^3)
0	17.60	17.03
50	14.10	12.28
100	3.23	4.21
150	3.87	3.05
200	2.21	2.66

Table 14
Study of Stem Designs and Metal Materials

Design	Femoral Head Metal	Irradiation (Mrads)	Initial Wear (mm/year)	Steady Wear	n
SOM	COP alloy*	100	.15	.076	19
T-28	Stainless steel	none	.37	.247	15
Bioceram	Alumina	none	.10	.098	71
Bioceram	Alumina	100	.072	.072	9

* COP alloy = stainless steel with 20% Cobalt added

Physical and Chemical Properties The physical properties, modulus, yield, elongation to break, creep, and fracture of cross-linked UHMWPE can be significantly changed due to irradiation or postirradiaton treatments. Table 16 presents the changes in properties with one particular cross-link treatment.

Table 17 demonstrates the changes in modulus and yield strength as a function of irradiation dose and posttreatment. The posttreatment was conducted to quench the free radicals formed during the irradiation process. The treatment involved melting the cross-linked UHMWPE for 5 hours.

The modulus always decreased after stabilization, but not all differences were statistically significant. The yield stress was consistently lower after stabilization ($p < .05$).

Fracture Toughness Figure 28 shows a plot of selected J integral curves for gamma in air-sterilized, melt-stabilized samples. All irradiated samples demonstrated a drop in fracture toughness over unirradiated controls. This indicates that the amount of energy to propagate a crack in cross-linked UHMWPE materials can be lower than the amount of energy to propagate the same crack length in a non-cross-linked material.

In summary, different forms of UHMWPE have been in clinical use since the early 1970s. However, their clinical performance was not as good as expected based on laboratory wear data.

In the 1990s, cross-linked UHMWPE products are irradiated at a much lower dose than the earlier treatments and usually involve a posttreatment to quench free radicals generated during the irradiation process. Although low laboratory wear can be achieved via cross-linking, yield, elongation to break, and fracture toughness properties are also reduced. It remains to be seen if this newest generation of cross-linked UHMWPE can provide an overall patient benefit.

Poly II

In the late 1970s, an effort to reduce creep (cold flow) and decrease wear of UHMWPE led to the development of a composite of carbon fibers and UHMWPE. This composite, Poly II, was made by directly molding the fibers and polyethylene powder into tibial inserts, patellas, and acetabular components. The addition of carbon fibers increased compressive yield strength, flexural yield strength, tensile properties, and creep resistance. However, these carbon-reinforced materials were found to have lower fatigue resistance compared to UHMWPE and suffered from manufacturing problems associated with incomplete molding. Surface damage scores of Poly II components were also higher than those of unreinforced UHMWPE components. Its use was discontinued approximately 7 years after its introduction into the marketplace.

Table 15
Cross-Linking Methods

Cross-Link Source	Environments	Dose (Mrads)	Posttreatments
Gamma	Air	5–10	None
	Nitrogen	5–10	50°–150°C for 5–10 hours
	Vacuum	5–10	50°–150°C for 5–10 hours
Electron beam	Air	5–10	None
	Nitrogen	5–10	50°–150°C for 5–10 hours
	Heat (melt)	5–10	50°–150°C for 5–10 hours

Table 16
Changes in Properties

Property	Unirradiated Control	20 Mrad Irradiation	% change
Modulus (GPa)	941	201	-78
Ultimate tensile strength (MPa)	46	15	-67
Yield (MPa)	23	14	-39
Elongation (%)	954	547	-42
Hardness	66	55	-17

Resorbable Polymers

The final polymer type to be discussed is bioresorbable polymers. The terms biodegradable and bioresorbable are often used interchangeably and in orthopaedic applications have the same meaning. These are polymers synthesized so that they will degrade chemically and physically over time.

Bioresorbable polymers are desirable in orthopaedic applications for several reasons. They may be used to provide immediate primary fixation or support as a suture, screw, anchor, or pin and then resorb once the tissue is healed, alleviating the need for a second surgical procedure to remove the device. Resorbable polymers may also be used as the support matrix for drug delivery. A drug mixed into a resorbable polymer matrix would be released as the polymer degrades.

A bioresorbable polymer must be strong enough at implantation for its intended use. The rate of degradation must be appropriate for either providing support for a sufficient length of time or releasing the drug at an appropriate rate and time. In addition, the bioresorbable polymer and its degradation products must be biocompatible.

The main types of resorbable polymers used in orthopaedics today are presented in Table 18. They include variations of polylactic acid (PLA), polyglycolic acid (PGA), polydioxanone (PDS), and polycaprolactone (PCL).

The properties of resorbable polymers are not easily provided, as they can span an enormously large range (eg, modulus values from .1–30 MPa and strength values from 3 to 290 MPa). These properties are a function of the type of polymer, copolymers, mixtures, molecular weights, fabrication, and reinforcing materials used.

Table 17
Average Modulus and Yield Stress Values

Post treatment	Irradiation Dose (Mrads)	Average Modulus		Average Yield	
		Not Treated	Quenched	Not Treated	Quenched
Gamma in air irradiated	2.5	939	740	23.5	20.7
	10	975	874	23.4	20.6
	20	1,015	749	23.7	19.6
	50	1,219	711	24.0	18.0
	100	1,056	663	24.6	17.6
Electron beam sterilized	2.5	952	834	23.2	20.0
	10	986	874	23.8	20.2
	20	1,003	7.3	24.1	19.3
	50	1,087	n/a	24.9	n/a

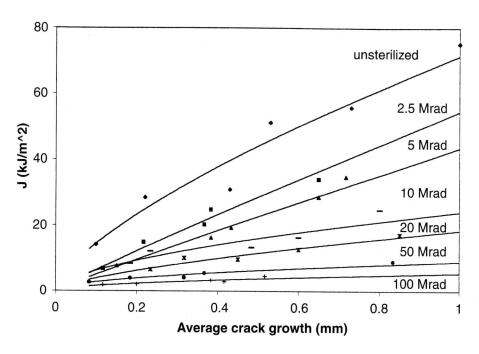

Figure 28
Plot of selected J integral curves for gamma in air-sterilized, melt-stabilized samples.

Table 18

Resorbable Polymers Used in Orthopaedics

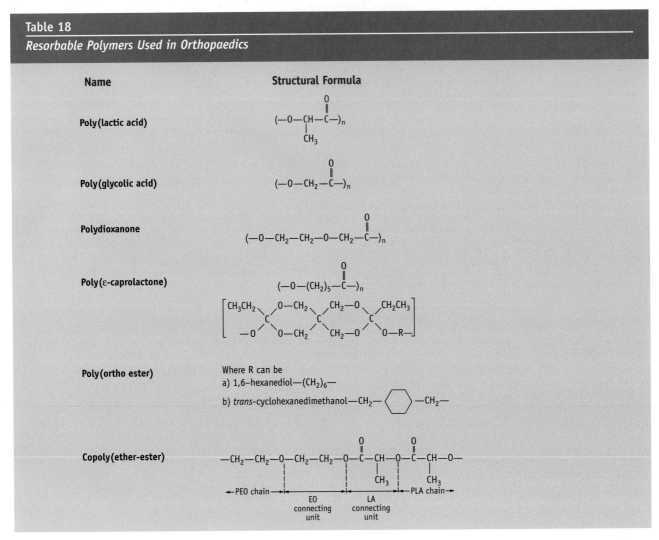

Name	Structural Formula
Poly(lactic acid)	
Poly(glycolic acid)	
Polydioxanone	
Poly(ε-caprolactone)	
Poly(ortho ester)	
Copoly(ether-ester)	

The 2 most common resorbable polymers used are derivatives of PLA and PGA. Lactic acid and glycolic acid differ by 1 hydrogen atom per monomer.

$$\begin{array}{c} COOH \\ | \\ H-C-R \\ | \\ CH_3 \end{array}$$

When R = H it is glycolic acid, and when R = CH$_3$ it is lactic acid. However, this subtle change provided significant differences in degradation rates, physical properties, and biologic activity.

One of the key differences is that lactic acid has a chiral center. As discussed previously, this is a central carbon atom with 4 different groups around it. One enantiomer is the D (dextrorotatory) and other the L (levorotatory) form, indicating the direction in which a sample rotates plane-polarized light. If a polymer is made from D lactic acid, then the polymer is designated poly-D-lactic acid (PDLA). Similarly, it is termed poly-L-lactic acid (PLLA) if it is made from L lactic acid. Figure 29 compares the structures of PDLA and PLLA. A polymer that contains a combination of both D and

L monomers is a PDLLA. All of these forms of material have appeared in the orthopaedic literature.

PLA has long been considered a desirable choice as the basis for a bioresorbable polymer because the degradation product is lactic acid, a "natural" Krebs cycle constituent that is already present. However, the form of the lactic acid (D or L) and the high concentration of lactic acid released to the surrounding region of the device may nonetheless present biocompatibility problems. Care should be exercised in oversimplifying the material aspect of these devices.

The final properties of the polymer are dependent on the monomers used, the molecular weight, and the manner in which the polymers are fabricated into the final device.

Table 19 illustrates the effect of molecular weight of PDLLA on resorption rates as expressed by mass loss. It should also be noted that mechanical properties often decrease faster than the mass loss rate. It is likely, in most of these cases, that there is virtually no strength left in these materials in just a 2- to 3-week period.

The use of heat during any fabrication process for a resorbable polymer presents difficulties because heat causes degradation of these materials. Table 20 demonstrates the effect of processing on the molecular weight of a resorbable PLLA polymer after molding at 200°C and 6.9 MPa. Note that the molecular weight decreases and the polydispersity changes. The final properties of a device made in this manner are substantially different from those of the starting PLLA polymer.

Ceramics

Ceramic materials are most commonly solid, inorganic compounds consisting of metallic and nonmetallic elements held together by ionic or covalent bonding. Ceramics include compounds such as silica (SiO_2), formed from oxygen (a nonmetallic element) and silicon (an element that falls along the boundary between metals and nonmetals), and alumina (Al_2O_3), formed from a nonmetallic and a metallic element. As with metals, ceramics have tightly packed atomic structures that are dictated by requirements of spatial coordination for covalent bonds and of charge neutrality for ionic bonds.

Ceramic materials are very stiff and brittle. When processed appropriately to high purity, they possess excellent biocompatibility (a function of their insolubility and chemical inertness) and exceptional wear resistance (with hard, hydrophilic surfaces). The brittle nature of ceramics limits their use in high load demand applications.

In orthopaedics, ceramics have gained favor as biomaterials for 2 quite different applications. The first involves their use in total joint replacement components as fully dense ceramics, such as alumina and zirconia, that possess inertness and high wear resistance superior to those of metallic alloys. The second involves the use of ceramics as bone graft substitutes and as coatings for metallic implants of less dense (even porous) ceramics, such as calcium phosphate and bioglass (SiO_2-Na_2O-CaO-P_2O_5), that are osteoconductive, providing surfaces to which bone will bond. The success and the limitations of ceramics in these applications can be understood by considering their bonding, structure, and properties.

Ionic and Covalent Bonding

Ceramics are typically 3-dimensional arrays of positively charged metal ions and negatively charged nonmetal ions, often oxygen. Positively charged ions formed from elements that readily release outer electrons and negatively charged ions formed from elements that readily accept electrons in their outer atomic shells are strongly attracted to one another by coulombic forces. Positively charged ions surround themselves with as many negatively charged ions as possible, and vice versa, resulting in a closely packed arrangement of strongly bonded nuclei for which the total charge is zero. This localization of the sharing of electrons between nuclei makes most ceramics excellent insulators, both electrical and thermal.

Other ceramic materials are held together by covalent bonds. Covalent bonds are formed through the mutual sharing of electrons between adjacent atoms so that the shared electrons complete the outer valence shell of each atom. As with materials that are ionically bonded, materials that are covalently bonded are also good insulators. The potential high strength of covalent bonds can be understood by considering diamond, a material composed of only covalently bonded carbon atoms.

Ceramic Microstructures

Most ceramic materials have polygranular microstructures similar to metals and metallic alloys. As with metals, the properties of ceramics are dictated to a large extent by the characteristics of the microstructure, including the grain size, the phases and their distribution within each grain, and porosity. The microstructures of ceramic materials result from the thermal processing used to produce them.

Table 19
Effect of PDLLA Molecular Weight on Rate of Mass Loss

Molecular Weight, Mw	% Mass Loss	Time Period
5,200	50	8 weeks
89,000	21	48 weeks
199,000	15	
266,000	10	
294,000	7	

PDLLA=poly-dextrorotatory-levorotatory lactic acid

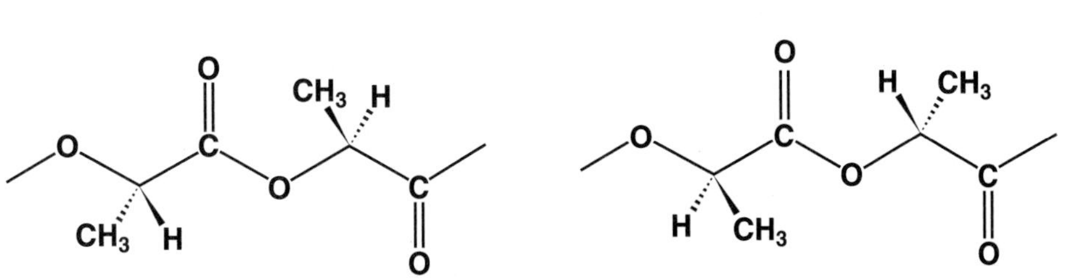

Figure 29

29 D- and L-forms of polylactic acid.

And again as with metals, the microstructure can be significantly altered by thermal processing techniques.

A common technique for fabricating ceramic materials is to mix fine particulates of the material with water and an organic binder and press them into a mold of the desired shape. The resulting part is dried by heating to evaporate the water and burn away the binder. The part is then fired or sintered at a much higher temperature. This process results in densification as the particles come into close contact driven by mechanisms such as diffusion, evaporation, and condensation that reduce the total surface energy in the part. As with the casting of metallic alloys, the resulting microstructure (and therefore properties) of the ceramic part will depend on the control of key variables in the processing. For example, strength is inversely proportional to both grain size and porosity. Grain size can be controlled by the starting size of the particles used to form the part; the smaller the particles, the smaller the grain size. However, grain size will increase during processing with longer sintering times. Porosity, on the other hand, will be reduced by longer sintering times. A trade-off exists, therefore, in choosing appropriate processing procedures to create a ceramic with the desired properties.

Alumina

Aluminum oxide (Al_2O_3) has excellent abrasion resistance and when highly polished creates a very low coefficient of friction surface articulating against both UHMWPE and itself.

Because of the excellent wettability of an alumina surface, better lubrication of the surface is possible. Wettability can be assessed through contact angle measurements, most commonly performed by placing a liquid drop on the surface and measuring the angle between the plane of the surface and a line tangent to the edge of the liquid drop where it intersects the surface. The contact angle for alumina is about 45°, in comparison to those of polyethylene and metallic alloys (stainless steel and cobalt alloy), which are in the range of 70° to 85°.

Because of its excellent wear resistance, alumina has gained favor as a material for femoral heads of total hip replacements. Because of its brittle nature, it is not used for the stem portion of the component; instead, alumina femoral heads are attached to metallic stems through a taper connection. Early clinical experience showed fracture of alumina femoral heads to be a significant complication, with an incidence of more than 5% in some reported series. Improvements and standardization in alumina processing, including refinement of the grain size and hot isostatical pressing of the material after sintering to further densify the material, and in manufacturing taper connections have led to a dramatic improvement in performance. Grain sizes for alumina, for example, typically exceeded 4 μ in the 1970s with densities of about 4 g/mm^3; grain sizes are now maintained at about 0.5 μ with densities of about 6 g/mm^3. The resulting refinement creates a 45% increase in strength.

Typical properties for alumina are given in Table 21. Because alumina is chemically inert, biocompatibility is excellent. However, recent reports of periprosthetic osteolysis secondary to alumina debris reinforce the concern that small particles ingested by cells can elicit an adverse biologic reaction regardless of their chemical nature.

Zirconia

Zirconium oxide (ZrO_2) is also used for femoral heads of total joint replacements, again because of its ability to create a low friction, wear resistant surface against UHMWPE. Unlike alumina, which relies on purity for its excellent properties, zirconia in pure form is unstable, changing phases between tetragonal, monoclinic, and cubic arrangements of molecules. The phase changes result in large volume changes that affect the mechanical properties considerably, often leading to internal cracks within the material. To avoid the instability and maintain the tetragonal phase (the toughest of the 3 phases), zirconia is stabilized (typically with yttrium oxide) to maintain the tetragonal phase.

To prevent detrimental transformations from occurring

Table 20
Effects of Manufacturing Processes on PLLA Molecular Weight

	Molecular Weight M_w	Average Molecular Weight M_n	Polydispersity M_w / M_n
Start	48,000	27,000	1.78
After molding in vacuum	30,400	11,400	2.67
After molding in air	26,900	9,300	2.89

Table 21
Properties of Orthopaedic Ceramics*

Property	Alumina	Zirconia
Strength (MPa)	580	900
Grain size (μ)	≤ 1.8	≤ 0.5
Density (g/cc)	3.98	6.0
Elastic modulus (GPa)	380	210

*   Data obtained from Heros RJ, Willmann G: Ceramics in total hip arthroplasty. *Semin Arthroplasty* 1998;9:114–122.

during the sterilization process, zirconia implants are often sterilized by exposure to ethylene oxide, a room temperature process. Resterilization at the time of operation of zirconia femoral head components for total hip replacement has been shown to lead to surface roughening. The elevated temperatures cause a phase transformation that results in the roughening and the possibility of increased wear on the opposing polyethylene acetabular component.

Tougher than alumina with a much smaller grain size (less than half a micron), zirconia has found clinical use as an alternative bearing material to metallic alloys for articulating against UHMWPE. Zirconia does not, however, wear well against itself or against other ceramics such as alumina.

Bioceramics and Glasses

The second application of ceramic materials is in the area of bone substitute materials. Certain ceramic and glass materials have been found to be osteophilic in nature, such that osteoblasts form bone with the mineral phase in direct contact with the ceramic surface. The chemical or physical bond that forms between the ceramic and the bone is not well understood, but results in sufficient interfacial strength that applications such as ceramic coatings on implants have been used in an attempt to improve implant fixation to bone. Most applications of bioceramics are aimed at the eventual resorption or removal of the bioceramic through substitution with remodeled bone.

The mineral phase of bone is hydroxyapatite, a calcium phosphate $(Ca_{10}[PO_4]_6[OH]_2)$. The stability of calcium phosphate ceramics depends on the temperature and the environment, and can be affected by substitution (for example, of a carbonate for a phosphate). Hydroxyapatite coatings for fixation of load-bearing implants have been in clinical use for more than a decade, though the true composition of these coatings can be quite variable because of differences in manufacturing processes and changes with time in vivo. Studies of coatings on retrieved implants show that the coatings are often osteoconductive, but bonding with bone is not uniform and the coatings themselves may not in fact be true hydroxyapatite, but a mixture of phases, including calcium oxide, tricalcium phosphate, and amorphous calcium phosphate. Coatings have been shown to dissolve and fracture from the implant substrate, as well as to be removed by an osteoclastic remodeling process.

Hydroxyapatite cements (either alone or in combination with PMMA bone cement) have also been developed. Injectable cements that cure isothermally to an apatite similar to that in bone and with a strength comparable to cancellous bone have been tested in animal models and are in clinical trials. The cement appears to maintain its strength as it is remodeled, making it a candidate bone graft material.

Bioactive glasses are based typically on combinations of SiO_2, CaO, NaO, and P_2O_5. These materials partially solubilize in vivo, forming a surface hydrogel that is rich in calcium and phosphate ions. Crystallization leads to the formation of apatite and thus a bond with the bone. The brittleness and inherent stability of these materials restrict their use to nonstructural applications such as coatings and fillers.

Materials for Orthotics and Prosthetics

Orthoses are constructed from polymers and metals with a single device often being made from a combination of both types of materials. The metals most suitable for orthotic fabrication are steel and aluminum alloys; the choice depends on the application. Steels are stronger and stiffer than aluminum alloys, but aluminum alloys are considerably lighter. A clinical example of this would be the upright of a lower extremity orthosis in which deformation under bending stresses is very important. The alignment of the patient's lower extremity, the patient's weight, and the patient's activity level, together with the loading pattern on the upright, are considered before selecting either a steel or an aluminum component.

The major advantage of steel in orthotics is its low cost, abundance, and relative ease of fabrication. Steel is fatigue-resistant and combines high strength with high rigidity or ductility depending on the alloy used. Steel is widely used in prefabricated joints, metal uprights, metal bands and cuffs, springs, and bearings. The main disadvantage of steel is its weight.

The main advantage of aluminum in orthotics is its high strength-to-weight ratio. Thus, aluminum is used whenever light weight is a major consideration, as in upper extremity orthoses. Aluminum does, however, have a lower fatigue strength than steel. Therefore, if high-magnitude, cyclic loading conditions are anticipated, steel is a better choice than aluminum.

Polymers play an important role in orthotics, with 2 major groups, thermoplastics and thermosets, both being used for orthotic design. Low temperature thermoplastics, those classified as requiring temperatures no higher than 80°C to become workable, may be molded directly to the body. These materials are popular for upper extremity applications in which the rapid provision of an assistive or protective orthosis is desirable. Minimal equipment is required: a source of hot water, scissors, and a heat gun. Low-temperature thermoplastics, however, are typically ineffective when high loads are anticipated because they are not very strong.

High-temperature thermoplastics require higher temperatures to become workable and are usually molded under vacuum to the prescribed shape of a plaster model prepared by the orthotist. Polyethylene and polypropylene are the most widely used high-temperature thermoplastics. Low-, medium-, and high-density polyethylenes are used, depending on the required mechanical properties. Low-density polyethylene is a good option for nonweightbearing applications, such as a supportive wrist and hand orthosis. High-density polyethylene is commonly used in spinal orthotic treatments where greater strength and elastic modulus are required. Polypropylene's unique flexing capability together with its excellent fatigue resistance is particularly useful for lower extremity orthotics. However, the plastic most often used for orthotic design is a copolymer of polyethylene and polypropylene. This copolymer is mostly polypropylene with 5% to 25% polyethylene and has much better fatigue resistance than either constituent polymer. The range of material properties possible with the copolymers together with the ability to alter structural properties by changing the shape and thickness of the device provides a very wide range of possible stiffnesses and strengths for orthotic designs.

The design of foot orthoses is an area in which the choice of materials is of paramount importance. Weight, for example, is important because of its effect on the moment of inertia of the lower extremity and thus on the amount of muscle power required to move the lower extremity. Shock absorption and comfort are required to relieve pain. If the function of the orthosis is to support, leather or felt with or without a more sturdy underliner are appropriate; if the function is to reduce shear force, a viscoelastic polymer may be used. Commonly, foot orthoses are required to cushion or absorb shock; closed-cell polyethylene foams and nitrogen-filled rubbers have proved successful. As is the case in most areas of prosthetic and orthotic design, clinical devices typically are manufactured from more than 1 material because the functional requirements demand varying characteristics from each component; for example, the diabetic patient with significant tissue loss and adherent scar tissue will require both shock absorption and reduction of shear.

Many of the most significant advances in prosthesis development have been related to new materials and the improved design features that they permit. Throughout the 19th century, prostheses designers used such readily available materials as leather, steel, tin, and wood to construct limbs. Today's wider selection of materials allows amputees to be fit with lightweight functional limbs constructed from thermoplastics, improved acrylic resins, titanium, graphite, and carbon fiber composites. The choice between an exoskeletal and an endoskeletal prosthesis should be made after reviewing the patient's lifestyle. The exoskeletal design provides strength via the hard laminated surface of the prosthesis; the endoskeletal system provides strength through a central pylon, which commonly is constructed of aluminum alloy or a graphite composite to give the patient a very strong, lightweight prosthesis. Cost and durability are advantages of the exoskeletal design. However, with the endoskeletal system it is possible to interchange modular components, to use soft cosmetic coverings, and to conveniently make alignment changes.

Typically only the socket of the prosthesis is custom fabricated; the other components are premanufactured in an array of sizes and varying levels of sophistication. Components and their materials are selected by the prosthetist to match the biomechanical and functional needs of each patient. Prosthetic sockets can be manufactured from either thermoplastic materials or fiber-reinforced thermosetting plastics. The use of thermoplastics for this important part of the prostheses has gained wider acceptance as both patient and prosthetist come to appreciate the advantages, including reduced manufacturing time.

Selected Bibliography

General

Black J (ed): *Orthopaedic Biomaterials in Research and Practice.* New York, NY, Churchill Livingstone, 1988.

Burstein AH, Wright TM (eds): *Fundamentals of Orthopaedic Biomechanics.* Baltimore, MD, Williams & Wilkins, 1994.

Frymoyer JW (ed): *Orthopaedic Knowledge Update 4: Home Study Syllabus.* Rosemont, IL, American Academy of Orthopaedic Surgeons, 1993.

Ratner BD, Hoffman AS, Schoen FJ, Lemons JE (eds): *Biomaterials Science: An Introduction to Materials in Medicine.* San Diego, CA, Academic Press, 1996.

Von Recum A, Jacobi JE (eds): *Handbook of Biomaterials Evaluation: Scientific, Technical and Clinical Testing of Implant Materials,* ed 2. Philadelphia, PA, Taylor & Francis, 1999.

Metals

American Society for Testing and Materials: *1998 ASTM Book of Standards, Volume 13.01 Medical Devices and Services.* West Conshohocken, PA, American Society for Testing and Materials, 1998.

Ceramics

Horowitz E, Parr JE (eds): Characterization and performance of calcium phosphate coatings for implants. West Conshohocken, PA, American Society for Testing and Materials, 1994, Series: ASTM STP 1196.

Li P: Bioactive ceramics: State of the art and future trends. *Semin Arthroplasty* 1998;9:165–175.

Willmann G: Ceramics for total hip replacement: What a surgeon should know. *Orthopedics* 1998;21:173–177.

Orthotics and Prosthetics

Goldberg B, Hsu JD (eds): *Atlas of Orthoses and Assistive Devices*, ed 3. St. Louis, MO, Mosby-Year Book, 1997.

Cross-Linked UHMWPE

Grobbelaar CJ, du Plessis TA, Marais F: The radiation improvement of polyethylene prostheses: A preliminary study. *J Bone Joint Surg* 1978;60B:370–374.

Oonishi H, Kotani T, Shikita T: *Proceedings of the 12 SICOT.* Amsterdam, Holland, Excerpta Medica, 1972, pp 107–123.

Oonishi H, Ishimaru H, Kato A: Effect of cross-linkage by gamma radiation in heavy doses to low wear polyethylene in total hip prostheses. *J Mater Sci* 1996;7:753–63.

Oonishi H, Saito M, Kadoya Y: Wear of high-dose gamma irradiated polyethylene in total joint replacement: Long term radiological evaluation. *Trans Orthop Res Soc* 1998;23:97.

Oonishi H, Shikita T: Alumina ceramic total hip prostheses. *Bessatsu Seiki-Geka Nankodo* 1983;3:264–279.

Oonishi H, Takayama Y: The low wear rate of cross-linked polyethylene socket in total hip prosthesis, in *Encyclopedic Handbook of Biomaterials and Bioengineering.* New York, NY, Marcel Dekker, 1995, vol 2, 1853–1868.

Premnath V, Merrill EW, Jasty M, Harris WH: Melt irradiated UHMWPE for total hip replacements: Synthesis and properties. *Trans Orthop Res Soc* 1997;22:91.

Rose RM, Cimino WR, Ellis E, Crugnola AN: Exploratory investigations on the structure dependence of the wear resistance of polyethylene. *Wear* 1982;77:89–104.

Streicher RM: Ionizing radiation for sterilization and modification of high molecular weight polyethylenes. *Plast Rubb Proc Appl* 1988;10:221–229.

Streicher RM: Investigation on sterilization and modification of high molecular weight polyethylenes by ionizing radiation. *Beta-Gamma* 1989;1:34–43.

Wroblewski BM, Siney PD, Dowson D, Collins SN: Prospective clinical and joint simulator studies of new total hip arthroplasty using alumina ceramic heads and cross-linked polyethylene cups. *J Bone Joint Surg* 1996;78B:280–285.

monitor peak and trough levels as well as perform vestibular and auditory function examination at frequent intervals to prevent renal and auditory toxicity. Gentamycin, tobramycin, and amikacin can be administered systemically. Neomycin is used topically in wound irrigation. Streptomycin is usually used to treat tuberculosis infections by intramuscular injection.

The antibiotics that interfere with transcription and translation of bacterial DNA include the quinolones, rifampin, and metronidazole. The quinolones inhibit the enzyme DNA gyrase. The orthopaedically useful quinolones are the fluoroquinolones, which are synthetic derivatives of nalidixic acid. Nalidixic acid is not able to achieve systemic antibacterial levels after oral intake and thus is useful only for urinary antisepsis. The fluorinated derivatives (ciprofloxacin, ofloxacin) have greater antibacterial activity. Ciprofloxacin is probably the most commonly used fluoroquinolone in managing orthopaedic infections. It is active against both gram-positive and gram-negative microorganisms. Perhaps the greatest advantage of this antimicrobial agent is its equal efficacy in both its oral and intravenous preparations. Tendon ruptures, namely Achilles tendon, have been reported following quinolone administration. Rifampin inhibits bacterial DNA-dependent RNA polymerase, thereby blocking the synthesis of RNA. It has a broad activity against gram-positive and gram-negative bacteria, mycobacteria, chlamydiae, and poxviruses. Metronidazole is useful against anaerobic organisms because it forms oxygen radicals, which are toxic to these organisms because they lack the protective enzymes superoxide dismutase and catalase. The oxygen radicals cause loss of the helical structure of DNA and result in breakage of DNA strands.

Clinical Applications

The role of antibiotics in orthopaedic surgery is multifold. They can be used to prevent infection in elective surgery cases and to treat open fractures and established infections. To prevent or treat infections most effectively, the orthopaedist must be familiar with the microbiology, pharmacology, toxicity, and cost of antibiotics. Agents should be chosen based on the efficacy against the most likely organisms to be encountered. Antibiotics are most effective when they are directed against a single pathogen for a short period of time, and are least effective (and even harmful) when directed against multiple pathogens for a long period of time. In general, the least toxic, least expensive, and most effective drug with the narrowest spectrum and best penetration should be used.

Surgical Prophylaxis

Surgical antibiotic prophylaxis refers to the administration of antibiotics to patients without clinical evidence of infection in the surgical field. Currently, 25% to 50% of all antimicrobial usage is for the prevention rather than the treatment of infection. In most elective musculoskeletal procedures, the pathogens that are likely to cause infection are actually relatively limited: S aureus, S epidermidis, aerobic streptococci, and anaerobic cocci. When considering prophylactic administration of antimicrobial agents, it must be decided if the indication is appropriate. In general, antibiotic prophylaxis is indicated in procedures with a high inherent infection rate or when the prevalence of infection is low but such an infection would have catastrophic results. The latter is best validated with prosthetic joint surgery. Several prospective, randomized, double-blind studies have demonstrated that preventive antibiotic therapy reduces the occurrence of infection in total joint arthroplasty to less than 1%, compared with approximately 4% when placebo was used. Similar studies have been performed examining hip fracture surgery, and again decreased occurrence of postoperative wound infections was documented in patients receiving perioperative preventive antibiotics. The value of routine administration of prophylactic antibiotics to patients who will have a foreign body implanted, a bone graft procedure, or extensive dissection resulting in residual dead space or hematoma is well accepted. The routine use of prophylactic antibiotics in soft-tissue procedures or diagnostic arthroscopy is not well studied and thus controversial.

When prophylactic antibiotic treatment is desirable, it should be administered in the most effective way. There is ample evidence to support that antibiotics must be present in the tissues at the time of surgery in order to prevent infection. It has become fairly standard to administer prophylactic antimicrobial agents as the patient is being transported to the operating room or during the induction of anesthesia. When these agents are started after the surgical procedure, infection rates are not significantly changed by their administration. Conversely, if they are started several hours prior to the procedure, their efficacy is decreased. Antibiotic prophylaxis started 1 or more days prior to surgery does not provide any additional protection and should be strongly discouraged because it alters the patient's normal flora. The duration of preventive antibiotic administration is somewhat controversial. In early reports of prosthetic surgery, antibiotics were frequently administered for 14 days. Many studies since then have found no difference in infection for patients receiving antibiotics for 1 day versus 7 to 10 days. In fact, a recent study demonstrated that a single dose of cefazolin administered at the beginning of total joint arthroplasty surgery resulted in no greater rate of infection than when the drug was continued for 48 hours postoperatively. Certainly, unique situations may require prolonged administration of postoperative antibiotics, such as in a compromised host or when an operation is performed in a contaminated wound. As for the selecting out of resistant organisms, there are studies to both support and refute this hypothesis. Nonetheless, it is generally accepted that an antibiotic of narrow range administered for the shortest duration possible will best avoid the selection of resistant strains of pathogenic organisms.

In most major centers, cephalosporins are the perioperative prophylactic antibiotic of choice. The cephalosporins are attractive for many reasons: they afford protection against the majority of bacteria that are associated with postoperative infection in orthopaedic surgery; they are relatively nontoxic, with the exception of hypersensitivity reactions, which are rare; and they are relatively inexpensive. It is desirable to administer only a single antibiotic for surgical prophylaxis, which makes cephalosporins ideal. At the present time, cefazolin is the initial drug of choice in the prevention of infection in total joint arthroplasty. Surgeons must be cautious, however, not to routinely use 1 or 2 agents in every situation, and to evaluate each patient individually. For example, patients who have been hospitalized for long periods of time may be colonized with nosocomial pathogens and require additional coverage. Also, specific antibiotic-bacterial susceptibilities vary from hospital to hospital and the surgeon must be aware of the indigenous bacteria and their susceptibility patterns at his or her respective institution.

Open Fractures

The recommendations made by Gustilo and Anderson in 1976 regarding the prevention of infection in open fractures: immediate and repeated irrigation and debridement, fracture stabilization, timely wound coverage, and empiric antibiotics, remain the standard by which most orthopaedists treat this condition. They considered the routine use of antibiotics in open fractures therapeutic rather than prophylactic. Infection following open fracture can have devastating results including nonunion, amputation, and even death secondary to sepsis. Both clinical and basic investigations over the past 2 decades have helped form the guiding principles by which open fractures are currently treated. All open fractures should be considered contaminated with both gram-positive and gram-negative organisms. The risk of infection in open fractures is dependent on the severity of soft-tissue injury. Antibiotic administration should be initiated as soon as possible following the identification of an open fracture. S aureus and gram-negative bacilli are the most common pathogens causing infections in open fractures. Originally, a first-generation cephalosporin such as cefazolin was believed to be adequate for the management of minimally contaminated fractures (grade I, II). Interestingly, over the past 20 years there has been an increase in the prevalence of gram-negative organisms that have been isolated from infected fractures. Whether this is the result of an actual change in the prevalence of infecting organisms or improved laboratory methods to isolate such organisms is unclear. As such, the use of a first-generation cephalosporin alone has been largely replaced in many centers by a regimen that combines an antistaphylococcal agent, such as a first-generation cephalosporin, with an aminoglycoside, or for single-agent coverage, a second-generation cephalosporin, such as cefamandole. Replacing the first-generation cephalosporin with a second-generation cephalosporin, in combination with an aminoglycoside, does not appear to improve clinical outcomes. In grade III injuries, the addition of an aminoglycoside is required in order to provide adequate gram-negative coverage. In a randomized, prospective study of type III open fractures, an infection rate of 29% was reported when using a cephalosporin alone, compared to 9% when using a cephalosporin in combination with an aminoglycoside.

Specific environmental exposures are associated with certain pathogens and should be covered accordingly. Farm-related exposures are often associated with Clostridium perfringens and necessitate the addition of penicillin. Contamination with soil increases the risk of infection from anaerobic microorganisms, which can be covered with clindamycin or metronidazole. Possible contamination with Pseudomonas as might occur in a freshwater environment should be covered with a third-generation cephalosporin such as ceftazidime or ciprofloxacin.

The optimal duration of therapy continues to be a subject of debate. In a double-blinded, prospective study, there was no difference between a 1-day course of a second-generation cephalosporin compared to a 5-day course in the prevention of open fracture-site infections. No such similar studies have been published for combination therapy. Certainly therapy must be continued long enough to prevent clinical infection. However, an unnecessarily prolonged course is associated with wound colonization with nosocomial pathogens, greater cost, and increased adverse drug reactions. It is important to note that despite optimal antibiotic therapy, a certain number of infections may be inevitable.

Bone and Joint Infections

The treatment of osteomyelitis and septic arthritis remains one of the most challenging problems in orthopaedic practice. In both the surgical and nonsurgical management of orthopaedic infections, antibiotics have an important role. The principles of treating musculoskeletal infections with antibiotics include identifying the organism, selecting the appropriate antibiotic, determining the optimum route of delivery, and planning the duration of therapy.

When antibiotic therapy is first initiated in patients with bone and joint infections, often the offending pathogen has not been identified. Empiric antibacterial therapy is based on the clinician's suspicion of the most likely organism (Table 2). Occasionally, a patient may present with a rapidly progressive infectious process requiring agents that will cover all possible pathogens. Once the offending organism has been identified and in vitro susceptibility studies performed, the appropriate antimicrobial agent is chosen. It is important that material for culture be obtained prior to the administration of antibiotics. Even resistant organisms can fail to grow once antibiotics have been administered.

Once the appropriate antibiotic is chosen, it is delivered either systemically or locally. The effectiveness of systemically delivered antibiotics requires adequate concentrations of the drug at the site of the drug-microorganism interaction to inhibit or kill the microorganism. At the same time, the concentration must be below levels that are toxic to the patient. Systemic levels of potentially toxic antibiotics are monitored by determining peak and trough concentrations. Peak concentrations are determined from blood concentration at 30 minutes after intravenous administration, and adjusted by changing the amount of drug. Trough levels are determined from blood concentration just prior to administration of intravenous antibiotics, and adjusted by adjusting the time interval between doses. If the trough level is 4 times the mean inhibitory concentration (MIC) of the antibiotic for the specific pathogen, the pathogen is considered to be sensitive to the antibiotic. The bone interstitial fluid concentration depends on plasma concentration, protein binding, and the ability of the antibiotic to cross the capillary membrane. In theory, the concentration in viable bone equals serum concentration once a steady state has been achieved.

The use of bacteriostatic agents (tetracycline, erythromycin, clindamycin) versus bactericidal agents (penicillin, cephalosporins, aminoglycosides, vancomycin, trimethoprim-sulfamethoxazole) continues to be controversial. Experiments have demonstrated that the beta-lactam agents, aminoglycosides, and tetracyclines are all able to achieve serum-level concentrations in both normal and acute osteomyelitic bone (Fig. 1). However, in patients with chronic bone infections in whom vascularity and hence drug penetration may be compromised, it would be prudent to use a bactericidal agent. Three antibiotics (clindamycin, quinolones, and rifampin) can penetrate macrophages and kill already ingested bacteria. This property extends their usefulness because *S aureus* can survive within the macrophages, protected from the actions of other antimicrobials.

The standard length of systemic treatment remains con-

Table 2

*Empiric Antibacterial Therapy for Osteomyelitis on Clinical Grounds**

Clinical Setting	Etiologies	Suggested Therapy
Newborn	*S aureus* Enterobacteriaceae Group A, B streptococci	Pencillinase resistant Synthetic penicillin
Child ≤ 4 years	*H influenzae* Streptococci *S aureus*	Parenteral 3rd generation cephalosporin
Child > 4 years	*S aureus* Streptococci *H influenzae*	Clindamycin or vancomycin
Adult (including history of drug abuse)	*S aureus* (occasional Enterobacteriaceas, *Streptococcus* sp)	Pencillinase resistant synthetic penicillin (if Gram negative bacilli on smear, add parenteral 3rd generation cephalosporin)
Postoperative or posttrauma	*S aureus* Enterobacteriaceae *Pseudomonas* sp	2nd generation cephalosporin, vancomycin + parental 3rd generation cephalosporin or imipenem cilastatin
Nail puncture, foot	*Pseudomonas* sp	Ciprofloxacin, ticarcillin Clavulanate, imipenim or 3rd generation cephalosporin
Contiguous with decubitis ulcer, diabetic foot	Polymicrobic: aerobic cocci, bacilli + anaerobes	Clindamycin, cephalexin

* Optimal antimicrobial therapy is based on accurate identification and in vitro susceptibility testing of causal agents; these are only initial guidelines.
(Reproduced with permission from Perry CR: *Bone and Joint Infections*. St. Louis, MO, CV Mosby, 1996.)

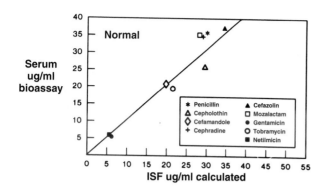

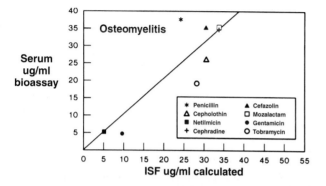

Figure 1

The relationship of the serum and bone interstitial fluid concentrations of antimicrobials for normal and osteomyelitic bone in a canine model. (Reproduced with permission from Fitzgerald RH Jr: Current concepts of antimicrobial therapy, in Greene WB (ed): *Instructional Course Lectures XXXIX*. Park Ridge, IL, American Academy of Orthopaedic Surgeons, 1990, pp 465–470.)

troversial but has been arbitrarily determined to be 4 to 6 weeks. The duration of treatment is largely based on trends as opposed to experimental evidence. Perhaps the most important aspect in determining the length of treatment is the clinical response of the patient, noted by changes in the physical examination, defervescence, and laboratory values such as C-reactive protein or erythrocyte sedimentation rate. It is currently believed that patients who respond to an initial parenteral course can be transferred to oral therapy in 1 to 2 weeks without adverse consequences as long as the infecting organism has been demonstrated to be sensitive to the oral agent, the antibiotic can achieve adequate serum levels without toxicity, and patient compliance can be reasonably assured. To date, there are no controlled studies documenting the optimal length of treatment or the appropriate time to transition from intravenous to oral therapy.

Infections associated with orthopaedic implants present a complex challenge. Organisms centered on biomaterials are often resistant to antibiotic therapy and often necessitate removal of the implant to irradiate the infection. Local

factors such as the material's surface composition and characteristics, the bacteria's ability to elaborate a protective polysaccharide coating, and the medium's composition have been reported to affect bacterial antibiotic sensitivity and host defense systems. When comparing the minimal bactericidal concentrations of certain antibiotics for biomaterial-adherent bacteria to bacteria in suspension, concentrations of twofold to 250-fold or higher were required. When specifically examining stainless steel, ultra-high molecular weight polyethylene, and polymethylmethacrylate (PMMA), bacteria adhering to PMMA were significantly more resistant. These killing kinetic studies indicate that a sensitivity testing technique will be needed to guide the management of biomaterial-related infections.

Local antibiotic therapy has the potential advantage of reducing the morbidity associated with prolonged systemic therapy. The most commonly employed delivery vehicle for local antibiotics is the bone cement PMMA. Since its introduction in the 1970s, the properties of antibiotic-containing bone cement have been extensively investigated. These drug-polymer composites were originally studied in the treatment of infected cemented total hip replacement. A salvage rate of 70% was reported for infected total hip arthroplasty (THA) with direct-exchange arthroplasty using gentamycin-containing PMMA. Since then, numerous thermostable antibiotics have been shown to have predictable elution kinetics from PMMA, and the applications for antibiotic-loaded cement have grown. The primary advantages of the antibiotic-cement composite are that high local concentrations can be achieved with minimum serum concentrations, and the material from which the antibiotic elutes occupies the dead space created by debridement.

Numerous studies have demonstrated that many commonly used antibiotics are eluted from PMMA in quantities that vastly exceed the MIC needed to treat most susceptible pathogens, far higher than possible with systemic antibiotics. Elution kinetics vary among antibiotics and are dependent on the integrity and porosity (surface area) of the bone cement. Most studies confirm that antibiotics are eluted from cement in large amounts in the first 2 or 3 days, after which there is low concentration in the surrounding fluid. The mechanical strength of the cement once impregnated with antibiotic powder is also well studied. The degree of cement weakening correlates with the amount of antibiotic added (Fig. 2). The use of 2 g or less of antibiotic powder per 40-g pack of cement does not appear to compromise the compressive strength of bone cement to any degree, obviating concerns of early mechanical failure resulting from antibiotic-impregnated cement.

For the treatment of infected THA, antibiotic-impregnated cement appears to improve the salvage rate regardless of the treatment philosophy adopted. For the treatment of osteomyelitis, animal studies have demonstrated that treatment with antibiotic-containing cement alone is equivalent

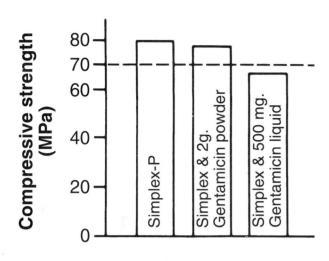

Figure 2

Compressive strength of cement versus amount of antibiotic. Compressive strength is reduced to below 70 MPa when more than 4.5 g is added to 40 g of powdered polymethylmethacrylate. (Reproduced with permission from Murray WR: Use of antibiotic-containing bone cement. *Clin Orthop* 1984;190:89–95.)

to systemic antibiotics alone. Some protocols employ antibiotic beads after thorough debridement in conjunction with perioperative intravenous antibiotics. The beads are usually removed 2 to 7 weeks after implantation. In the setting of trauma, antibiotic beads have been used as therapeutic spacers in severely comminuted open fractures until definitive fixation, grafting, and coverage can be completed. In addition, antibiotic-cement spacers have a role in infected nonunions.

Alternative local delivery systems have been investigated. Biodegradable carriers using bioerodible polymers impregnated with antibiotics have been studied. In addition, an implantable pump has also been described for the treatment of osteomyelitis and infected total joint arthroplasty.

The pharmacologic principles of treating septic arthritis closely mimic those of osteomyelitis. Empiric parenteral antibiotic therapy should be initiated as soon as cultures have been obtained and then replaced by the appropriate drug based on in vitro susceptibility studies. Drug concentrations in synovial fluid equivalent to plasma have been well documented for almost all antibiotics with the exception of erythromycin. Selection of empiric therapy must be tailored for each patient and is dependent on factors such as immunocompetence and suspected source of infection. Recent studies suggest that the use of nonsteroidal anti-inflammatory medications in conjunction with antibiotics may be beneficial in retarding glycosaminoglycan and collagen loss in articular cartilage. The mechanism for this phenomenon remains unclear.

Anticoagulation

Venous thromboembolism is a potentially life-threatening postoperative complication in patients who undergo orthopaedic procedures. In the orthopaedic literature, anticoagulation therapy has been primarily focused on patients who undergo elective THA and total knee arthroplasty (TKA). The American Academy of Orthopaedic Surgeons® recommends some form of prophylaxis for all patients who undergo total hip surgery. A 1992 survey of practicing orthopaedic surgeons revealed that 92% use a pharmacologic agent following elective THA as part of their management strategy for the prevention of thromboembolic disease. Fatal pulmonary embolism rates of 1% to 3% of untreated patients and asymptomatic pulmonary embolism rates of 10% to 15% have traditionally been used as the rationale for administering thromboembolic prophylaxis. As experience with joint arthroplasty has grown, so has the data available for analysis. More recent reports suggest that the rates of fatal pulmonary embolism and asymptomatic pulmonary embolism are much lower than previously suspected. Fatal pulmonary embolism probably occurs more on the order of 0.1% to 0.2%. Furthermore, it has been recently suggested by a number of authors that these percentages are unaffected by thromboprophylaxis. While there is no question that thromboprophylaxis will decrease the rates of deep venous thrombosis (DVT), the connection between reducing DVT rates and decreasing the overall death rate has not been equivocally established. To add to the controversy, reports of complications associated with anticoagulation therapy are becoming increasingly common. Death following elective surgery is a tragedy and no doubt a certain number of patients will die suddenly following total joint arthroplasty. However, the role of pharmaceutical intervention is unclear as the benefits versus disadvantages of thromboembolic therapy become increasingly difficult to decipher.

Patients at increased risk for the development of thromboembolism should be treated. Risk factors include prior episode of thromboembolism, prior venous surgery or orthopaedic surgery, advanced age, malignancy, congestive heart failure, immobilization, obesity, use of oral contraceptives, and excessive blood loss with transfusion. The ideal pharmacologic prophylactic regimen has yet to be established. Several options are available for primary prophylaxis against thromboembolic disease. The most commonly used agents are aspirin, warfarin, low-dose and adjusted-dose heparin, and low molecular weight heparin.

Aspirin

The beneficial effects of aspirin in thromboembolic disease are thought to be the result of the inhibition of thromboxane-A_2 synthesis by irreversibly inhibiting cyclooxygenase (COX) in platelets as well as megakaryocytes. Thromboxane-A_2 is a powerful inducer of platelet aggregation. It acts on cell surface receptors and activates phospholipase C, causing the formation of second messengers and subsequently a rise in intracellular calcium, which triggers aggregation.

The effectiveness of aspirin in the prevention of DVT and pulmonary embolism following orthopaedic procedures has yet to be established, though numerous studies have been performed. Initially, low-dose aspirin (1.2 g/day) was found to be efficacious in proximal DVT prevention compared to dextran and warfarin. Subsequent investigations cited the prevalence of DVT as high as 80% in patients receiving aspirin following THA. Higher doses of aspirin (3.6 g/day) also failed to provide adequate protection against thrombi formation. In other investigations, however, aspirin prophylaxis in patients undergoing THA prevented symptomatic DVT in up to 100% of these patients. Approximately 5% of the patients had asymptomatic DVT as detected by ultrasound and 12% had high-probability ventilation-perfusion (V-Q) lung scans, though no fatal pulmonary embolism occurred.

In the prevention of DVT following TKA, high-dose regimens were associated with fewer DVT than low-dose regimens. In one study, female patients undergoing TKA demonstrated less satisfactory responses to aspirin compared to their male counterparts.

Aspirin does not provide the best protection against thromboembolic disease following total joint replacement. There is some evidence to support its efficacy in the prevention of proximal thrombi in low-risk male patients. When looking at pulmonary embolism alone, however, aspirin is comparable to other methods of prophylaxis. The efficacy of aspirin in the prevention of DVT and pulmonary embolism following nonprosthetic joint replacement operations has not been studied sufficiently to draw conclusions.

Warfarin

Warfarin is a vitamin K antagonist that prevents the reductive metabolism of vitamin K epoxide back to its active form, hydroquinone, by inhibiting the enzymes responsible for the reaction. Stepwise oxidation to the epoxide form is coupled to carboxylation of several glutamate residues in prothrombin and factors II, VII, IX, and X, as well as the endogenous anticoagulants, protein C and protein S. Its anticoagulation effect results from the replacement of normal clotting factors with the decarboxylated factors. The missing carboxylated glutamyl residues are essential for normal activation of prothrombin. The half-life for these factors ranges from 6 to 60 hours. As such, there is an 8- to 12-hour delay in the action of warfarin, with full effect in 72 to 96 hours. The dose response of warfarin is difficult to predict because it depends on many factors. The anticoagulation effect of warfarin is measured by prothrombin time (PT). This test uses thromboplastin to promote factor X activation in the intrinsic pathway. Thromboplastins extracted from various tissues of various preparations have

variable responses to warfarin. The international normalized ratio (INR) standardizes the values for measuring the anticoagulation effects of warfarin.

Warfarin has been used in both prophylaxis and treatment of thromboembolism for almost 40 years and currently is the most commonly used agent. Initially, warfarin was used at higher doses to achieve PTs 1.5 to 2 times normal. This overanticoagulation resulted in bleeding complications. Since then several studies have documented the efficacy and safety of low-dose warfarin. The current recommended dosing protocol maintains the PT at 15 to 17 seconds and an INR of 1.8 to 2.5. This range is achieved by daily dose adjustments based on PT and INR, which require daily phlebotomy. Using the low-dose warfarin protocol, the prevalence of nonfatal pulmonary embolism is reportedly 0.5% to 3.2%, and major bleeding complications 1.5% to 2.4%. In a study of 3,700 hip arthroplasty procedures, no fatal pulmonary embolisms occurred with the low-dose warfarin protocol. The use of a fixed low-dose regimen has also been investigated. A randomized study comparing a fixed dosage (2 mg/day) with a daily adjusted dose found no difference in the prevalence of thrombi. The safety, efficacy, and cost effectiveness of low-dose warfarin after discharge have also been established. In a series of 268 patients who had undergone THA, warfarin was maintained for 12 weeks and resulted in no fatal pulmonary embolisms or major bleeding complications. Because the response to warfarin is hard to predict, careful patient monitoring is required, probably best achieved in an outpatient setting.

Heparin

Heparin is a heterogeneous mixture of sulfated mucopolysaccharide chains composed of alternating residues of glucosamine and uronic acid. These chains vary in molecular weight, averaging about 15,000 d. Commercially available heparin is extracted from bovine and porcine tissues and is referred to as unfractionated heparin. Its biologic activity is dependent on pentasaccharide sequences randomly distributed along the heparin chain. The pentasaccharide sequence on heparin binds antithrombin III and causes a conformational change in the structure of antithrombin III, exposing its active site (arginine). By exposing its active site, the affinity of antithrombin III for the proteases of the activated clotting factors, namely thrombin and Xa, increases its binding 1,000-fold. This inhibition of the proteases results in decreased clot formation.

Heparin is administered intravenously or subcutaneously because poor gastrointestinal absorbance precludes its oral administration. It is administered in an adjusted dose or a fixed low dose. Fixed low-dose heparin is given as 5,000 U every 8 to 12 hours. This regimen lessens the hypercoagulable state by inactivating thrombin and factor Xa. Higher molecular weight heparin also inhibits the aggregation of platelets. The efficacy of heparin in the general surgical population has been well established. In the orthopaedic population, however, fixed-dose heparin has failed to provide comparable thromboembolic protection, leading to the use of adjusted-dose heparin to maintain the partial thromboplastin time (PTT) between 31.5 and 36 seconds. This requires monitoring PTT several times per day and adjusting the dose accordingly. The dose-adjusted heparin protocol demonstrated a DVT rate of 14% to 22% diagnosed by venography, an almost threefold decrease in some studies compared to fixed-dose heparin. However, a significant rate of wound hematoma, up to 24%, was reported. Although dose-adjusted heparin is effective, alternative anticoagulation methods can result in fewer bleeding complications and permit greater ease of use.

Low Molecular Weight Heparin

The low molecular weight heparins (LMWH) are derived from unfractionated heparin by chemical or enzymatic depolymerization resulting in chains averaging 5,000 d. Several of these preparations have been investigated. The only Food and Drug Administration (FDA)-approved LMWH is enoxaparin (Lovenox). Like heparin, LMWH exerts its effects by binding antithrombin through its pentasaccharide sequence. Unlike heparin, LMWH has relatively low

inhibitory activity against thrombin. To inactivate thrombin, heparin must bind to antithrombin and thrombin simultaneously, which can only be accomplished if the heparin chain is a certain length (Fig. 3). The majority of LMWH chains are of insufficient lengths to bind both factors. The net result is fewer bleeding complications.

Enoxaparin for DVT prophylaxis is attractive for many reasons. First, its pharmacokinetic properties after subcutaneous injection are highly predictable. Unfractionated heparin binds to many endogenous proteins, thereby reducing its availability to interact with antithrombin III. In addition, because of variability in plasma concentration of heparin-binding proteins, including certain acute-phase reactants that increase in ill patients, an anticoagulation response of heparin is difficult to predict. Second, LMWH produces less bleeding effects compared to unfractionated heparin. Higher molecular weight heparins bind platelets, increase microvascular permeability, and bind endothelial cells, interfering with the interaction between platelets and blood vessel walls. Third, LMWH does not prolong PTT, obviating the need for monitoring by phlebotomy.

Clinically, the LMWH have proved to be both safe and effective for prophylaxis against DVT for orthopaedic procedures. For THA, LMWH have been shown to be superior in preventing DVT compared to both low-dose and adjust-

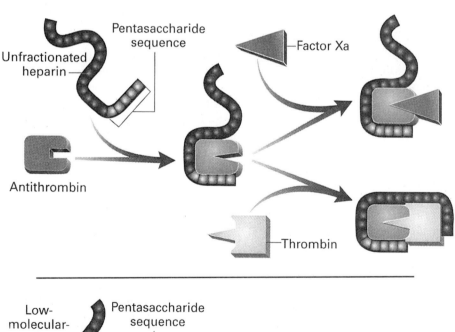

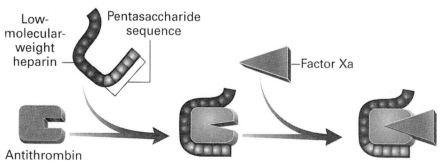

Figure 3

Catalysis of antithrombin-mediated inactivation of thrombin or factor Xa by unfractionated heparin or low molecular weight heparin (LMWH). The interaction of unfractionated heparin and LMWH with antithrombin is mediated by the pentasaccharide sequence of the drugs. Binding of either to antithrombin causes conformational change at its reactive center that accelerates its interaction with factor Xa. Consequently, both unfractionated heparin and LMWH catalyze the inactivation of factor Xa by antithrombin. In contrast to factor Xa inhibition, thrombin inactivation requires the formation of a ternary heparin-antithrombin-thrombin complex. This complex can only be formed by chains at least 18 saccharide units long. This explains why LMWH has less inhibitory activity against thrombin than unfractionated heparin. (Reproduced with permission from Weitz JI: Low-molecular-weight heparins. *N Engl J Med* 1997;337:688–698.)

ed-dose heparin preparations. When comparing LMWH to warfarin, LMWH is at least as efficacious as warfarin in prevention of DVT. For TKA, LMWH has been shown to be superior to warfarin in the prevention of the number of total DVTs, but does not decrease the number of proximal DVTs. A small increase in postoperative bleeding was reported using LMWH compared to warfarin. This was attributed to untimely initiation of therapy as the recommendations are not to start LMWH until at least 12 hours after operation. Small trials have also shown LMWH to decrease DVT rates in hip fracture surgery, acute spinal cord injury patients, and multitrauma patients.

Inhibitors of Bone Resorption

Metabolic bone diseases are generalized disorders of skeletal homeostasis caused by impairment of hormonal control of bone formation, mineralization, or remodeling. The most common metabolic bone diseases are osteoporosis and Paget's disease. Both of these diseases result from abnormal remodeling. Other conditions associated with abnormal bone metabolism include metastatic disease, corticosteroid usage, rickets, osteomalacia, and renal osteodystrophy.

Whereas remodeling is a coupled process involving both the osteoblast and osteoclast, the osteoclast is the cell that initiates and sustains bone remodeling. Osteoclasts are responsible for bone resorption. Osteoclastic bone resorption consists of several complicated processes: osteoclast differentiation and development; attachment of osteoclasts to calcified tissues; polarization of the cell in relation to the calcified tissue leading to development of the ruffled border and clear zone; secretion of acids and enzymes in the sub-osteoclastic space; mineral dissolution; and matrix degradation. Intense investigation has revealed several regulators of osteoclast function, varying from molecular transduction signals to the mechanism of osteoblast activation via cell-to-cell contact. This knowledge assists in both the understanding and development of therapeutic agents to treat diseases characterized by increased bone turnover.

Bisphosphonates

Bisphosphonates, formerly called diphosphonates, are synthetic analogs of inorganic pyrophosphate in which the P-O-P bond has been replaced with a nonhydrolyzable P-C-P bond (Fig. 4). Clinically, the most important action of the bisphosphonates is the inhibition of osteoclast-mediated bone resorption. As such they are used to treat diseases such as Paget's, hypercalcemia of malignancy, and primary osteoporosis. Treatment of secondary osteoporosis (bone loss secondary to known causes such as corticosteroid use,

tumors, immobilization) with bisphosphonates has also been investigated but to a lesser degree. Since their first description nearly a century ago, over 1,000 bisphosphonates have been synthesized, with a dozen or so investigated in humans. Approximately 6 are commercially available for the treatment of metabolic bone diseases in 1 or more countries.

The bisphosphonate compounds exert their effects on both a biochemical and cellular level. They have a strong affinity for calcium phosphate precipitates, inhibiting the formation and dissolution of this mineral in vitro. In vivo, this results in an inhibition of bone loss by preventing the formation of hydroxyapatite crystals in bone. However, its corollary, impairment of bone mineralization, is also an effect. The activity of the bisphosphonates varies greatly from compound to compound, making it virtually impossible to extrapolate data from one compound to another. For example, therapeutic doses of etidronate, when administered continuously, have been shown to inhibit the mineralization of calcified tissues leading to osteomalacia and fractures. However, alendronate, an aminobisphosphonate, has been shown to be one of the most potent inhibitors of bone resorption at doses that do not adversely affect bone mineralization.

On a cellular level, bisphosphonates are believed to inhibit osteoclasts directly by inducing changes in morphology. In vitro, the bisphosphonates bind exposed hydroxyapatite sites in areas of bone resorption. Osteoclasts bind these surfaces. During the acidification process, bisphosphonates are locally released, leading to an increased local concentration under the osteoclast within the space defined by the clear zone. This results in loss of the ruffled membrane function and the cessation of resorption. Pharmacokinetically, because the backbone of the molecule is a P-C-P bond as opposed to a P-O-P bond, the compounds are resistant to metabolism by endogenous phosphatases and therefore are absorbed, stored, and excreted unaltered by the body. Its intestinal absorption is low (approximately 1%) and further diminished by the presence of food, especially those high in calcium and iron. Once absorbed, the compounds

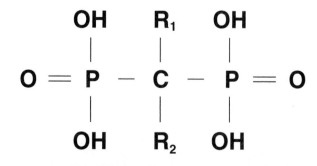

Figure 4

The structure of bisphosphonates.

are rapidly taken up by bone where they have a very long half-life (6 to 11 years).

The clinical efficacy of the bisphosphonate compounds is becoming well established. They are the drug of choice for the treatment of Paget's disease. The indications for pharmacologic intervention in Paget's are: bone pain, preparation for orthopaedic surgery, treatment of spinal stenosis, prevention of fractures or skeletal deformity in rapidly progressive phases of the disease, and treatment of high output congestive heart failure. Bisphosphonates have been shown to relieve symptoms, improve the appearance of radiographic lesions, and suppress biochemical and histologic indices of disease activity.

The current dose of etidronate (5 to 10 mg/kg/day for 3 to 6 months) provokes a varied response in patients. The more optimal dose (10 to 20 mg/kg/day) for suppression of disease activity is associated with an increased occurrence of fractures secondary to impairment of mineralization. An intermittent, cyclic dosing pattern helps to retard etidronate's untoward effects. Inhibition of bone resorption in Paget's using alendronate, however, has been shown to be equivalent if not superior to etidronate without impairment of bone mineralization. The optimal dose of alendronate in treatment of Paget's disease is 40 mg/day. Disadvantages of the aminobisphosphonates are mostly limited to their adverse gastrointestinal effects, which seem to be dose-dependent.

In the treatment of osteoporosis, there is strong support in the medical literature for the use of etidronate and alendronate therapy although only alendronate is FDA-approved for marketing in the treatment of osteoporosis. For etidronate, studies have shown a higher bone mineral density in the spine and hips of postmenopausal women taking cyclical regimens (1 week on treatment alternating with 13 weeks off treatment) compared to placebo. For alendronate, a recent 3-year investigation using a dose of 10 mg/day demonstrated a decrease in the incidence of fractures in patients on therapy. Alendronate use led to a decrease in vertebral and nonvertebral fractures as well as a decrease in loss of stature in postmenopausal women. Furthermore, an actual increase in bone mineral density was observed.

The bisphosphonates are an important part of the pharmacologic possibilities for the prevention and treatment of both Paget's disease and osteoporosis. In addition, successful treatment of steroid-induced osteopenia has been reported. Questions that remain unanswered concerning this therapeutic option include the status of bone metabolism once these drugs are discontinued.

Calcitonin

Calcitonin is a single-chain, 32-amino acid polypeptide hormone produced by the parafollicular cells of the thyroid gland. The principal effect of calcitonin is to lower serum calcium and phosphate by its action on bone and kidney. In bone, calcitonin inhibits osteoclastic resorption through its receptors, inducing changes in the cytoskeleton. This is accomplished by disruption of structures known as actin rings. Actin rings correspond to the clear zone in vivo, which is responsible for the formation of bone resorption pits, or Howship's lacunae.

Several molecular forms of calcitonin are available for therapeutic use. The first commercially available calcitonin was extracted from salmon. Salmon calcitonin is more potent than human calcitonin. It differs from human calcitonin by 1 amino acid. Although this difference is significant enough to be immunogenic, true allergic reactions consisting of anaphylaxis and urticaria are rare. Antibodies to salmon preparation do develop in a significant number of patients undergoing long-term treatment, but without clinical consequences. In the past, a test dose of calcitonin with medical monitoring was recommended. However, this approach has been shown to be unnecessary because anaphylaxis is rare.

The traditional route of administration has been via subcutaneous or intramuscular injection. Recent formulations for intranasal delivery are available. Both the injectable and nasal preparations are FDA-approved for the treatment of Paget's disease and osteoporosis. The FDA-approved doses are 100 units/day for injection and 200 units/day for nasal spray. Animal studies have demonstrated comparable activity of both forms. Nasal calcitonin has demonstrated fewer side effects than the injectable form and as such seems to be better tolerated as evidenced by the number of patients who discontinue therapy (a small fraction compared to up to a third, respectively). Side effects include gastrointestinal disturbance, vascular flushing, and local rash or nasal irritation. The side effects seem to be dose-related.

For the treatment of osteoporosis, calcitonin has been shown to be effective in relieving fracture pain, increasing bone density, and decreasing fracture rate. It has been shown to significantly alleviate the acute pain that results from osteoporotic vertebral fractures. Although the exact mechanism of pain relief is unknown, calcitonin is thought to act in part by stimulating the endogenous opioid system. Numerous studies have demonstrated a range of responses in bone density in postmenopausal women. Some studies have demonstrated that bone density was maintained after starting therapy. The majority of studies show that calcitonin results in significant increases in bone density, as much as 5% to 10% over 2 years of therapy. Benefits have been seen as early as 3 months after initiating therapy. Calcitonin is most effective in patients who have increased bone turnover. A minimal effect on bone density is observed in patients with low bone turnover. Fracture rates have been shown to be reduced in calcitonin-treated postmenopausal women. The prevalence of lumbar vertebral fractures decreased in women with established osteoporosis using both injectable and nasal preparations of calcitonin. The data on hip fractures suggests a similar trend. The long-term effects in the treatment of osteoporosis are not well established, with the longest controlled study being 3 years.

In the treatment of Paget's disease, calcitonin has been shown to be effective in decreasing bone pain; that is, pain associated with areas of pagetic bone thought to result from the stretching of periosteal pain fibers or by elaboration of pain mediators within the marrow. However, calcitonin is not effective in treating the pain of associated joint disease. It has shown to be of benefit in improving neurologic symptoms in spinal stenosis by decreasing soft-tissue vascularity and edema, as opposed to affecting bony structures. Calcitonin has not been shown to be effective in improving lytic lesions seen radiographically. There has been some suggestion of the benefits of perioperative calcitonin, particularly as it pertains to reducing blood loss associated with highly vascular pagetic bone. Dosing is dependent on the severity of symptoms. A typical dose is 50 IU daily until symptoms start to resolve and then decreasing to 3 times per week for maintenance.

Calcitonin has not been extensively investigated in secondary osteoporosis. A beneficial effect on steroid-induced osteoporosis has been reported as well as evidence to suggest prevention of disuse osteoporosis. In addition, hypercalcemic states, secondary to metastatic tumors, for example, treated with calcitonin have been shown to lower serum calcitonin.

Vitamin D and Estrogen

Although vitamin D and estrogen are not truly antiosteoclastic agents, they are important regulators of bone metabolism and are an important part of the pharmacologic armamentarium in treating metabolic bone disease.

Vitamin D is a unique steroid hormone that can modulate calcium homeostasis directly or through its effects on the differentiation and development of the various calcium-regulating cell systems. Several active metabolites of vitamin D have been identified (Table 3). Of these, the most important is 1,25-dihydroxyvitamin D_3 (1,25-$(OH)_2D_3$), also known as calcitriol. In order for vitamin D_3 to become functional it must first be 25-hydroxylated in the liver, and the resulting product must then be 1α-hydroxylated in the kidney to produce the functional form 1,25-$(OH)_2D_3$.

Bone, kidney, and intestine are the major target tissues for the active form, 1,25-$(OH)_2D_3$. In the kidney, it increases proximal tubular reabsorption of phosphate as well as acts as feedback regulator of its own resorption. In the intestine, it is responsible for active calcium transport. In bone, its physiologic role is not well understood. At pharmacologic doses, vitamin D has been shown to potentiate the activity of osteoclasts via osteoblast regulation. In osteoblasts, it is

known that 1,25-$(OH)_2D_3$ stimulates the synthesis of osteocalcin and osteopontin. Vitamin D stimulates osteoblasts to secrete an osteoclast-activating substance called osteoprotegerin ligand (OPGL). OPGL has been shown to activate osteoclasts in vitro and induce bone resorption in vivo.

Numerous clinical trials have investigated the possible role of vitamin D metabolites in the treatment of several metabolic bone disorders, including various forms of osteomalacia related to abnormalities of vitamin D metabolism, bone disease associated with chronic renal failure, and osteoporosis. The value of calcitriol in the treatment of the first 2 conditions is well established.

The treatment protocols for vitamin D-dependent rickets type I (VDD1) uses 1,25-$(OH)_2D_3$. In the treatment of x-linked hypophosphatemic vitamin D-resistant rickets (HPDR), 1,25-$(OH)_2D_3$ has demonstrated a more varied response pattern. VDD1, as its name implies, responds to pharmacologic doses of vitamin D. The disease is characterized by low plasma concentration of 1,25-$(OH)_2D_3$. In contrast, vitamin D-dependent rickets type II is characterized by elevated levels of 1,25-$(OH)_2D_3$ and results from end-organ resistance to this molecule. The basic abnormality on VDD1 appears to be altered activity of the renal enzyme 1α-hydroxylase enzyme, which is responsible for hydroxylation of 25$(OH)D_3$ into 1,25$(OH)_2D_3$. Replacement therapy with physiologic amounts of 1,25-$(OH)_2D_3$ results in correction of the abnormal phenotype, eliminating both the hypocalcemia and radiographic evidence of the disease in most individuals. If treatment is started shortly after birth, hypoplasia of tooth enamel that can occur in rickets may also be prevented. The therapeutic doses (25,000 to 75,000 IU/day) are close to maximum doses and place the patient at risk for nephrocalcinosis and impaired renal function. As such, these patients need to be monitored for signs of toxicity.

In the treatment of osteoporosis, several investigators have found favorable results using 1,25-$(OH)_2D_3$. It has

Table 3		
Vitamin D and Its Metabolites		
Abbreviation	**Vitamin**	**Drug Name**
	Provitamin D_3	7-dehydrocholesterol
D_2	Vitamin D_2	Ergocalciferol
D_3	Vitamin D_3	Cholecalciferol
25$(OH)D_3$	25-hydroxyvitamin D_3	Calcifediol
1,25$(OH)_2D_3$	1,25-dihydroxyvitamin D_3	Calcitriol
24,25$(OH)_2D_3$	24,25-dihydroxyvitamin D_3	

(Reproduced with permission from Kasser JR: *Orthopaedic Knowledge Update 5.* Rosemont, IL, American Academy of Orthopaedic Surgeons, 1996, p 1200.)

been demonstrated that patients with osteoporosis have reduced calcium absorption as well as reduced levels of physiologically active vitamin D compared to normal patients. Furthermore, a decline in calcitriol levels has been implicated in the pathogenesis of osteoporosis. There are studies, however, to support and refute the efficacy of calcitrol as part a treatment plan. Certainly those patients with impaired calcium absorption and low serum $1,25(OH)_2D_3$ are most likely to benefit from calcitriol intervention. The exact percentage of patients with low levels of vitamin D_3 is unknown, but it is probably as high as 10%.

The role of estrogens in the prevention and treatment of osteoporosis has been studied extensively. Many studies have shown that bone loss is accelerated after menopause and when ovarian hormone production ceases and circulating levels fall to 20% of previous levels. This bone loss can be reversed by the administration of estrogen. Although estrogens are known to inhibit bone resorption, the mechanisms responsible for this effect are poorly understood. Only recently has the presence of a specific estrogen receptor in osteoblasts and osteoclasts been confirmed. Although the level of such receptors is low, the fact that they appear to be active in osteoblasts, osteoblast-like cells, and osteoclasts provides the first real evidence that bone is a target tissue for estrogen action. Not only does estrogen block bone loss secondary to the postmenopausal state, but a decrease in fracture rates in the appendicular skeleton has also been documented. When used alone, 0.625 mg of conjugated estrogen per day is the lowest effective dose for retarding bone loss. When combined with calcium supplementation, some studies have suggested that 0.3 mg may be equally effective.

Corticosteroids

Corticosteroids are naturally-occurring, 21-carbon steroid hormones produced by the adrenal glands. They exert effects on most tissues in the body by alteration of gene expression because these hormones have the ability to cross the cell membrane and enter the nucleus to interact with DNA and RNA. Most of the therapeutically important steroids are synthesized from cholic acid or steroid sapogenins, and the many derivative combinations possible may result in a multitude of metabolic and pharmacodynamic effects. In orthopaedic practice, corticosteroids are used for their anti-inflammatory properties to palliate a variety of musculoskeletal disorders. These anti-inflammatory effects result from an inhibition of the synthesis of several classes of molecules, namely the leukotrienes, prostaglandins, and thromboxanes. This action is accomplished by inhibition of both the COX and lipoxygenase pathways of arachidonic acid metabolism secondary to the inhibition of phospholipase A_2 (Fig. 5).

In a survey of orthopaedists conducted by the American Academy of Orthopaedic Surgeons, 90% reported that they used steroid injections in the treatment of various musculoskeletal conditions (Table 4). Corticosteroid injections can be administered in an intra-articular, intrabursal, and intratendon sheath fashion. Even though injectable steroids are used extensively, very little is known about the exact mechanism of action in each of the different conditions treated.

Several injectable corticosteroids of varying solubility and half-life are commercially available (Table 5). There are no firm guidelines with regard to choice and dosage of

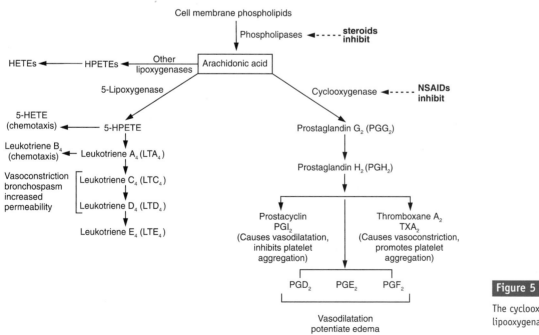

Figure 5

The cyclooxygenase and lipooxygenase pathways.

Table 4

Extra-articular Conditions Treated with Corticosteroid Injection by 233 Orthopaedists

Condition	Number of Orthopaedists	(%)
Elbow epicondylitis	217	93
Shoulder bursitis	211	91
Greater trochanteric bursitis	211	91
De Quervain tenosynovitis	203	87
Shoulder bicipital tendinitis	188	81
Pes anserinus bursitis	181	78
Plantar fasciitis	170	73
Myofascial trigger points	163	70
Carpal tunnel syndrome	131	56
Finger tenosynovitis	120	52
Tarsal tunnel syndrome	86	37
Achilles tendinitis	78	33
Back pain (epidural space injection)	57	24

(Reproduced with permission from Hill J, Trapp R, Colliver N: Survey on the use of corticosteroid injections by orthopaedists. *Contemp Orthop* 1989;18:39.)

steroids. Choice is largely determined by the clinician's previous experience or office inventory. In general, short- or intermediate-acting preparations (more water soluble) may be selected for acute conditions, whereas longer-acting preparations (water insoluble) are preferred for chronic conditions. A mixture of both short- and long-acting compounds is often administered regardless of the type of inflammatory process.

Dosage is commonly chosen based on the surface area that will receive the injection with a dose-equivalent of a specific steroid. For estimating dosage, a useful guide is as follows (using prednisolone tebutate suspension as a reference): for small joints of the hand and foot, 2.5 to 10 mg; for medium-sized joints such as the elbow and wrist, 10 to 25 mg; for the knee, ankle, and shoulder, 20 to 50 mg; and for the hip 25 to 40 mg. The longer time between dosing intervals, the better. A minimum of 4 weeks between intra-articular injections is usually recommended.

Intra-articular Injection

Intra-articular corticosteroid injections are designed to maximize local effects and minimize systemic effects pri-

marily in the adjunctive management of osteoarthrosis and rheumatoid arthritis. Several mechanisms of action of intra-articular steroids have been proposed: suppression of angiogenesis; diminished neutrophil migration into the joint; and diminished production of inflammatory mediators.

Results of therapy depend on the joint treated. Despite extensive anecdotal reports, a limited number of controlled studies suggest there is no long-term benefit from the use of intra-articular corticosteroids in hip and knee osteoarthrosis. In arthritic knees, steroid injection compared to placebo has been shown to provide greater pain relief at 1 week. At 4 weeks, however, results were similar for both groups. Some short-term benefit may be obtained in the patient waiting to undergo joint arthroplasty by temporary relief of pain and swelling. Smaller joints, such as the carpometacarpal, metacarpophalangeal, and acromioclavicular joints appear to have a better response as measured by sustained pain relief. This response is likely because of their nonweightbearing status. Corticosteroids have also been traditionally used for the treatment of chronic low-back pain by injection into the lumbar facet joints. A recent randomized, prospective study failed to show any therapeutic difference after injection with steroid compared to normal saline placebo.

Intra-articular steroids seem to entail a small risk of significant adverse effects. These include corticosteroid arthropathy, effects from systemic absorption, facial flushing, detrimental effects on intra-articular ligaments, iatrogenic infection, dermatologic changes, and hyperglycemia in diabetics. There is no firm evidence in the literature to support corticosteroid-induced arthropathy because numerous experiments demonstrate both protective and deleterious effects on articular cartilage following injection. This is largely because of the difficulty delineating whether arthropathy is secondary to an actual cause and effect or the natural progression of the primary disease process. Judicious use of intra-articular therapy dictates that repetitive joint injections should be avoided and weight-bearing joints should be rested approximately 24 hours after injection. Although intrasynovial steroids can cause suppression of the hypothalamic-pituitary-adrenal axis, true clinical adrenal insufficiency has not been reported. To avoid adrenal suppression, only 1 large joint should be injected at a time, with injections spread out over as long a time as possible. Adverse ligamentous effects will be discussed elsewhere in this chapter.

Iatrogenic septic arthritis is a rare complication if sterile technique is employed. Occupational Safety and Health Administration (OSHA) regulations mandate sterile gloves be worn when joint fluid is aspirated. The skin should be generously cleansed with an antiseptic agent to allow for the palpation of bony landmarks. In a series of 3,000 injections at a single institution, no instances of soft-tissue or joint sepsis were reported. These results suggest that this complication can be avoided by following rigid aseptic precautions, and avoiding the use of multiple-dose vials. Skin atrophy and hypopigmentation have been described following steroid injection. Suggested mechanisms for these dermatologic effects include leakage of the drug along the needle track, injection under pressure, and improper needle placement. Both reversible and permanent lesions may result. Absolute contraindications to intra-articular injection are presence of a known or suspected infection (articular, cellulitic, or systemic), known hypersensitivity reaction, osteochondral fracture, joint arthroplasty, presence of an uncontrolled bleeding disorder, and immediate preoperative status for joint arthroplasty of up to a few days.

Para-articular Injection

Inflammation of ligaments, tendons, and bursae are frequently idiopathic, self-limited afflictions that by clinical experience seem to respond favorably to local corticosteroid therapy. Satisfactory results seem to be site-dependent.

The most common sites for steroid injection of ligament injuries are the medial collateral ligament of the elbow, the extra-articular knee ligaments, and the ankle ligaments. Controlling inflammatory-mediated pain theoretically allows for earlier range of motion and presumably faster healing. The injections are ideally made into the peritendinous tissue as opposed to directly into the substance of the tendon itself. The main complication associated with ligamentous steroid injections is rupture of the ligament. Because inflammation is the first phase of the normal healing process, it has been proposed that the anti-inflammatory effects of steroid could be detrimental. In addition, steroids have been shown to interfere with collagen synthesis, lending yet another inhibitory mechanism of tendon healing because the majority of the dry weight of tendons is collagen. Biomechanical studies demonstrated that steroid-treated, acutely injured ligaments possessed the same tensile strength as nonsteroid-treated tendons but failed at lighter loads. The same effects were observed if the injection was delayed for 7 days following the end of the inflammatory phase for healing. This proposes that there must be other detrimental mechanisms outside of inhibition of the inflammatory stage. Clinically, the response of ligamentous injuries to treatment with steroid injection is quite variable. There are clinical studies to both support and condemn the use of steroids for ligamentous injury.

Tendinitis and tenosynovitis also show a varied response to steroid injection. As with ligaments, the steroid should be injected into the peritendinous structures or sheath, not directly into the substance of the tendon itself. Tenosynovitis of the thumb and finger flexors has been one of the most extensively studied conditions. Reports have shown

Table 5
Injectable Corticosteroids Commonly Used in Orthopaedic Practice

Solubility	Generic Name	Trade Name	Equivalent Dose, mg*
Most soluble	Betamethasone sodium phosphate	Celestone	0.6
Soluble	Dexamethasone sodium phosphate	Decadroim	0.75
	Prednisolone sodium phosphate	Hydeltrasol	5
Slightly soluble	Prednisolone tebutate	Hydeltra-T.B.A.	5
	Triamcinolone diacetate	Aristospan Forte	4
	Methylprednisolone acetate	Depo-Medrol	4
Relatively soluble	Dexamethasone acetate	Decadron-LA	0.75
	Hydrocortisone acetate	Hydrocortisone	20
	Prednisolone acetate	Prednalone	5
	Triamcinolone acetonide	Kenalog	4
	Triamcinolone hexacetonide	Aristospan	4
Combination	Betamethasone sodium phosphate-betamethasone acetate†	Cele	0.6

* For example, 0.6 mg of betamethasone sodium phosphate is equivalent to 0.75 mg of dexamethasone sodium phosphate, which is equivalent to 5 mg of prednisolone.

† Betamethasone acetate is slightly soluble.

(Reproduced with permission from Fadale PD, Wiggins ME: Corticosteroid injections: Their use and abuse. *J Am Acad Orthop Surg* 1994;2:133–140.)

satisfactory responses to injection, with positive results in up to 95% of patients. The best results are seen when there is single-digit involvement of less than 4 months' duration. In patients with De Quervain tenosynovitis, satisfactory results have been demonstrated in over 60%. Lateral epicondylitis has demonstrated a more variable response pattern. The initial course following injection has demonstrated a high positive response pattern, which is frequently followed by recurrence. The use of local steroids in the treatment of Achilles tendinitis is controversial. The only randomized controlled study showed no benefit of corticosteroids over placebo. As with ligaments, the complication of tendon rupture is real. However, again there are no published rigorous studies that evaluate the risk of rupture with or without steroid injection. Treatment of rotator cuff tendinitis has shown steroid injections to be effective in relieving pain in some series and in other series no difference between treated and placebo groups was observed.

The most common sites for bursal injection are subacromial, greater trochanteric, olecranon, prepatellar, and retrocalcaneal. Trochanteric and olecranon bursitis have demonstrated a favorable response to steroid injection, whereas prepatellar and retrocalcaneal bursitis have demonstrated a less favorable response pattern.

Special Considerations

Unicameral bone cysts (UBCs) represent an atrophic osteolytic process occurring in the metaphysis of long bones, usually in the first 2 decades of life. Although UBCs are most often asymptomatic, they may cause pain and pathologic fracture. The pathogenesis of UBCs has not been fully elucidated; however, bone resorptive factors, including prostaglandins, have been identified in the cystic fluid. One of the treatment options for UBCs is injection with methylprednisolone. Success rates as high as 96% have been reported with this method. Cysts often require more than 1 injection, usually spaced by 2-month intervals. Steroid injection seems to be as efficacious as curettage and bone grafting following a single trial of therapy.

Spinal cord injury patients may reap some potential benefit with pharmacologic intervention. The use of steroids in these patients is based on the assumption that edema plays a significant role in the physiology of spinal cord impairment. The clinical use of corticosteroids was initially based on the observation that cerebral edema around brain tumors was significantly reduced. In a prospective, randomized, double-blind multicenter study, spinal trauma patients who received methylprednisolone within 8 hours of injury and continued for 24 hours demonstrated better neurologic function than those who did not. An initial loading dose of 30 mg/kg followed by an hourly dose of 5.4 mg/kg for 23 hours is the regimen recommended by the National Acute Spinal Cord Injury Study (NASCIS).

Nonsteroidal Anti-Inflammatory Drugs

Nonsteroidal anti-inflammatory drugs (NSAIDs) are used to treat rheumatic and regional soft-tissue conditions in which pain is related to the magnitude of the inflammatory process. These drugs are heterogeneous in their chemical structure and diverse in their mechanism of action. A list of currently available NSAIDs is listed in Table 6. NSAIDs are the most frequently prescribed medications, accounting for about 4.5% of all prescriptions written in the United States.

One mechanism by which NSAIDs exert their effectiveness is by inhibiting the enzyme COX. COX catalyzes the reaction of arachidonic acid to physiologically important compounds, including prostaglandins and thromboxane. It is the inhibition of prostaglandin synthesis that is largely responsible for both the analgesic and anti-inflammatory therapeutic effects of NSAIDs. Prostaglandins produce small amounts of pain by themselves, but potentiate the pain caused by other mediators of inflammation. Prostaglandins also produce vasodilatation and increased vascular permeability. Although NSAIDs do not inhibit other mediators of the inflammatory response, they can attenuate this response enough to provide some relief from the clinical manifestations of inflammation.

Recently, 2 isoforms of COX have been identified, termed COX-1 and COX-2. COX-1 is a primarily constitutively expressed enzyme in many tissue types. Its role in maintaining gastric mucosa, regulating renal blood flow, and influencing platelet aggregation has been well established. COX-2, in contrast, is primarily an inducible enzyme involved in mediating pain and the inflammatory response. This discovery led to considerable interest in developing compounds that could selectively block inflammation and pain without disturbing normal homeostatic functions. The different activity of the 2 COX enzyme isoforms is thought to reside in a single amino acid substitution at the active site: isolucine in COX-1 for valine in COX-2. This amino acid difference leads to a conformational change resulting in the ability of the uniquely larger COX-2 specific inhibitor to gain access.

Agents now referred to as COX-2 inhibitors have been developed and successfully tested. In this section, the conventional anti-inflammatory drugs that inhibit both COX-1 and COX-2 functions will be referred to as NSAIDs. Drugs that selectively inhibit COX-2 will be referred to as COX-2 inhibitors.

NSAIDs inhibit COX by several different mechanisms. For example, aspirin binds covalently with a serine residue of the enzyme, leading to irreversible steric hindrance of the active site. Ibuprofen and piroxicam, however, are reversible competitive inhibitors of COX. Others, such as indomethacin and diclofenac, have the ability to also act on the lipooxygenase side of the arachidonic metabolism

Table 6

Dosage Data of Currently Available NSAIDs

Generic Name	Proprietary Name	Largest Unit Dose	Half-Life (Hrs)	Dosing Frequency
Aspirin		325 mg	0.25	2 q4h
Diclofenac	Voltaren	75 mg	2	bid
Diflunisal	Dikibud	500 mg	19	bid
Etodolac	Lodine	300 mg	6	qid
Fenoprofen	Nalfon	600 mg	2-3	quid
Flurbiprofen	Ansaid	100 mg	6	tid
Ibuprofen	Motrin	800 mg	2	qid
Indomethacin	Indocin	50 mg	4	tid
Ketoprofen	Orudis	75 mg	3	tid
Ketorolac	Toradol	10 mg	5	qid
Meclofenamate	Meclomen	100 mg	2	tid
Mabumetone	Reklafeb	500 mg	20-30	2 qd
Nabumetone	Relafen	750 mg	24	qd
Mabumetone	Reklafeb	500 mg	20-30	2 qd
Naproxen	Naprosyn	500 mg	14	bid
Oxaprozin	Daypro	600 mg	40-50	2 qd
Piroxicam	Feldene	20 mg	30-86	qd
Salicysalicylic acid	Disalcid	750 mg	1	qid
Sodium salicylate		650 mg	0.5	q4h
Sulindac	Clinoril	200 mg	8-14	bid
Tolmetin	Tolectin	400 mg	1-2	tid

(Reproduced with permission from Berger RG: Nonsteroidal anti-inflammatory drugs: Making the right choices. *J Am Acad Orthop Surg* 1994;2:255–260.)

pathway, leading to the inhibition of leukotriene inflammatory mediators.

Adverse Effects

Toxicity is the major contraindication for NSAID usage. About 20% of patients who use NSAIDs will experience some form of toxicity. Adverse side effects are common partly because these drugs are often given in high doses for extended periods of time, and they are widely used in the elderly population (> 65 years). The most common side effect is gastrointestinal disturbance. Damage to the mucosa of the gastrointestinal tract occurs by inhibition of prostaglandin synthesis, rather than by a direct erosive action of the NSAID. Prostaglandins inhibit gastric acid secretion, increase blood flow in the gastric mucosa, and express cytoprotective action. As such, prostaglandin inhi-

bition may lead to mucosal ischemia, and expose the mucosa to the damaging effects of acid by altering the protective mucosal barrier. Furthermore, NSAIDs diminish the function of thromboxane A-2, leading to disturbance in platelet aggregation and vasoconstriction. In patients with known gastrointestinal disease, the potentially synergistic disaster of bleeding can occur, further constricting their clinical utility of these drugs. Of those who experience NSAID-induced peptic ulceration, almost 30% require hospitalization. In persons older than 65 years, 20% to 30% of hospitalizations and deaths resulting from peptic ulceration are attributable to NSAID therapy.

Another major side effect is nephrotoxicity. Prostaglandins are synthesized in the renal medulla and glomeruli and are powerful vasodilators of the efferent and afferent arterioles. They are important in the regulation of renal blood flow and glomerular filtration. In patients with heart, liver, or intrinsic renal disease, NSAIDs can lead to acute renal failure. Other reported adverse effects include bronchospasm, rashes, decreased platelet function, tinnitus, headache, and hepatitis. In addition, selected NSAIDs have a variable effect on articular cartilage degradation in vitro. Many NSAIDs have been found to have adverse effects, a few have no effects, and a few have been shown to prevent cartilage degradation. Further studies to elucidate these effects are needed. There is evidence that toxicity associated with the use of more than 1 NSAID is additive.

Clinical Uses

The principal current indication for an NSAID prescription is for the management of degenerative osteoarthritis. There are numerous studies to demonstrate the efficacy of each available NSAID. When analyzing the data collectively, the following conclusions can be drawn: (1) all NSAIDs have proved to be superior to placebo in the treatment of osteoarthritis as measured by range of motion, pain scores, and ambulatory status; (2) there are no major objective differences in efficacy among the different NSAIDs. Responses to these drugs and the doses at which they are effective vary considerably from patient to patient. NSAID choice is largely based on patient and doctor preference and trial and error. They should be tried at least 2 to 4 weeks before switching. Dosing frequency also plays a role in NSAID choice. The intervals between drug doses usually approximate the plasma half-life. The more frequent dosing schedules probably decrease patient compliance and thus the beneficial effects of the drug. Of interest, acetaminophen was recently shown to be equally effective as and safer than ibuprofen for the management of osteoarthritis of the knee.

NSAIDs are also extensively used for the treatment of a variety of soft-tissue complaints, both acute and chronic, ranging from rotator cuff tendinitis to plantar fasciitis. Although some patients report relief of symptoms, the mechanism of action in treating these entities remains ambiguous. Some conditions such as tenosynovitis and bursitis demonstrate histologic evidence of inflammatory tissue. In contrast, muscle or tendon pain associated with overuse or a direct stretch injury for the most part has little or no inflammatory tissue response. As such, these conditions could display a similar response to purely analgesic agents. In fact, it has been suggested that inhibiting inflammation is detrimental to the natural healing process. Animal studies have demonstrated a delay of muscle regeneration in experimental muscle strains resulting in a decreased maximum failure load.

In the treatment of heterotopic ossification, NSAIDs, namely indomethacin, have traditionally been regarded as effective prophylaxis. Recent studies, however, have questioned the effectiveness of indomethacin in the prevention of heterotopic ossification associated with the treatment of acute acetabular fractures.

COX-2 Inhibitors

COX-2 metabolites are intimately involved in regulating pain and inflammation. COX-2 is generally considered an inducible enzyme. This means that COX-2 has the ability to regulate its expression in response to certain stimuli because of regions on the gene and mRNA coding for this protein. These characteristic regions allow for upregulation (increased expression) in response to cytokines in cells, such as chondrocytes macrophages, synoviocytes, and fibroblasts, where COX-2 is produced, and downregulation (decreased expression) in response to anti-inflammatory agents. COX-2 is also expressed constitutively (at basal rates) in the kidney and brain where it plays an important role in the normal development of these organs. In addition, there is strong evidence to support its function in the pathophysiology of Alzheimer's disease and colon cancer.

To date, there are 2 FDA-approved COX-2 inhibitors: celecoxib (Celebrex) and rofecoxib (Vioxx). In Phase II and Phase III trials, the efficacy of COX-2 inhibitors in relieving the signs and symptoms of osteoarthritis and rheumatoid arthritis has been demonstrated. The analgesic and anti-inflammatory effects seem to be comparable to those of conventional NSAIDs. In these same trials, COX-2 inhibitors demonstrated a favorable adverse events profile. Gastrointestinal toxicity, platelet function, and renal function in response to these drugs is similar to that of placebo.

These new anti-inflammatory drugs look promising as part of the pharmaceutical armamentarium for treating patients with degenerative and inflammatory arthritis without the untoward side effects of gastrointestinal and platelet dysfunction. It appears that these drugs will likely have a large impact on clinical practice, providing safer treatment for arthritis patients. Clearly, the full physiologic importance of the COX-2 inhibitors has yet to be discovered, necessitating judicious usage and close monitoring.

Desensitizing Agents

Reflex sympathetic dystrophy (RSD) syndrome is defined as an excessive or exaggerated response of an extremity to injury. RSD is characteristically manifested by certain constant characteristics: intense or unduly prolonged pain, vasomotor disturbances, delayed functional recovery, and various associated trophic changes. For those who do not routinely treat this condition, it may be surprising to discover that the inciting event may be a very small or even trivial injury or "small" surgical procedure that would normally be expected to resolve quickly without any sequelae. Pain that is out of proportion to the inciting cause is the hallmark of this condition. The terminology of sympathetic nervous system dysfunction is confusing. Major and minor causalgia, Sudek's atrophy, shoulder-hand syndrome, and reflex algodystrophy, among others, are terms that have been used in the literature to refer to RSD, although they differ with regard to clinical manifestations and response to treatment.

The true pathophysiology of RSD is not well understood because many of the actions of the sympathetic nervous system remain unknown. This has led to confusion in the diagnosis and treatment of RSD. The sympathetic nervous system innervates many structures, affecting many body functions. This occurs via alpha and beta receptors, which can be both excitatory and inhibitory at the end organ. It is believed that sensitization of the peripheral mechanoreceptors and nociceptors is mediated by alpha-adrenergic receptors. Norepinephrine is released from the sympathetic terminals, stimulating peripheral sensory nerves of the afferent spinothalamic tract, and resulting in transmission of pain and temperature signals to the neocortex. Another accepted theory suggests there is a decrease in afferent signals from decreased use of the extremity when it is painful. This decrease in afferent activity limits normal inhibition of the sympathetic system, leading to increased sympathetic discharge.

Treatment of RSD resistant to physical therapy is directed toward interruption of the abnormal reflex mediated by the autonomic nervous system. Surgical interruption via sympathectomy is usually a procedure of last resort. Sympathetic blockade is a valuable diagnostic and therapeutic tool. If complete sympathetic blockade does not relieve the pain, RSD can be ruled out as the cause in most cases. Blockade can be achieved centrally or regionally. Systemically, intravenous administration of an alpha blocker such as phentolamine is useful for diagnostic purposes, but its short duration limits its therapeutic use. Intravenous corticosteroids have also been shown to relieve symptoms of RSD, although the mechanism by which this is accomplished remains an enigma. Proposed mechanisms of their actions are decreased prostaglandin-mediated inflammation in the area of injury and decreased concentration of spinal prostanoids that facilitate the transmission of pain fibers in the spinal cord. Methods for spinal sympathetic blockade include paravertebral, epidural, and differential blockades. Of these, paravertebral blockade is considered the method of choice. A local anesthetic, such as lidocaine or bupivacaine, is injected outside the spinal column near sympathetic ganglia. Advantages of this method include avoidance of sensory or motor blockade and the ability to be done on an outpatient basis. Regional blockade has also been described using adrenergic neuron-blocking agents, such as guanethidine and reserpine. These agents block the normal release of norepinephrine from sympathetic neurons. They are delivered to an extremity via intravenous infusion through routes such as modified Bier blocks.

Oral pharmacologic therapy has been shown to be useful in the treatment of RSD as well. These drugs are used more commonly to control the symptoms associated with the chronic stages of this condition. Oral alpha-blockade agents such as phenoxybenzamine, prazosin, terazosin, and clonidine have been shown to be beneficial for causalgias. Oral corticosteroids can be effective in relieving symptoms if used in the first 2 weeks after injury in patients who present with early RSD. NSAIDs may have some benefit by minimizing inflammation, and hence pain, associated with injury. Antidepressants and narcotics are unfortunately routinely used to manage patients with RSD. These medications often lead to drug dependence and increased pain, making management even more difficult. Calcium channel blockers such as nifedipine, diltiazem, verapamil, and nicardipine have been used with some success in patients whose symptoms result from peripheral nerve injury. Intravenous bisphosphonates have recently been proposed as a therapeutic option, as some preliminary reports show rapid relief of pain. The proposed mechanism is decreased bone loss inciting the break in the cascade of events mediated in some way by cytokines. Interestingly, the bone mineral content of the affected extremity increased by a significant degree whereas change did not occur in the contralateral unaffected extremity. Although some of the oral medications can be easily administered by the orthopaedist, other medications can be more difficult and dangerous to use because of their side effects and drug interactions. As such, most of these drugs should be prescribed and monitored by a physician who is experienced in their use.

Selected Bibliography

Antibiotics

Burnett JW, Gustilo RB, Williams DN, Kind AC: Prophylactic antibiotics in hip fractures: A double-blind, prospective study. *J Bone Joint Surg* 1980;62A:457–462.

Duncan CP, Masri BA: The role of antibiotic-loaded cement in the treatment of an infection after a hip replacement, in Jackson DW (ed): *Instructional Course Lectures 44.* Rosemont, IL, American Academy of Orthopaedic Surgeons, 1995, pp 305–313.

Fitzgerald RH Jr: Current concepts of antimicrobial therapy, in Greene WB (ed): *Instructional Course Lectures XXXIX.* Park Ridge, IL, American Academy of Orthopaedic Surgeons, 1990, pp 465–470.

Fitzgerald RH Jr, Thompson RL: Cephalosporin antibiotics in the prevention and treatment of musculoskeletal sepsis. *J Bone Joint Surg* 1983;65A:1201–1205.

Perry C (ed): *Bone and Joint Infections.* London, England, M Dunitz, 1996.

Quintiliani R, Nightingale C: Principles of antibiotic usage. *Clin Orthop* 1984;190:31–35.

Silver A, Eichorn A, Kral J, et al: The Antibiotic Prophylaxis Study Group: Timeliness and use of antibiotic prophylaxis in selected inpatient surgical procedures. *Am J Surg* 1996;171:548–552.

Tsukayama DT, Gustilo RB: Antibiotic management of open fractures, in Greene WB (ed): *Instructional Course Lectures XXXIX.* Park Ridge, IL, American Academy of Orthopaedic Surgeons, 1990, pp 487–490.

Williams DN, Gustilo RB: The use of preventive antibiotics in orthopaedic surgery. *Clin Orthop* 1984;190:83–88.

Worlock P, Slack R, Harvey L, Mawhinney R: The prevention of infection in open fractures: An experimental study of the effect of antibiotic therapy. *J Bone Joint Surg* 1988;70A:1341–1347.

Anticoagulation

Ansari S, Warwick D, Ackroyd CE, Newman JH: Incidence of fatal pulmonary embolism after 1390 knee arthroplasties without routine prophylactic anticoagulation, except in high-risk cases. *J Arthroplasty* 1997;6:599–602.

Fender D, Harper WM, Thompson JR, Gregg PJ: Mortality and fatal pulmonary embolism after primary total hip replacement: Results from a regional hip register. *J Bone Joint Surg* 1997;79B:896–899.

Hull RD, Raskob GE, Pineo GF, et al: Subcutaneous low-molecular-weight heparin vs warfarin for prophylaxis of deep vein thrombosis after hip or knee implantation: An economic perspective. *Arch Intern Med* 1997;157:298–303.

Hull RD, Raskob GE: Prophylaxis of venous thromboembolic disease following hip and knee surgery. *J Bone Joint Surg* 1986;68A:146–150.

Janku GV, Paiement GD, Green HD: Prevention of venous thromboembolism in orthopaedics in the United States. *Clin Orthop* 1996; 325:313–321.

Leclerc JR, Geerts WH, Desjardins L, et al: Prevention of venous thromboembolism after knee arthroplasty: A randomized, double-blind trial comparing enoxaparin with warfarin. *Ann Intern Med* 1996;124:619–626.

Weitz JI: Low-molecular-weight heparins. *N Engl J Med* 1997;337: 688–698.

Zimlich RH, Fulbright, BM, Friedman RJ: Current status of anticoagulation therapy after total hip and total knee arthroplasty. *J Am Acad Orthop Surg* 1996;4:54–62.

Inhibitors of Bone Resorption

Adachi JD, Bensen WG, Brown J, et al: Intermittent etidronate therapy to prevent corticosteroid-induced osteoporosis. *N Engl J Med* 1997;337:382–387.

Bockman RS, Weinerman SA: Medical treatment for Paget's disease of bone, in Heckman JD (ed): *Instructional Course Lectures 42.* Rosemont, IL, American Academy of Orthopaedic Surgeons, 1993, pp 425–433.

Cauley JA, Seeley DG, Ensrud K, Ettinger B, Black D, Cummings SR: Estrogen replacement therapy and fractures in older women: Study of Osteoporotic Fractures Research Group. *Ann Intern Med* 1995; 122:9–16.

Einhorn TA: Bone metabolism and metabolic bone disease, in Kasser JR (ed): *Orthopaedic Knowledge Update 5.* Rosemont, IL, American Academy of Orthopaedic Surgeons, 1996.

Fleisch HA: Bisphosphonates: Preclinical aspects and use in osteoporosis. *Ann Med* 1997;29:55–62.

Glorieux FH: Calcitriol treatment in vitamin D-dependent and vitamin D-resistant rickets. *Metabolism* 1990;39(suppl 1):10–12.

Khan SA, Vasikaran S, McCloskey EV, et al: Alendronate in the treatment of Paget's disease of bone. *Bone* 1997;20:263–271.

Lacey DL, Timms E, Tan HL, et al: Osteoprotegerin ligand is a cytokine that regulates osteoclast differentiation and activation. *Cell* 1998;93:165–176.

Liberman UA, Weiss SR, Broll J, et al: The Alendronate Phase III Osteoporosis Treatment Study Group: Effect of oral alendronate on bone mineral density and the incidence of fractures in postmenopausal osteoporosis. *N Engl J Med* 1995;333:1437–1443.

Patel S, Lyons AR, Hosking DJ: Drugs used in the treatment of metabolic bone disease: Clinical pharmacology and therapeutic use. *Drugs* 1993;46:594–617.

Sato M, Grasser W, Endo N, et al: Bisphosphonate action: Alendronate localization in rat bone and effects on osteoclast ultrastructure. *J Clin Invest* 1991;88:2095–2105.

Shinoda H, Adamek G, Felix R, Fleisch H, Schenk R, Hagan P: Structure-activity relationships of various bisphosphonates. *Calcif Tissue Int* 1983;35:87–99.

Siminoski K, Josse RG: Consensus statements from the Scirentific Advisory Board of the Osteoporosis Society of Canada: 9. Calcitonin in the treatment of osteoporosis. *CMAJ* 1996;155:962–965.

Suda T, Nakamura I, Jimi E, Takahashi N: Regulation of osteoclast function. *J Bone Miner Res* 1997;12:869–879.

Steroids

Caldwell JR: Intra-articular corticosteroids: Guide to selection and indications for use. *Drugs* 1996;52:507–514.

Fadale PD, Wiggins ME: Corticosteroid injections: Their use and abuse. *J Am Acad Orthop Surg* 1994;2:133–140.

Gray RG, Gottlieb NL: Intra-articular corticosteroids: An updated assessment. *Clin Orthop* 1983;177:235–258.

Shrier I, Matheson GO, Kohl HW III: Ahilles tendonitis: Are corticosteroid injections useful or harmful? *Clin J Sport Med* 1996;6:245–250.

Neustadt DH: Intraarticular steroid therapy, in Moskowitz RW, Howell DS, Goldberg VM, Mankin HJ (eds): *Osteoarthritis: Diagnosis and Medical/Surgical Management*, ed 2. Philadelphia, PA, WB Saunders, 1992, pp 493–510.

Blair B, Rokito AS, Cuomo F, Jarolem K, Zuckerman JD: Efficacy of injections of corticosteroids for subacromial impingement syndrome. *J Bone Joint Surg* 1996;78A:1685–1689.

Nonsteroidal Anti-Inflammatory Drugs

Almekinders LC, Gilbert JA: Healing of experimental muscle strains and the effects of nonsteroidal antiinflammatory medication. *Am J Sports Med* 1986;14:303–308.

Berger RG: Nonsteroidal anti-inflammatory drugs: Making the right choices. *J Am Acad Orthop Surg* 1994;2:255–260.

Blackburn WD: Management of osteoarthritis and rheumatoid arthritis: Prospects and possibilities. *Am J Med* 1996;100:24S–30S.

Hawker G: Editorial: Prescribing nonsteroidal antiinflammatory drugs: What's new? *J Rheumatol* 1997;24:243–245.

Hochberg MC, Altman RD, Brandt KD: American College of Rheumatology: Guidelines for the medical management of osteoarthritis. Part I: Osteoarthritis of the hip. *Arthritis Rheum* 1995;38:1535–1540.

Lipsky PE: The clinical potential of cyclooxygenase-2-specific inhibitors. *Am J Med* 1999;106:51S–57S.

Simon LS: Role and regulation of cyclooxygenase-2 during inflammation. *Am J Med* 1999;106:37S–42S.

Towheed TE, Hochberg MC: A systematic review of randomized controlled trials of pharmacological therapy in osteoarthritis of the hip. *J Rheumatol* 1997;24:349–357.

Desensitizing Agents

Adami S, Fossaluzza V, Gatti D, Fracassi E, Braga V: Bisphosphonate therapy of reflex sympathetic dystrophy syndrome. *Ann Rheum Dis* 1997;56:201–204.

Lindenfeld TN, Bach BR Jr, Wojtys EM: Reflex sympathetic dystrophy and pain dysfunction in the lower extremity, in Springfield DS (ed): *Instructional Course Lectures 46*. Rosemont, IL, American Academy of Orthopaedic Surgeons, 1997, pp 261–268.

O'Brien SJ, Ngeow J, Gibney MA, Warren RF, Fealy S: Reflex sympathetic dystrophy of the knee: Causes, diagnosis, and treatment. *Am J Sports Med* 1995;23:655–659.

Schutzer SF, Gossling HR: The treatment of reflex sympathetic dystrophy syndrome. *J Bone Joint Surg* 1984;66A:625–629.

Chapter 8

Infections in Orthopaedics

Kevin L. Garvin, MD

James V. Luck, Jr, MD

Mark E. Rupp, MD

Paul D. Fey, PhD

This chapter at a glance

This chapter provides the reader with information to better understand how to prevent infection, how the process may occur, and current treatment. Tuberculin infections, immunosuppression, prophylactic antibiotic therapy, and viral diseases are also discussed.

One or more of the authors or the department with which they are affiliated has received something of value from a commercial or other party related directly or indirectly to the subject of this chapter.

Introduction

Musculoskeletal infections remain one of the most challenging and serious complications in orthopaedic surgery. The variation in clinical presentation further complicates the management of these patients because of the potential for a delay in diagnosis. Empiric or injudicious use of oral antibiotic therapy and the subtle nature of prosthetic-associated infection have added to the difficulty in prompt bacterial identification and definitive treatment of these patients. Although newer diagnostic tools and innovative treatments have been developed, the emergence of resistant bacteria continues to challenge even the most astute clinician. The purpose of this chapter is to provide the reader with information to better understand how to prevent infection, how the process may occur, and the current treatment. The chapter is also devoted to tuberculin infections, immunosuppression, prophylactic antibiotic therapy, and viral diseases.

Pathogenesis/Pathophysiology

The initial event of infection occurs when bacteria successfully lodge in the musculoskeletal system. The easiest and most common access for the bacteria is through a surgical wound. The bacteria are able to flourish in this environment because the tissues have been sufficiently traumatized by the surgery, with resultant compromised blood flow, hematoma formation, and foreign material (such as plates, screws, prostheses, or cement) that often remains in place. Direct inoculation of bacteria can also occur during open trauma. The final 2 routes bacteria may take to reach the musculoskeletal system are via hematogenous seeding and contiguous spreading from adjacent areas of infection.

One of several scenarios may occur once bacteria have gained entry to the soft tissues or bone. Bacteria may be destroyed by the host, live in symbiosis with the host, or flourish and cause host sepsis and possibly death. In any event, the first response to bacterial invasion involves an acute inflammatory reaction. A myriad of components, including polymorphonuclear cells, chemotactic factors, and the immune system, are involved in this process. Leukocyte diapedesis occurs, followed by infiltration of polymorphonuclear cells to the area. The process by which polymorphonuclear cells are attracted to the area by chemical substances is known as chemotaxis. Boyden originally discovered that chemotaxis occurred if serum was incubated with precipitates of antigens and antibiodies.

The immune system comprises cell-mediated and humoral components. Both the cell-mediated and the humoral responses are typically involved in bacterial infections. Once the polymorphonuclear cells attack bacteria, some may be damaged, thus releasing additional chemotactic molecules and attracting larger numbers of polymor-

phonuclear cells. When the polymorphonuclear cells are in proximity to the bacteria, the bacterial particles are ingested or phagocytized. For phagocytosis to occur, opsonins or components in the serum must coat the bacteria, making them more attractive for the macrophages.

This nonspecific immune response can be affected not only by the complement system activation but also by certain medications. Nonsteroidal anti-inflammatory agents, steroids, and aspirin are common medications that affect this process. An investigation was performed with Sprague-Dawley rats that were divided into 2 groups: one group received steroids, and the other was not treated. Osteomyelitis was then created in the tibia of both groups of animals. The polymorphonuclear cells of the group not receiving steroids exhibited greater chemotaxis ($p = 0.046$), but both groups exhibited comparable phagocytosis.

The more benign form of osteomyelitis or bone infection is called a Brodie's abscess. In a Brodie's abscess, the infection is located within the cortical contents of the bone and may be isolated by a thin reactive area of bone. It is common for pain to be the only presenting symptom of these patients. If the infectious process is less active or quiescent, the patient may be asymptomatic.

Acute hematogenous osteomyelitis has a predilection for the metaphyseal area of bone because of increased venous pooling, diminished blood supply, sluggish blood flow, and the cellular composition at this level. Once bacteria land in the metaphyseal region, the infection quickly progresses, allowing replication of bacteria and further compromising blood flow. Morrissey and associates and Whalen and associates were able to successfully create a model of acute hematogenous osteomyelitis. Young rabbits were divided into groups and, using a combination of trauma in the metaphyseal region of the tibia and intravenous *Staphylococcus aureus*, osteomyelitis was predictably produced in the metaphyseal region. In contrast, the same amount of *S aureus* injected into a second group of rabbits without trauma failed to cause an infection. In the affected limb, change occurred by 24 hours after the injection of bacteria and was represented by a small mass of neutrophils (2×2 mm). Phagocytized bacteria were also in the region. After 48 hours, the infection extended from the lower part of the metaphysis to the growth plate and epiphysis. The zone of necrosis in the lower part of the metaphysis was surrounded by inflammatory cells distally, but the proximal site of injury contained only fragmented cells, necrotic debris, and free bacteria. By 7 days, the inflammatory process involved the entire metaphysis, and it had also spread to the physeal and epiphyseal regions.

Although the investigators cautioned against direct extrapolation of their information to children, important questions were raised. Why did the trauma increase the susceptibility for infection? Did decreased tissue oxygen tension compromise phagocytosis of bacteria? The hypothetical explanation for this is a reduction of host defenses of the metaphysis caused by regional ischemia. The second important finding in the study was that bacteria were distributed along the region of the nutrient artery in the posteromedial aspect of the tibia and not in the terminal vessels near the metaphysis and physis. These findings indicate that factors other than circulation are involved in the infection process. It is postulated that among these factors are a deficiency of tissue-based macrophages and a mechanical or physical barrier by the calcified cartilage septa, which prevent leukocytes from gathering near bacteria. Although controversy still exists as to the exact pathophysiology of hematogenous osteomyelitis, these studies help make this complex process more understandable.

The process of infection often leaves behind a zone of necrosis and necrotic debris. The necrotic debris, called a sequestrum, provides the bacteria with a favorable milieu. The host attempts to isolate this sequestrum, or dead bone, by forming a wall of new bone. The new reactive bone surrounding the sequestrum is called an involucrum (Fig. 1).

The body contains several joints in which the metaphysis is intra-articular and therefore, a decompressed metaphyseal infection may result in septic arthritis. Classically, this occurs in the proximal femur in the child. Alternatively, as the metaphyseal infection progresses and exits through the cortex it may enter soft tissues, ultimately forming a tract to the skin or a sinus tract. The tract does not follow a predictable route and may exit near the joint or at a more distant point. Another site of infection is in the joints of the lower extremity in children, where septic arthritis occurs, but this occurs less often in the joints of the upper extremities.

Numerous different bacteria cause musculoskeletal infections. The pathogen varies according to the patient's age, circumstances relating to the infection, and host immune response. In neonates and infants, *Staphylococcus, Streptococcus,* and gram-negative bacteria are the predominant organisms. In patients 6 months up to 3 years of age, *Haemophilus influenzae* type B must also be strongly considered as well as *Staphylococcus* and *Streptococcus* species. After age 3, *Staphylococcus* and *Streptococcus* again dominate as the most pathogenic until adolescence. During adolescence, *Neisseria gonorrhoeae* is occasionally associated with musculoskeletal infections. *Staphylococcus epidermidis* or coagulase-negative *Staphylococcus* are the dominant organisms if an implant or prosthesis is involved.

Septic arthritis can afflict people of all ages and regardless of the type of bacteria, the potential for cartilage destruction, sepsis, and even death is always present. As bacteria thrive in the joint, their initial destructive forces take place by dissolution of the glycosaminoglycan units of cartilage. The glycosaminoglycan units include chondroitin-4-sulfate, chondroitin-6-sulfate, keratin sulfate, and marrow dramatin sulfate. Hyaluronate is also a glycosaminoglycan, but unlike the other units it is not bound to a protein core. The glycosaminoglycans function as subunits of the proteoglycan molecule, in part giving rise to its physical

properties of fluid retention or swelling pressure of the cartilage. Following the destruction of the glycosaminoglycan units, collagen breakdown ensues and is evident by gross physical alteration of the cartilage.

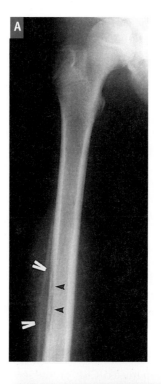
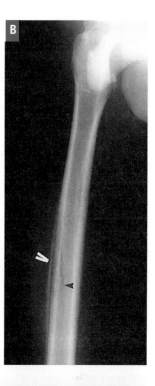

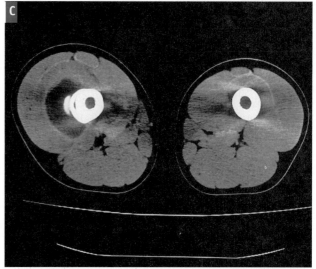

Figure 1

A and **B**, Radiographs of the femur of a 16-year-old boy who developed pain and swelling of the thigh and fever of several days' duration after bruising his thigh while sliding during a baseball game. Periosteal new bone formation (solid arrows) and resorption of the cortical bone (arrowheads) are shown. **C**, Computed tomography scan demonstrating the involucrum or new bone formation around the site of infection.

Diagnosis

Diagnosis of musculoskeletal infection can be established easily in the majority of patients. Infrequently the diagnosis requires sophisticated studies, but even in the most straightforward presentations, the clinician must always culture fluid and tissues to firmly establish the diagnosis and identify the pathogen. Patients suspected of having musculoskeletal infection often present with complaints of pain localized to the site of infection. Rarely will patients not include pain as a complaint when they are suffering with an infectious process. Localized warmth, swelling, and redness further suggest an infectious etiology. Additional findings of fever, chills, loss of joint motion, and unwillingness to use an extremity strongly support the diagnosis of infection.

Although the identification of bacteria associated with these symptoms secures the diagnosis, the difficulty is in localizing the precise site of infection. For example, in the infant or toddler, the history and physical examination may not point to any specific site. In contrast, the patient with chronic osteomyelitis and a draining sinus provides the physician with a path to the site of infection. The basic evaluation of these patients includes a complete blood count with differential, erythrocyte sedimentation rate (ESR), and C-reactive protein (CRP). CRP is present in only minimal concentration in plasma and is an acute phase protein. Unlike ESR, CRP concentrations rise within a few hours of the onset of infection, reaching extremely high values (up to 400 mg/L) within 48 hours and can return to normal a few weeks after the infection has been treated. CRP is more sensitive than ESR and is commonly used to evaluate patients with infection.

In patients suspected of musculoskeletal infection, the first imaging study is a radiograph of the affected limb. The earliest changes evident on the radiograph are soft-tissue swelling and loss of tissue planes. Bone changes normally do not occur until 1 to 2 weeks after the onset of infection. When present, the hallmark features of osteomyelitis on radiograph are bone resorption, bone destruction, and periosteal elevation. Bone loss of up to 30% to 40% is necessary before radiographic changes can be detected. Bone repair occurring near the infection is within the bone and along the periosteum. Periosteal new bone forms nearly parallel to the cortex, tapering to the cortex further from the nidus of infection (Fig. 1, B). If the infection continues to be active, intramedullary and periosteal new bone adjacent to the dead or necrotic bone that is being resorbed gives the typical appearance of chronic osteomyelitis. This typical picture can easily be confused with neoplasia and ultimately may necessitate biopsy to distinguish the 2 diseases.

In the early phase of infection, when radiographs are normal but infection is still suspected, bone imaging studies are performed. The 3-phase bone scan is typically the first study performed to evaluate patients. Technetium Tc 99m diphosphonate labels bone and is related to the blood flow and osteoblast activity. The first phase of the bone scan is a flow phase consisting of 2- to 5-second images performed while the radioactive material is injected. The second phase, the blood pool phase, occurs approximately 5 minutes after the radioactive material is injected. The third phase, the bone image phase, occurs approximately 3 hours after injection. Bone infection is strongly suspected when the radioactive material localizes in the bone after 3 hours. If a fourth phase were to be performed to diagnose infection, it would be based on the uptake of technetium Tc 99m methylene diphosphonate that is no longer bound to the lamellar bone after 4 hours but continues in woven bone at the site of infection up to 24 hours.

Triphasic technetium Tc 99m diphosphonate bone scanning is the most frequently used scan. It is sensitive for detecting acute hematogenous osteomyelitis and septic arthritis. In some neonates, the scans are less useful, with false negative or "cold" scans identified in an unacceptably high percentage. In other patients with underlying disease, bone scans can be positive but not because of the infection. This scenario is particularly true in patients with sickle cell disease.

The gallium citrate Ga 67 scan has also been used but is more time-consuming. Delayed imaging as late as 2 days after injection may be needed to detect the infection. The leukocyte-labeled nuclear imaging studies are also labor-intensive. To perform this scan, it is necessary to obtain the patient's blood and label the white cells with radioisotopes. The labeled white cells are reinjected into the patient, and then the patient is scanned. The reinjected white blood cells are given up to 24 hours to migrate to the site of inflammation and the scan is repeated. The cost and time necessary to perform the test and the rare indication have discouraged frequent use of radiolabeled imaging for these patients.

Magnetic resonance imaging (MRI) has the advantages of high sensitivity, specificity, and no radiation exposure. The disadvantages of an MRI scan are its cost and inaccuracy if a prosthetic device or internal fixation is present. Because marrow normally has high-signal intensity on T1-weighted images, the low signal of the inflammatory process on T1-weighted images is indicative of infection. The T2-weighted images have a high signal because the fatty marrow has been replaced by the inflammatory process. The MRI scan is also helpful to identify sequestra, areas of abscess formation, and sinus tracts. The purpose of these scans is to map the location of infection. Once this is performed, aspiration of the area is necessary to identify the bacterial organism. Chapter 9, MRI of the musculoskeletal system, presents a more detailed discussion.

Treatment

Once the correct diagnosis has been established and the bacteria identified, appropriate treatment can promptly be initiated. The treatment of a patient with osteomyelitis or septic arthritis requires a thorough understanding of the disease process. The mainstay of treatment is surgical debridement of infected and necrotic tissues. Rarely can successful treatment of osteomyelitis and septic arthritis be achieved without the surgical treatment of the infection. In the very acute presentation of acute hematogenous osteomyelitis, medical treatment may be the only treatment necessary to eradicate the infection.

It is possible to forego surgical treatment if the infection is acute in presentation with little tissue necrosis and minimal purulence. The nonsurgical treatment of this group of patients is enhanced with the prompt initiation of antibiotic therapy specific for the bacteria. The antibiotic therapy should begin immediately after cultures have been obtained. The selection of antibiotics is geared toward the pathogen most likely to be present. For example, a 3-year-old child suspected of having hematogenous osteomyelitis is likely to be infected with *S aureus,* but *H influenzae B* may also be present. On the other hand, a 9-year-old child with sickle cell disease is also likely to be infected with *S aureus,* but the presence of encapsulated organisms such as *Salmonella* should be considered, and the antibiotic therapy must include this organism as well.

The recommended duration of antibiotic treatment is shorter than previous recommendations. Rarely is more than 4 weeks of antibiotic treatment prescribed, but when it is, the patients are likely to receive 1 to 2 weeks of parenteral therapy followed by 4 to 5 weeks of oral therapy, for a total antibiotic duration of approximately 4 to 6 weeks. This is based on bacterial sensitivity to the antibiotic, the patient's response to treatment, and when necessary, the decreasing values of ESR, complete blood count with differential, and CRP. Rarely, if the infection has not responded, the antibiotics may be continued for a longer period. Long-term antibiotic therapy is used only when it is certain that the infection has been adequately debrided, the antibiotics are appropriate for the bacteria, and the host does not have a correctable problem contributing to the infection.

If the infectious process has become more advanced with necrotic material, sequestra, or gross purulence, then surgical debridement is indicated. Orr was one of the first surgeons to emphasize the importance of wide drainage in surgical debridement. This technique preceded the discovery of penicillin and was the main aspect of treatment. Surgical debridement with wide drainage for removal of all necrotic bone, grossly infected tissue, and foreign material is the most important aspect of treatment for patients with osteomyelitis.

If a large volume of tissue and foreign material is removed, a tissue void remains at the site. When soft tissue has been debrided, it is normally replaced with a local or free muscle, or muscle and skin composite flap. Biologic tissues have the advantage of obliterating the dead space and providing vascularity to an area previously filled with necrotic tissue. If bone is removed at the site of debridement, it is often necessary to replace it using bone graft or other techniques (Ilizarov) to stimulate new bone formation. Local antibiotics are used in these situations as well, with the advantage of high local concentrations directly at the site of infection and low systemic concentrations, thus avoiding toxicity. It is hoped that local antibiotics released in a controlled manner can replace the need for systemic antibiotics in these patients. Antibiotic delivery systems include implantable pumps, bioresorbable polymers, nonbiodegradable pellets of polymethylmethacrylate, sebaceous fatty acid dimers, and bone graft-type materials. Local antibiotic delivery systems have gained popularity despite some question of their effectiveness. Research does support their use as being equal to or better than parenteral antibiotics without local antibiotic delivery.

Infections and Total Joint Replacement

Infection after total joint arthroplasty shares many of the same features as acute hematogenous osteomyelitis, septic arthritis, and chronic osteomyelitis. In each of these situations the underlying infectious process causes pain at rest. This classic symptom represents the underlying inflammatory process. Associated symptoms of fever or chills are rarely present in patients with infected total joints. Physical examination of total joint patients may also lack positive signs of infection, such as warmth, redness, drainage, or sinus tracts. However, if any of these clinical findings are present, there is a very high likelihood of an underlying infectious process. Despite the lack of these positive findings, a strong clinical suspicion in the patient with persistent pain after total joint replacement could lead to further studies to assist in identifying the infection. The basic laboratory studies include ESR, CRP, and a complete blood count with a differential. The usefulness of these laboratory tests individually has been questioned, because they are all nonspecific for the infectious process. Further invasive tests, such as aspiration or obtaining tissue intraoperatively, are much more sensitive and specific for the infection. The fluid and tissues can be analyzed via Gram stains, cultures, and frozen section analyses. Aspiration of the hip joint on a routine basis before revision is of questionable benefit, but when indicated based on other evidence it is an excellent procedure to help determine whether infection is present.

If the aspiration leads to detection of infection, the joint is treated with debridement and particular attention given to removal of all foreign materials and infected, necrotic tissue. If the aspiration fails to yield fluid, or if the culture of aspirated fluid is negative, the patient may still have an infection and be a candidate for surgery. A surgical revision in this patient is for septic or aseptic loosening of the implant. At the time of surgical treatment, tissue is obtained for histologic frozen section analysis and culture. These tissue specimens are obtained from granulation tissue adjacent to the prosthesis between the bone and acetabular component, or between the bone and femoral component. The tissue is analyzed under high-power magnification and the number of polymorphonuclear cells is quantified. Frozen section analysis of at least 1 polymorphonuclear cell under a high-power field (average of 1 per 10 high-powered fields) lowers the threshold for infection, increases the sensitivity, and possibly does not reduce the specificity. Using more than 10 polymorphonuclear cells per high-powered field lowers the sensitivity but is more specific and has a higher positive predictive value.

It is critical that the surgeon select grossly inflamed granulation tissue because a sampling error can occur if tissues from less inflamed areas not in contact with the joint are examined. In addition to the analysis of tissues in the search for polymorphonuclear cells, mononuclear inflammatory cells are prominent and characterized in cellular histologic overview in patients with purulent endoprosthetic infections. Additional research will need to be conducted in this area to confirm results from chronically infected joint implants. However, it is suggested that the absence of these neutrophils does not contribute to the pathologic events in the pseudocapsular area, but instead a mononuclear inflammatory cell reaction occurs, which is a macrophage-dependent foreign body-type response. The orthopaedic surgeon should have a working relationship with a pathologist experienced in the interpretation of frozen section analysis of tissues about implants.

Histopathologic analysis of the tissue may result in false negative results because of sampling error. False-positive results rarely occur. It is possible to obtain acutely inflamed tissue near a fracture and have a false-positive result.

Polymerase chain reaction (PCR) is a technique that uses the 16S ribosomal units of DNA, which are preserved in all phylogeny. Vector ribonucleic acid (RNA) or DNA and bacterial DNA are amplified by the PCR, which allows for visual detection and further evaluation. PCR has been limited because of the vast numbers of bacteria, each of which has a specific RNA and DNA, making the routine use of PCR an extremely onerous task. As these sequences for bacterial genus and species are developed, it will be possible to test all tissue samples against known primers for each bacteria.

The definitive diagnostic test for periprosthetic infection remains culture of tissue obtained at the time of surgery.

The positive culture must be supported by the clinical probability of infection and based on other positive signs, symptoms, laboratory, or radiographic findings. These positive signs may include any of the above-mentioned tests, signs, or symptoms.

Abnormal radiographic findings of the prosthesis loosening are nonspecific for the process being aseptic or septic. Radiographic findings suggestive but not specific for septic loosening are aggressive nonfocal osteolysis, periosteal bone formation, or focal lysis.

Nuclear scanning to confirm the diagnosis of infection when suspected is less well established. Technetium Tc 99m mdp scans require injection of an isotope followed by scans at various intervals after the nuclear isotope has been injected. A scan is performed immediately after the injection for evaluation of blood flow to the soft tissues adjacent to the implant, an intermediate scan a few minutes after the injection as the blood flows to the deeper tissues, and a delayed scan (2 to 3 hours after injection) to evaluate the uptake of the isotope by the bony tissue. These scans are sensitive, but lack specificity, and therefore have been combined with other types of scans such as leukocyte scans to help increase the specificity.

Leukocyte scintigraphy is a frequently used method of scanning to detect total joint infections. Leukocyte scans require taking blood from the patient and labeling it with specific radioisotopes. It may be repeated up to 24 hours later. Two of the most commonly used types of leukocyte scintigraphy are Indium In 111 or technetium Tc 99m mdp complex to hexamethyl prophyelamine oxide. Scans hold promise with 80% to 90% sensitivity and 85% to 100% specificity. Major drawbacks to the routine use of these scans are the labor necessary to complete them and their high cost.

The newest types of nuclear imaging studies are immunoscintigraphy labeling of immunoglobulins. Indium In 111 labeled human nonspecific immunoglobulin G (indium In 111 IgG) is a type of immunoscintigraphy that has been studied clinically to evaluate infection and inflammation. Early results are promising for this technique as well as other immunoscintigraphy (^{123}I, ^{111}In, ^{99m}Tc). As implied by the name, polyclonal or monoclonal antibodies are labeled with iodine I 123, indium In 111, or technetium Tc 99m. The success of the scans has varied, reportedly between 67% and 100% for specificity and 88% to 100% sensitivity. Radiotracer-labeled chemotactic peptides have also been recently used, but clinical studies on humans are currently not available.

Once the diagnosis has been established, the treatment of the patients with periprosthetic or infected hip and knee arthroplasty relies on the same basic principles for treatment as infection elsewhere in the body. The infected site must be surgically debrided to remove infected and necrotic tissue and foreign material. Once the surgical procedure is completed, final cultures of this debrided tissue are obtained and parenteral antibiotic therapy is initiated to treat any microscopically retained bacteria. If any of these forms of treatment are not successfully performed, the infection has an excellent chance of persisting or recurring. Retention of the components may be possible in the early infection (less than 3 months) or if the patient's symptoms have been present for a short period of time (less than 1 to 2 weeks). Even with these strict criteria the failure rate may approach 50%. More standard treatment as listed above can be performed in 1 stage, where the prosthesis is replaced at the time of the surgical debridement, in 2 stages, where an interval ranges from 6 weeks to several years, or even 3 stages, where all of the surgical debridement is followed by reconstruction with bone graft at a second surgery, and a final prosthesis placement at a third surgery.

Antibiotic Prophylaxis for Patients With Total Joint Replacement

The number of joint replacements performed annually will continue to increase over the next several years. It has been estimated that 450,000 to 500,000 joint replacements are performed annually, and literally millions of patients have a joint already replaced. The prevention of infection is paramount to the long-term success of the implant in these patients. In 1997, a panel of orthopaedic surgeons, infectious disease specialists, and dentists met and developed an advisory statement to help determine the best means of antibiotic prophylaxis for these patients. At the time of the advisory statement there was no evidence to support routine antimicrobial prophylaxis in joint replacement patients prior to dental treatment. The antimicrobial prophylaxis statement included 3 outlines identifying patients at potentially increased risk of hematogenous infection

(Outline 1), dental procedures stratified and based on the likelihood that the procedure would cause a bacteremia (Outline 2), and the type of antibiotic recommended (Outline 3). Surgeons must realize that the advisory statement and content of the outlines are guidelines and should not be used to replace sound clinical judgment by the dentist or orthopaedic surgeon when treating these patients.

Emerging Resistant Strains of Bacteria

Mechanisms of Antibiotic Action and Resistance

The mechanism of action of commonly used antimicrobial agents is summarized in Table 1. Antibiotics are active against targets present in bacteria that are either not found

---

Outline 1

Patients at Potential Increased Risk of Hematogenous Total Joint Infection

Immunocompromised/immunosuppressed patients
Inflammatory arthropathies: rheumatoid arthritis, systemic lupus erythematosus
Disease, drug, or radiation-induced immunosuppression

Other patients
Insulin-dependent (type 1) diabetes
First 2 years following joint placement
Previous prosthetic joint infections
Malnourishment
Hemophilia

(Reproduced with permission from the American Academy of Orthopaedic Surgeons Advisory Statement: Antibiotic Prophylaxis for Dental Patients with Total Joint Replacements. Copyright © 1997 American Dental Association and American Academy of Orthopaedic Surgeons.)

Outline 2

Incidence Stratification of Bacteremic Dental Procedures

Higher Incidence*
Dental extractions
Periodontal procedures including surgery, subgingival placement of antibiotic fibers/strips, scaling and root planing, probing, recall maintenance
Dental implant placement and reimplantation of avulsed teeth
Endodontic (root canal) instrumentation or surgery only beyond the apex
Initial placement of orthodontic bands but not brackets
Intraligamentary local anesthetic injections
Prophylactic cleaning of teeth or implants where bleeding is anticipated

Lower Incidence†
Restorative dentistry§ (operative and prosthodontic) with/without retraction cord¶
Local anesthetic injections (nonintraligamentary)
Intracanal endodontic treatment; postplacement and buildup
Placement of rubber dam
Postoperative suture removal
Placement of removable prosthodontic/orthodontic appliances
Taking of oral impressions
Fluoride treatments
Taking of oral radiographs
Orthodontic appliance adjustment

(Reproduced with permission from the American Academy of Orthopaedic Surgeons Advisory Statement: Antibiotic Prophylaxis for Dental Patients with Total Joint Replacements. Copyright © 1997 American Dental Association and American Academy of Orthopaedic Surgeons.)

* Prophylaxis should be considered for patients with total joint replacement that meet the criteria in Outline 1. No other patients with orthopaedic implants should be considered for antibiotic prophylaxis prior to dental treatment/procedures.

† Prophylaxis not indicated.

§ This includes restoration of carious (decayed) or missing teeth.

¶ Clinical judgment may indicate antibiotic use in selected circumstances that may create significant bleeding.

in human cells or are selectively more susceptible to the effect of the antimicrobial agent. Briefly, antibiotics can be divided into the following groups based on their site and mechanism of action: (1) inhibition of cell wall synthesis; (2) alteration of cell membrane permeability; (3) inhibition of bacterial metabolism; (4) inhibition of protein synthesis; and (5) interference with nucleic acid synthesis or activity.

Unfortunately, bacteria have demonstrated a remarkable ability to develop resistance to the effects of antibiotics. There are 3 basic resistance mechanisms: alteration of the target of the antibiotic; prevention of access of the drug to the target; and inactivation of the drug. Many strains of bacteria possess more than one of these resistance mechanisms against many different classes of antibiotics. Table 2 summarizes some of the major mechanisms of resistance to antimicrobial agents. Figure 2 illustrates resistance mechanisms that are commonly encountered in the use of β-lactam antibiotics against aerobic gram-negative bacilli.

The development of antimicrobial resistance in *S aureus* aptly shows how microbes adapt to antimicrobial selective pressure. This is a particularly significant example for orthopaedic surgeons because *S aureus* is frequently encountered in orthopaedic wound infections, osteomyelitis, and prosthetic joint infections. When penicillin was introduced into medical practice in the mid 1940s, *Staphylococci* were almost universally susceptible. Within a few years, isolates of *Staphylococci* were described that hydrolyzed penicillin. Today, approximately 90% of clinically encountered strains produce β-lactamases that destroy early-generation penicillins.

Outline 3
Suggested Antibiotic Prophylaxis Regimens*

Patients not allergic to penicillin: cephalexin, cephradine or amoxicillin: 2 grams orally 1 hour prior to dental procedure

Patients not allergic to penicillin but unable to take oral medications: cefazolin 1 gram or ampicillin 2 grams intramuscularly/intravenously 1 hour prior to the procedure

Patients allergic to penicillin: clindamycin: 600 mg orally 1 hour prior to the dental procedure

Patients allergic to penicillin and unable to take oral medications: clindamycin 600 mg intramuscularly/intravenously 1 hour prior to the procedure

*No second doses are recommended for any of these dosing regimens

(Reproduced with permission from the American Academy of Orthopaedic Surgeons Advisory Statement: Antibiotic Prophylaxis for Dental Patients with Total Joint Replacements. Copyright © 1997 American Dental Association and American Academy of Orthopaedic Surgeons.)

Table 1
Mechanisms of Action of Common Antibiotics

Antibiotic Class	Mechanism of Action	Site of Action
Beta-Lactams (penicillins and cephalosporins)	Inhibition of cell wall production by prevention of peptidoglycan cross linkage	Cell wall
Glycopeptides (vancomycin)	Inhibition of cell wall production by interference with addition of cell wall subunits	Cell wall
Bacitracin	Inhibition of cell wall production by interference with cell wall subunit carrier lipid	Cell wall
Aminoglycosides (gentamicin)	Inhibition of protein synthesis by binding with 30S ribosomal subunit	Protein synthesis
Macrolides (erythromycin)	Inhibition of protein synthesis by binding with 50S ribosomal subunit	Protein synthesis
Lincosamides (clindamycin)	Inhibition of protein synthesis by binding with 50S ribosomal subunit	Protein synthesis
Chloramphenicol	Inhibition of protein synthesis by binding with 50S ribosomal subunit	Protein synthesis
Tetracycline	Inhibition of protein synthesis by binding with 50S ribosomal subunit	Protein synthesis
Mupirocin	Inhibition of protein synthesis by interference with isoleucine t-RNA synthetase	Protein synthesis
Streptogrammin (synercid-investigational)	Inhibition of early and late stages of protein synthesis at ribosomal level	Protein synthesis
Oxazolidinones (linezolid-investigational)	Inhibition of protein synthesis by binding to 50 ribosomal subunit	Protein synthesis
Rifamycins (Rifampin)	Inhibition of DNA-dependent RNA polymerase	FDNA synthesis
Quinolones (Ciprofloxacin)	Inhibition of DNA gyrase	DNA synthesis
Novobiocin	Inhibition of DNA gyrase	DNA synthesis
Metronidazole	Inhibition of DNA synthesis by generation of short-lived reactive intermediates by electron transfer system	DNA synthesis
Sulfonamides and trimethroprim	Inhibition of enzymes involved in folic acid biosynthesis	Cell metabolism
Everinomicin (Ziracin-investigational)	Unknown	Unknown

(Reproduced with permission from the Centers for Disease Control and Prevention.)

Table 2

Mechanisms of Antibiotic Resistance

Antibiotic Class and Type of Resistance	Specific Resistance Mechanism
Altered Target	
β-Lactam Antibiotics	Altered penicillin binding proteins
Vancomycin	Altered peptidoglycan subunits
Aminoglycosides	Altered ribosomal proteins
Macrolides	Ribosomal RNA methylation
Quinolones	Altered DNA gyrase
Sulfonamides	Altered dihydropteroate
Trimethoprim	Altered dihydrofolate reductase
Rifampin	Altered RNA polymerase
Detoxifying Enzymes	
Aminoglycosides	Phosphotransferase, acetyltransferase, Nucleotidyltransferase
β-Lactam Antibiotics	β-Lactamase
Chloramphenicol	Acetyltransferase
Decreased Uptake	
Diminished permeability	
β-Lactam antibiotics tetracycline, quinolones, trimethoprim	Alteration in outer membrane porins
Active efflux pumps	
Erythromycin	Membrane transport system
Tetracycline	Membrane transport system

(Reproduced with permission from the Centers for Disease Control and Prevention.)

In 1959 the semisynthetic, penicillinase-stable, anti-staphylococcal penicillins were introduced. Methicillin was the first such antibiotic, followed by drugs more commonly used today such as nafcillin and oxacillin. Strains of *S aureus* resistant to methicillin (MRSA) were identified almost immediately, and nosocomial outbreaks caused by MRSA were soon observed. Currently, in the United States, approximately 25% of nosocomially-acquired *S aureus* isolates are resistant to methicillin. Staphylococci are resistant to methicillin by virtue of production of an altered penicillin-binding protein (PBP2a) that has a low affinity for β-lactam antibiotics. The PBPs are membrane-bound peptidases that catalyze the transpeptidation reaction that cross-links the peptidoglycan that makes up the staphylococcal cell wall. PBP2a is encoded by the gene *mecA*, which probably originated in a coagulase-negative species of staphylococci. It appears that the *mecA* gene was acquired by a few strains of *S aureus* and that all subsequent MRSA are clonal descendants from the first progenitors. They have now successfully circumnavigated the globe, and MRSA can be found throughout the world. MRSA are resistant to all β-lactam antibiotics even if automated in vitro susceptibility tests indicate otherwise. Strains of MRSA have acquired many of the resistance mechanisms outlined in Table 2 and are often resistant to a host of antibiotics including aminoglycosides, macrolides and lincosamides, tetracyclines, sulfonamides, and quinolones.

To combat these multiresistant staphylococci, vancomycin, which was first introduced in 1956, has been increasingly employed. The first strains of intermediately-

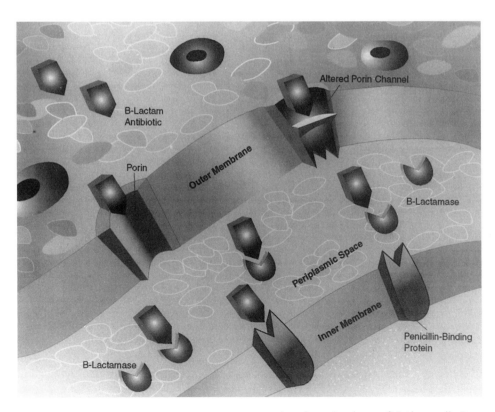

Figure 2

Resistance mechanisms encountered in the use of β-lactam antibiotics against gram-negative aerobic bacilli. Commonly encountered resistance mechanisms include: detoxifying enzymes (such as β-lactamase) and decreased uptake because of alterations in the outer membrane porin channels. Other resistance mechanisms, not shown here, that may be active in other bacteria against a variety of antibiotics include alterations in the target site (such as altered penicillin binding proteins) and active transport efflux pumps.

susceptible *S aureus* have recently been described, and many experts believe that the number of vancomycin-resistant strains will inexorably spread. This pattern of antibiotic discovery, exuberant use, and emergence of resistance has been repeated for many antibiotics and species of bacteria.

Acquisition and Transfer of Resistance Traits

Although many questions regarding how bacteria acquire and transfer antibiotic resistance determinants remain unanswered, a number of aspects of this problem are clear. Bacteria acquire resistance traits by both mutation and gene acquisition. During the process of DNA replication, random mutational events occasionally occur that escape the proofreading function of DNA polymerase. Usually these mutations result in a weakened or metabolically less efficient bacteria that is selected out in the competitive struggle with its brethren and the mutation is not passed on. However, occasionally a mutational event will result in a survival advantage allowing the organism to propagate. If the mutational event occurs in an antibiotic target and then the bacteria is subjected to that antibiotic, it may be the only strain that can reproduce and thus will become the dominant strain. Then, often because of poor infection control practices and modern-day travel and transport of humans, this strain may be passed from person to person. Examples of single mutational events rendering a bacteria resistant to an antibiotic include rifampin resistance in staphylococci because of a mutation in the β-subunit of DNA-dependent RNA polymerase or quinolone resistance in staphylococci because of mutations in *gyrA* resulting in a Ser 84 to Leu change.

Many species of bacteria and fungi naturally produce antibiotics (presumably to inhibit other competing species) and have developed mechanisms to modify their own inhibitory biochemical products as a form of self-protection. Thus, many of the antibiotic resistance determinants that are clinically important today may have existed at a low level in nature for millions of years — long before humans started to use these compounds medically. However, humans have markedly altered the degree of selective pressure to develop and transfer these resistance determinants by producing literally kilotons of antibiotics.

Bacteria have also developed numerous mechanisms to exchange genetic material both intraspecies and interspecies. Bacterial species such as pneumococci and menigococci can take up foreign DNA from the environment and incorporate it into their chromosomes. Many resistance determinants are located on transposons or plasmids that can be transferred from one bacterium to another by conjugation. Plasmids and transposons are mobile, extrachromosomal pieces of DNA that can insert themselves into the bacterial chromosome. Some of these mobile genetic elements have loci known as integrons or insertion sequences that enable them to capture exogenous genes. Therefore, a number of resistance genes can be grouped on the same plasmid or transposon, allowing for the transfer of multiple resistance traits. Unfortunately, in most instances, once acquired, resistance traits appear to remain stable in the bacteria even if the selective pressure for such a trait is lifted.

Treatment of Antibiotic-Resistant Bacteria

A comprehensive review of antibiotic treatment of resistant pathogens is beyond the scope of this chapter. However, a few comments will be offered regarding the treatment of staphylococcal infections, as staphylococci are the most frequently encountered pathogens in orthopaedic surgery and have become increasingly resistant to antibiotics. Parallels between antibiotic-resistant staphylococci and other resistant bacteria with regard to the increased complexity of care can be inferred from the following discussion.

Clinically encountered strains of both *S aureus* and coagulase-negative staphylococci, primarily species *S epidermidis,* produce an inducible β-lactamase that renders early generation penicillins inactive. Antistaphylococcal penicillins such as nafcillin or oxacillin are unsurpassed by other antibacterial agents and should be considered the treatment of choice for susceptible strains of staphylococci (penicillin should be used for the few strains that do not produce β-lactamase). Animal studies and clinical data suggest that antistaphylococcal cephalosporins, such as cefazolin, are less efficacious than antistaphylococcal penicillins and should therefore be used only in patients who do not tolerate therapy with a penicillin. Unfortunately, approximately 25% of strains of *S aureus* and 75% of strains of coagulase-negative staphylococci (MRSA and methicillin-resistant *Staphylococcus epidermis*) are resistant to semisynthetic antistaphylococcal penicillins.

As previously mentioned, MRSA strains should be regarded as resistant to all β-lactam antibiotics despite what might appear to be contrary information derived from in vitro susceptibility testing. This warning is based on the difficulty with which heterotypic expression of methicillin resistance is detected, the results from studies using large inocula for testing, and the well-described clinical failures when other β-lactam antibiotics have been used to treat infections due to MRSA. The only currently available antibiotic that shows consistent activity against MRSA strains is vancomycin. However, because vancomycin has been used extensively for treatment of infections due to MRSA and MRSE, many physicians are mistaken in believing that vancomycin is therapeutically equivalent to β-lactam antibiotics for the treatment of methicillin-susceptible strains of staphylococci. Animal studies and clinical experience demonstrate convincingly that vancomycin is less effective than β-lactam agents against methicillin-susceptible staphylococci.

Combinations of drugs are sometimes used in the treatment of patients with staphylococcal infections. The role of rifampin in combination with another antistaphylococcal agent is controversial. In vitro tests with *S aureus* have revealed contradictory results. However, for treatment of serious infections caused by coagulase-negative staphylococci, most data support the use of rifampin in combination with other agents. At times, methicillin-resistant strains of staphylococci will remain susceptible to other agents such as trimethoprim/sulfamethoxazole or fluoroquinolones. Although clinical experience is largely lacking, many clinicians choose to use combinations of these drugs with more traditional antistaphylococcal agents in patients with particularly severe infections or those not responding to single drug therapy.

Although aminoglycosides are not useful alone against staphylococci, they have been used in combination with vancomycin or an antistaphylococcal β-lactam. In such combinations aminoglycosides have demonstrated synergistic activity. The use of aminoglycosides must be balanced against their potential for nephrotoxicity, other side effects, and added cost. Some clinicians choose to use aminoglycosides in combination with another agent only during the first 3 to 5 days of therapy to give initial synergistic activity while avoiding nephrotoxicity associated with longer use.

A number of investigational drugs hold promise against MRSA/MRSE and other antibiotic resistant gram-positive pathogens such as vancomycin-resistant enterococci. These drugs include: synercid (a streptogrammin), linezolid (an oxazolidinone), Ziracin (an everinomicin), and glycylcyclines (tetracycline derivatives). In addition, some of the more recently introduced quinolones, such as trovafloxacin and clinafloxacin, appear to have better activity versus gram-positive pathogens than earlier generation quinolones.

The above discussion is not meant to diminish the importance of surgical care in the patient with an orthopaedic infection. Indeed, removal of osseous sequestra and foreign bodies remains an extremely important part of care. In fact, most authorities recognize that the probability of curing a patient suffering from osteomyelitis or a prosthetic implant infection is quite low without adequate surgical debridement.

Tuberculosis

Tuberculosis has been a serious threat to society for thousands of years. During the middle of this century until 1985, tuberculosis was becoming much less prevalent in the United States. This so-called control of tuberculosis was achieved by a combination of medical treatment, public health coordination, and society's willingness to participate in the public health coordinating process (Tables 3 and 4).

In 1986, the prevalence of this disease increased, primarily because of the immigration of individuals from countries where the disease was more common, contraction of the disease by immunosuppressed individuals with viral disease (human immunodeficiency virus, HIV; acquired immunodeficiency syndrome, AIDS), institutional transmission of the disease, and poorer public health control. During the time of increase (1986-1992), the majority (60%) of new cases of tuberculosis were diagnosed in persons born outside of the United States. Those individuals were predominantly born in Asia (47%) or Central or South America (44%). In 1993, the number of tuberculosis cases again began to decline and by 1995, the case rate (8.7/100,000 population) was the lowest since 1953.

Tuberculosis is commonly caused by *Mycobacterium tuberculosis* but may also be caused by *M africanum* (endemic to NW Africa) and *M bovis*. *M tuberculosis* is known as an acid-fast bacillus because it resists decolorization with strong mineral acids after it has been stained with carbol fuschsin or Ziehl-Neilsen methods. Once cultured, it grows very slowly with visible colonies forming in 2 to 4 weeks. *M tuberculosis'* rate of growth is dependent on oxygen tension; hence, in the lung *M tuberculosis* may multiply quickly. The Centers for Disease Control and Prevention (CDC) reported in 1991 that one fifth of newly diagnosed cases in the United States were extrapulmonary. Clearly, the pulmonary area is the most common site of tuberculosis. Sites of extrapulmonary tuberculosis include the spine and extremities.

Spinal tuberculosis with subsequent paraplegia was first described by Percival Pott in the late 18th century. The thoracic spine continues to be the most common skeletal area of disease, and surgical treatment is often necessary to prevent severe spinal deformity.

Table 3

Recommendation for Treatment of Adults With Musculoskeletal Tuberculosis

Medication	Dosage
Isoniazid	300 mg/day
Rifampin	600 mg/day
Pyrazinamide	30 mg/kg/day (for 2 months)
Ethambutol	Should be included in the initial regimen until the results of drug susceptibility studies are available
Pyridoxine	10 mg/day (given as prophylaxis against isoniazid-induced neuropathy)

(Reproduced with permission from the Centers for Disease Control and Prevention.)

Diagnosis

The diagnosis of tuberculosis can usually be made with little difficulty provided the clinician has a high index of suspicion and proceeds with the appropriate tests. The skin test with controls uses a purified protein derivative of tuberculin injected subcutaneously, and the skin reaction to the protein injection is quantitative. False-positive results may occur in those patient who were previously vaccinated with bacille Calmette-Guérin. False-negative results may occur in some patients, for example, the elderly, HIV-positive individuals, and the chronically ill, who are immunosuppressed or malnourished and unable to mount an immune response.

Culture of tissue from the site of infection is the definitive test to document the presence of tuberculosis. Culture is especially important at this time because many of the patients at risk (immigrants, HIV-positive individuals) may harbor other infections or have multidrug-resistant strains of tuberculosis. Once appropriate specimens have been obtained, treatment should be initiated. One problem is that the tuberculosis culture may take weeks to become positive, yet treatment should be initiated promptly after diagnostic tissue is obtained. At this time, treatment is tailored to the most likely type of infection. For example, multidrug-resistant tuberculosis is likely to be present in an immunocompromised HIV patient and the appropriate treatment regimen must be used to treat these high-risk patients.

Treatment

Medical treatment of tuberculosis has been extremely effective. Streptomycin, para-amino-salicylic acid, and isoniazine were responsible for lowering the prevalence of the disease from 1952 until 1985. As the prevalence of tuberculosis increased from 1985 to 1992, so did its drug resistance. The CDC has revised guidelines for the prevention and treatment of tuberculosis as a result of resistant organisms.

Surgical treatment of tuberculosis is necessary to drain large abscesses of major joints and in patients with progressive spinal disease. If the disease has destroyed the articular cartilage of a major joint, reconstruction of that joint may be possible by arthrodesis or arthroplasty. Most surgeons favor arthrodesis but effective chemotherapeutics have made arthroplasty possible with promising short-term and intermediate results

Spinal tuberculosis is a challenging problem because of bone and soft-tissue destruction that can lead to deformity and paraplegia (Fig. 3). It is also possible to spare the bony elements but develop neurologic impairment from abscesses or local tuberculosis infiltration of the neural structures.

The role of surgery for spinal tuberculosis is controversial except in patients with neurologic impairment and severe kyphosis or in patients who have compromise of the neural canal because of the infection.

Table 4	
Tuberculosis Control Program *	
Control Type	**Control Sections**
Administrative controls	Annual risk assessment
	Written TB infection control plan
	Education program for health care workers
	Protocols for:
	Screening patients for suspected TB
	Diagnostic evaluation of patients with suspected TB
	Isolation and initiation of treatment
	TST program for health care workers:
	Routine TST at intervals established by risk assessment
	Protocol for evaluating health care workers with positive TST
	Protocol for identifying health care workers with possible TB
	Protocol for investigating TST conversions in health care workers
Engineering controls	Expert evaluation of ventilation system
	Isolation rooms in accordance with CDC guidelines
	Additional air cleaning devices (HEPA filtration, UVGI) if indicated
Respiratory protection program	Protocol for situations requiring personal respiratory protection
	Education for health care workers
	NIOSH-certified respirators
	Fit testing program for health care workers

*   TB = tuberculosis; TST = tumor skin test; CDC = Centers for Disease Control and Prevention; HEPA = high efficiency particulate air; UVGI = ultraviolet; NIOSH = National Institute for Occupational Safety and Health

(Reproduced with permission from the Centers for Disease Control and Prevention.)

Viral Diseases

Viral diseases have played a major role in the practice of orthopaedic surgery since its origin, when the primary focus was the crippled child, often a victim of poliomyelitis or birth defects from maternal viral diseases. Despite the elimination of most of these diseases through vaccination programs, viral diseases continue to play a critical although much different role in the practice of orthopaedic surgery. Today, the HIV, hepatitis B virus (HBV), and hepatitis C virus (HCV) represent potential hazards for patients and health care personnel through transmission in the health care setting. In addition, these chronic diseases in their advanced states may present increased risk of postoperative complications.

Human Immunodeficiency Virus

HIV is a member of the Lentivirus subfamily of the Retroviridae family. Retroviruses are enveloped RNA viruses that are dependent on a DNA polymerase termed reverse transcriptase. HIV is a single-strand RNA composed of 9,300 nucleotide base units, genetic encoding segments, and a replication promoter region. Two major types have been identified. HIV-1 is prevalent worldwide. HIV-2 is still principally found in people from West Africa. There are 9 currently classified HIV-1 subtypes based on variations in the envelope gene *(env)* of which the largest portion (48%) are subtype B. HIV mutates at an extremely rapid rate, creating "swarm" or "quasispecies" within the same individual host. The *env* gene mutates much more frequently than the gene responsible for encoding reverse transcriptase *(pol)*, which accounts for the relatively large number of patients responsive to reverse transcriptase inhibitor therapy. Mutation frequency and strain variation have additional significance on the validity of screening and confirmatory diagnostic tests for HIV.

Highly sensitive screening tests for HIV became available in 1985. They are based on antibody to the virus. The principal screening test is enzyme-linked immunosorbent assay (ELISA), which is performed by mixing the patient's serum with HIV antigen made from purified viral lysate. If the initial ELISA is positive, it is repeated. If both are positive, the result is confirmed with an immunoelectrophoresis or immunoblot procedure such as Western blot or immunofluorescence assay. Sensitivity and specificity for the ELISA alone is over 98% for HIV-1. Combining the ELISA and the Western blot, the false positive rate is no more than 0.00006%. Synthetic peptide-based enzyme immunoassays have been used for subtypes of HIV. Home collection kits for highly confidential testing are now available. There is a window of infectivity between exposure and seroconversion that may extend for several months. Some investigators have attempted to determine the applicability of the polymerase chain reaction test (PCR) as a screening test to detect HIV during this period. The PCR amplifies proviral DNA to make it detectable. However, the specificity of the HIV PCR is not high because cross-reaction with other DNA contaminates the specimen. One study reported an average sensitivity of 99% but a specificity of 94.7%.

It has been estimated that 0.5% of the United States population is HIV-positive. The distribution of these patients is uneven and is most highly concentrated in coastal, urban areas. In high endemic areas, trauma centers report that up to 10.4% of their emergency trauma patients are HIV-positive. In anonymous serosurveys conducted by the CDC at multiple institutions, 0.2% to 8.9% of emergency room patients and 0.1% to 7.8% of all hospital admissions were found to be HIV-positive. Orthopaedic surgeons practicing in high endemic areas may anticipate that 3% to 10% of their acute trauma cases are HIV-positive. In an emergent situation the patient's status is often unknown but could be critical in management of the case.

Surgery on the HIV-positive patient, elective or emergent, involves some special risks, which may be divided into 2 categories: risk to the patient and risk to health care personnel. Because of concern about these issues, some orthopaedic surgeons may pursue nonsurgical management of fractures usually treated surgically and are reluctant to recommend elective surgery in the HIV-positive patient. Both of these risks must be understood and considered in making a decision regarding the appropriateness of surgery for these patients.

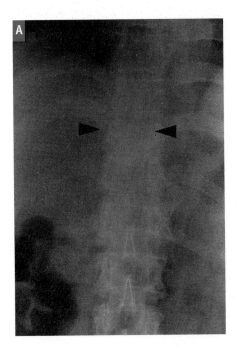

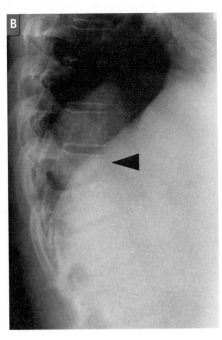

Figure 3

A and **B**, Radiographs of the spine of a 35-year-old man who had persistent pain and fever despite medical treatment for tuberculosis. There is kyphosis with the apex at T9 (black arrows). The ninth through eleventh thoracic vertebrae have been eroded by the tuberculosis.

Pathophysiology of Immunity Impairment

The CD4 lymphocyte, which is responsible for cellular immunity, is the primary target cell in HIV infection. However, differentiation of the B lymphocyte, responsible for humoral immunity, is indirectly impaired. Additional derangements occur in the monocyte/macrophage cell line and the production of gamma interferon and lymphokines, which are products of antigenically stimulated lymphocytes.

As the disease progresses, the absolute polymorphonuclear leukocyte count drops to a level that impairs phagocytosis. This level may be further reduced by marrow-suppressing drugs such as zidovudine used to treat AIDS. Malnutrition, which may be the consequence of both the disease process and therapeutic medications, causes hypoalbuminemia, which may further impair lymphocyte function and phagocytosis. In addition to the crucial role they play in the immune system, CD4 lymphocytes and lymphokines are important in wound healing.

Autoimmune dysfunction also occurs with AIDS. One manifestation of this phenomenon is platelet deficiency which, if uncorrected, can result in excessive bleeding at surgery. Immunodeficiency-associated thrombocytopenic purpura may be the result of an autoimmune globulin directed against platelet antigens similar to the IgG produced in idiopathic thrombocytopenic purpura. This platelet deficiency is treated initially with steroids and, if persistent, with splenectomy. The former further reduces host resistance to infection and the latter is associated with an increased risk of septicemia.

Several groups have studied neutrophil bactericidal capacity in HIV-positive patients. This capacity is dependent on chemotaxis, phagocytosis, and secretion of oxygen-dependent and -independent microbicides and is reduced in serum of HIV-positive patients compared to that of normal controls in vitro.

As a result of this complex and widespread immune system impairment, patients with advanced HIV infection have increased susceptibility to common pathogens as well as to opportunistic infections. These cases often present with minimal inflammatory response and appear deceptively benign.

Surgical Complications and Outcome

Impaired defenses to common surgical pathogens and delayed wound healing are causes for concern about the outcome of orthopaedic procedures on the HIV-positive patient, in terms of both early and late complications.

Earlier surgical outcome studies reviewed complications in critically ill AIDS patients undergoing emergency procedures. At that time, treatment of AIDS was very limited and the 30-day postoperative mortality rate for these patients was in the range of 30% to 50%. Later studies include the asymptomatic and symptomatic HIV-positive group of patients as well as those with AIDS as defined by the revised CDC criteria. These studies may be divided into those reporting early postoperative infections, mostly involving surgical wounds, and those describing late infections of hematogenous origin.

Early Postoperative Infections

Diettrich and associates reported a series of 120 major surgical cases performed between 1986 and 1990. The 30-day mortality for the emergent group was 0/24 in the HIV-positive patients and 7/30 (23%) in the AIDS patients. For the elective procedures it was 0/40 in the HIV-positive patients and 1/26 (4%) in those with AIDS. The risk of morbidity or mortality was higher if the patient had a history of opportunistic infection and a serum albumin level below 25 g/l. Results in the HIV-positive group without AIDS, 0% mortality and 4% postoperative complications, are roughly comparable to the HIV-negative population.

Buehrer and associates studied surgical wound infection rates in HIV-positive and HIV-negative hemophiliacs; of the 169 procedures reviewed, 53 were orthopaedic. There were 2 wound infections but no statistically significant difference in the wound infection rate between the HIV-positive group (1.4%) and the HIV-negative group (0). There were no wound infections in the 7 procedures performed on patients with AIDS. Paiement and associates reported on 476 orthopaedic surgical trauma patients treated with at least 1 open procedure at San Francisco General Hospital. The study groups were divided into HIV-negative patients (444) and HIV-positive patients without AIDS (30). In the clean and clean contaminated category, there were 15/364 infections in the HIV-negative group and 0/21 in the HIV-positive group. In the open fracture category, deep infections occurred in 3/80 in the HIV-negative group and 1/9 in the HIV-positive group. Because of the retrospective nature of this study, CD4 counts and other immune parameters were not available.

Late Hematogenous Infections

To date there has been much speculation but few studies on the effect of HIV infection on the incidence of late prosthetic joint infection. Two studies involving hemophiliacs have been presented at national meetings and are outlined below. In the first study, the incidence of infection was studied in 93 joint replacements performed in 62 hemophiliacs between 1968 and 1991. At the time of surgery, 25 patients were HIV-negative and 25 were HIV-positive. The status of the 12 patients who had surgeries performed between 1978 and 1985 was unknown. There were no early postoperative infections in any of these patients. The incidence of late postoperative infection in the HIV-negative group was 8%, which is similar to the average in other studies on HIV-negative hemophiliacs (10%). This high incidence of late hematogenous prosthetic joint infection in hemophiliacs prior to HIV infection may be a consequence of bacteremia from frequent intravenous self-administration of clotting factor concentrate. The incidence of late prosthetic joint infection in the patients known to be HIV-positive at surgery was 18%. Because of the small numbers in each group this difference is not statistically significant but may represent a trend. It seems likely that the already high risk of infection in hemophiliacs is magnified by the immune impairment caused by HIV infection. This hypothesis should not be assumed to be true for the nonhemophiliac HIV-positive patients who do not possess the other risk factors found in hemophilia.

In a second study, 26 total knee replacements in hemophiliacs performed between 1984 and 1991 with 1 to 9 years of follow-up were reviewed. Despite the fact that all patients were HIV-positive, there were no early or late deep infections reported.

Opportunistic infections, common in patients with AIDS, very rarely cause orthopaedic implant infection despite the fact that *Mycobacterium* infections, including atypical strains, are common in patients with advanced HIV infection. Hawkins and associates found disseminated *M avium-intracellulare* (MAI) infection in 53% of patients dying from AIDS at the Sloan-Kettering Cancer Center. The same authors reported positive blood cultures in 98% and bone marrow aspirations in 100% of patients with MAI. McLaughlin and associates reported 1 patient who developed MAI infection in both prosthetic hips. Both sides had demonstrated prosthetic loosening for many years. The patient had clinical AIDS at the time of apparent *Mycobacterium* infection. The prostheses in this patient could have become infected through either hematogenous seeding or from the adjacent bone. Loosening with hyperemic interface membrane would predispose to this complication. Fungal infections are also common in HIV-positive patients but, to the best of our knowledge, there have been no reports of fungal prosthetic joint infection related to HIV infection.

Pharmacologic management of HIV infection has improved dramatically in recent years. Advancements in antiretroviral therapy have resulted in significant reduction in viral load, often to undetectable levels, and improvement in immune status as evidenced by elevation in the CD4 count. In many cases, this has reversed disease progression and improved the candidacy of HIV-infected patients for needed elective surgery. Three drug regimens, including 2 nucleoside analog reverse transcriptase inhibitors such as zidovudine and lamivudine, and 1 protease inhibitor such as indinavir should be considered for all patients with detectable viral RNA in plasma. Restoration of CD4 cells in patients with moderately advanced disease is incomplete. Therefore, voluntary testing of all patients with risk factors for HIV is recommended so that treatment may commence before the immune system begins to show significant impairment that may not be completely reversible.

Transmission of HIV in the Surgical Setting

Transmission of HIV from patient to health care worker has been reported in 151 instances, 49 of which are well documented. Of these 49, 42 resulted from percutaneous injury, 5 from mucocutaneous exposure, 1 from both, and 1 from unknown transmission. Forty-four of these exposures involved blood. To date, there have been no documented seroconversions resulting from puncture by suture needles, which is the most common cause of percutaneous exposure in surgery. Seroconversions have resulted from injuries by solid, sharp implements including scalpels, glass, and lancets. The absence of seroconversion from suture needle injury may relate to the low inoculum carried by this solid needle and its further reduction as it passes through one or more layers of surgical gloves. The risk of seroconversion after a percutaneous injury of any type is estimated at 0.3% based on an extensive ongoing surveillance study conducted by the CDC.

The prevalence of occupational seroconversion among surgeons has been estimated in 2 studies, one of orthopaedic surgeons and the other of general, obstetrics/gynecology, and orthopaedic surgeons. None of the 3,267 orthopaedic surgeons reporting only occupational risk factors in the first study was HIV-positive. One out of the 740 in the second group was HIV-positive. The frequency of percutaneous injury in orthopaedic procedures has been studied in multiple investigations and is typically 3% to 4%. The risk of puncture increases with the length of the procedure, amount of blood lost, and the presence within the surgical site of sharp objects such as bone fragments, wires, and pins.

In a prospective observational study of blood contacts in the surgical setting, Tocars and associates reported 99 percutaneous injuries in 1,382 procedures; 77% of these injuries were related to suturing. The injury rate during orthopaedic procedures was 4%. In 28 cases (32%) the implement causing the injury recontacted the patient's tissues, thus creating a potential mechanism for surgeon-to-patient transmission. Transmission of bloodborne viruses from surgeon to patient in the health care setting has been reported. There have been well-documented clusters of cases of HBV and HCV transmission from a single surgeon to multiple patients. In 1997, the first case of HIV transmission from surgeon to patient was reported in France. This case involved a French HIV-positive orthopaedic surgeon who performed 2 lengthy hip procedures lasting 10 and 4 hours, respectively, on a female patient with no other risk factors. Gene sequencing of the surgeon's virus matched the infected patient. All transfused blood and blood donors tested negative. This differential in transmissibility between HIV, HBV, and HCV probably relates, in part, to the differing risk of seroconversion between these diseases as well as the relative prevalence among surgeons.

The risk of HBV seroconversion from a single percutaneous injury has been estimated to be as high as 30% or approximately 100 times that for HIV. Studies of HCV transmission following percutaneous injury in the surgical setting are very limited but have been reported at 2.7% to 10%. Patient-to-patient transmission of HIV in the clinical setting has been reported in a dental office, a newborn nursery, and an outpatient surgical office. Transmission in these instances appears to have resulted from breakdown in sterile technique, such as the sterilization of instruments or contamination of multidose medication vials.

Recommendations for the prevention of viral transmission in the health care setting with emphasis on operating room precautions have been published by the American Academy of Orthopaedic Surgeons® (AAOS), the CDC, and the Occupational Safety and Health Administration. Methodologies to completely prevent surface contamination of skin or conjunctiva are available and include impervious gowns, high-top shoe covers, face shields, and space suits. The potential for aerosol transmission of HIV-infected particles has been studied. One laboratory simulation demonstrated blood aerosolization by the use of power surgical tools. HIV carried on these particles was culturable. However, multiple serosurveys of surgeons and dentists failed to show a clinical manifestation of this phenomenon.

Cut-resistant cloth gloves can greatly reduce the likelihood of injuries from bone spicules, wires, and pins but cannot prevent suture needle punctures. This must be accomplished by meticulous technique and may be further facilitated by the use of semisharp needles. There is compelling evidence that significant inoculum reduction occurs for punctures through multiple layers of gloves. In the event of a significant exposure, recent data supports the use of zidovudine to reduce the risk of seroconversion. Third-generation antiretrovirals and protease inhibitors may be of additional benefit and are recommended for higher risk exposures such as a deep puncture with an implement visibly contaminated with HIV-infected blood, especially in a patient with a high viral load (Table 5).

Hepatitis B and C

Despite the availability of a safe, effective recombinant hepatitis B vaccine, hepatitis B remains the most common occupationally acquired bloodborne disease in the health care setting. In a recent study of surgeons, 17% were HBV-positive. Fourteen percent of those still susceptible to HBV had not received the vaccine. Several studies have reported a range of 0.5% to 5% HBV carriers among hospitalized patients. The CDC estimated that 5,100 health care workers in the United States acquired HBV on the job in 1991 and that 125 of these would die from consequences of this disease.

HCV was identified in 1989 as the probable cause of most non-A, non-B hepatitis. It is a small single-stranded RNA virus and part of the Flaviviridae family. HCV genomes are heterogeneous but closely related. A portion of the cloned genome has been used to develop an immunoassay to detect antibodies against HCV (anti-HCV) in the serum.

HCV is transmitted principally through the blood. It is estimated that 90% of recipients of blood from an HCV-positive donor will contract the disease. Transmission via transplanted organs and musculoskeletal allografts has been reported. Sexual transmission is much less likely than for HIV but remains controversial and poorly defined. It is estimated that nearly 4 million Americans are infected with HCV, with moderately increased prevalence in minorities: 3.2% of blacks, 2.1% of Hispanics, and 1.5% of non-Hispanic whites. The incidence appears to be declining since 1989. In 1997 it was estimated that 30,000 new cases occurred annually. Most infections are subclinical but virtually all patients demonstrate liver cell damage as evident from elevation of the serum aminotransferase. Approximately 85% of infected individuals have chronically elevated liver enzymes and chronic active hepatitis. At least 20% will go on to develop cirrhosis within 2 decades after exposure. The incidence of hepatocellular carcinoma is elevated and estimated to be 1% to 5% after 20 years' infection. The incidence is highest in those with cirrhosis. HCV is responsible for 8,000 to 10,000 deaths annually, a rate that is estimated to triple over the next 10 to 20 years. Persistent infection with intermittent viremia appears to occur in all infected individuals.

Screening tests for HCV use enzyme immunoassays to detect anti-HCV. The assays contain core HCV antigens. PCR tests detect HCV RNA and are used as a reference standard. The second generation enzyme immunoassay (EIA-2) is 92% to 95% sensitive but specificity has yet to be precisely established. Positive EIA-2 tests should be confirmed with a recombinant immunoblot assay. Even with a positive RIBA the specificity is only 70% to 75% in low-risk donors. Positive individuals may require PCR testing. However, a single negative PCR does not mean the patient is not infected and intermittently viremic. Viral load can be determined by quantitative PCR. Treatment for hepatitis C is limited. Alpha-interferon has been the primary form of therapy with an end of treatment response rate of 40% to 50% and a sustained response rate of 15% to 20%. Treatment is recommended for those with persistently elevated serum alanine aminotransferase who are at increased risk of developing cirrhosis.

Serosurveys among health care personnel have demonstrated rates ranging from 0% to 1.7%. One such survey, performed at the AAOS Annual Meeting in 1991, showed 0.8% of surgeons tested were positive. This compares to 0.09% to 0.36% among United States blood donors. The percentage of surgeons testing positive in this study correlated with age (years in practice): 30 to 39 years old were 0.4% positive; 40 to 49, 0.8%; 50 to 59, 1.2%; and 60 or older, 1.4%. In addition to parenteral transmission from patient to health care personnel in the health care setting, transmission from surgeon to patient has been described as well.

The risk of seroconversion following a percutaneous injury contaminated with HCV-positive blood has been estimated from 2.7% using EIA-1 to 10% in a study using EIA-2 and PCR testing for HCV RNA.

Viral Transmission From Musculoskeletal Allografts

There are an estimated 150,000 musculoskeletal allografts implanted in the United States annually. Two documented cases of HIV transmission from infected donor to recipient have been reported. The first graft was donated prior to the availability of an HIV antibody screen. The second case involved a donor who tested negative and was probably in the window of infectivity between exposure and seroconversion. Transmission in the first case was via fresh-frozen femoral head. The second case involved the donation of multiple organs, fresh-frozen bone and soft-tissue allografts, and the preparation of processed, freeze-dried bone chips and soft tissues. All organs and 3 of 4 fresh-frozen allografts transmitted the virus. There were no transmissions from the processed freeze-dried material. During the processing, blood and marrow elements were removed. In addition, freezing, defatting with ethanol, and lyophil-

---

Table 5

Provisional Public Health Service Recommendations for Chemoprophylaxis After Occupational Exposure to Human Immunodeficiency Virus (HIV)

Type of Exposure	Source Material*	Antiretroviral Prophylaxis†	Antiretroviral Regimen§
Percutaneous	Blood¶		
	Highest risk	Recommend	ZDV plus 3TC plus IDV
	Increased risk	Recommend	ZDV plus 3TC ± IDV**
	No increased risk	Offer	ZDV plus 3TC
	Fluid containing visible blood, other potentially infectious fluid, or tissue	Offer	ZDV plus 3TC
	Other body fluid (eg, urine)	Do not offer	
Mucous membrane	Blood	Offer	ZDV plus 3TC ± IDV**
	Fluid containing visible blood, other potentially infectious fluid, or tissue	Offer	ZDV ± 3TC
	Other body fluid (eg, urine)	Do not offer	
Skin††	Blood	Offer	ZDV plus 3TC ± IDV**
	Fluid containing visible blood, other potentially infectious fluid, or tissue	Offer	ZDV ± 3TC
	Other body fluid (eg, urine)	Do not offer	

(Adapted from Centers for Disease Control and Prevention: Update: Provisional Public Health Service recommendations for chemoprophylaxis after occupational exposure to HIV. *MMWR Morb Mortal Wkly Rep* 1996;45:458–472.)

* Any exposure to concentrated HIV (eg, in a research laboratory or production facility) is treated as percutaneous exposure to blood with highest risk. "Other potentially infectious fluid" is defined as including semen, vaginal secretions, and cerebrospinal, synovial, pleural, peritoneal, pericardial, and amniotic fluids.

† Recommendations are defined as follows: "Recommend" indicates that postexposure prophylaxis (PEP) should be recommended to the exposed worker with counseling. "Offer" indicates that PEP should be offered to the exposed worker with counseling. "Do not offer" indicates that PEP should not be offered because these are not occupational exposures to HIV.

§ Regimens are as follows: ZDV = zidovudine, 200 mg 3 times a day; 3TC = lamivudine, 150 mg twice daily; IDV = indinavir, 800 mg 3 times a day (if IDV is not available, saquinavir may be used, 600 mg 3 times a day). Prophylaxis is given for 4 weeks. For full prescribing information, see package inserts.

¶ "Highest risk" is defined as both a larger volume of blood (eg, deep injury with large-diameter hollow needle previously in source patient's vein or artery, especially involving an injection of source patient's blood) and the presence of blood containing a high titer of HIV (eg, source patient with acute retroviral illness or end-stage AIDS; viral load measurement may be considered, but its use in relation to PEP has not been evaluated). "Increased risk" is defined as either exposure to a larger volume of blood or the presence of blood with a high titer of HIV. "No increased risk" is defined on the basis of there being neither exposure to a larger volume of blood nor the presence of blood with a high titer of HIV (eg, solid suture-needle injury from source patient with asymptomatic HIV infection).

** Possible toxicity of additional drug may not be warranted.

†† For skin, risk is increased for exposures involving high titer of HIV, prolonged contact, an extensive area, or an area in which skin integrity is visibly compromised. For skin exposures without increased risk, the risk of drug toxicity outweighs the benefit of PEP.

ization may sterilize any remaining virus. Fresh-frozen allografts have also been reported to transmit HCV.

There is experimental evidence that bone-derived cell lines are difficult to infect with HIV. Therefore, both clinical and laboratory evidence make it probable that HIV and HCV infection are transmitted via contaminating blood elements rather than osseous cell lines or hydroxyapatite structure in musculoskeletal allografts. Today, cadaver allograft screening includes PCR testing as well as antibody testing for HIV, HBV, and HCV. The risk of HIV transmission from musculoskeletal allografts is probably less than that for a unit of transfused blood, which is currently estimated at 1 in 440,000 to 600,000.

Summary

HIV, HBV, and HCV play a critical role in the practice of orthopaedic surgery. It is essential that the practicing orthopaedic surgeon understand the risks associated with these diseases in terms of candidacy for surgery, both elective and emergent, as well as the risks of transmission in the health care setting. HIV infection does impair the immune system and increase the patient's susceptibility to infection from both opportunistic organisms and normal surgical pathogens. However, most of the clinical studies available to date do not demonstrate an increased incidence of early postoperative complications in the asymptomatic HIV-positive patients compared to the HIV-negative group. Furthermore, most of the orthopaedic studies and the more recent general surgery studies do not show an increased incidence of early complications in the symptomatic HIV-positive patients with CD4 counts above 200 undergoing elective procedures.

The risk of complications following emergent surgery is consistently higher in patients with AIDS. The basic science work establishes some impairment of defenses against common orthopaedic pathogens and wound healing as well. As the disease progresses and these impairments increase, the hazard of early complications increases. The risk of late prosthetic implant infection, although not yet quantified, may be somewhat increased as well, especially in hemophiliacs. Implant infection with opportunistic organisms, although rare, has been reported. Dramatic improvement in pharmacologic management of HIV infection has resulted in viral load reduction to undetectable levels and elevation of the CD4 count. This stable condition may continue indefinitely, greatly improving these patients' candidacy for elective surgery.

Despite the ready availability of a safe and effective vaccine, hepatitis B remains a greater occupational threat to health care personnel than AIDS or hepatitis C because of its greater transmissibility. The obvious solution to this problem is universal utilization of the vaccine by those potentially at risk. Hepatitis C is more prevalent than HIV and about 10 times more transmissible by needle stick. A vaccine is not on the horizon. Appropriate surgical precautions remain the best defense.

Transmission of the viral diseases in the surgical setting from patient to surgeon, surgeon to patient, and patient to patient has been described. Appropriate precautions, developed by the AAOS and CDC, if followed universally, can minimize this risk. Testing for the presence of these viruses is well developed. When testing and preparation are properly performed the risk of patient-to-patient transmission via skeletal allografts is within an acceptable range.

Selected Bibliography

Bacterial Infections

Barrack RL, Harris WH: The value of aspiration of the hip joint before revision total hip arthroplasty. *J Bone Joint Surg* 1993;75A:66–76.

Chambers HF: Parenteral antibiotics for the treatment of bacteremia and other serious staphylococcal infections, in Crossley KB, Archer GL (eds): *The Staphylococci in Human Disease*. New York, NY, Churchill Livingstone, 1997, pp 583–601.

Fitzgerald RH Jr, Jacobson JJ, Luck JV Jr, et al: Antibiotic prophylaxis for dental patients with total joint replacements. *AAOS Bull* 1997;45:9–11.

Gustilo RB, Merkow RL, Templeman D: The management of open fractures. *J Bone Joint Surg* 1990;72A:299–304.

Hanssen AD, Osmon DR, Nelson CL: Prevention of deep periprosthetic joint infection. *J Bone Joint Surg* 1996;78A:458–471.

Jacoby GA, Archer GL: New mechanisms of bacterial resistance to antimicrobial agents. *N Engl J Med* 1991;324:601–612.

Lachiewicz PF, Rogers GD, Thomason HC: Aspiration of the hip joint before revision total hip arthroplasty: Clinical and laboratory factors influencing attainment of a positive culture. *J Bone Joint Surg* 1996;78A:749–754.

Lonner JH, Desai P, Dicesare PE, Steiner G, Zuckerman JD: The reliability of analysis of intraoperative frozen sections for identifying active infection during revision hip or knee arthroplasty. *J Bone Joint Surg* 1996;78A:1553–1558.

Nijhof MW, Oyen WJ, van-Kampen A, Claessens RA, van der Meer JW, Corstens FH: Evaluation of infection of the locomotor system with indium-111-labeled human IgG scintigraphy. *J Nucl Med* 1997;38: 1300–1305.

Ostermann PA, Seligson D, Henry SL: Local antibiotic therapy for severe open fractures: A review of 1085 consecutive cases. *J Bone Joint Surg* 1995;77B:93–97.

Perry CR, Hulsey RE, Manner FA, Miller GA, Pearson RL: Treatment of acutely infected arthroplasties with incision, drainage, and local antibiotics delivered via an implantable pump. *Clin Orthop* 1997; 281:216–223.

Rupp ME: Coagulase-negative staphylococcal infections: An update regarding recognition and management. *Curr Clin Top Infect Dis* 1997; 17:51–87.

Sochacki M, Garvin KL: An immunocompromised osteomyelitis model. *Trans Orthop Res Soc* 1995;20:258.

Infections and Total Joint Replacement

Aalto K, Osterman K, Peltola H, Rasanen J: Changes in erythrocyte sedimentation rate and C-reactive protein after total hip arthroplasty. *Clin Orthop* 1984;184:118–120.

Davenport K, Traina S, Perry C: Treatment of acutely infected arthroplasty with local antibiotics. *J Arthroplasty* 1991;6:179–183.

Emerging Resistant Strains of Bacteria

Archer GL, Scott J: Conjugative transfer genes in staphylococcal isolates from the United States. *Antimicrob Agents Chemother* 1991; 35:2500–2504.

Barber M: Methicillin-resistant Staphylococci. *J Clin Pathol* 1961; 14:385–393.

Benner EJ, Kayser FH: Growing clinical significance of methicillin-resistant Staphylococcus aureus. *Lancet* 1968;2:741–744.

Bryant RE, Alford RH: Unsuccessful treatment of staphylococcal endocarditis with cefazolin. *JAMA* 1977;237:569–570.

Carrizosa J, Kobasa WD, Kaye D. Effectiveness of nafcillin, methicillin, and cephalothin in experimental Staphylococcus aureus endocarditis. *Antimicrob Agents Chemother* 1979;15:735–737.

Chambers HF: Methicillin resistance in staphylococci: Molecular and biochemical basis and clinical implications. *Clin Microbiol Rev* 1997;10:781–791.

Collis CM, Hall RM: Expression of antibiotic resistance genes in the integrated cassettes of integrons. *Antimicrob Agents Chemother* 1995;39:155–162.

Davies J: Inactivation of antibiotics and the dissemination of resistance genes. *Science* 1994;264:375–382.

Reduced susceptibility of Staphylococcus aureus to vancomycin: Japan, 1996. *Morb Mortal Wkly Rep* 1997;46:624–626.

Salyers AA, Amabile-Cuevas CF: Why are antibiotic resistance genes so resistant to elimination? *Antimicrob Agents Chemother* 1997;41: 2321–2325.

Spratt BG: Hybrid penicillin-binding proteins in penicillin-resistant strains of Neisseria gonorrhoea. *Nature* 1988;332:173–176.

Sreedharan S, Peterson LR, Fisher LM: Ciprofloxacin resistance in coagulase-positive and negative staphylococci: Role of mutations at serine 84 in the DNA gyrase A protein of Staphylococcus aureus and Staphylococcus epidermidis. *Antimicrob Agents Chemother* 1991;35: 2151–2154.

Pathogenesis/Pathophysiology

Boyden S: The chemotactic effect of mixtures of antibody and antigen on polymorphonuclear leukocytes. *J Exp Med* 1962:115:453–466.

Kenten JH, Casadei J, Link J, et al: Rapid electrochemiluminescence assays of polymerase chain reaction products. *Clin Chem* 1991; 37:1626–1632.

Morrissy RT, Haynes DW, Nelson CL: Acute hematogenous osteomyelitis: The role of trauma in a reproducible model. *Trans Orthop Res Soc* 1980;5:324.

Whalen JL, Fitzgerald RH Jr, Morrissy RT: A histological study of acute hematogenous osteomyelitis following physeal injuries in rabbits. *J Bone Joint Surg* 1988;70A:1383–1392.

Tuberculosis

Recommendations of the Advisory Council for the Elimination of Tuberculosis: Screening for tuberculosis and tuberculosis infection in high-risk populations. *Morb Mortal Wkly Rep* 1995;44:19–34.

Human Immunodeficiency Virus

AAOS Task Force on AIDS and Orthopaedic Surgery: *Recommendations for the Prevention of Human Immunodeficiency Virus (HIV) Transmission in the Practice of Orthopaedic Surgery.* Park Ridge, IL, American Academy of Orthopaedic Surgeons, 1989.

Barbul A, Damewood RB, Wasserkrug HL, Penberthy LT, Efron G: Fluid and mononuclear cells from healing wounds inhibit thymocyte immune responsiveness. *J Surg Res* 1983;34:505–509.

Centers for Disease Control and Prevention: Case-control study of HIV seroconversion in health-care workers after percutaneous exposure to HIV-infected blood: France, United Kingdom, and United States, January 1988-August 1994. *MMWR Morb Mortal Wkly Rep* 1995;44:929–933.

Center for Disease Control and Prevention: Recommendations for HIV testing services for inpatients and outpatients in acute-care hospital settings. *MMWR Morb Mortal Wkly Rep* 1993;42:1–6.

Centers for Disease Control and Prevention: Update: Provisional Public Health Service recommendations for chemoprophylaxis after occupational exposure to HIV. *MMWR Morb Mortal Wkly Rep* 1996; 45:468–480.

Centers for Disease Control: Update: Universal precautions for prevention of transmission of human immunodeficiency virus, hepatitis B virus, and other blood-borne pathogens in health-care settings. *MMWR Morb Mortal Wkly Rep* 1988;37:377–382, 387–388.

Cheingsong-Popov R, Lister S, Callow D, Kaleebu P, Beddows S, Weber J: WHO Network for HIV Isolation and Characterization: Serotyping HIV type 1 by antibody binding to the V3 loop. Relationship to viral genotype. *AIDS Res Hum Retroviruses* 1994;10:1379–1386.

Diettrich NA, Cacioppo JC, Kaplan G, Cohen SM: A growing spectrum of surgical disease in patients with human immunodeficiency virus/acquired immunodeficiency syndrome: Experience with 120 major cases. *Arch Surg* 1991;126:860–866.

Essary LR, Kinard SJ, Butcher A, et al: Screening potential corneal donors for HIV-1 by polymerase chain reaction and a colorimetric microwell hybridization assay. *Am J Ophthalmol* 1996;122:526–534.

Fishel R, Barbul A, Wasserkrug HL, Penberthy LT, Rettura G, Efron G: Cyclosporine A impairs wound healing in rats. *J Surg Res* 1983; 34:572–575.

Ganesh R, Castle D, McGibbon D, Phillips I, Bradbeer C: Letter: Staphylococcal carriage and HIV infection. *Lancet* 1989;2:558.

Hu DJ, Dondero TJ, Rayfield MA, et al: The emerging genetic diversity of HIV: The importance of global surveillance for diagnostics, research, and prevention. *JAMA* 1996;275:210–216.

Johnson GK, Robinson WS: Human immunodeficiency virus-1 (HIV-1) in the vapors of surgical power instruments. *J Med Virol* 1991;33:47–50.

Karon JM, Buehler JW, Byers RH, et al: Projections of the number of persons diagnosed with AIDS and the number of immunosuppressed HIV-infected persons: United States, 1992–1994. *MMWR Morb Mortal Wkly Rep* 1992;41:1–29.

Kelen GD, Fritz S, Qaqish B, et al: Unrecognized human immunodeficiency virus infection in emergency department patients. *N Engl J Med* 1988;318:1645–1650.

Krumholz HM, Sande MA, Lo B: Community-acquired bacteremia in patients with acquired immunodeficiency syndrome: Clinical presentation, bacteriology, and outcome. *Am J Med* 1989;86:776–779.

McGrath MS: HIV: Overview and General Description, in Cohen PT, Sande MA, Volberding P (eds): *The AIDS Knowledge Base: A Textbook on HIV Disease from the University of California, San Francisco, and the San Francisco General Hospital.* Waltham, MA, Medical Publishers Group, 1990, Section 3.1.1, pp 1–3.

Murphy PM, Lane HC, Fauci AS, Gallin JI: Impairment of neutrophil bactericidal capacity in patients with AIDS. *J Infect Dis* 1988;158: 627–630.

Onorato IM, McCray E: Prevalence of human immunodeficiency virus infection among patients attending tuberculosis clinics in the United States. *J Infect Dis* 1992;165:87–92.

Pau CP, Kai M, Holloman-Candal DL, et al: WHO Network for HIV Isolation and Characterization: Antigenic variation and serotyping

of HIV type 1 from four World Health Organization-sponsored HIV vaccine sites. *AIDS Res Hum Retroviruses* 1994;10:1369–1377.

Ravikumar TS, Allen JD, Bothe A Jr, Steel G Jr: Splenectomy: The treatment of choice for human immunodeficiency virus-related immune thrombocytopenia? *Arch Surg* 1989;124:625–628.

Schneider PA, Abrams DI, Rayner AA, Hohn DC: Immunodeficiency-associated thrombocytopenic purpura (IDTP): Response to splenectomy. *Arch Surg* 1987;122:1175–1178.

Tao G, Kassler WJ, Branson BM, Peterman TA: Home Collection Kits for HIV Testing: Evaluation of three strategies for dealing with insufficient dried blood specimens. *J Acquir-Imm Defic Syndr Hum Retrovirol* 1997;15:312–317.

Wilber JC: HIV Antibody Testing: Methodology, in Cohen PT, Sande MA, Volberding P (eds): *The AIDS Knowledge Base: A Textbook on HIV Disease from the University of California, San Francisco, and the San Francisco General Hospital.* Waltham, MA, Medical Publishers Group, 1990, Section 2.1.2, pp 1–8.

Pathophysiology of Immunity Impairment

Burack JH, Mandel MS, Bizer LS: Emergency abdominal operations in the patient with acquired immunodeficiency syndrome. *Arch Surg* 1989;124:285–286.

Ellis M, Gupta S, Galant S, et al: Impaired neutrophil function in patients with AIDS or AIDS-related complex: A comprehensive evaluation. *J Infect Dis* 1988;158:1268–1276.

Grant IH, Armstrong D: Management of infectious complications in acquired immunodeficiency syndrome. *Am J Med* 1986;81(suppl 1A):59–72.

Surgical Complications and Outcome

Buehrer JL, Weber DJ, Meyer AA, et al: Wound infection rates after invasive procedures in HIV-1 seropositive versus HIV-1 seronegative hemophiliacs. *Ann Surg* 1990;211:492–498.

Carpenter CC, Fischl MA, Hammer SM, et al: Antiretroviral Therapy for HIV Infection in 1997: Updated recommendations of the International AIDS Society. USA panel. *JAMA* 1997;277:1962–1969.

Goldberg VM, Heiple KG, Ratnoff OD, Kurczynski E, Arvan G: Total knee arthroplasty in classic hemophilia. *J Bone Joint Surg* 1981;63A: 695–701.

Hawkins CC, Gold JW, Whimbey E, et al: Mycobacterium avium complex infections in patients with the acquired immunodeficiency syndrome. *Ann Intern Med* 1986;105:184–188.

Luck JV Jr, Hansraj KK, Griffin MD, Kasper CK: Risk factors for late infection with total hip and knee arthroplasties. Proceedings of the American Academy of Orthopaedic Surgeons 61st Annual Meeting, New Orleans, LA. Rosemont, IL, American Academy of Orthopaedic Surgeons, 1994, p 241.

Luck JV Jr, Kasper CK: Surgical management of advanced hemophilic arthropathy: An overview of 20 years' experience. *Clin Orthop* 1989; 242:60–82.

Luck JV Jr, Logan LR, Benson DR, Glasser DB: Human immunodeficiency virus infection: Complications and outcome of orthopaedic surgery. *J Am Acad Orthop Surg* 1996;4:297–304.

McCollough NC III, Enis JE, Lovitt J, Lian EC, Niemann KN, Loughlin EC Jr: Synovectomy or total replacement of the knee in hemophilia. *J Bone Joint Surg* 1979;61A:69–75.

McLaughlin JR, Tierney M, Harris WH: Mycobacterium avium intracellulare infection of hip arthroplasties in an AIDS patient. *J Bone Joint Surg* 1994;76A:498–499.

Paiement GD, Hymes RA, LaDouceur MS, Gosselin RA, Green HD: Postoperative infections in asymptomatic HIV-seropositive orthopedic trauma patients. *J Trauma* 1994;37:545–551.

Robinson G, Wilson SE, Williams RA: Surgery in patients with acquired immunodeficiency syndrome. *Arch Surg* 1987;122:170–175.

Wilson SE, Robinson G, Williams RA et al: Acquired immune deficiency syndrome (AIDS): Indications for abdominal surgery, pathology, and outcome. *Ann Surg* 1989;210:428–434.

Transmission of HIV in the Surgical Setting

Division of HIV/AIDS Prevention: HIV/AIDS Surveillance Report: Year-end edition, Vol 7, No. 2. Atlanta, GA, Centers for Disease Control and Prevention, 1995, p 21.

Dorozynski A: French patient contracts AIDS from surgeon. *BMJ* 1997;314:250.

Esteban JI, Gomez J, Martell M, et al: Transmission of hepatitis C virus by a cardiac surgeon. *N Engl J Med* 1996;334:555–560.

Harpaz R, Von Seidlein L, Averhoff FM, et al: Transmission of hepatitis B virus to multiple patients from a surgeon without evidence of inadequate infection control. *N Engl J Med* 1996;334:549–554.

Hussain SA, Latif AB, Choudhary AA: Risk to surgeons: A survey of accidental injuries during operations. *Br J Surg* 1988;75:314–316.

Reseau National de Sante Publlique: Evaluation de risque de transmission du V.I.H. par un chirurgien a l'hospital de Saint Germain en Lay (Yvelines): Rapport a la Direction Generale de la Sante. Reseau National de Sante Publique. St. Maurice, France. Decembre 1996.

Tokars JI, Bell DM, Culver DH, et al: Percutaneous injuries during surgical procedures. *JAMA* 1992;267:2899–2904.

Tokars JI, Chamberland ME, Schable CA, et al: A survey of occupational blood contact and HIV infection among orthopedic surgeons: The American Academy of Orthopaedic Surgeons Serosurvey Study Committee. *JAMA* 1992;268:489–494.

Tokars JI, Marcus R, Culver DH, et al: Surveillance of HIV infection and zidovudine use among health care workers after occupational exposure to HIV-infected blood: The CDC Cooperative Needlestick Surveillance Group. *Ann Intern Med* 1993;118:913–919.

Hepatitis B and C

Grady GF, Lee VA, Prince AM, et al: Hepatitis B immune globulin for accidental exposures among medical personnel: Final report of a multicenter controlled trial. *J Infect Dis* 1978;138:625–638.

Kiyosawa K, Sodeyama T, Tanaka E, et al: Hepatitis C in hospital employees with needlestick injuries. *Ann Intern Med* 1991; 115:367–369.

Marranconi F, Mecenero V, Pellizzer GP, et al: HCV infection after accidental needlestick injury in health-care workers. *Infection* 1992;20:111.

Maynard JE: Nosocomial viral hepatitis. *Am J Med* 1981;70:439–444.

Mitsui T, Iwano K, Masuko K, et al: Hepatitis C virus infection in medical personnel after needlestick accident. *Hepatology* 1992;16:1109–1114.

Panlilio AL, Shapiro CN, Schable CA, et al: Serosurvey of human immunodeficiency virus, hepatitis B virus, and hepatitis C virus infection among hospital-based surgeons. Serosurvey Study Group. *J Am Coll Surg* 1995;180:16–24.

Seeff LB, Wright EC, Zimmerman HJ, Alter HJ, Dietz AA, Felsher BF, et al: Type B hepatitis after needlestick exposure: Prevention with hepatitis B immune globulin. Final report of the Veterans Administration Cooperative Study. *Ann Intern Med* 1978;88:285–293.

Centers for Disease Control: Evaluation of blunt suture needles in preventing percutaneous injuries among health-care workers during gynecologic surgical procedures: New York City, March 1993-June 1994. *MMWR Morb Mortal Wkly Rep* 1997;46:25–29.

Kelen GD, Green GB, Purcell RH, et al: Hepatitis B and hepatitis C in emergency department patients. *N Engl J Med* 1992;326:1399–1404.

National Institutes of Health Consensus Development Conference Panel Statement: Management of hepatitis C. *Hepatology* 1997;26 (suppl 1):2S–10S.

Alter MJ: Epidemiology of hepatitis C. *Hepatology* 1997;26(suppl 1): 62S–65S.

McQuillan G, Alter MJ Moyer L, et al: Abstract: A population based serologic study of hepatitis C virus infection in the United States. Proceedings of the IX International Symposium on Viral Hepatitis and Liver Disease, Rome; 1996:8A.

Seeff LB: Natural history of hepatitis C. *Hepatology* 1997;26(suppl 1): 21S–28S.

Viral Transmission From Musculoskeletal Allografts

Campbell DG, Li P, Oakeshott RD: HIV Infection of human cartilage. *J Bone Joint Surg* 1996;78-B:22–25.

Tomford WW: Current Concepts Review: Transmission of disease through transplantation of musculoskeletal allografts. *J Bone Joint Surg* 1995;77A:1742–1754.

Chapter 9

Magnetic Resonance Imaging of the Musculoskeletal System: Advances in Musculoskeletal Imaging

Charles G. Peterfy, MD, PhD

Timothy P.L. Roberts, PhD

Harry K. Genant, MD

This chapter at a glance

This chapter provides an introduction to the fundamentals of magnetic resonance imaging (MRI), discusses the diversity of MRI capabilities in musculoskeletal imaging, and offers a review of the developments of dedicated-extremity MRI and imaging in arthritis.

One or more of the authors or the department with which they are affiliated has received something of value from a commercial or other party related directly or indirectly to the subject of this chapter.

The past 2 decades have seen remarkable advances in medical imaging. The advent of magnetic resonance imaging (MRI), in particular, has brought unprecedented power to the study of musculoskeletal disorders. Musculoskeletal indications presently account for approximately 20% to 30% of referrals for MRI. Advances in MRI technology continue to improve the quality of images and expand the range of pathologies that can be evaluated, and a growing awareness among clinicians of the unique and unprecedented capabilities of MRI continues to extend the use of MRI for an increasing number of costly and frustrating medical problems.

Two recent advances that deserve special attention are (1) the emergence of special-purpose MRI technology and (2) the growing role of MRI in the evaluation of arthritis and its treatment. This chapter will give an introduction to the fundamentals of MRI, discuss the diversity of MRI capabilities in musculoskeletal imaging, and offer a review of the developments of dedicated-extremity MRI (E-MRI) and imaging in arthritis, describing how they are changing the way musculoskeletal disease is being evaluated.

MRI: Background and Implications for the Musculoskeletal System

MRI has emerged as a powerful tomographic tool and diagnostic modality in contemporary radiology. The nuclear magnetic resonance (NMR) signal from which cross-sectional images are ultimately derived is particularly sensitive to a number of characteristics of the physicochemical microenvironment, such as water mobility, macromolecule (predominantly protein) content, and microstructure. As such it can allow differentiation of different soft tissues, and identification, delineation, and description of pathologically-abnormal tissues in a fashion unrivaled by other imaging techniques (such as conventional radiography, computed tomography [CT], and the techniques of nuclear medicine: single photon emission CT and positron emission tomography). Such sensitivity and differential power are accompanied by the diagnostically confounding factor of image misinterpretation and susceptibility to image degrading or confusing artifact. Recognition of the complexity of the NMR signal and the techniques by which a degree of specificity to tissue physicochemical microenvironmental features can be obtained allows unimagined diagnostic and prognostic utility in the early detection, grading, and characterization of disease processes. Consideration of MRI as a technique with physiologic sensitivity as well as morphologic or anatomic quality extends its application in the identification, study, and follow-up of disease processes; quantifica-

tion of tissue characteristics offers enhanced diagnostic and prognostic markers as well as provides a tool for the monitoring of the efficacy of therapeutic intervention.

MRI Primer: The Origin of the NMR Signal

The origin of the NMR signal used in the generation of magnetic resonance images is the proton, or hydrogen nucleus, primarily found in water and lipid molecules. Other biologically-relevant nuclei such as 23Na and 31P offer NMR opportunities, but imaging applications have to date been limited, largely because of the low sensitivity of the NMR technique to these nuclei and the low concentrations in which they are commonly encountered. The magnetic moment or "spin" property of the hydrogen nucleus, when placed in a strong external magnetic field, is the feature that is exploited in exciting and detecting an NMR response from tissue. Unlike conventional radiography or CT, no ionizing radiation is used; rather, the NMR effect is excited by applying a radio wave of appropriate frequency using a dedicated transmitter coil that surrounds the body part under investigation. The precise frequency varies with the magnitude of the external magnetic field and is approximately 25 MHz for systems operating at 0.2 T and approximately 64 MHz for systems at 1.5 T. The response of the excited protons, the NMR signal, is detected after the radio wave (or radiofrequency [RF] pulse) is turned off: individual nuclear magnetic moments (from each proton) precess, or rotate, about the external magnetic field axis and induce a signal in a pick-up (receiver) coil. In practice, these moments tend to precess at slightly different rates (as they experience slightly different local magnetic fields) and so dephase; thus the detected signal (being proportional to the vector sum of individual proton moments) decays. This decay is normally quite rapid and is characterized by the time constant T2*, reflecting all forms of loss of phase coherence, from all forms of regional magnetic field variation (Fig. 1). Such variation in the magnetic field may arise from inhomogeneity associated with magnet construction, or from differences in the magnetic susceptibility (the degree to which the tissue becomes magnetized when placed in an external magnetic field) of neighboring tissues (such as soft tissue and bone), as well as from random fluctuations in each proton's local magnetic field caused by the very interactions of proton nuclear magnetic moments themselves.

The Spin Echo

Construction-related inhomogeneity of magnetic field as well as field variations from the different magnetic susceptibilities of different tissues are spatially fixed; that is, they do not vary over time. On the other hand, the fluctuations in local magnetic field induced by the presence of a single diffusing water molecule approaching another are random. This feature allows the first category of spin-dephasing mechanisms to be somewhat predicted and reversed. The technique by which this can be achieved is referred to as the spin-echo: if a second RF pulse is applied some time after the first RF pulse has been turned off, the loss of phase coherence can be partially reversed. Essentially, the second RF pulse causes the spin magnetic moment vectors, which have precessed out of phase, by virtue of their different precession rates, to be reflected in the rotation plane. Subsequent precession continues with each spin precessing at the same rate as before (because its spatial position and local effective magnetic field have not altered). However, the different precession rates that were previously causing dephasing of the precessing spin population now act to "rephase" the nuclear magnetic moments, until eventually a so-called "echo" forms at an equal time after application of the second (often called "refocusing" RF pulse). The total time between the initial RF pulse and the echo formation is called the echo time (TE), and is simply twice the time between the initial and second RF pulses. As such, TE is a user-controllable parameter, because the second RF pulse can be applied at will.

Image Contrast: T2 and the Influence of Echo Time

Although the spin echo technique causes rephasing of spatially-dependent dephasing mechanisms (such as those associated with construction-related inhomogeneity or the magnetic susceptibilities of different tissues), the echo is still attenuated in amplitude by the irreproducible "interac-

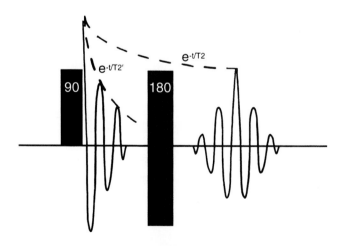

Figure 1

Free induction decay and spin echo refocusing. Signal decays after initial (90°) radiofrequency excitation with a time constant T2*, which describes the rate of loss of phase coherence of the excited spin population (signal, S, as a function of time, t, is given by the equation: $S[t] \propto \exp^{-t/T2^*}$).

tion"-based dephasing, described by the time constant T2. This T2-related dephasing cannot be reversed by the application of a second RF pulse because there is no expectation that each spin will experience the same magnetic fields during the second period as it did prior to the second RF pulse. Practically, the amount of echo attenuation then depends on 2 factors: T2 (reflecting water interactions) and TE (the echo time), reflecting the "opportunity" for such dephasing to occur. Although T2 is a property of the tissue, TE is completely under the control of the investigator (some hardware and signal-to-noise ratio limitations apply, but TEs are commonly varied in the range 2 to 100 ms). Thus, by appropriate choice of the parameter, TE images can be made either insensitive (short TEs) or highly sensitive (long TEs) to differences in T2 between tissues under study. Such short TE images, insensitive to T2 differences, merely reflect the abundance of protons (and so are commonly called proton density-weighted images). Images with long TE (and thus great sensitivity to differing T2 parameters of different tissues) are termed T2-weighted.

In general, all tissues will show decreasing signal intensity with increasing TE, but tissues with short T2 values (such as bone and ligaments) will appear black, and tissues with longer T2 values (such as synovial fluid) will remain hyperintense, even on T2-weighted images with long TE values. There are a number of factors that influence the characteristic T2 value of different tissues and the physiologic origins of T2 differences are complex. However, in simple terms, it can be considered that sustained interactions (that is, proximity) of protons on water molecules leads to rapid loss of phase coherence and a short T2 value. On the other hand, in tissues with high water mobility, such as synovial fluid, the interactions between the highly mobile water molecules are brief and little effective dephasing is induced; thus, T2 values are relatively long. An example of the usefulness of such physiologic interpretation is given by the T2 prolongation observed in chondromalacia leading to focal hyperintensity in cartilage in areas of disease, reflecting the increased water mobility and decrease in sustained water proton interactions arising from the loss of matrix structure. Thus, hyperintensity on T2-weighted image indicates a high water content, which is a marker of pathology, but also can be interpreted physiologically in terms of changes in the tissue microenvironment.

Image Contrast: T1 and the Influence of Repeat Time

What is the role of sequence repeat time (TR) on image contrast? Why not just use the shortest method possible (to obtain images quickly)? Between successive applications of RF pulses, the excited nuclear magnetic moments must recover to their equilibrium (preexcitation) state. This process (called longitudinal or spin-lattice relaxation) can be thought of as the mechanism by which energy absorbed during RF application (excitation) is redistributed to the proton's surroundings (or lattice). In general, this process depends on the ability of the surroundings to readily absorb this energy and thus reflects another property of the physicochemical microenvironment, namely the availability of large macromolecules (proteins) and microstructures (collagen/proteoglycan matrix) to interact with the excited proton on the water molecule.

Typical T1 values vary widely between different tissues (and also with external field strength) but as a rule of thumb, 5 times the T1 value should be allowed between successive applications of the RF pulses if a fully-relaxed image is required (that is, TR >5 × T1). The term fully-relaxed implies that each species is then being sampled during imaging with equal and full efficiency. With T1-values for fluids typically measured in hundreds of milliseconds, or even seconds, this would imply long TR times and consequently long image acquisition times. Further, although fully-relaxed images have high signal-to-noise ratio (because all proton populations are being sampled with near 100% efficiency), their appearance reflects proton density alone and lacks any form of soft-tissue contrast not directly related to proton abundance. T2-weighted images, as discussed above, are generally acquired with long TR values to give all tissues maximum sampling efficiency, with physiologically-relevant contrast introduced by the use of long TE values, sensitive to differences in tissue T2 values (Table 1).

If images are acquired with shorter TR values, protons in different tissues may not achieve fully-relaxed status in the TR interval and so will be inefficiently sampled by subsequent RF pulses. Thus, they will contribute less amplitude to subsequent echoes and in general will be represented with diminished image intensity. Tissues with short T1 values (such as lipids) may nevertheless recover fully (or at least substantially) and will thus appear relatively hyperintense. Such images are called T1-weighted, because image intensity (and contrast) depends on the tissue T1 values (with short T1 tissues appearing relatively bright). Again,

this contrast information is obtained at a price of diminished signal-to-noise ratio, compared to the proton-density weighted image; however, because TR is shorter, T1-weighted images may be acquired faster. Thus, signal averaging techniques (repeating the entire scan) may be employed to improve signal-to-noise ratio and image quality.

In general, choice of the parameters TR and TE in the spin echo imaging sequence allow images with differing soft-tissue signal intensities, or contrast, to be obtained. These signal intensity differences, arising from different tissue proton density and T1 and T2 values, can be interpreted in terms of the physicochemical microenvironment of water in the tissues and thus offer insight into the underlying physiology and pathophysiology. In general, structures with a high water content are bright on T2-weighted images, and those with a high fat content are bright on T1-weighted images.

MRI Primer: Image Formation

MRIs are formed from the above basic RF application and echo collection, along with the use of spatial coordinate labeling, which is achieved through the appropriate use of 3 magnetic field gradients. These fields are generated by additional electromagnetic coils inside the scanner, which have the property of linearly varying the local magnetic field along the x-, y-, or z- directions, when electric current is applied to them. The 3 processes integral to most MRI techniques are the steps of slice-selection, frequency encoding, and phase encoding. Each process is associated with 1 dimension of the 3-dimensional (3-D) Cartesian space.

Slice-selection is achieved by application of a magnetic field gradient (in the slice direction) synchronously with the application of the RF excitation pulses. In this manner, a narrow band (or slice) of protons is selected from within the entire coil volume. Frequency encoding refers to the collection of the spin echo in the presence of a magnetic field gradient (perpendicular to the slice-select gradient). Thus, the spin echo collected consists of signals from spin ensem-

Table 1

General Rules for Different Spin-Echo Image Contrasts: Influence of TR and TE* Image Description

	TR	TE	Appearance
Proton density	Long (> 5 x T1)	Short (< T2)	High signal to noise ratio Poor soft-tissue contrast
T1-weighted	Short (< ~ T1)	Short (< T2)	Signal higher for tissues with short T1 values
T2-weighted	Long (> 5 x T1)	Long (> ~ T2)	Signal higher for tissues with long T2 values
Mixed (rarely used)	Short	Long	Low signal to noise ratio

*   Use of "long" and "short" descriptors are relative to the T1 and T2 values of tissues under investigation. TR=sequence repeat time; TE=echo time

bles precessing at different rates (according to their coordinate in the direction of the frequency-encoding, or readout, gradient). The distribution of spins in this direction can be obtained from a frequency analysis or single dimensional Fourier transformation of the collected echo. However, while a projection of the spin distribution along this axis from a restricted "slice" of the volume is obtainable from this single echo, it is not possible to construct an entire 2-D image from a single collected echo. In fact, in order to generate MRI, it is necessary to have repeated application of the RF excitation pulses and thus collection of many spin echoes. Each of these spin echoes is acquired having been slightly modified by the application of a magnetic field gradient pulse in the phase-encoding direction between the initial RF excitation pulse and the echo collection.

Upon 2-D Fourier transformation of the array of collected echoes, the image is revealed, with a pixel matrix equivalent to the number of data points sampled per echo, multiplied by the number of different echoes (or phase-encoding steps) employed. Typically this number is in the range 128 to 256, although some applications call for higher spatial resolution; therefore, a 512×512 pixel matrix is employed (requiring 512 separate applications of the RF pulses and thus 512 separate echoes to be collected). The time between successive RF pulse applications, and thus between successive echo collections, is called the sequence TR. It is clear that the image acquisition time is related to the product of TR and the number of phase-encoded echoes collected. Typical values for TR range from 10 ms to several seconds. Thus, typical MRI procedures vary in length from approximately 1 second to many minutes.

Fat Suppression: FATSAT and STIR

The MRI signal originates from protons in the body. Although the primary source of these is water molecules, protons from liquid-state lipid moieties also can contribute signal. This signal may contaminate MRIs, particularly on T1-weighted images, in which lipid signal appears hyperintense by virtue of its short T1 value. Two principal methods of preparing MRI sequences such that lipid contribution to signal is suppressed are available: chemical shift selective saturation (CHESS or FATSAT) and STIR (short tau inver-

sion recovery). For both techniques, some physical property helps in distinguishing water-proton-originating signal from lipid-proton-originating signal.

The FATSAT technique exploits the fact that the lipid molecular environment is chemically somewhat different from water. The presence of double bonds and the multiple oxygen moieties in particular give rise to a magnetic field shielding effect, causing the protons to experience a different local magnetic field, to that of water protons in the same position. Thus, lipid-protons precess, as a group, at a different rate to water protons. This precession frequency offset is referred to as chemical shift and has a magnitude of about 3 parts per million (ppm) (that is, it scales in absolute frequency difference with increasing external magnetic field). Using frequency selective excitation techniques (modulated RF excitation pulses), followed by gradient pulses to induce complete loss of phase, or scrambling, of excited protons, the lipid signal can be excited and destroyed prior to image formation, yielding images containing signal only from water protons. (The converse technique can also be applied to generate fat-only images.) (Fig. 2). Another way in which the different chemical shift of water and lipid protons can be exploited relies on the relative phase of the water and lipid spin populations, during precession after excitation. After RF excitation in a gradient-recalled-echo imaging sequence, lipid-proton spins and water-proton spins precess at different rates according to their chemical shift. Progressively they dephase. If a voxel contains a 50%/50% mixture of water-protons and lipid-protons, it is clear that at a certain time after excitation, the dephasing will lead to complete cancellation (opposed or anti-phase). If this time is chosen as the imaging echo time, no signal will result. This fat-water opposed approach can be used to attenuate signal in bone marrow, while not attenuating signal from nearby cartilage, thereby enhancing contrast. At 1.5T this critical fat-water opposed echo time is approximately 2.5 ms. After 5 ms the fat and water protons will again be in phase and signals will reinforce. After 7.5 ms they will again cancel, etc. At lower field strengths, such as 0.2T, where precession rate (frequency) differences are much smaller, the critical TE for cancellation of signal is 20 ms and for reinforcement, 40 ms. These times are rather long compared with T2* times and therefore both fat and water signals are attenuated by transverse relaxation processes over such a long TE. Hence, the choice

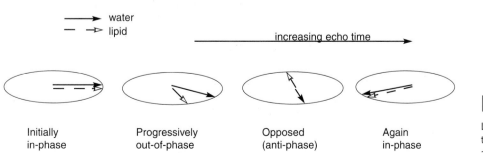

water
lipid

increasing echo time

Initially
in-phase

Progressively
out-of-phase

Opposed
(anti-phase)

Again
in-phase

Figure 2

Lipid and water proton magnetization vectors precess at different rates and thus may oppose or reinforce.

of fat-water opposed or in-phase is not so readily available at low fields. In some environments (particularly where local field variations are rampant by virtue of local susceptibility variations such as in the ankle joint) and at low magnetic field strengths (where the frequency difference between water proton precession and lipid proton precession is too small to allow appropriate selectivity of excitation), this FATSAT technique is inappropriate.

An alternative strategy, based on exploiting the different T1 values of water and lipid protons, is employed in the STIR approach. Prior to imaging, an RF pulse of sufficient intensity to effect a 180° rotation, or inversion of the nuclear magnetic moments, is applied to all species. After this pulse the magnetic moment vector recovers by T1 (longitudinal) relaxation processes toward its equilibrium alignment (see above description of T1-weighted images). However, because the starting position was 180° rotated rather than 90° (as in imaging), at some point the z-component of magnetization passes through zero (on its progression from inverted -1 to recovered +1). At that point, if an imaging sequence is commenced then these magnetic moments will contribute zero signal to subsequent echoes (sampling efficiency equals zero). Therefore, species satisfying that condition (having reached the null point) will appear black on subsequent images. Arriving at the null point will depend on tissue T1 values and on the interval, tau, allowed between the inversion pulse and the subsequent imaging. If tau is made short, species with relatively fast recovery (short T1 values) may arrive at the null point, and other species will have progressed only a little from their initial inverted positions, and still contribute strongly to the subsequent echo formation and thus appear bright in images. This is the basis of the STIR technique. Because lipids have short T1 values, allowing a short tau after inversion causes the lipids to recover just to the null point, whereas water protons are still near their initial inverted state and thus contribute efficiently to the image, which will appear fat-suppressed (the negative near-inverted state of the water proton magnetization is irrelevant because magnitude images are observed). The precise tau value required to cause tissue to be "nulled" can be calculated according to the expression: tau = 0.69 * T1.

Magnetization Transfer Contrast

Another contrast mechanism that can be harnessed by MRI is magnetization transfer contrast (MTC). The magnetic resonance signal that is observed originates primarily in protons of free water (and lipid) molecules in tissue, and is characterized by a relatively sharp resonance line shape (typically with a line width of 10 to 50 Hz) corresponding to a relatively long T2 (tens of ms). However, protons also exist in or are closely associated with the molecules of larger structures such as proteins. These protons are bound more rigidly in their macromolecular structure and consequently have much shorter T2 values and correspondingly broad resonance line shapes (tens of kHz). As such they are practically invisible to conventional MRI approaches. These protons may, however, exchange with protons of free water molecules that approach and interact with them.

This process of exchange depends on local chemical interactions and differs between different types of macromolecules, but is especially pronounced if exposed hydroxyl (-OH) groups are present. It is not possible to observe this effect directly, as the signal detected depends on the current free water contribution. If, however, the protons of the macromolecular structure are magnetically labeled, then it might be possible to detect the amount of exchange with free water that has taken place by the amount of labeled protons that contribute to the free water signal. This magnetic labeling is achieved by saturation of the bound (macromolecular) protons. In practice this is achieved by preceding the MRI sequence with an off-resonance excitation that does not affect the narrow line of the free water but does saturate the protons of the broader resonance line (the macromolecular protons). Saturation may be achieved with low power off-resonance excitation (2 to 4 kHz typically) or by the use of on-resonance "binomial" excitation pulses (for example, $90_x 180_{-x} 90_x$) that cause a net rotation of zero near nominal resonance (the free water) but generate periodic excitation at frequencies away from it.

In practice, signal loss will be observed relative to a control image (with no saturation prepulse) in areas where there is a substantial exchange between free and bound pools of protons. Where this exchange is reduced (because of the reduction in availability of macromolecular structures, for example), the signal loss is correspondingly attenuated. Subtraction images thus appear hyperintense in regions of pronounced magnetization transfer effect, such as in healthy cartilage. Quantification may be achieved by constructing the magnetization transfer ratio (MTR): MTR = $(M_0 - M_S)/M_0$. This ratio has been employed particularly in the study of cartilage collagen/proteoglycan matrix destruction in the early stages of osteoarthritis, because the intact matrix shows a particularly pronounced MTC effect (and thus high MTR), which becomes progressively attenuated as it is destroyed. Thus, MTC may provide useful physiologic insight into the physicochemical microenvironment and offer an early marker for disease and a quantitative measure of recovery or therapeutic efficacy (Table 2).

Faster Imaging— Gradient-Recalled Echo

As an alternative to generating a spin-echo with the use of a second 180° refocusing RF pulse, a gradient-recalled echo can be formed using only a single excitation pulse and reversing the polarity of the frequency-encoding gradient in such a way that spins are intentionally dephased and then precisely rephased at the center of the signal acquisition period. This echo amplitude will depend on T2* (rather than T2 as for the spin-echo) because any spatially-fixed dephasing processes (such as those arising from magnetic susceptibility differences or field inhomogeneities) have no mechanism to be refocused. Imaging using gradient-recalled echoes is performed analogously to conventional spin-echo imaging by the collection of a series of echoes, each with a different phase-encoding gradient amplitude. Although using a lower flip angle generates less signal amplitude (because signal is obtained only from the horizontal component of the precessing magnetic moments vectors; that is, is proportional to the trigonometric sine of the flip angle), this effect is more than compensated for by the fact that recovery to the fully-relaxed state can be achieved more quickly (because the vertical component of magnetization has been attenuated only according to the cosine of the flip angle). For example, with a flip angle of 30°, the amplitude of the detected signal is reduced to $\sin(30°) = 50\%$, but the z-component of magnetization is attenuated to only $\cos(30°) = 86.7\%$, thus having only 13.3% left to recover to achieve the fully-relaxed condition. Therefore, much shorter TR values can be used, resulting in much shorter image acquisition times. This result can be exploited in dynamic imaging, or in the generation of 3-D high-resolution images, in clinically reasonable time frames.

Rapid Imaging: Fast Spin Echo

Fast spin echo (FSE) imaging (also known as RARE, or turbo spin echo, TSE) allows rapid high-resolution imaging by the acquisition of multiple spin echoes after each excitation. Because each echo is separately phase-encoded, fewer excitations are thus required to complete the data acquisition required for image construction. These images can readily be made to exhibit T2-weighting, useful for pathologic identification. Because of their spin-echo nature, FSE images have an additional advantage of showing little sensitivity to magnetic susceptibility (field variation-dependent) artifact. Indeed, on low field scanners, use of the FSE imaging sequence has allowed MRI to be diagnostically useful, even in the presence of some metal prosthetics.

The timesaving capability of FSE compared to that of conventional spin echo is clearly related to the number of echoes collected per excitation. Typically this number is chosen to be 8 to 16. However, in principle, the entirety of k-space could be sampled from a single excitation to yield a single-shot ultra-fast imaging sequence. Variants using reduced flip angle refocusing pulses have been developed (U-FLARE being the most prominent acronym). The time saved can be reinvested in a number of ways. First, the reduced scan time permits increased patient throughput. Second, because the number of excitations (and therefore

Table 2
General Appearance of Various Tissues With Different Magnetic Resonance Sequence Parameters*

Tissue	Appearance			
	T2-weighted image	T1-weighted image	Fat-suppressed T1-weighted image	Magnetization transfer subtraction image
Cortical bone	Black	Black	Black	Black
Ligaments	Black	Black	Black	Black
Healthy cartilage	Gray	Gray	Gray (good contrast to bone marrow)	White
Chondromalacia (diseased cartilage)	White	Gray	Gray	Gray
Bone marrow	Gray	White	Black	Black
Normal fluid	White	Black	Black	Black
Abnormal fluid (pus)	White	Gray	Black	Black
Muscle	White	Gray	Gray	Gray

*   At high field strength (~1.5T), the following parameters would be typical: T2-weighted: TR ~2-3 s, TE > 80 ms. T1-weighted: TR ~50 to 500 ms, TE < 20 ms. Fat-suppressed: using either FATSAT (frequency offset ~3 ppm) or STIR (TI~100 to 150 ms). Magnetization transfer subtraction image generated by difference between identical proton-density or T1-weighted images with and without off-resonance radiation (frequency offset = 1 to 2 kHz).

TR intervals) is reduced, the duration of TR can be increased to properly satisfy the ideal (5 × T1) requirement to eliminate the effects of partial saturation due to incomplete longitudinal recovery between successive excitations. Particularly for long T1 species this effect may be substantial. Having thus increased the basic signal available for imaging by eliminating partial saturation effects, it is then feasible to employ longer TE times to achieve greater T2-weighting without prohibitively poor signal-to-noise ratios.

The choice of echo train length (ETL), the number of echoes per excitation, brings with it some compromise. Fundamentally, although a long ETL yields a more rapid image, it is clear that different echoes (different lines of k-space) will have different T2-weighting, because they have different TEs. It is possible that this additional weighting of k-space may give rise to artifacts, particularly blurring in the image. Of course, shorter ETLs have fewer different TEs and therefore reduced artifact. The source of the artifact can be viewed in terms of the relevance of the different portions of the k-space map. Sometimes referred to as a map of "spatial frequency", the k-space map carries essentially low spatial frequency information (gross form and contrast) nearer the center and high spatial frequency information (needed for sharpness and image detail) toward its edges. Because T2-weighting is defined in terms of the contrast observed and conventional spin echo with its relation to the sequence echo time is familiar, an effective TE in FSE is defined as the echo time of the echoes that make up the central (low spatial frequency and therefore contrast-influencing) portion of k-space. Neighboring lines of k-space are collected at identical echo times by collecting one from each excitation. For example, in the collection of a "short effective echo time" FSE image (for approximately proton density contrast) the first echo of each echo train might be phase-encoded to be near the center of k-space, with other echoes filling the periphery of the k-space map. Conversely, for a "long effective TE image (for T2-weighting), the early echoes would be allocated high-phase encoding values and fill the extremes of k-space, while the center lines of k-space would be filled with later (longer TE) echoes. The source of the blurring artifact often seen in proton density FSE images may at least in part be attributed to the fact that the edges of k-space are being acquired with long echo times (because the short TE echoes fill the center of k-space) and so have poor signal-to-noise ratios. This leads to a poor definition of high spatial frequency image components such as edges and small objects.

In general, the appearance of FSE images resembles a conventional spin-echo image with a TE equal to the effective TE of the FSE sequence. This has led to widespread adoption of the faster variant. One confounding drawback remains: the appearance of relatively hyperintense lipid signal on otherwise T2-weighted FSE scans. Several explanations for this paradoxical lipid signal have been offered, including (but not limited to) enhanced loss of signal on spin echo (but not FSE) scans arising from the J-coupling of protons on the lipid moiety. Additionally, the use of multiple slice-selective high flip angle (~180º) RF pulses may engender magnetization transfer signal suppression in tissue, but not lipid, again leading to lipid relative hyperintensity. Whatever the underlying explanation, the lipid signal, if considered undesirable, can be eliminated, or attenuated, using FATSAT prepulses, or the STIR inversion recovery approach.

In summary, the versatility of MRI, its dependence on multiple contrast mechanisms, each with physiologic and pathophysiologic interpretations, and its noninvasive character lie at the heart of its increasing application in musculoskeletal radiology. Elevation of its status from a merely anatomic technique to a technique with physiologically-based diagnostic, grading, and prognostic capabilities will serve to increase further its utility and application. The remainder of this chapter deals with 2 specific examples of newer applications in musculoskeletal imaging.

Dedicated-Extremity MRI

Up to the present day, clinical MRI has been dominated by a single configuration of imaging hardware: the whole-body scanner. In order to obtain an image of a knee or wrist with such a system, the entire body has to be placed within the bore of the magnet. This circumstance has a number of important implications. First of all, some patients experience feelings of claustrophobia. Although only 5% to 10% of patients cannot complete the examination because of claustrophobia, a larger percentage of patients find the whole-body scanner experience unpleasant, and sometimes require sedation to cope. For children who require heavy sedation or anesthesia, supervision by an anesthesiologist may be necessary.

Exposing the entire body to the magnetic field within the bore of even relatively low-field strength magnets poses a potential health risk to patients with pacemakers, vascular clips, cochlear implants, or various other metallic implants. Relatively high stray fields associated with most MRI magnets extend this risk to include metallic objects such as oxygen tanks, wheelchairs, or intravenous poles inadvertently brought into the examination room.

Moreover, the purchase price, maintenance costs, and space requirements of these systems are high, and siting often necessitates expensive renovations, such as structural reinforcement, air conditioning, special power sources, and variable degrees of shielding. High cost has been a principal impediment to the use of MRI in a number of important clinical applications, such as the evaluation of acute extremity trauma and osteomyelitis, and as a screening tool for diseases such as osteoarthritis during which morphologic changes may develop long before clinical symptoms emerge.

Until very recently, the only alternative to this classic circumferential whole-body design has been the so-called "open" configuration, which uses low-field permanent magnets to eliminate the need for complete enclosure of the patient. However, although these open systems are somewhat less claustrophobic and less expensive than high-field superconducting magnets, they remain relatively expensive, and still engender many of the original drawbacks of circumferential, whole-body imagers with respect to patient discomfort and health risk. The recent development of new metal alloys that allow permanent magnets to be constructed in a smaller size than before has spawned a new type of MRI system: the dedicated extremity scanner.

E-MRI represents a radical departure from the conventional whole-body design. With this technology, only the extremity of interest is placed within the magnet bore while the rest of the body remains outside (Fig. 3). This unique design offers a number of practical and economic advantages, including lower cost, facilitated siting, improved patient comfort, and reduced patient risk. The following discussion examines some of these features and looks at how this technology is affecting musculoskeletal imaging in today's environment of cost containment and health care reform.

Increased Patient Comfort and Safety

With E-MRI, only the patient's limb is inserted into the small scanner bore; the rest of the body remains outside of the scanner. This technique obviates feelings of claustrophobia, eliminates the need for sedation, and affords greater comfort to the patient. Additionally, patients can have direct contact with the technician seated in the same room with them during the examination. Because the torques and eddy currents generated by low-field E-MRI are lower than those of conventional MRI, E-MRI is theoretically safer.

Limitations of E-MRI

One potential limitation of E-MRI is that only the distal two thirds of an extremity can be evaluated. This excludes the shoulder and hip, which presently account for a significant proportion of the musculoskeletal volume. Future magnet designs, however, may accommodate these joints as well.

There are also restrictions in the maximum field of view available. For example, the Artoscan™ (Esaote, Genoa, Italy/Lunar, Madison, WI) provides 11 cm of effective field of view and is capable of evaluating most intra-articular abnormalities or highly focal trauma. However, extensive injuries may require multiple scans with repositioning to adequately cover the anatomy. In a series of 2,437 consecutive examinations, however, Passariello reported that only 2% could not be successfully completed.

Technical Performance/Image Quality

In any discussion of diagnostic utility it is important to acknowledge the fundamental difference between intermediate measures of "image quality" and more clinically meaningful measures of "diagnostic power." Difficulty in coming to grips with this distinction has been a major stumbling block in the long-standing and sometimes acrimonious debate over which field strength is optimal for MRI. Arguments in support of high-field strength MRI often focus on technical parameters that scale with field strength (for example, signal-to-noise ratio) or on subjective qualities tied to image aesthetics. Of the small handful of studies that have formally compared the diagnostic power of high-field MRI with that of low-field MRI, most have failed to find any significant difference.

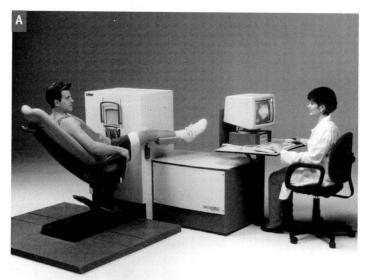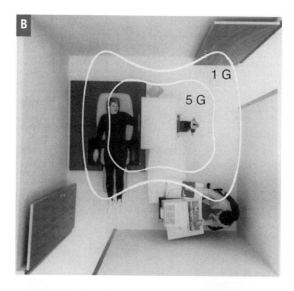

Figure 3

Dedicated-extremity MRI (E-MRI). **A,** Example of a circumferential small-bore 0.2T E-MRI system. **B,** The fringe magnetic field of the Artoscan™. E-MRI scanner is 4 ft from the center of the bore of the magnet. This makes E-MRI imaging safer to operate and easier to site. (Reproduced with permission from Artoscan™, Esaote, Genoa, Italy, distributed in the United States by Lunar Corp, Madison, WI.)

Despite the fact that E-MRI has been available for several years, very little formal assessment of the diagnostic power of this modality has reached the literature. The preliminary evidence, however, is encouraging and the diagnostic power of E-MRI appears to have parity with conventional MRI. Several studies in the knee, for example, have demonstrated high sensitivity and specificity of E-MRI for both meniscal tear and cruciate ligament tear (Fig. 4).

New Clinical Applications

Even more intriguing than lowering the cost of imaging conditions for which the indications are already well established is the prospect that E-MRI may allow this modality to be extended to conditions that for practical or economic reasons have not benefited greatly from MRI thus far. Fractures of the extremities, for example, particularly those involving the scaphoid, talus, or the tibial plateau, are often occult on initial radiographs despite additional special views (Fig. 5). In order to avoid the sometimes serious consequences of missing these fractures (such as nonunion, malunion, and osteonecrosis), clinically suspected cases are often unnecessarily immobilized and subjected to serial reevaluations. This results in increased costs and greater patient morbidity. Moreover, with the growing popularity of rollerblading, skateboarding, and snowboarding, the incidence of these injuries is on the rise.

MRI is currently the most sensitive technique for detecting nondisplaced fractures, but in many cases, cost is prohibitive. Low cost and high diagnostic accuracy make E-MRI well suited to service this large population. Because of its small size and easy siting, an E-MRI system could easily be placed in or very close to a busy emergency room or in a physician's office. Not only could E-MRI identify fractures that would otherwise have been missed with conventional radiography, it could rule out fractures in the much larger percentage of patients who had clinically suspected fractures, eliminating unnecessary immobilization and follow-up examinations.

In a recent study of 45 consecutive patients with upper extremity trauma and negative initial radiographs, E-MRI identified 25 fractures in 20 patients (44%), including 4 scaphoid fractures that subsequently became evident on follow-up radiography. Twenty-three of the 45 cases (51%) showed no evidence of fracture. E-MRI showed a diagnostic accuracy for fracture of 100%. As expected, fractures were most conspicuous on STIR images. However, T1-weighted 3-D gradient echo, which could be acquired in as little as 4 minutes, was equally accurate (100%). In each case, a fracture line could be delineated.

Heller and associates recently completed a cost effectiveness study of MRI in suspected scaphoid fracture using decision-tree analysis and 3-way sensitivity testing. Based on probabilities derived from a 10-year meta-analysis of the literature on scaphoid fracture, and cost values derived from 1995 USA Medicare reimbursement rates, MRI was found to be more cost effective than immobilization with follow-up clinical examination and radiography, as long as the cost of MRI was kept below $240. Parity with serial radiography and clinical examination was reached if the prevalence of scaphoid fracture rose above 46% (the true probability based on the meta-analysis was only 20%), the sensitivity of radiography rose above 86% (the true probability was only 40%), or the cost of clinical evaluation and immobilization dropped below $86 (the Medicare reimbursement was $144). Conversely, as the prevalence of scaphoid fracture decreased and that of associated injuries increased, the threshold value for MRI increased. If intangible benefits to the patient are factored in, such as alleviation of anxiety associated with uncertainty about the diagnosis of a condition with potentially serious low-stream implications, and freedom from unnecessary immobilization and repeat visits to the physician and imaging center, the actual value of MRI increases further. Similar methods could be used to help establish guidelines for managing other types of injuries, such as suspected tibial plateau fracture or fracture of the ankle.

A particularly frustrating situation in imaging trauma is the patient with persistent or recurrent pain following internal fixation with metallic orthopaedic hardware. Because of the likelihood of excessive image degradation by metallic artifacts on either CT or MRI, such patients are often denied any cross sectional imaging whatsoever (Fig. 6). Evaluation of postoperative complaints in these patients must thus rely on clinical evaluation or conventional radiography. The severity of metallic artifacts, however, depends on a number of technical factors, and can be reduced significantly when appropriate measures are taken.

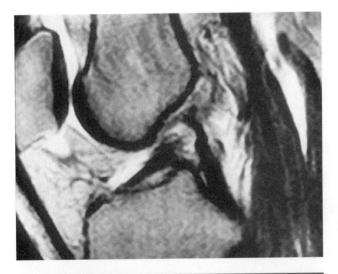

Figure 4

Sagittal T2-weighted dedicated-extremity MRI of the knee shows discontinuity of the cruciate ligament, diagnostic of a complete tear. (Reproduced with permission from Peterfy CG, Roberts T, Genant HK: Dedicated extremity MRI: An emerging technology. *Radiol Clin North Am* 1997;35:1–20.)

Image artifacts created by nonferromagnetic implants include spatial distortions because of misregistration in the frequency encoding direction, and loss of signal intensity caused by intravoxel dephasing. Loss of phase coherence within the voxel is a time-dependent phenomenon, and therefore worsens as TE is prolonged, an effect sometimes referred to as blooming. This mechanism of dephasing is corrected by the 180° rephasing pulse used in spin echo techniques. Metallic artifacts are, thus, most severe on gradient-echo images, which combine both mechanisms of image distortion, and minimal on FSE images.

Metallic artifacts also scale directly with the main magnetic field strength and inversely with the gradient field strength. Artifacts are, therefore, less severe on low-field images acquired with strong gradients. Metallic artifacts are further reduced when the long axis of the hardware is aligned with the static magnetic field (B_0), and the direction of phase encoding. Knowledge of the relationship between the anatomy in question and the relative orientation of the metal hardware, B_0, and phase encoding is therefore useful for planning an imaging protocol for a patient with orthopaedic hardware. As stated above, the orientation of B_0 in E-MRI is horizontal to the long axis of the magnet bore. Consequently, screws in a buttress plate on the lateral tibial plateau of the knee, for example, cause minimal artifacts when the limb is rotated to align the screws with B_0, whereas the buttress plate itself, which is perpendicular to

B_0, produces larger artifacts. In a superconducting high-field magnet, B_0 is aligned with the long axis of the bore; therefore, the reverse is true: the buttress plate is always aligned with B_0 and the screws are always perpendicular to B_0. The screws thus cause the largest artifacts in such a magnet and are relatively indifferent to limb rotation. In a typical open whole-body permanent magnet, B_0 is vertically oriented so that the screws cause minimal artifact with the patient lying on the side and the leg rotated approximately 90°. These considerations should be kept in mind when imaging a patient with hardware.

Other conditions that may benefit from E-MRI are osteomyelitis and arthritis. Applications in arthritis are particularly intriguing, as this is an area undergoing explosive clinical development.

Applications of MRI in Arthritis

Cartilage thickness can be indirectly inferred from the width of the joint space on radiographs, but these measurements have repeatedly been shown to be inaccurate and imprecise. Joint space width is only valid as a measure where cartilage surfaces are in direct contact. In the knee this requires axial loading, which is easily accomplished by having the patient stand during filming. However, because

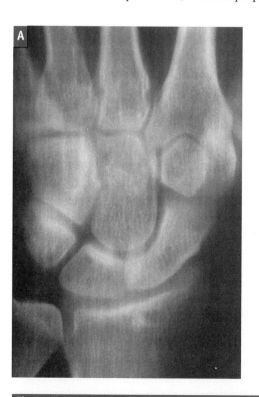

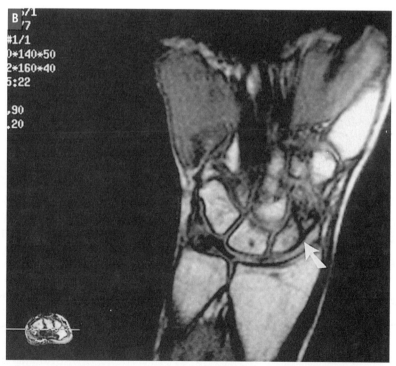

Figure 5

Dedicated-extremity MRI of scaphoid fracture. **A,** Coronal tomography of the scaphoid of a patient who fell off her bicycle shows no evidence of fracture. **B,** Coronal T1-weighted 3-dimensional gradient echo image of the same wrist shows a fracture line (*arrow*) traversing the waist of the scaphoid. (Reproduced with permission from Peterfy CG, Roberts T, Genant HK: Dedicated extremity MRI: An emerging technology. *Radiol Clin North Am* 1997;35:1–20.)

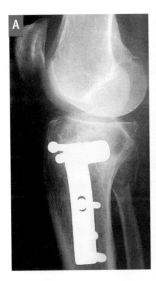
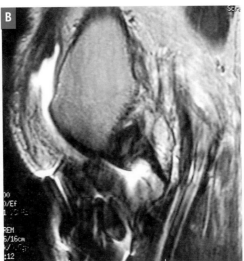
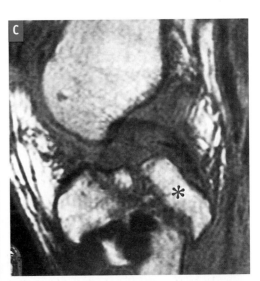

Figure 6

Reduced metallic artifacts with low-field dedicated-extremity MRI. **A,** Lateral radiograph of the knee shows metallic fixation hardware for remote tibial plateau fracture but no other specific abnormalities to explain persistent pain in this patient several months postsurgery. **B,** Sagittal fast spin-echo image of the same knee acquired at 1.5T (Signa, General Electric) is too distorted by metallic artifacts to delineate articular anatomy. **C,** Sagittal 3-dimensional gradient echo image acquired at 0.2T (Artoscan, Esaote, Genoa, Italy) shows markedly less metallic artifacts from the fixation hardware and reveals a large nonunited fracture fragment (*asterisk*) of the tibial plateau at the insertion of the posterior cruciate ligament. (Reproduced with permission from Peterfy CG, Roberts T, Genant HK: Dedicated extremity MRI: An emerging technology. *Radiol Clin North Am* 1997;35:1–20.)

only a small area of the normally incongruent surfaces of the femur and tibia articulate in any single position, reproducibility of the radiographic joint space width is very sensitive to variations in the flexion among serial images.

MRI, on the other hand, is ideally suited for evaluating arthritic joints. It provides multiplanar and 3-D image data without superimposition and offers unparalleled soft-tissue contrast that allows direct visualization of all components of the joint simultaneously. This capacity for whole-organ evaluation of the joint is entirely unprecedented in medical imaging and cogent to current models of arthritis as a disease of organ failure, akin to heart failure, in which damage to a single component leads to injury of other components and ultimately pain and joint dysfunction. Moreover, because MRI is nondestructive, several parameters can be evaluated in the same specimen and frequent serial examinations can be performed in even asymptomatic joints. With more than 4,000 units in the United States and over 9,000 units worldwide, the availability of MRI is sufficient to support large multicenter, multinational clinical studies. Finally, the cost of MRI continues to decrease, not just because of market forces, but also because of technical advances such as E-MRI. All of these factors are facilitating the growth of this application of MRI.

Imaging Articular Cartilage With MRI

MRI is unique in its ability to allow direct visualization of the articular cartilage. It is the high water content of articular cartilage that forms the basis for MRI signal in this tissue. This base signal, however, is modulated through a vari-

ety of mechanisms by interactions between the tissue water and the collagen and proteoglycan matrix in cartilage. These mechanisms include T1 relaxation, T2 relaxation, magnetization transfer, water diffusion, and magnetic susceptibility. The multiplicity of tissue characteristics that affect image contrast on MRI is the key to this modality's unparalleled capacity for soft-tissue discrimination. The extent to which each of these mechanisms contributes to the overall image contrast depends on exactly how the MRI parameters are assigned.

T2 relaxation results in a loss of signal as hydrogen nuclei in water fall out of phase with each other in the presence of collagen. Accordingly, T2-weighted images depict articular cartilage as a low signal intensity tissue, whereas synovial fluid, which lacks collagen or other constituents that promote T2 relaxation, is depicted with high signal intensity. Cartilage-fluid interfaces are thus well delineated with this pulse sequence (Fig. 7). T2-weighted images are also useful for identifying areas of chondromalacia, as the loss of collagen reduces the degree of T2 relaxation and thus signal loss in cartilage. Accordingly, areas of increased signal intensity in cartilage on T2-weighted images are indicative of matrix damage (Fig. 8). In addition to subjective assessments of signal intensity, T2 relaxation in cartilage can be quantified and mapped onto images; however, this information is currently used only in clinical research.

Another marker of matrix damage in articular cartilage is imbibition of anionic contrast media into regions of proteoglycan loss. Gadolinium-diethylenetriamine penta-acetic acid ($Gd-DTPA^{-2}$) enhances the T1 relaxation of nearby water molecules and thus raises their signal inten-

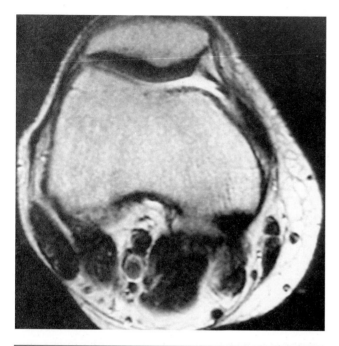

Figure 7

Harnessing T2 contrast to delineate normal articular cartilage. Axial T2 weighted fast spin-echo image of the patella depicts the cartilage as a homogeneously low-signal intensity structure sharply contrasted against adjacent high-signal intensity joint fluid.

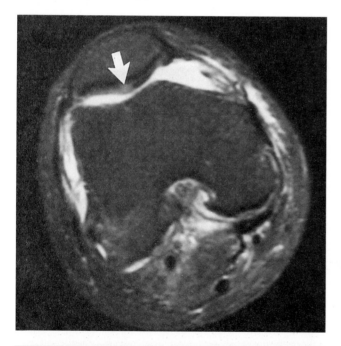

Figure 8

Magnetic resonance imaging appearance of chondromalacia. Axial T2-weighted fast spin-echo image with fat suppression shows elevated signal intensity (*arrow*) in the cartilage over the ridge of the patella indicative of collagen matrix damage.

sity on T1-weighted images. Under normal circumstances, the fixed negative charge of proteoglycan molecules in cartilage repel anionic Gd-DTPA^{-2}, so that only the synovial fluid is affected by the compound. This delineates the fluid-cartilage interface on T1-weighted images and is the basis for magnetic resonance arthrography. However, as proteoglycans are lost and the fixed negative charge in cartilage decreases, Gd-DTPA^{-2} is allowed to penetrate this tissue and raise the signal intensity on T1-weighted images. Although this technique shows considerable promise for identifying and monitoring early degenerative changes in cartilage, the optimal conditions for its use have yet to be worked out in detail.

In the absence of Gd-DTPA^{-2} intrinsic differences in T1 relaxation between articular cartilage and fat are sufficiently high to delineate cartilage-bone and cartilage-adipose interfaces on conventional T1-weighted images. However, T1 differences between cartilage and joint fluid are considerably smaller, and so these interfaces are poorly delineated. T1 contrast between cartilage and adjacent joint fluid can be augmented by suppressing the signal from fat. Combining this technique with thin-section 3-D gradient echo produces extremely high contrast and high resolution images of the articular cartilage (Fig. 9). In a recent study of 41 knees by Recht and associates, this technique demonstrated a sensitivity of 81% and specificity of 97% for identifying cartilage surface defects visible on arthroscopy. Other studies have reported similar results. The

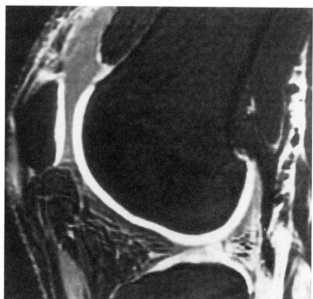

Figure 9

Harnessing T1 contrast to delineate articular cartilage. Sagittal fat-suppressed T1-weighted gradient echo image of the knee depicts articular cartilage as an isolated high signal intensity band in sharp contrast to adjacent low-signal intensity joint fluid and suppressed marrow and adipose fat. (Reproduced with permission from Peterfy CG, Majumder S, Long P, van Dijke CF, Sach K, Genant HK: MR imaging of the arthritic knee: Improved discrimination of cartilage, synovium, and effusion with pulsed saturation transfer and fat-suppressed T1-weighted sequences. *Radiology* 1994;191: 413–419.)

technique is easy to use and available on most high-field (1.5T) clinical MRI systems around the world. For these reasons, fat-suppressed 3-D MRI is usually the technique of choice for morphometric analyses of articular cartilage.

Another relaxation mechanism that can be harnessed to increase contrast between cartilage and adjacent articular structures is magnetization transfer. This approach is most useful when combined with high-resolution T2*-weighted 3-D gradient-echo images, which otherwise offer poor cartilage contrast (Fig. 10), or when operating at low magnetic field strengths (for example, most E-MRI scanners) that cannot support spectral fat suppression. Magnetization transfer, however, offers only limited contrast between hyperplastic synovial tissue and cartilage in rheumatoid arthritis. Whether this is also true at low-field strength is not yet known, but it is at least 1 reason why fat-suppressed T1-weighted imaging is preferred over magnetization transfer when high-field strength MRI is used.

Regardless of whether T1-weighted fat-suppressed imaging or magnetization transfer subtraction is used, the 3-D image data can be used to perform a variety of sophisticated morphometric analyses. For example, by summing the voxels (pixel area × slice thickness) comprising a segmented image of the cartilage, the exact volume of this complex structure can be quantified with accuracy and reproducibility errors of less than 5% (Fig. 11). Moreover, it is possible to construct thickness maps of individual cartilage plates using techniques adapted from stereophotogrammetry (Fig. 12). Similar techniques can also be used to analyze contact patterns between articulating cartilage plates in studies of patellofemoral tracking.

Bone Changes in Osteoarthritis

Because of its relative lack of hydrogen nuclei, bone tissue does not generate any signal on conventional MRI. Cortical and trabecular bone is, therefore, depicted as curvilinear signal voids silhouetted on either side by signal-producing tissues, such as marrow and adipose. MRI thus has an inherent contrast for bone. Despite this, the contours of

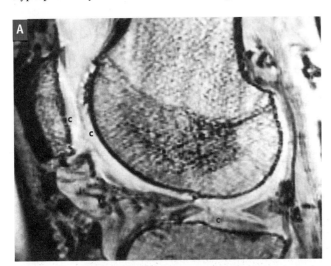

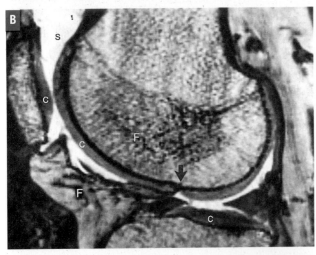

Figure 10

Harnessing magnetization transfer for imaging articular cartilage. **A,** Conventional T2*-weighted, thin-partitioned sagittal 3-dimensional gradient-echo image shows poor contrast between cartilage (c) and joint fluid. **B,** Addition of pulsed magnetization transfer to the same imaging sequence markedly decreased signal intensity in cartilage (C) but had significantly less effect on effusion (S), bone, or adipose tissue (F). This combined high cartilage fluid contrast with sufficient spatial resolution to allow delineation of small surface defects in the cartilage (long arrow).

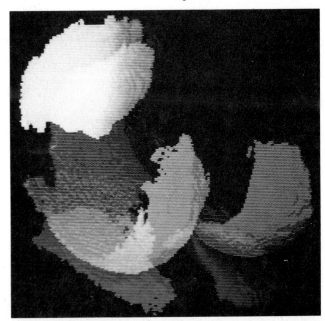

Figure 11

Composite 3-dimensional rendering of individual cartilage plates segmented from magnetization transfer subtraction images of the knee of a patient with osteoarthritis. Patellar, tibial, and femoral cartilages are viewed from a posteromedial vantage point.

Anterior

Lateral

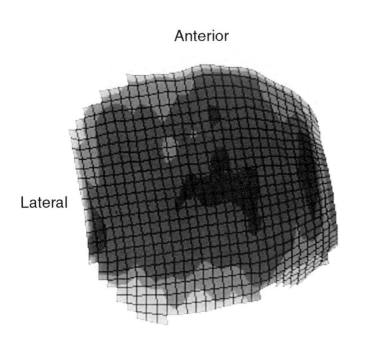

Thickness

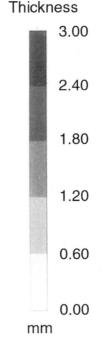

3.00

2.40

1.80

1.20

0.60

0.00

mm

Figure 12

Mapping articular cartilage thickness with magnetic resonance imaging. B-spline geometric model of the patellar cartilage was generated from a fat-suppressed T1-weighted 3-dimensional gradient echo image data set. Regional cartilage thickness (perpendicular to the cartilage-bone interface) is depicted in intervals of 1 mm. (Reproduced with permission from Ateshian GA, Cohen A, Kwak SD, et al: *Determination of In Situ Contact Areas in Diarthroidial Joints By MR Imaging*. (San Franscisco, CA, American Society of Mechanical Engineers, 1995.)

individual cortices and trabeculi are generally less sharp on conventional MRI scans than on routine clinical radiographs. This is because clinical MRI typically has lower spatial resolution than does clinical radiography (at least, along the 2 dimensions of the radiographic film). This potential advantage of radiography, however, must be balanced against its problem with projectional superimposition, which can transform a complex 3-D network of trabeculi in the cancellous bone into a haystack of overlapping linear shadows. The relative weakness of MRI in 2-point discrimination is, thus, offset by the advantages of its tomographic viewing perspective, as mentioned previously. MRI is thus well suited for examining the marginal osteophytes (Fig. 13) in osteoarthritis, and especially helpful in delineating central osteophytes (Fig. 14) that can be extremely difficult to see with conventional radiographs, and that may have a different pathogenesis.

The most intriguing capability of MRI when dealing with the bones, however, is the capacity of this modality for detecting abnormalities involving the marrow space. Conditions arising in this compartment generally remain occult on radiographs until the cortical and trabecular bones themselves are affected. MRI, on the other hand, can directly visualize any excess water in the marrow space, and thus identify hemorrhage and edema from even mild bone trauma, exudate from early osteomyelitis, and cellular material from infiltrating neoplasms.

Areas of "marrow edema" are often seen in joints with osteoarthritis (Fig. 15). Usually, these areas develop beneath defects in the articular surface, presumably from pulsion of synovial fluid through the defect, or from microtrauma associated with biomechanical incompetence of the load-bearing surface. Occasionally, however, marrow edema is seen some distance from the articular surface as well. There is speculation that the development of marrow edema in osteoarthritis is associated with local pain. This hypothesis, however, has never been carefully tested. Whether areas of marrow edema correlate directly with increased uptake of technetium-labeled radiotracer in bone scintigraphy, and/or accelerated disease progression,

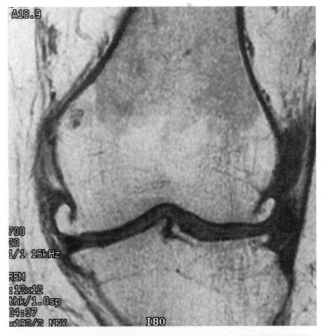

Figure 13

Marginal osteophytes are delineated with magnetic resonance imaging (MRI). Coronal T1-weighted MRI scan of the knee of a patient with osteoarthritis provides regional delineation of marginal osteophytes of the femorotibial joint.

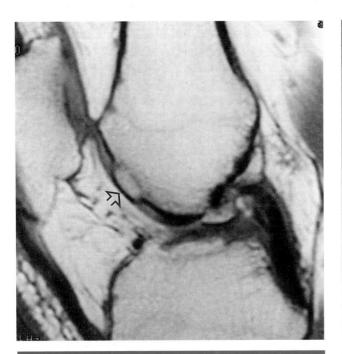

Figure 14

Delineating central osteophytes with magnetic resonance imaging. Sagittal T1-weighted MRI scan of the knee shows a central projection of articular bone (*arrow*) through a focal defect in the articular cartilage of the trochlear groove in a 33-year-old patient with anterior knee pain and remote football injury to the patellofemoral joint. Posttraumatic basal delamination of articular cartilage at this site, with subsequent cartilage breakdown and focal proliferation of subchondral bone, is a potential mechanism of such lesions.

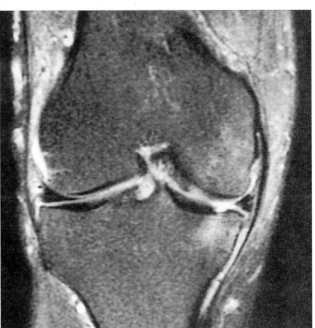

Figure 15

Bone marrow edema is depicted with magnetic resonance imaging. Coronal fat-suppressed T2-weighted MRI scan of the knee of a patient with osteoarthritis shows an area of marrow edema beneath a focal defect in the articular cartilage over the medial tibial plateau. A more diffuse area of marrow edema is also present in the medial femoral condyle. (Reproduced with permission from Peterfy CG, Majumder S, Long P, van Dijke CF, Sach K, Genant HK: MR imaging of the arthritic knee: Improved discrimination of cartilage, synovium, and effusion with pulsed saturation transfer and fat-suppressed T1-weighted sequences. *Radiology* 1994;191: 413–419.)

or inversely with the response to treatment, has yet to be determined. Nevertheless, this is a feature of osteoarthritis that only MRI can elucidate.

Conclusion

Exciting changes are occurring in the area of musculoskeletal MRI. Fueled by the need for cost containment and the demands of a rapidly aging population, new technologies have emerged that greatly extend the capabilities of this diagnostic imaging tool. E-MRI, although still in its early stages, offers a convenient and cost-effective alternative to conventional MRI for imaging already established clinical indications, while also expanding the envelope of MRI to include disorders that thus far have not benefited greatly from this modality. The increasing prevalence of arthritis in our society and the prospect of more effective therapies on the horizon that are directed at altering the disease process itself rather than simply palliating its symptoms, have increased the importance of imaging all components of the joint, particularly the articular cartilage, and have promoted the rapid development of MRI for this clinical application.

Selected Bibliography

Ateshian GA, Kwak SD, Soslowsky LJ, Mow VC: A stereophotogrammetric method for determining in situ contact areas in diarthrodial joints, and a comparison with other methods. *J Biomech* 1994;27: 111–124.

Barile A, Masciocchi C, Mastantuono M, Passariello R, Satragno L: The use of a "dedicated" MRI system in the evaluation of knee joint diseases. *Clin MRI* 1995;5:79–82.

Barnett MJ: MR diagnosis of internal derangements of the knee: Effect of field strength on efficacy. *Am J Roentgenol* 1993;161: 115–118.

Bell RA: Economics of MRI technology. *J Magn Reson Imaging* 1996;6:10–25.

Chan WP, Lang P, Stevens MP, et al: Osteoarthritis of the knee: comparison of radiography, CT, and MR imaging to assess extent and severity. *Am J Roentgenol* 1991;157:799–806.

Cohen ZA, McCarthy DM, Ateshian GA, et al: In vivo and in vitro knee joint cartilage topography, thickness, and contact areas from MRI. *Trans Orthop Res Soc* 1997;22:625.

Disler DG, McCauley TR, Wirth CR, Fuchs MD: Detection of knee hyaline cartilage defects using fat-suppressed three-dimensional spoiled gradient-echo MR imaging: Comparison with standard MR imaging and correlation with arthroscopy. *Am J Roentgenol* 1995;165:377–382.

Eckstein F, Gavazzeni A, Sittek H, et al: Determination of knee joint cartilage thickness using three-dimensional magnetic resonance chondro-crassometry (3D MR-CCM). *Magn Reson Med* 1996;36: 256–265.

Fife R, Brandt K, Braunstein E, et al: Relationship between cartilage damage and radiographic joint space narrowing (JSN) in early osteoarthritis (OA) of the knee. *Arthritis Rheum* 1990;33:S117.

Franklin PD, Lemon RA, Barden HS: Accuracy of imaging the menisci on an in-office, dedicated, magnetic resonance imaging extremity system. *Am J Sports Med* 1997;25:382–388.

Heller D, Peterfy C, Genant HK: Conceptual framework for cost-effectiveness of imaging tests. *Acad Radiol* 1998;5 (Suppl 2):340–343.

Jack CR Jr, Berquist TH, Miller GM, et al: Field strength in neuro-MR imaging: A comparison of 0.5 T and 1.5 T. *J Comput Assist Tomogr* 1990;14:505–513.

Kim DK, Ceckler TL, Hascall VC, Calabro A, Balaban RS: Analysis of water-macromolecule proton magnetization transfer in articular cartilage. *Magn Reson Med* 1993;29:211–215.

Masciocchi C, Barile A, Navarra F, et al: Clinical experience of osteoarticular MRI using a dedicated system. *MAGMA* 1994;2:545.

Orrison WW Jr, Stimac GK, Stevens EA, et al: Comparison of CT, low-field-strength MR imaging, and high-field-strength MR imaging: Work in progress. *Radiology* 1991;181:121–127.

Passiarello R, Masciocchi C, Barile A, Mastantuono M, De Bac S, Satragno L: Niche MR unit shows promise in extremities. *Diagn Imaging Eur* 1995, pp. 17–20.

Peterfy CG, Majumdar S, Lang P, van Dijke CF, Sack K, Genant HK: MR imaging of the arthritic knee: Improved discrimination of cartilage, synovium, and effusion with pulsed saturation transfer and fat-suppressed T1-weighted sequences. *Radiology* 1994;191:413–419.

Peterfy CG, Roberts T, Genant HK: Dedicated extremity MR imaging: An emerging technology. *Radiol Clin North Am* 1997;35:1–20.

Peterfy CG, van Dijke CF, Janzen DL, et al: Quantification of articular cartilage in the knee with pulsed saturation transfer subtraction and fat-suppressed MR imaging: Optimization and validation. *Radiology* 1994;192:485–491.

Recht MP, Kramer J, Marcelis S, et al: Abnormalities of articular cartilage in the knee: Analysis of available MR techniques. *Radiology* 1993;187:473–478.

Recht MP, Piraino DW, Paletta GA, Schils JP, Belhobek GH: Accuracy of fat-suppressed three-dimensional spoiled gradient-echo FLASH MR imaging in the detection of patellofemoral articular cartilage abnormalities. *Radiology* 1996;198:209–212.

Rutt BK, Lee DH: The impact of field strength on image quality in MRI. *J Magn Reson Imaging* 1996;6:57–62.

Steinberg HV, Alarcon JJ, Bernardino ME: Focal hepatic lesions: Comparative MR imaging at 0.5 and 1.5 T. *Radiology* 1990;174: 153–156.

Wolff SD, Chesnick S, Frank JA, Lim KO, Balaban RS: Magnetization transfer contrast: MR imaging of the knee. *Radiology* 1991;179: 623–628.

Chapter 10

Bone Densitometry

Harry K. Genant, MD

Cornelis van Kuijk, MD, PhD

This chapter at a glance

This chapter presents an overview of bone densitometry techniques such as conventional radiography, radiogrammetry, quantitative computed tomography, and single and dual x-ray absorptiometry and discusses the advantages and disadvantages of these techniques.

Introduction

Bone densitometry is a general term encompassing all techniques used to quantify the amount of bone in the skeleton. Many techniques are currently available for clinical and/or experimental use, ranging from simple to complex in nature and from relatively inexpensive to very expensive. All technical modalities as applied routinely in radiology are represented, from conventional radiology to computed tomography (CT), ultrasound, and magnetic resonance imaging.

Bone densitometry is used primarily to assess bone status in primary and secondary osteoporosis as well as to monitor treatment of these diseases. Bone densitometry provides a fracture risk assessment and is used to evaluate preventive interventions for bone loss due to aging and other metabolic diseases besides osteoporosis. The measurement of periprosthetic bone loss is a new application of bone densitometry.

Overview of Bone Densitometry Techniques

This chapter will discuss the different techniques available for bone densitometry, and outline some of the technical differences between the techniques. Several features of these techniques are described in Table 1. In general, distinction can be made among ultrasound technology, magnetic resonance technology, and techniques that use an x-ray or radionuclide source. Equipment using an isotope source is now virtually obsolete, having gradually been replaced by similar equipment using an x-ray source. Furthermore, distinction can be made among techniques that measure bone status in the peripheral skeleton (hand, forearm, lower leg) or in the central skeleton (spine, hip). These skeletal sites differ in both function (weightbearing versus nonweightbearing) and composition (trabecular/cortical bone ratio). Trabecular bone, because of its high surface area, is more active metabolically than cortical bone, and changes in bone status are usually identified earlier in bones with a high trabecular content. Techniques also differ in measured regions of interest such as area projection or true volumetric assessments.

Techniques providing an area (2-dimensional) measurement, such as single or dual energy x-ray absorptiometry (SXA, DXA), are in fact measuring an apparent density that is not a true density. Still the output of these measurements is called bone mineral density (BMD; measured in g/cm^2) of bone mineral content (BMC; measured in grams). Only techniques providing a volumetric (3-dimensional) measurement, such as quantitative computed tomography (QCT), have a true density output in g/cm^3. Area measurements are therefore influenced by changes in bone dimensions such as those occurring during normal bone maturation and growth.

Conventional Radiography

Cortical thinning and increased intracortical porosity in tubular bones are well-known radiologic features of diminished bone mass, or osteopenia. Visibly apparent loss of specific trabecular structures in the femoral neck and vertebral bodies is another well-recognized feature. However, it has been estimated that at least 30% of the skeletal calcium is lost before even the experienced eye can detect osteopenia on conventional radiographs. Several grading methods have been developed to assess and evaluate visibly apparent features of osteopenia. One example is the well-known Singh index, by which the appearance of the

Table 1
Overview of Different Techniques*

Technique	Anatomic Site of Interest (%)	Precision In Vivo	Accuracy Error (%)	Estimated Effective Dose Equivalent (μSv)
Radiogrammetry	Metacarpals, radius, femur	1 to 3	—	<1
Radiographic absorptiometry	Phalanges, metacarpals	1 to 3	5	<1
Single x-ray absorptiometry	Radius, calcaneus	1 to 2	4 to 6	<1
Dual x-ray absorptiometry	Spine, femur, radius, total body	1 to 3	3 to 10	1 to 20
Quantitative computed tomography	Spine, femur	2 to 4	5 to 15 (single-energy)	50 to 100
Peripheral quantitative computed tomography	Radius, tibia	1 to 2	2 to 8	1 to 2
Quantitative ultrasound	Calcaneus, tibia, patella, phalanges	1 to 4	?	NA
Quantitative magnetic resonance imaging	Calcaneus, spine	4 to 10	?	NA

* Precision refers to reproducibility of the measurement technique in vivo and is given as coefficient of variation (%). Dose refers to the effective dose equivalent given in μSv (micro-Sievert). For comparison, the annual natural dose is approximately 3,000 μSv. NA, not applicable.

trabecular structure in the femoral neck is graded. Although this and other "visual" methods certainly can provide some information, there is a substantial interobserver variability and their use in daily clinical practice is questionable. Consequently, more objective and precise techniques for quantifying the amount of bone have been developed.

Radiogrammetry

In radiogrammetry, predefined dimensions at one or different skeletal sites are measured. Several dimensions can be measured, such as total bone width, cortical thickness, ratio of cortical width to total bone width, and cortical area. These measurements are usually performed on radiographs of tubular bones such as the metacarpals and the radius. The bone dimensions usually are measured with rulers and calipers. Recently, however, computer-aided techniques have been developed in which image processing and analysis tools are used to perform these measurements in a semiautomated fashion. Radiogrammetry provides bone dimensions only and does not provide real density or related measurements. As such, it is considered a crude method with limited use in clinical practice.

A recent addition to this field is the measurement of the hip-axis length on standard radiographs of the hip as well as on images acquired by bone densitometers. The hip-axis length seems to be a prognostic factor for future hip fractures, independent of bone density at the hip.

Radiographic Absorptiometry

In radiographic absorptiometry a standardized radiograph of the hand is made along with an aluminum reference wedge. In general, the radiographic density of the metacarpals or phalanges is determined and compared with that of the wedge using a densitometric technique after digitizing the radiograph. The results are given in aluminum equivalent values. No distinction is made between the cortical and trabecular compartments of bone. Currently, several methods, all based on the same principle, are in use, and some of them are commercialized in several countries. One of them, the Osteogram (CompuMed; Manhattan, CA), collects phalangeal measurements (Fig. 1). Other systems include the Osteoradiometer (NIM; Verona, Italy), which provides metacarpal bone and radius measurements; the Bonalyzer (Teijin; Tokyo, Japan), for radius measurements and one (Chugai; Tokyo, Japan) for metacarpal measurements.

Single X-Ray Absorptiometry

In single x-ray absorptiometry (SXA) a highly collimated photon beam from an x-ray source is used to measure the photon attenuation of the measurement site (usually the radius or the os calcis), which is converted to BMC in grams

or (projectional) areal BMD in g/cm² using a known standard. SXA measurements are confined to the peripheral skeleton, and the cortical and trabecular compartments of bone cannot be measured separately. Single photon absorptiometry is the older nuclear version of this technique, now virtually obsolete.

SXA is relatively simple to perform, is comfortable for the patient, and, therefore, has gained widespread acceptance. In general, it can be stated that measurements at specific bone sites predict fracture risk at that specific site very well and are moderate to reasonably good predictors at other skeletal sites. SXA measures at peripheral sites. Hip fractures are the most relevant osteoporotic fractures because they cause extensive morbidity and mortality. In addition, the prevalence of vertebral fractures is quite high in osteoporosis. Many physicians, therefore, prefer density measurements at the hip and/or the spine.

Dual X-Ray Absorptiometry

Dual x-ray absorptiometry (DXA) is the modern, upgraded version of dual-energy photon absorptiometry (DPA). The radionuclide source in DPA has been replaced by an x-ray tube in DXA. A dual-energy spectrum is generated by rapid switching of the tube voltage supply or by K-edge filtering.

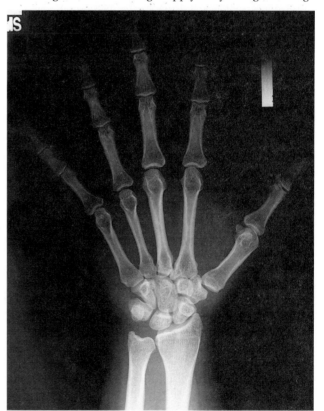

Figure 1

Example of a hand x-ray made for radiographic absorptiometry with the aluminum wedge in place. (Reproduced with permission from the Osteoporosis and Arthritis Research Group.)

DXA is used for bone mass measurements in the central skeleton (femur, spine) and can be used for fat content assessment (total body composition assessments). As with SXA, bone mass estimates are given as BMC or as BMD. DXA cannot differentiate between cortical and trabecular bone.

Measurements of photon attenuation at 2 different energies are necessary to separate bone and soft-tissue attenuation. Bone mass measurements can then be made at the central skeleton. Examination times are reduced, and the reproducibility of the measurements has improved in DXA as compared with DPA. Different DXA systems are available from different manufacturers. There are pencil-beam systems that use a highly collimated x-ray beam to measure the attenuation on a point-by-point basis. Scanning times are longer than with systems using a fan-beam geometry and multiple detectors. DXA-technology has gained widespread acceptance and distribution. Examples of DXA scans are shown in Figure 2.

DXA measurements of the spine in the anteroposterior projection are influenced by (intervertebral) osteoarthrosis, which falsely increases the measured BMC. This problem is a major disadvantage when elderly patients are evaluated, and lateral DXA scanning of the spine has been developed as a potential solution. The patient is placed in a lateral position, or the x-ray tube and detector unit are rotated in those systems equipped with a C-arm. The spinal measurement is usually less precise in the lateral projection. Another pitfall with spinal DXA measurements is the falsely high density value in fractured vertebrae and the falsely low density value after posterior element resection. Femoral DXA has become very popular because it provides measurements at a site prone to fractures in the osteoporotic population.

Recently, new software has made it possible to evaluate bone mass (g) and areal density (g/cm²) at the forearm and the calcaneus on regular DXA equipment. In addition, dedicated equipment for peripheral DXA has been developed.

Special orthopaedic software that allows the assessment of periprosthetic bone density is primarily used in evaluating bone changes around hip and knee implants.

Quantitative Computed Tomography

QCT is the only method that can estimate bone density separately in the trabecular and cortical bone compartments and can provide a true density (g/cm³) estimate. The vertebral body usually is the site of measurement. A reference standard made of different concentrations of hydroxyapatite in plastic is placed under the lumbar spine of the patient and scanned simultaneously. On a lateral localization view, a slice selection is made at the midvertebral levels of 3 to 4 consecutive vertebral bodies. The average CT value of the trabecular region within the vertebral body is measured in the image and compared with that of the reference standard. An example of a spinal QCT-examination is shown in Figure 3.

Single-energy QCT is the technique most widely used and recommended, although it has been argued in the literature

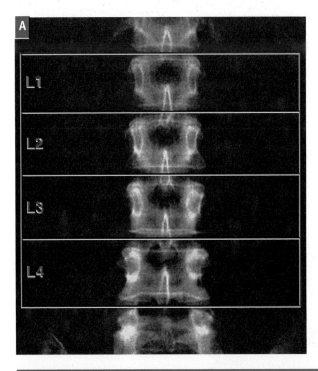
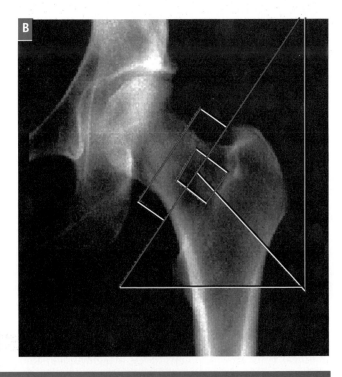

Figure 2

A, Dual-energy x-ray absorptiometry of the spine (anteroposterior projection). **B,** Dual-energy x-ray absorptiometry of the femur. (Reproduced with permission from the Osteoporosis and Arthritis Research Group.)

that the intravertebral fat falsely lowers the measured BMD. However, this is also true for DXA measurements. For both single-energy QCT and DXA, appropriate calibration can partially correct the systematic offsets related to the intravertebral fat.

Dual-energy QCT is used to improve the accuracy of the bone density assessment because it potentially can compensate for the fat error. The reproducibility of measurements with dual-energy QCT is less than with single-energy QCT and the radiation dose is doubled. Single-energy QCT, therefore, remains the generally recommended QCT technique.

Although primarily used for bone mass measurements in the spine, femoral QCT has been reported. Furthermore, newer CT systems capable of spiral (helical) CT scanning allow a volumetric acquisition of imaging data from which a highly accurate 3-dimensional reconstruction of vertebral bodies or femora can be made. This capability as well as the use of advanced image analysis tools allows for sophisticated density measurements in several regions of interest as well as for measurements of geometric dimensions of the object of interest. The clinical applicability of the volumetric QCT technique, however, is still under investigation.

QCT can be done on regular clinical CT systems because most manufacturers provide a QCT option on their systems. In addition, special purpose CT systems have been developed for peripheral QCT (pQCT) of the radius and tibia. The first generation of these pQCT systems used a nuclear source. Newer systems use an x-ray source.

Quantitative Ultrasound

More recently, ultrasound velocity and attenuation measurements have been developed for noninvasive measurement of bone quantity. Measurements are confined to the peripheral skeleton and can be made at the calcaneus, tibia, patella, and phalangeal bones.

Parameters measured are ultrasound transmission velocity and broadband ultrasound attenuation. These parameters generally are postulated to be determined by both bone density and bone architecture, although the latter claim is still somewhat controversial. Most studies show a convincing correlation between ultrasound parameters and bone mass measurements, indicating that with current equipment the ultrasound parameters reflect bone mass only.

A clear advantage of quantitative ultrasound in clinical practice is its absence of radiation exposure. Quantitative ultrasound is popular in Europe and Japan. The Food and Drug Administration (FDA) recently approved 2 different quantitative ultrasound devices for the US market. One measures the speed of sound and broadband attenuation in the calcaneus, a skeletal area rich in trabecular bone. The other measures speed of sound at the cortical surface of the tibia. It is expected that other systems will be approved soon.

These systems are used to identify patients with an increased risk of osteoporotic fracture. Current data are insufficient to recommend these measurements for longitudinal monitoring of disease or therapy.

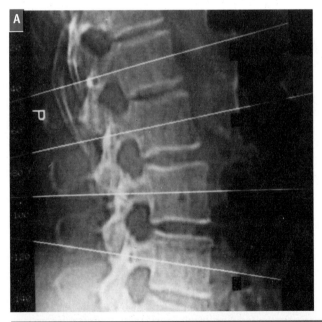

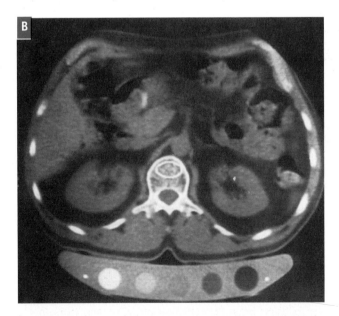

Figure 3

Typical quantitative computed tomography examination of the spine. **A,** Lateral scout view (also called scanogram) of the lumbar spine. This scout view is used to plan midvertebral slices typically through 3 or 4 consecutive vertebral bodies. **B,** Typical axial slice through a vertebral body. Note the calibration material underneath the patient that is used to convert the measurements within the region of interest (usually an ellipse-shaped region within the trabecular part of the vertebral body) from Hounsfield units to bone-equivalent values (usually g/cm³ calcium hydroxyapatite). (Reproduced with permission from the Osteoporosis and Arthritis Research Group.)

Quantitative Magnetic Resonance Imaging

As a research tool, (high-resolution) MRI is used to quantify the amount of bone as well as to study trabecular architecture. In quantitative MRI, the T2* relaxation time is measured. T2* is theoretically related to the density of the trabecular network and its geometry. Furthermore, high-resolution MRI is used to study trabecular architecture. The costs and availability of MRI magnets prohibit the use of this technique in routine clinical practice.

Which Technique to Use?

The choice of technique is generally influenced by scientific proof, clinical validation, cost, and availability. Several researchers have tried to determine the distinct values of these techniques. When these techniques are compared in terms of their discriminative power between normal healthy patients and those with (spinal) osteoporosis or between those patients with mild and severe osteoporosis, QCT has reportedly been the best technique, followed by DXA, SXA, radiographic absorptiometry, and quantitative ultrasound. However, all techniques show considerable overlap between normal patients and those with osteoporosis. Some investigators have objected to this way of validating these techniques and have argued that their real value lies in their ability to predict future fractures. As such, each general class of techniques should be validated in large population-based longitudinal studies, and data are now available from such studies. These studies generally show that the ranking of tests based on prospective data parallels the results of cross-sectional studies. BMC assessment with radiographic absorptiometry, SXA, DXA, QCT, and quantitative ultrasound all seem to have predictive power for future osteoporotic fractures in the spine and hip.

The correlation between the different techniques is modest (typically between r = 0.6 to 0.7), precluding prediction of bone mass at one site by bone mass measurement at another site for the individual patient. The modest correlation is the result of technical differences between the techniques and differences in measurement sites, which have a different composition (ratio cortical/trabecular bone) and differ in metabolic activity. The various techniques are, therefore, complimentary rather than competitive. Priority could be given to measuring sites of biologic relevance (for example, the spine for vertebral osteoporosis, the hip for fracture risk assessment at that site). Precision (or reproducibility) is important when discussing these techniques, as well as the rate of bone change expected in the skeletal part under investigation. If there is an expected change of bone mass of 1% a year, it takes 5.6 years to detect a significant bone change with a technique having a 2% reproducibility. If the expected change is 2%, detection takes 2.8 years with the same technique. However, a technique with 1% reproducibility will detect this 2% change in 1.4 years. Usually changes (both losses and gains) have been found to be higher in the central trabecular compartments with much more bone surface and active red marrow for metabolic activity than in cortical compartments of bone. Therefore, the vertebral bodies in the spine with their large trabecular compartments are often chosen as the sites for serial measurement.

In summary, identifying those at risk for fracture can be done with most densitometry techniques. Monitoring the disease or treatment over time should preferably be done with techniques that can measure sites such as the spine that are rich in trabecular content and are known to respond quickly. Preference should be given to QCT over DXA in the elderly population in whom degenerative disease causes DXA of the spine to be unreliable. Alternatively, the femur can be measured with DXA.

Apart from these valid scientific reasons, in daily clinical practice, the choice of technique will depend on the local availability of equipment and physician expertise. Worldwide DXA is currently the technique used most often for density measurements in clinical practice and in clinical drug trials. The FDA guidelines for drug evaluation, as well as diagnostic guidelines such as provided by the World Health Organization (WHO), are based on DXA-data.

Which Patients Need Bone Densitometry?

There is now a general consensus that bone mass measurements are very useful. In concept it has been suggested that low bone mass in the asymptomatic patient predicts fracture risk, just as high cholesterol or high blood pressure predicts the risk of heart disease or stroke. There are several clinical situations in which an assessment of bone mass and consequently fracture risk affects therapeutic decisions. The best known is probably the use of hormonal replacement therapy in estrogen deficiency (either because of ovariectomy or menopause), because estrogen deficiency is well known to cause bone loss. Other situations are monitoring bone loss caused by corticosteroid use (secondary osteoporosis) and monitoring drug efficacy for treatment or prevention of osteoporosis. As previously mentioned, a new emerging application is the measurement of periprosthetic bone status in hip arthroplasty. In general, bone densitometry is indicated in those patients with suspected low bone mass (and therefore increased fracture risk) to confirm the diagnosis and to quantify its severity. It is also indicated to monitor preventive and therapeutic interventions with an effect on bone mass.

Interpretation of the Bone Densitometry Report

Interpretation of the data provided by bone densitometry techniques is problematic. The results are usually given in BMC, BMD, speed of sound, broadband ultrasound attenuation, etc, with a range of units used. Because bone density decreases in aging, and difference in bone density exists between sexes and races, bone density measurements should be compared with those of age-, sex-, and race-matched healthy controls. Therefore, a normative data base is mandatory for interpreting the level of BMC. Usually, the estimated bone density is given as a Z-score and a T-score. The Z-score is a measure of the patient's results as the deviation from the mean of age-matched controls divided by the standard deviation of this mean, which is an indication of the biologic variability. To obtain the T-score, the bone density of a patient is compared to the peak bone mass of young normal adults. The T-score gives the patient's results as a deviation from the mean of young normal adults divided by the standard deviation of the mean.

Still, for most clinicians these data are confusing. The WHO generated a document to aid clinicians in their interpretations of bone densitometry results. This information provides working definitions for the use of bone densitometry and is presented in Outline 1. These guidelines are helpful in clinical practice so that the clinician can provide patients with the necessary information to discuss any therapeutic decisions. It has, however, been argued that this threshold-based diagnosis is not the best way to use bone densitometry techniques because there is a gradient of fracture risk that increases with decreasing BMD values. Furthermore, the WHO criteria are based on DXA data. Whether the same standards can be used for data acquired with other techniques, such as quantitative ultrasound systems, is questionable.

Summary

Some insight in the advantages and disadvantages of bone densitometry techniques as well as some knowledge about these techniques is necessary in order to use them to their full extent in clinical practice. Several refresher courses are provided by different scientific and other nonprofit organizations. Local expertise and interest will usually dictate the availability and proper use of these techniques.

Outline 1
World Health Organization Guidelines for Interpretation of Bone Densitometry Results*

Normal: A value for BMD or BMC not more than 1 SD below the average value of young adults.

Low Bone Mass or Osteopenia: A value for BMD or BMC more than 1 SD below the young adult average, but not more than 2.5 SD below.

Osteoporosis: A value for BMD or BMC more than 2.5 SD below the young adult average.

Severe osteoporosis: A value for BMC or BMD more than 2.5 SD below the young adult average value and the presence of one or more fragility fractures.

BMD, bone mineral density
BMC, bone mineral content
SD, standard deviation

*   1 SD change in BMD equals a 10% to 12% change in bone density; for every SD of decrease in BMD in the elderly, the relative risk of fracture increases by a factor of 1.5 to 1.8.

Selected Bibliography

Conventional Radiography

Ardran GM: Bone destruction not demonstrable by radiography. *Br J Radiol* 1951;24:107–109.

Finsen V, Anda S: Accuracy of visually estimated bone mineralization in routine radiographs of the lower extremity. *Skeletal Radiol* 1988;17:270–275.

Kawashima T, Uhthoff HK: A pattern of bone loss of the proximal femur: A radiologic, densitometric, and histomorphometric study. *J Orthop Res* 1991;9:634–640.

Mayo-Smith W, Rosenthal DI: Radiographic appearance of osteopenia. *Radiol Clin North Am* 1991;29:37–47.

Mirsky EC, Einhorn TA: Current concepts review: Bone densitometry in orthopaedic practice. *J Bone Joint Surg* 1998;80A:1687–1698.

Singh M, Nagrath AR, Maini PS: Changes in trabecular pattern of the upper end of the femur as an index of osteoporosis. *J Bone Joint Surg* 1970;52A;457–467.

Radiogrammetry

Barnett E, Nordin BEC: The radiological diagnosis of osteoporosis: A new approach. *Clin Radiol* 1960;11:166–174.

Bloom RA, Pogrund H, Libson E: Radiogrammetry of the metacarpal: A critical reappraisal. *Skeletal Radiol* 1983;10:5–9.

Faulkner KG, Cummings SR, Black D, Palermo L, Glüer CC, Genant HK: Simple measurement of femoral geometry predicts hip fracture: The study of osteoporotic fractures. *J Bone Miner Res* 1993; 8:1211–1217.

Glüer CC, Cummings SR, Pressman A, et al: Prediction of hip fractures from pelvic radiographs: The study of osteoporotic fractures. *J Bone Miner Res* 1994;9:671–677.

Horsman A, Simpson M: The measurement of sequential changes in cortical bone geometry. *Br J Radiol* 1975;48:471–476.

Kalla AA, Meyers OL, Parkyn ND, Kotze TJvW: Osteoporosis screening: Radiogrammetry revisited. *Br J Rheumatol* 1989;28:511–517.

Meema HE: Improved vertebral fracture threshold in postmenopausal osteoporosis by radiogrametric measurements: Its usefulness in selection for preventive therapy. *J Bone Miner Res* 1991;6:9–14.

Meema HE, Meindok H: Advantages of peripheral radiogrametry over dual-photon absorptiometry of the spine in the assessment of prevalence of osteoporotic vertebral fractures in women. *J Bone Miner Res* 1992;7:897–903.

Radiographic Absorptiometry

Cosman F, Herrington B, Himmelstein S, Lindsay R: Radiographic absorptiometry: A simple method for determination of bone mass. *Osteoporos Int* 1991;2:34–38.

Seo GS, Shiraki M, Aoki C, et al: Assessment of bone density in the distal radius with computer assisted X-ray densitometry (CXD). *Bone Miner* 1994;27:173–182.

Trouerbach WT, Hoornstra K, Birkenhäger JC, Zwamborn AW: Roentgendensitometric study of the phalanx. *Diagn Imaging Clin Med* 1985;54:64–77.

Yang SO, Hagiwara S, Engelke K, et al: Radiographic absorptiometry for bone mineral measurement of the phalanges: Precision and accuracy study. *Radiology* 1994;192,857–859.

Yates AJ, Ross PD, Lydick E, Epstein RS: Radiographic absorptiometry in the diagnosis of osteoporosis. *Am J Med* 1995;98:41S–47S.

Single X-ray or Photon Absorptiometry

Bjarnason K, Nilas L, Hassager C, Christiansen C: Dual energy X-ray absorptiometry of the spine: Decubitus lateral versus anteroposterior projection in osteoporotic women. Comparison to single energy X-ray absorptiometry of the fore-arm. *Bone* 1995;16:255–260.

Cameron JR, Sorenson J: Measurement of bone mineral in vivo: An improved method. *Science* 1963;142:230–232.

Cheng S, Suominen H, Sakari-Rantala R, Laukkanen P, Avikainen V, Heikkinen E: Calcaneal bone mineral density predicts fracture occurrence: A five-year follow-up study in elderly people. *J Bone Miner Res* 1997;12:1075–1082.

Glüer CC, Vahlensieck M, Faulkner KG, Engelke K, Black D, Genant HK: Site-matched calcaneal measurements of broad-band ultrasound attenuation and single X-ray absorptiometry: Do they measure different skeletal properties? *J Bone Miner Res* 1992;7:1071–1079.

Kelly TL, Crane G, Baran DT: Single X-ray absorptiometry of the forearm: Precision, correlation, and reference data. *Calcif Tissue Int* 1994;54:212–218.

Dual X-ray or Photon Absorptiometry

Drinka PJ, DeSmet AA, Bauwens SF, Rogot A: The effect of overlying calcification on lumbar bone densitometry. *Calcif Tissue Int* 1992;50:507–510.

Glüer CC, Steiger P, Selvidge R, Elliesen-Kliefoth K, Hayashi C, Genant HK: Comparative assessment of dual-photon absorptiometry and dual-energy radiography. *Radiology* 1990;174:223–228.

Hagiwara S, Engelke K, Yang S-O, et al: Dual X-Ray absorptiometry forearm software: Accuracy and intermachine relationship. *J Bone Miner Res* 1994;9:1425–1427.

Jaovisidha S, Sartoris DJ, Martin EM, de Maeseneer M, Szollar SM, Deftos LJ: Influence of spondylopathy on bone densitometry using dual energy X-ray absorptiometry. *Calcif Tissue Int* 1997;60:424–429.

Jergas M, Breitenseher M, Glüer CC, et al: Which vertebrae should be assessed using lateral dual-energy X-ray absorptiometry of the lumbar spine? *Osteoporosis Int* 1995;5:196–204.

Jergas M, Genant HK: Lateral dual X-ray absorptiometry of the lumbar spine: Current status. *Bone* 1997;20:311–314.

Kelly TL, Slovik DM, Schoenfeld DA, Neer RM: Quantitative digital radiography versus dual photon absorptiometry of the lumbar spine. *J Clin Endocrinol Metab* 1988;67:839–844.

Lilley J, Walters BG, Heath DA, Drolc Z: In vivo and in vitro precision for bone density measured by dual-energy X-ray absorption. *Osteoporos Int* 1991;1:141–146.

Orwoll ES, Oviatt SK: Longitudinal precision of dual-energy X-ray absorptiometry in a multicenter study: The Nefarelin Bone Study Group. *J Bone Miner Res* 1991;6:191–197.

Peppler WW, Mazess RB: Total body bone mineral and lean body mass by dual-photon absorptiometry: I. Theory and measurement procedure. *Calcif Tissue Int* 1981;33:353–359.

Rand T, Seidl G, Kainberger F, et al: Impact of spinal degenerative changes on the evaluation of bone mineral density with dual energy X-ray absorptiometry (DXA). *Calcif Tissue Int* 1997;60:430–433.

Yamada M, Ito M, Hayashi K, Ohki M, Nakamura T: Dual-energy X-ray absorptiometry of the calcaneus: Comparison with other techniques to assess bone density and value in predicting risk of spine fractures. *Am J Roentgenol* 1994;63:1435–1440.

Quantitative Computed Tomography

Cann CE, Genant HK: Precise measurement of vertebral mineral content using computed tomography. *J Comput Assist Tomogr* 1980; 4:493–500.

Genant HK, Cann CE, Ettinger B, Gordan GS: Quantitative computed tomography of vertebral spongiosa: A sensitive method for detecting early bone loss after oophorectomy. *Ann Intern Med* 1982;97:699–705.

Kalender WA, Klotz E, Suess C: Vertebral bone mineral analysis: an integrated approach with CT. *Radiology* 1987;164:419–423.

Kuiper JW, van Kuijk C, Grashuis JL, Ederveen AG, Schütte HE: Accuracy and the influence of marrow fat on quantitative CT and dual-energy X-ray absorptiometry measurements of the femoral neck in vitro. *Osteoporos Int* 1996;6:25–30.

Lang TF, Keyak JH, Heitz MW, et al: Volumetric quantitative computed tomography of the proximal femur: Precision and relation to bone strength. *Bone* 1997;21:101–108.

Mazess RB: Errors in measuring trabecular bone by computed tomography due to marrow and bone composition. *Calcif Tissue Int* 1983;35:148–152.

Müller A, Rüegsegger E, Rüegsegger P: Peripheral QCT: A low-risk procedure to identify women predisposed to osteoporosis. *Phys Med Biol* 1989;34:741–749.

Rüegsegger P, Elsasser U, Anliker M, Gnehm H, Kind H, Prader A: Quantification of bone mineralization using computed tomography. *Radiology* 1976;121:93–97.

Schneider P, Borner W: Peripheral quantitative computed tomography for bone mineral measurement using a new special QCT-scanner: Methodology, normal valgus, comparison with manifest osteoporosis. *Roto Fortschr Geb Rontgenstr Neuen Bildgeb Verfahr* 1991;154:292–299.

van Kuijk C, Grashuis JL, Steenbeek JCM, Schütte HE, Trouerbach WT: Evaluation of postprocessing dual-energy methods in quantitative computed tomography: Part 2. Practical aspects. *Invest Radiol* 1990;25:882–889.

Quantitative Ultrasound

Glüer CC: International Quantitative Ultrasound Consensus Group: Quantitative ultrasound techniques for the assessment of osteoporosis. Expert agreement on current status. *J Bone Miner Res* 1997;12:1280–1288.

Njeh CF, Boivin CM, Langton CM: The role of ultrasound in the assessment of osteoporosis: A review. *Osteoporosis Int* 1997;7:7–22.

Gregg EW, Kriska AM, Salamone LM, et al: The epidemiology of quantitative ultrasound: A review of the relationship with bone mass, osteoporosis and fracture risk. *Osteoporos Int* 1997;7:89–99.

Orgee JM, Foster H, McCloskey EV, Khan S, Coombes G, Kanis JA: A precise method for the assessment of tibial ultrasound velocity. *Osteoporos Int* 1996;6:1–7.

Roux C, Fournier B, Laugier P, et al: Broadband ultrasound attenuation imaging: A new imaging method in osteoporosis. *J Bone Miner Res* 1996;11:1112–1118.

Ventura V, Mauloni M, Mura M, Paltrinieri F, de Aloysio D: Ultrasound velocity changes at the proximal phalanxes of the hand in pre-, peri- and postmenopausal women. *Osteoporos Int* 1996;6:368–375.

Quantitative Magnetic Resonance Imaging

Jergas M, Majumdar S, Keyak JH, et al: Relationships between young modulus of elasticity, ash density, and MRI derived effective transverse relaxation time T2* in tibial specimens. *J Comput Assist Tomogr* 1995;19:472–479.

Ouyang X, Selby K, Lang P, et al: High resolution magnetic resonance imaging of the calcaneus: Age-related changes in trabecular structure and comparison with dual X-ray absorptiometry. *Calcif Tissue Int* 1997;60:139–147.

Rosenthal H, Thulborn KR, Rosenthal DI, Kim SH, Rosen BR: Magnetic susceptibility effects of trabecular bone on magnetic resonance imaging of bone marrow. *Invest Radiol* 1990;25:173–178.

DXA (Orthopaedic Applications)

Kröger H, Miettinen H, Arnala I, Koski E, Rushton N, Suomalainen O: Evaluation of periprosthetic bone using dual-energy X-ray absorptiometry: Precision of the method and effect of operation on bone mineral density. *J Bone Miner Res* 1996;11:1526–1530.

Kröger H, Vanninen E, Overmeyer M, Miettinen H, Rushton N, Suomalainen O: Periprosthetic bone loss and regional bone turnover in uncemented total hip arthroplasty: A prospective study using high resolution single photon emission tomography and dual-energy X-ray absorptiometry. *J Bone Miner Res* 1997;12:487–492.

Marchetti ME, Steinberg GG, Greene JM, Jenis LG, Baran DT: A prospective study of proximal femur bone mass following cemented and uncemented hip arthroplasty. *J Bone Miner Res* 1996;11:1033–1039.

Comparison of Methods/Reviews

Cummings SR, Black DM, Nevitt MC, et al: Bone density at various sites for prediction of hip fractures: The Study of Osteoporotic Fractures Research Group. *Lancet* 1993;341:72–75.

Genant HK, Engelke K, Fuerst T, et al: Noninvasive assessment of bone mineral and structure: State of the art. *J Bone Miner Res* 1996;11:707–730.

Genant HK, Guglielmi G, Jergas M (eds): *Bone Densitometry and Osteoporosis*. Heidelberg, Germany, Springer, 1998.

Grampp S, Genant HK, Mathur A, et al: Comparisons of noninvasive bone mineral measurements in assessing age-related loss, fracture discrimination, and diagnostic classification. *J Bone Miner Res* 1997;12:697–711.

Ito M, Hayashi K, Ishida Y, et al: Discrimination of spinal fracture with various bone mineral measurements. *Calcif Tissue Int* 1997;60: 11–15.

Lafferty FW, Rowland DY: Correlations of dual-energy X-ray absorptiometry, quantitative computed tomography, and single photon absorptiometry with spinal and non-spinal fractures. *Osteoporos Int* 1996;6:407–415.

Ravn P, Overgaard K, Huang C, Ross PD, Green D, McClung M: EPIC Study Group: Comparison of bone densitometry of the phalanges, distal forearm and axial skeleton in early postmenopausal women participating in the EPIC study. *Osteoporos Int* 1996;6:308–313.

Seeley DG, Browner WS, Nevitt MC, Genant HK, Scott JC, Cummings SR: Which fractures are associated with low appendicular bone mass in elderly women? The Study of Osteoporotic Fractures Research Group. *Ann Intern Med* 1991;115:837–842.

Wasnich RD: Does current bone mass predict future fractures?, in Christiansen C, Overgaard K (eds): *Osteoporosis*. Copenhagen, Denmark, Osteopress, 1990, pp 442–445.

Yu W, Glüer CC, Grampp S, et al: Spinal bone mineral assessment in postmenopausal women: A comparison between dual X-ray absorptiometry and quantitative computed tomography. *Osteoporos Int* 1995;5:433–439.

Applications

Consensus Development Conference: Who are candidates for prevention and treatment for osteoporosis? *Osteoporos Int* 1997;7:1–6.

Genant HK, Block JE, Steiger P, Glüer CC, Ettinger B, Harris ST: Appropriate use of bone densitometry. *Radiology* 1989;170:817–822.

Johnston CC Jr, Slemenda CW, Melton LJ III: Clinical use of bone densitometry. *N Engl J Med* 1991;324:1105–1109.

Kanis JA, Geusens P, Christiansen C: Guidelines for clinical trials in osteoporosis: A position paper of the European Foundation for Osteoporosis and Bone Disease. *Osteoporos Int* 1991;1:182–188.

Miller PD, Bonnick SL, Rosen CJ: Consensus of an international panel on the clinical utility of bone mass measurements in the detection of low bone mass in the adult population. *Calcif Tissue Int* 1996; 58:207–214.

World Health Organization: Assessment of osteoporotic fracture risk and its role in screening for postmenopausal women. Geneva, Switzerland, WHO Technical Reports Series 843, 1994.

Chapter Outline

Chapter 11

Radioisotopes in Orthopaedics

Robert Schneider, MD

Bruce Rapuano, PhD

This chapter at a glance

This chapter presents a discussion of radioisotopes, which are currently being used in orthopaedics for diagnosis, research, and therapy.

Introduction

Shortly after the discovery of radioactivity it was recognized that some radioactive materials could localize in bone. The first use of radioisotopes was to treat malignant neoplasms. In 1935, bone was shown to be metabolically active and not an inert tissue by using phosphorus 32, a beta emitter, to study phosphorus metabolism. Other radioisotopes were also used to study bone mineral, collagen, cartilage, and bone blood flow. After the advent of nuclear reactors, more radioisotopes became available for research, eventually leading to their clinical use for diagnosis. It was shown that increased uptake of radioisotopes occurred in fractures, tumors, arthritis, and other conditions even before abnormalities could be seen on radiographs. Geiger counters and other probes were used initially to localize the radioactivity, but these mechanisms were cumbersome and their clinical value was limited. Rectilinear scanners, and later, gamma cameras, made localization of the radioactivity easier and provided anatomic detail that enabled bone scanning for diagnostic imaging.

Radioisotopes are currently being used in orthopaedics for diagnosis (to detect and follow conditions that may be the cause of bone and joint abnormalities), research (to study bone and cartilage metabolism), and therapy (to treat malignant neoplasms and for radionuclide synovectomy).

Radioisotopes and the Scanning Process

Radioisotopes of many elements such as calcium, strontium, magnesium, gallium, indium, fluorine, tin, and lead have been found to localize in the skeleton. Compounds that localize in bone include phosphate and phosphonate complexes, alizarin, and tetracycline. Only a few of these have been used on a regular basis in clinical practice for diagnosis. Emission scanning is used, meaning that the radioisotope is injected or ingested into the body and the gamma radiation from within the body is imaged. Some of the important factors in a radionuclide scanning agent are as follows:

(1) Energy of the radioisotope—gamma energy levels that are too high will penetrate the crystal detector and collimators of the gamma camera too easily, and gamma energies that are too low will not penetrate the body. Only gamma emissions can be used for scanning. Alpha and beta emissions do not penetrate the body and increase the radiation dose.

(2) Bone to soft-tissue ratio—high bone uptake and high soft-tissue clearance allow better anatomic resolution of the skeleton.

(3) Lesion to background ratio—the higher the uptake of radioisotopes by the abnormality, the more easily the lesion can be identified.

(4) Radiation dose—shorter physical and biologic half-lives allow a higher dose to be injected, with less radiation exposure to the patient. A sufficient number of photons must be available for imaging without too high a radiation dose. The half-life of the isotope, however, must be long enough that sufficient time is allowed for the radioisotope to be localized in the target tissue so that scanning can be done.

(5) Availability—radioisotopes with short half-lives, such as technetium Tc 99m, may be available from on-site generators. Radioisotopes that have longer half-lives can be shipped.

Strontium 85, introduced in 1961, was the first radioisotope to be used clinically for bone scanning. It replaces calcium in the calcium hydroxyapatite crystal and is excreted in the bowel. It has an energy of 572 keV, higher than ideal for gamma cameras. It has a long half-life of 65 days and a biologic half-life of 100 days, which cause a high radiation dose and limit the amount that can be injected. Because of the high radiation dose, ^{85}Sr was initially reserved for patients with known malignancy, and scans had poor anatomic resolution because of the limited amount injected. However, scans done 2 days to 2 weeks after injection allowed good soft-tissue clearance.

Strontium Sr 87m has a short half-life of 2.7 hours and a better energy (388 keV) for scanning than does ^{85}Sr. However, soft-tissue clearance is poor, leading to poor image quality, so clinical use is limited.

Fluorine 18, a positron emitter with an energy of 511 keV, was the next radioisotope used clinically and replaces the hydroxyl group in the hydroxyapatite crystal of bone. It has a short half-life of 1.85 hours, excellent and rapid uptake by bone, and rapid soft-tissue clearance. Its energy of 511 keV is higher than ideal for use with a gamma camera. Fluorine 18 is produced by a cyclotron, which limits its availability, and its short half-life limits the ability to transport the isotope long distances. It was the radioisotope of choice for bone scanning until the advent of technetium Tc 99m labeled phosphate complexes. Fluorine 18 is one of the radioisotopes now used in positron emission tomography (PET) scanning.

In 1971, Tc 99m-labeled phosphate complexes were introduced for bone scanning. Technetium Tc 99m is an excellent agent for scanning; it has a relatively short half-life of 6 hours, and its energy of 140 keV makes imaging with a gamma camera ideal. Stannous tin is used to reduce the ^{99m}Tc pertechnetate so that it can form a chelate with a phosphate or phosphonate complex. These complexes are taken up by the skeleton. The first of the phosphate complexes to be used were polyphosphate and pyrophosphate.

These organic phosphates, which have P-O-P bonds, have been replaced for bone scanning by the diphosphonate complexes, which have P-C-P bonds that are more stable and have a more rapid blood clearance. Initially, ethylene diphosphonate (EHDP) was used but now methylene diphosphonate (MDP) or hydroxymethane diphosphonate (HMDP) are used. Although HMDP has a more rapid blood clearance than MDP, scans done at 2 to 4 hours with either of these radionuclides provide virtually identical results.

The exact method of localization of the ^{99m}Tc phosphonate complex is not completely understood. It is thought that ^{99m}Tc is transported to the bone crystal surface by the phosphonate complex, which adsorbs onto the bone crystal surface. Transport into the bone crystal is relatively slow and probably not complete by the time of the scanning at 2 to 4 hours. Technetium Tc 99m pertechnetate is not taken up by the bone, indicating that the phosphonate complexes must carry the ^{99m}Tc to the bone. It is still unclear as to whether the ^{99m}Tc phosphonate complexes enter the bone intact into the mineral phase, or whether the complexes separate with the ^{99m}Tc going into the organic phase, especially newly formed osteoid. There has been experimental evidence for both hypotheses.

Increased bone turnover is thought to be the most important factor producing increased uptake of the radionuclide. Microradiographic studies have shown higher localization of the radionuclide in mineralization fronts of newly formed bone in areas that were undergoing bone repair due to surgical defects. Areas of bone undergoing less rapid turnover, such as normal cortical bone, have uptake of radionuclide but quantitatively less than in more metaboli-cally active areas such as the metaphyses or areas around active epiphyseal growth plates.

Blood flow is another factor involved in the uptake of radionuclide. In areas where there is no blood flow, there is no uptake. Increased blood flow leads to increased uptake, however, only to a limited extent. Increased vascularity from reactive hyperemia may cause a twofold to threefold increase in uptake of ^{99m}Tc phosphonate complexes, while considerably higher levels are obtained in conditions in which there is new bone formation. The percentage increase in uptake in the skeleton, in fractures, and with other pathologic conditions with increased bone turnover is usually far greater than the increase in blood flow.

Uptake in immature collagen has also been thought by some authors to be responsible for high radioisotope uptake found in pathologic conditions. The high uptake found in osteomalacia, hyperparathyroidism, and Paget's disease may be due to the presence of large amounts of osteoid. Other authors, however, dispute the presence of radioisotope in collagen on bone scans. High bone turnover with these conditions may be responsible for the high uptake.

With ^{99m}Tc diphosphonate agents, about 50% of the injected dose is taken up by the skeleton within 3 hours. Most of the rest of the dose is excreted into the urine with only a small amount remaining in the blood at about 3 to 4 hours after injection. Hydrating the patient helps increase extraction and excretion of the radioisotope from the blood and soft tissues. Image quality is worse in elderly or obese patients, and in those with renal failure, hypercalcemia, and on various medications such as bisphosphonates.

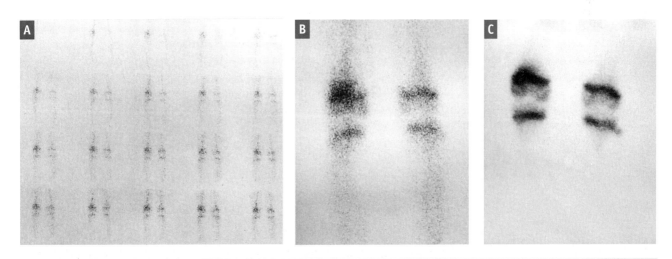

Figure 1

Three-phase bone scan of the knees in a child shows increased vascularity on the the dynamic flow (**A**) and blood pool (**B**) scans and increased uptake on the delayed static images (**C**) in the metaphyseal region of the right femur due to osteomyelitis.

Radioisotopes in the Diagnosis of Musculoskeletal Abnormalities

Radioisotopes are used in the diagnosis of orthopaedic conditions to detect abnormalities and to determine the extent of disease. Diagnosis with radioisotopes is based on differences in physiologic activity between normal and abnormal areas of the skeleton. Thus, lesions may be detected with radioisotope scanning even when anatomic abnormalities cannot be detected radiographically. When abnormalities are detected with bone scans, more anatomic detail can be obtained with radiographs, computed tomography (CT), and magnetic resonance imaging (MRI). Abnormalities such as recent fractures, tumors, and osteomyelitis show increased vascularity on images obtained immediately after injection of radioisotopes. Delayed images show increase in uptake of radioisotope over time in these lesions. New and rapid bone turnover as seen in fractures, tumors, and osteomyelitis produce woven bone that tightly binds the ^{99m}Tc phosphonate complexes to the bone.

Bone scans are performed with intravenous injection of 20 to 30 mCi (740 to 1010 MBq) of ^{99m}Tc-labeled phosphonate complex. For localized abnormalities, 3-phase bone scans are done (Fig. 1). The first phase is a dynamic flow study, a radionuclide angiogram in which scans are done every 2 to 5 seconds after injection for 1 to 2 minutes. This shows the radionuclide in the blood vessels, including the arterial, capillary, and venous phases. The second phase of the bone scan is a blood pool scan, or a static image done immediately after the flow study and within 5 minutes after injection, which shows radionuclide in the extravascular space before bone uptake occurs. The dynamic flow and blood pool scans are known as the early phases of the bone scan. They are helpful in evaluating inflammatory lesions such as cellulitis and osteomyelitis, in detecting vascular soft-tissue abnormalities such as tumors, and in dating traumatic lesions such as fractures or myositis ossificans in which increased blood flow occurs. Vascularity increases early in these lesions and returns to normal with successful treatment before the increased bone uptake does. The third phase of the bone scan consists of static images done 2 to 4 hours after injection that show radionuclide uptake by the bone.

A fourth stage is a scan that may be helpful when there is poor image quality in the third phase due to prolonged soft-tissue clearance or radionuclide in the bladder, which obscures portions of the pelvic bones. It is done 24 hours after injection, and these delayed images have better bone to soft-tissue ratio and often better lesion to background ratio, but are rarely needed for diagnosis.

A gamma camera containing a sodium iodide detector crystal is the instrument used routinely in bone scanning. Scans are done as either whole body images using a moving camera or table, or as multiple spot images. Whole body images are usually done for screening of metastatic disease (Fig. 2). Whole body bone scanning allows screening the entire skeleton at relatively low cost and time to search for abnormalities. Spot images, including anterior, posterior, and lateral images, provide better resolution for interpreting focal skeletal abnormalities. The choice of collimators affects image quality. High resolution, ultra-high resolution, and pinhole collimators increase the resolution, but a longer scanning time is the result. Pinhole collimators provide magnification and better detail of small areas

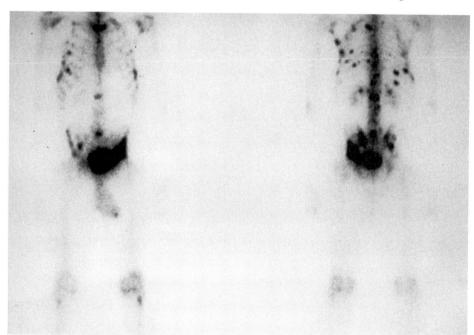

Figure 2

Whole body bone scan. Anterior and posterior scans show multiple areas of high uptake in the axial skeleton in a random pattern typical of metastatic disease.

(Fig. 3). This is especially helpful in imaging children's hips where the growth plates may obscure the epiphyses. Single photon emission computed tomography (SPECT) is a method of obtaining tomographic images on a bone scan. The scans are obtained with an arc of 360° or 180° around the patient. The images can be reconstructed into axial, coronal, or sagittal planes. SPECT scans are especially helpful for detecting abnormalities in the posterior elements of the spine that may be obscured by the vertebral bodies (Fig. 4).

In some cases, stress fractures of the pars may be visualized only on the SPECT scan and not on the planar images. SPECT scanning has also been used to look for areas of decreased uptake in osteonecrosis. PET is done using positron emitting isotopes such as ^{18}F. Dedicated PET scanners are expensive and, although increasing in quantity, have only limited availability at this time because of the

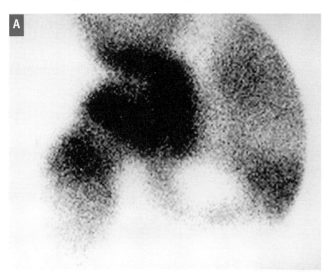
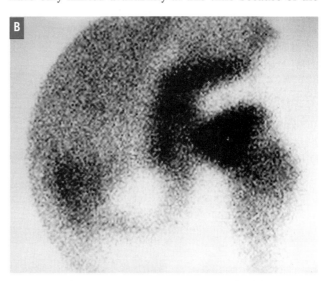

Figure 3

Pinhole collimator scans of the right (**A**) and left (**B**) hips in a child show absent uptake in the epiphysis of the left femoral head indicating avascularity from Legg-Calvé-Perthes disease.

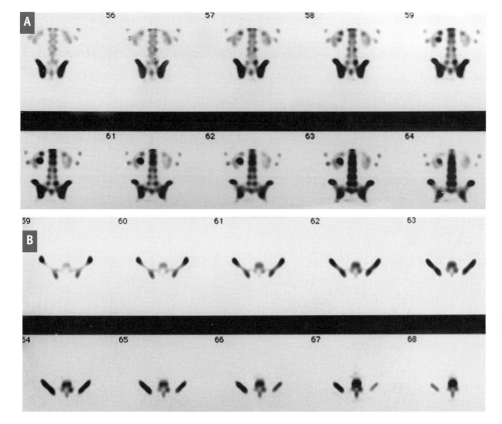

Figure 4

Single photon emission computed tomography scan of the lumbar spine with (**A**) coronal and (**B**) axial reconstructions. There is a focal area of increased uptake in the left pars of L-5 from a stress fracture.

expense. Access to a cyclotron is needed to provide the short-lived radioisotopes. Modifications in dual-head gamma cameras may allow PET scans. Improved image quality can be obtained with bone scanning with ^{18}F using PET as compared with planar or SPECT bone scanning; however, the clinical use of PET for bone scanning has not been widespread. PET scanning is used mainly for tumor imaging with the use of ^{18}F fluoro-2-deoxy-glucose (FDG), which is a glucose analog. FDG is transported into the cells in a manner similar to that of glucose but is not metabolized, so there is a high accumulation in cells with high metabolic activity.

Trauma

Fractures can usually be detected within 24 hours to 3 days of injury (Fig. 5). In a small percentage of cases, the scan may be negative and only become positive at 72 hours or even up to 2 weeks after injury. Fractures in the axial skeleton and in the long bones may take longer to show increased uptake as compared with fractures around the

area of joints. Fractures of the skull may be negative on bone scans. Although some authors have suggested that fractures in the elderly may take longer to become positive on bone scans, most studies show that age is not an important factor in diagnosis by bone scan. After fracture, the dynamic flow study is positive for 2 to 3 weeks before reverting to normal. The blood pool scan is positive for approximately 8 weeks. In the third phase of the bone scan, the delayed static images stay positive for 6 months to 2 years after injury because of continued bone healing and remodeling. If malalignment or malposition occurs, bone remodeling may continue, and the bone scan may remain positive indefinitely after the injury.

Bone bruises are fractures of trabecular bone that occur without interruption of the cortex. Bone bruises show increased vascularity and uptake of radionuclide on bone scan. The bone scan may revert to normal earlier than with fractures through the cortex, because bone healing and bone remodeling terminate earlier. Osteochondral injuries and osteochondritis dissecans also show increased uptake on bone scans. Delayed static images may show increased

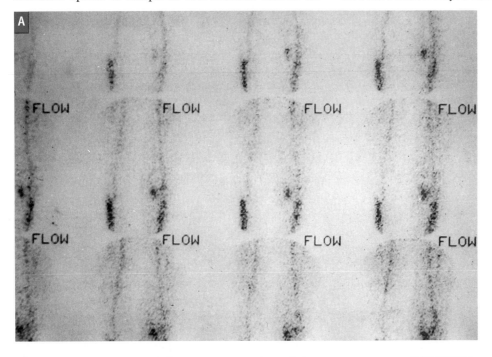

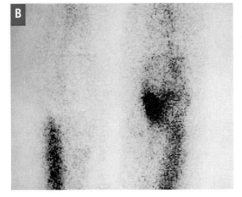

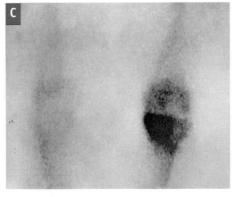

Figure 5

There is increased vascularity on the flow (**A**) and blood pool (**B**) and increased uptake on the delayed static images (**C**) in the left medial tibial plateau, consistent with a fracture or bone bruise.

uptake indefinitely as a result of ongoing repair; complete healing often does not occur.

Stress fractures may occur without abnormal stress in osteopenic bone (insufficiency fractures), or with excessive stress on normal bone (fatigue fractures). Insufficiency fractures tend to occur in areas of trabecular bone such as the sacral ala, tibial plateau, and calcaneus (Fig. 6). At these sites, lucent fracture lines and periosteal reaction are usually not seen on radiographs, and the radiographic finding of sclerosis from bone repair may take 2 weeks or more to become visible after the onset of symptoms. Usually the bone scan is positive at the onset of pain. As with traumatic fractures, increased vascularity is seen early in these conditions on the flow and blood pool scans, returning to normal on these scans sooner than delayed static images. Sacral ala insufficiency fractures often occur in conjunction with pubic ramus fractures.

When multiple bilateral symmetric insufficiency fractures occur, osteomalacia should be considered. These insufficiency fractures may be seen in the ribs, pubic rami, tibial plateaus, femoral condyles, and inferior aspect of the scapulae.

Fatigue fractures in runners are most common in the diaphysis of the tibia in the posterior and medial aspect, metatarsals, calcanei, and femoral necks; the latter two are also common sites of insufficiency fractures.

Stress fractures of the pars interarticularis in the spine are common in athletes, especially with activities involving hyperextension. Spondylolysis or defects in the pars that have occurred earlier during childhood do not show increased uptake on bone scans. Recent stress or traumatic fractures of the pars show increased uptake (Fig. 4). SPECT scanning is helpful in detecting increased uptake on bone scan in pars stress fractures; in some cases the planar images may be normal due to the overlying normal vertebral bodies obscuring the increased uptake in the pars.

Osteoporotic compression fractures of the spine can be detected even before vertebral collapse occurs. Compression fractures return to normal on bone scans in 6 months or longer after the fracture, depending on whether continued bone remodeling is occurring. Multiple vertebral compression deformities that show varying degrees of uptake on bone scan are consistent with osteoporotic compression fractures as opposed to pathologic compression fractures from metastatic disease.

Heterotopic bone formation or myositis ossificans shows increased vascularity and later increased uptake on bone scan before radiographs are abnormal. A normal bone scan shows that the heterotopic bone formation is in an inactive state and can safely be resected. However, the bone scan may stay positive for many years. Decreasing ratios of uptake of radionuclide in heterotopic bone to background on serial scans suggests that the heterotopic bone formation is quiescent and that surgery can be performed.

Neoplastic Disease

Increased uptake of ^{99m}Tc phosphonate complexes in bone scanning in neoplastic lesions is caused mainly by osteoblastic response with new bone formation. With lytic metastatic disease, an osteoblastic response occurs in reaction to bone destruction in an attempt at a repair process. This occurs especially in lesions in which the cortex and periosteum are involved. Small lytic lesions entirely within the medullary cavity may not cause increased uptake on a bone scan and may not be detected. SPECT scanning has a higher sensitivity for visualizing metastatic lesions within the vertebral bodies than does planar imaging. Increased uptake from malignant lesions has to be differentiated from benign processes such as degenerative and posttraumatic disease. This is not always possible on the bone scan alone, and correlation with other imaging modalities such as radiographs, CT scans, and MRI scans may be necessary. Untreated malignant lesions tend to grow and show more intense increased uptake over time on serial scans; this may help distinguish them from fractures that show decreasing uptake on serial scanning. A paradoxical increase in uptake and size of the metastatic lesions seen on bone scans, known as the flare phenomenon, may occur after treatment with chemotherapy for up to 6 months after the start of chemotherapy, despite clinical improvement. It is the result of bone repair after successful therapy. Malignant neoplastic lesions may show increased uptake in the bone beyond the actual site of the lesion due to hyperemia and bone

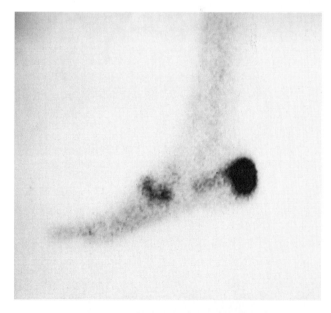

Figure 6

High uptake is present in the posterior aspect of the calcaneus due to a stress fracture. There is moderate increased uptake in tarsometatarsal joints from degenerative disease.

marrow edema occurring beyond the site of the tumor. This condition is known as an extended pattern of uptake and limits the ability of bone scans to show the exact anatomic extent of malignant lesions. In some lytic metastases, no osteoblastic response may occur either because of the very rapid bone destruction or because of limited response of the bone to the lesion. In these instances, a cold area of decreased uptake may occur. Decreased uptake is more difficult to detect than areas of increased uptake. The cold lesions account for well under 5% of metastatic lesions seen on a bone scan. In multiple myeloma, about 50% of the lesions do not show abnormal increased uptake. In the patient with multiple lesions, however, some of them can usually be detected on a bone scan.

There is a tendency for malignant lesions to show high uptake while benign lesions show less intense or normal uptake; however, an overlap occurs with some benign lesions showing high uptake. On bone scans, Paget's disease (Fig. 7) and fibrous dysplasia (Fig. 8) show high uptake that may be mistaken for metastatic disease; however, characteristic diagnostic patterns of uptake in these conditions may be seen on bone scan, unlike metastatic disease, which tends to show a random pattern of multiple areas of increased uptake in the axial skeleton (Fig. 2). Virtually all enchondromas show some increased uptake, so no differentiation can be made from low grade chondrosarcoma. Nonossifying fibromas and fibrous cortical defects that are healing show increased uptake. Benign bone cysts do not show abnormal increased uptake unless a fracture is present. Osteoid osteomas are often diagnostic on a bone scan showing a small focal area of high uptake in the nidus and increased uptake in surrounding bone sclerosis.

Gallium Ga 67 citrate scanning has been used to evaluate musculoskeletal tumors. Most malignant tumors show increased uptake of gallium. Gallium scanning, however, is limited by its lack of specificity as fractures and other benign lesions also show increased uptake.

Scanning has been done with thallium Tl-201 and with ^{99m}Tc methoxyisobutyl isonitrile (MIBI), radionuclides originally used as myocardial perfusion imaging agents in order to determine the response to the chemotherapy and to differentiate malignant tissue from postoperative changes after therapy in patients with malignant bone tumors. Thallium Tl 201 chloride acts as an analog to potassium chloride. The mechanism of uptake of ^{99m}Tc MIBI is most likely related to mitochondrial activity and plasma membrane potential. With increasing grades of malignancy there is a tendency toward higher uptake of these agents. In areas of absent perfusion in the necrotic portions malignant tumors there will be absent uptake. PET with FDG is being used in a similar manner to distinguish malignant from metabolically inactive tissue after treatment. The uptake of FDG is related to the amount of glycolysis in the lesion, with high grades of malignancy tending to have higher uptake. Successful chemotherapy will cause a decrease in the uptake of these radionuclides on the posttreatment scans as compared with the pretreatment scans. Malignant tissue may be distinguished from posttreatment fibrosis.

Infection

A wide range of radionuclide scanning agents may be used for diagnosing bone and soft-tissue infections. Three-phase

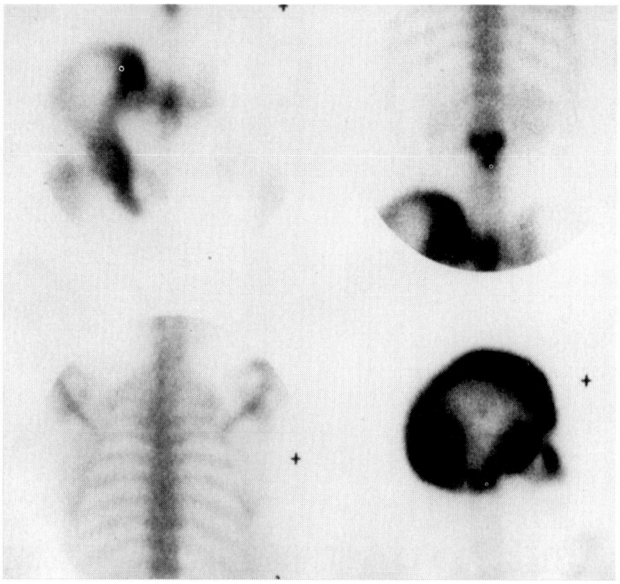

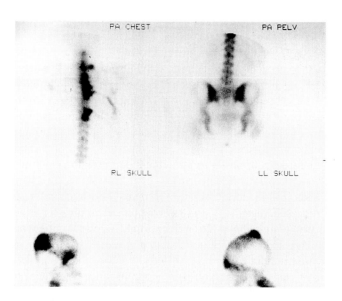

Figure 7

There is high uptake in the entire skull, in the left hemipelvis, and in the L-3 vertebral body and spinous process, in a pattern typical of Paget's disease.

Figure 8

There is high uptake in the right side of multiple vertebral bodies, in a right rib, in the skull, and in the frontal bone due to fibrous dysplasia.

bone scanning with ^{99m}Tc phosphonate complexes can detect bone and joint infections before radiographs are positive. With osteomyelitis, 3-phase bone scans show increased vascularity on the dynamic flow and blood pool phases and increased uptake in the bone on the delayed static images done 2 to 4 hours after the injection (Fig. 1). When necessary, a scan can be done 24 hours after injection, which may show an increasing ratio of bone to background uptake. If the dynamic flow and blood pool scans show increased vascularity and the delayed static images do not show increased uptake within the bone, the diagnosis may be cellulitis without osteomyelitis. Soft-tissue infections, ulcers, and inflammation can produce edema or even periostitis in the adjacent bone, causing increased uptake on delayed images simulating osteomyelitis. Limiting the specificity of the bone scan for infection is the fact that numerous conditions, including fractures and tumors, also show similar increases in vascularity and uptake on a 3-phase bone scan. In septic arthritis, there is diffuse increased vascularity on the dynamic flow and blood pool phases and increased uptake on delayed static images around the entire joint. The diffuse increased uptake within

the bone may be due to hyperemia or to bone reaction due to early destructive changes in the bone from the infection.

Various radionuclides have been developed in an attempt to increase the specificity of diagnosing infection. Gallium 67 localizes in infection due to a number of factors, including uptake in neutrophils and bacteria, binding to lactoferrin, increased capillary permeability, and increased vascularity. Unfortunately, ^{67}Ga also localizes in tumors, fractures, and in other areas of increased bone turnover similarly to but less intense than on bone scans. To improve the specificity of the gallium scan it should be compared with a bone scan. Mismatch, that is, incongruity between areas of increased uptake on the gallium scan that are not present on the bone scan, or higher uptake on the gallium scan than on the bone scan are evidence of infection (Fig. 9). However, these findings are only present in about 25% to 33% of the cases of infection.

White blood cell or leukocyte scanning with indium 111 or ^{99m}Tc hexamethyl propylene amine oxine (HMPAO) can be used to scan for infection. These scans require obtaining a sample of the patient's blood, labeling the white blood cells or leukocytes in vitro, and then reinjecting them into the

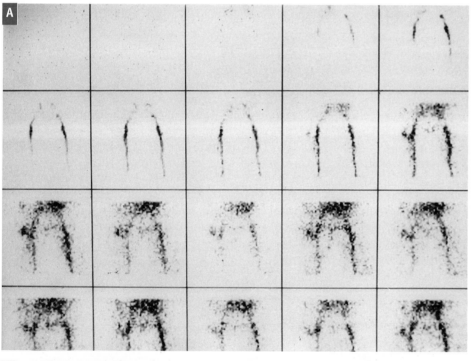

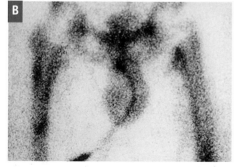

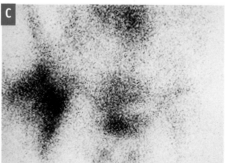

Figure 9

A bone scan in an infected right total hip prosthesis shows increased vascularity on the flow (**A**) and increased uptake diffusely around the right hip prosthesis on the delayed static image (**B**). A gallium scan showed high uptake in the right hip that was not matched by the bone scan (**C**).

patient. The white blood cells with the radioisotope label migrate to the site of the infection. Indium-labeled white blood cell scanning is done 24 hours after injection. Technetium-labeled white blood cell scanning is done 3 or 4 hours after injection. Unlike bone scans and gallium scans, in the absence of infection white blood cells generally do not show increased uptake at the site of increased bone turnover. However, there is uptake in bone marrow. If a white blood cell scan shows an area of increased uptake, a ^{99m}Tc sulfur colloid bone marrow scan may be done and compared with the white blood cell scan to look for areas of incongruity or mismatch. Sites that show increased uptake of white blood cells but do not show uptake on the colloid scan are indicative of infection. The combination of white blood cell scanning with bone marrow scanning with colloids increases the specificity for infection.

In cases of acute infection or abscess where there is an accumulation of white blood cells, a diagnosis of infection can be made more readily than in chronic infections, where there are relatively few neutrophils or white cells. Increasing ratios of white blood cell uptake to background in a 24-hour scan as compared with a 4-hour scan may help in diagnosis of infection. Infections of the spine may show either normal, increased, or commonly decreased uptake of radiolabeled white blood cells.

New radionuclide techniques in which infectious processes can be localized with radioisotopes in vivo without the need for labeling autologous blood in vitro have been developed but have not yet been approved for clinical use in the United States. These agents are labeled with either ^{111}In or ^{99m}Tc. Radiolabeled chemotactic peptides show high uptake at the site of infection shortly after injection, most likely due to binding to receptors in the locally present leukocytes. Technetium ^{99m}Tc nanocolloid accumulates in infection through increased capillary permeability and capillary leakage. The nanocolloid will continue to leak into the extra capillary space even in cases of long-standing infection, so nanocolloid may be superior to white blood cell imaging in chronic infection. Radioisotope-labeled monoclonal anti-granulocyte antibodies, polyclonal immunoglobulins (Ig) G and M, localize in the site of infection, also because of increased capillary permeability and capillary leakage. These agents have relatively slow accumulation into the lesion, and relatively slow clearance from the soft tissues and blood. This scenario may cause a delay in the time in which the scan will be positive, in turn delaying a diagnosis. None of the radionuclide imaging methods can differentiate infection from noninfectious inflammatory processes. Different imaging methods may be necessary for different types of infections, whether acute or chronic, peripheral or axial.

Osteonecrosis

Bone scanning with ^{99m}Tc phosphonate complexes has been shown to be more sensitive than radiography but less sensitive than MRI in the diagnosis of osteonecrosis. Paradoxically, increased vascularity on flow and blood pool phases and increased uptake on delayed static images are common in osteonecrosis. In nontraumatic osteonecrosis, revascularization and a repair process are occurring by the time the patient is symptomatic. Hyperemia during revascularization causes increased radiotracer activity in the early phase. New bone is formed as a result of creeping substitution. This new bone is deposited on the dead trabeculae of the necrotic bone, causing increased uptake on the delayed static images (Fig. 10). Osteonecrosis may lead to bone marrow edema, which causes marked increased vascularity and uptake on the bone scan in an area larger than the actual zone of necrosis. The condition may have an appearance similar to other causes of bone marrow edema, such as transient osteoporosis, bone bruise, insufficiency fracture infection, and neoplasm. Collapse of the bone due to fracture through the necrotic area also leads to increased uptake on the bone scan. Areas of decreased uptake or photopenic areas may be present, surrounded by a rim of increased uptake. This condition is best seen in the femoral head and is diagnostic of osteonecrosis (Fig. 11).

With fractures of the femoral neck, scaphoid, and talus, the blood supply may be interrupted, leading to posttraumatic osteonecrosis. The avascularity can be detected on ^{99m}Tc phosphate complex bone scans; vascular flow and uptake are absent, as interruption of the blood supply from the fracture prevents the radioisotope from reaching the area (Fig. 12). Radiographic and even MRI changes typical of osteonecrosis may be apparent only months later.

Bone marrow imaging with ^{99m}Tc or ^{111}In colloid has been used in the past in the diagnosis of posttraumatic osteonecrosis, as an adequate blood supply is needed for colloid to reach the bone marrow. The colloid scans are difficult to interpret because the amount of bone marrow varies in each patient. Image quality on bone marrow scans is poor because most of the radiocolloid is taken up in the

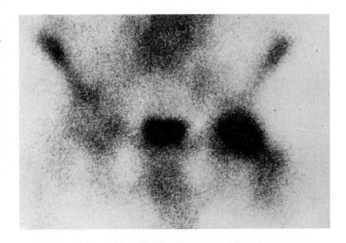

Figure 10

There is high uptake in the left femoral head due to osteonecrosis.

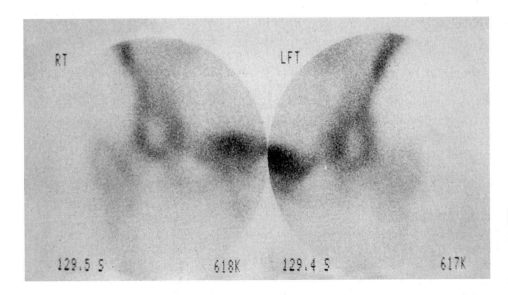

liver and spleen, and relatively little radionuclide enters the bone marrow.

Legg-Calvé-Perthes (LCP) disease may be recognized on bone scans before radiographs are considered abnormal. In early LCP disease, the bone scan shows decreased vascularity and uptake in the entire femoral head (Fig. 3). In later stages of the disease, revascularization occurs and increased uptake may be seen in the metaphyseal region of the femoral neck with normal uptake restored in the femoral head. In most instances, LCP disease can be distinguished from transient synovitis by bone scan; however, in some cases, transient synovitis may cause decreased vascularity and uptake in the femoral head due to compression of the blood vessels. This condition may be relieved by aspiration of the joint.

Arthritis

Early attempts at evaluating arthritis with radioisotope scanning involved the use of radiolabeled albumin and ^{99m}Tc pertechnetate. Synovitis, especially the acute proliferative type, causes increased vascularity that can be detected by the blood pool markers taken up in inflamed synovium. These vascular markers are seldom used clinically now because they have been replaced by routine bone scanning with ^{99m}Tc phosphonate complexes, which have been shown to be more sensitive, although not specific for arthritis. In arthritis, the flow and blood pool phases of a bone scan demonstrate the increased vascularity present with synovitis. Delayed static images show diffuse increased uptake due to hyperemia and increased bone turnover from bony erosions, or from proliferative changes in seronegative spondylopathies or osteoarthritis. In osteoarthritis, the early vascular phases may be normal if synovitis or hypermia is not present. Synovitis, however, may occur in osteoarthritis and cause abnormality in all 3 phases. Osteoarthritis has a tendency to show asymmetric uptake of radioisotope in the joint, reflecting the sites of involvement; inflammatory arthritis tends to show diffuse increased uptake around the entire joint (Fig. 13). In conditions such as lupus erythematosus in which arthralgia is present without acute proliferative synovitis, bony erosions, or proliferative changes, the bone scan is normal. The hallmark of arthritis that helps distinguish it from other conditions such as fractures and tumors is uptake on both sides of the joint on the bone scan.

The sacroiliac joints normally show higher uptake of radio-

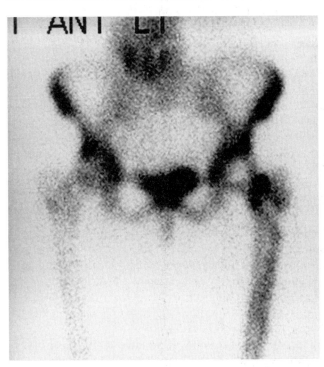

In a patient with an ununited fracture of the femoral neck that has been pinned, there is absent uptake of radionuclide in the femoral head, indicating avascularity.

nuclide than other areas of the skeleton. Asymmetric increased uptake due to unilateral sacroiliitis can be readily detected visually or by quantitative evaluation with regions of interest over the 2 sacroiliac joints. Symmetrical increased uptake may be difficult to determine visually. Quantitative studies have been done with regions of interest placed over the right and left sacroiliac joints and the body of the sacrum with ratios of number of counts taken from each site. Overlap in these ratios between normal and abnormal patients have been shown in some studies, making diagnosis of symmetrical sacroiliitis by quantitative sacroiliac bone scanning not reliable.

In the acute phase of reflex sympathetic dystrophy syndrome (RSDS), there is diffuse increased vascularity and uptake of radionuclide in all 3 phases of the bone scan. In the subacute phase, blood flow may be normal with increased uptake seen on delayed images. In the late or atrophic phase of RSDS, there may be normal or decreased vascularity and uptake on the bone scan.

Pain With Joint Prostheses

Three-phase radionuclide scanning may be done to evaluate painful prosthetic joint replacement. Pain may be caused by infection, mechanical loosening, or fracture, all of which may be detected by bone scans.

Increased vascularity is present for several months after surgery, and increased uptake of radionuclide on delayed static images occurs for approximately 1 year or more. Studies of cemented hip prostheses have shown that uptake usually returns to normal in about 1 year; however, in about 20% of the cases there is continued increased uptake around portions of the femoral component, including the distal stem and greater and lesser trochanters, for

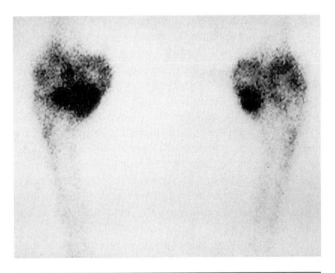

Figure 13

There is increased uptake in the medial compartments of the right and left knees that is most intense in the medial tibial plateaus, representing osteoarthritis.

more than 1 year. In noncemented femoral components, there is often increased uptake at the distal stem for many years after the surgery. With knee prostheses, there may be continued increased uptake around the medial and lateral tibial plateau for more than 1 year after surgery.

Early during the course of infection, radiographs are usually normal because it takes time for infectious loosening to occur. With infection, there is increased vascularity on the flow and blood pool scans and increased uptake on delayed static images around the prosthesis (Fig. 14). This pattern of diffuse increased vascularity and uptake around a painful prosthesis more than 1 year after surgery is suggestive of infection, especially if radiographs are normal. Focal increased uptake may also occur in infected prostheses, similar to that which occurs with mechanical loosening.

In mechanical loosening, motion of the prosthesis causes increased bone turnover, which is most likely caused by bone resorption resulting in localized increased uptake of radionuclide. Blood flow and blood pool scans are often normal. When a femoral component of a total hip prosthesis comes loose, increased uptake occurs around the tip of the distal stem of the prosthesis as a result of motion that causes reactive bone formation. Increased uptake around the greater and lesser trochanters alone may be a normal postoperative change and is not a sign of loosening. When mechanical loosening is advanced, radiographs show extensive abnormalities and the bone scan may show diffuse increased vascularity and uptake around the entire prosthesis. This condition may appear identical to infectious loosening.

Stress transmitted through the prosthesis to the bone causes new bone formation at the site. This is seen as a localized area of increased uptake on the bone scan, and is most common on the lateral aspect of the distal stem of the femoral component of the hip prosthesis. Radiographs will usually show cortical thickening at the site, indicating stress rather than mechanical loosening. Stress changes may occur in other sites around femoral components, especially with noncemented components indicating sites of stress transmission. Stress fractures also show focal increased uptake.

Insufficiency stress fractures may be the cause of pain around joint prostheses in patients who are osteopenic. These fractures may occur in the pubic rami in patients who have hip replacements, and cause pain in the groin simulating pain from the hip joint. Posterior pain may be caused by insufficiency fractures of the sacrum. These fractures may not be readily detectable on radiographs, but bone scanning assists in diagnosis.

Although bone scanning is sensitive for diagnosing infection around total joint prostheses, it is not specific. As discussed previously, infectious scanning agents such as ^{67}Ga citrate or radiolabeled white blood cells are more specific for infection than bone scans, but these agents have limitations.

Radionuclide arthrography has been shown to be useful

for detecting mechanical loosening of prostheses, especially femoral components of total hip prostheses and tibial components of total knee prostheses. Technetium 99m sulfur colloid is injected into the joint and scans are done at least 1 hour later, so that there is ample time for the radionuclide to dissect into the cement-bone or metal-bone interface around the prosthetic component. The radiolabeled colloid does not have significant uptake in the bloodstream and is not deposited in the bone as in a bone scan. The evaluation of acetabular components of total hip prostheses and femoral components of total knee prostheses is made difficult by radionuclide in the joint pseudocapsule. Radionuclide arthrography, however, is not widely used in clinical practice.

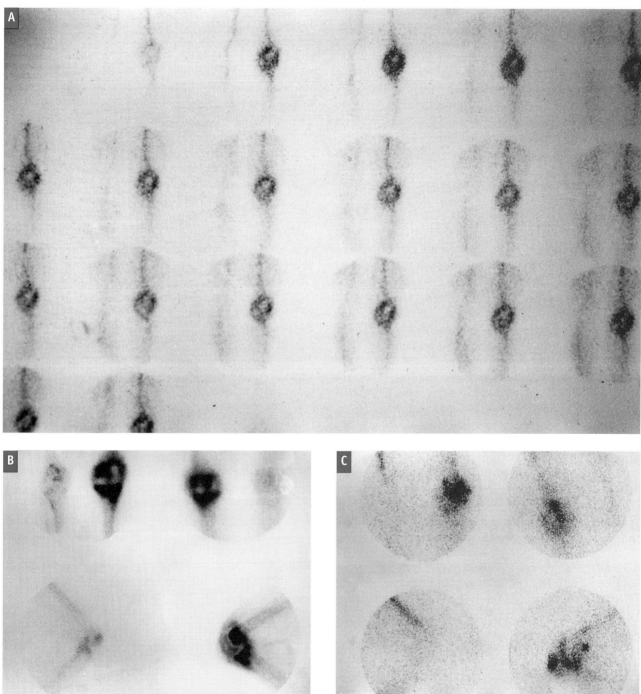

Figure 14

In a patient with an infected left total knee prosthesis, there is increased vascularity on the flow (**A**) and increased uptake diffusely around the left total knee prosthesis on the delayed static images (**B**), even though the patient's radiographs were normal. An indium-111 white blood count scan (**C**) shows high uptake around the prosthesis not matched by the bone scan.

Use of Radioisotopes in Orthopaedic Research

Both long- and short-lived radioisotopes are used in the basic science and clinical study of orthopaedic disorders. Compounds labeled with radioisotopes possessing half-lives of 12.33 (tritium) and 5730 years (carbon 14) are used most often in orthopaedic research to monitor the synthesis and breakdown of extracellular matrix components of cartilage and bone, including collagen, proteoglycans, and glycosaminoglycans, either in vitro or in tissue explants (ex vivo). Calcium 45 with a half-life of 6 months is used to assess hydroxyapatite mineral formation as well as its breakdown. Sulfur 35 is an isotope with a comparatively short radioactive half-life (87.4 days) that is used to quantitate the sulfation of 1 class of proteoglycans in vitro or ex vivo. Each of these isotopes is a weak beta emitter (Table 1) with a distinct energy spectrum that can facilitate double labeling studies (see below). Isotopes in this group are thus safe to handle with minimal external exposure to the investigator, because only the most energetic beta particles in the decay spectrum of ^{45}Ca (>0.2 MeV) are capable of penetrating skin. In contrast, ^{32}P, a moderate to strong beta emitter often used in other areas of biomedical research (such as the labeling of DNA for gene expressions studies), produces radiation with average and maximum energies that are each 10 times those of other isotopes listed in Table 1.

Tritiated proline has been routinely used to measure collagen, an important component of the extracellular matrix, with the latter serving primarily as a supporting element in both skeletal and connective tissue. As such, pathologic changes that occur in vivo in the turnover (formation and breakdown) of matrix constituents, including the major types of collagen present in bone (type I) and cartilage (type II), are characteristic of degenerative orthopaedic disorders such as osteoporosis, osteoarthritis, and rheumatoid arthritis. Radiotracer studies done in vitro of the biochemical and genetic mechanisms underlying these conditions are facilitated by the comparatively high hydroxyproline/proline ratio found among the collagen family of proteins. This

enrichment of hydroxyproline in the collagen molecule can be exploited by using radiotracer studies with [^{3}H] proline, which, following cellular uptake into cultured cells or tissue explants, is incorporated into newly synthesized collagen and converted by prolyl hydroxylase into [^{3}H] hydroxyprolyl collagen formation or degradation, respectively. In such studies, labeled hydroxyproline in acid hydrolysates of the labeled cells or tissues is counted via liquid scintillation following purifications by chromatography on a Dowex-50 column (rat femur and costal cartilage). Alternatively, tritiated or [^{14}C] hydroxyproline in an acid hydrolysate can first be oxidized to a pyrole in the presence of chloramine and then separated from labeled proline by either toluene extraction (labeled human bone tissue) or silica gel chromatography (chick embryo).

Although hydroxyproline is a more specific marker for collagen, its formation can also be quantified as the content of [^{3}H] proline in collagenase digestible protein (rat calvarium). One study has shown that the newly synthesized collagen labeled with radioactive proline can be isolated by NaCl precipitation of proteins in (human bone) tissue culture medium, digestion of noncollagenous proteins in the precipitate with 10% pepsin, and NaCl precipitation of soluble collagen. Labeled intact collagen obtained in this manner can then be purified by sodium dodecyl sulfate polyacrylamide gel electrophoresis (SDS-PAGE), quantitated by liquid scintillation counting of gel slices, and typed following autoradiography using specific purified collagen standards as markers. This latter method requires ^{14}C proline instead of an isotope of lower energy to obtain optimal imaging on x-ray film. A more recently developed method is based on the trichloroacetic acid precipitation of ^{3}H proline-labeled proteins onto polyvinylidene difluoride membranes in a 96-well plate using bovine adult articular chondrocytes. This technique facilitated the rapid handling of a large number of samples and avoided undesired steps that are characteristic of other precipitation-based methodologies, such as multiple centrifugations and the use of carrier albumin that often interferes with subsequent analyses (such as SDS-PAGE). Because this method provides a relatively nonspecific measure of collagen that can only be

Table 1

Energies and Research Applications of Beta-emitting Radioisotopes

Isotopes	Avg. Energy (MeV)	Max. Energy (MeV)	Use in Orthopaedic Research	Labeled Precursor
H-3	0.005	0.018	Collagen, proteoglycans	Proline, acetate, glucosamine
C-14	0.0049	0.058	Collagen, proteoglycans	Proline, acetate, glucosamine
S-35	0.048	0.167	Proteins, proteoglycans	Sulfate, methionine
Ca-45	0.077	0.257	Mineralization/resorption	Calcium
P-32	0.694	1.71	—	—

applied to the analysis of cartilage, in which 40% to 80% of all proline is found in collagen, more specific methods such as those described above must be used for other tissues.

The content of extracellular matrix constituents of articular cartilage can also be measured through the use of radiolabeled precursor molecules. Other than collagen, whose quantification has already been discussed, these extracellular components of cartilage include nonglycosylated proteins, proteoglycans, and hyaluronic acid, one of several hexosamines or acidic glycosaminoglycans (AGAGs) that is found in connective tissue. Because individual molecules of AGAGs, including hyaluronate, constitute subunits for the assembly of carbohydrate side chains in proteoglycans, AGAG formation is a critical step in the biosynthesis of proteoglycans. As such, AGAGs provide several potential radiolabeling sites for studying both proteoglycan metabolism and the content of free hyaluronic acid.

The major cartilage AGAGs are synthesized as alternating copolymers of β-glucuronic acid (Gluc) and N-acetyl-β-glucosamine (Glu-NH, hyaluronic acid) or N-acetyl-β-galactosamine-6-sulfate; the remainder is sulfated at the 4 position (chondroitin sulfate A). The process of polymerization is catalyzed by glycosyl transferases, and the wide range of molecular weights found for the 2 predominant hexosamines in cartilage may be related either to random chain termination and/or cleavage of a larger molecule after synthesis. The radiolabeled precursors used to measure proteoglycans and AGAGs can be extracted with 4M guanidinium chloride/0.05M sodium acetate buffer in the presence of Triton X-100 detergent and proteinase inhibitors (bovine articular cartilage). AGAGs can also be released from proteoglycans by digestion with pronase or by β-elimination by alkaline borohydride treatment (smooth muscle cells). Proteoglycans and hyaluronic acid can then be purified and separated from other AGAGs on diethylaminoethyl-Sephacel and size determined by gel filtration on Sepharose CL-2B and Sephacryl-1000 (Pharmacia Biotech, Uppsala, Sweden), respectively. Alternatively, hexosamine-containing substances, after an initial solvent extraction, can be further fractionated with cetylpyridinium chloride to separate AGAGs and proteoglycans, followed by separation of chondroitin-6 sulfate from hyaluronic acid and other AGAGs by 2-dimensional electrophoresis (fibroblasts). Radiolabeled glucosamine can also be used to successfully label chondroitin sulfates (presumably by isomerization to galactosamine after cellular uptake). In the latter study, the activity of hyaluronic acid synthetase released by fibroblasts made permeable by 1 freeze-thaw cycle was also measured by incubation with uridine diphosphate (UDP)-[^{14}C]-N-acetylglucosamine in the presence of UDP-glucuronic acid. In addition, the AGAG content of extracted labeled proteoglycans can be quantified by treatment with AGAG-degrading enzymes such as hyaluronidase or chondroitin lyase and measurement of the soluble radioactivity in trichloroacetic acid

precipitates of the undigested proteins.

Direct comparisons between the effects of a given treatment on the synthesis of each species of AGAG can be made by labeling control cultures with [^{14}C] glucosamine and treated cultures with tritiated glucosamine, combining the 2 cultures, and measuring the [^{3}H]/[^{14}C] ratios in the various AGAG fractions. This double-label technique corrects for differences in overall basal turnover between different AGAGs to allow direct comparisons using [^{14}C] radioactivity as an internal standard. Other types of experiments that measure proteoglycan breakdown to release AGAGs use techniques involving a labeling period, wash of cultures to remove label, and incubation of cultures in label-free media (often in the presence of some physiologic or pharmacologic stimulus to breakdown) and measurements of the individual radioactivities of proteoglycans and free AGAGs in both the tissue and medium (bovine calf cartilage). Routine labeling of the protein core of proteoglycans with [^{3}H; ^{35}S] methionine and size characterization by gel chromatography can be performed. It is even possible to use double labeling techniques with glucosamine and methionine tagged with distinct isotopes differing enough in energy (^{3}H versus ^{14}C or ^{45}S) to allow comparisons between the size distribution of the proteoglycan core proteins and that of the carbohydrate side chains in the same sample by gel filtration.

Finally, both the processes of mineralization and resorption are routinely assessed by measuring the uptake or release of calcium 45 in the skeleton, explants of bone, and cell cultures. By combining radiotracer techniques with total calcium measurements by atomic absorption spectophotometry, both formation and resorption can be quantified. Following the bolus injection of laboratory animals with ^{45}Ca and the long-term daily administration of drug treatment, bones from sacrificed animals were harvested, defatted, dehydrated, and ashed in a muffle furnace. In this manner, effects of treatments in vivo on the total mass of calcium resorbed could be computed by multiplying basal mean calcium (atomic absorption) by the percentage of basal ^{45}Ca release from prelabeled bone. Bone formation (total calcium deposition) is then quantified as the sum of the mass of calcium resorbed (calculated as above) and the net increase in the calcium mass of each bone (atomic absorption).

Alternatively, effects of treatments in vitro on the resorptive process can be measured in incubations with calvaria prelabeled by injection of fetal rats with ^{45}Ca. Using this method, the release of ^{45}Ca into the calvaria culture media is calculated as a percentage of total radioactivity in the bone (after digestion overnight in the trichloroacetic acid). Bone formation in vivo has also been measured as the incorporation of injected ^{45}Ca into rat tibia in the absence of total mass measurements. In a more recent study, calvaria bone cells were isolated, pulsed in vitro with ^{45}Ca in the presence of a pharmacologic agent and repeatedly washed-chased to allow the release of the rapidly exchangeable fraction of cellular ^{45}Ca. The remaining radioactivity incorporated into the cell layers was then quantified as an index of mineral deposition.

The most frequent experimental method of measuring blood flow to bone in animals is the use of radioisotope-labeled microspheres. The microspheres are resin particles with a cross-sectional diameter slightly greater than the diameter of capillaries. The radioactive microspheres are injected into the left heart and are trapped by the tissue in the first passage. Blood is extracted from an artery at a known rate. The number of microspheres in bone tissue samples and in the extracted blood can be determined by the amount of radioactivity. The number of microspheres in the bone tissue is related to the blood flow to the tissue. Blood flow can be calculated by the following equation:

$$\text{Blood flow} = \frac{\text{Microspheres in tissue} \times \text{withdrawal rate of blood}}{\text{Microspheres in blood}}$$

Radioisotopes for Therapy

Treatment of Pain From Bone Metastases

Intravenous injection of radioisotopes can be used to palliate the pain from bone metastases. The radioisotope concentrates in the bone metastasis and delivers a high dose of beta radiation to the tumor, with much lower doses to normal tissue. The maximum range in mm in soft tissue is approximately equal to the maximum energy in MeV times 5, which gives a range of up to several mm. The radioisotopes used are either directly taken up by bone, or are tagged to carriers that are taken up by bone. Radiopharmaceuticals that have been used include phosphorus P 32 orthophosphate, strontium Sr 89 chloride, samarium Sm 153 EDTMP, rhenium Re 186 HEDP, and Tin Sn 117m DTPA. A bone scan is used to determine if the bone metastases have increased uptake of radioisotope. Only those lesions that show increased uptake on a bone scan can be treated with this therapy. The treatment is only for reduction in pain and not for cure or destruction of the lesion. Reduction in pain occurs within several days to several weeks after treatment, and lasts for up to 6 months. Pain relief is often short-term, however, with an increase in pain sometimes occurring for several days after treatment. Pain from pathologic fractures or sources other than the metastatic lesions themselves can not be treated with this method. Temporary myelosuppression to some degree occurs with the use of most of these radioisotopes.

Radioisotope Synovectomy

Intra-articular injection of radioisotopes can be used for synovectomy with results that are thought to be comparable with those obtained from open surgical and arthroscopic synovectomy (Table 2). Radiation synovectomy is especially applicable in conditions that have not responded to conservative therapy or where the costs and risks of surgery are high. Radioisotope synovectomy has been shown to reduce synovitis and bleeding in over 70% of cases in which it has been used. Clinical improvement occurs approximately 3 months after injection. Synovectomy is most useful in the early stages of arthritis. It is not helpful in relieving pain because of arthritic destruction of articular cartilage. Radioisotopes that are predominantly beta emitters are preferred because they produce radiation with a soft-tissue penetrance of less than 1 cm that can radiate the synovium but does not radiate the whole body. There is, however, potential for leakage out of the joint after intra-articular injection, into lymph nodes and, to a lesser degree, into blood vessels and the liver.

Table 2		
Radioisotopes Used for Synovectomy		
Radionuclide	Half-life (days)	Range (mm)
P-32	14	7.9
Dy-165	0.1	5.7
Y-90	2.7	11.1
Au-198	2.7	3.8
Re-186	3.7	4.5
Sm-153	1.9	0.8

The radioisotopes are injected in colloid or particulate form to decrease leakage out of the joint. Larger particles have less leakage than smaller ones. Gold 198 was the first radioisotope used for synovectomy; however, up to 48% of injected activity was found to leak into draining lymph nodes. Phosphorus P 32 chromic phosphate, dysprosium Dy 165 ferric hydroxide macroaggregates, and samarium Sm 153 and rhenium Re 186 particulate hydroxyapatite have larger particles than gold Au 198 and yttrium Y 90 colloids and have low levels of extra-articular leakage.

Summary

Radioisotopes provide methods for studying the physiology of the musculoskeletal system for research and for clinical diagnosis. Bone scanning is a sensitive method for detecting many of the abnormalities affecting bones and joints, including neoplastic disease, infection, fracture, osteonecrosis, and arthritis. Specificity, however, is more limited because many of these abnormalities cause similar findings on a bone scan. Specificity can be improved by interpreting the findings on bone scanning in a clinical context of history, physical examination, and radiographic findings. The pattern of abnormal uptake can also help in diagnosis in some cases. Radionuclides developed for diagnosing infection are still limited in differentiating infection from noninfectious inflammatory disease. MRI provides sensitivity as good as or better than radionuclide bone scanning in many of the abnormalities of bones and joints, and usually better specificity as there is good anatomic detail of bones, joint, and soft-tissue structures. Bone scanning, however, is still useful because it can provide a whole body study to detect abnormalities that may not be included in the area scanned by MRI.

Radioisotopes have a relatively small role in therapy for musculoskeletal disease. Radioisotope synovectomy can be used as an alternative to open surgical or arthroscopic synovectomy. Radioisotope therapy can lead to temporary palliation of pain in some patients with bony metastases.

Selected Bibliography

Radioisotopes in Orthopaedic Diagnosis

Christensen SB: Osteoarthrosis: Changes of bone, cartilage and synovial membrane in relation to bone scintigraphy. *Acta Orthop Scand* 1985;214(suppl):56:1–43.

Collier BD Jr, Fogelman I, Rosenthall L (eds): *Skeletal Nuclear Medicine*. St. Louis, MO, Mosby Year Book, 1996.

Gosfield E III, Alavi A, Kneeland B: Comparison of radionuclide bone scans and magnetic resonance imaging in detecting spinal metastases. *J Nucl Med* 1993;34:2191–2198.

Holder LE, Schwarz C, Wernicke PG, Michael RH: Radionuclide bone imaging in the early detection of fractures of the proximal femur (hip): Multifactorial analysis. *Radiology* 1990;174:509–515.

Magnuson JE, Brown ML, Hauser MF, Berquist TH, Fitzgerald RH Jr, Klee GG: In-111-labeled leukocyte scintigraphy in suspected orthopedic prosthesis infection: Comparison with other imaging modalities. *Radiology* 1988;168:235–239.

Merkel KD, Brown ML, Dewanjee MK, Fitzgerald RH Jr: Comparison of indium-labeled-leukocyte imaging with sequential technetium-gallium scanning in the diagnosis of low-grade musculoskeletal sepsis: A prospective study. *J Bone Joint Surg* 1985;67A:465-476.

Miniaci A, Bailey WH, Bourne RB, et al: Analysis of radionuclide arthrograms, radiographic arthrograms, and sequential plain radiographs in the assessment of painful hip arthroplasty. *J Arthroplasty* 1990;5:143–149.

O'Connor MK, Brown ML, Hung JC, Hayostek RJ: The art of bone scintigraphy: Technical aspects. *J Nucl Med* 1991;32:2332–2341.

Palestro CJ, Kim CK, Swyer AJ, Capozzi JD, Solomon RW, Goldsmith SJ: Total-hip arthroplasty: Periprosthetic indium-111-labeled leukocyte activity and complementary technetium-99m-sulfur colloid imaging in suspected infection. *J Nucl Med* 1990;31:1950–1955.

Palestro CJ, Kim CK, Swyer AJ, Vallabhajosula S, Goldsmith SJ: Radionuclide diagnosis of vertebral osteomyelitis: Indium-111-leukocyte and technetium-99m-methylene diphosphonate bone scintigraphy. *J Nucl Med* 1991;32:1861–1865.

Rupani HD, Holder LE, Espinola DA, Engin SI: Three-phase radionuclide bone imaging in sports medicine. *Radiology* 1985;156:187–196.

Spitz J, Lauer I, Tittel K, Wiegand H: Scintimetric evaluation of remodeling after bone fractures in man. *J Nucl Med* 1993;34:1403–1409.

Tsan MF: Mechanism of gallium-67 accumulation in inflammatory lesions. J Nucl Med 1985;26:88–92.

Radioisotopes in Orthopaedic Research

Anagnostou F, Plas C, Forest N: Ecto-alkaline phosphatase considered as levamisole-sensitive phosphohydrolase at physiological pH range during mineralization in cultured fetal calvaria cells. *J Cell Biochem* 1996;60:484–494.

Bockman RS, Guidon PT Jr, Pan LC, Salvatori R, Kawaguchi A: Gallium nitrate increases type I collagen and fibronectin mRNA and collagen protein levels in bone and fibroblast cells. *J Cell Biochem* 1993;52:396–403.

Deudon E, Berrou E, Breton M, Picard J: Growth-related production of proteoglycans and hyaluronic acid in synchronous arterial smooth muscle cells. *Int J Biochem* 1992;24:465–470.

Firschein HE, Alcock NW: Rate of removal of collagen and mineral from bone and cartilage. *Metabolism* 1969;18:115–119.

Juva K, Prockop DJ: Modified procedure for the assay of H-3- or C-14-labeled hydroxyproline. *Anal Biochem* 1966;15:77–83.

Koyano Y, Hammerle H, Mollenhauer: J. Analysis of 3H-proline-labeled protein by rapid filtration in multiwell plates for the study of collagen metabolism. *Biotechniques* 1997;22:706-708, 710–712, 714.

Krishnamra N, Seemoung J: Effects of acute and long-term administration of prolactin on bone 45Ca uptake, calcium deposit, and calcium resorption in weaned, young, and mature rats. *Can J Physiol Pharmacol* 1996;74:1157–1165.

Murota S, Abe M, Otsuka K: Stimulatory effect of prostaglandins on the production of hexosamine-containing substances by cultured fibroblasts (3) induction of hyaluronic acid synthetase by prostaglandin F2 alpha. *Prostaglandins* 1977;14:983–991.

Ng CK, Handley CJ, Mason RM, Robinson HC: Synthesis of hyaluronate in cultured bovine articular cartilage. *Biochem J* 1989;263:761–767.

Rocher W, Hostert E, Dietz G, Bartholmes P: De novo synthesis of type-I collagen in bone biopsy material. *J Orthop Res* 1995;13:649–654.

Sah RL, Doong JY, Grodzinsky AJ, Plaas AH, Sandy JD: Effects of compression on the loss of newly synthesized proteoglycans and proteins from cartilage explants. *Arch Biochem Biophys* 1991;286:20–29.

Shaughnessy SG, Young E, Deschamps P, Hirsh J: The effects of low molecular weight and standard heparin on calcium loss from fetal rat calvaria. *Blood* 1995;86:1368–1373.

Svanberg M, Knuuttila M: Dietary xylitol retards bone resorption in rats. *Miner-Electrolyte-Metab* 1994;20:153–157.

Radioisotopes for Therapy

Clunie G, Lui D, Cullum I, Edwards JC, Ell PJ: Samarium-153-particulate hydroxyapatite radiation synovectomy: Biodistribution data for chronic knee synovitis. *J Nucl Med* 1995;36:51–57.

Newman AP: Synovectomy, in Kelley WN, Harris ED Jr, Ruddy S, Sledge CB (eds): *Textbook of Rheumatology*, ed 4. Philadelphia, PA, WB Saunders Co; 1993, pp 649–670.

Papatheofanis FJ: Quantitation of biochemical markers of bone resorption following strontium-89-chloride therapy for metastatic prostatic carcinoma. *J Nucl Med* 1997;38:1175–1179.

Silberstein EB: Treatment of the pain of bone metastases, in Collier BD Jr, Fogelman I, Rosenthall L (eds): *Skeletal Nuclear Medicine*. St. Louis, MO, Mosby Year Book, 1996, pp 469–474.

Sledge CB, Atcher RW, Shortkroff SA, Anderson RJ, Bloomer WD, Hurson BJ: Intra-articular radiation synovectomy. *Clin Orthop* 1984;182:37–40.

Chapter 12

Pulmonary Distress and Thromboembolic Conditions Affecting Orthopaedic Practice

Carol D. Morris, MD, MS

William S. Creevy, MD

Thomas A. Einhorn, MD

This chapter at a glance

This chapter will discuss the pathophysiology, prevention, and treatment of conditions that commonly lead to pulmonary distress in orthopaedic surgical practice.

Introduction

Respiratory deterioration is a well-recognized complication following orthopaedic trauma and orthopaedic operations. Venous thromboembolism and fat embolism syndrome are major causes of morbidity and mortality after long bone fractures and certain orthopaedic procedures. This chapter will address the basic scientific principles that underlie the interactions between the pulmonary and musculoskeletal systems. Specifically, the pathophysiology, prevention, and treatment of conditions that commonly lead to pulmonary distress in orthopaedic surgical practice will be discussed.

Fat Embolism Syndrome

Fat embolism syndrome (FES) refers to a distinct entity in which there is unanticipated respiratory compromise secondary to the mechanical and biochemical effects of fat emboli to the lungs. It can occur in the traumatic setting as well as in nontraumatic conditions, including diabetes mellitus, burns, severe infections, inhalation of anesthesia, chronic pancreatitis, osteomyelitis, cardiopulmonary bypass, sickle cell anemia, renal infarction, fatty liver, acute decompression sickness, liposuction, and parenteral lipid infusion. In addition, FES has been observed following certain orthopaedic procedures that involve instrumentation of the medullary canal, such as total hip and knee arthroplasty and intramedullary fracture stabilization.

It is important to distinguish between fat embolism and FES because the mere presence of intravascular fat is not synonymous with FES. Fat embolism refers to the presence of fat globules in the lung parenchyma and peripheral circulation, most commonly following long-bone fractures or other major trauma. Fat embolism itself is quite common and can be detected in over 90% of patients with long-bone fractures. Classic FES is a multisystem disorder that represents the most serious manifestation of fat embolism. The pathoclinical triad for FES occurs as respiratory distress, neurologic decompensation, and skin petechia, usually occurring 12 to 24 hours after skeletal trauma. Most series report the prevalence of FES in up to 3% of patients with isolated lower extremity fractures, 5% to 10% of patients with multiple long-bone or pelvic fractures, and less than 1% of patients after total hip or knee arthroplasty. It is likely that these numbers are representative of some part of the continuum of FES and not likely fulminant disease. The mortality of FES is estimated at 10% to 20%.

Pathophysiology

The understanding of the end-organ damage caused by fat embolism is incomplete. Mechanical and biochemical theories for the genesis of FES have been proposed, and it is likely that both contribute to this condition. The mechanical theory proposes that when fat cells are disrupted, such as in traumatic violation of the medullary canal, they are extruded into the venous circulation via nearby torn vessels. A transient rise in intramedullary pressure (IMP) above venous pressure allows the fat cells to enter the venous circulation where they travel to the pulmonary vascular bed, are deposited, and are trapped as emboli. It has been clearly demonstrated that the fat (as well as other marrow elements) found in the lungs resembles marrow fat. The smaller vessels of the lung, on the order of 20 μm, become mechanically occluded by fat emboli. The obstruction is made worse by the adherence of platelets and fibrin to the fat globule, causing a plug. Some fat droplets may pass through the lungs and reach the systemic circulation, causing embolic phenomena at distant sites such as the kidney, brain, or retina.

The biochemical theory proposes that lung lipases hydrolyze the innocuous neutral fat emboli to chemically toxic free fatty acids. The free fatty acids trigger an inflammatory cascade of mediator-related effects, leading to endothelial damage, inactivation of lung surfactant, and an increase in capillary permeability. These events lead to interstitial pulmonary edema, which provides an adult respiratory distress syndrome (ARDS)-like picture. The significance of the conversion to fatty acids is supported by numerous animal models in which the injection of neutral fats into the bloodstream increased pulmonary vascular resistance but failed to elicit alterations in parameters indicative of distributed gas exchange and, hence, pulmonary function. The biochemical theory is further supported by the release of various humoral factors (thromboxane, prostaglandins, catecholamines) after severe trauma that act to mobilize circulating and stored free fatty acids, exert vasoactive responses, and activate hemostatic pathways, which, in turn, directly assault lung tissues.

Why certain trauma patients develop FES and others do not remains unclear. A large number of trauma patients (30% to 50%) develop hypoxemia as evidenced by an arterial oxygen tension less than 980 mm Hg on room air. This transient hypoxemia is most likely caused by subclinical pulmonary fat emboli. It has been hypothesized that a predisposing or aggravating condition, such as shock, hypovolemia, disseminated intravascular coagulation, sepsis, or preexisting cardiopulmonary dysfunction, must exist for patients to develop FES.

FES after orthopaedic procedures in which the medullary canal is instrumented, such as total joint arthroplasty or prophylactic fixation of impending fractures, has also been studied extensively. Numerous animal and clinical studies in which various techniques such as transesophageal echocardiography and pulmonary hemodynamic monitoring were used, have demonstrated the presence of fat emboli to the lungs during such procedures. As previously stated, for marrow fat to enter the venous circulation, IMP must exceed venous pressure. The physiologic IMP of the femur is about 30 to 50 mm Hg. During reaming of the femoral canal for intramedullary (IM) nail insertion, insertion of the nail for unreamed nailing, or preparation for the canal for noncemented endoprosthetic replacement, IMP peaks of up to 800 mm Hg occur in the distal femur. Plug insertion, cement application, and prosthetic insertion during cemented hip arthroplasty can cause pressures of up to 1,400 mm Hg. As a consequence of the IM hypertension in the femur, fat marrow is released into the venous circulation.

Diagnosis

FES is a diagnosis of exclusion based on a collection of clinical symptoms in the setting of appropriate trauma. Prognosis depends largely on early diagnosis. No single clinical feature or laboratory test establishes the diagnosis of FES. Many of the clinical signs require a high index of suspicion because they can be transient and easily missed. Gurd's criteria for the diagnosis of FES are commonly used, with clinical signs subdivided into major and minor groups. The major criteria include hypoxemia ($PaO_2 < 60$ mm Hg), central nervous system depression, and petechial rash that most often is located in the axilla, conjunctiva, and palate. The minor criteria are tachycardia, pyrexia, fat presence in the urine or sputum, fat emboli in the retina, and unexplained sudden anemia or thrombocytopenia. The diagnosis of FES is made when 1 of the major signs and 4 of the minor signs are present.

Diagnostic studies are largely nonspecific. Electrocardiographic changes may show evidence of right heart strain but are usually absent. The chest radiograph may appear normal initially, with changes ensuing over the next 72 hours. Typically diffuse, bilateral infiltrates are seen that can display an alveolar or interstitial pattern. These patchy infiltrates, sometimes referred to as a snowstorm pattern, can progress until both lung fields are opaque. Laboratory studies such as the arterial blood gas (ABG), hematocrit, platelet count, serum lipase levels, and demonstration of fat globules in the sputum or urine can help establish the diagnosis of FES, although no definitive confirmatory test exists. Of these, the ABG is the most useful. A drop of the Po_2 to less than 50 mm Hg within 72 hours of admission is the most consistent finding in patients with FES. It is clearly important to exclude other treatable causes of hypoxemia including pneumothorax, hemothorax, volume overload, pneumonia, and pulmonary embolus. Most of these can be distinguished on physical examination and a chest radiograph.

More invasive techniques for detecting the presence of fat in lungs have been investigated. These include bronchoalveolar lavage and examination of pulmonary venous samples obtained from a pulmonary artery catheter. Although some small studies and case reports favor their usefulness, it is generally accepted that the presence of fat alone in alveolar tissues is not reliable diagnostic evidence of FES. In addition, serum protein electrophoresis has been studied as an early detection method demonstrating distinct patterns of serum lipoproteins in patients with FES. The usefulness of these more advanced diagnostic tools has yet to be determined.

In addition to the above clinical and laboratory findings, risk factors based on fracture patterns have been examined. There is a higher prevalence of FES in patients with multiple fractures compared to those with an isolated fracture. The distribution of fractures clearly favors the lower extremity, although there are case reports and series demonstrating occurrence of FES in patients with isolated upper extremity fractures. With respect to open versus closed fractures, the data are inconclusive. Historically, it was assumed there was increased risk in the closed fracture population because open fractures were presumed decompressed and, therefore, less likely to embolize. There are enough clinical and animal investigations to dispute this theory.

Prevention and Treatment

There is no specific therapy for FES. Treatment is largely supportive, directed at ensuring proper resuscitation, appropriate management of underlying trauma, and supportive pulmonary care. Perhaps the most important aspect of management is the identification of patients who are at risk for FES to ensure an early diagnosis and intensive symptomatic treatment. In severe cases in which patients exhibit decreasing pulmonary compliance and progressive hypoxemia, the onset of ARDS should be suspected. These patients often require mechanical ventilatory support and continuous positive end-expiratory pressure.

Few pharmacologic agents have been shown to be efficacious in preventing or treating FES. Steroids have been widely, although not universally, accepted as beneficial in treating high-risk patients. They are used on the premise that they decrease capillary permeability by stabilizing capillary and lysosomal membranes and by decreasing the inflammatory reaction caused by free fatty acids. The efficacy of methylprednisolone in the prophylactic treatment of FES has been studied in a number of prospective randomized studies. The data support the value of steroid treatment in reducing the risk of FES and pulmonary dysfunction. However, the safety of this therapy has not been fully elucidated. Life-threatening infection has been implicated as a possible detrimental effect of steroid therapy in patients who are already at increased risk for this complication.

Although it is the responsibility of the entire trauma team to aid in the diagnosis and treatment of FES, certain aspects of the patient's care are directly related to the orthopaedic management. The most investigated topics are early versus delayed fracture fixation and reamed versus unreamed IM nailing.

Numerous clinical investigations have clearly demonstrated the benefit of early pelvic and long-bone fracture stabilization as evidenced by decreased hospital and intensive care unit stays and decreased nonfracture complications, namely pulmonary complications. Most investigations report a several-fold increase in the prevalence of FES in patients treated with delayed fixation versus early fixation (less than 24 to 48 hours). The type of fixation is somewhat more controversial. Early reamed IM fixation in patients with pulmonary injury has been reported to increase the risk of pulmonary injury. These effects seem to be less severe if nailing is performed without reaming. Other authors have reported that patients treated by delayed reamed IM fixation suffered more pulmonary complications than those treated early by the same method even in the presence of blunt thoracic trauma. Regardless of the method of fixation chosen, the literature overwhelmingly supports early fixation in all patients including those with pulmonary contusion and high injury severity scores, regardless of age.

The notion that reaming the femoral canal places patients at an increased risk for the development of fulminant FES has received considerable attention. The pressure changes that take place when a closed portion of the femoral canal is cannulated are perhaps best understood using a hydraulic model. The pressure that the advancing reamer, nail, or alignment guide generates is related to the amount of decompression that can occur from back flow. This is calculated using the gap equation (Fig. 1). As the magnitude of back flow increases, the pressure generated by the device decreases. Two of the important variables can be controlled, namely the gap (h) and the length of the seal (L). The gap is defined as the distance between the endosteal surface and the outer diameter of the reamer, which, according to the equation, is proportional to the flow rate,

or back flow rate, to a power of 3. Simply stated, the design of the reamer has an effect on IM pressure. Short reamers with sharp, deep flutes will allow for greater back flow, less IM hypertension, and, hence, a decreased embolic fat load to the lungs. Another technical aspect of reaming that is under the control of the operating surgeon is the force of reaming. Biomechanical studies have demonstrated that reaming with less compression force can reduce IM pressures to a significant degree.

Taken collectively, the data regarding the outcome of reamed versus unreamed femoral nailing favors reamed nailing with respect to union and technical and implant-related complications. Nonetheless, there are physiologic disadvantages to reaming. Although various clinical investigations have suggested that reaming in multiple trauma patients may suppress pulmonary function, it is difficult at this time to identify a subset of patients whose pulmonary status is tenuous enough to warrant unreamed nailing.

Thromboembolic Disease

Venous thromboembolism remains a major cause of morbidity and mortality among adults after lower extremity orthopaedic surgery. In the United States, each year an estimated 700,000 people experience asymptomatic pulmonary embolism (PE), and 200,000 die from this complication. Approximately 70,000 of these deaths occur within 1 hour of the appearance of symptoms. The magnitude of thromboembolic risk has been well documented in the orthopaedic literature. Patients undergoing hip surgery have the greatest mortality; without anticoagulation therapy, up to 75% will show deep vein thrombosis (DVT) by radiographic criteria, and as many as 20% will develop clinically significant PE with a mortality of 1%. Patients having knee surgery are at significant risk as well. Without anticoagulation therapy, as many as 80% will show asymptomatic DVT by radiographic criteria, and asymptomatic PE will develop in 8% of cases. Fatal PE is less common after knee surgery, occurring in less than 1% of patients. The frequency of DVT and fatal PE in various clinical settings is outlined in Table 1.

Deep venous thrombosis is also a common complication following major trauma. Screening studies using venography found that the incidence of DVT in trauma patients was as high as 58%. This group includes patients whose only major trauma involved the face, chest, or abdomen. For patients with pelvic or long-bone fractures, the rate of DVT approaches 80%. Risk factors associated with DVT in trauma patients include older age, the need for surgery or blood transfusion, lower extremity fractures, and spinal cord injury.

Survival after a thromboembolic event depends heavily on whether the diagnosis is made early and therapy is started promptly. Most patients who die from PE will have had

Table 1
Frequency of Fatal Pulmonary Embolism (PE) and Deep Vein Thrombosis (DVT) (diagnosed by venography)

Unprotected Patients	DVT	Fatal PE
Total hip arthroplasty	70%	1% to 3.4%
Total knee arthroplasty	80%	<1%
Open meniscectomy	20%	?
Hip fracture	60%	3.5%
Spine trauma with paralysis	100%	1%
Polytrauma patients	35% to 58%	?
Pelvic fracture	20% to 60%	?

A

$$Qle = \frac{\pi \cdot dm \cdot h^3 \; \Delta p}{12 \; \eta \cdot L}$$

Qle = flow rate

dm = average diameter of bore and piston

h = gap

Δp = pressure difference

L = length of seal (cm)

η = dynamic viscosity (Ns/m^2)

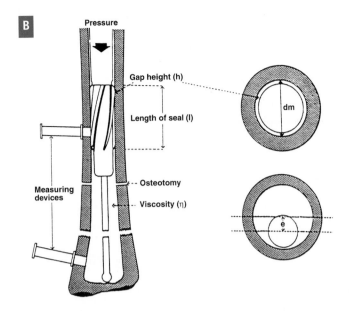

Figure 1

A, The gap equation. **B,** Schematic representation of the values to be entered in the gap equation. (Reproduced with permission from Stürmer K: Measurement of intramedullary pressure in an animal experiment and propositions to reduce the pressure increase. *Injury* 1993;24(suppl 3):S7–S21.)

an otherwise favorable prognosis for their preexisting medical condition, and in these cases, PE is a potentially preventable complication.

The pathophysiology by which venous thromboembolism develops depends on the interaction between biochemical and physiologic events within a specific anatomic milieu. Therefore, this complication must be discussed within the context of defined anatomic sites. Unless otherwise stipulated, this chapter will refer to venous thromboembolic events that occur in the lower extremities after total hip or knee arthroplasty or long-bone or hip fracture surgery.

Coagulation

The coagulation of blood entails the formation of fibrin through the interaction of more than a dozen proteins in a cascading series of proteolytic reactions (Fig. 2). At each step, a clotting factor undergoes limited proteolysis and itself becomes an active protease. Each clotting factor enzyme activates the next clotting factor until an insoluble fibrin clot is formed. Two initially independent pathways (the intrinsic and extrinsic pathways) for the initiation of clot formation converge to share a common clotting pathway. The extrinsic system is activated by the release of thromboplastin into the bloodstream during cell damage. This may occur in the dissection of bone and soft tissue. The intrinsic pathway is activated by the contact of factor XII with collagen on the exposed subendothelium of damaged vessels. Both the intrinsic and extrinsic pathways lead to the formation of factor X. Prothrombin (factor II) is converted to thrombin by activated factor X in the presence of factor V, Ca^{2+}, and phospholipid. Thrombin then catalyzes

the conversion of soluble circulating substrate, fibrinogen (factor I), to fibrin. The clotting cascade can therefore be simplified into 3 stages: (1) triggering of prothrombin converting activity through the intrinsic and extrinsic pathways; (2) converting prothrombin to thrombin; and (3) converting fibrinogen to fibrin by the catalyzing activity of the thrombin complex, during which an initially loose fibrin plug entangles to form a tight fibrin clot in the presence of factor XIII.

The fibrinolytic system prevents clot propagation and allows clot dissolution as healing takes place. In the normal state, there is a very delicate balance between the coagulation and fibrinolytic systems. Without the action of the fibrinolytic system, the fibrin clot would propagate indefinitely. The key element in the fibrinolytic mechanism is the conversion of plasminogen to plasmin. Plasmin dissolves the fibrin stroma and prevents the activation of certain coagulation factors.

Pathogenesis of Venous Thromboembolism

Many factors play a role in maintaining the delicate balance between the coagulation and fibrinolytic systems. Hypercoagulability, venous stasis, and endothelial damage, generally known as Virchow's triad of factors, lead to the generation of a venous thrombosis.

Hypercoagulability exists when coagulation dominates over fibrinolysis. Tissue trauma increases the levels of procoagulating substances, such as collagen fragments, tissue thromboplastin, and fibrinogen, in the plasma and enhances platelet activity and number. These changes tip

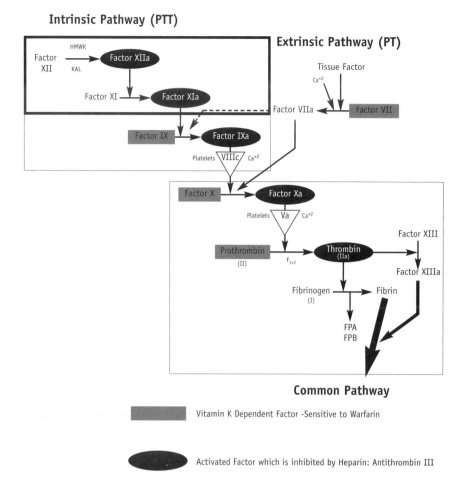

Intrinsic Pathway (PTT)

Extrinsic Pathway (PT)

Common Pathway

Vitamin K Dependent Factor -Sensitive to Warfarin

Activated Factor which is inhibited by Heparin: Antithrombin III

Figure 2

The coagulation pathway. Important features include the contact activation phase, vitamin K-dependent factors (affected by warfarin), and the activated serine proteases that are inhibited by heparin-antithrombin III. Prothrombin measures the function of the extrinsic and common pathways; the partial thromboplastin time measures the function of the intrinsic and common pathways. (Adapted with permission from Stead RB: Regulation of hemostasis, in Goldhaber SZ (ed): *Pulmonary Embolism and Deep Venous Thromboembolism*. Philadelphia, PA, WB Saunders, 1985, p 32.)

the coagulation-fibrinolytic system's balance toward coagulation and, eventually, venous thrombus formation. The patient is in a procoagulant state as soon as the surgical or traumatic event takes place, and thrombosis occurs during the surgical procedure. By measuring indices of thrombogenesis and fibrinolysis at various stages of total hip arthroplasty, the greatest activation of thrombosis was observed to occur during reaming of the femur and insertion of the femoral component, especially a cemented one. There was little activation of thrombosis during the femoral neck osteotomy and surgery on the acetabulum.

Both intrinsic and extrinsic coagulation systems have been implicated in studies concerning DVT and total hip replacement. A significant increase in the circulating levels of prothrombin F1.2, thrombin-antithrombin complexes, and fibrinopeptide A has been noted during preparation of the femur and in impaction of the prosthesis, implicating the activation of thrombin generation. When the femoral component is inserted, tissue thromboplastin from the bone marrow is forced into the venous circulation. This effect is more pronounced when cement is used as supported by a greater rise in mean pulmonary artery pressure during cemented component insertion. Furthermore, an acute drop in the circulating levels of antithrombin III dur-

ing and immediately after total hip replacement surgery has been reported. Antithrombin III is a naturally-occurring inhibitor of thrombin, activated factor X, and possibly other activated factors in the intrinsic system. The depletion of antithrombin III increases the amount of thrombin released during and immediately after surgery, thus creating a favorable environment for thrombus formation. Interestingly, the decrease in antithrombin III and increase in fibrinopeptide A and D-dimer is significantly greater during total hip arthroplasty surgery compared to nonorthopaedic surgery. This observation is consistent with the higher rates of DVT noted after orthopaedic procedures compared to procedures involving laparotomy.

Endothelial damage and venous stasis, the 2 remaining components of the triad, have been documented during hip surgery. Several investigators have demonstrated microscopic evidence of endothelial damage associated with total hip replacement. They postulated that endothelial tears are caused by excessive venodilation, which results from smooth muscle relaxation caused by blood-borne vasoactive substances. This leads to cell separation and exposure of subendothelial collagen. Filling of the long saphenous and femoral veins has been shown to increase during hip dislocation, suggesting a pressure differential across the twisted part of the vein and increasing vasodilation distally as a result of increased intraluminal pressure. This is supported by the observation that once the hip is reduced and hence venous occlusion released, desaturated blood entering the circulation is detectable as a transient reduction in venous oxygen partial pressure in the pulmonary artery. Routine anesthetics, inactivity, and positioning also can have a vasodilatory effect.

Platelets also play a central role in the development of a thrombus because their adhesiveness and activity are increased after tissue trauma. Platelets accumulate behind small valve cusps, where eddy currents arise. An aggregated nidus develops, over which fibrin forms. As fibrin accumulates across the vessel, a clot develops. Platelets also adhere and accumulate in the areas where the subendothelial portions of the veins have been damaged. In addition, fibrin formation is more easily triggered if blood contains procoagulant substances secondary to tissue trauma.

Once vascular damage has occurred and the vessel endothelium has been exposed, the clotting cascade is set into motion. Although clot development may be initiated by these events, it is not known how long a clot continues to propagate and enlarge. Moreover, it is unclear how the use of antithrombotic drugs and physical modalities alter this process. It is well known, however, that physical inactivity significantly favors clot propagation because venous perfusion tends to be reduced. Physical activity leads to increased blood flow. In an area that is perfused with fresh blood, there is a relative dilution in the concentration of activated coagulation and an exposure of these factors to their natural biochemical inhibitors.

Surgery, trauma, obesity, malignancy, myocardial infarction, congestive heart failure, older age, and oral contraceptive use are well-known risk factors for venous thrombosis. Table 2 lists intrinsic and extrinsic factors that cause vascular damage and activate the coagulation pathways. In hip surgery, for example, this may occur locally as a result of damage to the wall of the femoral vein. In patients with disseminated malignant disease, studies have shown that extracts of malignant tumor cells contain cysteine proteases, which may activate factor X directly, thus accelerating the conversion of prothrombin to thrombin.

Ninety-five percent of pulmonary emboli that achieve clinical attention arise from venous thromboses in the deep veins of the lower extremities. Venous thrombosis in the lower extremities can develop in the superficial leg veins, the deep veins of the calf (calf vein thrombosis), the deep veins above the knee (popliteal vein thrombosis), and the more proximal veins in the thigh (proximal vein thrombosis). The classic view of DVTs in the lower limb is that of a clot forming in the small veins of the calf, and then propagating proximally past the popliteal area into the larger veins of the thigh and pelvis. It has been demonstrated, however, that patients who undergo hip surgery often develop proximal thrombi de novo, and that these thrombi

Table 2	
Risk Factors for Thromboembolism After Surgery or Trauma	
Intrinsic Factors	**Extrinsic Factors**
Age	Increased blood viscosity
History of DVT	Extent of tissue trauma
Varicose veins	Immobility
Malignancy	Paralysis
Oral contraceptives	
Inherited factors	
Congestive heart failure	
Smoking	
Obesity	

may be more dangerous than those that occur in the calf. Thromboses of the superficial femoral veins generally occur in varicosities and are usually benign and self-limiting. Deep calf vein thrombosis is less serious than proximal vein thrombosis because the thrombi are smaller and less frequently associated with clinical impairment or major complications. When patients with venous thrombosis develop local symptoms, the symptoms usually occur as a result of large occlusive thrombi, and approximately 80% of these are located in the proximal veins of the thigh or extend into the popliteal region. PE occurs more frequently in patients with proximal vein thrombosis than in patients with calf vein thrombosis. Most clinically significant and fatal pulmonary emboli arise from thrombi in the proximal veins of the thigh.

Natural History of Thrombosis and Embolization

Once a thrombus has formed, it will evolve in 1 of 3 ways: (1) the thrombus will undergo partial or complete lysis, with complete or near-complete recannulization of the thrombosed blood vessel; (2) the thrombus will become more organized, resulting in further occlusion of the vessel; (3) the thrombus will become dislodged, in whole or in part, and escape to a proximal site in the vascular system as an embolus.

Changes that lead to eventual dissolution of a thrombus are already manifest within 48 hours of formation. In these situations, the platelet mass will become loose, fibrin will extend into the spaces between platelet remnants, and neutrophils and monocytes will invade the thrombus and begin phagocytosis. After 1 week, up to 10% patency may be reestablished. As the process continues and endothelial cells proliferate and begin to extend over the receding thrombus mass, 50% to 70% patency may be achieved after 12 weeks.

Diagnosis of Thromboembolic Disease

Commonly, a screening examination such as ultrasound imaging or venography is used to determine the existence and location of a DVT after a total joint replacement. Physical examination alone (Homan's sign, edema, palpable cord) has proved less reliable, with a specificity and sensitivity of less than 50%.

The sensitivity, specificity, and accuracy of the commonly used methods for the detection of DVT vary considerably. The interpretation of the examination is technician- and radiologist-specific. It has been suggested that each institution perform its own internal validity study to assess the sensitivity, specificity, positive predictive value, negative predictive value, and accuracy of the screening test used within that institution. Radiocontrast venography, ultrasonography, fibrinogen I 125 labeling, and impedance plethysmography have all been used as diagnostic tools. Fibrinogen labeling and impedance plethysmography have been largely abandoned because of unacceptably low specificity and sensitivity.

Venography remains the reference standard for the localization and characterization of DVT in the calf and thigh. The advantages of using venography include direct visualization and acute sensitivity in detection of DVT. The procedure, however, is invasive, expensive, and exposes the patient to radiation. In addition, a certain percentage of patients are not candidates for venography because of allergic hypersensitivity or poor venous access. Color-flow ultrasound is the most technically advanced ultrasonic technique. It combines conventional Doppler spectral analysis with high-resolution tissue imaging and simultaneous display of flow formation. It is noninvasive and provides little if any added risk to patient care.

The efficacy of venography compared to ultrasound has been studied by numerous investigators. The matrix in Figure 3 outlines how sensitivity, specificity, positive predictive value, negative predictive value, and accuracy are determined. The results from study to study vary considerably. Some authors assert that once technician expertise has been achieved, ultrasound screening approaches a sensitivity and accuracy near that of venography. Certainly this has been demonstrated for the detection of proximal thrombi in symptomatic patients. Beyond this specific clinical scenario, the sensitivity of ultrasound for detecting DVT, especially distal DVT, has yet to be demonstrated as an adequate surveillance method.

Pulmonary Embolism

PE is not a disease per se, but rather a complication of venous thrombosis. PE results from the obstruction of the pulmonary artery or 1 of its branches by a clot or foreign body that has been brought to the site of lodgment by blood current. After the embolus has lodged and interrupted pulmonary blood flow, the ratio of regional ventilation to perfusion increases. The lung responds with bronchoconstriction to reduce wasted ventilation. This response is mediated by a local reduction in CO_2 output. Other vasoactive substances, such as serotonin, histamine, and prostaglandins, may play a role in this process, but the net effect is to reduce the size of peripheral airways, the lung volume, and the static pulmonary compliance. The hypoxemia that is associated with this ventilation-perfusion imbalance may show some improvement after supplemental oxygen is administered; however, the effects are usually minimal. Pulmonary infarction, as a consequence of embolism, is relatively rare and is associated clinically with problems of poor systemic perfusion, such as shock and congestive heart failure.

The clinical findings in PE depend primarily on the size of the embolus and on the cardiopulmonary status of the patient and can involve any combination of broad, nonspe-

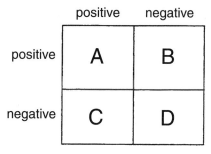

Reference standard

	positive	negative
positive	A	B
negative	C	D

A = true positive   B = true negative
C = false negative   D = true negative

Sensitivity = A / (A + C)

Specificity = D / (B + D)

Positive predictive value = A / (A + B)

Negative predictive value = D / (C + D)

Accuracy = (A + D) / (A + B + C + D)

Figure 3

Definitions of sensitivity, specificity, positive predictive value, negative predictive value, and accuracy. (Reproduced with permission from Westrich GH, Allen ML, Tarantino SJ, et al: Ultrasound screening for deep venous thrombosis after total knee arthroplasty: 2-year reassessment. *Clin Orthop* 1998;356:125–133.)

cific associated symptoms and signs. Dyspnea is the most frequent symptom followed by pleuritic chest pain. Tachypnea is the most common clinical sign followed by rales, tachycardia, and pyrexia. These symptoms and signs are nonspecific and must be interpreted in light of the risk factors for thromboembolism that each patient shows.

Diagnosis of Pulmonary Embolism

In any setting in which pulmonary embolism is suspected, an electrocardiogram (EKG) will address the possibility of concomitant myocardial infarction. The EKG tends to show abnormalities characteristic of PE only in patients with extensive embolization. Changes such as ST segment depression, T wave inversions in lead III, increased P waves, right bundle branch block, or right axis deviation occur in only 25% of patients with documented PE.

A chest radiograph must be obtained. A radiograph that is normal in a severely dyspenic patient is strongly suggestive of PE. Classic radiologic abnormalities associated with massive PE include a relative local hyperlucency in a region of segmental arterial occlusion or an enlarged hilar artery. The most common, highly nonspecific abnormalities include pleural effusion, atelectasis, or an elevated hemidiaphragm.

Arterial blood gas analysis measures pH, Pco_2, Po_2, HCO_3, the percent O_2 saturation, and the temperature of blood. These data can be helpful in the management of patients with suspected PE, but they are not useful for the diagnosis because the findings are nonspecific in patients who have preexisting pulmonary disease. Although an arterial Po_2 of less than 60 mm Hg is highly suggestive of respiratory distress, a normal Po_2 does not exclude the diagnosis of PE. Approximately 15% of patients with angiographically documented pulmonary emboli have a mean arterial Po_2 greater than 85 mm Hg.

Radionucleotide ventilation-perfusion scanning (V/Q scan) is currently the most widely used diagnostic test for the detection of PE. This study charts the perfusion of technetium Tc 99m-labeled human albumin isotope through the pulmonary tree. Areas of reduced perfusion as small as 2 cm in diameter can be detected. The specificity of this part of the test, however, is low, because disturbance in pulmonary flow from any cause can produce an abnormal scan. The test becomes more specific with the use of Tc 99-labeled microaerosols. When inhaled, these microaerosols disperse mainly to the peripheral airways. If the radioactive gas enters the areas of perfusion defects and then is cleared, this mismatch of ventilation and perfusion is characteristic of vascular obstruction. If, however, ventilation is also abnormal (ventilation-perfusion match), no reliable diagnostic conclusion can be reached and pulmonary angiography is required.

Pulmonary angiography is the reference standard by which the presence of PE can be established or excluded.

The technique is invasive and requires specialized personnel. A radiopaque material is injected through a cardiac catheter that has been advanced into the pulmonary artery, affording direct viewing of the filling defect or sharp cutoff in a vessel greater than 2.5 mm in diameter, both of which are diagnostic for PE.

Spinal CT scan has gained considerable interest as a method for the detection of pulmonary embolism. A number of studies have demonstrated superior sensitivity and specificity in the detection of PE for spiral CT scanning compared to scintigraphy. In patients without PE, this imaging modality has the added advantage of confirming an alternate diagnosis.

Treatment of Pulmonary Embolism

Most patients who have an acute episode of venous thrombosis and PE will be treated successfully by heparin followed by oral anticoagulant therapy with warfarin. The status of plasma coagulation is readily assessed by laboratory tests. Intravenous heparin therapy is monitored by the partial thromboplastin time (PTT). PTT screens the intrinsic limb of the coagulation system. After 7 to 10 days of heparin of therapy, 3 months of oral anticoagulant therapy with warfarin is administered. Anticoagulation achieved by warfarin is monitored by the prothrombin time (PT) and international normalized ratio (INR). PT screens the extrinsic or tissue-factor dependent pathway. INR corrects for the variability in the sensitivity of the different reagents used at various institutions to measure PT. The frequency of recurrence during this period is approximately 5%, and the risk of bleeding is between 2% and 20%. After 3 months, anticoagulation is discontinued. With this protocol, the risk of recurrence over the following 12 months has been shown to be between 6% and 10%. Pharmacologic agents used for the prevention of venous thrombosis and pulmonary embolism are discussed in Chapter 7.

Selected Bibliography

Fat Embolism

Amato JJ, Rheinlander HF, Cleveland RJ: Post-traumatic adult respiratory distress syndrome. *Orthop Clin North Am* 1978;9:693–713.

Behrman SW, Fabian TC, Kudsk KA, Taylor JC: Improved outcome with femur fractures: Early vs. delayed fixation. *J Trauma* 1990;30: 792–798.

Bone LB, Johnson KD, Weigelt J, Scheinberg R: Early versus delayed stabilization of femoral fracture: A prospective randomized study. *J Bone Joint Surg* 1989;71A:336–340.

Bulger EM, Smith DG, Maier RV, Jurkovich GJ: Fat embolism syndrome: A 10-year review. *Arch Surg* 1997;132:435–439.

Caillouette JT, Anzel SH: Fat embolism syndrome following the intramedullary alignment guide in total knee arthroplasty. *Clin Orthop* 1990;251:198–199.

Gurd AR: Fat embolism: An aid to diagnosis. *J Bone Joint Surg* 1970; 52B:732–737.

Hofmann S, Huemer G, Salzer M: Pathophysiology and management of the fat embolism syndrome. *Anaesthesia* 1998;53(suppl 2):35–37.

Kallenbach J, Lewis M, Zaltzman M, Feldman C, Orford A, Zwi S: "Low-dose" corticosteroid prophylaxis against fat embolism. *J Trauma* 1987;27:1173–1176.

Kropfl A, Berger U, Neureiter H, Hertz H, Schlag G: Intramedullary pressure and bone marrow fat intravasation in unreamed femoral nail. *J Trauma* 1997;42:946–954.

Levy D: The fat embolism syndrome: A review. *Clin Orthop* 1990; 261:281–286.

Lindeque BG, Schoeman HS, Dommisse GF, Boeyens MC, Vlok AL: Fat embolism and fat embolism syndrome: A double-blind therapeutic study. *J Bone Joint Surg* 1987;69B:128–131.

Muller C, Frigg R, Pfister U: Effect of flexible drive diameter and reamer design on the increase of pressure in the medullary cavity during reaming. *Injury* 1993;24(suppl 3):S40–S47.

Pape HC, Auf'm'Kolk M, Paffrath T, Regel G, Sturm JA, Tscherne H: Primary intramedullary femur fixation in multiple trauma patients with associated lung contusion: A cause of posttraumatic ARDS? *J Trauma* 1993;34:540–548.

Wolinsky PR, Banit D, Parker RE, et al: Reamed intramedullary femoral nailing after induction of an "ARDS-like" state in sheep: Effect on clinically applicable markers of pulmonary function. *J Orthop Trauma* 1998;12:169–176.

Deep Venous Thrombosis and Pulmonary Embolism

Dalen J, Hirsch J (eds): Fifth ACCP Consensus Conference on Antithrombotic Therapy. *Chest* 1998;114(suppl 5).

Kakkar VV, Howe CT, Flanc C, Clarke MB: Natural history of postoperative deep-vein thrombosis. *Lancet* 1969;2:230–232.

Lotke PA, Elia EA: Thromboembolic disease after total knee surgery: A critical review, in Greene WB (ed): *Instructional Course Lectures XXXIX*. Park Ridge, IL, American Academy of Orthopaedic Surgeons, 1990, pp 409–412.

Montgomery KD, Geerts WH, Potter HG, Helfet DL: Thromboembolic complications in patients with pelvic trauma. *Clin Orthop* 1996; 329:68–87.

Paiement GD: Prevention and treatment of venous thromboembolic disease complications in primary hip arthroplasty patients, in Cannon WD Jr (ed): *Instructional Course Lectures 47*. Rosemont, IL, American Academy of Orthopaedic Surgeons, 1998, pp 331–335.

Pellegrini VD Jr, Clement D, Lush-Ehmann C, Keller GS, Evarts CM: Natural history of thromboembolic disease after total hip arthroplasty. *Clin Orthop* 1996;333:27–40.

Westrich GH, Allen ML, Tarantino SJ, et al: Ultrasound screening for deep venous thrombosis after total knee arthroplasty: 2-year reassessment. *Clin Orthop* 1998;356:125–133.

Wolf LD, Hozack WJ, Rothman RH: Pulmonary embolism in total joint arthroplasty. *Clin Orthop* 1993;288:219–233.

Thromboembolic Disease

Ciccone WJ II, Fox PS, Neumyer M, Rubens D, Parrish WM, Pellegrini VD Jr: Ultrasound surveillance for asymptomatic deep venous thrombosis after total joint replacement. *J Bone Joint Surg* 1998; 80A:1167–1174.

Geerts WH, Code KI, Jay RM, Chen E, Szalai JD: A prospective study of venous thromboembolism after major trauma. *N Engl J Med* 1994; 331:1601–1606.

Gefter W, Hatabu H, Holland GA, Gupta KB, Henschke CI, Palevsky HI: Pulmonary thromboembolism: Recent developments in diagnosis with CT and MR imaging. *Radiology* 1995;197;561–574.

Mayo JR, Remy-Jardin M, Muller NL, et al: Pulmonary embolism: Prospective comparison of spiral CT with ventilation-perfusion scintigraphy. *Radiology* 1997;205:447–452.

Sharrock NE, Go G, Harpel PC, Ranawat CS, Sculco TP, Salvati EA: The John Charnley Award: Thrombogenesis during total hip arthroplasty. *Clin Orthop* 1995;319:16–27.

Stürmer K: Measurement of intramedullary pressure in an animal experiment and propositions to reduce the pressure increase. *Injury* 1993;24(suppl 3):S7–S21.

Section 2

Tissues and Pathophysiology

Chapter Outline

Chapter 13

Form and Function of Bone

Mathias P.G. Bostrom, MD

Adele Boskey, PhD

Jonathan K. Kaufman, MD

Thomas A. Einhorn, MD

This chapter at a glance

This chapter discusses the form and function of bone and covers a broad range of material from the basic structure of bone and its biomechanical properties to bone homeostasis and disease processes.

Introduction

Bone is an extremely dynamic and well-organized tissue, from the modulation of the apatite crystal arrangement at the molecular level to the strain pattern of the trabecular network at the organ level. The synergy of the molecular, cellular, and tissue arrangement provides a tensile strength nearly that of cast iron, with such an efficient use of material that the skeleton is of surprisingly low weight for such a supporting structure. At the microscopic level, bone consists of 2 forms: woven and lamellar (Fig. 1).

Woven bone is considered immature bone, or primitive bone, and normally is found in the embryo and the newborn, in fracture callus, and in the metaphyseal region of growing bone. This type of bone often is found in tumors, osteogenesis imperfecta, and pagetic bone. Woven bone is coarse-fibered and contains no uniform orientation of the collagen fibers. It has more cells per unit volume than does lamellar bone, its mineral content varies, and its cells are randomly arranged. The relatively disoriented collagen fibers of woven bone give it isotropic mechanical characteristics; when tested, the mechanical behavior of woven bone is similar regardless of the orientation of the applied forces.

Lamellar bone begins to form 1 month after birth. By 1 year of age, it is actively replacing woven bone, as the latter is resorbed. By age 4 years, most normal bone is lamellar bone. Thus, lamellar bone is a more mature bone that results from the remodeling of immature woven bone. Lamellar bone is found throughout the mature skeleton in both trabecular and cortical bone regardless of whether the bone was formed by intramembranous or endochondral ossification. The highly organized, stress-oriented collagen of lamellar bone gives it anisotropic properties; that is, the mechanical behavior of lamellar bone differs depending on the orientation of the applied forces, with its greatest strength parallel to the longitudinal axis of the collagen fibers.

Woven and lamellar bone are structurally organized into trabecular (spongy or cancellous) bone and cortical (dense or compact) bone (Fig. 1). Cortical bone has 4 times the mass of trabecular (cancellous) bone, although the metabolic turnover of trabecular bone is 8 times greater than that of cortical bone because of its extraordinarily high surface area for cellular activity. Bone turnover is a surface event and trabecular bone has a remarkably greater surface area than cortical bone.

Trabecular bone is found principally at the metaphysis and epiphysis of long bones and in cuboid bones such as the vertebrae. The internal beams or spicules of trabecular bone form a 3-dimensional (3-D) branching lattice aligned along areas of mechanical stress. Trabecular bone is subjected to a complex set of stresses and strains, although compression seems to predominate. Figure 2 illustrates new woven bone in a trabecular pattern with no discernible matrix orientation (A) compared to lamellar bone arranged in a trabecular pattern (B) with a layered arrangement of matrix fibers.

Cortical bone is found as the "envelope" in cuboid bones, and it composes the diaphysis in long bones. Cortical bone is subject to bending and torsional forces as well as to compressive forces. In small animals, there is no special arrangement of the vascular network in cortical bone; it consists simply of layers of lamellar bone, called compact bone. In larger animals that experience rapid growth, cortical bone is made up of layers of lamellar bone and woven bone, with the vascular channels located mainly in the woven bone. This bone is termed plexiform bone (Fig. 1). Such an arrangement of bone allows rapid growth and the accumulation of large amounts of bone over a short time.

TYPES OF BONE

MICROSCOPIC   **STRUCTURAL**

LAMELLAR

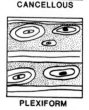
CANCELLOUS

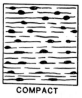
COMPACT

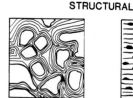
WOVEN

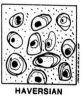
PLEXIFORM

HAVERSIAN

Figure 1

Diagrams of types of bone.

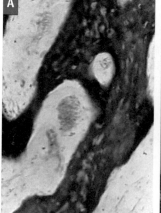
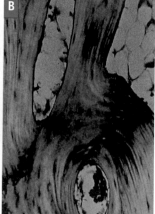

Figure 2

Photomicrographs of woven and lamellar bone.

Haversian bone is the most complex type of cortical bone. It is composed of vascular channels circumferentially surrounded by lamellar bone. This complex arrangement of bone around the vascular channel is called the osteon. The osteon is an irregular, branching, and anastomosing cylinder composed of a more or less centrally placed neurovascular canal surrounded by cell-permeated layers of bone matrix. Osteons are usually oriented in the long axis of the bone and are the major structural units of cortical bone. Cortical bone is, therefore, a complex of many adjacent osteons and their interstitial and circumferential lamellae. Figure 3 illustrates a single osteon surrounded by interstitial lamellae. Figure 4 shows a photomicrograph of cortical bone from a femoral shaft with inner circumferential lamellae next to the marrow cavity (lower left corner). Also shown are many osteons with their concentric lamellae, and the interstitial lamellae between osteons.

The central canal of an osteon, called the haversian canal, contains cells, vessels, and, occasionally, nerves and the canals connecting osteons called Volkmann's canals. Most vessels in the haversian canals have the ultrastructural features of capillaries, although some smaller-sized vessels may resemble lymphatic vessels. When examined histologically, these smaller vessels contain only precipitated protein; their endothelial walls are not surrounded by a basement membrane. Such features are characteristic of lymphatic vessels. The basement membrane of capillary walls may function as a rate-limiting or selective ion-limiting transport barrier, because all material traversing the vessel wall must go through the basement membrane. The presence of this barrier is particularly important in calcium and phosphorus ion transport to and from bone, and may play an important role in the response of bone to mechanical loads.

The capillaries in the central canals are derived from the principal nutrient arteries of the bone or the epiphyseal and metaphyseal arteries. Figure 5, *A*, shows the nutrient artery of a long bone entering the shaft and branching to form the vascular network in cortical bone. Using lower magnification and injecting India ink (Fig. 5, *B*) provides a better picture of the complexity of this vascular network.

Cortical and trabecular bone are distinguished from each other primarily by differences in porosity and, consequently, apparent density. Apparent density is the ratio of the mass of bone tissue in a specimen to the bulk volume of the specimen (bone plus bone marrow spaces). Typically, mean values for the apparent density of hydrated human femoral cortical bone and proximal tibial trabecular bone are 1.85 g/cm^3 and 0.30 g/cm^3, respectively. The respective standard deviations are typically 0.06 g/cm^3 (± 3% of the mean value) and 0.10 g/cm^3 (± 30% of the mean value). This indicates that almost 70% of the apparent density values for femoral cortical bone are in the range 1.80 to 1.90 g/cm^3, whereas almost 70% of the values for tibial trabecular bone are in the

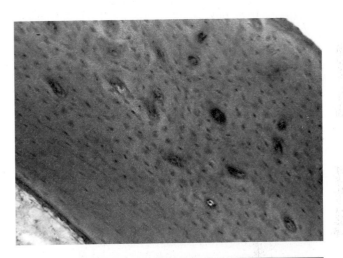

Figure 4

Photomicrograph of cortical bone.

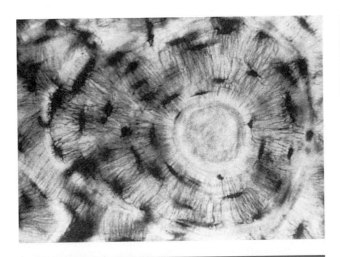

Figure 3

Photomicrograph of a bone osteon.

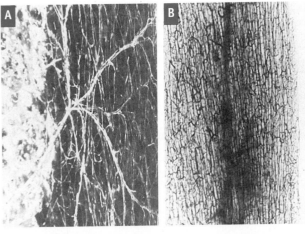

Figure 5

Photomicrograph showing vasculature of cortical bone.

range 0.20 to 0.40 g/cm^3. Although the magnitudes of these ranges are similar, the percentage deviations are much larger for trabecular bone. This distinction is important because the material properties of trabecular bone are very sensitive to apparent density.

Because the densities of trabecular and cortical bone can overlap, cortical bone is usually defined as bone with less than approximately 30% porosity. However, porosity is not the only difference between cortical and trabecular bone. Trabecular bone can also be distinguished from cortical bone by differences in bone architecture (Fig. 6). Cortical bone can be described architecturally as a solid containing a series of voids: haversian and Volkmann's canals and, to a lesser extent, lacunae and canaliculi. The porosity of cortical bone tissue (typically 10%) is primarily a function of the density of these voids. However, trabecular bone can be described architecturally as a network of small, interconnected plates and rods of individual trabeculae with relatively large spaces between the trabeculae. Individual trabeculae contain only some of the voids (canaliculi and lacunae and, very seldom, haversian canals) that are contained in cortical bone. Therefore, the porosity of trabecular bone (typically 50% to 90%) is dominated by the spaces between individual trabeculae. It is the combination of differences in porosity and architecture that primarily differentiates cortical from trabecular bone and that accounts for their characteristic material properties.

Bone Cell Morphology

Osteoblasts

The major types of bone cells are the osteoblasts, osteocytes, and osteoclasts. The bone-forming cells are the osteoblasts and osteocytes; while of the same lineage, these cells differ not only in location but also function. An osteoblast is defined as a cell that produces osteoid, or bone matrix. Osteoblasts make type I collagen, are responsive to parathyroid hormone (PTH), and produce osteocalcin and bone sialoprotein, extracellular matrix proteins specific to bone (and dentin). Osteoblasts line the surface of bone and follow osteoclasts in cutting cones. Osteocytes are osteoblasts encased in a mineralized matrix. Factors that induce the process of bone cell differentiation are currently under active investigation, and these include the bone morphogenetic proteins (BMPs) along with other growth factors and cytokines. The interleukins, insulin-derived growth factor, and platelet-derived growth factor, among others, all affect osteoblast differentiation in vitro.

The most distinctive features of the osteoblast are illustrated in the light and electron micrographs of osteoblasts adjacent to new bone (Fig. 7). At the light microscopic level (Fig. 7, A) the active osteoblast shows intense staining with basophilic stains, and appears to be polarized with the

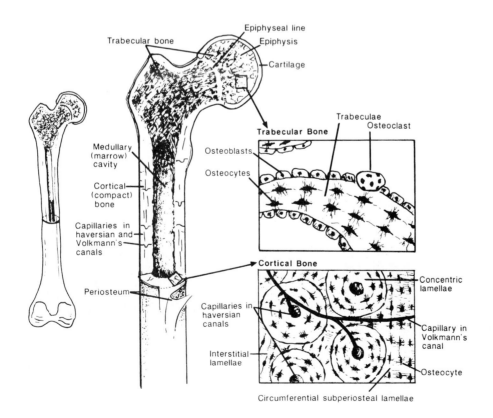

Figure 6

Schematic diagram of cortical and trabecular bone showing the different microstructures. (Reproduced with permission from Hayes WC: Biomechanics of cortical and trabecular bone: Implications for assessment of fracture risk, in *Basic Orthopaedic Biomechanics*. New York, NY, Raven Press, 1991, pp 93–142.)

nucleus located at the end of the cell away from the bone surface. The apparent shape of the osteoblast is a function of the orientation of the section being examined. Some of the osteoblasts shown in the electron micrograph (Fig. 7, *B*) appear rectangular with their long axes perpendicular to the osteoid (bone surface). The cytoplasm of the cell is occupied by 3 major components: the nucleus, the Golgi apparatus, and the rough endoplasmic reticulum. The nucleus in the osteoblast is large relative to that in other cell types. The abundant rough endoplasmic reticulum is characteristic of cells that manufacture protein for export. The Golgi apparatus, adjacent to the nucleus, is responsible for the secretion of these proteins. Mitochondria and cyto-skeletal elements are found throughout the cytoplasm.

Histochemical studies have demonstrated that alkaline phosphatase is distributed over the outer surface of the osteoblast cell membrane. As indicated by the electron photomicrograph, there is a layer of newly formed unmin-eralized bone matrix (osteoid) between the osteoblast cell membrane and the mineralized matrix of bone.

Osteocytes

Once an osteoblast becomes surrounded by bone matrix, which then becomes mineralized, the cell is characterized by a higher nucleus-to-cytoplasm ratio and contains fewer organelles. Such a cell is the osteocyte of bone, and although osteocytes are the most numerous of bone cells they seem to receive the least amount of attention. Light microscopy (Fig. 3) reveals osteocytes arranged concentri-cally around the central lumen of an osteon and between lamellae. They are uniformly oriented with respect to the longitudinal and radial axes of lamellae. Osteocytes have extensive cell processes that project through the canaliculi, and establish contact and "communication" between adja-cent osteocytes and the central canals of osteons via gap junctions. The canaliculi are oriented in a radial fashion around the central haversian canal. Electron micrography of mature osteocytes shows a decreased organelle content, a greater nucleus-to-cytoplasm ratio, and numerous cell processes extending outward through the canaliculi (Fig. 8).

Osteocytes can metabolically manipulate their environ-ment more or less independent of surface resorption and accretion. This ability is important to cellular regulation of calcium exchange. Bone crystals are extremely small and have a surface area of approximately 100 m^2/g or a total of 100 acres of surface area in the adult human body. Most of these crystals, buried away from the endosteal and periosteal bone surfaces, appear to be unavailable to effect the necessary mineral exchange with extracellular fluid, making it difficult to explain the immediate exchange of bone mineral with the extracellular fluid. There is, however, a vast surface area on the haversian canal and lacunar walls and an even larger area on the canalicular walls, which in the adult totals about 300 m^2, or 3 acres, where bone min-eral exchange with extracellular fluid can take place. The metabolic/structural role of osteocytes has not been identi-fied, but their intricate 3-D distribution and their intercon-necting cell processes (gap junctions) indicate that they are perfectly organized to serve as an intricate system to help communicate strain and stress signals and regulate the overall metabolism of the tissue.

Osteoclasts

Osteoclasts are the major resorptive cells of bone and are characterized by their large size (20 to 100 µm in diameter) and their multiple nuclei. Osteoclasts are derived from pluripotent cells of the bone marrow, which are the hematopoietic precursors that also give rise to monocytes and macrophages. Whereas monocytes are mononuclear cells, macrophages and osteoclasts are formed from the fusion of monocytes. Osteoclasts differ from macrophages

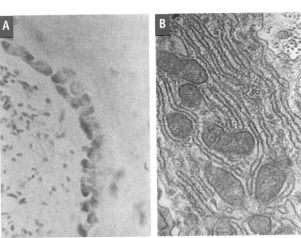

Figure 7

Light (**A**) and electron (**B**) photomicrographs of osteoblasts.

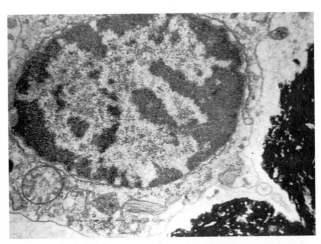

Figure 8

Electron photomicrograph of a mature osteocyte.

(foreign body giant cells) in that the osteoclasts produce tartrate-resistant acid phosphatase. Osteoclasts are also distinguished from macrophages by virtue of their abilities to resorb bone and express certain cell surface markers as well as by their acid phosphatase activity. It is presumed that at some point during mononuclear cell development, the cell becomes committed to form either a macrophage or an osteoclast. The cellular origin of the osteoclast is underscored by recent clinical trials in which new osteoclast populations of donor origin were found in patients with osteopetrosis who had received successful bone marrow allografts.

Osteoclasts lie in regions of bone resorption in pits called Howships lacunae (Fig. 9). The electron photomicrograph (Fig. 9, *B*) demonstrates a strongly polarized cell with a paucity of rough-surfaced endoplasmic reticulum, a moderate number of ribosomes, numerous smooth vesicles, and well-developed mitochondria. As shown in the histologic section (Fig. 9, *A*), the other major feature of the osteoclasts is the ruffled (brush) border, which results from extensive infoldings of the cell membrane adjacent to the resorptive surface. Osteoclasts appearing some distance from the surface of bone do not have ruffled borders and are called "inactive" or "resting" osteoclasts. Direct observations show that the ruffled border of the osteoclasts sweeps across the surface of bone. The infolds of the ruffled border end in numerous channels and vesicles in the cell cytoplasm, within which lie numerous mineral crystals. Osteoclast bind to the bone surface through cell attachment proteins called integrins, and they resorb bone by isolating an area of bone under the region of cell attachment. The osteoclasts then lower the pH of the local environment by production of hydrogen ions through the carbonic anhydrase system. The lowered pH increases the solubility of the apatite crystals, and after the mineral is removed, the organic components of the matrix are hydrolyzed through acidic proteolytic digestion.

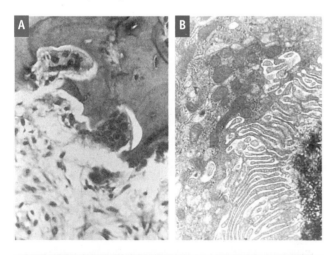

Figure 9

Light (**A**) and electron (**B**) photomicrographs of osteoclasts.

Cellular Mechanisms of Bone Modeling

All bone surfaces are continuous and typically are lined by resting osteoblasts called bone lining cells, with small intercellular gaps between the cells and their cytoplasmic processes. The endosteal surface is connected to the Volkmann's canals of the haversian systems via canaliculi. Although the cellular layer protects the bone from the extracellular fluid space, the osteoblasts on the bone surface are in direct chemical contact with the osteocytes within the mineralized bone by their cellular processes within the canaliculi. This organizational structure is consistent with the concept that bone cells are in intimate communication with each other and that osteoblasts receive the majority of systemic endocrine-based signals and then transmit them to other cells in bone. Conversely, strain-generated signals such as direct cell deformation, streaming potentials, or shear stress caused by fluid flow could be perceived by osteocytes, and their regulatory information passed on to the osteoblasts.

Depending on its functional activity, the osteoblast's structure or shape may change. The tall, plump osteoblasts that line bone surfaces are metabolically active and dedicated to the process of bone matrix (osteoid) synthesis. Among the matrix elements produced by osteoblasts are structural proteins, such as type I collagen; a variety of noncollagenous proteins, including osteocalcin and osteopontin, osteonectin, and proteoglycans (Table 1); and regulatory factors, such as cytokines, growth factors, and prostaglandins (Table 2). On other bone surfaces, where bone is not being actively formed, the osteoblasts appear elongated and flat and are relatively quiescent metabolically. These osteoblasts are often called resting bone lining cells. Evidence suggests that these osteoblasts may be producing enzymes and enzyme-regulating proteins such as collagenase, collagenase inhibitor, and plasminogen activator, which are involved in the process of bone matrix degradation. In addition to the above synthetic products, osteoblasts produce neutral proteases, alkaline phosphatase, and other enzymes that degrade the extracellular matrix and prepare it for calcification. The lining osteoblasts are in communication with osteocytes through cell processes within the canaliculi that form gap junctions. Rapid fluxes of bone calcium across these junctions may be involved in the transmission of information between osteoblasts on the bone surface as well as to osteocytes within the structure of bone itself.

The specific receptor-effector interactions in osteoblasts are best illustrated by responses to PTH, prostaglandins, 1,25-dihydroxyvitamin D, and glucocorticoids. PTH and prostaglandins bind to cell surface-associated receptors and then trigger intracellular second messenger pathways to bring about the cellular response. These mechanisms

Table 1

Bone Noncollagenous Matrix Proteins

Protein (Name in Other Tissues)	Other Sources*	Postulated Function	Basis for Postulate
Phosphorylated Glycoproteins			
Osteopontin—bone sialoprotein 1 (SPP, 2ar, pp69)	D, O	Cell binding; regulate mineral proliferation	Solution studies
Bone sialoprotein—bone sialoprotein 2	D	Cell binding; initiation of mineralization	Solution studies
Osteonectin (SPARC, BM-40)	D, BV	Ca binding; mineral-collagen interaction: regulation of cell shape; regulation of cell migration	Solution studies
BAG-75 (dentin matrix phosphorprotein)	D	Matrix interactions	Solution studies
Tetranectin	BV	Regulation of mineral deposition	Implant in nude mice
Thrombospondin	C, O	Modulation of cell metabolism; binding to collagen	Distribution in vitro studies
γ-Carboxyglutamic Acid-Containing Proteins			
Osteocalcin—bone Gla protein	D, BV	Regulates mineral maturation	Knockout mice and solution studies
Matrix GLa-protein—MGP	C	Regulates mineral deposition	Knockout mice
Glycosaminoglycan-Containing Proteins			
Aggrecan	C	Tissue hydration; inhibition of mineralization: remnant from cartilage	Solution studies
Veriscan	C, O	Space filling	Theoretical
Decorin—CS PGII (DS-PGII: PG-40)	C, D, O	Regulates collagen fibrillogenesis	Solution studies
Biglycan—SC-PGI	C, D, O	Binds growth factors, collagen, and cells; regulates mineralization	Solution studies; Turner's syndrome
Betaglycan (Heparan sulfate PG)	O	Binds growth factors	
Syndecan (Heparan sulfate PG)	O	Unknown	
Osteoglycan	C	Binds TGF-β	
HA-PG III		Binds to collagen and apatite	Solution studies
Fibromodulin	C, D	Interacts with types I and II collagen; binds growth factors	In vitro studies
Thrombomodulin	C, D	Interacts with types I and II collagen; binds growth factors	In vitro studies
Lumican	C, D	Interacts with types I and II collagen; binds growth factors	In vitro studies
Others			
Fibrillin	O	Anchors elastin fibrils	Marfan's syndrome
Vitronectin (complement S-protein)	O	Osteoclast adhesion	In vitro studies
Tenascin	C, D, O	Early mesenchyme differentiation	In vitro studies
Fibronectin	C, D, O	Cell-matrix interactions	In vitro studies

* The proteins shown are synthesized by bone cells. Other than bone, the protein indicated is made in: C = cartilage, D = dentin, BV = blood vessels, O = a wide variety of other tissues, TGF-β = transforming growth factor-β.

Table 2

Factors Regulating Bone Cell Metabolism

Factor*	Cells Acted Upon	Effects
Prostaglandins	Osteoblast; osteoclast	Resorption
Leukotrienes	Osteoclast	Resorption
Cytokines and Growth Factors (GF)		
TGF-α and -β	Osteoblast; osteoclast	Differentiation; protein synthesis
PDGF	Osteoblast	Differentiation
EGF	Osteoblast	Proliferation; differentiation; protein synthesis

FGF
    Acidic
    Basic
	Osteoblast	Differentiation

IL-1, -3, -4, -6, -8, -11	Osteoblast; osteoclast	Protein synthesis; differentiation resorption
LIF	Osteoblast	Protein synthesis
TNF	Osteoblast	Protein synthesis
Lipocortin II	Osteoclast	Differentiation
IGFs I and II	Osteoblast	Resorption
BMP 2-7	Precursor cells; osteoblast	Differentiation; maturation
MCSF	Osteoclast	Resorption
Hormones		

Peptide
    Calcitonin
    Parathyroid
    CGRP
	Osteoclast
	Osteoblast
	Osteoblast
		Formation; resorption
		Formation; resorption
		Formation; resorption

Steroid
    Vitamin A
    Vitamin D
	Osteoblast
	Osteoblast; osteoclast
		Differentiation
		Differentiation; protein synthesis; mineral homeostasis

Estrogen	Osteoblast; osteoclast	Formation; resorption
Testosterone	Osteoblast	Formation
Thyroid	Osteoblast	Resorption
Glucocorticoid	Osteoblast	Differentiation; resorption; protein synthesis

* Many of these factors have a variety of actions on the bone cells, depending upon concentration and maturity of cell affected. This table indicates the types of activity that have been shown to be directly affected. TGF = transforming growth factor; PDGF = platelet-derived growth factor; EGF = epidermal growth factor; FGF = fibroblast growth factor; IL = interleukin; LIF = leukemia inhibitory factor; TNF = tumor necrosis factor; IGF = insulin-like growth factor; BMP = bone morphogenetic protein; MCSF = macrophage colony stimulating factor; CGRP = calcitonin gene-related peptide.

include both the adenylate cyclase/cyclic adenosine monophosphate pathway and the phosphoinositol-calcium pathway. On the other hand, 1,25-dihydroxyvitamin D and glucocorticoids diffuse across the membrane and bind to cytosolic receptors, which then translocate to the nucleus of the cell and interact with nuclear DNA to modulate and regulate the transcription of DNA to messenger RNA. Recent evidence suggests that osteoblasts also contain receptors for estrogen, and that these function like other steroid hormone receptors. How these estrogen receptors and the resultant osteoblastic responses function to regulate osteoclastic bone resorption remains unknown, although it is recognized that the actions of osteoblasts and osteoclasts are coupled.

Osteoclasts at specific bone sites are activated only after disruption of the osteoid layer that covers the bone surfaces; an osteoblast-mediated effect. This exposure of the underlying mineralized matrix may be caused by the degradation of surface osteoid by collagenases elaborated by flat, elongated osteoblasts (resting bone lining cells), or by the contraction of osteoblasts in response to stimulation by PTH, 1,25-dihydroxyvitamin D_3, or prostaglandins of the E series. This contraction allows osteoclasts to gain access to the mineralized bone. What appears to be the degradation of the bone matrix also results in the activation of specific molecules buried within the bone matrix, for example, BMPs. These released signal molecules, which have mitogenic, differentiating, and chemoattracting properties, may be extremely important in the modulation of cellular events at specific regions in bone. Moreover, these molecules may be the key agents that regulate bone homeostasis by maintaining a coupling between bone formation and resorption. Other unreleased molecules in bone matrix may serve as anchoring molecules to which effector cells attach. Thus, as the bone is stimulated to resorb it may release from its matrix a substance that stimulates bone formation, transforming growth factor beta (TGF-β) or BMP, thereby maintaining bone homeostasis. PTH mediates bone resorption by stimulation of PTH receptors on osteoblasts, which in turn mediate osteoclastic bone resorption; osteoclasts do not have PTH receptors. While endogenous PTH generally acts as a catabolic agent, intermittent exogenous PTH may prove to be a useful agent in the treatment of osteoporosis.

As mentioned above, for an osteoclast to resorb bone, the osteoblast syncytium, or canopy, must first (1) contract somewhat, so that the osteoclast can gain access to the bone surface, and (2) elaborate neutral proteases to degrade the thin layer of unmineralized osteoid covering the bone. Evidence suggests that osteoclasts must be exposed to a mineralized bone surface as well as to certain matrix components in order for them to become active.

Two intracellular areas of the osteoclast are important for its bone resorbing function. These are the clear zone and the ruffled border areas of the cell that gained their name from their appearance under electron microscopy. The clear zone is that area of the osteoclast in which attachment of the cell to the bone surface takes place. Evidence suggests that attachment of the osteoclast to bone occurs through a receptor-mediated process (integrins). Once osteoclasts have attached to bone, the clear zone surrounds and seals off the area where bone is to be resorbed much the same as a saucer placed upside down on a table would seal off the area beneath it. This area of the bone is called the subosteoclastic space. Bone resorption then takes place in this space in a concerted fashion in which intracellular carbonic anhydrase degrades carbonic acid to produce free protons (hydrogen ions). These protons are released from the cell by means of a hydrogen ion-adenosine triphosphatase pump. Because this area of the bone has been isolated beneath the osteoclast, these protons accumulate until the pH of this microenvironment reaches a low enough level (approximately pH 4) to dissolve the mineral phase of the bone and promote the activity of the matrix-degrading osteoclastic hydrolytic enzymes. These matrix-degrading lysosomal enzymes, including cathepsin B and acid phosphatase, are then released across the ruffled border, a complex of plasma membrane infoldings, and are the actual agents that degrade the organic matrix and continue to dissociate the mineral phase of bone. Evidence suggests that some of the free mineral crystals and matrix components are phagocytized back into the cell, where they are degraded.

Because the remodeling of bone is a very specific spatial process, resorption must occur under close local control, possibly through the facility of other cells in bone and bone marrow. Because the predominant bone-resorbing hormones, such as PTH, 1,25-dihydroxyvitamin D, and prostaglandin E, do not have receptors on osteoclasts, their action to increase bone resorption must be mediated through another cell, such as the osteoblast, which does have receptors for these hormones. Other cells may also participate in the bone resorption process. For example, mast cells release heparin, an agent that enhances collagenase activity and may have a resorptive effect on bone matrix. Monocytes and lymphocytes may modulate bone remodeling through the release of local regulatory cytokines. At present, the specific cell and associated factors that regulate bone resorption are under active investigation.

Bone Matrix Composition

Bone is a composite material, consisting of mineral, proteins, water, cells, and other macromolecules (lipids, sugars, etc). Although bone cells are the principal regulators of bone metabolism, bone matrix and mineral participate in the control of cell-mediated processes. Therefore, the inorganic and organic components of bone have both structural and regulatory properties.

The composition of bone differs depending on anatomic site, age, dietary history, and the presence of disease. In general, however, the mineral or inorganic phase accounts for 60% to 70% of the tissue, water accounts for 5% to 8%, and the organic matrix makes up the remainder. Approximately 90% of the organic matrix is collagen; 5% to 8%, noncollagenous proteins. The mineral phase is an analog of the naturally-occurring mineral hydroxyapatite, $Ca_{10}(PO_4)_6(OH)_2$ (Fig. 10). The apatite crystals are small and contain abundant impurities (for example, carbonate, sodium, and citrate), some of which reflect dietary history (for example, fluoride and strontium).

Inorganic Phase

The inorganic component of bone is principally composed of a calcium phosphate mineral analogous to crystalline calcium hydroxyapatite (Fig. 10). This apatite is present as a plate-like crystal, which is 20 to 80 nm long and 2 to 5 nm thick. The small amounts of impurities in hydroxyapatite, such as carbonate, which can replace either the phosphate or the hydroxide groups, or chloride and fluoride, which can replace the hydroxyl groups, may alter certain physical properties of the crystal, such as solubility. These altered properties may impart important biologic effects that are critical to normal function. Newly formed woven bone, which is not as well mineralized as mature lamellar bone, contains particles with a smaller average crystal size, which may make resorption easier.

Organic Phase

The organic phase of the extracellular matrix of bone plays a wide variety of roles, determining the structure and the mechanical and biochemical properties of the bone. Approximately 90% of the organic matrix of bone is type I collagen; the remainder consists of noncollagenous matrix proteins, minor collagen types, lipids, and other macromolecules. Growth factors and cytokines, bone inductive proteins, and the more abundant matrix proteins such as osteonectin, osteopontin, bone sialoprotein, osteocalcin, bone proteoglycans, and other phosphoproteins and proteolipids make small contributions to the overall volume of bone and major contributions to its biologic function (Tables 1 and 2).

Collagen is a ubiquitous protein of extremely low solubility, which consists of 3 polypeptide chains composed of approximately 1,000 amino acids each. It is the major structural component of the bone matrix. Bone collagen is constructed in the form of a triple helix of 2 identical $\alpha1(I)$ chains and 1 unique $\alpha2$ chain stabilized by hydrogen bonding between hydroxyproline and other charged residues. This produces a fairly rigid linear molecule 300 nm long. Each molecule is aligned with the next in a parallel fashion in a quarter-staggered array to produce a collagen fibril (Fig. 11). The collagen fibrils are then grouped in bundles to

Hydroxyapatite:

$$Ca_{10} (PO_4)_6 (OH)_2$$

Mg^{+2} CO_3^{-2} CO_3^-

Sr^{+2} HPO_4^{-2} F^-

Na^+

K^+

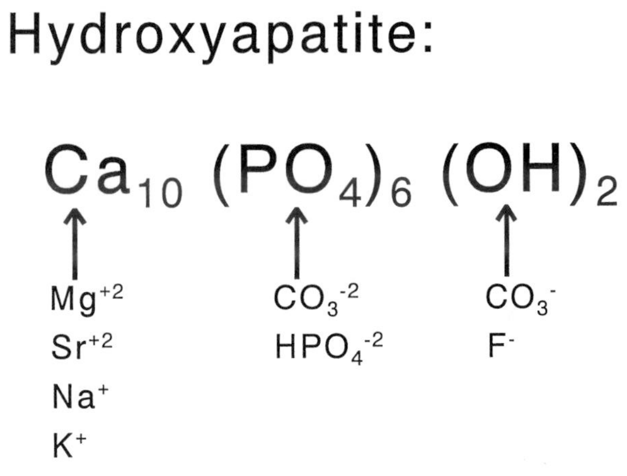

Figure 10

Bone mineral is an analog of the naturally occurring calcium phosphate, hydroxyapatite, whose chemical formula is shown here. In bone, as illustrated here, there may be substitutions for calcium, phosphate, and hydroxide groups, the extent of such substitutions varying with age, dietary history, tissue site, and health status.

form the collagen fiber. Within the collagen fibril, gaps, called "hole zones," exist between the ends of the molecules. In addition, "pores" exist between the sides of parallel molecules. Noncollagenous proteins or mineral deposits can be found within the holes and pores. Mineralization of the matrix is thought to commence in the hole zones.

Collagen synthesis is completed within the cell, and processing continues in the extracellular matrix, and involves both posttranslational and postsecretory processing. In the cell, almost half of the proline and 15% to 20% of the lysine residues are hydroxylated on the individual α chains, and these hydroxylations are followed by the glycosylation of the hydroxylysine residues in an intracellular, posttranslational process. This step leads to the formation of the triple

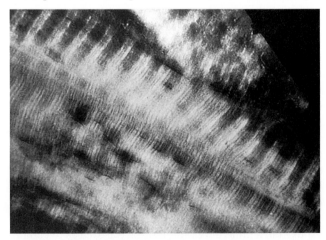

Figure 11

Electron photomicrograph of bone collagen.

helical procollagen molecule, which is the secreted form. Once outside the cell, the terminal nontriple helical propeptides are enzymatically cleaved to form the collagen molecule. The collagen molecules are stabilized by cross-links formed between reactive aldehydes on different chains. The reactive aldehydes are formed by oxidative deamination of both lysine and hydroxylysine. Urinary excretion of peptides with these unique cross-links is commonly used as a marker of bone resorption, because only extracellular collagen contains these cross-links.

The nature and postulated functions of several noncollagenous bone proteins have been described in Table 1. One of the more extensively studied noncollagenous proteins in bone is osteocalcin or bone γ-carboxyglutamic acid-containing protein (bone Gla protein). This is a small (5.8 kd) protein in which 3 glutamic acid residues are carboxylated as a result of the vitamin K-dependent posttranslational modification. The carboxylation of these residues converts this protein into a calcium- and mineral-binding protein. Osteocalcin accounts for 10% to 20% of the noncollagenous protein present in bone and is closely associated with the mineral phase. Although the precise function of this bone-specific protein is not known, it is thought to play some role in attracting osteoclasts to sites of bone resorption and in regulating the maturation of bone mineral crystals. The synthesis of osteocalcin is enhanced by 1,25-dihydroxyvitamin D and inhibited by PTH and corticosteroids. Osteocalcin is a synthetic product of osteoblasts, and the related dentin-forming cells, odontoblasts.

Animals treated with sodium warfarin (an agent that blocks the vitamin K-dependent carboxylation of glutamate residues in osteocalcin and other γ-carboxyglutamate containing proteins) have decreased amounts of carboxylated osteocalcin in their bones but few other significant changes in bone structure. Studies of patients who have been treated with sodium warfarin similarly show significant changes in osteocalcin biochemistry but no serious clinical effects. However, young animals treated with warfarin demonstrate premature epiphyseal closure, but no other long bone abnormalities. The appearance of warfarin embryopathy (nasal hypoplasia, stippled epiphyses, and distal extremity hypoplasia) in the offspring of women treated with warfarin during pregnancy suggests that osteocalcin, or more likely the γ-carboxylated matrix Gla protein, which is a component of both cartilage and bone, may play a role in bone development. Animals that lack osteocalcin because of genetic manipulation (knockout animals) have thickened hypermineralized bones with very small mineral crystals, yet apparently normal osteoclast activity. Animals in which the matrix Gla-protein has been knocked out show excessive cartilage calcification, verifying the suggestion from the warfarin-treated animals that this protein regulates cartilage calcification.

Gla proteins such as osteocalcin have been shown to be elevated in the serum and urine of patients with Paget disease, primary hyperparathyroidism, renal osteodystrophy, and high turnover osteoporosis. Although osteocalcin has been touted as being potentially useful as a clinical marker in patients with osteoporosis, this application is limited because the presence of osteocalcin in the serum or urine could be caused either by extensive bone resorption or by increased bone formation. The presence of bone-specific collagen cross-links has proved to be a more sensitive marker of remodeling.

Other noncollagenous proteins found in bone may also be important in relation to their calcium and mineral binding properties. Osteonectin, a 32-kd protein secreted by both osteoblasts and platelets, has been shown to bind both denatured collagen and hydroxyapatite. Although not entirely known, its role may be to regulate calcium concentrations or to potentiate nucleation or stabilization of calcium phosphate or the organization of mineral within the matrix framework. Phosphorylated sialoproteins, small proteoglycans, and other phosphoproteins synthesized by osteoblasts also play a role in matrix organization. Many of the phosphoproteins are believed to be localized in the hole zones of collagen fibrils. Their phosphate groups attract calcium to the area and may be responsible for the nucleation phenomena during the initial stages of mineralization. Of these proteins, bone sialoprotein has been found to nucleate mineral in solution, making it a likely in situ promoter of apatite formation.

Several of the bone matrix proteins (for example, osteopontin, bone sialoprotein, bone acidic glycoprotein, thrombospondin, and fibronectin) contain arginine-glycine-aspartic acid sequences. Such sequences, characteristic of cell binding proteins, are recognized by a family of cell membrane proteins known as integrins. The integrins span the cell membrane and provide a link between the extracellular matrix and the cytoskeleton of the cell. Integrins on osteoblasts, osteoclasts, and fibroblasts provide means for anchoring these cells to the extracellular matrix.

Present in very small amounts in the bone matrix are growth factors and cytokines such as TGF-β, insulin-like growth factor, the interleukins (IL-1, IL-6), and BMP 1-7. These proteins bind to both the bone mineral and matrix, and are released during the process of osteoclastic bone resorption. Such proteins have important effects regulating bone cell differentiation, activation, growth, regeneration, and turnover (Table 2). It is likely that these growth factors serve as the coupling factors that link the processes of bone formation and bone remodeling. Growth factor and hormone interaction with cell receptors regulate the flux of calcium ions into and out of the cell, an event that may be key in controlling matrix mineralization.

Bone Mineralization

Mineralization of the organic matrix of bone is a complicated process that is not fully understood. Osteoblasts regulate the concentration of calcium ions in the matrix through the release of calcium from intercellular compartments. Osteoblasts also secrete the macromolecules which, as indicated above, determine the site and rate of initial calcification.

Mineralization of skeletal tissues can be considered as having 2 distinct phases: (1) formation of the initial mineral deposits at multiple discrete sites (initiation); and (2) proliferation or accretion of additional mineral crystals on the initial mineral deposits (growth). Of the total body mineral, only a small fraction represents the initial deposit. The bulk of the mineral comes from growth of the initial crystalline material.

Initiation of mineralization requires a combination of events, including increases in the local concentration of precipitating ions, formation or exposure of mineral nucleators, and removal or modification of mineralization inhibitors. The vast majority of mineral in the body is an analog of the naturally occurring mineral, hydroxyapatite $(Ca_{10}[PO_4]_6[OH]_2)$ shown in Figure 10. The nature of the first mineral crystals deposited in bone and the site at which they are deposited is still unknown. Extracellular matrix vesicles, located at a distance from the collagen fibrils, have been identified as the site of initial mineral deposition in young, calcifying cartilage and in young bone; however, the bulk of the mineral in bone as well as much of the initial mineral is closely associated with collagen.

More energy is required to form the initial mineral crystals than is required to add ions or ion clusters to already existing crystals. Secondary nucleation, the growth of small crystallites in a branching manner from the surface of other small crystals, also requires less energy than does de novo initiation. To circumvent the large energy required of initial apatite formation, a less stable (or metastable) precursor phase may form first, and later either be converted directly to apatite or serve as a heterogenous nucleator of apatite. A heterogenous apatite nucleator is a foreign material that has 1 or more surfaces on which apatite crystals can grow. Once primary nucleation has occurred, there is an early, rapid increase in size from crystal nuclei to the first solid phase particles initially observed by electron microscopy. This process is termed crystal growth. Operationally, the 2 processes, primary nucleation and crystal growth, have been defined as multiplication.

Of the connective tissue collagens, only type I (bone, tendon, skin) collagen can support apatite deposition in vitro (Fig. 11). It has been shown that mineralized type I collagen contains cross-links that are chemically different from those in nonmineralized osteoid. Such collagen cross-linking may also affect the distribution of mineral within the collagen. What causes the orientation of matrix fibrils in lamellae is unknown; however, the pattern obviously forms prior to mineralization.

Some noncollagenous proteins, such as the bone sialoprotein, dentin phosphoproteins, and osteonectin-collagen complexes, seem to promote collagen mineralization in vitro. In addition, certain proteolipids and calcium acidic phospholipid phosphate complexes also can promote hydroxyapatite deposition in vitro. Extracellular matrix vesicles may facilitate calcification by (1) concentrating ions; (2) providing a protective environment free of mineralization inhibitors; and/or (3) providing enzymes involved in matrix modification. Table 1 shows the noncollagenous proteins found to modulate bone mineralization.

Figure 12 shows that initial mineral deposition may be promoted both by the formation or exposure of nucleators and/or by the removal or modification of inhibitors. In vitro, large proteoglycans extracted from both calcifying and noncalcifying cartilage inhibit apatite growth. The phosphoproteins that serve as in vitro nucleators can also regulate growth if present in sufficient concentrations. It is likely that initial mineralization of collagen is dependent on several matrix proteins; the events in this process are still being investigated intensely.

After deposition of initial calcium phosphate crystals into collagen (mineral nucleation of osteoid), more and more crystals must be added to give bone its rigidity. Although some of the new mineral added to osteoid is deposited by initial nucleation, most of the additional mineral is acquired by secondary nucleation, in which new crystals of apatite are deposited on nuclei of existing hydroxyapatite, by crystal growth of apatite already contained within the holes and pores of the collagen (Fig. 13), and by agglomeration (fusion) of these crystals. This accretion of new mineral continues until bone is fully mineralized; however, even fully mineralized mature bone is only 70% mineral, and the cells are always separated from the mineral by a

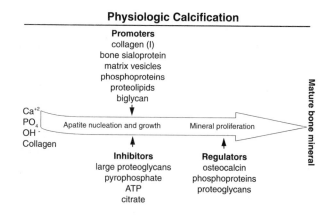

Figure 12

Bone mineral deposition consists of several stages, which are dependent on a variety of matrix proteins as illustrated here, and in Table 1.

Mineral accretion: *biological considerations*
Heterogeneity within a collagen fibril

Progressively increasing mineral mass due to:

1. Increased number of new mineral phase particles (nucleation)
    a. Heterogeneous nucleation by matrix in collagen holes (? pores)
    b. 2° crystal induced nucleation in holes and pores
2. Initial growth of particles to ~ 400 Å X 15-30 Å X 50-75 Å

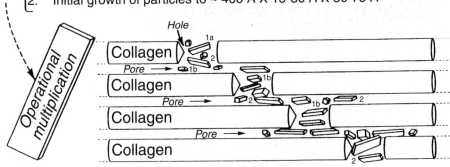

Figure 13

Diagram showing mineral accretion.

thin layer of osteoid. Certain matrix proteins are believed to be involved both in limiting the size to which crystals grow and in preventing mineral deposition in certain areas.

In summary, from the physical chemical standpoint, mineral accretion in tissues arises by (1) primary or heterogenous nucleation; (2) crystal growth; (3) secondary nucleation induced by previously formed crystals; and (4) aggregation of these mineral crystals.

The increase in the number of mineral phase particles in the collagen fibrils, which accompanies mineral accretion, can occur in either the holes or the pores (Fig. 11). Electron microscope studies reveal that from the spatial point of view, mineralization proceeds as a discontinuous process starting in the hole zones, and then proceeding to the pores. Discrete, physically separated loci within the osteoid fibrils become impregnated with mineral particles about the same time, forming a number of mineralization sites. It thus appears that initial mineralization takes place simultaneously at different locations within the collagen fibrils. Electron microscopy indicates that as crystal growth and secondary nucleation continue, the discrete growth areas enlarge and eventually coalesce. An understanding of how mineral accretion in bone as a whole proceeds, once nucleation begins in any single compartment, is integral to discussions of the influence of various metabolic and nutritional diseases on bone mineralization.

Bone Remodeling

Bone growth begins early in embryogenesis and continues throughout adolescence until skeletal maturity. Long bones grow by 2 mechanisms. They grow in length by a process of endochondral ossification, and in width by a process of intramembranous or subperiosteal new bone formation. Even following skeletal maturity, bone continues to remodel throughout life and adapt its material properties to the mechanical demands placed on it. The cellular and molecular mechanisms by which bone responds to mechanical stress (Wolff's law) are still poorly understood. These mechanisms are under intense investigation and may, in time, play an important role in the prevention and treatment of musculoskeletal disease. Investigation of the effects of biomechanics on bone remodeling is currently underway. See Chapter 5 for a more detailed discussion of this subject.

Cortical bone constitutes approximately 80% of the skeletal mass, and trabecular bone approximately 20%. Bone surfaces may be undergoing formation or resorption, or they may be inactive. These processes occur throughout life in both cortical and trabecular bone. Bone remodeling is a surface phenomenon, and it occurs on periosteal, endosteal, haversian canal, and trabecular surfaces. The rate of cortical bone remodeling, which may be as high as 50% per year in the midshaft of the femur during the first 2 years of life, eventually declines to a rate of 2% to 5% per year in the healthy elderly. Rates of remodeling in trabecular bone are proportionately higher throughout life and may normally be 5 to 10 times higher than cortical bone remodeling rates in the adult (Fig. 14).

Both cortical and trabecular bone are constantly remodeled by a specific cycle of cellular activity (Fig. 15). Flattened cells line the surfaces of bone and probably have a function similar to that of osteocytes. Under normal circumstances, the remodeling process of resorption followed by formation is closely coupled and results in no net change in bone mass. A bone modeling unit (BMU) consists of a group of all the linked cells that participate in remodeling a certain area of bone through a sequence of cell activity con-

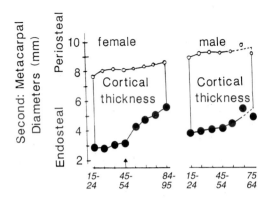

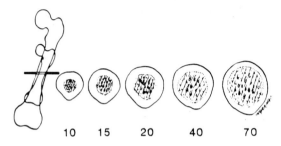

FEMORAL CROSS SECTIONS

10   15   20   40   70

Figure 14

Effects of age on metacarpal cortex and femoral diaphysis.

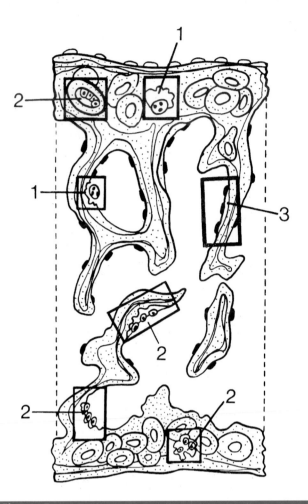

Figure 15

Schematic drawing showing principles of bone remodeling. Initially, bone is resorbed by osteoclasts both in the cortex and on the trabeculae (**1**). Bone formation by means of osteoblastic activity occurs at the site of the old resorbed bone (**2**). The osteoblasts themselves become incorporated into bone as osteocytes (**3**).

sisting of activation, resorption, and formation. It was originally thought that all cells in a BMU originate from a single cell line.

The dynamics of bone remodeling are illustrated in Figure 16, and the heterogeneity of adjacent bone caused by age and the continual internal remodeling of cortical bone is demonstrated.

Cortical bone remodeling proceeds via cutting cones (Fig. 17) and is similar to processes in other hard biologic tissues. Cutting cones, or sheets of osteoclasts, bore holes through the hard bone, leaving tunnels that appear in a cross section as cavities. The head of the cutting cone consists of osteoclasts that resorb the bone. Closely following the osteoclast front is a capillary loop and a population of osteoblasts that actively lay down osteoid to refill the resorption cavity. By the end of the process, a new osteon has been formed, which is the substance of the cortical bone.

Bone Blood Flow

Anatomic Features

Bone has 3 separate but interactive circulatory systems, which are described using the long bone as a model. The nutrient blood supply originates from a major artery of the systemic circulation and enters the diaphysis through a

nutrient foramen. The number of nutrient vessels differs for each long bone. Once in the medullary space, each nutrient vessel branches into ascending and descending medullary arteries and further subdivides into arterioles, which directly penetrate the endosteal surface and supply the diaphyseal regions. The metaphyseal complex is the second system that arises from the periarticular plexus (that is, the geniculate arteries); it penetrates the thin bone cortices to supply the metaphyseal regions. These vessels anastomose with the medullary arteries and with the epiphyseal arteries, after closure of the growth plate. Finally, the periosteal capillaries supply the outer layers of cortical bone where there are muscular attachments. Most researchers believe that the periosteal capillaries supply the outer 15% to 20% of the cortex (periosteal surface), even in the absence of muscular attachments. These 3 systems are interconnected; the watershed interconnections play a key role when the bone is injured. When the medullary system is taken

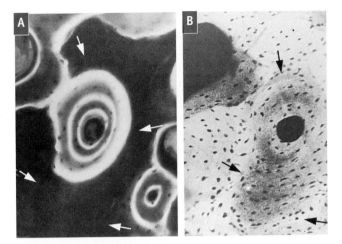

Figure 16

Microradiographs showing dynamics of bone remodeling. **A,** A thin section of cortical bone after tetracycline double labeling. Tetracycline is incorporated at sites of active mineralization of the bone matrix (concentric circles); by measuring time and distance between deposits, mineralization rates in bone remodeling can be assessed. The peripheral darker areas represent quiescent areas of the osteon. **B,** The most recently formed bone, which surrounds the haversian canal, is the least mineralized and appears dark. The oldest bone, which is the most highly mineralized, but quiescent from the standpoint of remodeling, appears quite light.

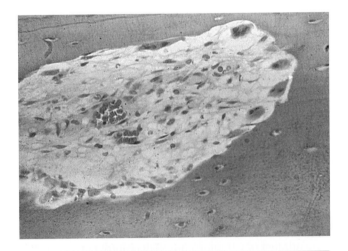

Figure 17

Photomicrograph showing cutting cones' mechanism.

away, for example, the periosteal system becomes dominant in the revascularization of the diaphyseal cortex.

The medullary arteries are thick-walled near their origin from the nutrient system. The walls thin down to 2 flattened layers of cells as the artery moves toward the metaphysis. All along the endosteal surface, side branches exit into the haversian system of capillaries, which ultimately return to venules in the medullary canal, which, in turn, drain into the central venous sinus and out the nutrient vein. The density of the venules is greater in the metaphyses and in areas where the hematopoietic marrow is active.

Clinical Relevance

Many clinical problems involving the musculoskeletal system have as their basis a disturbance of bone microcirculation. Osteomyelitis involves nonviable cortical or cancellous bone as the focus for bacterial adherence. Posttraumatic osteonecrosis involves an acute disruption of the arterial blood supply. Revascularization of these regions from metaphyseal sources, when the epiphyseal arteries cannot rapidly be recanalized, produces trabecular weakening and microfracture. Prosthetic joint devices generally devitalize endosteal surfaces; external fixation devices and bone plates affect both the endosteal supply (drilling into the medullary cavity) and the periosteal surface. The revascularization of these affected areas can produce pathologic bone resorption. Finally, fracture of bone, especially if it is a result of high-energy trauma, produces ischemic fragments that must be revitalized and are susceptible to infection. These topics are discussed in greater detail in future chapters.

Techniques for Studying Bone Vascularity

Current knowledge of the vascular anatomy of bone is based on angiographic studies. Large vessel structure is studied using barium perfusate and standard radiographs; the microcirculation is studied using thin-section (200 to 400 μm), high-resolution microradiographs. By changing the character of the perfusate, the distal vascular tree can be defined. Specimens perfused with methylsalicylate or glycerin (Spalteholtz method) reveal 3-D structure. These techniques provide no information on the function of the microcirculation.

The Fick indicator dilution technique involves injecting bone-seeking isotopes such as those of strontium and measuring the relative counts in bone effluent referable to segments of bone removed. This method has inherent inaccuracies because the isotope is not extracted completely on the first pass through the bone.

Hydrogen washout involves measuring the concentration of hydrogen ion with a platinum electrode; the hydrogen is breathed and the electrode must be placed into the bone. The concentration of the hydrogen at the electrode is proportional to the blood flow in the region. Xenon washout uses the same basic principles with locally injected xenon gas. These methods are problematic because of the need to insert electrodes into the region of interest, which affects the local microcirculation.

Use of radiolabeled microspheres is generally accepted to be the most accurate method for the experimental measurement of bone blood flow. Fifteen-μm spheres are labeled with 1 of 6 isotopes; this size is optimum for distal arteriolar trapping. The spheres are injected into the central arterial circulation, and peripheral arterial sampling is preferred. After flushing with heparin-saline, the reference organ (peripheral arterial) sampling is stopped. Because of the limited number of isotopes, only 6 measurements can be obtained per animal. At sacrifice, the bone area of interest and blood extracted are counted, and the blood flow is calculated using standard equations. Because it requires removal of bone, the method is not appropriate for clinical studies.

Laser Doppler flowmetry assesses the number and velocity of moving blood cells under the probe, which must contact the region of interest. This method assesses only small areas of bone at depths of 2.9 mm for cortical bone and 3.5 mm for cancellous bone. The values, provided in milli-Volts, are proportional to flow. This method is applicable to the clinical setting but multiple measurements must be made.

Finally, vital microscopy enables direct study of the microcirculation within titanium hollow screws. Using pulsed labels and video cameras, quantitative data can be generated.

Assessment of bone blood flow with these methods has clarified several factors. There is great heterogeneity of flow within cortical and cancellous bone. Moreover, arteriovenous shunts within bone can produce a source of error for some of the methods of measurement. Values are generally reported as milliliters per minute per gram of tissue (ml/min/g of bone) and vary from 1.6 to 7.0 ml/min/g in cortical bone and 10.0 to 30.0 ml/min/g in cancellous bone. Vasomotion, or rhythmic dilation and contraction of precapillary beds, has been identified in bone. Bone has the ability to autoregulate flow. Arterial inflow stops when systemic arterial blood pressure falls below 80 mm Hg and the arterial oxygen tension falls below 75 mm Hg. Finally, within different regions of the bone, hematocrit varies from 50% to 75% of the arterial hematocrit. The lowest hematocrits are found in regions with the highest perfusion rates.

Armed with these physiologic factors and the knowledge of how surgical manipulation influences bone flood flow, researchers can make progress in the development of new surgical techniques.

Biomechanics of Bone

Bone is the primary structural element of the human body. It protects vital internal organs, serves as a dynamic metabolic bank for the body's mineral resources, and provides a framework that allows skeletal motions. Bone differs from engineering structural materials in that it is self-repairing and can alter its properties and geometry in response to changes in mechanical and metabolic demand. Although the hypertrophy that occurs in skeletal muscle in response to heavy exercise or the atrophy that occurs in response to disuse is obvious, it is less apparent that bone is also remarkably responsive to mechanical demands. Bone density reductions are known to occur with aging, disuse, and certain metabolic conditions. Increased bone density occurs with heavy exercise and after treatment with certain therapeutic agents. Moreover, changes in bone geometry are observed during fracture healing, with aging, with exercise, and after certain surgical procedures. Understanding these phenomena, which appear to be adaptive, stress-related events, has been a central focus of bone physiology and biomechanics for over a century.

Many of these adaptive phenomena appear to be directed toward restoring and maintaining the structural integrity of the skeleton despite changes in the mechanical environment, a type of biomechanical homeostasis. Fracture healing and increased levels of bone density with severe exercise are obvious examples. Less obvious is the possibility that the cross-sectional geometry of long bones might change with aging in order to compensate for age-related reductions in bone density and mechanical properties. Epidemiologic evidence indicates that the reductions in bone density and strength known to occur in cortical bone with aging are not accompanied by dramatic increases in the incidence of shaft fractures among the elderly, suggesting that compensatory mechanisms are at work. However, such homeostatic, compensatory mechanisms do not appear to be sufficient to protect the aging skeleton against fracture at other skeletal sites such as the hip, spine, and distal radius.

In the United States alone, more than 250,000 hip fractures and 500,000 vertebral fractures occur each year among persons over age 45. As a result, there is an urgent need to improve understanding of fracture etiology, to identify patients most at risk, and to develop cost-effective interventions aimed at fracture prevention. To do so, however, requires an understanding of such mechanical factors as the relative importance of bone loss and trauma in fracture etiology, the role of trabecular versus cortical bone in the strength of the hip and spine, the importance of fatigue damage accumulation in the etiology of spontaneous fractures, and the relationships between fracture risk and the different load regimes that occur both during the activities of daily living and in response to traumatic events, such as a fall from standing height.

To address these issues and to provide an objective basis for a number of common clinical decisions, current knowledge on the mechanical behavior of bone is summarized here. By way of introduction, this text distinguishes between the behavior of bone tissue at the material level and the behavior of a whole bone at the structural level.

Material and Structural Behavior

The material behavior of bone describes how bone tissue behaves mechanically, regardless of where that tissue is located in any particular whole bone. To determine this fundamental material behavior, mechanical tests are performed on standardized specimens under controlled mechanical and environmental conditions. These tests are designed to eliminate any behavior associated with specimen geometry. The single requirement for the validity of the data obtained is that they be used only for bone with the same microstructure and in the same environment as the test specimens.

The simple equation for compression of a cylinder (Fig. 18, *A*) is:

$$F = (AE/l_0)\Delta l$$

where F is the force, Δl is the elongation of the cylinder, l_0 is the original length, A is the cross-sectional area, and E is Young's modulus.

A plot of force against deformation (Fig. 18, *B*) describes the structural behavior of the cylinder under axial loading.

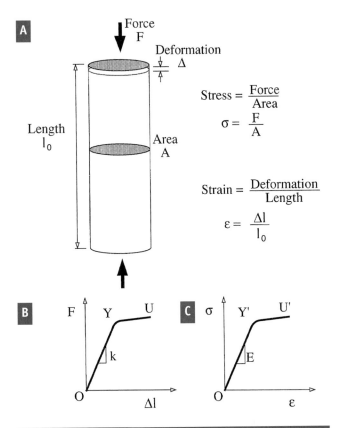

Figure 18

A, Cylindrical specimen used in uniaxial compression tests of human bone. Stress and strain are calculated from the force, deformation, and dimensions of the specimen. **B,** The force-deformation plot describes the structural behavior of the specimen. The linear region (also known as the elastic region) is from O to Y. At Y, "yielding" occurs, with internal rearrangement of the structure, often involving damage to the material. In the region Y-U (also known as the postyield region), nonelastic deformation occurs until finally, at U, fracture occurs. **C,** The stress-strain plot describes the material behavior of the tissue which makes up the specimen. The elastic behavior occurs up to Y´, and the postyield behavior occurs after Y´. The yield strength is at Y´ and the ultimate strength is at U´ where fracture occurs. The Young's modulus E is the slope of the linear region of this plot. (Reproduced with permission from Keaveny TM, Hayes WS: Mechanical properties of cortical and trevacular bone, in Hall BD (ed): *Bone*. Boca Raton, FL, CRC Press, vol 7, pp 285–344.)

The slope of the force deformation plot, the axial structural stiffness, is directly proportional to both the cross-sectional area and the Young's modulus (quantity E), and is inversely proportional to the length. Thus, in a test of 2 cylinders made from the same material (E constant), and of equal lengths (l constant) but with different cross-sectional areas (A different), the slopes of the force-deformation curves, and thus the structural stiffnesses, would be different for the 2 cylinders. Similarly, 2 bones of equivalent tissue properties (same E), but with different geometries, will display different structural stiffnesses. Conversely, because whole bones have different cross-sectional areas and lengths, it is not possible to use force deformation plots of whole bones to compare the material behavior of the bone tissue within the bones.

To eliminate these geometric effects, force is divided by cross-sectional area, F/A, and elongation is divided by original length, $\Delta l/l_0$, producing the geometrically normalized measures of force and elongation, known as stress σ and strain ε, respectively. Thus, the force deformation plot (Fig. 18, *B*) is transformed to a stress-strain plot (Fig. 18, *C*). Because the stress-strain relationship is independent of specimen geometry, this relationship describes only material behavior.

The initial slope of the stress-strain plot is Young's modulus E. For example, the 316L stainless steel commonly used with bone plates has a Young's modulus of 200 GPa; polymethylmethacrylate bone cement has a Young's modulus of approximately 2.3 GPa; cortical bone and relatively stiff trabecular bone have Young's moduli of approximately 17 GPa and 1 GPa, respectively. These numbers indicate that the stainless steel is an order of magnitude stiffer than cortical bone.

A typical stress-strain curve for wet cortical bone obtained from the femoral diaphysis and tested in uniaxial tension is shown in Figure 19. This stress-strain curve can be broken into 3 regions: the initial linear region, the yield region, and the postyield region. The modulus is the slope of the linear region. In contrast, the strength properties are obtained from the yield and postyield regions. Yielding, the onset of permanent deformation, occurs at the junction of the linear and postyield regions. This junction defines the yield strength σ_y, which, for bone, represents the stress when microstructural damage starts to occur. Fracture occurs when the ultimate strength σ_{ult} is reached.

The most basic mechanical properties of bone are obtained from tests where standardized specimens are progressively loaded in 1 direction until fracture. Such tests (as shown schematically in Figure 18) are called uniaxial, monotonic tests. If the bone is stretched, the test is called a tension test; if the bone is compressed, the test is a compression test. If the bone is twisted, the test is a torsion test. For a torsion test, the bone specimen shown in Figure 18 would be twisted about its longitudinal axis (Fig. 20). By recording the values of torsion and angular twist of the bone, it is possible to plot a torsion twist diagram, exactly analogous to the force deformation plot for a compression or tension test. Similarly, if the torsion and angular twist were normalized by the appropriate geometric parameters, it would be possible to derive a stress-strain plot, where stress is called the shear stress, and strain is called the shear strain. The slope of the shear stress-strain plot is the shear modulus G. Thus, the shear modulus, in units of MPa, is directly analogous to the Young's modulus.

Other, more complicated loading configurations may sometimes be used where loads act simultaneously in different directions. These are called multiaxial tests. The strength properties of bone are different for multiaxial loading from those for the simpler, uniaxial loading cases. Furthermore, the material properties of bone under multiple low amplitude loading cycles (fatigue) are different from those for single, monotonic loads. Finally, all these properties depend on the rate of loading (its viscoelastic properties), the amount of time the loads act on the bone (creep), and the age of the bone tissue.

Material Properties

Cortical Bone

Elastic Behavior

The elastic properties of isotropic materials do not depend on the orientation of the material with respect to the loading direction, and are characterized by a single modulus (Young's modulus). Most conventional engineering materials, such as 316L stainless steel, are isotropic. The other parameter necessary to fully characterize the elastic behavior of an isotropic material is Poisson's ratio. Poisson's ratio is a measure of how much a material bulges when compressed, or of how much a material contracts when stretched. This parameter, which typically is 0.3 for metals, also is found from a uniaxial test, and is the negative of the strain perpendicular to the loading direction divided by the strain along the loading direction.

The elastic properties of anisotropic materials depend on their orientation with respect to the loading direction. This is true for bone; however, the elastic properties of human cortical bone display a certain degree of symmetry, which reflects the bone's osteonal microstructure. The elastic properties of human cortical bone for loading in the plane transverse to the longitudinal axis are approximately isotropic and are substantially different from those for loading in the longitudinal direction, which is parallel to the axis of the osteons (along the longitudinal axis of the diaphysis). Therefore, human cortical bone usually is considered to be a transversely isotropic material. Transverse isotropy is a subset of anisotropy.

Two parameters, Young's modulus and Poisson's ratio, are used to describe the elastic properties of an isotropic material. The modulus of cortical bone in the longitudinal direction is approximately 1.5 times its modulus in the transverse direction and over 5 times its shear modulus. Its relatively high Poisson's ratios, with values up to 0.6, indicate that cortical bone bulges more than metals when subjected to uniaxial compression.

Strength

The strength properties of cortical bone also depend on the loading direction, making it transversely isotropic from both modulus and strength perspectives. The strength of cortical bone also depends on whether it is loaded in tension, compression, or torsion. This represents an asymmetry in the strength properties, adding further complexity to the description of these properties. Consequently, it is not precise to specify the strength of cortical bone with a single number.

Typical stress-strain curves for uniaxial, monotonic tension and compression loading of cortical bone, both in the longitudinal and transverse directions, show that cortical bone is stronger in compression than in tension (Fig. 21). For example, the tensile strength in longitudinal loading is approximately 130 MPa, whereas the corresponding compressive strength is 190 MPa. For transverse loading, the tensile strength is very low (50 MPa), whereas the compres-

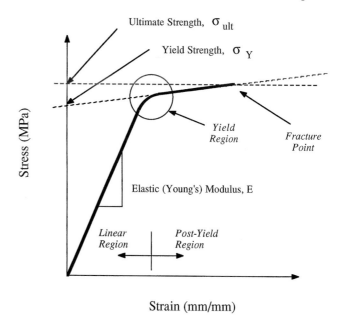

Figure 19

Typical stress-strain plot for cortical bone in tension, showing the linear, yield, and postyield regions. Note that the yield and ultimate strengths are similar. (Reproduced with permission from Keaveny TM, Hayes WC: Mechanical properties of cortical and trabecular bone, in Hall BK (ed): *Bone*. Boca Raton, FL, CRC Press, vol 7, pp 285–344.)

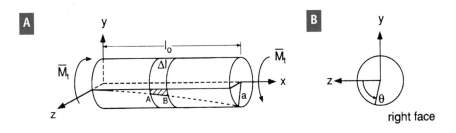

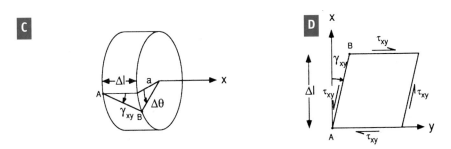

Figure 20

A, A circular shaft subject to twisting by a couple M_t at either end. The angle of twist θ between the right and left faces is given by $\theta = M_t l_0 / GI_p$ (**B**). **C,** The shear modulus G may be determined from the twist angle $\Delta\theta$ between two nearby surfaces separated by $G = (M_t \Delta 1)/(\Delta\theta I_p)$. **D,** In the pure shear state, the shear stresses τ_{xy} act on each face.

sive strength (130 MPa) is comparable to the tensile strength in longitudinal loading. These data suggest that cortical bone has adapted to a situation in which compressive loading is greater than tensile loading. This situation is consistent with the combined bending and axial compressive loads that are thought to act on the femoral diaphysis during everyday activities such as walking. Under these loading conditions, maximum compressive stresses are larger than maximum tensile stresses.

Because the tensile and compressive yield strengths of cortical bone are approximately equal to the respective ultimate strengths (Fig. 21), the maximum stresses that bone can sustain are close to its yield strength. Thus, when cortical bone is loaded close to its yield point, it is also close to fracture. Furthermore, bone loaded by stresses that are just above its yield strength will deform by a relatively large amount compared to its elastic behavior. Therefore, cortical bone undergoes relatively large deformations just prior to fracture.

Energy Absorption, Ductility, and Brittleness

Materials that absorb substantial energy before failure are classified as tough materials. Biomechanically, toughness is important in traumatic events, such as automobile accidents or falls, in which bone is forced to absorb energy. If the energy delivered to the bone is greater than the energy the bone can absorb, fracture occurs. Figure 21 indicates that, for both tensile and compressive loading in the longitudinal direction, the strains that occur in cortical bone at failure (ultimate strains) are much larger than those that occur at yielding (yield strains). Thus, for longitudinal loading, cortical bone is a tough material because it can absorb substantial energy before fracture. Furthermore, because the ultimate strain for longitudinal loading is substantially

larger than the yield strain, cortical bone can be classified as a relatively ductile material for longitudinal loading; that is, cortical bone can undergo a large amount of deformation prior to failure.

The stress-strain curve for transverse loading (Fig. 21) shows that bone is tougher under compressive loads than under tensile loads. Consequently, bone has the lowest resistance to loading regimens that cause tensile stresses in the transverse direction; for example, those that can arise as "hoop" stresses when cementless hip prostheses are press fit into the diaphyses of long bones. Because the ultimate strain is close to the yield strain for tensile loading in the transverse direction, bone is relatively brittle for transverse loading. Thus, cortical bone can behave in a relatively ductile or brittle fashion, depending on the loading direction and on whether tensile or compressive forces are applied.

Viscoelastic Behavior

Cortical bone displays viscoelastic behavior because its mechanical properties are sensitive to both the strain rate and the duration of the applied loads.

Strain Rate Sensitivity

The in vivo strain rate for bone can vary by more than an order of magnitude in the course of daily activities such as slow walking (strain rate ~ 0.001 per second), brisk walking (strain rate ~ 0.01 per second), and slow running (strain rate ~ 0.03 per second). Other activities, such as a jump from the height of 2 stairs or a fall from standing height, might result in strain rates as high as those encountered during slow and fast running, respectively. Generally, the strain rate increases as activity becomes more strenuous.

The mechanical properties of cortical bone are sensitive to strain rate. Figure 22 shows how the stress-strain behav-

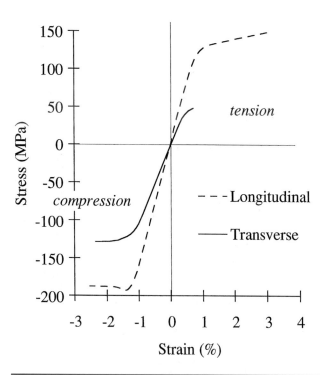

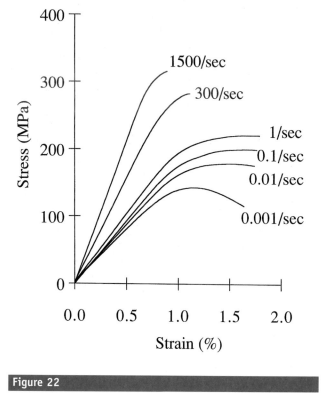

Figure 21

Stress-strain plots for human cortical bone for tensile and compressive loading. Data are shown for both longitudinal and transverse loading directions. (Adapted with permission from Gibson LJ, Ashby MF: *Cellular Solids: Structure and Properties.* Elmsford, NY, Pergamon Press, 1988, based on curves and data from Reilly DT, Burstein AH: The elastic and ultimate properties of compact bone tissue *J Biomech* 1975;B:393–405 and Currey JD: *The Mechanical Adaptations of Bones.* Princeton, NJ, Princeton University Press, 1984.)

Figure 22

Strain rate dependence of cortical bone material behavior. Both modulus and strength increase for increased strain rates. (Reproduced with permission from McElhaney JH: Dynamic response of bone and muscle tissue. *J Appl Physiol* 1966;21:1231–1236.)

ior for longitudinal compression of bovine bone is sensitive to strain rate. The increase in the initial slope of the stress-strain plot as the strain rate increases indicates that cortical bone has a higher modulus at higher strain rates. However, for typical daily activities (strain rates from 0.001 to 0.01 per second), the modulus changes only by approximately 15%.

Over the complete range of strain rates, the yield and ultimate strengths of cortical bone increase as the strain rate increases (Fig. 22), thereby indicating that cortical bone is stronger and stiffer for more strenuous activity. The same change in strain rate produces a relatively larger change in strength than in modulus (Fig. 23), indicating that ultimate tensile strength is slightly more sensitive to strain rate than is modulus. These data indicate that bone is approximately 20% stronger for brisk walking than for slow walking.

At very high strain rates (greater than 0.1 per second) representing high-impact trauma, cortical bone becomes more brittle (ultimate strain decreases) for loading in the longitudinal direction (Fig. 22). Thus, cortical bone exhibits a ductile to brittle transition as the strain rate increases. However, for the range of strain rates typical of more normal activity (less than 0.1 per second), ductility increases (ultimate strain increases) as the strain rate increases.

Based on the shapes of these stress-strain plots and the fact that energy per unit volume is equal to the area below the stress-strain curve, the optimal range of strain rates for maximum energy absorption is 0.01 to 0.1 per second. This range suggests that bone has adapted to absorb energy from the impact that arises from relatively strenuous activities such as running.

Creep Behavior

If bone tissue is subjected to a constant stress for an extended period of time, it will continue to deform. This phenomenon is called creep. A typical creep curve for adult human cortical bone under tensile loading (Fig. 24) is a plot of strain as a function of time for a constant stress level. Cortical bone exhibits the same 3 characteristic stages of creep behavior as do many conventional engineering materials. In the primary stage, specimen strain continues after loading and the creep (increase in strain) rate gradually decreases. In the secondary stage, there is a lower, usually constant creep rate. Finally, in the tertiary stage, there is a marked increase in the creep rate just before creep fracture. If cortical bone is loaded at certain levels for enough time, creep fracture will occur, although the stress level is well below the yield and ultimate strengths (Fig. 24). As shown in Figure 25, the time required for creep failure (fracture) to occur decreases as the stress increases, and resistance to creep fracture is greater for compressive than for tensile loading.

If creep occurs without fracture, and the bone is fully unloaded, permanent deformation results. For example, if creep is a result of relatively high tensile stresses held for several minutes, and the specimen is unloaded before creep fracture occurs, the specimen will be permanently deformed such that it is longer than its original length. This behavior is referred to as viscoplastic: "visco" from the creep behavior during loading, and "plastic" from the permanent deformation after unloading. Furthermore, if the applied constant stress is above a threshold level (70 MPa, or 55% of its ultimate strength, for human cortical bone loaded in longitudinal tension), the rate at which creep deformation occurs and the magnitude of the permanent deformation after unloading both increase sharply (Fig. 26). Creep studies have not yet been performed for loading in the transverse direction.

The mechanisms for creep behavior in cortical bone have not been determined. However, scanning electron micrographs of fractured surfaces have indicated that the creep mechanisms appear to be different for tensile and compressive loading. Osteon pullout is common for tensile loading, and fractures tend to cross through the osteons for compressive loading.

Age Effects
The modulus and strength properties of cortical bone progressively deteriorate with aging for both men and women. The longitudinal modulus and tensile yield strength of cortical bone taken from the femoral middiaphysis decrease by approximately 2% per decade after age 20 years (Fig. 27). For example, from the third to ninth decades, respectively, the ultimate tensile strength of bone, for longitudinal loading, decreases from approximately 130 MPa to 110 MPa, and the corresponding elastic moduli change from approximately 17 GPa to 15.6 GPa. The slope of the stress-strain curve after yielding increases by 8% per decade. Probably the most significant change from a fracture risk perspective

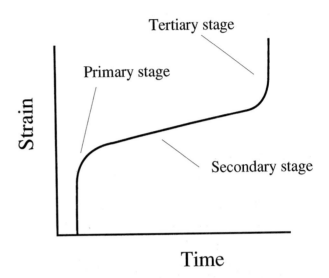

Figure 24

Schematic diagram showing the 3 stages of creep behavior of human cortical bone. (Reproduced with permission from Carter DR, Caler WE: A cumulative damage model for bone fracture. *J Orthop Res* 1985;3:84-90.)

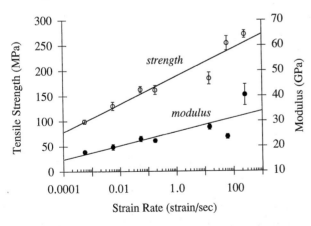

Figure 23

Comparison of strain rate sensitivities for modulus and ultimate tensile strength of human cortical bone for longitudinal loading. Over the full range of strain rates, strength increases by about a factor of 3, and modulus by a factor of 2. (Reproduced with permission from Wright TM, Hayes WC: Tensile testing of bone over a wide range of strain rates: Effect of strain rate, micro-structure and density. *Med Biol Eng Comput* 1976;14:671-680.)

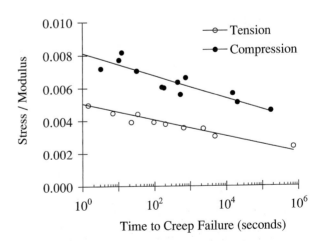

Figure 25

Creep fracture stress for human cortical bone as a function of the time to failure. To account for variations in modulus between specimens, stress values have been normalized (divided) by the initial modulus (measured at the beginning of the experiment). These data indicate that resistance to creep fracture is greater for compressive loading. (Reproduced with permission from Caler WE, Carter DR: Bone creep-fatigue damage accumulation. *J Biomech* 1989;22:625-635.)

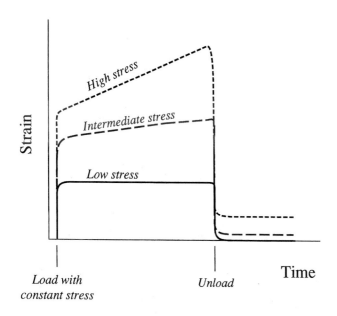

Figure 26

Schematic of typical strain-time curves, illustrating "viscoplastic" behavior of human cortical bone. In this experiment, the bone is loaded at a constant stress, and the strain is measured as a function of time. The specimen is then unloaded before creep fracture occurs. Typical behaviors are shown for different applied stresses. As the stress is increased, a creep threshold is reached, beyond which the creep rate (the slope in the second stage of creep behavior) increases. The permanent deformation (strain after unloading) also increases as the applied stress is increased. Interestingly, exactly similar behavior occurs for some chopped glass-fiber composite materials at elevated temperatures. (Reproduced with permission from Fondrk M, Bahniuk E, Davy DT, et al: Some viscoplastic characteristics of bovine and human cortical bone. *J Biomech* 1988;21:623–630.)

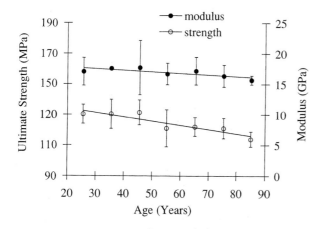

Figure 27

Age-related effects on longitudinal modulus and ultimate tensile strength of human femoral cortical bone. (Reproduced with permission from Burstein AH, Reilly DT, Martens M: Aging of bone tissue: Mechanical properties. *J Bone Joint Surg* 1976;58B:82–86.)

is the reduction in energy absorption (area under the stress-strain curve) that occurs with aging. The decrease in energy absorption by approximately 7% per decade results mainly from reductions in the ultimate strain. Taken together, these data indicate that cortical bone material in the human femur becomes less stiff, less strong, and more brittle with aging.

Microstructure and Mechanical Properties

Age-related changes in material properties vary for different bones. For example, decreases in ultimate tensile strength and modulus are greater for the femur than for the tibia, although decreases in ultimate strain are similar for each bone. One explanation for this is that the rate of bone turnover may be greater in the tibia than in the femur, and the mechanism that reduces both modulus and strength is inhibited as new osteons are formed. However, many parameters affect the mechanical properties of cortical bone.

Parameters that have been investigated as determinants of the mechanical properties of cortical bone are apparent density (proportional to porosity), ash density (total mineral content divided by bulk volume), histology (number of osteons, primary versus secondary bone), collagen composition and content, orientation of the collagen fibers and mineral, composition of the cement lines, bonding between the mineral and collagen phases, and accumulation of microcracks in the bone matrix and around osteons.

It is difficult to correlate these parameters with the mechanical properties of cortical bone because the ranges of modulus and strength values for this tissue are relatively small. Consequently, many of these issues remain equivocal, and this discussion is limited to the less controversial findings. Modulus and ultimate strength have been positively correlated with apparent density using a power law in which the reported exponents for modulus are in the range of 1.5 to 7.5. Both monotonic and fatigue strengths were found to be sensitive to the relative number of osteons in the bone. Correlation of density and microstructure suggests that haversian remodeling of primary bone is accompanied by a reduction in density. Nevertheless, microstructure has been shown to affect some mechanical properties after these changes in density were taken into account.

Probably the most important determinant of modulus and strength is the ash density or mineral content. In a study on properties of cortical bone from a wide range of species, multiple regression analysis demonstrated that almost 90% of the variance in modulus and strength can be explained using a power law model with both volume fraction (proportional to apparent density) and mineral content (proportional to ash density) as independent variables. Water content is also important in the mechanical properties of cortical bone. Wet bone, as found in situ, is less stiff, less strong, and less brittle than fully dried bone, although rewetting bone after it has been dried can almost fully restore its in situ behavior. Finally, collagen content has been shown to dominate the stiffness behavior after yielding has occurred.

Fatigue Properties

The strength properties just described characterize situations where there is a single application of force (monotonic loading). However, in vivo cortical bone is exposed primarily to repetitive, low intensity loading, which produces lower stress levels than those required to fracture a bone specimen during monotonic loading. This cyclic loading of bone can result in damage at the microstructural level. For example, during walking, the proximal femur is loaded cyclically with each step. The spine is loaded cyclically while a person is lifting objects, rising from a chair, and bending over. Not all loads result in damage to bone. If damage does occur, however, and if the damage accumulates over time, the strength of the bone is reduced. High levels of stress over shorter periods of time also may lead to fatigue damage, as shown by the relatively frequent incidence of stress fractures in military recruits, long distance runners, and race horses subjected to rigorous training programs. Thus, the major cause of these stress fractures appears to be fatigue damage accumulation. The mechanical properties of bone under the action of cyclic, repetitive loading are called the fatigue properties of bone.

Fatigue properties of cortical bone, besides being interesting for their role in stress fractures, are of interest as a potential stimulus for bone remodeling. Because the fatigue properties of cortical bone mainly have been measured in devitalized bone specimens, the effects of bone remodeling on the fatigue behavior of bone in vivo remain unknown. Physiologic levels of loading can induce fatigue damage and failure in vitro; therefore, bone remodeling, which occurs continuously in vivo, may repair the damage caused by relatively low intensity loading, such as occurs in walking. Studies have demonstrated that microcracks do occasionally occur in vivo. Thus, it has been hypothesized that one role of bone remodeling is to repair microcracks that form in bone as a result of the repetitive loading of daily activity.

Up to 10% of age-related hip and over 50% of age-related spine fractures are classified as spontaneous because they occur without any obvious trauma. If fatigue cracks continue to occur in bone with continued repetitive loading, and there are age-related reductions in the rate of bone turnover to repair these cracks, bone monotonic strength may progressively be compromised with age. Thus, the fatigue behavior of bone may be a causative factor in spontaneous fractures.

To determine the fatigue properties of bone using traditional engineering techniques, standard specimens of bone are cyclically loaded to fracture in controlled environments at a fixed level of stress (or, sometimes strain). The number of load cycles at fracture is recorded as the fatigue life corresponding to the specified stress level. Testing is performed at different stress levels, and results usually are presented as a σ-n plot of stress level (σ) versus the logarithm of the fatigue life, or number of cycles (n) (Fig. 28). This curve indicates that fatigue fracture will occur at any stress level above the endurance limit if the number of load cycles is large enough. The important concept is that fatigue fracture, like creep fracture, can occur at stress levels that are substantially lower than the monotonic strength.

The fatigue life of bone is better correlated with strains than with stresses, and in particular, with ranges of strains (defined as the difference between the maximum and minimum values of the applied cyclic strain). Figure 29 shows the in vitro fatigue life of human cortical bone for high cyclic strain ranges. Strain ranges representative of normal walking, mild exercise, and vigorous exercise are also shown. On average, approximately 5,000 cycles of loading correspond to the number of steps in 10 miles of running, whereas 1 million cycles correspond to 1,000 miles. The data in Figure 29 indicate that a total running distance of less than 1,000 miles could cause fracture of cortical bone tissue. The fatigue life of cortical bone also depends on temperature. Figure 30 shows the σ-n curve for bovine cortical bone for 2 different temperatures (21°C and 45°C). These data indicate that the fatigue life of cortical bone can be reduced considerably as the temperature increases from room temperature to body core temperature. Foot skin temperatures of up to 43°C have been recorded in subjects walking briskly in a warm environment. Because deep tissue temperatures in the extremities can be within 2°C of skin temperatures, bone temperatures in the foot may vary from less than room temperature to several degrees above body core temperature. The temperature dependence of fatigue properties may have physiologic consequences.

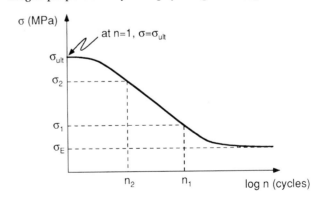

Cyclic fatigue failure will occur
at n_1 cycles of stress σ_1
or n_2 cycles of stress σ_2

Figure 28

Idealized fatigue σ-n curve for cortical bone. Fatigue fracture occurs at stress level σ_1 in n_1 cycles, or at stress level σ_2 at n_2 cycles. Note that the fatigue life n is shown on a log scale.

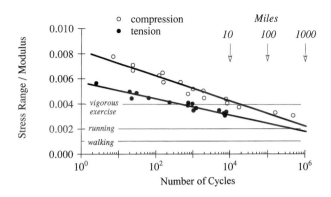

Figure 29

Fatigue life curve as a function of strain-range (stress range/modulus) for human femoral cortical bone for compressive and tensile loading. Typical strain-ranges for different activities are shown, and typical distances for walking and running are also shown. Behavior must be extrapolated for less strenuous activities. Note that, as with creep behavior, resistance to fatigue fracture is greater for compressive loading. (Reproduced with permission from Carter DR, Caler WE, Spengler DM, Frankel VH: Fatigue behavior of adult cortical bone: The influence of mean strain and strain range. *Acta Orthop Scand* 1981;52:481–490.)

Increases in strain rate result in increases in the monotonic strength of cortical bone; however, for a fixed stress level, fatigue damage increases with increasing strain rate. Therefore, more fatigue damage occurs for more strenuous exercise. Furthermore, for a fixed stress level, the fatigue life of cortical bone in uniaxial tension is less than in uniaxial compression, indicating that regions of cortical bone loaded in tension are at a higher risk of fatigue failure than regions loaded in compression by the same magnitude force. Studies have shown that the damage patterns for tensile and compressive loading are different, with mostly osteon debonding for tension and oblique cracking for compression. The curves shown in Figure 29 can be used to estimate the damage that accumulates in the bone as a result of a number of cycles of loading at a particular strain range level. One simple approach is to assume there is a linear rate of damage accumulation at each strain range level. Figure 29 indicates that the in vitro fatigue life at a tensile strain range of 0.002 is approximately 10^6 cycles. Therefore, a linear damage model (known as Miner's Rule) implies that 104 cycles at a strain range of 0.002 (10 miles of running) uses up $10^4/10^6$ (0.01) of the fatigue life. In the absence of a biologic repair process, 100 of these 10-mile runs would use up all the fatigue life and cause fracture. Similarly, a few cycles at very high loads could substantially reduce the fatigue life, so that subsequent activities such as walking could cause fatigue fracture after, say, 10^6 cycles (approximately 1 year). Therefore, fatigue damage accumulation is probably an important causative factor in stress fractures.

Mechanisms of Fatigue Damage Accumulation

Because fatigue behavior is so important, much interest has developed in the actual mechanism of fatigue damage accumulation in cortical bone. The fatigue mechanism for cortical bone has been shown to be similar to the mechanism for artificial, oriented, short-fiber composite materials. There are 3 characteristic stages of fatigue fracture, corresponding to crack initiation, crack growth (propagation), and final fracture. Because the modulus of the bone decreases as cracks form, these 3 stages can be demonstrated by a plot of stiffness versus number of cycles (Fig. 31). In the primary stage of crack initiation within the bone, a small decrease in the stiffness and strength would be experienced. In the secondary stage, crack propagation results in a slow but steady further decrease in these values. Finally, in the

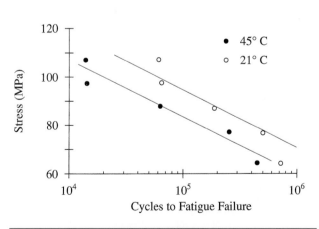

Figure 30

Temperature dependence of fatigue life for bovine femoral cortical bone. Each data point represents the mean value for six specimens tested at that stress level. Fatigue life is reduced by a factor of three when temperature is increased from 21°C to 45°C. (Reproduced with permission from Carter DR, Hayes WC: Fatigue life of compact bone: 1. Effects of stress, amplitude, temperature and density. *J Biomech* 1976;9:27–34.)

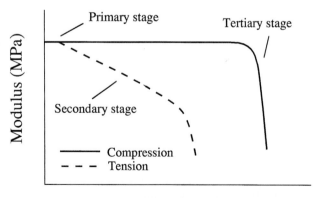

Figure 31

Schematic diagram of the modulus degradation which occurs for human cortical bone with fatigue loading. Note the different behaviors for tensile and compressive loading. The precise shape of these curves further depends on the magnitude of the applied stress. (Reproduced with permission from Pattin CAG: *Cyclic Mechanical Property Degradation in Bone During Fatigue Loading*. Palo Alto, CA, Stanford University, 1991. Thesis.)

tertiary stage, fracture is preceded by a rapid decrease in the ability to support load. The precise shape of these curves depends on the magnitude and sign (tension versus compression) of the applied load.

For cortical bone, haversian canals, lacunae, or canaliculi act as crack initiators because these discontinuities in the bone microstructure cause local increases in stress (stress concentrations). However, crack initiation, per se, is not necessarily detrimental to the structural integrity of cortical bone because cracks may induce bone remodeling. Cortical bone also has been shown to remodel such that stress concentrations about small holes are reduced. Bone not only repairs cracks, but also may remodel to reduce stresses about these cracks. What becomes important then, is how well bone can stop the growth of cracks so that they remain small enough to be repaired by remodeling.

The second and most important stage of fatigue failure is the slow propagation of these microcracks, which tend to join together once they progress beyond the initiation stage. The resulting larger cracks then run into weak material interfaces (cement lines) between the osteons in the secondary haversian systems, causing 2 things to occur. First, some osteons debond from the matrix, contributing to the osteon pullout phenomenon commonly observed on fractured surfaces of cortical bone. Second, the direction of crack propagation is changed from perpendicular to the loading direction to parallel to the loading direction. This change has the effect of producing a stress at the crack tip that, instead of opening the crack, is parallel to the crack and, therefore, harmless (does not open the crack).

These effects, and possibly others, tend to stop cracks from progressing across bone in the transverse direction, thereby increasing the bone's resistance to propagation of transverse cracks under longitudinal loading. Weak longitudinal interfaces in bone that stop the progression of transverse cracks include the interfaces between the osteons and the interstitial material, those between adjacent lamellae in the interstitial material, and those between the interfaces within single osteons. Therefore, even if cracks form easily because of bone's natural voids, other imperfections in the microstructure, namely the weak interfaces in the haversian system, tend to stop their progression under loads typical of normal activity.

This second stage of fatigue damage results in a slight reduction of modulus in bone; however, because damage accumulates, it reduces the fatigue life of bone. The final stage of fatigue fracture occurs because cracks coalesce and become so large that the weak interfaces can no longer absorb them. The specimen then fails as the final crack travels across the specimen, resulting in a sharp decrease in modulus followed by its fracture.

Trabecular Bone There is a large variation in density for trabecular bone. Both spatial and temporal variations in trabecular bone density can occur as a result of changes in anatomic location and age, respectively. For example, trabecular bone material properties within the proximal tibia can vary by up to 2 orders of magnitude because of changes in density alone. Material properties for trabecular bone have been reported for most anatomic sites. In addition, noninvasive densitometric studies have shown that trabecular bone mineral density in the hip and spine decreases with age, reaching lower levels in women than men. Because in vitro biomechanical studies of cadaveric material have shown that the material properties of trabecular bone are very sensitive to apparent density, discussion of these properties requires reference to the anatomic location and the age of the tissue.

To further complicate matters, material properties of trabecular bone also depend on its architecture, which, like its density, depends on the anatomic site and, to a lesser extent, on age. While cortical bone is essentially a low porosity solid, trabecular bone is best described as an open-celled porous foam. Made up of a series of interconnecting trabeculae, trabecular bone can be idealized as a combination of rod-rod, rod-plate, or plate-plate basic cellular structures where rods and plates represent thin and thick trabeculae, respectively (Fig. 32). Depending on the type and orientation of these basic cellular structures, the mechanical properties can vary by at least an order of magnitude.

Elastic Behavior

In general, the modulus of trabecular bone can vary from approximately 10 MPa to 2,000 MPa, depending on the anatomic site and age. Trabecular bone is much less stiff than cortical bone, which has a modulus of approximately 17,000 MPa. However, there are regions in the skeleton, such as the cranium, the subchondral plate in the proximal tibia, the metaphyseal shell in the proximal femur, and the end plates in vertebral bodies, where the distinction between cortical and trabecular bone is less clear. Mean values of the modulus in these regions have been measured in the range of 1,150 MPa to 9,650 MPa. Because most research has focused on the material properties of the trabecular bone that is found in the metaphyses of long bones, attention is limited to these regions.

Dependence on Apparent Density

As mentioned above, the material properties of trabecular bone are very sensitive to apparent density. In particular, it has been demonstrated that the modulus E of trabecular bone in any loading direction is related to its apparent density ρ by a power-law relationship of the form:

$$E = a + b\,\rho^c$$

where a, b, and c are constants that depend on the architecture of the tissue.

As with any power law, the most important parameter in this relationship is the exponent c, which directly affects

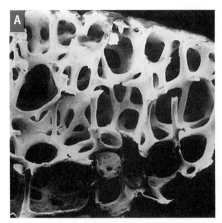
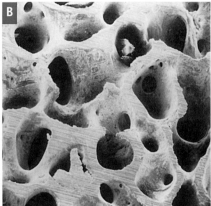
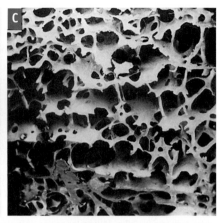

Figure 32

Scanning electron micrographs showing the various basic cellular structures of human trabecular bone: **A,** The rod-rod basic cellular structure, from the femoral head; **B,** The more dense plate-plate cellular structure, also from the femoral head; **C,** The plate-rod cellular structure, from the femoral condyle. (Reproduced with permission from Gibson JL: The mechanical behavior of cancellous bone. *J Biomech* 1985;18:317–328.)

how density affects the modulus. In general, the exponent has a value of approximately 2 (Fig. 33). Statistical analyses have shown that the best fit for the modulus of specimens pooled from a wide range of anatomic sites is obtained by a squared exponent. Consequently, a 25% reduction in density, as has been observed in elderly cadaveric vertebrae, results in a 56% decrease in modulus.

Dependence on Architecture

When the architecture is controlled, the variation in apparent density of trabecular bone can explain most of the variation in modulus. However, as can be seen from the scatter in modulus values for any particular value of apparent density (Fig. 33), other variables, namely the architecture, can also affect modulus. Scanning electron microscopes have been used successfully to illustrate the large variation in trabecular bone architecture over different anatomic sites.

The architecture of trabecular bone describes both the shape of the bone and its orientation. The basic structure describes the general connectivity of the trabeculae, the mean thickness of individual trabeculae, the mean spacing between trabeculae, and the number of trabeculae. There is a clear relationship between the density of the bulk trabecular bone and both the number and mean thickness of individual trabeculae. For the lumbar spine, there is a strong linear relationship between density and these variables (Fig. 34). In the subcapital region of the proximal femur, however, the relationship between mean trabecular thickness and density is highly nonlinear (Fig. 34).

The different architectures that exist for trabecular bone result in an anisotropy of elastic properties. In contrast to cortical bone, trabecular bone is nearly isotropic at some anatomic sites (proximal humerus), and highly anisotropic at others (elderly lumbar spine). Because trabecular bone is both anisotropic and heterogeneous, it is difficult to generalize about its elastic properties.

Uniaxial Strength

Much research has focused on the compressive strength of trabecular bone because its in vivo failure is believed to be dominated by compressive loads. Figure 35 shows typical stress-strain plots for specimens of trabecular bone with different apparent densities under uniaxial compressive

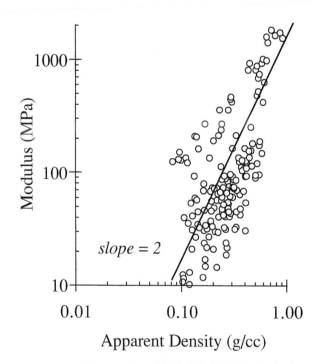

Figure 33

Compressive modulus as a function of apparent density for trabecular bone. The orientation of the specimen is not controlled. In general, the modulus of trabecular bone, when taken from a wide range of species and anatomic locations, varies as a power-law function of density with an exponent of approximately 2. (Reproduced with permission from Keaveny TM, Hayes WC: Mechanical properties of cortical and trabecular bone, in Hall BK (ed): *Bone.* Boca Raton, FL, CRC Press, 1993, vol 7, pp 285–344.)

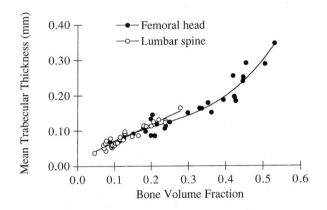

Figure 34

Mean thickness of the trabeculae in the lumbar spine and the subcapital region of the proximal femur as a function of bone volume fraction, which is proportional to apparent density. (Reproduced with permission from Snyder BD, Hayes WC: Multiaxial structure-property relations in trabecular bone, in Mow VC, Ratcliffe A, Woo SL-Y (eds): *Biomechanics of Diarthrodial Joints*. New York, NY, Springer-Verlag, 1990, pp 31–59.)

loading. Both the elastic and postyield behaviors are sensitive to apparent density. These characteristics are also displayed by artificial and natural porous foam materials such as aluminum honeycombs, cork, and balsa wood.

The stress-strain plots in Figure 35 have 3 regions that represent distinct phases of material behavior. In the first stage, the material is in the linear region, in which individual trabeculae bend and compress as the bulk tissue is compressed. In the second stage, failure occurs by fracture of some trabeculae and buckling of others. As more and more trabeculae fail, the strain increases until broken trabeculae begin to fill the pores, causing the specimen to stiffen in stage 3. Lower density specimens can deform more before the final stiffening phase than can higher den-

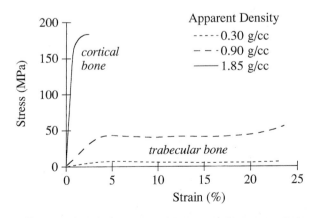

Figure 35

Example of typical compressive stress-strain behaviors of trabecular and cortical bone for different apparent densities. (Reproduced with permission from Keaveny TM, Hayes WC: Mechanical properties of cortical and trabecular bone, in Hall BK (ed): *Bone*. Boca Raton, FL, CRC Press, 1993, vol 7, pp 285–344.)

sity specimens (Fig. 35). This ability to deform to compressive strains of over 50% highlights a unique feature of trabecular bone: it can absorb considerable energy (area under the stress-strain curve) for large compressive loads while maintaining a minimum mass.

The compressive strength of trabecular bone also is related to its apparent density by a squared power-law relationship (Fig. 36). Many studies have demonstrated strong linear relationships between compressive strength and modulus. Thus, stiffer trabecular bone is proportionally stronger, which suggests that the main parameter that may control failure in trabecular bone is not the maximum level of stress, but the maximum level of strain (strain = stress divided by modulus). This supposition is supported by the evidence that trabecular bone yields at strains in the range of 1% to 4%, with only a weak dependence on density.

These relationships between apparent density and both modulus and strength have important physiologic and clinical consequences. First, bone can easily regulate its strength and stiffness can easily be regulated by adjusting its apparent density. Second, subtle changes in bone apparent density result in large changes in strength and modulus, indicating that an order of magnitude reduction in both trabecular bone strength and modulus can occur by the time density reductions of 30% to 50% are visible radiographical-

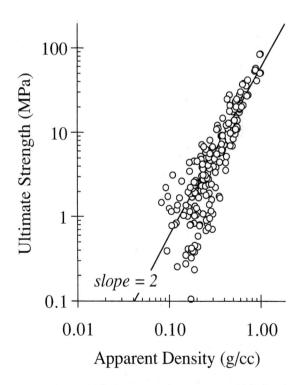

Figure 36

Ultimate compressive strength as a function of apparent density for trabecular bone. In general, compressive strength varies as a power-law function of density with an exponent of approximately 2. (Reproduced with permission from Keaveny TM, Hayes WC: Mechanical properties of cortical and trabecular bone, in Hall BK (ed): *Bone*. Boca Raton, FL, CRC Press, vol 7 pp 285–344.)

ly. Thus, conventional radiographic techniques used to assess fracture risk of whole bones are poor indicators of bone tissue strength.

The tensile behavior of a block of trabecular bone is much different from its compressive behavior (Fig. 37). Although the linear behavior is similar to that for compressive loading, the postyield behavior is completely different. For tensile loading, failure occurs by fracture of the individual trabeculae. As more trabeculae fracture, the specimen can take less and less load, until finally complete fracture occurs. This behavior is similar to that for fiber-reinforced concrete, and is typical of engineering materials designed to resist primarily compressive forces.

Comparison of the compressive and tensile behaviors of trabecular bone (Figs. 35 and 37) indicates that the postyield load-carrying capacity of trabecular bone is high for compression and almost negligible for tension. Thus, trabecular bone loaded beyond the ultimate strength in compression can still carry substantial load; it will not significantly overload surrounding trabecular bone, and failure will not spread to the surrounding tissue. However, for tension loading beyond the ultimate strength, no load can be carried by the tissue because it fractures. In this case, the surrounding tissue must carry the full load, and thus may be overloaded. If subsequent failure of that material occurs, a cascade effect could result in which a crack could propagate across a whole bone, causing fracture. Although local failure of trabecular bone in compression is not likely to lead to failure of a whole bone, local failure in tension could have catastrophic consequences.

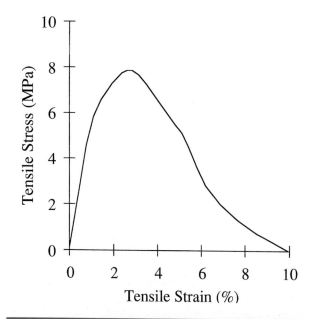

Figure 37

Tensile stress-strain behavior of trabecular bone. Compare this with the compressive behavior shown in Figure 36. (Reproduced with permission from Carter DR, Schwab GH, Spengler DM: Tensile fracture of cancellous bone. *Acta Orthop Scand* 1980;51:733–741.)

Age Effects

Age-related fractures are an enormous clinical and social problem in the United States, particularly for the spine, distal radius, and proximal femur, which are largely trabecular bone structures. The ways in which both density and architecture can affect the material properties of trabecular bone have been discussed. Both of these parameters change with aging, resulting in age-related trabecular bone fragility, which has been associated with the large incidence of hip, spine, and radial fractures in the elderly. Although absolute bone density is not a particularly good predictor of hip and spine fracture risk, changes (decreases) in bone density and the resulting increase in bone fragility are good predictors of spine fracture. Thus, a major research area in trabecular bone biomechanics is quantification of age-related changes in trabecular bone density and architecture, particularly for the spine.

Figure 38 shows typical age-related changes in human trabecular bone from the lumbar spine. As the bone loses mass, its density diminishes and its architecture changes. The reductions in density depend on a number of factors, including gender and anatomic site. In general, bone mineral "density" (which reflects the areal density of both trabecular and cortical bone for a particular cross-section) declines with age, reaching lower levels in females than males. To reflect these gender-specific bone mineral "density" reductions, osteoporosis has been categorized as senile or postmenopausal. Senile osteoporosis affects both females and males, resulting in equal reductions in cortical and trabecular bone mass. Postmenopausal osteoporosis is thought to affect a relatively small subset of females, and it is characterized by excessive and disproportionate trabecular bone loss. In the lumbar spine, direct measurements have shown a decrease in trabecular bone density of approximately 50% from ages 20 to 80 years.

Results of histomorphometric studies also have shown that aging results in changes in trabecular bone architecture. These studies have demonstrated that, with decreasing density, the number and thickness of the trabeculae decrease, while the size of the intertrabecular spaces increases. Data from 3-D stereologic studies have demonstrated that, regardless of density, the number of horizontal trabeculae in the lumbar spine is less than the number of vertical trabeculae, and that the number of vertical trabeculae decreases with decreasing density at twice the rate of the horizontal trabeculae (Fig. 39). Thus, contrary to the evidence from earlier 2-D histomorphometric studies, vertical trabeculae do not become thicker with aging, and preferential loss of horizontal trabeculae does not appear to occur in the lumbar spine. In fact, these data from 3-D studies suggest that preferential loss of vertical trabeculae occurs with increasing age. This loss of trabeculae may be more damaging to the structural integrity of trabecular bone than mere thinning because lamellar new bone can be formed only on existing surfaces, making complete loss

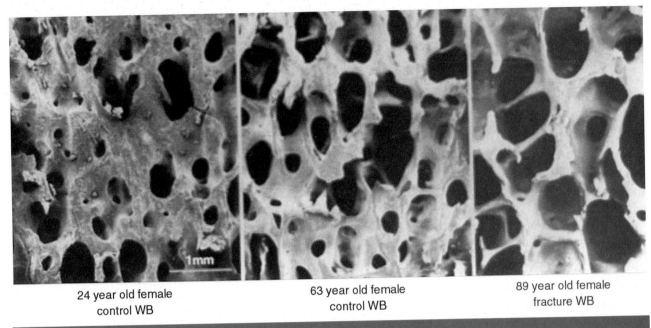

24 year old female
control WB

63 year old female
control WB

89 year old female
fracture WB

Figure 38

Age-related changes in apparent density and architecture of human trabecular bone from the lumbar spine. (Courtesy of Marc D. Grynpas, PhD.)

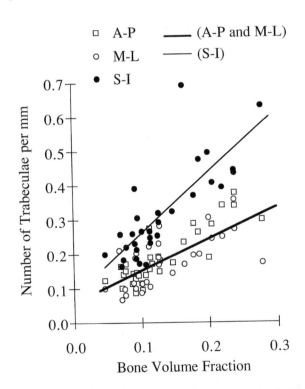

Figure 39

Decrease in the number of vertical (S-I) and horizontal (M-L, A-P) trabeculae with decreasing bone volume fraction (proportional to apparent density) for the human lumbar spine. The rate of loss of vertical trabeculae is twice that of the horizontal trabeculae. Even so, there are always more vertical than horizontal trabeculae (M-L, medial-lateral direction; S-I, superior-inferior direction; A-P, anteroposterior direction). (Reproduced with permission from Snyder BD, Hayes WC: Multiaxial structure-property relations in trabecular bone, in Mow VC, Ratcliffe A, Woo SL-Y (eds): *Biomechanics of Diarthrodial Joints*. New York, NY, Springer-Verlag, 1990, pp 31–59.)

of a single trabeculum irreversible.

Because the strength of trabecular bone depends on both apparent density and architecture, these age-related changes can substantially weaken it. For example, failure caused by buckling of individual trabeculae is more likely when trabeculae become fewer, thinner, and longer. This reduced resistance to failure caused by buckling of individual trabeculae has been referred to as a "triple jeopardy," because 3 independent factors—reduction in number, decrease in thickness, and increase in length—contribute to the weakening mechanism. In addition, failure of individual trabeculae may occur by fracture. The weakening mechanism for fracture is reduction in the number and thickness of the trabeculae, which might be referred to as a "double jeopardy."

The observed reductions in trabecular bone density are manifested as changes in the architecture, which can be quite subtle. Because of the double and triple jeopardy mechanisms, the accompanying reductions in strength may be greater than those suggested by reductions in density alone. Obviously, the accelerated bone loss that occurs with postmenopausal osteoporosis further reduces the strength of trabecular bone. Thus, normal, age-related changes, coupled with pathologic processes, can produce substantial changes in the strength of trabecular bone. This weakening must play a significant role in the etiology of age-related fractures of the hip and, particularly, of the spine.

Structural Properties

Bones of the appendicular skeleton are long, slender, and slightly curved. They are loaded primarily by compressive contact forces applied at the joint surfaces and by tensile muscle forces applied about the articulating surfaces. The contact forces are generally larger in magnitude than the muscle forces. The diaphysis, therefore, is loaded by a net compressive force. The combined action of the compressive and tensile forces about the joint result in a net bending moment acting on the diaphysis. This bending moment also can exist in the absence of muscle forces because of the curvature of the bone. Moreover, torque about the longitudinal axis can result in a net torsional moment about the diaphyseal axis. Therefore, long bones are subjected to a combination of axial compressive forces, bending moments, and torsion. Review of the behavior of simple structures (see Chapter 5) is suggested before continuing with examination of the structural properties of bones.

Bending of Bone

A bone can be subjected to bending loads in a number of ways, including the application of 2 sets of forces near the ends (Fig. 40). This loading configuration, known as 4-point bending, often is used in the laboratory for studying the biomechanics of bone, and it subjects the central section of the bone to a constant bending moment M. Increasing the moment of inertia and modulus will increase the bending (structural) stiffness of a bone; increasing the length will decrease the stiffness.

Whereas the cross-sectional area is the most important geometric parameter for axial loading, the moment of inertia is the most important geometric parameter for bending. The moment of inertia describes how the material is distributed with respect to a specified reference axis, called the neutral axis. A region of material that is at a greater distance from the neutral axis is much more efficient in resisting bending about that axis than a region of material coincident with it. For example, consider the bending behavior of a long, slender meterstick. The bending stiffness is lower when the meterstick is bent on the flat surface than when it is bent on the narrow edge because more of the material is located coincident with the neutral axis for the former case.

Long bones are hollow, with most bone tissue located away from the neutral axis, which is the centroid of the cross section. The long bone's hollow tubular structure has a physiologic role, which includes providing a bone marrow reservoir and a medullar blood supply. However, from a mechanical perspective, this geometry represents an excellent design to resist primarily bending loads in both frontal and sagittal planes and torsional loads about the diaphyseal axis.

Combined Axial and Bending Loads on Bone

The stress in the femur resulting from a combination of axial and bending loads is simply the sum of the stresses caused by each loading mode. The femur behaves as follows under combined axial and bending loads. Bending in the frontal plane causes tensile stresses along the lateral aspect and com-

pressive stresses along the medial aspect. On the lateral side, by contrast, the stresses resulting from axial loading and bending are of opposite signs. Either tensile or compressive stresses could occur here, depending on the relative magnitudes of the axial and bending stresses. Because bending stresses at the periosteal surfaces in the femoral diaphysis are generally much greater than axial stresses, tensile stresses occur on the lateral aspect of the femur.

Bending of the femur in the sagittal plane as a result of posteriorly directed loads also results in tensile and compressive stresses in the anterior and posterior aspects, respectively. Similar situations occur in most long bones. In general, compressive stresses are higher than tensile stresses throughout the appendicular skeleton. The compressive strength of cortical bone is greater than the tensile strength, indicating that cortical bone tissue has adapted to the higher compressive stresses that occur in long bones because of the combined compressive and bending loads commonly encountered during daily activities.

Age-Related Remodeling of the Diaphysis

Age-related remodeling of cortical bone can result in large changes in the areal moment of inertia. These geometric changes also

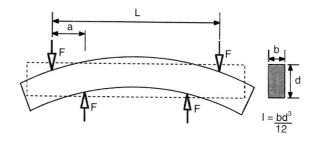

Mid-span deflection, $\delta = Fa(3L^2 - 4a^2) / 24EI$

I = Areal moment of inertia
E = Modulus

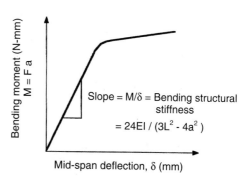

Figure 40

Beam in four-point bending, showing the undeformed shape in dashed lines and the deformed shape in solid lines. The midspan deflection δ depends on the applied bending moment, M = Fa; the geometry, L and I; and the material properties, E. The quantity I is called the areal moment of inertia.

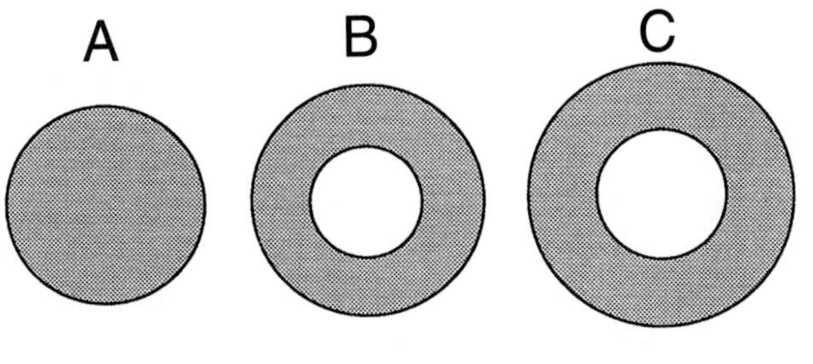

	A	B	C
Area (cm²)	2.77	2.85	3.09
Relative axial strength	1.00	1.03	1.11
Moment of inertia (cm⁴)	0.61	1.06	1.67
Relative bending strength	1.00	1.49	2.05

Figure 41

Relative axial and bending strengths for cylinders B and C with respect to a solid cylinder A. Cylinder B represents a young diaphysis; cylinder C represents an elderly diaphysis, with enlarged endosteal and periosteal diameters. Axial strengths are relatively similar. Bending strengths, however, are progressively higher for cylinders B and C, respectively. This indicates that age-related diaphyseal expansions increase the strength of the diaphysis, which, in turn, may offset the age-related decreases in tissue strength that are known to occur for cortical bone.

can influence the bending stresses and, therefore, the strength of a long bone (Fig. 41).

Axial stresses are relatively insensitive to age-related geometric changes, but bending stresses are quite sensitive. Age-related endosteal and periosteal expansions of the diaphysis, therefore, can reduce bending stresses (if the external loads are identical) by over 25% with respect to younger bones. Because age-related changes also result in reductions in the strength of cortical bone tissue, the age-related geometric remodeling process may serve to compensate for these tissue-level strength reductions. Evidence in support of this mechanism comes from the lack of an exponential increase in diaphyseal fracture incidence in the elderly. This is in contrast to the high rate of fracture in the proximal femur and spine, where this age-related compensatory geometric remodeling does not occur.

Combined Axial, Bending, and Torsional Loads Stresses resulting from axial loading and bending can be combined by simple addition when the stresses act in the same direction. When shear stresses resulting from torsion are superimposed, the axial, bending, and shear stresses are combined in a more complex manner to give a tensile or compressive stress, called a principal stress, which acts in the principal direction. When there is no torsion, the principal stress is the sum of the axial and bending stresses, and the principal direction is in the direction of the axial and bending stresses. For combined axial, bending, and shear stresses, the principal stress will be greater than the sum of the axial and bending stresses, and the principal direction will differ from the direction of the axial and bending stresses. Thus, the effect of imposing a torsional load on combined axial and bending loads is to increase the principal stress and change the principal direction.

In Vivo Fracture Prediction

Quantitative computed tomography (QCT) generates a cross-sectional image of the vertebral body. This image allows preferential measurement of trabecular bone density. Because QCT presents a number of significant research advantages in the development of objective fracture risk predictors for the hip and spine, this section provides a summary of knowledge on the development and in vitro validation of regional fracture risk predictors for these 2 sites. The results are discussed in light of available evidence on in vivo loads associated both with the activities of daily living and with trauma. The findings are then compared against comparable estimates of fracture risk for diaphyseal regions. While this discussion stresses the importance of bone density on in vivo fracture prediction, Cummings has demonstrated that smoking, low body weight, and a personal or first relative with a low energy fracture clearly increases the risk of hip fracture. In addition, bone turnover is highly correlated with the risk of fracture.

Factor of Risk

In engineering, the design of failure-resistant structures requires 3 important pieces of information: (1) the geometry of the structure; (2) the mechanical properties of the materials from which the structure is made; and (3) the location and direction of the loads to which the structure is subjected. Engineering theories based on this information can be used to estimate the stresses in the structure for various imposed loads. These stresses then can be compared against the known strengths of the materials within the structure to test for failure. The ratio of the material strength to the imposed stress at each point is called the safety factor. An alternative definition of the safety factor is expressed in terms of forces, and is the ratio of the force required to cause failure of the entire structure to the imposed force.

The inverse of the safety factor, called the risk factor, also provides a convenient measure of fracture risk for a structure under a particular set of loading conditions. The risk factor r is given by

$$r = F_{service}/F_{failure}$$

where $F_{service}$ is the imposed load and $F_{failure}$ is the magnitude of the imposed load that would cause failure for the structure. When the risk factor is low (for example, much less than 1), the force required to cause failure is much greater than the imposed force, and the structure can be expected to be at low risk of failure under the imposed loads. Conversely, when the risk factor is high (for example, close to or greater than 1), the structure is at high risk of failure. In engineering design, it often is possible to decrease the risk factor by increasing the size of the structure, using a stronger material, or, in some cases, reducing the magnitude of the imposed loads. Most engineering structures operate with risk factors in the range of approximately 0.15 to 0.20. Fracture prediction in the human skeleton is complicated because there is considerable uncertainty about the magnitudes and directions of the imposed loads at the hip and spine during typical daily activities. Even less is known about the forces generated as a result of a traumatic event such as a fall. Skeletal regions at high risk of age-related fractures exhibit far more complex geometries than most engineering structures, and these geometries can change with bone remodeling. In addition, bone density, microstructure, and morphology not only exhibit marked spatial heterogeneity but also change dramatically as a consequence of aging and disease. In view of these complexities, it is not surprising that very little is known regarding the risk factors that exist in skeletal regions such as the hip and spine under the imposed loads associated with either normal daily activity or traumatic events.

QCT and Material Properties of Trabecular and Cortical Bone

To establish correlations between QCT data and the compressive material properties of trabecular bone, scans are taken at defined locations and then small specimens are removed and tested in vitro to determine elastic modulus and uniaxial compressive strength. Experiments have shown relatively strong correlations between the QCT density and modulus ($R^2 \approx 0.70$) and compressive strength ($R^2 \approx 0.70$, Fig. 42). Thus, QCT can be used to estimate the modulus and strength of trabecular bone tissue. However, only poor correlations have been found between QCT data and both modulus and strength of cortical bone tissue. Presumably, this lack of correlation is due to the very narrow range in cortical bone densities coupled with the inability of QCT to differentiate between these densities (poor resolution). Research in this area is still in progress.

QCT and Vertebral Body Failure

Numerous studies have been performed to correlate the load required to fracture an isolated lumbar vertebral body (posterior elements removed) in vitro and some integral measure of its QCT density as measured in a typical clinical scan. Strong correlations have been found between the fracture load and the (directly measured apparent) density

of trabecular bone within the vertebral body ($R^2 \approx 0.80$), but correlations between the fracture load and the mean QCT density ($R^2 \approx 0.50$, Fig. 43) are only moderate. The mean value of the fracture loads for uniaxial compression of intact, elderly lumbar vertebrae is approximately 3,100 to 3,400 N. To calculate risk factors, these mean values must be compared against estimates of the in vivo loads imposed on the lumbar spine during normal daily activities. Using a variety of experimental and theoretical techniques, in vivo lumbar spine compressive loads have been predicted, which range from 440 to 700 N for relaxed standing, 1,100 N for coughing, 1,800 N for sit-up exercises, 1,850 N for forward flexion of 20° while lifting a 20-kg mass, and 3,400 N for lifting 20 kg with the back bent and knees straight. Some mathematical models have predicted lumbar forces as high as 5,400 N during lifting of a 50-kg mass with the legs straight. Predictions have also been made of lumbar compressive loads in the range 18,800 to 36,400 N during power lifting by highly trained athletes.

Fracture Risk Factors for the Spine

Although such large forces would be unlikely to occur in the elderly subjects who might be candidates for fracture risk

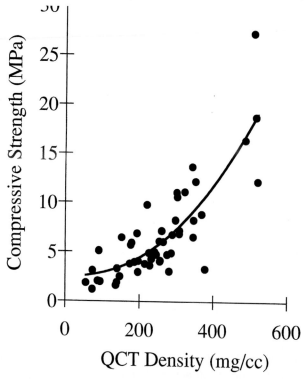

Figure 42

Ultimate compressive strength of femoral subcapital trabecular bone and quantitative computed tomography (QCT) equivalent density. $Y = 8.9 \times 10^{-6} X^{2.31} + 2.78$; $R^2 = 0.70$. (Reproduced with permission from Lotz JC, Gerhart TN, Hayes WC: Mechanical properties of trabecular bone from the proximal femur: A quantitative study. *J Comput Assist Tomogr* 1990;14:107–114.)

prediction, they indicate that dynamic activities and the lifting of heavy objects are likely to increase spinal forces well above the average vertebral fracture loads measured in vitro using elderly cadaveric subjects. Note that all in vitro failure experiments have been conducted using isolated vertebral bodies (for example, with the posterior elements removed and without the potential of load carrying by intra-abdominal pressure). Current evidence suggests, however, that intra-abdominal pressure reduces spinal compressive forces only by about 15% and that the facet joints carry only between 3% to 25% of lumbar spine loads. Thus, even if additive maximum contributions (40%) from intra-abdominal pressure and the facet joints are assumed, estimated lumbar spine loads from common daily activities (such as forward flexion of 20° with a 10-kg mass in each hand) are about 1,100 N. For lifting a 50-kg mass with the knees straight, estimated forces are 3,200 N. Based on the in vitro failure data for elderly spines, these 2 loading cases would involve risk factors of about 0.33 for forward flexion with 20 kg in each hand to about 1 for lifting 50 kg with the knees straight. With reported in vitro fracture loads for lumbar vertebrae ranging from less than 2,000 N to over 5,000 N (Fig. 43), it is not surprising that vertebral compression fractures are such a common occurrence among the elderly.

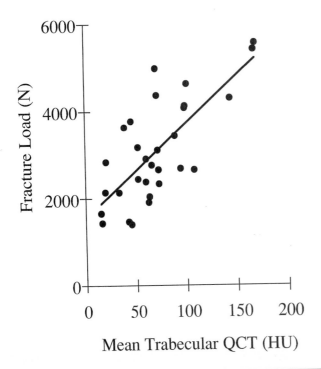

Figure 43

Failure load for an isolated lumbar vertebral body (posterior elements and end plates removed) under uniaxial compression and mean quantitative computed tomography value (in Hounsfield units, HU) of the trabecular bone within the vertebral body. Y = 21.5 X + 1540; R²= 0.54. (Reproduced with permission from Mosekildel L, Bentzen SM, Ørtoft G, et al: The predictive value of quantitative computed tomography for vertebral body compressive strength and density. *Bone* 1989;10:465–470.)

QCT and Proximal Femur Failure

To investigate relationships between QCT densitometric parameters and spontaneous fractures of the proximal femur, proximal femora have been scanned with QCT and then mechanically loaded in vitro using forces typical of single-legged stance. In one such study, fracture forces were in the range of approximately 2,000 to 8,500 N. Work to fracture (area under the force-deformation curve, which is a measure of the energy absorbed during the fracture process) was in the range of approximately 20 to 100 joules (J). In these experiments, moderate positive correlations were observed between the force required to cause in vitro fracture and the mean QCT number (reported in Hounsfield units, HU) from the trabecular bone within the subcapital region ($R^2 \approx 0.60$, Fig. 44). Slightly improved correlations were obtained using the sum of the intertrochanteric trabecular and cortical HU values multiplied by their respective cross-sectional areas. Fracture forces for simulated normal gait measured in various other in vitro experiments were in the range 1,000 to 12,750 N.

All these data relate to loading conditions for normal gait, and, therefore, are applicable only to hip fractures that occur during activities such as single-legged stance and normal gait. Spontaneous hip fractures associated with these activities represent less than 10% of the more than 250,000 hip fractures that occur annually in the United States. More than 90% of all hip fractures are associated with trauma caused by a fall, usually from standing height or lower. Under such traumatic conditions, the magnitudes and directions of the forces applied to the hip are probably much different from those that occur during normal gait. To investigate the ability of QCT data to predict fracture for these traumatic conditions, mechanical tests must be performed in vitro using loads typical of such trauma as a fall from standing height directly onto the side of the greater trochanter. For these experiments, fracture loads range from approximately 800 to 4,000 N. These loads are much lower than those required to fracture the femur in vitro for simulated gait loads (1,000 to 12,750 N). Similarly, work to fracture values range from approximately 5 to 500 J for a simulated fall from standing height, and are relatively low compared to gait values (20 to 100 J). The most significant relationships between the magnitude of the traumatic fracture loads and QCT indices of bone strength occur in the intertrochanteric region. Very significant positive correlations have been found between mean intertrochanteric trabecular QCT value and whole bone strength ($R^2 \approx 0.90$, Fig. 45). Even stronger correlations have been observed between whole bone strength and the mean intertrochanteric trabecular QCT value multiplied by the total intertrochanteric cross-sectional area. These findings indicate that QCT can provide an excellent predictor of the strength of the proximal femur whole bone as measured in vitro for certain assumed traumatic loading conditions.

These studies on whole bone strength and QCT, although

preliminary, provide first-order estimates of the strength of the proximal femur for loads representing normal gait and one type of fall. In elderly cadaver specimens, both the upper end of the range and the mean values for fracture load were about twice as high for gait loads as for loads representing a fall. These differences are probably the consequence of differences in whole bone strength when the approximately elliptical femoral neck is loaded against its geometrically weak axis (relatively low areal moment of inertia) for a fall instead of against its strong axis (relatively high areal moment of inertia) for normal gait. Lower cortical and trabecular bone tissue strengths for transverse loading may also account for lower whole bone strengths for loading to the side of the hip.

Fracture Risk Factors for the Hip

To estimate fracture risk factors for the hip, the in vitro measurements of whole bone strength must be compared with estimates of in vivo loading on the proximal femur for different activities. A variety of mathematical models for single-legged stance have predicted in vivo forces that range from as low as 1.8 times body weight (BW) to 6 times BW. During normal gait, predictions are in the range of approximately 3 to 8 times BW. Hip joint forces of 7 to 8

times BW have been predicted for stair ascent and of approximately 3 times BW for rising from a chair. In vivo forces at the hip joint for total hip arthroplasty patients have been measured directly using instrumented prostheses. For normal, quiet gait, various studies have consistently reported in vivo hip joint forces of approximately 3 times BW; forces as high as 5.5 times BW have been reported for dynamic loading associated with periods of instability during single-legged stance.

For the 55-kg individual, typical of elderly populations, at high risk of hip fracture, forces of 3 times BW for single-legged stance correspond to values of about 1,600 N. Forces of 6 times BW (representative of stair ascent and more dynamic activities) correspond to values of about 3,200 N. A typical mean value for in vitro failure load (5,250 N, for example) would then indicate risk factors of approximately 0.30 and 0.60 for single-legged stance and more dynamic activities, respectively. Using the entire range of reported in vitro failure loads (1,000 to 12,750 N) would suggest a range of risk factors of 0.13 to 1.6 for single-legged stance and 0.25 to 3.2 for stair ascent. Thus, these predictions confirm what is known clinically that some spontaneous fractures of the hip occur in response to habitual activities such as single-legged stance, normal gait, and stair ascent.

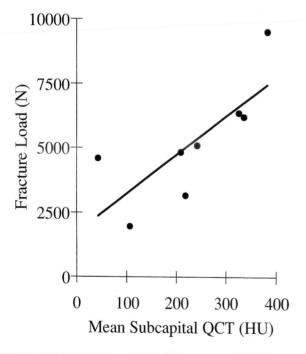

Figure 44

Force required to fracture the proximal femur under single-legged stance loading conditions and mean quantitative computed tomography (QCT) value (in HU) of the trabecular bone within the subcapital region of the proximal femur. These data relate to prediction of spontaneous hip fractures. $Y = 15.0 X + 1750$; $R^2 = 0.59$. (Reproduced with permission from Esses SI, Lotz JC, Hayes WC: Biomechanical properties of the proximal femur determined in vitro by single-energy quantitative computed tomography. *J Bone Miner Res* 1989;4:5715–5722.)

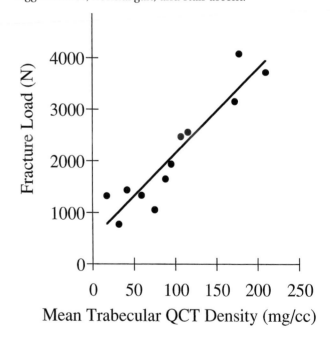

Figure 45

Force required to fracture the proximal femur under loading conditions representative of a fall to the side of the hip and mean quantitative computed tomography (QCT) value (in equivalent density, mg/cc) of the intertrochanteric trabecular bone. These data relate to prediction of traumatic hip fractures. Note that the range of forces required to cause fracture is much lower for traumatic fractures than for spontaneous fractures (see Figure 44). $Y = 16.2 X + 495$; $R^2 = 0.87$. (Reproduced with permission from Lotz JC, Hayes WC: The use of quantitative computed tomography to estimate risk of fracture of the hip from falls. *J Bone Joint Surg* 1990;72B:689–700.)

It is far more difficult to estimate risk factors for falls because in vivo forces on the hip during impact from a fall have not yet been measured. However, it is possible to compare the work to fracture values for femora tested in vitro against the potential energy available during a fall from standing height. Epidemiologic studies have indicated that the available potential energy for individuals who fall and fracture a hip (500 J) significantly exceeds the energy for individuals who fall and do not fracture (450 J). These energies are an order of magnitude greater than the maximum work to fracture in the in vitro experiments simulating a fall to the side of the hip, and nearly 20 times the reported mean work to fracture. Therefore, much less energy is needed to fracture the proximal femur than is available in a simple fall from standing height. It follows that a fall to the side of the hip from standing height involves substantial trauma to the skeleton.

Other potentially important factors that can influence the force delivered to the proximal femur during impact from a fall include energy absorption processes in soft tissues overlying the greater trochanter, the state of muscle contraction, and the position of the trunk and extremities at impact. Preliminary experiments have predicted peak impact forces ranging from approximately 5,000 to 9,000 N in the muscle-relaxed state and from approximately 7,000 to 15,500 N in the muscle-active state. In females, threefold increases in soft-tissue thickness cause a 20% reduction in predicted peak impact force. More significantly, falling in a muscle-relaxed state reduces peak forces by more than half. Comparing these estimates of fall impact force with the average in vitro failure load data described above indicates risk factors in the range of 2.5 to 7.1. The inescapable conclusion is that in elderly individuals, any fall with direct impact to the greater trochanter has a high probability of fracturing the hip. This is true regardless of the thickness of the soft tissue overlying the hip, the state of muscle activity at impact, or, more interestingly, the fragility of the bone within the proximal femur.

In Vivo Fracture Risk Prediction

A final step toward the development of clinical fracture risk predictors is to test their discriminatory and predictive power in clinical populations. Women with vertebral fractures generally have lower spinal bone mass than controls. Approximately 90% of women with vertebral fractures have spinal bone mineral density values of less than 0.97 g/cm^2. In older women, however, there is substantial overlap in QCT equivalent mineral density between individuals with atraumatic vertebral fractures and age-matched controls. This overlap reduces the predictive power of spinal QCT for an individual patient; it also is consistent with the concept that loading conditions are important in spine fracture etiology. For the hip, densitometric evidence suggests that the frequency of femoral neck fractures increases as bone mineral density declines below a densitometric threshold of about 0.95 g/cm^2. However, for those over age 70 years (who represent 90% of hip fracture patients), there is considerable overlap in densitometric measures between hip fracture patients and controls. Thus, as with the spine, densitometric estimates of proximal femoral strength are not good predictors of fracture risk.

For both the spine and hip, loading histories such as repeated bending and lifting of objects, chronic coughing, frequent stair ascent, or the single incidence of a fall are not accounted for in simple densitometric comparisons to fracture thresholds or in approaches that rely on densitometric comparisons with age- and gender-matched controls. Without data on the activity (and thus the force) precipitating a spontaneous fracture, little can be said about the relative importance of loading factors and bone fragility in the etiology of these fractures. A comparable situation exists for hip fractures that result from falls, although in this case it appears that for elderly individuals at greatest risk, factors related to the mechanics of the fall dominate the etiology, while factors related to densitometric measures alone have much less significance. Until better data are available on the activities and loading parameters that cause fracture, it will be difficult to establish and reliably test densitometric fracture risk predictors.

Bone Metabolism and Mineral Homeostasis

Bone mineral homeostasis is tightly controlled by the synchronized action of the vitamin D_3 metabolites, PTH, and calcitonin. Together these hormones regulate the dietary absorption of calcium, bone mineral resorption and deposition, and renal secretion and reabsorption of calcium and phosphorus. In this way, the vital control of serum calcium concentration is an integral part of the control of bone mineral homeostasis.

Vitamin D Pathways

The active vitamin D metabolites are potent calcitropic hormones. Their primary function is to enhance calcium and phosphorus absorption across the lumen of the small intestine and to enhance calcium and phosphorus resorption from bone. Ultraviolet light acting on the skin transforms 7-dehydrocholesterol into vitamin D_3 (cholecalciferol). In whites, 1 hour of direct sunlight produces the daily requirement of 400 units of vitamin D. In blacks and other dark-skinned individuals, more direct sunlight is required. Vitamin D occurs rarely in natural foods (cod-liver oil) and, consequently, is added to some foods as vitamin D_2 (radiated ergosterol). Vitamin D (D_2 or D_3) is hydroxylated in the liver to 25-hydroxyvitamin D (25(OH)vitamin D_3). Both vitamin D_3 and 25(OH)vitamin D_3 are inactive precursor vitamins. A serum 25(OH) vitamin D_3 level is the best indication of body stores of vitamin D_3. In the presence of elevated levels of PTH, or hypocalcemia or hypophosphatemia, an enzyme in the mitochondria of the kidney's proximal tubules hydroxylates the 25(OH)vitamin D_3 into the active hormone metabolite 1,25-dihydroxyvitamin D_3 (1,25(OH_2) vitamin D_3). In the presence of decreased levels of PTH, or hypercalcemia or hyperphosphatemia, 25-hydroxyvitamin D is converted into the inactive metabolite 24,25-dihydroxyvitamin D. Figures 46 and 47 illustrate the metabolic pathways of vitamin D.

Calcium Homeostasis: Vitamin D, PTH, and Calcitonin

The maintenance of a stable calcium gradient between the extracellular and intracellular environments is essential for life. Normally, the extracellular concentration of calcium is about 5 orders of magnitude (10^5) greater than the intracellular concentration of calcium. A number of complex intracellular systems are responsible for the microregulation of intracellular calcium homeostasis. Of total body calcium, 99% is sequestered in the skeleton, leaving approximately 1% to circulate in the extracellular fluid. It is this 1% that is so assiduously controlled and regulated by the PTH-vitamin D-calcitonin endocrine system. These 3 calcitropic hormones, in conjunction with other paracrine factors, not only modulate the concentration of serum calcium in the extracellular fluid, they control the fluctuation of the calcium from the outside to the inside of the cell. The endocrine

control of cytosolic and extracellular calcium and associated phosphorus metabolism are outlined in Table 3.

Calcium Nutritional Requirements

Proper calcium nutrition is critical to bone maintenance. Chronic mild dietary deficiency of calcium will lead to a negative calcium balance and gradual loss of bone mass. In young individuals, approximately 15% to 25% of ingested calcium is absorbed. In elderly persons, this percentage declines; consequently, the elderly require more dietary calcium to achieve the same net calcium transport across the intestinal lumen because of the less efficient transformation of 25-(OH)vitamin D to the active metabolite 1,25-(OH_2)vitamin D in the aging kidney. Augmented dietary calcium also may be necessary during the adolescent growth spurt, during early adulthood when maximum bone mass is being achieved, during pregnancy, and, especially, during lactation.

Table 4 provides guidelines for minimum daily calcium requirement by age and activity level.

Elaborate endocrine feedback loops exist to prevent dangerous and life-threatening hypocalcemia. A reduction in ionized serum calcium levels engenders a host of protective mechanisms, which serve to restore the serum calcium level to normal through more efficient absorption from the gastrointestinal tract, reabsorption from the kidney, and

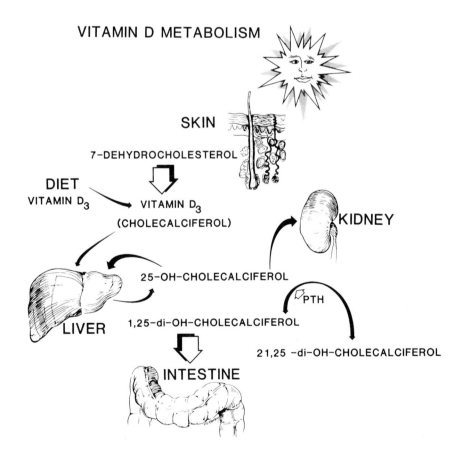

Figure 46

Diagram showing the metabolic pathways of vitamin D.

resorption from bone. Primary disorders of this regulatory system may lead to chronic hypocalcemia or hypercalcemia and promote symptomatic clinical disease. The major metabolic pathways involved in the maintenance of a normal concentration of calcium in the extracellular fluid are outlined in Figure 48.

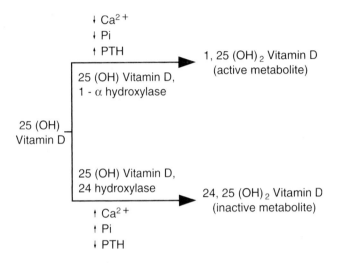

Figure 47

Vitamin D metabolism in renal tubular cell.

Age-Related Changes in Bone Mass and Morphology

Figure 49 illustrates the relationship between age, bone mass, and gender. Much anabolic skeletal activity occurs during the adolescent growth spurt. Early in adolescence, the skeleton undergoes rapid longitudinal growth with only moderate increase in mineral content. The addition of layers of bone at the periosteum and endosteum is balanced by an increase in the porosity of the bone. Increased bone turnover provides some of the minerals needed for the new bone. Not until late adolescence, when longitudinal growth slows, does bone mineral content rapidly increase. Bone mass peaks after skeletal maturity some time during the third decade.

In the period between the onset of adolescence and skeletal maturity, dietary habits and hereditary factors play a large role in determining the ultimate size of the bone mineral bank. The size of this bank stays nearly constant throughout most of adult life, with the body redistributing its assets according to structural needs. Until adolescence, bone mass is equal for blacks and whites; thereafter, bone mass increases to a greater level in blacks. The factors responsible for this are unknown. By the fifth decade, bone mass begins to decline, with dramatic gender differences in bone loss. Both men and women lose cortical bone at the same rate; however, trabecular bone mass decreases more rapidly in women with the onset of menopause and thereafter. Local bone loss

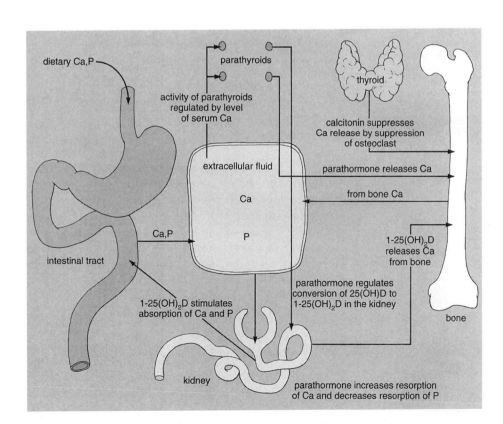

Figure 48

A schematic model of calcium and phosphorous metabolism. (Reproduced with permission from Bullough PG: *Atlas of Orthopedic Pathology.* Hampshire, England, Gower Press, 1992, p 7.5.)

Table 3
Regulation of Calcium and Phosphate Metabolism

	Parathyroid hormone (PTH) (peptide)	1,25 (OH)$_2$D* (steroid)	Calcitonin (peptide)
Origin	Chief cells of parathyroid glands	Proximal tubule of kidney	Parafollicular cells of thyroid gland
Factors stimulating production	Decreased serum CA^{2+}; Decreased serum P_i	Elevated PTH	Elevated serum CA^{2+}
Factors inhibiting production	Elevated serum CA^{2+}; Elevated 1,25 (OH)$_2$D	Decreased PTH; Elevated serum CA^{2+}; Elevated serum P_i;	Decreased serum CA^{2+}
Effect on end organs for hormone action			
Intestine	No direct effect; Acts indirectly on bowel by stimulating production of 1,25 (OH)$_2$ in kidney	Strongly stimulates intestinal absorption of CA^{2+} and P_i	?
Kidney	Stimulates 25 (OH)D $-1\alpha - OH_{ase}$ in mitochondria of proximal tubular cells to convert 25 (OH)D to 1,25 (OH)$_2$D; Increases fractional resorption of filtered CA^{2+}; Promotes urinary excretion of P_i	?	?
Bone	Stimulates osteoclastic resorption of bone; Stimulates recruitment of preosteoclasts ?	Strongly stimulates osteoclastic resorption of bone	Inhibits osteoclastic resorption of bone; Role in normal human physiology
Net effect on calcium and phosphate concentrations in extracellular fluid and serum	Increased serum calcium; Decreased serum phosphate	Increased serum calcium; Increased serum phosphate	Decreased serum calcium (transient)

* 1,25 (OH)$_2$D = 1,25-dihydroxyvitamin D; PTH = parathyroid hormone; 25 (OH)D = 25-hydroxyvitamin D; ? = unknown.

Table 4
Guidelines for Calcium Requirements

Group	Daily Elemental Calcium Requirements*
Children	500-700 mg
Growth spurt to young adult (10 to 25 years of age)	1,300 mg
Adult male (25 to 65 years of age)	750 mg
Adult female (25 to 65 years of age)	
Postmenopausal	1,500 mg
Elderly	1,200 mg
Pregnancy	1,500 mg
Lactation	2,000 mg
Healing long-bone fracture (women and men)	1,500 mg

* One daily equivalent of calcium is equal to 250 mg of elemental calcium. One equivalent is equal to an 8-oz glass of milk.

is variable throughout the skeleton. Evidence from kinetic studies indicates that after age 40 years, formation rates remain constant while resorption rates increase. Over several decades, the skeletal mass may be reduced to 50% of peak trabecular and 25% of peak cortical mass.

Outline 1 illustrates the 4 major mechanisms of bone mass regulation. In the healthy young adult skeleton, bone formation and resorption are tightly coupled. Uncoupling leads to changes in bone density in adults. Increased bone formation without elevated resorption will result in increased bone mass; an unchecked increase in osteoclast activity will cause an overall loss of bone mass.

Metabolic Bone Disease

Metabolic bone diseases are generalized disorders of skeletal homeostasis and comprise some of the most common and some of the most esoteric disorders seen by the

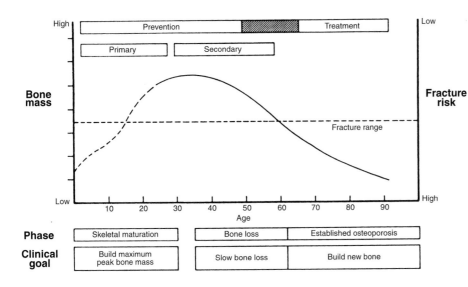

Figure 49

Graph showing the relationship among bone mass, age, and sex. (Reproduced with permission from Wasnich RD: Epidemiology of osteoporosis, in Favus MJ (ed): *Primer on the Metabolic Bone Diseases and Disorders of Mineral Metabolism*, ed 3. Philadelphia, PA, Lippincott Raven, 1996, pp 249–252.)

orthopaedist. Over the past decade, great progress has been made in the understanding and treatment of metabolic bone disease. A few basic definitions are essential. Osteopenia is a generic word used to describe the radiographic picture of decreased bone density. Osteopenia is neither a disease nor a diagnosis and conveys no information about the underlying etiology of the condition. Osteoporosis, on the other hand, is a more specific term referring to a state of decreased mass per unit volume (density) of normally mineralized bone matrix. When this decrease leads to increased skeletal fragility, a pathologic state of osteoporosis exists. Osteomalacia refers to an increased, normal, or decreased mass of insufficiently mineralized bone matrix (Fig. 50).

Osteomalacia

Deficient or impaired mineralization of bone matrix (osteoid) is the diagnostic feature of all osteomalacic syndromes, regardless of etiology. Rickets, the juvenile counterpart of osteomalacia, refers to the impaired mineralization of cartilage matrix (chondroid) and a resultant arrest in formation of primary spongiosa. Osteomalacia can be present at any age, once lamellar bone has formed. Rickets is exclusively a disorder of children.

The single most important causative factor in the development of osteomalacia is the failure to maintain a serum calcium-phosphorus level sufficient to promote mineralization of newly-formed osteoid. The etiologies of osteomalacia are numerous but may easily be classified into 5 major categories (Outline 2). The serum, urine, and bone biopsy findings in the various metabolic bone diseases are detailed in Table 5. The management of the individual osteomalacic condition depends on the specific pathophysiology. The unifying theme in the treatment of all rachitic and osteomalacic conditions is the restoration of the serum calcium-phosphorus level to normal so that normal mineralization

Outline 1
Four Mechanisms of Bone Mass Regulation

Stimulation of Osteoblasts
  Weight-bearing activity
  Growth
  Fluoride
  Intermittent PTH/PTHrP*
  Ultrasound

Inhibition of Osteoblasts
  Lack of weight-bearing activity
  Alcoholism
  Chronic disease
  Normal aging
  Hypercortisolism

Inhibition of Osteoclasts
  Weight-bearing activity
  Estrogen
  Testosterone
  Bisphosphonates
  Calcitonin
  Adequate vitamin D intake
  Adequate calcium intake

Stimulation of Osteoclasts
  Lack of weight-bearing activity
  Hyperparathyroidism
  Hypercortisolism
  Hyperthyroidism
  Estrogen deficiency
  Testosterone deficiency
  Acidosis
  Myeloma
  Lymphoma
  Inadequate calcium intake
  Normal aging

*   PTH = parathyroid hormone; PTHrP = parathyroid hormone-related protein

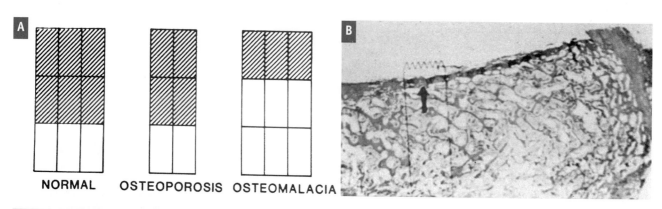

Figure 50

A, Diagram showing amount (number of sections) of normally mineralized (cross-hatched sections) and insufficiently mineralized (blank sections) bone matrix. **B,** Photomicrograph of transcortical bone biopsy specimen, demonstrating sparse trabeculae with cortical resorption.

of cartilage and bone matrix can occur. Vitamin D deficiency states may be treated by providing the vitamin, which is a fat-soluble sterol that has a long half-life, or providing its metabolites, 25(OH) vitamin D or 1,25(OH$_2$) vitamin D, just distal to any metabolic block. Vitamin D-resistant conditions are treated by providing inorganic phosphate and 1,25-(OH$_2$)vitamin D$_3$, which is essential in suppressing PTH, which will rise with phosphate treatment alone. All therapy must be carefully monitored to prevent hypercalcemia or an excess of vitamin D. Calcitriol therapy should be stopped 24 hours prior to corrective osteotomies, and may be resumed following surgery when the patient is mobile.

Renal Osteodystrophy

Renal osteodystrophy is a common complication of chronic renal failure and is one of the most common causes of osteomalacia. Chronic glomerular disease leads to renal insufficiency, azotemia, and acidosis. The resulting metabolic changes often produce profound skeletal effects. These skeletal changes can include rickets or osteomalacia, osteitis fibrosa, osteoporosis, osteosclerosis, and metastatic calcification (Fig. 51).

The mechanism of the bone changes in renal osteodystrophy is complex (Fig. 52). The major abnormalities are phosphate retention secondary to uremia and insufficient renal synthesis of 1,25(OH)$_2$ vitamin D. These 2 abnormalities result in hypocalcemia leading to secondary hyperparathyroidism, with bone changes of osteitis fibrosa. In some cases of secondary hyperparathyroidism, the solubility of serum calcium and phosphorus is exceeded, and ectopic calcification may occur in the conjunctivae, blood vessels, periarticular tissues, and skin. As the renal failure progresses and the glomerular filtration rate falls below 20 ml/min, the persistent acidosis further aggravates the negative calcium balance.

During the past 2 decades, a form of renal osteodystrophy has been identified, which is characterized by pure osteo-

malacia. The commonly accepted cause is aluminum from the aluminum-containing phosphate binders that are prescribed for the treatment of hyperphosphatemia in renal failure. Aluminum is readily absorbed in the gastrointestinal tract and normally is excreted by the kidneys. However, in the presence of renal failure, aluminum may accumulate and be deposited in the brain, leading to dementia, and in the bone, leading to osteomalacia. The mechanism by which aluminum deposition causes osteomalacia is unclear, but evidence suggests that the aluminum inhibits mineralization either by inhibiting calcium (cation) deposition or by toxicity to osteoblastic mitochondrial function. Attempts to eradicate this problem have included the investigational substitution of calcium carbonate, an alternate phosphate binder, and chelation of aluminum with desferoxamine.

The skeletal manifestations of renal osteodystrophy are similar to those of other forms of rickets/osteomalacia. Most patients have severe bone pain and tenderness and may have pathologic fractures. The radiographic findings of renal osteodystrophy reflect the clinical and biochemical

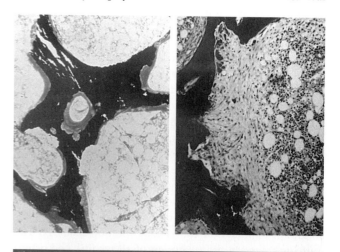

Figure 51

Photomicrographs showing hyperparathyroidism.

Table 5
Serum and Urine Findings in Various Metabolic Bone Diseases*

Disorder	[Ca]	[Pi]	AP	PTH	25 (OH) Vitamin D	1,25 (OH)₂ Vitamin D	Urinary Calcium	Bone Biopsy Findings	Associated Findings
Postmenopausal osteoporosis (type I)	N	N	N	N,↓	N	N	↑,N	Variable	Osteopenia
Age-related osteoporosis (type II)	N	N	N	↑, N	N	N	N	Variable	Osteopenia
Chronic glucocorticoid-associated osteoporosis	N	N	N	↑, N	N	N	↑, N	Inactive turnover	Severe osteopenia
Primary hyperparathyroidism	↑	N, ↓	N, ↑	↑	N	↑, N	↑	Active turnover; peritrabecular fibrosis	Variable, depending on degree of hyper-calcemia
Cancer with bony metastases	↑	↑, N	↑, N	N, ↓	N	N, ↓	↑↑	Tumor	History of primary tumor; bony destruction: + bone scan
Multiple myeloma; lymphoma	↑	↑, N	↑, N	N, ↓	N	N, ↓	↑↑	Comfirmatory for tumor	Destructive lesions on radiographs; abnormal protein electrophoresis
Primary carcinoma not involving bone	↑	↓	↑, N	↓	N	↓	↑↑	Variable	Osteopenia, ↑ PTH-related peptide
Sarcoidosis	↑	↑, N	↑, N	N, ↓	N	↑	↑	Active turnover	Hilar adenopathy
Hyperthyroidism	↑	N	N	N, ↓	N	N	↑	Active turnover	↓ TSH; osteopenia; tachycardia tremor, systemic hyperthyroid changes
Vitamin D intoxication	↑	↑, N	↑, N	N, ↓	↑↑↑	N	↑	Active turnover	History of excessive vitamin D intake
Milk-alkali syndrome	↑	↑, N	↑, N	N, ↓	N	N, ↓	↑	Variable	History of excessive calcium and alkali ingestion (anatacids)
Severe generalized immobilization	↑	↑, N	↑, N	N, ↓	N	N, ↓	↑↑	Active turnover	Osteopenia; multiple fractures; neurologic dysfunction
Vitamin D deficiency (dietary; gastrointestinal)	N, ↓	↓	↑	↑	↓	↓	↓	Osteomalacia	
Dietary phosphate deficiency (Rare)	N	↓	↑	N	N	↑	N	Osteomalacia; absence of hyper-parathyroid changes	Phosphate-binding antacid abuse with normal renal function

* Ca, calcium; Pi, phosphate; AP, alkaline phosphatase; PTH, parathyroid hormone; 25(OH) Vitamin D, 25 hydroxyvitamin D; 1,25 (OH)₂ vitamin D, 1,25 dihydroxyvitamin D. N = Normal; ↓ = Decreased; ↑ = Increased; TSH = thyroid stimulating hormone.

Table 5 (continued)

Serum and Urine Findings in Various Metabolic Bone Diseases*

Disorder	[Ca]	[Pi]	AP	PTH	25 (OH) Vitamin D	1,25 (OH)$_2$ Vitamin D	Urinary Calcium	Bone Biopsy Findings	Associated Findings
Mesenchymal tumor producing phosphaturic factor	N	↓	↑	N	N	N	N	Osteomalacia; absence of hyperparathyroid changes	Normal 1,25 (OH)$_2$ vitamin D level but inappropriately low considering degree of phosphaturia
Vitamin D resistance (X-linked dominant-Albright's syndrome)	N	↓	↑	N	N	N	N	Osteomalacia; absence of hyperparathyroid changes	Normal 1,25 (OH)$_2$ vitamin D level but inappropriately low considering degree of phosphaturia
Fanconi-type II	N	↓	↑	N	N	N	N	Osteomalacia; absence of hyperparathyroid changes	Normal 1,25 (OH)$_2$ vitamin D level but inappropriately low considering degree of phosphaturia; glyosuria
Fanconi-type III	N	↓	↑	N	N	N	N	Osteomalacia; absence of hyperparathyroid changes	Normal 1,25 (OH)$_2$ vitamin D level but inappropriately low considering degree of phosphaturia; aminoaciduria
Vitamin D dependent rickets (type I) rare	↓	↓	↑	↑	N	↓↓	↓	Osteomalacia hyperparathyroid changes	Defect in renal converting enzyme from 25 (OH) vitamin D to 1,25 (OH)$_2$ vitamin D
Vitamin D dependent rickets (type II) rate	↓	↓	↑	↑	N	↑↑	↓	Osteomalacia; hyperparathyroid changes	Probable 1,25 (OH)$_2$ vitamin D receptor defect
Renal tubular acidosis	↓	↓	↑	↑	N	↑, N	↑	Osteomalacia; hyperparathyroid changes	Elevated blood urea nitrogen and creatinine
Renal osteodystrophy (mixed)	N, ↓	↑↑	↑	↑↑	N	↓↓	—	Pure osteomalacia; aluminum at mineralization front	Elevated blood urea nitrogen and creatinine
Renal osteodystrophy (predominant aluminum-associated osteomalacia)	↑, N	↑, N	↑	↑	N	↓↓	—	Pure osteomalacia; aluminum at mineralization	Elevated blood urea nitrogen and creatinine
Hypophosphatasia	↑	↑	↓↓	N	N	N	↑	Pure osteomalacia	Elevated urinary physphoethanol amine early loss of teeth

*   Ca, calcium; Pi, phosphate; AP, alkaline phosphatase; PTH, parathyroid hormone; 25(OH) Vitamin D, 25 hydroxyvitamin D; 1,25 (OH)$_2$ vitamin D, 1,25 dihydroxyvitamin D. N = Normal; ↓ = Decreased; ↑ = Increased; TSH = thyroid stimulating hormone.

changes seen and vary widely, with most patients exhibiting a mixed disease pattern (Fig. 53).

Osteosclerosis may be present in 20% of renal osteodystrophy patients; it may be eccentrically located in the long bones or seen as dense and lucent bands in the spine ("rugger-jersey" spine). Hyperparathyroidism can result in osteosclerosis through an increase in osteoid deposition and osteoblastic activity. Slipped capital femoral epiphyses may be indicative of renal osteodystrophy in children (Fig. 54).

Laboratory findings include elevated blood urea nitrogen and creatinine levels, normal or low serum calcium, and a serum inorganic phosphate that is usually over 5.5 mg%. The alkaline phosphatase and PTH levels are almost invariably elevated. Approximately 20% of patients with renal osteodystrophy have relatively normal calcium and phosphorus levels, have only slightly increased PTH levels, and suffer from profound osteomalacia. These findings probably are related to extremely high levels of phosphate-binder related aluminum deposits in the bone of some of these patients.

Although the diagnosis of renal osteodystrophy is usually obvious, a tetracycline-labeled bone biopsy is used for the best evaluation of the individual components of this disease. Analysis of a bone biopsy currently is the only reliable means of determining bone aluminum deposition. This evaluation is needed to guide treatment of the variable components (that is, osteomalacia, hyperparathyroidism, and aluminum deposition).

Medical treatments for renal osteodystrophy include (1) adjusting the serum calcium and phosphorus levels to normal; (2) suppressing secondary hyperparathyroidism; (3) chelating bone aluminum in patients with aluminum-associated osteomalacia; and (4) renal transplantation. Overall management of the renal disease includes chronic dialysis or renal transplantation. Additional measures include

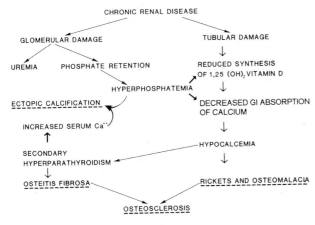

MECHANISM OF BONE CHANGES
IN RENAL OSTEODYSTROPHY

Figure 52

Pathogenesis of bone changes in renal osteodystrophy.

Outline 2
Causes of Rickets and Osteomalacia

Nutritional Deficiency
  Vitamin D deficiency
  Dietary chelators (rare) of calcium
    Phytates
    Oxalates (found in spinach)
  Phosphorus deficiency (unusual)
      Antacid (aluminum-containing) abuse leading to severe
        dietary phosphate binding

Gastrointestinal Absorption Defects
  Postgastrectomy (rare today)
  Biliary disease (interference with absorption of fat-soluble
    vitamin D)
  Enteric absorption defects
      Short bowel syndrome
      Rapid transit (gluten-sensitive enteropathy) syndromes
      Inflammatory bowel disease
        Crohn's disease
        Celiac disease

Renal Tubular Defects (Renal Phosphate Leak)
  X-linked dominant hypophosphatemic vitamin D-resistant
    rickets or osteomalacia
  Classic Albright's syndrome or Fanconi's syndrome-type I
  Fanconi's syndrome-type II
  Phosphaturia and glycosuria
  Fanconi's syndrome-type III
  Phosphaturia, glycosuria, and aminoaciduria
  Vitamin D-dependent rickets (or osteomalacia)-type I*
  Vitamin D-dependent rickets (or osteomalacia)-type II†

Renal Tubular Acidosis
  Acquired (associated with many systemic diseases)
  Genetic:
      Debre-De Toni-Fanconi syndrome
      Lignac-Fanconi syndrome (cysteinosis)
      Lowe's syndrome

Renal Osteodystrophy
Miscellaneous Causes
  Soft-tissue tumors secreting putative factors
      Fibrous dysplasia
      Neurofibromatosis
      Other soft-tissue and vascular mesenchymal tumors
  Anticonvulsant medication. Induction of hepatic P450
    microsomal enzyme by some anticonvulsants (phenytoin,
    phenobarbital, mysoline) causes increase in Vitamin D
    metabolites
  Heavy metal intoxication
      Hypophosphatasia
      High-dose diphosphonates
      Sodium fluoride

* A genetic or acquired deficiency of renal tubular 25-hydroxyvitamin D
  1-alpha enzyme prevents conversion of 25 hydroxyvitamin D to active
  polar metabolite 1,25 dihydroxyvitamin D

† This represents enteric and organ insensitivity to 1,25 dihydroxyvitamin D
  and is probably caused by an abnormality in the 1,25 dihydroxyvitamin D
  nuclear receptor

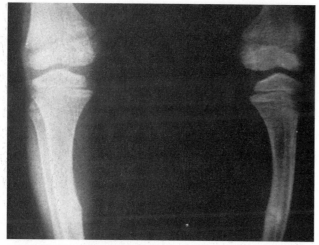

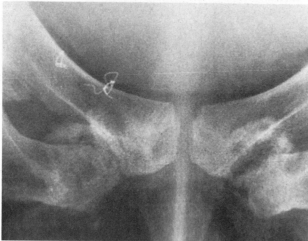

Figure 53

Radiographs showing osteomalacia.

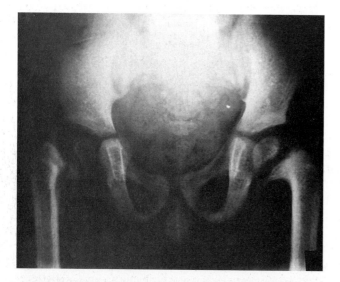

Figure 54

Radiograph of renal osteodystrophy.

administration of calcium carbonate to diminish hyperphosphatemia, administration of $1,25(OH)_2$ vitamin D to increase calcium absorption and to decrease PTH secretion, and parathyroidectomy to control the occasional autonomous hyperparathyroidism. Because, in the presence of bone aluminum deposition, parathyroidectomy may actually worsen bone changes by decreasing bone remodeling rates, a bone biopsy is suggested in patients who have renal osteodystrophy before consideration of parathyroidectomy. Desferoxamine, a chelator of trivalent cations, has proved to be an effective chelator of aluminum in patients in whom a biopsy has documented aluminum-associated osteomalacia.

Endocrinopathies Affecting Bone

A large number of endocrinopathies affect bone formation or resorption and lead to impaired bone metabolism. Some of these endocrinopathies include PTH excess, thyroid hormone excess, glucocorticoid excess (Cushing's disease), juvenile-onset diabetes mellitus (type I), and estrogen deficiency (Fig. 55). PTH enhances both bone resorption (osteoclastic activity) and bone formation (osteoblastic activity). With continuous production or administration of PTH, overall metabolism is enhanced and resorption surpasses formation, leading to net bone loss. However, recent studies indicate that pulsed administration of PTH may enhance formation over resorption. Thyroid hormone excess leads to excessive bone turnover and results in gradual net bone loss. Free thyroxin index is the best serum assay for monitoring thyroid replacement to prevent iatrogenic hyperthyroidism.

Excessive cortisol, either endogenous or exogenous, is most deleterious to bone mass. Corticosteroids decrease calcium absorption across the intestinal lumen, enhance calcium loss from the kidney, inhibit bone matrix formation, and cause secondary hyperparathyroidism with concurrent enhancement of bone resorption, resulting in marked loss of bone mass. An alternate-day treatment regimen with 1 day at physiologic levels may be less damaging. Administration of calcium, vitamin D, and calcitonin or a bisphosphonate (to prevent bone resorption) may counter some of the deleterious effects of cortisol administration.

Juvenile-onset diabetes mellitus (type I) may lead to bone loss. Poorly controlled diabetes mellitus leads to diuresis of calcium. Bone formation is decreased and secondary hyperparathyroidism compensating for urinary calcium loss leads to net bone loss.

Osteoporosis

With advancing age everyone loses bone mass, but not everyone develops osteoporosis. The 2 most important determinants in the development of osteoporosis are peak bone mass and the rate of bone loss thereafter.

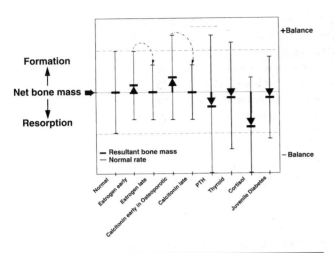

Figure 55

Bone mass regulation by hormones.

Peak bone mass generally is achieved in the early part of the fourth decade of life. Thereafter, bone is lost at a rate that depends on several factors. These factors include (1) the normal aging process; (2) the accelerated bone loss associated with menopause; and (3) genetic, environmental, and nutritional conditions and chronic disease states.

The mechanism of bone loss resulting from normal aging is poorly understood. Based solely on normal aging, the rate of bone loss in women is nearly equivalent to that of men. This bone loss is independent of menopausal bone mass loss. Factors that contribute to bone loss include decreased activity, a calcium-deficient diet, inherited characteristics, and factors related to childbirth, premature menopause, and alcoholism (Outline 3).

Estrogen deficiency is directly implicated in the etiology of osteoporosis. Although postmenopausal women produce estrogen, the levels are below those of premenopausal women and age-matched men. Twenty percent of postmenopausal women have a marked paucity of estrogen. In addition, smoking enhances estrogen degradation and low body fat results in insufficient estrogen production.

The primary consequences of postmenopausal bone loss are fractures of the hip, distal radius, and vertebrae. Calcium intake and absorption have been identified as key factors in fracture incidence. Individuals ingesting physiologic levels of calcium have one fourth to one third the rate of hip fractures experienced by individuals with low calcium intake. Excess calcium intake may be harmful and is less effective than estrogen in preventing osteoporosis.

Recent attention has also demonstrated that eating disorders such as anorexia and excessive exercise leading to amenorrhea may also result in profound osteoporosis. This particular type of osteoporosis is especially worrisome because it affects women at a relatively early age, when their bone mass should be reaching its peak. Excessive loading or overuse can also lead to stress fractures, a special problem in military recruits as well as athletes. Whether the cause of these fractures is purely structural such as decreased moment of inertia of the bone or also the result of poor calcium intake and decreased bone mass is not known.

Treatment of Osteoporosis

Treatments for osteoporosis have had variable success because of inaccurate diagnosis and insufficient understanding of the disease process. Calcium, physiologic vitamin D, and mild exercise appear to decrease bone resorption and to mineralize osteoid, but do not increase total bone mass (Fig. 56).

Estrogen receptors have been identified in bone-forming cells. It appears that estrogen acts to block the action of PTH on osteoblasts and marrow stromal cells. Clinically, estrogen supplementation decreases bone loss by acting to counter the effect of unopposed PTH activity. Without the action of estrogen, osteoblasts and marrow stromal cells secrete increased levels of IL-6, which stimulates the osteoclasts to resorb bone. Estrogen does not appreciably alter bone formation rates. Consequently, the primary effect of estrogen therapy is the maintenance of bone mass. Recently, selective estrogen receptor modulators such as Raloxifene (Evista) have been introduced and may prove to be useful in the treatment of osteoporosis without many of the unwanted side effects associated with estrogen supplementation.

Calcitonin is another treatment option for osteoporosis. It can be administered either via subcutaneous injection or nasal spray. It decreases osteoclastic bone resorption and, for the short term, enhances bone formation, leading to slight net bone accretion. In long-term treatment, osteoblastic activity slows and bone mass becomes stabilized.

Recent clinical studies show that almost all bisphosphonates have dramatic effects in suppressing bone resorption, and in preventing fractures of the hip and vertebral bodies. These drugs (biphosphonates) act in 2 ways to inhibit bone resorption: they directly stabilize the bone crystal, thus making it more resistant to osteoclastic bone resorption, and they directly inhibit the activity of the osteoclast. The net effect is a profound inhibition of bone resorption. This class of antiresorptive drugs promises to have widespread application in the inhibition of bone resorption and in the prevention and treatment of a vast array of osteopenic conditions. In addition, these agents may prove to be useful in the prevention and inhibition of particulate-induced osteolysis of total joint arthroplasties.

As mentioned earlier, intermittent administration of PTH appears to be anabolic and PTH as well as PTHrP analogs are currently undergoing clinical trials for osteoporosis with early dramatic increases in bone mass especially in areas of trabecular bone. The safety and efficacy of these agents are not yet established.

Finally, a number of combination therapies have been proposed linking an anabolic agent with an antiresorptive agent along with calcium and vitamin D supplementation. Once again the safety and efficacy of these therapies remains uncertain.

Differential Diagnosis of Osteoporosis and Osteomalacia

These 2 osteopenic conditions seen in adults are commonly confused. Osteoporosis is characterized by a decreased apparent density of normally mineralized bone matrix. Osteomalacia refers to an increased, normal, or (most commonly) decreased mass of insufficiently mineralized bone matrix (Table 6). Insufficient mineralization includes unmineralized osteoid and delayed mineralization of osteoid.

Osteoporosis, which is much more common than osteomalacia, is age-related and occurs most often following menopause and in the elderly of both sexes. Occasionally, onset may result from rare genetic and less common determinants such as hypercortisolism, hyperthyroidism, hyperparathyroidism, alcohol abuse, tumors, immobilization, chronic disease, and expression of abnormal collagen or bone matrix genes.

Unlike its more easily diagnosed childhood counterpart, rickets, adult osteomalacia may be difficult to diagnose clinically. Incidence is evenly distributed throughout all age groups. The most common causes are chronic renal failure, vitamin D deficiency (found in approximately 30% of institutionalized elderly persons), abnormalities of the vitamin D pathway, and hypophosphatemic syndromes. Rarer causes are renal tubular acidosis, aluminum intoxication, hypophosphatasia, and mesenchymal tumors that lead to hypophosphatemic conditions.

Symptoms of osteoporosis are not usually evident until spontaneous fractures occur, when pain is felt at the fracture site. The most common sites for symptomatic osteoporosis are the spine, ribs, hips, and wrists. Osteomalacia, in contrast, may cause generalized bone pain and bone tenderness, predominantly in the appendicular skeleton.

The radiographic features of the 2 diseases are often similar, but axial changes predominate in osteoporosis and appendicular changes in osteomalacia. Osteomalacia should be suspected in anyone with symmetric pathologic features, atraumatic fractures, or pseudofractures (Looser's zones), which are small, incomplete cortical fractures perpendicular to the long axis of a bone and often bilaterally symmetric. Common areas of involvement include the medial borders of the scapulae, ribs, ischiopubic rami, femoral necks, lateral borders of the femurs, and distal radii.

Results of routine laboratory studies are normal in osteoporosis but may be abnormal in osteomalacia. Osteomalacia should be suspected when the product of the serum calcium level multiplied by the serum phosphate level is chronically below 25 $(mg/dl)^2$, especially if accompanied by an elevated bone-specific alkaline phosphatase level and a 24-hour urinary calcium excretion of less than 50 mg. Osteomalacia caused by vitamin D deficiency should be suspected both in a person who has bone pain or pathologic fracture and is taking anticonvulsants or has a history of

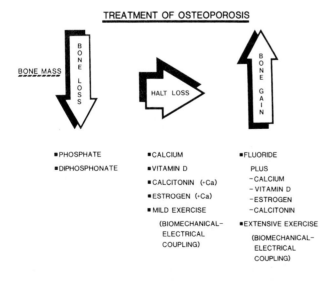

TREATMENT OF OSTEOPOROSIS

BONE MASS

BONE LOSS

HALT LOSS

BONE GAIN

- PHOSPHATE
- DIPHOSPHONATE

- CALCIUM
- VITAMIN D
- CALCITONIN (+Ca)
- ESTROGEN (+Ca)
- MILD EXERCISE
  (BIOMECHANICAL-ELECTRICAL COUPLING)

- FLUORIDE
  PLUS
  – CALCIUM
  – VITAMIN D
  – ESTROGEN
  – CALCITONIN
- EXTENSIVE EXERCISE
  (BIOMECHANICAL-ELECTRICAL COUPLING)

Figure 56

Recommended treatments for osteoporosis.

Table 6

Comparison of Osteoporosis and Osteomalacia

	Osteoporosis	Osteomalacia
Definition	Bone mass decreased Mineralization normal	Bone mass variable Mineralization decreased
Age of onset	Generally elderly, postmenopausal	Any age
Etiology	Endocrine abnormality Age Idiopathic	Vitamin D deficiency Abnormality of vitamin D pathway Hypophosphatemic syndromes Renal tubular acidosis Hypophosphatasia
Symptomatology	Pain referable to fracture site	Generalized bone pain
Signs	Tenderness at fracture site	Tenderness at fracture site and generalized tenderness
Laboratory findings		
Serum Ca++	Normal	Low or normal (high in hypophosphatasia)
Serum P_1	Normal	Low or normal (high in renal osteodystrophy)
Alkaline phosphatase	Normal	Elevated, except on hypophosphatasia
Urinary Ca++	High or normal	Normal or low (high in hypophosphatasia)
Bone biopsy	Tetracycline labels normal	Tetracycline labels abnormal

malabsorption syndrome, and in an elderly person who has a fracture of the femoral neck. The serum level of 25(OH)vitamin D is an excellent indicator of total body reserves of vitamin D.

Because these 2 diseases are very similar, a diagnosis of osteomalacia should be excluded by means of a transiliac bone biopsy following a 2-course administration of tetracycline. In 50% of patients, osteomalacia cannot be diagnosed by laboratory values and can be distinguished from osteoporosis only by bone biopsy. However, the diagnosis of osteomalacia will be expedited if the physician is familiar with the causes and has a high index of suspicion.

Paget Disease

In 1877, Sir James Paget described a bone disease that he called "osteitis deformans." Autopsy studies have yielded a 3% prevalence in a population age 40 years and older and a 10% prevalence in those patients older than 90 years of age. The disease is more common in North America, England, Australia, New Zealand, and Germany than elsewhere; it is rare in Scandinavia. In 15% to 25% of cases, a familial incidence has been clearly documented. Clinically, a large number of patients are asymptomatic.

The radiographic features of Paget disease are illustrated in Figure 57. The distal tibia demonstrates the advancing osteolytic front, whereas thickening of the cortices with loss of normal architectural configuration and deformity is seen in the proximal portion of the tibia.

In the initial phase of Paget disease, the dominant feature is osteoclasis (Fig. 57). Pagetic bone is remodeled at a higher rate than that required by the mechanical forces applied to it. In the active phase, both osteoclastic destruction and osteoblastic formation (the 2 phases of bone remodeling) occur in the same area of the bone. The inactive or "burnt out" phase is characterized by a dense mosaic bone pattern and little cellular activity. Paget disease engenders a unique radiographic feature of osteosclerosis with bone enlargment and helps distinguish the sclerotic phase of Paget disease from other osteoclerotic lesions. Often all 3 phases of Paget disease may be seen in the same bone biopsy specimen. Although the remodeling of pagetic bone is abnormal, the process of mineralization is normal.

Multiple resorbing and forming surfaces are characteristic of pagetic bone. This chaotic process leads to reorganization of the large plates of oriented lamellar bone into small areas of disorganized bone segments (Fig. 57).

In a biopsy of a pagetic vertebral body (Fig. 58), multiple resorbing lacunae are visualized. When the same slide is viewed under polarized light, there is evidence for disorganization of the collagen fibrils. The consequence of disorganization of the matrix is the enhanced brittle nature of the pagetic matrix and the high incidence of pathologic fracture and deformity. Fractures heal in pagetic bone at a slower rate than normal, and the remodeling process never restores the strength of the fracture site to that of normal bone.

Besides the classic radiographic and morphologic characteristics of Paget disease, the hypermetabolic state gives rise to scintiphotographic and chemical abnormalities. Alkaline phosphatase, a hallmark of bone formation, and urinary hydroxyproline, an indicator of bone resorption, are both elevated in active Paget disease. The coupling that exists between osteoblastic bone formation and osteoclastic bone resorption causes this elevation.

Although the etiology of Paget disease is unknown, growing evidence points to a possible slow viral infection as the cause of the disease. Measles and paramyxovirus-like inclusion bodies have been found in the nuclei of pagetic osteoclasts. Current treatment is directed at controlling osteoclast activity either with calcitonin or more recently with newer generation of bisphosphonates.

The indications for pharmacologic intervention in Paget disease are: (1) bone pain; (2) preparation for orthopaedic surgery; (3) treatment of pagetic spinal stenosis; (4) prevention of fractures or skeletal deformity in patients with rapidly progressive osteolytic lesions or in young patients; and (5) treatment of high output congestive heart failure.

Noninvasive Bone Density Measurement

Although plain radiographs are useful in the initial evaluation of osteopenia, they are the least accurate, least precise method of assessing bone density. In general, a decrease in bone mass of at least 30% is necessary to be detected on plain films. Other noninvasive radiographic and radioisotope techniques have been developed to determine skeletal mass. These methods are more precise, sensitive, and safe.

Noninvasive bone densitometry provides information about the density of bone at a specific site being measured. Density measurements of the lumbar spine have correlated relatively well with the incidence of spontaneous vertebral

fractures (R = 0.6 to 0.8). However, bone densitometry does not provide information about current rates of bone remodeling, and it offers no predictive information on future bone loss rates. Current rates of bone remodeling can be determined using various indirect serum and urine biochemical determinations, although day-to-day variability may limit their clinical usefulness. Baseline and serial bone density measurements are useful in assessing osteopenia and in monitoring the progress of therapeutic regimens.

Although bone mass is a major determinant of fracture threshold, other factors, such as cardiovascular status, medications, neuromuscular disorders, body habitus, and falls, may play an important role in the incidence of fractures.

Presently, 1 method is widely available and accepted for clinically relevant bone densitometry: dual energy x-ray absorptiometry (DEXA) for assessment of integral (cortical and trabecular) bone mineral in the spine, hip, or total body. Ultrasound studies of bone density and quality show much promise for the future, but are not currently in widespread use.

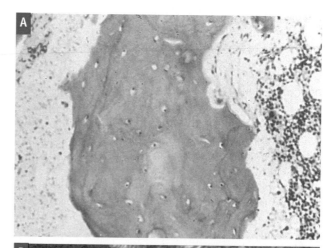

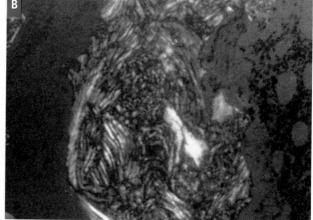

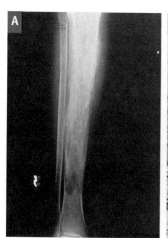
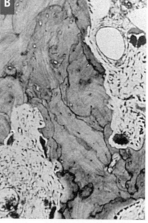

Figure 57

Radiographic features (**A**) and osteoclasis (**B**) in Paget disease.

Figure 58

Photomicrograph showing biopsy of a pagetic vertebral body viewed under normal (**A**) and polarized (**B**) light.

Dual Photon Absorptiometry and Dual-Energy X-ray Absorptiometry

Dual photon absorptiometry (DPA) originally allowed for the measurement of axial skeletal bone mineral density by accounting for the attenuation of the signal by the soft tissues. In the last decade, an X-ray-based, rather than isotope-based, dual-energy projectional system (DEXA) has been developed. This technology initially was applied to measurement of bone density in the proximal femur, and it has shown excellent correlation with DPA in the spine. DEXA has significant advantages over the old DPA techniques, including superior precision, lower radiation dose, shorter examination time, higher image resolution, and greater technical ease. The method is safe, quick, and readily available. DEXA can be used to assess baseline bone density in a patient at risk for osteoporosis, and it can be used safely and accurately to follow prevention regimens or the course of therapy.

Quantitative Computed Tomography

As noted in the section on fracture prediction, QCT generates a cross-sectional image of the vertebral body. This image allows preferential measurement of trabecular bone density. Because the rate of turnover in trabecular bone is nearly 8 times that in cortical bone, QCT provides a uniquely sensitive indicator of bone density in a region of the skeleton that is highly vulnerable to early metabolic changes. This technique involves the simultaneous scanning of a phantom composed of tubes containing standard solutions of a bone mineral equivalent. This phantom is used to calculate a standard calibration curve from which the vertebral trabecular bone density can be extrapolated. Measurements taken from the centers of vertebral bodies T12 to L4 are averaged to yield a mean bone density. Because the central portion of the vertebral body (trabecular bone) can be measured selectively, osteophytes and aortic calcifications are excluded. As with DEXA, precision is excellent, but it may be reduced in severely osteopenic and kyphotic individuals as a result of difficulty in relocating the exact sites of previous measurements. Accuracy is within 5% to 10%. A further decrease is possible because of the variable fat content of the bone marrow, especially in older patients. The radiation dose is higher than with the DEXA techniques.

Ultrasound

As noted previously, ultrasound is currently being studied as a means for assessing mechanical properties of bone. Ultrasound is attractive because it does not expose a patient to ionizing radiation (as occurs with x-ray scanners), and because it is noninvasive, safe, and relatively inexpensive. It is also viewed as having the potential for measuring the strength and stiffness of bone directly, in contrast to x-ray densitometric techniques, which measure bone mass only.

Bone Biomarkers

In addition to bone mass measurements such as DEXA, a new group of biochemical tests has been developed for clinical use that are increasingly being used to study patients with osteoporosis. There are several markers of bone formation, including bone-specific alkaline phosphatase (an osteoblast enzyme) and osteocalcin (a bone matrix protein). Levels of both these markers can be determined in the serum. Collagen degradation products in the urine, particularly the cross-linked telopeptides and pyridinolines, have the highest specificity to bone resorption activity. The telopeptides markers (NTx and CTx) appear to be the most specific and responsive markers of systemic osteoclast activity. The biochemical indices of bone turnover just described provide different yet complementary information that can aid in predicting risk of future bone loss and osteoporotic fracture. In addition, bone resorptive markers can be used to monitor effectiveness of therapy.

Transiliac Bone Biopsy

Before the advent of bone biomarkers, accurate information concerning rates of bone turnover and mineralization could be determined only from direct sampling of bone. Thus, historically, transiliac bone biopsies were done frequently to determine the diagnosis of metabolic bone diseases. Although not performed as frequently, this method remains a useful technique in understanding the nature of metabolic bone problems

The iliac crest is a readily accessible biopsy site and reflects changes at other clinically relevant sites. A 5- to 8-mm diameter core is obtained through a small 1-cm biopsy incision under local anesthesia. Time-spaced dynamic tetracycline labeling permits the determination of mineralization rates in specimens that have not been decalcified. Tetracycline binds to newly mineralized osteoid. Two weeks before a bone biopsy, the tetracycline is administered twice each day for 3 days; this procedure is then repeated in the 3 days immediately prior to the bone biopsy. The mean distance between the tetracycline labels, as seen and measured using fluorescent microscopy, is divided by the number of days between the 2 courses of tetracycline to determine the mineral apposition rate. Abnormal patterns of fluorescent label deposition are the diagnostic hallmark of osteomalacia. When normal mineralization is present, as in osteoporosis, 2 distinct bands will result from the 2 doses of tetracycline. When mineralization is impaired, as in the case of osteomalacia, a single band of fluorescence will result.

Bone histomorphometry involves the quantitative analysis of undecalcified bone in which the parameters of skeletal remodeling are expressed in terms of volumes, surfaces, and cell numbers. Clinical and biochemical studies often fail to predict histologic changes. In addition, histologic changes vary regionally and are strongly influenced by local factors, including weightbearing stress (magnitude and direction), blood supply, marrow environment, and type of bone (cortical versus trabecular).

Bone biopsy is not necessary for evaluation of most patients with metabolic bone disease. However, biopsy is an important diagnostic tool in men and women younger than age 50 years who have idiopathic osteopenia, in any patient in whom osteomalacia is highly suspected, and in patients with chronic renal failure with skeletal symptoms. Because of the inherent problem of regional sample error, bone biopsy should not be used to establish the diagnosis of osteoporosis; rather, it should be used to exclude a diagnosis of osteomalacia in a patient with osteopenia. In the evaluation of a patient with renal failure, bone biopsy can provide information to distinguish osteomalacia from osteitis fibrosa from aluminum-associated bone disease.

Summary

This chapter on the form and function of bone covers a broad range of material from the basic structure of bone and its biomechanical properties to bone homeostasis and disease processes that perturb this homeostasis. While the technology involved in the treatment of orthopaedic patients continues to evolve rapidly, understanding these basic principles remains crucial. Not only do these principles allow the orthopaedic surgeon to predict how bone will behave clinically but serves as the necessary foundation of knowledge for the rational practice of orthopaedic surgery.

Acknowledgments

The authors wish to thank Frederick S. Kaplan, MD, Wilson C. Hayes, PhD, Tony M. Keaveny, PhD, and Joseph P. Iannotti, MD, PhD, for previous work on this chapter.

Selected Bibliography

Bone Cell Morphology

Baron R, Ravesloot JH, Neff L, et al: Cellular and molecular biology of the osteoclast, in Noda M (ed): *Cellular and Molecular Biology of Bone.* San Diego, CA, Academic Press, 1993, pp 445–495.

Hall BK (ed): *Bone: The Osteoclast,* ed 2. Boca Raton, FL, CRC Press, 1991, vol 2.

Hall BK (ed): *Bone: The Osteoblast and Osteocyte.* Caldwell, NJ, Telford Press, 1990.

Bone Blood Flow

Brookes M (ed): *The Blood Supply of Bone: An Approach to Bone Biology.* London, England, Butterworths, 1971.

Hall BK (ed): *Bone: Fracture Repair and Regeneration.* Boca Raton, FL, CRC Press, 1992, vol 5.

Hellem S, Jacobsson LS, Nilsson GE, Lewis DH: Measurement of microvascular blood flow in cancellous bone using laser Doppler flowmetry and 133Xe-clearance. *Int J Oral Surg* 1983;12:165–177.

Rhinelander FW: Tibial blood supply in relation to fracture healing. *Clin Orthop* 1974;105:34–81.

Tondevold E: Haemodynamics of long bones: An experimental study on dogs. *Acta Orthop Scand Suppl* 1983;205:9–48.

Tothill P: Bone blood flow measurement. *J Biomed Eng* 1984;6:251–256.

Bone Mechanics

Bone Mineralization

Aubin JE, Turksen K, Heersche JNM: Osteoblastic cell lineage, in Noda M (ed): *Cellular and Molecular Biology of Bone.* San Diego, CA, Academic Press, 1993, pp 1–45.

Boskey AL: Matrix proteins and mineralization: An overview. *Connect Tissue Res* 1996;35:357–363.

Boskey AL: Mineral-matrix interactions in bone and cartilage. *Clin Orthop* 1992;281:244–274.

Boskey AL: Osteopontin and related phosphorylated sialoproteins: Effects on mineralization. *Ann NY Acad Sci* 1995;760:249–256.

Ducy P, Desbois C, Boyce B, et al: Increased bone formation in osteocalcin-deficient mice. *Nature* 1996;382:448–452.

Eyre DR: The collagens of musculoskeletal soft tissues, in Leadbetter WB, Buckwalter JA, Gordon SL (eds): *Sports-Induced Inflammation: Clinical and Basic Science Concepts.* Park Ridge, IL, American Academy of Orthopaedic Surgeons, 1990, pp 161–170.

Hall BK (ed): *Bone: Bone Matrix and Bone Specific Products.* Boca Raton, FL, CRC Press, 1991, vol 3.

Hall BK (ed): *Bone: Bone Metabolism and Mineralization.* Boca Raton, FL, CRC Press, 1992, vol 4.

Hardingham TE, Fosang AJ: Proteoglycans: Many forms and many functions. *FASEB J* 1992;6:861–870.

Heinegard D, Oldberg A: Structure and biology of cartilage and bone matrix noncollagenous macromolecules. *FASEB J* 1989;3:2042–2051.

Hruska KA, Rolnick F, Duncan RL, Medhora M, Yamakawa K: Signal transduction in osteoblasts and osteoclasts, in Noda M (ed): *Cellular and Molecular Biology of Bone.* San Diego, CA, Academic Press, 1993, pp 413–444.

Hynes RO: Integrins: Versatility, modulation, and signaling in cell adhesion. *Cell* 1992;69:11–25.

Luo G, Ducy P, McKee MD, et al: Spontaneous calcification of arteries and cartilage in mice lacking matrix GLA protein. *Nature* 1997;386:78–81.

Mundy GR, Boyce BF, Yoneda T, Bonewald LF, Roodman GD: Cytokines and bone remodeling, in Marcus R, Feldman D, Kelsey J (eds): *Osteoporosis*. San Diego, CA, Academic Press, 1996, pp 301–313.

Reddi AH, Sampath TK: Bone morphogenetic proteins: Potential role in osteoporosis, in Marcus R, Feldman D, Kelsey J (eds): *Osteoporosis*. San Diego, CA, Academic Press, 1996, pp 281–287.

Robey PG, Boskey AL: The biochemistry of bone, in Marcus R, Feldman D, Kelsey J (eds): *Osteoporosis*. San Diego, CA, Academic Press, 1996, pp 95–183.

Calcium Homeostasis

Boden SD, Kaplan FS: Calcium homeostasis. *Orthop Clin North Am* 1990;21:31–42.

Einhorn TA, Levine B, Michel P: Nutrition and bone. *Orthop Clin North Am* 1990;21:43–50.

Eriksen EF, Colvard DS, Berg NJ, et al: Evidence of estrogen receptors in normal human osteoblast-like cells. *Science* 1988;241:84–86.

Ettinger B, Genant HK, Cann CE: Postmenopausal bone loss is prevented by treatment with low-dosage estrogen with calcium. *Ann Intern Med* 1987;106:40–45.

Martin TJ, Findlay DM, Moseley JM: Peptide hormones acting on bone, in Marcus R, Feldman D, Kelsey J (eds): *Osteoporosis*. San Diego, CA, Academic Press, 1996, pp 185–204.

Reichel H, Koeffler HP, Norman AW: The role of the vitamin D endocrine system in health and disease. *N Engl J Med* 1989;320:980–991.

Metabolic Bone Disease

Bullough PG, Bansal M, DiCarlo EF: The tissue diagnosis of metabolic bone disease: Role of histomorphometry. *Orthop Clin North Am* 1990;21:65–79.

Chapuy MC, Arlot ME, Duboeuf F, et al: Vitamin D_3 and calcium to prevent hip fractures in elderly women. *N Engl J Med* 1992;327:1637–1642.

Cumming RG, Nevitt MC, Cummings SR: Epidemiology of hip fractures. *Epidemiol Rev* 1997;19:244–257.

Favus MJ, Christakos S, Kaplan F, et al (eds): *Primer on the Metabolic Bone Diseases and Disorders of Mineral Metabolism*, ed 3. Philadelphia, PA, Lippincott-Raven, 1996.

Genant HK, Block JE, Steiger P, Glueer CC, Ettinger B, Harris ST: Appropriate use of bone densitometry. *Radiology* 1989;170:817–822.

Horowitz MC: Cytokines and estrogen in bone: Anti-osteoporotic effects. *Science* 1993;260:626–627.

Hortobagyi GN, Theriault RL, Porter L, et al: Efficacy of pamidronate in reducing skeletal complications in patients with breast cancer and lytic bone metastases: Protocol 19 Aredia Breast Cancer Study Group. *N Engl J Med* 1996;335:1785–1791.

Kaplan FS, Singer FR: Paget's disease of bone: Pathophysiology, diagnosis, and management. *J Am Acad Orthop Surg* 1995;3:336–344.

Kelsey JL, Hoffman S: Risk factors for hip fracture. *N Engl J Med* 1987; 316:404–406.

Komm BS, Terpening CM, Benz DJ, et al: Estrogen binding, receptor mRNA, and biologic response in osteoblast-like osteosarcoma cells. *Science* 1988;241:81–84.

Liberman UA, Weiss SR, Bröll J, et al: Effect of oral alendronate on bone mineral density and the incidence of fractures in postmenopausal osteoporosis: The Alendronate Phase III Osteoporosis Treatment Study Group. *N Engl J Med* 1995;333:1437–1443.

Lindsay R (ed): *Osteoporosis: A Guide to Diagnosis, Prevention, and Treatment*. New York, NY, Raven Press, 1992.

Mankin HJ: Rickets, osteomalacia, and renal osteodystrophy: An update. *Orthop Clin North Am* 1990;21:81–96.

Mazess RB: Bone densitometry of the axial skeleton. *Orthop Clin North Am* 1990;21:51–63.

Pak CY, Sakhaee K, Adams-Huet B, Piziak V, Peterson RD, Poindexter JR: Treatment of postmenopausal osteoporosis with slow-release sodium fluoride: Final report of a randomized controlled trial. *Ann Intern Med* 1995;123:401–408.

Ultrasound

Alves JM, Ryaby JT, Kaufman JJ, Magee FP, Siffert RS: Influence of marrow on ultrasonic velocity and attenuation in bovine trabecular bone. *Calcif Tissue Int* 1996;58:362–367.

Gluer CC: Quantitative ultrasound techniques for the assessment of osteoporosis: Expert agreement on current status. The International Quantitative Ultrasound Consensus Group. *J Bone Miner Res* 1997; 12:1280–1288.

Kaufman JJ, Einhorn TA: Ultrasound assessment of bone. *J Bone Miner Res* 1993;8:517–525.

Chapter Outline

Chapter 14

Bone Injury, Regeneration, and Repair

Susan M. Day, MD

Robert F. Ostrum, MD

Edmund Y.S. Chao, PhD

Clinton T. Rubin, MD

Hannu T. Aro, MD

Thomas A. Einhorn, MD

This chapter at a glance

This chapter discusses bone injury along with the ways in which the organ system as a whole responds to injury.

Introduction

Injury to bone can occur by a multitude of causes. In addition to physical injury (trauma), infection, tumor, genetic disorders, and many other conditions can produce changes in bone that could be considered injurious. Bone injury from any cause must be viewed in terms of its effect on the cellular content of bone, the ability of such cells to produce extracellular matrix, and the structure and organization of the organic and inorganic components of bone itself. This chapter describes those injuries to bone caused by circulatory loss and physical injury. Such injuries jeopardize cell viability and structural integrity. Injury to one affects the other; loss of cell viability will directly and indirectly affect the structural organization of bone. Similarly, structural repair necessitates cellular changes. In the strictest sense, bone repair is a regenerative process that brings about changes in all aspects of the organ system. In this chapter, bone injury is discussed along with the ways in which the organ system as a whole responds to injury.

Depending on the nature of the injury and the proposed method of repair, certain aspects of the process play a predominant role, but the underlying reactions and principles remain the same and need to be understood if normal functioning bone is to be maintained.

Osteonecrosis

Osteonecrosis can arise from a variety of disorders. The term itself, defined as the death of a segment of bone in situ, actually refers to the death of the cells within bone from lack of circulation, not from disease. Unless secondary effects occur, the organic and inorganic matrices of the structural components of bone are not affected; dead bone refers to dead cells. Such cells include osteocytes, whether they are in cortical or cancellous bone, and usually include the cells of the hematopoietic and fatty marrow contents as well. The term osteonecrosis is preferred to such commonly used terms as avascular necrosis and aseptic necrosis because (1) it is the most appropriate description of the histopathologic process seen, and (2) it doesn't suggest any specific etiology.

Etiology

Osteonecrotic bone is not avascular; the vessels are still present. However, in all causative mechanisms of osteonecrosis, the circulation within the vessels is compromised. Such compromise may be grouped into 4 possible mechanisms: (1) mechanical disruption of the vessels; (2) occlusion of the arterial vessels; (3) injury to or pressure on the arterial wall; and (4) occlusion to the venous outflow vessels. Mechanical vascular disruption may result from a fracture or dislocation, or from such atraumatic events as stress or fatigue fractures. Arterial occlusion can arise from

thrombosis, embolism, circulating fat, nitrogen bubbles, or abnormally shaped cells (sickle cell crises). Temporary or permanent damage to an intact vessel wall can arise from within the wall as in vasculitis or radiation injury, from within the vessel as in the release of materials that can cause angiospasm, or from external pressure or chemical reaction on the wall as in extravasated blood, fat, or cellular elements in the marrow cavity. In a closed system, if the circulation in the venous outflow is compromised by any of these mechanisms so that venous pressure exceeds arterial pressure, circulation to the cells supplied by this source will be compromised. If a sufficient collateral circulation is present at any site where such compromise occurs, cells remain viable. Although bone has a rich blood supply, it may vary from site to site; therefore, it is likely that only cells in certain locations are susceptible to becoming nonviable.

Osteonecrosis can be the result of trauma. A displaced fractured femoral neck, dislocation of the femoral head, displaced fracture of the scaphoid, displaced fracture of the talar neck, and a 4-part fracture of the humeral head are the most common traumatic injuries leading to osteonecrosis and its clinically significant secondary complications of collapse of the subchondral bone and adjacent articular surface. The osteonecrosis associated with infection (osteomyelitis or pyarthrosis) is thought to be produced by the combination of increased intramedullary pressure and arterial occlusion. In cases in which osteonecrosis is associated with Gaucher's disease, the marrow cavity is packed with Gaucher's cells (macrophages filled with cerebroside). In cases in which it is associated with sickle-cell disease, the marrow cavity is packed with sickled red blood cells. The osteonecrosis in these last 2 diseases seems to result from direct occlusion of the intraosseous arteries. The osteonecrosis associated with decompression sickness, so-called caisson disease, probably is caused by vascular occlusion by nitrogen bubbles that come out of solution with the rapid drop in barometric pressure. Osteonecrosis after irradiation of bone probably occurs as a result of radiation damage to the capillaries. It also occurs in association with ethanol abuse, corticosteroid administration, hyperlipidemia, and pancreatitis, and, very often, in otherwise normal individuals (those with idiopathic osteonecrosis).

Idiopathic osteonecrosis and osteonecrosis associated with ethanol or corticosteroids account for the vast majority of cases of nontraumatic osteonecrosis. The mechanisms that cause osteonecrosis in these patients are unknown. In fact, there is some evidence to suggest that the use of corticosteroids in renal transplant subjects may not be the causative agent related to the osteonecrosis. One proposed mechanism is arterial occlusion by fat emboli (Fig. 1); it is postulated that the fat emboli arise from a fatty liver, from plasma lipoproteins, or directly from marrow fat. There is experimental evidence supporting this mechanism, but whether it is the cause of osteonecrosis in a significant percent of humans is not known. A popular explanation for idiopathic osteonecrosis, especially that seen in the femoral head, is intraosseous hypertension. The theory is that the intraosseous vessels are occluded secondary to excessive pressure within the medullary space. The cause of the suspected intraosseous hypertension is not known. Although measurement of the intraosseous pressure of bones with early osteonecrosis reveals increased pressure, it is not clear whether this pressure is a cause or an effect. The only conclusion that should be made is that the cause of osteonecrosis in the majority of cases still is not adequately understood.

Cellular Bone Injury

Regardless of the inciting disorder, the morphologic processes of osteonecrosis are very similar. Animal studies have demonstrated that in the first few days to 1 week after vascular compromise has been initiated, there are no histologic changes. During the second week, the marrow contents begin to show evidence of necrosis, including death of hematopoietic cells, capillary endothelial cells, and

lipocytes. The shrinking of the osteocytes produces the empty lacunae typical of necrotic bone. The death of cells within the fatty marrow causes the release of lysosomes, and the tissue becomes acidified. Released calcium forms an insoluble soap with saponified, free fatty acids released from dead lipocytes. Normal fatty marrow has little water; however, after it becomes necrotic, the early changes are associated with increased water. It is this change in water content that is the first abnormality that can be detected clinically. This change can be seen on a magnetic resonance imaging (MRI) scan. The MRI scan measures the alignment of hydrogen ions and, because water is the principal source of these hydrogen ions in humans, it is quite sensitive to the water content of tissues (Fig. 2).

Repair of Osteonecrotic Bone

The remaining events associated with osteonecrosis are related to replacement of the acellular bone and the time it takes for this process to occur. The initiation of repair can occur only if the surrounding viable cellular tissues receive some signal to suggest that such a process is needed. In some sites and where the area of cell death is small, no signal appears to be generated to initiate this process; the bone infarct remains for life. If they are small enough and in an area that does not compromise the structural integrity of the bone, such lesions will be clinically silent, nonprogressive, and may be detected only as incidental findings on an MRI or bone scan related to intramarrow fluid changes or mild peripheral reactive changes, respectively. Commonly, this situation occurs when necrosis of cells involves only the medullary bone with no involvement of the subchondral plate; no symptoms and no functional abnormalities result. The necrotic tissues, especially the saponified fats, calcify and may be seen on plain radiographs forever.

If osteonecrosis involves cortical cancellous bone and a reparative response is initiated, a reactive hyperemia and vascular fibrous repair are first noted in the adjacent bony tissues. The subsequent events appear identical to those that occur with the incorporation of a bone graft and are commonly referred to as creeping substitution. Revascularization of the necrotic bone from the adjacent fibrous tissue is noted within a few weeks. Vessels grow into the medullary canal to revascularize the cancellous bone and into the haversian canals of the cortex. In the cortical bone their histologic appearance is that of so-called cutting cones, and is similar to what is seen at the metaphyseal end of the growth plate (Fig. 3). At both sites, primitive mesenchymal cells accompany the vessels and differentiate into osteoblasts and osteoclasts. It is not known what stimulates the differentiation of the undifferentiated mesenchymal cells, but it is likely to be one or several cytokines released from the necrotic bone. Other local factors, including pH, oxygen tension, and mechanical stress, also influence the differentiation of the mesenchymal cells.

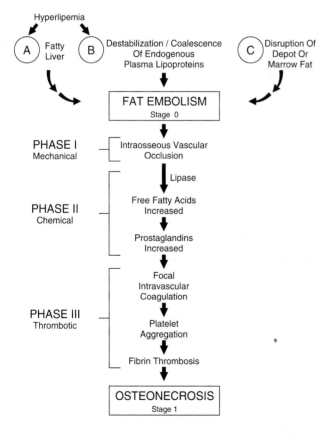

MECHANISMS OF LIPID METABOLISM RESULTING IN FAT EMBOLISM AND OSTEONECROSIS

Figure 1

Schematic representation of 3 mechanisms potentially capable of producing intraosseous fat embolism and triggering a process leading to focal intravascular coagulation and osteonecrosis. (Reproduced with permission from Jones JP Jr: Fat embolism and osteonecrosis. *Clin Orthop* 1985; 16:595–633.)

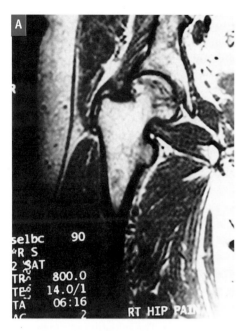

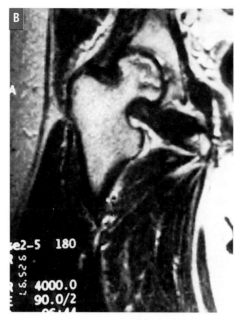

Figure 2

T1-weighted (**A**) and T2-weighted (**B**) magnetic resonance images of osteonecrotic bone in the femoral head.

In cancellous bone, the next event is the production of osteoid on the scaffolding of the necrotic trabeculae (Fig. 4). The trabeculae are thickened by the new viable bone, and, as a result, the early repair of the cancellous bone increases the density of the bone. This density, which is the result of new bone applied to existing old bone, may not reflect the strength of a similarly dense bone undergoing normal remodeling. Although calcification of necrotic marrow may account for some of the increased density seen within the osteonecrotic bone in the early stages of osteonecrosis, the majority of the changes seen on plain radiographs of osteonecrotic subchondral bone are caused by the increased thickness of the individual trabeculae. The appearance of the increased density requires a substantial amount of new bone formation that is not obvious on plain radiographs until between 6 and 12 months after the onset of necrosis.

In necrotic cortical bone, the bone in the haversian canals is resorbed before new bone is produced. Osteoclasts are formed by the fusion of mononuclear cells, and resorption of the necrotic haversian bone begins just after vascular invasion. Resorption continues until the majority of the haversian bone, but almost none of the interlamellar bone, has been removed. Then osteoblasts begin the process of replacing the haversian system (Fig. 3). Thus, cortical bone first becomes osteoporotic and regains its original density only after it has been repaired. This resorption weakens the cortical bone, which explains the fractures observed at 18 to 24 months after the onset of necrosis. It takes that long to resorb enough bone for a pathologic fracture to occur. As the repair of the necrotic bone continues, the density, as seen on the radiograph, and the strength return to normal. This process takes at least 2 years.

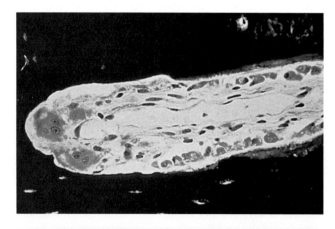

Figure 3

Photomicrograph showing a cortical cutting cone.

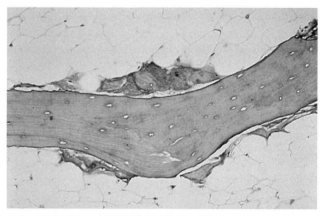

Figure 4

Photomicrograph of a cancellous bone graft undergoing creeping substitution. Note lamellar bone with empty lacunae and the presence of woven bone with basophilic staining osteoblasts which appears to be "creeping" on this dead bone.

Structural Sequelae

Necrotic bone initially has no alteration in its mechanical properties; osteonecrosis directly affects only the cells, and structurally the bone functions normally. If, however, the osteonecrosis involves the subchondral bone, the eventual fracture and collapse of the bone leads to irregularities in the articular surface and, subsequently, to degenerative arthritis. All evidence indicates that this scenario is a secondary mechanical phenomenon that occurs over time as a result of the absence of cells to respond to the effects of the continuation of normal daily activities. The fracture and collapse appear to be the result of multiple fatigue fractures that are caused by repetitive loading of the bone and cannot be repaired. They seem to be initiated in areas of bone where: (1) the remaining avascular subchondral trabeculae oriented perpendicular to the joint surface lack the means to repair small microfractures; (2) the resorption of the subchondral bone at the periphery, where there is vascular invasion of the necrotic bone, results in osteoporotic, weakened bone; or (3) the junction of increased bone density at the front of revascularization results in a stress riser between it and adjacent avascular bone. Prior to complete fracture and collapse, the microfractures can elicit a pain response. If functional activities are reduced, viable bone within or surrounding the osteonecrotic bone area undergoes a reduction in bone mass. The relative increased density of unresorbed necrotic bone compared to the adjacent viable osteoporotic bone permits the recognition of necrotic bone on plain radiographs. When the necrotic bone collapses, leading to loss of subchondral support, the result is the appearance of the crescent sign. In the talus, Hawkins' sign the subchondral radiolucency seen in the talar bone, represents the resorption of necrotic bone and suggests that the bone is revascularized. When subchondral radiolucency is not seen, the bone is not being resorbed and vascularization is not present.

Clinical Effects

The severity and significance of the clinical syndrome in osteonecrosis depends on the size and site of its occurrence. If the lesion is small enough and the area can be revascularized, then it is likely no effect will be seen. If the area of involvement is large and blood supply cannot be restored, then the area remains necrotic, fracture within the necrotic area can occur and the result is progressive collapse. When the area becomes incongruous, joint destruction results. Bones that are often affected include the femoral head, humeral head, talus, medial femoral condyle and scaphoid. Because the treatment will differ at sequential intervals in the course of the syndrome, various staging systems have been proposed for assessing the progression of osteonecrosis. These have focused mainly on the femoral head. Ficat originally described a staging classification

based on plain radiographs in which stage I disease is a symptomatic hip in which no radiographic change is evident. In stage II, radiographs demonstrate patchy areas that are radiolucent and radiodense. The "crescent sign" represents the transition between stage II and stage III. Subchondral collapse is the hallmark of stage III. By stage IV the articular surface has collapsed. The radiographic classification most familiar and most commonly used is the Cruess modification of the Ficat classification, which defines stage III as the appearance of the crescent sign, stage IV as collapse of the femoral head and adds stage V, narrowing and arthrosis of the joint. Stage 0 is defined as the asymptomatic, radiographically normal hip in the patient at risk.

Bone Repair and Regeneration

Fracture healing is a complex, highly ordered, physiologic process. Unlike other tissues that heal by the formation of a scar, in fracture healing the original tissue (bone) is regenerated and the properties of the preexisting tissue are restored. This complex process involves a cascade of regenerative events that begins at the moment of fracture.

Biomechanics of Fractures

Fractures can be classified according to the characteristics of the force that causes them. A fracture may arise from forces of low magnitude that are cyclically repeated over a long period of time or from a force having sufficient magnitude to cause failure after a single application. The susceptibility of bone to fracture under fluctuating forces or stresses of low magnitude is related to its crystal structure and collagen orientation, which reflect the viscoelastic properties of the bone. Cortical bone is vulnerable to both tensile and compressive fluctuating stresses. Under each cycle of loading, a small amount of strain energy may be lost through microscopic cracks along the cement lines. Fatigue load under certain strain rates can cause progressive accumulation of microdamage in cortical bone. When such a process is prolonged, bone may eventually fail through fracture-crack propagation. However, bone is a living tissue and can undertake a repair process simultaneously. Periosteal callus and new bone formation near the microscopic cracks can arrest crack propagation by reducing the high stresses at the tip of the crack. This phenomenon is commonly seen in stress fractures.

Fractures caused by a single application or injury can be classified according to the magnitude and area distribution of the force, as well as to the rate at which the force acts on the bone. When the trauma is direct, soft-tissue injury and fracture comminution are related to the loading rate. When force is applied to the bone at a distance from the fracture site, strong muscle contractions across a joint with a fixed distal segment may result in separated, distracted, fracture fragments. Fractures of the olecranon and patella are examples of this type of injury.

Regardless of where the force is applied, such forces may generate compressive, tensile, or shear stresses or some combination thereof in the bone. Whether each type of stress generated acts independently or with the others in various combinations, the failure patterns of long bones follow some basic rules. In general, the combination of the bone's material strength and anisometric properties, particularly its 3 principal planes of stress (tension, compression, and shear), dictate when, how, and along which path the fracture will occur (Fig. 5). Cortical bone, as a material, is generally weak in tension and shear, particularly along the longitudinal plane; therefore, the area where tensile stresses arise fails first. The closer the majority of such tensile stresses are oriented to the long axes of the bone, the less force will be needed to break the bone. Studies on dog tibias have shown that the maximum load to failure is 3 times higher for the production of a transverse fracture than for that of a spiral fracture.

Transverse fractures are the result of pure tensile forces or bending. Failure of bone from a pure tensile force occurs progressively across the bone, creating a transverse fracture without comminution. Similarly, the pattern of fracture arising from pure bending is a simple transverse line because failure stresses are almost pure tensile in type. Uneven bending is more apt to produce an oblique fracture line. Occasionally, the cortex under compression breaks as a result of existing shear stress before the tension failure progresses all the way across the bone; in this situation, comminution occurs on the compression side, and a single butterfly fragment or multiple fragments may be created. In contrast, spiral fractures are the result of pure torsional injuries, and have 2 different types of fracture lines: an angled line turning around the circumference of the bone, and a more or less longitudinal line linking the proximal and distal portions of the spiral. In experimental conditions, the average angled line of a spiral fracture is approximately 30° off the longitudinal axis, and the total angle of ascent of each spiral fracture clinically has been noted to vary from 30° to 70° and is never transverse. To a certain

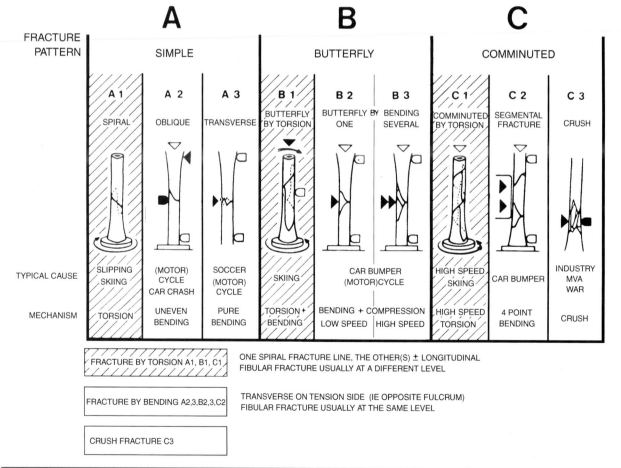

Figure 5

The 9 main fracture groups; fractures are classified according to degree of comminution and etiology. (Reproduced with permission from Johner R, Wruhs O: Classification of tibial shaft fractures and correlation with results after rigid internal fixation. *Clin Orthop* 1983;178:7–25.)

degree, a bending moment always exists when torsional forces are applied. Its presence is the reason for the line linking the ends of the spiral and prevents the endless propagation of the spiral fracture. Under certain circumstances it produces a butterfly fragment rather than a single linking line. In contrast, combining an axial load with torsional forces has little effect on the failure pattern of the resulting spiral fracture.

The susceptibility of a bone to fracture from a single injury is related not only to its modulus of elasticity and anisometric properties but to its energy-absorbing capacity as well. Bone undergoing rapid loading must absorb more energy than bone loaded at a slower rate. The kinetic energy of the impacting object is defined as $1/2 \, MV^2$, where M is the mass and V is the velocity of the impacting object. Energy absorbed by the bone during loading is released when the bone is fractured. This phenomenon helps to explain why injuries with rapid loading involving higher velocities dissipate energy and result in more significant structural changes, that is, greater fracture comminution and displacement. Thus, gunshot wounds inflicted by high-velocity bullets result in considerably more bone comminution and soft-tissue damage than gunshot wounds from low-velocity bullets. This same phenomenon is seen with the application of indirect forces as well. At low speeds, bending plus tensile stress will cause a fracture with a single butterfly fragment, whereas the same mechanism of injury at high speeds will cause several butterfly fragments. High-speed torsion alone, that is, without an associated bending moment, can cause a spiral fracture with comminution. The most common etiology of segmental fractures is 4-point bending, which is commonly seen when a tibia is hit by a car bumper, considered a high-velocity injury.

How the pattern of bone injury relates to the types of forces applied to bone is not merely of concern to the bone's structural integrity, but to its healing capacity as well. The importance of soft-tissue injury and cell viability has been stressed by many authors. The time to union is greatly prolonged in fractures that have more soft-tissue stripping. Experimental studies have demonstrated the retarding effect of muscle damage on bone healing. The larger load under bending failure may cause the surrounding soft tissues and periosteum to sustain more damage and, thus, may affect the fracture healing potential. Long-bone shaft fractures resulting from high-energy injuries have a higher rate of bone healing complications than fractures from low-energy injuries. In addition, open fractures have a higher incidence of nonunion than closed fractures in most large series.

Fracture Healing Responses

In order to understand the different processes that contribute to fracture healing, it is useful to view these healing events in terms of 4 distinct responses, which include those that take place in the bone marrow, cortex, periosteum, and external soft tissues. Depending on the type of fracture, its location, and the method by which it is treated, 1 or several of these responses can occur simultaneously.

At the moment of impact, the energy absorbed by the bone leads to mechanical and structural failure. Besides the actual break in continuity of the bone, there is a disruption of the blood supply to the bone at the fracture site. Within a few hours after a fracture is sustained, normal architecture of the bone marrow elements is lost, blood vessels in the region adjacent to the fracture callus clot and the cellular complement of the bone marrow are reorganized into regions of high and low cellular density. In the region of high cellular density, there appears to be a transformation of endothelial cells to so-called polymorphic cells; by 24 hours after fracture, these cells already express an osteoblastic phenotype and begin to form bone.

In classic histologic terms, fracture healing has been divided into so-called primary fracture healing and secondary fracture healing. Primary healing, or primary cortical healing, involves a direct attempt by the cortex to reestablish itself when continuity has been disputed. In order for a fracture to become united, bone on one side of the cortex must unite with bone on the other to reestablish mechanical continuity. This process seems to occur only when there is anatomic restoration of the fracture fragments and when the stability of fracture reduction is ensured by rigid internal fixation and a substantial decrease in interfragmentary strain. After stable fixation has been achieved, gaps will remain along with contact points. Healing within the gaps first occurs by the ingrowth of blood vessels, which begins soon after injury. Mesenchymal cells differentiate into osteoblasts, which begin to lay down osteoid on exposed bone surfaces. This generally occurs without osteoclast resorption. The edges of necrotic bone as well as fracture callus within the fracture gap then undergo resorption. Osteoclasts in cutting cones on one side of the fracture exhibit a tunneling resorptive response whereby they reestablish new haversian systems, providing pathways for the penetration of blood vessels. These new blood vessels are accompanied by endothelial cells, perivascular mesenchymal cells, and osteoprogenitor cells. This process leads to the callus being replaced by new osteons. The contact areas provide stabilization for the gaps. This direct contact prevents the ingrowth of blood vessels seen early in gap healing. Healing in contact areas is the result of cutting cones crossing the contact area, which then allows the passage of blood vessels.

Secondary healing involves responses in the periosteum and external soft tissues. Perhaps the most important response in fracture healing takes place in the periosteum. Here, both committed osteoprogenitor cells and uncommitted undifferentiated mesenchymal cells contribute to the process of fracture healing by a recapitulation of embryonic intramembranous ossification and endochondral bone formation. The response from the periosteum is a fundamental reaction to bone injury and is enhanced by motion and inhibited by rigid fixation. It has been shown to be rapid, capable of bridging gaps as large as half the diameter of the bone.

The bone formed by intramembranous ossification is found peripheral to the site of the fracture, results in the formation of a socalled hard callus, and forms bone directly without first forming cartilage. Consequently, structural proteins in the hard callus appear very early in the healing process. On the other hand, the callus that forms by endochondral ossification is found adjacent to the fracture site, involves the development of a cartilage anlage that becomes calcified and then replaced by bone, and is characterized by the production of a litany of molecules related to a variety of musculoskeletal tissue types.

The response of the external soft tissues is also an important process in the fracture healing sequence, involving rapid cellular activity and the development of an early bridging callus that stabilizes the fracture fragments. This process depends heavily on mechanical factors and may be depressed by rigid immobilization. The type of tissue formed from the external soft tissues evolves through a process of endochondral ossification in which undifferentiated mesenchymal cells are recruited, proliferate, and eventually differentiate into cartilage-forming cells.

Stages of Fracture Healing

Most fractures are either left untreated, or are treated with a form of management that results in some degree of motion (sling immobilization, cast immobilization, external fixation, intramedullary fixation). Thus, the majority of fractures heal by a combination of intramembranous and endochondral ossification. These 2 processes participate in the fracture repair sequence by means of at least 6 discrete stages of healing. These stages include an initial stage in which a hematoma is formed and inflammation occurs, a subsequent stage in which angiogenesis develops and cartilage begins to form, and then 3 successive stages of cartilage calcification, cartilage removal, and bone formation, and ultimately a more chronic stage of bone remodeling.

According to several textbooks published before the age of molecular biology, the presumed contribution of the initial blood clot formed at the fracture site was to develop into a scaffold made of fibrin, which was to provide some early mechanical stability. It is now generally well accepted that the function of the clot is to serve as a source of signaling molecules with the capacity to initiate the cascades of cellular events critical to fracture healing. For example, inflammatory cells secreting cytokines, such as interleukins-1 and -6 (IL-1, IL-6), may be important in regulating the early events in the fracture healing process. In addition, degranulating platelets in the clot may release signaling molecules, such as transforming growth factor-beta (TGF-β) and platelet-derived growth factor (PDGF), which are important in regulating cell proliferation and differentiation of committed mesenchymal stem cells. Moreover, some of these cytokines or signaling molecules may be involved in other processes, such as chemotaxis or angiogenesis, and may also serve as competence and progression factors in many of the cellular responses.

In a rat fracture model, over the first 7 to 10 days of fracture healing, intramembranous and endochondral bone formation is initiated. By the middle of the second week after fracture healing, abundant cartilage overlies the fracture site and this chondroid tissue initiates biochemical preparations to undergo calcification. At this time, the callus can be divided into hard callus, where intramembranous ossification is taking place, and soft callus, where the process of endochondral ossification is proceeding.

Calcification of fracture callus cartilage occurs by a mechanism almost identical to that which takes place in the growth plate. Approximately 9 days after fracture, there is an abundance of elongated proliferative chondrocytes that undergo mitosis and divide. By 2 weeks after fracture, cell proliferation declines and hypertrophic chondrocytes become the dominant cell type in the chondroid callus. Electron microscopic examination of the hypertrophic chondrocytes shows the budding of membrane structures to form vesicularized bodies. These bodies, known as matrix vesicles, migrate to the extracellular matrix where they participate in the regulation of calcification. These matrix vesicles possess the enzyme complements needed for proteolytic modification of the matrix, a necessary step in the preparation of the cells for calcification. In addition, matrix vesicles possess phosphatases needed to degrade matrix phosphodiesters in order to release phosphate ions for precipitation with calcium. Quantitative expression of protease activity shows a peak in all types of proteases at approximately 14 days after fracture with the peak in alkaline phosphatase occurring approximately 3 days later. This temporal distribution of enzymes is consistent with the concept that large proteins and proteoglycans in the extracellular matrix of the callus may inhibit calcification until they are biochemically modified.

Once cartilage is calcified, it becomes a target for the ingrowth of blood vessels. These vessels bring with them perivascular cells, which are the progenitors of osteoblasts. Thus, the calcified cartilage in fracture callus is nearly identical to the primary spongiosa found in the growth plate and, as it becomes resorbed by calcified tissue-resorbing cells (chondroclasts, osteoclasts), the woven bone that replaces it is nearly identical to the secondary spongiosa of the growth plate. At this stage in the healing process, the fracture is considered to be united.

Vascular Response

The healing of a fracture is greatly dependent on blood flow to the injured area throughout the healing process. The 3 major blood supplies to the long bone are the nutrient artery, the metaphyseal arteries, and the periosteal arteries (Fig. 6). The nutrient arteries penetrate the cortex of the shaft and then divides into ascending and descending medullary arteries. These endosteal blood vessels are the ones that are destroyed during introduction of a reamed intramedullary nail. The metaphyseal arteries supply blood to the metaphysis and anastomose with the medullary arteries. The metaphyseal arteries, therefore, continue to feed the medullary arteries when they have been disrupted by a fracture. The periosteal arteries, which enter the cortex along heavy muscle and fascial attachments, supply blood to the outer one third of the cortex, whereas the medullary arteries supply blood to the inner two thirds of the cortex. However, normal periosteal blood vessels appear unable to contribute any significant blood supply to the medullary circulation after it has been disrupted. The vascular response to a fracture varies with time. Initially, the blood flow rate decreases because of disruption of vessels at the fracture site. Within hours to a few days, this decrease is followed by a great increase in the blood flow rate, which peaks at 2 weeks. The blood flow then gradually returns to normal in approximately 12 weeks (Fig. 7).

How the fracture is manipulated, reduced, and immobilized can have a great effect on fracture site vascularity. Internal fixation of any type may disrupt vessels, especially the microvasculature. Reaming the medullary canal and inserting a tight-fitting rod significantly lowers the blood flow when compared to that of plated fractures in dogs. In the dog, blood flow is decreased in both plated and rodded tibias at 42 and 90 days postfracture, with a greater decrease in the rodded tibia. At 120 days, blood flow in the rodded

and plated tibias is equal. Thus, the initial decrease in blood flow following endosteal reaming is compensated, by 90 days, by development of collateral periosteal vessels.

Accompanying the above-described changes in blood flow to the fracture are rather profound changes in the local tissue PO_2. Oxygen tension is very low in the fracture hematoma, low in newly formed cartilage and bone, and highest in fibrous tissue (Fig. 8). Despite the great ingrowth of capillaries into the fracture callus, the increase in cell proliferation is such that the cells exist in a state of hypoxia. This hypoxic state is favorable for cartilage formation.

Biochemistry of Fracture Healing

During endochondral bone formation, 2 main types of proteoglycans are expressed in the extracellular matrix of the callus. Dermatan sulfate is expressed by fibroblasts in the early fracture callus and, during the second week, chondroitin 4-sulfate is expressed in large amounts by the chondrocytes. By the third week, the amount of proteoglycans and their aggregates decreases, and mineralization of the fracture callus begins. Collagenase, gelatinase, and stromelysin are proteindegrading enzymes that cleave components of the extracellular matrix and prepare the fracture callus for calcification. Alkaline phosphatase activity also increases prior to mineralization. IL-1 and IL-6 may also regulate fracture callus matrix modification and stimulate mineralization of the callus.

Histochemical localization of calcium in the fracture callus suggests that mitochondria play an important role in matrix calcification of the cartilaginous fracture callus. These intracellular organelles may serve as calcium reservoirs in callus

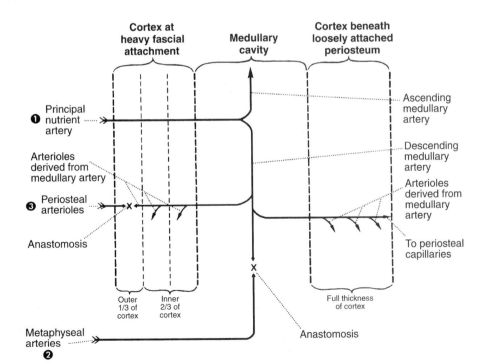

chondrocytes. As the cartilage matrix progressively mineralizes, chondrocyte mitochondria lose progressively more calcium. The initial site of matrix calcification in the fracture callus may be within or on matrix vesicles, collagen fibrils, or proteoglycan disaggregates or collapsed aggregates.

Approximately 9 days after fracture in the rat, there is abundant expression of type II collagen, the major structural protein of cartilage, by the proliferative chondrocytes in the soft callus and periosteum. By day 14 after fracture, although the predominant collagen type found at the fracture site is type II, expression of messenger RNA (mRNA) for this molecule is essentially absent. Almost all chondrocytes are present as hypertrophic cells, and there is no expression of the type II procollagen chain. Thus, by day 14, there has been a switching off of events involved in the production of cartilage, probably because the tissue is undergoing preparation for cartilage calcification and chondrocyte removal. Type I collagen, the predominant collagen of bone, is present in low quantities during the initial stages of fracture healing and increases steadily as cartilage is transformed by osteoblasts into woven bone.

The minor fibrillar collagens also play an important role in fracture healing. Type III collagen, expressed by fibroblasts, is found along the periosteal surface, serving as a substrate for migration of osteoprogenitor cells and capillary ingrowth. Type V, found in areas of fibrous tissue formation and associated with blood vessels, is expressed in both soft and hard callus throughout the fracture healing period, beginning at the time of initial callus formation and maintained throughout the remodeling phase. The highest accumulation of type V collagen is detected in cells in the subperiosteal callus where intramembranous ossification is occurring. Types V and XI collagens have a closely related structure and share the same function in a variety of tissues. It has been suggested that these minor collagens regulate the growth and orientation of types I and II collagen fibrils

in noncartilaginous and cartilaginous tissues, respectively. Type IX collagen has been localized to the surface of type II collagen fibrils and is thought to contribute to the mechanical stability of the type II collagen framework. Type X collagen, a nonfibrillar collagen, is expressed by hypertrophic chondrocytes as the extracellular matrix undergoes calcification. Type XI collagen heterotrimer molecules are composed of 3 different chains that copolymerize with molecules of types II and IX collagens. It has been suggested that the diameter of these collagen fibrils is determined by the ratio of type XI to type II collagen molecules in the fibers, and that increasing the ratio results in thinner fibers, whereas decreasing the ratio results in thicker fibers. It has also been determined that minor fibrillar collagen heterotrimers of types XI and V have been found in fracture callus. Therefore, it is possible that type XI collagen participates in the formation of tissue- and stage-specific heterotrimers with distinct functional properties, and may regulate the tridimensional assembly of fibrillar macroaggregates by varying the biochemical composition of the collagen trimers.

Three noncollagenous extracellular matrix proteins, osteonectin, osteopontin, and osteocalcin, are involved in bone repair and regeneration. Osteonectin peaks in expression in the soft callus on day 9 and has a prolonged peak in expression in the hard callus from days 9 to 15. Osteonectin is expressed at the onset of both intramembranous and endochondral ossification, which suggests that it may play a role in the early stages of ossification. This protein is expressed at the same time as fibril-forming collagens (types I and V), which indicates that it may regulate tissue morphogenesis in conjunction with other matrix components. Osteonectin has been found in proliferating and hypertrophic chondrocytes but not in cartilage matrix, which suggests a regulatory role in cell function rather than matrix stabilization.

Osteocalcin, a bone-specific, vitamin K-dependent pro-

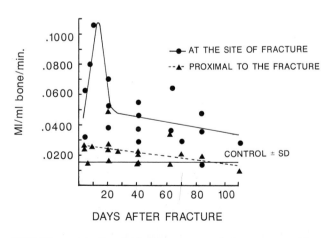

Figure 7

Blood flow rate at a fracture site as determined by a ^{125}I-labeled 4-iodoantipyrine washout technique.

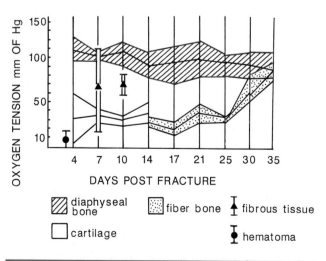

Figure 8

Changes in oxygen tension at fracture site.

tein, contains 3 γ-carboxyglutamic acid residues that allow it to bind calcium ions and hydroxyapatite surfaces. In a closed fracture healing model in the rat, osteocalcin is expressed in fracture callus only by osteoblastic cells in subperiosteal new bone formed by intramembranous ossification. Initiation of the expression of this protein occurs between days 9 and 11, and the peak in expression is observed at approximately day 15.

Osteopontin, an extracellular matrix protein known to be important in cellular attachment, is detected in osteocytes as well as osteoprogenitor cells in subperiosteal hard callus. This protein is also known to interact with the CD44 multifunctional cell surface glycoprotein that binds to hyaluronic acid, type I collagen, and fibronectin. The presence of CD44 has been detected in bone cells in adult and growing rat tibiae, suggesting that it may play a role in normal bone remodeling. These findings of the coexistence of CD44 and osteopontin in some osteocytes and osteoclasts in fracture callus suggest a receptor-ligand interaction between CD44 and osteopontin in fracture healing.

Fibronectin, a molecule that mediates adhesion and migration, is important in tissue growth and repair. This molecule has several roles in the healing process and is produced by such cell types resident in the fracture callus as fibroblasts, chondrocytes, and osteoblasts. Fibronectin has been found in the fracture hematoma within the first 3 days after fracture, in the fibrous portions of the provisional matrices, and, to a lesser extent, in cartilage matrix. Although fibronectin is present throughout the fracture repair process, its production by cells associated with the callus appears to be greatest in the earliest stages of healing, consistent with a potential role for this molecule in the establishment of provisional fibers in cartilaginous matrices.

Biomechanical Properties of Fracture Callus

The mechanical properties of a healing fracture depend on both the material and geometric properties of the uniting callus. The restoration of fracture strength and stiffness is related to the amount of new bone connecting the fracture fragments. The stiffness (hardness) of the fracture callus closely correlates with its calcium content (Fig. 9). The tensile strength of the fracture site during callus formation correlates to the ratio of callus/cortical bone area (Fig. 10). The change from a low stiffness, rubbery quality to a hard tissue type of resiliency occurs during a rather short period of time and progresses through 4 distinct stages (Outline 1).

Fracture healing, during all stages of the reparative process, is highly susceptible to mechanical factors directly related to the amount of interfragmentary motion. In any form of fracture fixation, bone fragments under load will experience a certain amount of relative motion which, by unknown mechanisms, determines the morphologic patterns of fracture repair. The interfragmentary strain result-

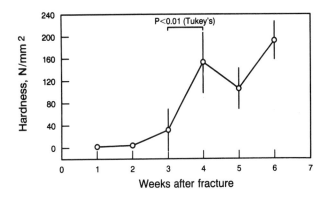

Figure 9

Compressive behavior (hardness) of fracture cells. (Adapted with permission from Aro HT, Wipperman BW, Hodgson SF, et al: Prediction of properties of fracture callus by measurement of mineral density using micro-bone densitometry. *J Bone Joint Surg* 1989;71A:1020–1030.)

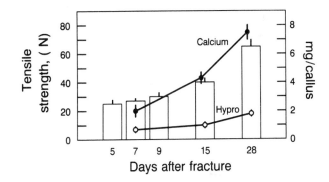

Figure 10

Breaking strength of fracture callus in tensile stressing. (Adapted with permission from Chao EYS, Aro HT: Biomechanics of fracture fixation, in Mow VC, Hayes WC (eds): *Basic Orthopaedic Biomechanics*. New York, NY, Raven Press, 1991, pp 293–335.)

Outline 1

The Four Biomechanical Stages of Fracture Repair

Stage I	The bone fails through the original fracture site with a low stiffness, rubbery pattern
Stage II	The bone fails through the original fracture site with a high stiffness, hard tissue pattern
Stage III	The bone fails partially through the original fracture site and partially through the intact bone with a high stiffness, hard tissue pattern
Stage IV	The site of failure is not related to the original fracture site and occurs with a high stiffness pattern

ing from this motion is believed to govern the type of tissue that forms between the fracture fragments. Fracture healing results in a gradual decrease in interfragmentary motion. Different tissues can sustain different maximum tensile stresses before failure. Granulation tissue can tolerate 100% strain, fibrous tissue and cartilage tolerate appreciably less strain, and compact bone can resist only 2% strain. Therefore, granulation tissue is best able to tolerate the changes in interfragmentary motion that occur at the fracture site early in the course of healing. Interfragmentary strain is inversely proportional to the fracture gap size. When the fracture gap is small, even slight interfragmentary motion can increase the strain to the extent that granulation tissue may not be able to form. To circumvent this situation, small sections of bone near the fracture gap may undergo resorption, thereby making the fracture gap larger and reducing the overall strain. As the fracture becomes more stable, the presence of cartilage and new bone reduces the strain, and fracture healing proceeds.

The nature of the cellular response directly correlates with the degree of bony stability at the fracture site during repair. When mechanical stability is present and the bone ends are in intimate contact, very little cartilage will form, and a thin layer of hard callus will eventually be produced by direct haversian remodeling. When a more mechanically unstable condition exists, hard callus cannot, early on, bridge the bone ends; exuberant cartilaginous callus must first form and then, if stability is sufficient, proceed to be transformed to bone by endochondral ossification. During calcification of the soft callus, if insufficient immobilization exists in conjunction with the presence of an excessive fracture gap, a nonunion may occur because of the persistence of fibrous tissue or a failure of the fibrocartilaginous callus between the fracture fragments to transform into osteogenic callus tissue.

Biology and Biomechanics of Fracture Fixation

If a fracture is inherently stable, because of direct impaction of the bony ends or adjacent ligamentous and bony support, little additional effort is needed to maintain a minimal amount of interfragmentary motion. Cast or brace immobilization or no immobilization may be all that is needed. However, many fractures require additional internal or external support. Such support alters the normal biologic process and mechanics during and after fracture repair. This section provides a review of the healing mechanisms of long bones and a discussion of the influence of stable and unstable fixation on fracture biomechanics.

Compression Plating

Rigid compression plating of an osteotomy inhibits callus formation; the bone ends unite directly by haversian remod-

eling. This type of healing has been referred to as contact healing in contact areas and as gap healing in noncontact areas. It is considered primary bone healing in contradistinction to the previously described secondary fracture healing, which includes callus formation and the 5 stages of fracture union. The haversian remodeling seen in primary fracture healing has 2 main functions: the revascularization of necrotic fracture ends and reconstitution of the intercortical union. The 3 requirements for haversian remodeling across the fracture site are the performance of an exact reduction, the production of stable fixation, and the existence of a sufficient blood supply.

When a dynamic compression plate is applied to an osteotomy in bone, the compression at the osteotomy site diminishes slowly over a period of time, and it is reduced by approximately 50% within 2 months. This same phenomenon also is seen when there is no osteotomy and a dynamic compression plate is applied to an intact bone. Therefore, this slow decrease in compression is not caused by shortening of the fragments and resorption, but instead is a result of haversian remodeling under the plate and screws.

The use of a dynamic compression plate in an osteotomy model has been shown to lead to primary bone healing. When there are no gaps and the fracture fragments are rigidly held together, there is no ingrowth of mesodermal cells from the periosteum or endosteum. Active haversian remodeling is seen at approximately the fourth week of fixation via proliferation of haversian canals along the longitudinal axis of the bone. If a gap exists, which often is seen opposite the plate even if there is rigid fixation, new blood vessels and osteoblasts deposit osteoid into this gap in the first 8 days of fixation. The lamellar bone that is formed in this gap is oriented 90° to the longitudinal axis. Axially oriented osteons then bridge across this perpendicularly oriented osteoid by haversian remodeling. The growth of these secondary osteons starts 4 weeks after fracture fixation in the dog and later in humans; thus, there is always a lag period before the activation of haversian remodeling. This delay in activation has been postulated to be related to the clearance of damaged tissue at the fracture site.

The growth of secondary osteons from one fracture fragment to another does not occur only at sites of macroscopic gaps; it will occur in areas that seem to have intimate contact between the fracture fragments. After reduction and compression plating, incongruencies remaining at the fracture site will result in small gaps. Within weeks after fracture, these gaps are filled by direct lamellar or woven bone formation; that is, appositional bone formation. Woven bone formed within the gap acts as a spacer but does not unite the fracture ends. Secondary osteons use the gap tissue as a scaffold to grow from one fragment to another.

Although primary bone healing refers to union without callus formation and secondary bone healing to union by means of callus formation, this distinction represents an oversimplification that is not always seen in vivo. The production of a small amount of callus opposite a dynamic compression plate indicates that there is sufficient interfragmentary motion opposite the plate to allow for a slight amount of callus healing. If this motion is excessive or continues so that bony union is not achieved, the plate will fail through cyclic loading. However, a small amount of motion and subsequent callus formation opposite the plate can be advantageous, leading to earlier and stronger union. Fractures also exist that heal without callus formation and, nevertheless, go through the stages previously described for secondary bone healing, which include both endochondral and intramembranous bone formation. Examples include fractures of the scaphoid and talus, which are not heavily endowed with periosteum.

When applying a plate for fixation, the appropriate number of screws must be used to minimize stresses and achieve optimal results. A plate with less than adequate fixation and a decreased working length is at risk for failure. Recommendations are for at least 6 cortices on each side for the forearm and 6 to 8 cortices on each side at the humerus. For the tibia and femur, 8 or more cortices on each side are preferred. Such screws traversing the medullary cavity do not significantly disturb the circulation; medullary vessels curve closely around tight screws. By 1 week after fracture fixation, the arterioles and capillaries of the medullary canal cross an osteotomy site, thereby effecting a medullary osseous union. At 6 weeks after tight plate application, vascularization of the cortex under the plate is greatly reduced.

External Fixation

Although primary bone healing can be seen with plate fixation, it can also be seen with external fixation. In a study of osteotomies in canine tibias held in place with half-frame external fixators placed in the mediolateral plane, compression was applied across the osteotomy site in one group and not in another. Both groups showed a significantly greater amount of periosteal new bone formation in the anteroposterior plane than in the mediolateral plane where there was more rigidity. Primary bone healing of both the contact and gap type was seen in both groups. However, the existence of primary bone healing with external fixation does not indicate that it is the preferred method of healing. Less rigid fixation has been shown to lead to controlled interfragmentary motion and, therefore, to more periosteal callus and new bone formation, which may produce equally good union.

The mechanical strength of a fracture augmented by an external (or internal) fixation device must be considered to be based not solely on the mechanical properties of the fixator, pins, and their connections, but on a composite structure in which load sharing and motion occur between the device and the fracture site. It has been shown that for an external fixator applied to a canine tibial fracture in which the fragment ends are not in contact, the stiffness of the composite is low and varies between 2,000 and 4,000 N/cm. In such situations, partial weightbearing of about 20 kg causes 0.5 to 1.0 mm of axial cyclic movement of fracture fragments. Thus, to avoid failure, the decision of how much weightbearing is appropriate depends not only on the frame and pin configuration but also on whether fracture reduction can yield such ideal contact. Too rigid a construct also may not be ideal. When external fixation with controlled micromovement was compared to osteotomies after static rigid external fixation, vast improvement in healing was reported. More elastic fixation allows the bone to bear weight without the external fixation acting as a stress-shielding device. Making the frame more elastic by decreasing the number of pins from 6 to 4 led to an increase in the amount of periosteal callus seen in radiographs; however, there also was increased loosening of the pins as a result of the additional motion at the pin-bone junction. Thus, it is difficult to determine how rigid a frame is necessary and when a frame becomes too rigid.

According to the 2-column theory, if the bone is in contact, a simple anterior unilateral frame will act as a second column, and will be sufficient to allow some weightbearing and to result in union. If there is no bony contact, 2 columns of external fixation are necessary initially. These columns would be provided by using either a stacked anterior frame or an anterior frame combined with an anteromedial frame. Others believe that a very rigid frame is necessary initially and that disassembly of the external fixation device with a sequential decrease in the stiffness is the way to achieve union.

Many factors determine the rigidity of a frame. The pin holes should be less than 30% of the bone diameter to decrease the risk of open section fracture. It has been shown that a 5-mm stainless steel pin is 144% more rigid than a 4-mm pin. The difference in rigidity is so large because the bending stiffness of the pin is proportional to the areal moment of inertia, which is half the radius to the fourth power. Tubular rods with an 11-mm diameter are approximately twice as stiff as solid connecting rods with an 8-mm diameter. Increasing the pin spread within each bone segment to 9 cm triples the resistance to anteroposterior bending, and decreasing the bone rod distance to 2.5 cm leads to a threefold increase in resistance to transverse bending. Another way to increase stiffness of the frame is to separate half pins by greater than 45° when applying anterior and anteromedial frames together (Outline 2).

Pin and pin tract complications are often difficult to avoid; however, there appear to be several distinct factors that can improve the performance of the pin-bone interface. Half pins are subjected primarily to bending loads. Some stress can be reduced by using a larger pin diameter, reducing the sidebar separation, reducing the distance between the sidebar and the bone, and applying transfixation pins rather than half pins to increase the bending rigidity of the pin. As

Increased pin diameter

Increased pin number

Decreased bond-rod distance

Increased pin group separation

Half pins separated > 45°

noted, weightbearing should be avoided in patients with fractures without cortical contact. In such cases, studies have shown that the location of maximum stress is within a pin group. The site varies according to loading mode, but pin-bone failure is mainly at the entry near the cortex. Pin insertion technique is also important. Thermal necrosis, which may occur if the pin is placed intracortically or if a power drill is used to place the pin, can result in pin loosening. Preloading in either the radial or axial direction may decrease the incidence of pin-bone loosening. Axial dynamization as the fracture heals restores the cortical contact in stable fractures and, therefore, decreases the pin-bone stresses (Table 1).

Circular External Fixation

Circular external fixation configurations have become popular for the treatment of fractures, posttraumatic deformities, osteomyelitis, and congenital anomalies. Circular rings are connected to 1.8- or 2-mm wires that are fixed to the ring at tensions of 90 to 130 kg. The optimum orientation of the wires on the ring is 90° to each other to provide the most stability; however, because of anatomic considerations this is not always possible. Because of the circular configuration, the bending stiffness of the frame is independent of the loading direction. When compared to the Hoffmann-Vidal frame, which has 4-mm transfixation pins applied medial to lateral and attached to half pins applied through the anterior area and is very rigid, the Ilizarov frame was half as rigid in compression. In anteroposterior bending and in torsion, the frames are comparable in rigidity. However, with lateral-medial bending, the Hoffmann-Vidal frame had a rigidity of 800 N/cm versus 80 N/cm for the Ilizarov frame. This decreased rigidity of the frame in bending resulted from bowing of the transverse wires and slippage of the bone along the smooth-tensioned wires. In torsion, the primary cause of laxity in the system was wire deflection. The most critical factors in frame stability are the number, tension, and size of the cross wires. The factors that are available to increase the stability of the circular external fixator include: (1) larger wire diameter; (2) decreased ring size; (3) use of olive wires; (4) increased number of wires; (5) crossing wires at right angles at the center of the bone; (6) increased wire tension; (7) positioning of the center rings close to the fracture or nonunion site; and (8) closer distance between adjacent rings. However, as is the case with monoplanar and biplanar external fixation, the appropriate amount of stability and stiffness is not known. The lower rigidity of this frame, especially in compression and lateral-medial bending when compared to the Hoffmann-Vidal frame, may be advantageous in providing the appropriate amount of axial loading to the regenerate bone in order to allow it to become structurally sound.

Intramedullary Nails

In 1940, Kuntscher introduced the technique of closed intramedullary nailing of the femur, and in 1950 he added reaming of the medullary canal to improve contact between the nail and the cortical wall for more stable fixation. In the 1970s, Klemm and Schellmann added interlocking to the nail, which broadened indications for its use and allowed treatment of nonmidshaft fractures by closed nailing techniques. Closed intramedullary nailing with interlocking is currently the treatment of choice for fractures

Table 1	
Types of Axial Stimulation at the Fracture Site Under External Fixation	

Type	Description
Passive dynamization	Load transmission through fracture site due to pin bending under weightbearing (rigid sidebar)
	Removal of additional sidebar or pins results in reduction of axial, torsional, and bending stiffness, proportionally
Active axial dynamization	Load transmission through fracture site under weightbearing without pin bending (telescoping sidebar)
	Relaxation of the axial constraint in the fixator does not affect the torsional and bending stability of the fixation
Controlled axial micromovement	Load transmission through fracture site using controlled force/displacement actuator (telescoping sidebar)

from the lesser trochanter to the supracondylar area of the femur. In addition, modification of the intramedullary tibial nail to allow interlocking has led to its use for fractures of the tibia that go from just below the plateau to just above the supramalleolar region.

With the addition of a loose-fitting intramedullary rod into the medullary canal, the endosteal circulation is able to regenerate rapidly and completely where space has been left between the nail and the endosteal surface. When reaming is used for placement of an intramedullary nail, the results are different. The damage following reaming is similar to an experimental situation in which there is simultaneous ligation of the nutrient artery and interruption of the metaphyseal blood supply. Because of the anatomy of the medullary blood supply, the essential damage is caused by the first reaming, and there is necrosis of the inner 50% to 70% of the cortex. Subsequent reaming has little effect on cortical vascularity; therefore, the amount of reaming actually performed is of minor importance. After reaming and the application of a tight-fitting intramedullary nail at the 4-week stage of repair, there appear to be 3 paths for blood supply: (1) through a regenerative endosteal membrane; (2) through the external callus at its junction with the cortex; and (3) through the substance of the cortex itself. Six weeks after medullary reaming and tight nailing, the significant regenerative blood supply to all the bony tissue appears by microangiography to be endosteal. Thus, the overall regenerative blood supply at 6 weeks follows the same 3 pathways as it did at 4 weeks, with a notable increase in the size of the posterior intracortical (from the nutrient artery) arteries.

It has been suggested that reaming, with its concomitant increase in intraosseous pressure, is responsible for the generation of medullary content emboli, and should, therefore, be avoided in traumatized patients with pulmonary contusion. However, a recent study found that in a sheep model, most pulmonary emboli occurred when the medullary canal is first opened, and there was no substantial difference in the outcome of animals that had undergone reaming and those that did not.

Revascularization of the necrotic cortex comes from 2 sources. One is the regenerative medullary circulation through small arterioles in the new endosteal membrane that has been able to form within the crevices around the intramedullary nail. The other is a new extraosseous circulation supplied by large arteries derived from the surrounding soft tissues with branches traversing the full thickness of the external callus to support the osteoclastic removal of the necrotic cortex. This periosteal blood supply is not the same as the periosteal circulation of a normal long bone. These new periosteal arterioles enter the cortex where the periosteum is only loosely attached, and this new extraosseous blood supply is a transitory phenomenon assisting with cortical repair. After its disruption at the endosteal surface, the principal nutrient artery turns back

and produces intracortical branches that supply blood to the femoral cortex.

By 12 weeks after reaming, a thick, highly vascular endosteal membrane surrounds the entire nail tract, and large intracortical arteries appear in the posterior cortex at this time. It has been shown in dog and sheep long bones that it takes 8 to 12 weeks to achieve total revascularization; in humans, this time is even longer. This would suggest that there would be a higher risk of nonunion with intramedullary reaming of an open fracture that has been stripped of its periosteal blood supply. However, clinical studies have shown that in the tibia, rates of union and infection were similar for reamed and unreamed nails. Tibia fractures treated with unreamed nails may, however, have a higher occurrence of hardware failure. Data from recent experimental studies in which microsphere and laser Doppler techniques were used following intramedullary reaming and nailing show that perfusion to the cortex at the fracture site is diminished during the early phase of fracture healing, but by 90 days, the collateral blood supply to the endosteal cortex has overcome this deficit.

Comparison of Fixation Methods

Plate Fixation Versus Intramedullary Fixation

When plate fixation was compared with intramedullary rod fixation in dogs, blood flow reached higher levels and remained elevated longer in osteotomies that were fixed with the rods than those fixed with the plates (Fig. 11). Rod-fixed osteotomies healed by periosteal callus, whereas plate-fixed osteotomies showed predominantly endosteal callus formation (Fig. 12). There were no significant differences in bone porosity between the fixation methods. The plated osteotomies displayed higher torsional stiffness values than the rod-fixed osteotomies at 90 days, but this difference was no longer apparent at 120 days.

These data show that bone heals by different mechanisms with different types of fixation. Rigid plate fixation promoted early recovery of mechanical properties, although this method inhibited periosteal callus formation. The time needed for return of normal strength and stiffness was, however, the same for both methods, indicating that the end result of the different healing patterns was the same.

Plate Fixation Versus External Fixation

In animal studies, characteristics of the union of bone osteotomies achieved by means of compression plating (8-hole prebent dynamic compression plate) were compared with those achieved by unilateral external fixation. In

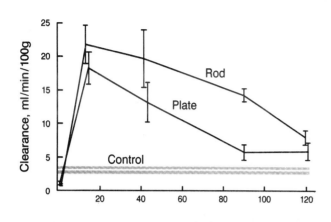

Figure 11

Fracture site clearance: mean values. (Adapted with permission from Rand JA, An KN, Chao EYS, Kelly PJ: A comparison of the effect of open intramedullary nailing and compression-plate fixation on fracture site blood flow and fracture union. *J Bone Joint Surg* 1981;63A:427–442.)

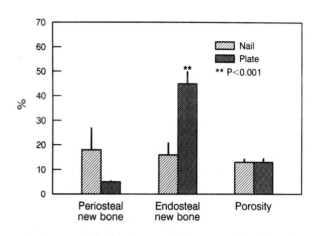

Figure 12

Callus formation in rod- and plate-fixed osteotomies. (Adapted with permission from Chao EYS, Aro HT: Biomechanics of fracture fixation, in Mow VC, Hayes WC (eds): *Basic Orthopaedic Biomechanics*. New York, NY, Raven Press, 1991, pp 293–335.)

vitro mechanical testing showed that the plate-bone system was significantly more rigid than the external fixator-bone system in all testing modes other than lateral bending in the plane of the external fixator. The use of both methods in vivo led to osteotomy union by 120 days. However, the maximum torque and stiffness of the plated osteotomies were significantly higher than those of the osteotomies treated with external fixation.

It should again be emphasized that the rigidity of the composite fixation system, rather than the type of device used, is an important factor in early bone healing. Data indicate that the rigidity of fixation governs not only whether the fracture will heal, but also the mechanism through which bone union will take place. Biologic and biomechanical pathways to osseous union can be changed by manipulating the rigidity of fixation during the treatment course. It has been well established that internal and external fixation devices both lead to fracture union, but do so through slightly different biologic processes, as dictated by their biomechanical characteristics. Plate fixation favors endosteal healing, whereas intramedullary nailing and less rigid external fixation encourage periosteal healing. Rigid external fixation of osteotomy prevents periosteal callus formation; thus, it relies on osteonal cortical reconstruction with minimal endosteal healing. Axially dynamized external fixation facilitates direct cortical reconstruction with periosteal new bone formation.

The occurrence of pin loosening can be decreased by improved initial pin torque resistance accomplished by preloading pins. Careful pin insertion technique, by using low speed drills and inserting the pins by hand, may protect against thermal necrosis. A stable fixator construct and limited loading of the frame may also lessen the dynamic stress, which may contribute to pin loosening.

Factors Influencing Fracture Repair

When bony bridging does not progress at an expected pace, the patient is said to have a delayed union or nonunion, depending on time since fracture and other factors such as the site and severity of the injury, and host and/or local factors.

Host Factors

Common host factors implicated in delayed fracture healing include diabetes mellitus, smoking, and nutritional status. Although the pathophysiology has not been well explained, diabetes has been associated with defects in collagen, with most studies reporting a decrease in total collagen content, defects in collagen cross-linking, or alterations in collagen ratios. In an experimental animal model, streptozotocin-induced diabetes led to decreased collagen in fracture callus, which negatively influenced fracture healing.

The deleterious effect of cigarette smoking on fracture healing and bone graft incorporation is well known, although the mechanism of this effect is not. Cigarette smoke has been shown to directly interfere with osteoblastic function. In addition, nicotine has vasoconstrictive properties that may diminish blood flow at the fracture site. Although good basic science research in this area is lacking, the fact that tobacco use has been found to be associated with decreased bone mineral density suggests an effect on bone metabolism that may also influence fracture healing.

Malnutrition, a serious problem affecting nearly half of all patients undergoing an orthopaedic procedure, may cause a variety of detrimental effects in both inpatient and outpatient populations. Malnourished patients may have prolonged hospital stays complicated by loss of immuno-competence, wasting of skeletal muscle mass, and generalized weakness. Furthermore, in a patient with a fracture, malnourishment is likely to be exacerbated because long bone fractures are associated with increased rates of catabolism and significant urinary nitrogen loss that may lead to a negative protein balance.

Like the other generally recognized host factors, the pathophysiology of the effect of protein deprivation on fracture healing is not well understood. The influence of chronic protein malnutrition on bone, but not fracture callus, has been previously described. Poor proliferation of cartilage cells and reduced osteoblast activity have been demonstrated in protein-deficient animals. These observations indicate reduced osteoblast and chondroblast activities, suggesting diminished capabilities for both membranous and endochondral bone formation. Inasmuch as the activity of osteoblasts is involved in periosteal callus formation and that of chondroblasts is involved in external callus formation, callus formation in a state of protein deprivation is likely to be affected in the immediate postfracture period.

Studies evaluating fracture healing in animals on a low protein diet prior to and after fracture have demonstrated diminished periosteal and external callus formation at the fracture site. This callus, when mechanically tested, displays neither the strength or stiffness of normal fracture callus; it is not clear why this occurs. It has not been determined whether a specific lack of a crucial amino acid leads to the delay in healing or if some other factor is responsible. It is possible that because cellular proliferation and activity are affected, the activity of a growth factor necessary for fracture repair is diminished. Interestingly, diminished levels of insulin-like growth factor-I (IGF-I), which have been associated with decreased levels of albumin and transferrin in malnourished patients, have been associated with impaired growth in patients with anorexia nervosa. As cel-lular responses for growth are similar to those of fracture healing, it is possible that diminished levels of IGF-I play a role in the pathophysiology of protein deprivation.

Local Factors

Local factors that may impede fracture healing include extensive injury to the bone or surrounding soft tissue, interruption of the local blood supply, imposition of soft tissue between fracture fragments, inadequate reduction and/or immobilization, and bone death caused by avascularity, radiation, thermal or chemical burns, or infection.

In general, if there is motion at the fracture site, callus will form. The larger the stress, the greater the amount of callus. If the motion is excessive, however, the increased strain may result in tissue proliferation but may also damage the vascularization, resulting in delayed union or nonunion. Intermittent hydrostatic compression across the fracture site and poor vascularity may result in a fibrocartilaginous callus. Intermittent shear stresses are thought to encourage ossification (Fig. 13).

Augmentation of Fracture Healing

When fracture healing is delayed (arbitrarily from 3 to 9 months), spontaneous healing may occur, with time, for a certain percentage of patients or intervention may be required. Generally, if the initial insult was not severe and if the area has good blood supply, it is likely a delayed union will heal only with careful management of intrinsic biomechanical factors. A fracture can be labeled as a nonunion after no progress in healing has been carefully documented for 6 to 8 months after the original injury. Anatomically, a

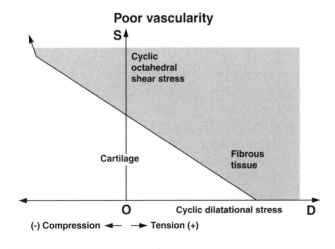
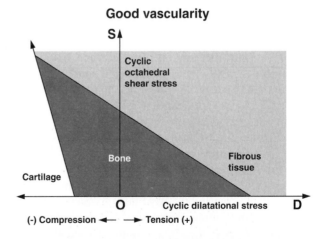

Figure 13

Influence of intermittent stresses and vascularity on differentiation of mesenchymal tissue. (Adapted with permission from Carter DR, Blenman PR, Beaupré GS: Correlations between mechanical stress history and tissue differentiation in initial fracture healing. *J Orthop Res* 1988;6:736–748.)

nonunion is a fracture bridged with soft tissue. It must be differentiated from a synovial pseudarthrosis, in which a fluid-filled gap exists. In nonunion, the gap usually contains interposed cartilage, fibrous tissue, or both. Gap tissue characteristics reflect the local mechanical and nutritional factors that dominate in the first weeks of repair. Furthermore, these characteristics should dictate the type of therapeutic interaction necessary to produce bony union.

The goal in treating a nonunion is to stimulate a process of bone regeneration. Nonunions may be divided into 2 groups: those that have a good blood supply and are hypertrophic, and those that have a poor blood supply and become atrophic. Hypertrophic nonunions generally require stabilization only, often without surgical invasion of the nonunion site. Atrophic nonunions require both stabilization and a means to restart the repair process. Fracture healing may be enhanced locally or systemically and by biologic or mechanical methods.

Osteogenic Methods

Osteogenic methods to enhance fracture healing include the use of naturally-occurring materials, such as autogenous or allogeneic bone grafts or autogenous bone marrow grafts, that have been shown to induce or support the formation of bone.

Tissue obtained from and implanted within the same individual is an autograft. Tissue obtained from a donor of the same species is an allograft. Tissue obtained from a donor of a different species is a xenograft. An orthotopic transplantation is implantation of tissue into an identical anatomic site; implantation into a distant anatomic site is called a heterotopic transplantation. Cancellous and cortical grafts are currently in common clinical use as autografts or allografts.

Autogenic bone usually is used as a fresh graft. Allogeneic bone usually is stored frozen, lyophilized, or chemically sterilized; no viable cells remain. Each of these storage procedures substantially decreases the immunogenicity of allogeneic bone. The biologic host response is also different between autogenic and allogeneic bone and, as in osteonecrosis, is different depending on whether the graft is composed of cancellous or cortical bone. Therefore, it is important to understand the biologic process of revascularization and graft incorporation not only as it relates to the type of bone needing to be regenerated but also to the source of the graft material.

The incorporation of a bone graft, whether it is autogenic or allogeneic in origin, involves a partnership between the transplanted tissue and the host bed into which it is placed. The graft contributions start with a passive osteoconduction, whereby the tissue acts as a trellis or scaffold for bony ingrowth of the host tissues. The graft then stimulates bone formation by a process of osteoinduction. Although a small fraction of the osteoblastic cells survive the transplant

(more with cancellous than with cortical bone and more with rapid transplantation than with delayed), most cells that participate in the healing accompany the recruitment of host blood vessels, which invade the graft. A bone graft dies after harvesting, but may undergo a process of revascularization in its host bed.

Cancellous Grafts

For nonvascularized autogenous cancellous bone grafts, graft repair or regeneration is similar to that noted in osteonecrosis of cancellous bone. The first phase is vascular ingrowth and progenitor mesenchymal cell invasion. In a dog model, this occurs during the first 3 weeks after implantation (Fig. 14, A). The second phase, which occurs in the dog model between 3 and 12 weeks after implantation, is a combination of osteoblastic appositional new bone formation onto the dead trabeculae of the graft and osteoclastic resorption of the graft trabeculae (Fig. 14, B). The third phase, between 3 and 6 months after implantation, is that of remodeling and reorientation of the trabeculae to a mature pattern. This phase is influenced by the mechanical factors acting on the host bed. In this animal model, the process of remodeling becomes quiescent at 1 year after grafting (Fig. 14, C).

In a canine model, fresh cancellous bone allogeneic grafts (allografts), which do not cross major histocompatibility barriers, progress through the same sequence of incorporation steps, but twice as slowly (Fig. 15). The initial phase, which consists of hemorrhage and necrosis corresponding to the surgical placement of the graft, is identical to that for the autograft. The fibrin clot develops and the same inflammatory response ensues. As in the autograft, increased vascularity in the adjacent tissues, dilation of the blood vessels, transudation, and exudation are noted, but perhaps are greater in extent and degree.

At this point, however, the response appears to differ. The fibrin clot, clearly of great importance to the system, breaks down, and the loosely structured granulation tissue that serves as a source of cellular elements for repair becomes filled with chronic inflammatory cells rather than fibroblasts and blood vessel elements. The numbers of lymphocytes, plasma cells, and mononuclear elements markedly increase. The major portion of the delay appears to occur in osteoclastic resorption and new bone formation. Final graft incorporation with remodeling may remain incomplete.

The use of these data in the clinical setting of patient care must be done with caution. In humans, clinical data and occasional histologic evaluation of cancellous grafts suggest that the same sequence of steps occurs, but the process takes place at approximately half the rate seen in canine studies, and large grafts may remodel even more slowly. The incorporation of allograft corticocancellous bone and osteochondral segments has resulted in incomplete remodeling and incorporation of subchondral allogeneic bone as late as 7 years after implantation.

Cortical Grafts

There are 3 major differences in incorporation of autogenous nonvascularized cortical bone in animal models as compared to that of cancellous bone grafts. First, the vascularization of cortical grafts is much slower, taking 8 weeks

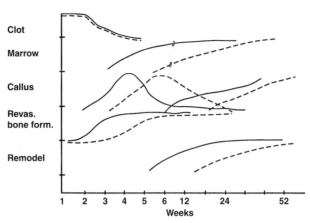

Figure 15

Time line for cancellous bone incorporation of autografts and allografts. Dashed lines are allografts.

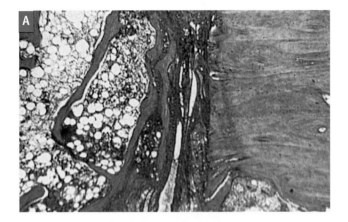

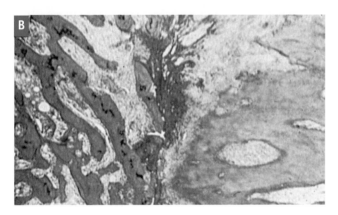

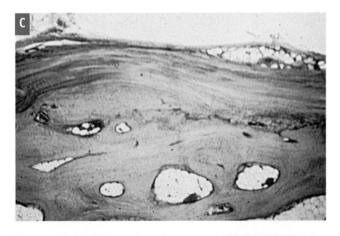

Figure 14

Composite photomicrograph showing transition from cancellous bone graft to reconstituted bone in a dog model. **A,** At 1 week the cancellous graft (*left*) is adjacent to the host cortex, and premature mesenchymal cells are accumulated at the junction. **B,** At 2 weeks, new bone formation is noted in both the graft and the host. **C,** By 1 year the autograft has been completely incorporated.

for completion. Second, osteoclastic resorption must precede the osteoblastic new bone formation. In a manner similar to the repair or regeneration in osteonecrosis, creeping substitution occurs. Osteoclasts form cutting cones within the donor bone and new bone is formed behind the cutting cones. Third, during the process, autogenous cortical grafts generally do not demonstrate complete substitution with viable bone and, thus, are an admixture of necrotic graft bone and viable new host bone. The healing process begins at the host-graft cortical junction, with bridging external endochondral bone formation from the host tissue during the first 4 to 6 weeks, followed by interstitial cortical osteoclasis and creeping substitution.

An allograft functions as an osteoconductive system. Similarly, with allogeneic tissues, the transplanted bone graft acts as a trellis or scaffold for bony ingrowth of the host tissues. The function of either type of graft as a stimulator of host bone formation by the process of osteoinduction, however, is poorly understood.

Allograft cortical bone undergoes the same qualitative sequence of steps during graft incorporation as does autograft cortical bone. The length of time for creeping substitution is greatly prolonged when allogeneic cortical bone is used. The factors that stimulate host blood vessels to proliferate, invade the graft, and develop into cutting cones appear to be diminished, absent, or severely suppressed. Recruitment and differentiation of cellular elements to become both vascular invaders and the osteoblastic and osteoclastic elements essential to creeping substitution are reduced in extent and degree. Replacement of tissue by host bone is slow, and the stimulatory effect exerted on the host is virtually absent. New bone formation in either the host or the donor part is limited in degree, and repair of the host-donor junction site is prolonged when compared to the use of autogenous bone. Healing of a delayed or nonunion site in the host bone may respond to the mechanical aspects of the insertion of the graft, but most authorities consider that the allogeneic donor part contributes little in the form of osteoinduction. The proportion of necrotic graft bone to viable host bone is much greater in allogeneic grafts, and the active process of graft substitution may last several years.

On rare occasions, 2 special patterns of healing, or the lack thereof, are encountered after implantation of an allogeneic graft. Under well-defined circumstances, the host soft tissues wall off the allogeneic part for an extended period of time, possibly years, and the tissues show little or no vascular proliferation or attempt at invasion of the graft. Under other conditions, presumably immune-directed, the graft is surrounded by inflammatory cells, invaded rapidly by numerous blood vessels, and destroyed. Following such a dissolution, the donor site may show no remnants of the implanted graft.

Structural Properties of Cancellous Versus Cortical Grafts

The qualitative differences in graft incorporation between cancellous and cortical bone result in substantial biomechanical differences. The incorporation of cancellous bone grafts with osteoblastic new bone formation onto the necrotic trabeculae of the graft tissue leads to an early increase in graft strength. Cortical bone grafts first undergo osteoclastic bone resorption, which substantially increases graft porosity and weakens the graft. The quantitative temporal interrelationships between the physical integrity and the biologic processes of repair within a segmental autogenous cortical bone transplant are summarized in Figure 16. In the canine model, cortical grafts show the greatest compromise in mechanical strength at 12 weeks. Although complete cortical graft incorporation does not occur, the biomechanical strength returns to normal between 1 and 2 years posttransplantation.

In the clinical setting, histologic evaluation of nonvascularized autogenous cortical grafts in humans demonstrates that the same repair process occurs as in canine models, but takes approximately twice as long. These data suggest that human segmental cortical grafts should lose approximately half their biomechanical strength during the first 6 months. This process, which is related to osteoclastic resorption, is slowly reversed during the second year after implantation. These observations correlate with the highest incidence of mechanical graft failure between 6 and 8 months after transplantation. The process of graft incorporation and creeping substitution is substantially prolonged with allogeneic bone grafts.

Autogenous Bone Marrow

It has been suggested that autogenous bone marrow, independent of cancellous or cortical bone, can be used for an effective osteogenic graft. This hypothesis is based on the

fact that autogenous bone marrow contains osteogenic precursor cells that could contribute to the formation of bone. Autogenous bone marrow has been used to augment the osteogenic response to allografts and xenografts. There have also been reports that autogenous bone marrow used alone may be effective for the stimulation of fracture repair, although this hypothesis has not been fully tested.

It is possible that methods will be developed to allow the isolation, purification, and cultural expansion of marrow-derived mesenchymal cells. With methods that will allow the isolation and removal of cells that have osteogenic potential, these cells may be added to a culture medium that will stimulate the replication of cells, ultimately yielding a supply of highly osteogenic cells. A series of studies on animals has shown that cells prepared in this manner may be combined with a calcium-phosphate-ceramic delivery system to regenerate bone or to enhance the repair of skeletal defects.

Osteoconductive Methods

Osteoconduction is a process that supports the ingrowth of capillaries, perivascular tissues, and osteoprogenitor cells from the recipient host bed into the 3-dimensional structure of an implant or graft. The rationale for use of osteoconductive materials is that normal osteoblastic or osteoblast-like cells have the ability to form bone on an appropriate surface. Such a surface is able to support the

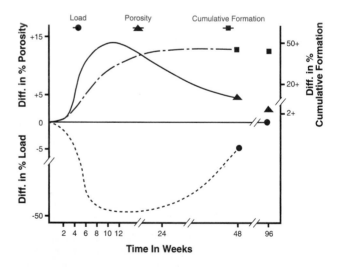

Figure 16

The quantitative temporal interrelationships between the physical integrity and the biologic processes of repair within a segmental autogenous cortical bone transplant. (Reproduced with permission from Burchardt H: Biology of cortical bone graft incorporation, in Friedlaender GE, Mankin HJ, Sell KW (eds): *Osteochondral Allografts*. New York, NY, Little, Brown, 1981.)

attachment, spreading, division, and differentiation of cells and is also able to support the growth, vascularization, and remodeling of bone. Examples of osteoconductive materials include ceramic materials, bioactive glasses, and synthetic polymers.

Ceramics

Most ceramics are calcium phosphate-based and are composed of hydroxyapatite, tricalcium phosphate, or a combination of the two substances, which is usually used because each has its own advantages. Biodegradation is dependent on the chemical composition and porosity of the compound. Tricalcium phosphate is resorbed and remodeled more quickly than hydroxyapatite.

The first calcium phosphate-based bone graft substitute to be approved for use was Interpore (Interpore International, Irvine, CA). Interpore, composed predominantly of hydroxyapatite biomatrix, is formed by the conversion of a marine coral calcium phosphate to crystalline hydroxyapatite. This substrate becomes a template for host bone, sustains living tissues, and has been shown to be as efficacious as autogenous bone graft. Collagraft (Collagen Corporation, Palo Alto, CA) is a mixture of hydroxyapatite, tricalcium phosphate, and fibrillar collagen. It is to be used in conjunction with autogenous bone marrow as a composite bone graft substitute. Collagraft has been shown to be as effective as autogenous bone graft in augmentation of fracture healing.

Recently, a process has been developed for the in situ formation of the mineral phase of bone. This involves the combination of inorganic calcium and phosphate to form Norian SRS (Norian Corporation, Cupertino, CA) a paste that can be injected into the site of a fracture. Under physiologic conditions, the material begins to harden within minutes, forming the mineral dahllite. After 12 hours, the dahllite formation is nearly completed, giving the material an ultimate compressive strength of 55 mPa. As a result, treatment of certain fractures with this calcium-phosphate material can augment the fixation that is achieved with a cast or surgically. Studies of animals have shown that the material is remodeled in vivo and in many cases is completely resorbed and replaced by host bone.

Bioactive Glasses

Bioactive glasses are silicophosphatic chains that may bond ionically to compounds. These compounds can undergo ionic translocations, allowing an exchange of ions with the physiologic milieu. This property may make these substances useful as delivery systems for growth factors.

Synthetic Polymers

Synthetic polymers of the family of polyhydroxy acids such as polylactic acid (PLA) and polyglycolic acid (PGA) have been used for many years as suture material, and are now used as resorbable plates and screws. Use of these compounds as delivery systems for growth factors has been explored. Biodegradation of the polyhydroxy acids has been found in the past to be unpredictable, which in turn may result in inconsistent delivery.

Osteoinductive Methods

Osteoinduction is a process that supports the mitogenesis of undifferentiated perivascular mesenchymal cells, leading to the formation of osteoprogenitor cells with the capacity to form new bone. Unlike osteoconductive materials, osteoinductive substances lead to the formation of bone at extraskeletal sites, and the osteoinductive capacity of a specific molecule may be potentiated by other factors that influence cellular responses, such as those that enhance cellular proliferation, migration, attachment to extracellular matrix molecules, and differentiation. Osteoinductive substances, because of this ability to regulate cellular activity, are being intensely investigated as potential adjuncts to fracture healing.

Growth-Promoting Proteins

Growth factors are osteoinductive signaling molecules that have the capacity to initiate the cascades of cellular events that are critical to fracture healing. Several growth factors that have been associated with healing fractures include the TGF-β family, bone morphogenetic protein (BMP), insulin-like growth factors (IGFs), fibroblastic growth factors (FGFs), and PDGFs.

TGF-β, which exists in 3 mammalian isoforms, is found in the fracture hematoma as early as 24 hours after fracture has occurred. TGF-β is present in platelets, mesenchymal cells, osteoblasts, and young and mature chondrocytes in the callus, as well as in hypertrophic chondrocytes adjacent to the ossification front. This factor induces the synthesis of cartilage-specific proteoglycans and type II collagen by mesenchymal cells, and stimulates collagen synthesis and proliferation by osteoblasts. Based on the high concentrations found in bone, its effect on protein synthesis by chondrocytes and osteoblasts in vitro, and its release into the fracture hematoma by platelets, TGF-β may be responsible for regulating cartilage and bone formation in the fracture callus. TGF-β has a broad range of activity, including cellular differentiation and proliferation of many skeletal cell types, and in many studies has been found to enhance the healing of osseous wounds. Subperiosteal injection of TGF-β has been shown to stimulate cellular differentiation and proliferation of mesenchymal precursor cells. It has also been found to be autoregulatory, increasing the production of TGF-β in osteoblasts and chondrocytes. TGF-β has also been found to induce the healing of critically-sized defects in the skulls of rabbits, suggesting potential therapeutic applications for nonhealing osseous defects. In an animal model of fracture healing, this growth factor was found to increase callus cross-sectional area.

BMP, a low molecular weight hydrophobic glycoprotein discovered in demineralized bone material (DBM), can induce bone formation ectopically. Purification of DBM has led to the isolation of several members of the BMP family. BMPs are able to enhance cell differentiation, directing undifferentiated mesenchymal cells to differentiate along the osteochondrogenic lineage. BMP-3 is a bone-inductive protein also known as osteogenin. Osteogenin is extremely potent in its capacity to induce the rapid differentiation of extraskeletal mesenchymal tissue into bone. Recombinant human BMP-2, when combined with a demineralized bone matrix carrier, and recombinant human BMP-7 (also known as OP-1), when combined with a bovine collagen carrier, have been found to induce endochondral bone formation in segmental defects in a number of species. The BMPs are not only involved in cell differentiation, but also in matrix regulation. BMP-1 does not actually act as a growth factor; rather, it is a procollagen C-proteinase with the ability to cleave the carboxy termini of procollagens I, II, and III.

FGF exists in acidic (FGF-1) and basic (FGF-2) forms, both present in and acting on bone. In vivo studies have shown that although both forms are mitogenic for endothelial cells, fibroblasts, chondroblasts, and osteoblasts, FGF-2 is the more powerful of the two. Both forms have been shown to increase fracture callus in a rat fracture model. FGF-2 has been shown to improve fracture healing in streptozotocin-induced diabetic rats.

PDGF consists of 2 polypeptide chains; it stimulates replication in bone cell cultures in vitro and increases type I collagen synthesis. PDGF also stimulates bone resorption in vitro by a mechanism that involves prostaglandin synthesis. The main functions of PDGF are chemotactic; it attracts inflammatory cells to the fracture site and induces mesenchymal cell proliferation. PDGF is released from platelets and monocytes in the earliest stages of wound healing and may play a role in initiating fracture repair. Multiple subperiosteal injections of PDGF have been shown to induce subperiosteal bone formation. In a rabbit fracture model, it has been shown to increase callus formation without demonstrating an increase in mechanical strength.

Systemic Approaches

It has been demonstrated that direct or indirect injury to bone marrow enhances osteogenesis at distant skeletal sites. While the mechanism remains unknown, this response suggests the possibility that a systemic factor may enhance fracture healing.

IGF-I, a low molecular weight polypeptide, is produced by the liver in response to growth hormone (GH), and circulates bound to a carrier protein. IGF-I is known to have an important regulatory effect on endochondral ossification at the growth plate and it is therefore presumed to have a similar effect on fracture healing. Animal studies have shown an enhancement of intramembranous bone formation;

however, endochondral bone formation has yet to be demonstrated. Because IGF-I production is GH-dependent, it has been hypothesized that GH could stimulate fracture repair. This has never been proven, however, with some studies demonstrating an enhancement and others failing to show any effect.

IGF-II is closely related to IGF-I and is one of the most prevalent growth factors in bone. Although it is found in higher concentrations, IGF-II binds with a lower affinity than IGF-I to the IGF receptor. In vitro studies have demonstrated that IGF-II stimulates bone cell proliferation and cartilage matrix production in a dose-dependent manner. IGF-II also stimulates type I collagen and type I procollagen mRNA. IGF-II is produced by bone cells derived from a number of species, including humans. Parathyroid hormone (PTH) and 1,25 dihydroxy vitamin D_3 (1,25 $(OH)_2$ vitamin D_3) stimulate production of IGF-II in vitro cultures.

There are studies to suggest that PTH and parathyroid hormone related peptide (PTHrP) may improve fracture healing. In a rat model, it has been demonstrated that PTH increases the concentration of IGF-I and TGF-β in bone. It is possible that these growth factors mediate the effect of PTH on fracture healing. In vitro studies have shown that PTHrP induces IL-6 production by human osteoblastic cells and plays a role in chondrocyte differentiation.

An important class of compounds that may eventually be used in the systemic enhancement of fracture healing is the prostaglandins. Prostaglandins have several functions in bone, and at times these functions may seem contradictory. When prostaglandins are released from traumatized bone and soft tissues, they increase intracellular cyclic adenosine monophosphate (cAMP) and stimulate production of IGF. Several in vitro studies have shown that they stimulate type I collagen synthesis. However, their effect on regulating the fracture callus in the presence of nonsteroidal anti-inflammatory agents is still unclear. Indomethacin has been reported to inhibit prostaglandin synthesis, thereby producing fracture callus weakness. Contrary to these findings, ibuprofen has been shown to have no effect on fracture healing despite being a potent inhibitor of prostaglandin synthesis.

Electromagnetic Fields

The potential role of electricity in the regulation of bone tissue was first considered over 40 years ago with the report of electric currents being generated with the loading of dry bone. The discovery of load-induced piezoelectric potentials in bone provided a means by which stress or strain could intrinsically alter the biophysical environment of the bone cell, and thus influence proliferation and differentiation. This mechanoelectric hypothesis became even more attractive when it was demonstrated that, in wet bone, 2 sources of electrical current existed in parallel: piezoelectric currents induced by the deformation of collagen, and the relatively large electrokinetic currents (streaming potentials) produced by the strain-induced flow of charged constituents of extracellular fluids flowing past the mineral phase of the matrix.

The interdependence of electric fields and functional load bearing is critical in establishing a physiologic justification for exogenously inducing fields in the absence of strain. Measurement of the electric potentials generated by functional levels of strain shows the average field intensities in bone are quite small, on the order of 1 $\mu V/\mu e$ (1 microvolt per microstrain). Considering the adult skeleton is seldom subject to strains exceeding 4,000 μe, if endogenous fields are to influence bone morphology they must do so at field intensities below 4 mV/cm. This field intensity, in and of itself, is certainly sufficient to perturb a membrane potential of an osteoblast to the point of having some biologic effect. However, a large percentage of bone tissue is rarely subject to strains greater than 500 μe, yet bone mass is retained in these areas. Therefore, if each cell at each site of the bone is responsible for its own assessment of the physical milieu in its adjacent matrix, fields of 500 $\mu V/cm$, 50% below the 1 mV/cm threshold often considered the low end of biologic "relevance," must represent some regulatory role. It is important to keep these biophysical thresholds in mind when considering the intensities of the biophysical interventions currently available.

When exogenously applied, microamperes, direct electrical currents, capacitively coupled electrical fields, and alternating, pulsed electromagnetic fields (PEMF) affect bone cell activity in various ways in culture, in living bone tissue, and clinically, in fracture nonunion. In addition, PEMFs appear to affect endochondral bone formation, connective tissue repair, osteoporosis, and a variety of other conditions. At the same time, negative results of electromagnetic stimulation tested on several animal models have been reported, and there is the continuing question of how specific waveform characteristics affect the biologic results. It is important to emphasize that the use of electricity in the clinic remains extremely controversial, with some physicians strongly in support of its use and many who remain unconvinced of its benefit. Principal issues in the pro/con electricity feud include inconsistent efficacy, weak scientific arguments justifying the use of a complex waveform, and, at the level of the cell, the poor experimental support for any of the proposed mechanisms of field interaction.

Bassett and associates were the first to report the efficacy of oscillating electromagnetic fields to treat nonunions. The use of PEMFs was shortly thereafter approved by the Food and Drug Administration (FDA) for clinical use in treating human nonunions. These devices, based on the principle that bone responds to mechanical stress (Wolff's Law), were intended to noninvasively induce electrical currents to replace the endogenous currents in the absence of the nor-

mal mechanical loading. In the more common form of treatment, a magnetic field is produced by forcing electric current through a wound wire coil placed over the fracture. Electrical currents proportional to the time rate of change of the magnetic flux traverse the fracture as a result of Faraday induction. Another method of producing time-varying electric currents in a fracture uses capacitive coupling, in which a time-varying electric field is applied to the limb by means of capacitor plates placed on the skin overlying the fracture.

Inducing electric fields to mimic the fields that arise during functional activity (on the order of 4 mV/cm, at frequencies below 10 Hz) is not practical. This is because of the strong relaxation processes that occur in the surrounding tissue and attenuate the signal before it reaches the bone. However, it is possible to mimic the higher frequency potentials recorded during impact loading of bone tissue. As a result, developers of clinical devices use induction waveforms consisting of relatively high frequency (1 to 10 kHz) pulses, gated at a relatively low frequency (1 to 100 Hz). These pulsed or pulseburst type waveforms (commonly known as PEMFs) have become the standard of the industry for electromagnetic bone healing devices.

In attempts to identify the biologically relevant component of the induced fields, numerous studies have been directed toward describing the spectral content of the electric fields induced in the bone and surrounding tissue by PEMF devices. The earliest studies confirmed that most of the induced electric field energy was in the first 10 to 20 harmonics of the pulse repetition rate, and it was suggested that this range (under 100 kHz) must be the range of physiologic importance. On the other hand, there remains a contingent of investigators who suggest that even though the energy content above 100 kHz is small, it may in fact possess the maximum biologic efficacy. To address this issue, Rubin and associates used an in vivo animal model of disuse osteoporosis to correlate the spectral content of PEMF devices to bone formation and resorption activity. Calculating the changes in the induced spectra arising from alterations in the pulse waveforms, they concluded that bone remodeling activity is maximally responsive to induced electric fields at frequencies below 120 Hz. This analysis also strongly suggested that the tissue responded to the induced electric field and not to the imposed magnetic flux density, which has been independently confirmed.

To further characterize the frequency response characteristics of this same adaptation model, McLeod and Rubin used sinusoidally varying fields to stimulate bone remodeling activity. They found that extremely low frequency (ELF) sinusoidal electric fields (below 150 Hz) are quite effective at preventing bone loss and inducing new bone formation. In addition to a strong frequency selectivity, with field effectiveness peaking in the range of 15 to 30 Hz, bone tissue showed a remarkable sensitivity to induced ELF fields. At 15 Hz, induced electric fields of no more than 1 $\mu V/cm$ affected remodeling activity. At both higher and lower frequencies, bone tissue sensitivity to induced electric fields was substantially reduced, consistent with reports of the responses of connective tissue cells in vitro.

The maximal sensitivity of bone tissue to induced electric fields in the 15 to 30 Hz range has interesting implications. Although very high frequency electric fields (10 kHz and above) do not naturally occur in bone tissue during normal physiologic function, externally applied high frequency fields might couple into specific molecular processes within bone cells, thereby affecting tissue activity. McLeod and Rubin's results, however, indicate that the ELF field components of the clinical PEMF signals that reside within the 15 to 30 Hz band are far more capable of stimulating bone remodeling activity than either the very high frequency components or the very low frequency components (below 1 Hz). This observation seems to support the contention that the endogenous electric fields arising through electrokinetic or piezoelectric processes are an integral aspect of bone homeostasis. Furthermore, these results may suggest the particular character of physical activity that would accelerate bone healing. Although activities such as walking induce mechanical strains and endogenous currents primarily below 10 Hz, postural muscle activity (for example, quiet standing) relies on higher frequency (20 to 30 Hz) muscle contractions to ensure stability and so may be more important in the maintenance of bone mass. The same conclusion, that postural muscle activity can affect bone healing, seems to have been reached by many physicians through unrelated clinical observation, for it is now common for orthopaedic surgeons to promote postural weight-bearing on a fracture to ensure rapid healing.

Three double-blinded clinical trials have been undertaken to assess the efficacy of PEMF treatment of fracture healing. In the earliest of these trials, PEMF treatment was found to be no more effective than conservative treatment in promoting union in patients with fractures that had not healed in 52 weeks. In a subsequent trial in a small number of patients, Sharrard showed that for delayed unions with incomplete healing after 16 to 32 weeks, PEMF provided a substantial and significant benefit, albeit smaller than that of surgical intervention. A double-blinded trial of PEMF treatment following tibial osteotomies showed a doubling of the number of patients at stage 3 or 4 (50% to 100% healed) within the first 60 days of treatment, an outcome consistent with an earlier double-blinded trial on femoral intertrochanteric osteotomies. The successes of PEMF treatment of fractures and osteotomies have led to other applications of PEMF technology. These include the treatment of hip prostheses (in order to more rapidly stabilize the implants), spinal fusion, and osteonecrosis of the femoral head. A randomized, double-blinded placebo-controlled clinical trial established the therapeutic benefit of PEMF in painful osteoarthritis of the knee or cervical spine. Eyre and associates reported that PEMFs did not affect the

regenerate bone during limb lengthening but did prevent bone loss adjacent to the distraction gap, in a double-blinded study. Capacitive coupling has also been shown, in another double-blinded prospective study, to have a significant effect on healing of nonunion of long bones.

The frequencies and field intensities that are most effective in regulating tissue modeling and remodeling in vivo or in modulating cell activity in vitro are similar to those achieved in bone during normal functional activity. This is strong evidence that endogenously produced electric fields serve an important role in regulating normal bone modeling and remodeling processes. Isolation of the optimal signal characteristics for regulating bone cell activity and tissue regeneration will greatly improve understanding of the physiologic basis of the skeletal healing response.

Low-Intensity Ultrasound

The sole intervention approved by the Food and Drug Administration to augment the healing of fresh fractures is low-intensity ultrasound. Although the approval was largely based on 2 double-blinded, placebo-controlled trials, substantive evidence at the basic science level shows that ultrasound has a strong influence on biologic activity. Ultrasound, a form of mechanical energy that can be transmitted in biologic organisms as high-frequency acoustic pressure waves, has been widely used in medicine as a therapeutic, surgical, and diagnostic tool. Therapeutic ultrasound and some surgical ultrasound use intensities as high as 1 to 3 W/cm^2, and can cause considerable heating in living tissues. Use of ultrasound as a surgical instrument employs even higher intensity levels (5 to 300 W/cm^2), to fragment caliculi, ablate diseased tissues such as cataracts, and even to remove methylmethacrylate cement during revision of total joints.

Much lower magnitudes of ultrasound (1 to 50 mW/cm^2) are used to drive diagnostic devices that noninvasively image vital organs, fetuses, peripheral flow, ophthalmic echography, and even osteoporosis. This intensity level, 5 orders of magnitude below that used in surgery, studiously avoids the energy levels that cause heating of tissues, and is considered nonthermal and nondestructive. Considering the mechanical basis of ultrasound, it should come as no surprise that these acoustic pressure waves, at least in theory, represent a reasonable means of influencing the healing of fractures, that is, the noninvasive surrogate for Wolff's Law.

Xavier and Duarte were the first to report that the normal fracture repair process in humans could be accelerated by as much as 35% by brief (20 minutes per day) exposure to very low-intensity ultrasound (30 mW/cm^2). In an effort to optimize the signal parameters, Duarte in 1983 used histology and radiographs to demonstrate that ultrasound signals identical to those used in the human successfully accelerated the healing of a rabbit fibular osteotomy (28% faster than controls).

Using mechanical integrity as a critical endpoint, Pilla and colleagues used the midshaft fibula osteotomy model of the rabbit to demonstrate that brief periods (20 minutes/day) of low pulsed ultrasound (200 ms burst of 1.5 MHz sine waves repeated at 1 kHz) with an intensity of 30 mW/cm^2 was capable of accelerating the recovery of torsional strength of a midshaft fibula osteotomy of the rabbit. Results from this study showed that by day 17, each fracture treated with ultrasound was as strong as the intact, contralateral fibula. In contrast, it took 28 days for the osteotomized fibulas that did not receive treatment to reach the strength of their intact, contralateral controls. This study indicates that biomechanical integrity was achieved in essentially half the time in the stimulated group.

Wide-ranging studies at both the in vitro and in vivo level have been made to probe the biologic mechanism(s) responsible for the observed ultrasound influence on osteogenesis and fracture healing. Ryaby and colleagues have reported that low-intensity ultrasound increased calcium incorporation in both differentiating cartilage and bone cell cultures. This increased second messenger activity was paralleled by the modulation of adenylate cyclase activity and TGF-β synthesis in osteoblastic cells. Work published by Bolander's group at the Mayo Clinic demonstrated that exposure of cultured chondrocytes to low-intensity ultrasound stimulates an upregulation of aggrecan gene expression. During endochondral ossification, this large chondroitin sulfate molecule aggregates with hyaluronan, decorin, and biglycan, creating key proteoglycan scaffolding elements for type II collagen. These investigators used an in vivo model to validate that aggrecan gene expression was elevated under conditions of wound healing in response to low-intensity ultrasound. Making the necessary link back to the structural level, this study also found higher mechanical strength (increased torsional strength) in the treated calluses in comparison to their contralateral untreated controls.

There is significant evidence, at the basic science level, that low-intensity ultrasound can modulate gene expression, influence second messenger activity of chondroblasts and osteoblasts, enhance blood flow, and accelerate and augment the fracture healing process (histologically, radiographically, and biomechanically) in various animal models. However, the greatest test of ultrasound must be at the clinical level. The clinical evaluation of ultrasound has been done via a series of double-blinded, placebo-controlled multicenter trials. In the first such study, which focused on cortical bone, 67 closed or grade I open tibial fractures were evaluated by Heckman and associates (1994). Ultrasound treatment of 20 minutes per day at 30 mW/cm^2 led to a significant (24%) reduction in the time of clinical healing (86 ± 5.8 days in the active treatment group compared with 114 ± 10.4 days in the control group; $p = 0.01$). Using both

clinical and radiographic criteria, a 38% decrease in the time to overall healing was apparent (96 ± 4.9 days in the active treatment group compared with 154 ± 13.7 days in the control group; $p = 0.0001$). This study also reported that the patients' compliance with the daily use of the ultrasound device was excellent, and that there were no serious complications related to its use. Importantly, this study also showed that several of the untreated patients went on to delayed union, while no patients who were treated suffered this complication, suggesting that ultrasound exposure not only accelerates healing, but helps to ensure healing.

In the second study, to determine the efficacy of ultrasound to heal fractures in areas that consist primarily of trabecular bone, a multicenter, prospective, randomized, double-blinded, placebo-controlled clinical trial of 61 dorsally angulated fractures of the distal radius was performed. This 1997 study performed by Kristiansen and colleagues showed that the time to union was 38% shorter for the ultrasound-treated fractures (61 ± 3 days) as compared to those treated with placebo (98 ± 5 days: $p < 0.0001$). In addition to the accelerated rate of healing, this study showed that ultrasound treatment was associated with a significantly smaller loss of reduction (20% ± 6% for active compared with 43% ± 8% obtained with the placebo treatment), an important criteria in return to function of many fracture sites.

Because of the nature of the study design, the type of injury that is going to be treated must be rigorously defined. Therefore, the 2 studies described above excluded many patients because their injuries did not meet the classification (for example, open type II fracture versus type I fracture), or because the patients had extenuating circumstances such as diabetes that might have hindered the healing process. Ironically, it is just these patients that are often the ones in greatest need of intervention.

Although healing may be optimized in the young healthy patient with a closed fracture and a normal healing response, it is more likely that the real benefit of biotechnology and/or bioengineering will be seen in those patients in whom the healing response is overwhelmed, such as in those with severe injuries, or in those patients in whom the healing response is normally impaired, such as in those who smoke. A recent study by Cook and associates (1997) compared the effects of low-intensity ultrasound in the acceleration of tibial and distal radius fracture healing in smokers, and they were able to show a statistically significant reduction in healing time in this high-risk group. The healing time for tibial fractures in smokers was 175 days ± 27 days, but with ultrasound treatment the healing time was reduced by 41%, to 103 days ± 8.3 days. Smokers with distal radius fractures had a healing time of 164 days ± 22.5 days, which was reduced by 51% to 98 days ± 6 days with ultrasound treatment. This finding is important from 2 distinct viewpoints. First, it suggests that low level biophysical stimuli can "reestablish" the normal rate and stages of healing that habits such as smoking typically disrupt. This is encouraging as it is often these "delayed" processes that result in nonunions. Second, suggesting that ultrasound can normalize healing in systemic circumstances that are often impaired may provide insight into the mechanisms whereby this biophysical stimulus interacts with the biologic system (that is, counteracting the diminished efficiency of oxygen transport in the smoker or angiogenesis in the diabetic).

In summary, ultrasound represents an effective combination of conservative and aggressive treatment to ensure that the normal process of healing is followed, and meets several of the criteria that suggest its application be seriously considered for complex fractures or patients who are likely to have compromised healing. Ultrasound influences several stages of the healing process, including signal transduction, gene expression, blood flow, tissue modeling and remodeling, and the mechanical attributes of the callus. Although the specific aspect of healing that is most important in the acceleration of the process may not be understood, the fact that ultrasound influences several aspects at several different stages may be an attribute.

Summary

Bone fracture union may follow any one of many combinations of pathways. Clinical factors such as the patient's expectations, compliance with treatment, degree of tolerance, the physician's experience, and other socioeconomic considerations are likely to play important roles in the selection of fixation methods. The best treatment modality and fixation device must be selected according to the fracture morphology and the clinical condition of the patient. A thorough knowledge of the device's biomechanical function and expected biologic response will optimize its effectiveness. Understanding the role of cell mediators and biophysical factors in the healing process may ultimately allow the modulation of fracture healing regardless of the fixation technique used.

Selected Bibliography

Osteonecrosis

Boettcher WG, Bonfiglio M, Hamilton HH, Sheets RF, Smith K: Non-traumatic necrosis of the femoral head: I. Relation of altered hemostasis to etiology. *J Bone Joint Surg* 1970;52A:312–321.

Catto M: Pathology of aseptic bone necrosis, in Davidson JK (ed): *Aseptic Necrosis of Bone.* Amsterdam, The Netherlands, Excerpta Medica, 1976, pp 3–100.

Chryssanthou CP: Dysbaric osteonecrosis: Etiological and pathogenetic concepts. *Clin Orthop* 1978;130:94–106.

Cruess RL: Osteonecrosis of bone: Current concepts as to etiology and pathogenesis. *Clin Orthop* 1986;208:30–39.

Fisher DE: The role of fat embolism in the etiology of corticosteroid-induced avascular necrosis: Clinical and experimental results. *Clin Orthop* 1978;130:68–80.

Glimcher MJ, Kenzora JE: The biology of osteonecrosis of the human femoral head and its clinical implications: I. Tissue biology. *Clin Orthop* 1979;138:284–309.

Glimcher MJ, Kenzora JE: The biology of osteonecrosis of the human femoral head and its clinical implications: II. The pathological changes in the femoral head as an organ and in the hip joint. *Clin Orthop* 1979;139:283–312.

Glimcher MJ, Kenzora JE: The biology of osteonecrosis of the human femoral head and its clinical implications: III. Discussion of the etiology and genesis of the pathological sequelae: Comments on treatment. *Clin Orthop* 1979;140:273–312.

Hawkins LG: Fractures of the neck of the talus. *J Bone Joint Surg* 1970;52A:991–1002.

Hungerford DS, Lennox DW: The importance of increased intraosseous pressure in the development of osteonecrosis of the femoral head: Implications for treatment. *Orthop Clin North Am* 1985;16:635–654.

Jones JP Jr: Fat embolism and osteonecrosis. *Orthop Clin North Am* 1985;16:595–633.

Jones JP Jr: Concepts of etiology and early pathogenesis of osteonecrosis, in Schafer M (ed): *Instructional Course Lectures 43.* Rosemont, IL, American Academy of Orthopaedic Surgeons, 1994, pp 499–512.

Steinberg ME: Early diagnosis, evaluation, and staging of osteonecrosis, in Schafer M (ed): *Instructional Course Lectures 43.* Rosemont, IL, American Academy of Orthopaedic Surgeons, 1994, pp 513–518.

Smith SR, Bronk JJ, Kelly PJ: Effect of fracture fixation on cortical bone blood flow. *J Orthop Res* 1990;8:471–478.

Bone Repair and Regeneration

Brighton CT: Principles of fracture healing: Part I. The biology of fracture repair, in Murray JA (ed): *Instructional Course Lectures XXXIII.* St. Louis, MO, CV Mosby, 1984, pp 60–82.

Einhorn TA, Majeska RJ, Rush EB, Levine PM, Horowitz MC: The expression of cytokine activity by fracture callus. *J Bone Miner Res* 1995;10:1272–1281.

Einhorn TA, Hirschman A, Kaplan C, Nashed R, Devlin VJ, Warman J: Neutral protein-degrading enzymes in experimental fracture callus: A preliminary report. *J Orthop Res* 1989;7:792–805.

Hiltunen A, Aro HT, Vuorio E: Regulation of extracellular matrix genes during fracture healing in mice. *Clin Orthop* 1993;297:23–27.

Iwaki A, Jingushi S, Oda Y, et al: Localization and quantification of proliferating cells during rat fracture repair: Detection of proliferating cell nuclear antigen by immunohistochemistry. *J Bone Miner Res* 1997;12:96–102.

Jingushi S, Joyce ME, Bolander ME: Genetic expression of extracellular matrix proteins correlates with histologic changes during fracture repair. *J Bone Miner Res* 1992;7:1045–1055.

Kopman CR, Boskey AL, Lane JM, Pita JC, Eaton B II: Biochemical characterization of fracture callus proteoglycans. *J Orthop Res* 1987; 5:7–13.

Liu SH, Yang RS, al-Shaikh R, Lane JM: Collagen in tendon, ligament, and bone healing: A current review. *Clin Orthop* 1995;318:265–278.

McKibbin B: The biology of fracture healing in long bones. *J Bone Joint Surg* 1978;60B:150–162.

Pau WT, Einhorn TA: The biochemistry of fracture healing. *Curr Orthop* 1992;6:207–213.

Weber GF, Ashkar S, Glimcher MJ, Cantor H: Receptor-ligand interaction between CD44 and osteopontin (Eta-1). *Science* 1996;271: 509–512.

Yamazaki M, Majeska RJ, Moriya H, Einhorn TA: Role of osteonectin during fracture healing. *Trans Orthop Res Soc* 1997;22:254.

Yamazaki M. Majaeska RJ, Nakajima F, Ogasawasa A, Moriya H, Einhorn TA: Spatial and temporal distribution of CD44 and osteopontin in fracture callus. *Trans Orthop Res Soc* 1997;22:604.

Biology and Biomechanics of Fracture Fixation

Brumback RJ, Uwagie-Ero S Lakatos RP, Poka A, Bathon GH, Burgess AR: Intramedullary nailing of femoral shaft fractures: Part II. Fracture-healing with static interlocking fixation. *J Bone Joint Surg* 1988;70A:1453–1462.

Bucholz RW, Ross SE, Lawrence KL: Fatigue fracture of the interlocking nail in the treatment of fractures of the distal part of the femoral shaft. *J Bone Joint Surg* 1987;69A:1391–1399.

Duwelius PJ, Huckfeldt R, Mullins RJ, et al: The effects of femoral intramedullary reaming on pulmonary function in a sheep lung model. *J Bone Joint Surg* 1997;79A:194–202.

Johnson KD, Tencer AF, Sherman MC: Biomechanical factors affecting fracture stability and femoral bursting in closed intramedullary

nailing of femoral shaft fractures, with illustrative case presentations. *J Orthop Trauma* 1987;1:1–11.

Kessler SB, Hallfeldt KK, Perren SM, Schweiberer L: The effects of reaming and intramedullary nailing on fracture healing. *Clin Orthop* 1986;212:18–25.

Perren SM: Physical and biological aspects of fracture healing with special reference to internal fixation. *Clin Orthop* 1979;138:175–196.

Perren SM, Cordey J, Rahn BA, Gautier E, Schneider E: Early temporary porosis of bone induced by internal fixation implants: A reaction to necrosis, not to stress protection? *Clin Orthop* 1988;232:139–151.

Rhinelander FW: Effects of medullary nailing on the normal blood supply of diaphyseal cortex, in American Academy of Orthopaedic Surgeons *Instructional Course Lectures XXII*. St. Louis, MO, CV Mosby, 1973, pp 161–187.

Sarmiento A: Functional fracture bracing: An update, in Griffin PP (ed): *Instructional Course Lectures XXXVI*. Park Ridge, IL, American Academy of Orthopaedic Surgeons, 1987, pp 371–376.

Winquist RA, Hansen ST Jr, Clawson DK: Closed intramedullary nailing of femoral fractures: A report of five hundred and twenty cases. *J Bone Joint Surg* 1984;66A:529–539.

White AA III, Panjabi MM, Southwick WO: The four biomechanical stages of fracture repair. *J Bone Joint Surg* 1977;59A:188–192.

External Fixation

Hart MB, Wu JJ, Chao EY, Kelly PJ: External skeletal fixation of canine tibial osteotomies: Compression compared with no compression. *J Bone Joint Surg* 1985;67A:598–605.

Kummer FJ: Biomechanics of the Ilizarov external fixator. *Bull Hosp Jt Dis Orthop Inst* 1989;49:140–147.

Lewallen DG, Chao EY, Kasman RA, Kelly PJ: Comparison of the effects of compression plates and external fixators on early bone-healing. *J Bone Joint Surg* 1984;66A:1084–1091.

Weber BG: On the biomechanics of external fixation, in Weber BG, Magerl F (eds): *The External Fixator: AO/ASIF-Threaded Rod System Spine-Fixator*. Berlin, Germany, Springer-Verlag, 1985, pp 27–53.

Wu JJ, Shyr HS, Chao EY, Kelly PJ: Comparison of osteotomy healing under external fixation devices with different stiffness characteristics. *J Bone Joint Surg* 1984;66A:1258–1264.

Factors Influencing Fracture Repair

Carter DR, Blenman PR, Beaupré GS: Correlations between mechanical stress history and tissue differentiation in initial fracture healing. *J Orthop Res* 1988;6:736–748.

Einhorn TA, Levine B, Michel P: Nutrition and bone. *Orthop Clin North Am* 1990;21:43–50.

Golden NH, Kreitzer P, Jacobson MS, et al: Disturbances in growth hormone secretion and action in adolescents with anorexia nervosa. *J Pediatr* 1994;125:655–660.

Guarniero R, de Barros Filho TE, Tannuri U, Rodrigues CJ, Rossi JD: Study of fracture healing in protein malnutrition. *Rev Paul Med* 1992;110:63–68.

Hessov I: Energy and protein intake in elderly patients in an orthopedic surgical ward. *Acta Chir Scand* 1977;143:145–149.

Jensen JE, Jensen TG, Smith TK, Johnston DA, Dudrick SJ: Nutrition in orthopaedic surgery. *J Bone Joint Surg* 1982;64A:1263–1272.

Jha GJ, Deo MG, Ramalingaswami V: Bone growth in protein deficiency: A study in rhesus monkeys. *Am J Pathol* 1968;53:1111–1123.

Kawaguchi H, Kurokawa T, Hanada K, et al: Stimulation of fracture repair by recombinant human basic fibroblast growth factor in normal and streptozotocin-diabetic rats. *Endocrinology* 1994;135:774–781.

Kwiatkowski TC, Hanley EN Jr, Ramp WK: Cigarette smoking and its orthopedic consequences. *Am J Orthop* 1996;25:590–597.

Macey LR, Kana SM, Jingushi S, Terek RM, Borretos J, Bolander ME: Defects of early fracture-healing in experimental diabetes. *J Bone Joint Surg* 1989;71A:722–733.

Augmentation of Fracture Healing

Einhorn TA: Enhancement of fracture-healing. *J Bone Joint Surg* 1995;77A:940–956.

Osteoconduction

Hollinger JO, Brekke J, Gruskin E, Lee D: Role of bone substitutes. *Clin Orthop* 1996;324:55–65.

Gazdag AR, Lane JM, Glaser D, Forster RA: Alternatives to autogenous bone graft: Efficacy and indications. *J Am Acad Orthop Surg* 1995;3:1–8.

Osteoinduction

Beck LS, Ammann AJ, Aufdemorte TB, et al: In vivo induction of bone by recombinant human transforming growth factor beta 1. *J Bone Miner Res* 1991;6:961–968.

Bolander ME: Regulation of fracture repair by growth factors. *Proc Soc Exp Biol Med* 1992;200:165–170.

Bostrom MP, Lane JM, Berberian WS, et al: Immunolocalization and expression of bone morphogenetic proteins 2 and 4 in fracture healing. *J Orthop Res* 1995;13:357–367.

Centrella M, McCarthy TL, Canalis E: Transforming growth factor-beta and remodeling of bone. *J Bone Joint Surg* 1991;73A:1418–1428.

Goldring MB, Goldring SR: Skeletal tissue response to cytokines. *Clin Orthop* 1990;258:245–278.

Goldring SR, Goldring MB: Cytokines and skeletal physiology. *Clin Orthop* 1996;324:13–23.

Horowitz MC: Cytokines and estrogen in bone: Anti-osteoporotic effects. *Science* 1993;260:626–627.

Joyce ME, Jingushi S, Bolander ME: Transforming growth factor-beta in the regulation of fracture repair. *Orthop Clin North Am* 1990;21:199–209.

Joyce ME, Roberts AB, Sporn MB, Bolander ME: Transforming growth factor-beta and the initiation of chondrogenesis and osteogenesis in the rat femur. *J Cell Biol* 1990;110:2195–2207.

Joyce ME, Terek RM, Jingushi S, Bolander ME: Role of transforming growth factor-beta in fracture repair. *Ann N Y Acad Sci* 1990;593:107–123.

Khouri RK, Koudsi B, Reddi H: Tissue transformation into bone in vivo: A potential practical application. *JAMA* 1991;266:1953–1955.

Mohan S, Baylink DJ: Bone growth factors. *Clin Orthop* 1991;263:30–48.

Mustoe TA, Pierce GF, Thomason A, Gramates P, Sporn MB, Deuel TF: Accelerated healing of incisional wounds in rats induced by transforming growth factor-beta. *Science* 1987;237:1333–1336.

Noda M, Camilliere JJ: In vivo stimulation of bone formation by transforming growth factor-beta. *Endocrinology* 1989;124:2991–2994.

Sporn MB, Roberts AB: Peptide growth factors are multifunctional. *Nature* 1988;332:217–219.

Sporn MB, Roberts AB: Transforming growth factor-β: Multiple actions and potential clinical applications. *JAMA* 1989;262:938–941.

Trippel SB, Coutts RD, Einhorn TA, Mundy GR, Rosenfeld RG: Growth factors as therapeutic agents. *J Bone Joint Surg* 1996;78A:1272–1286.

Urist MR: Bone: Formation by autoinduction. *Science* 1965;150:893–899.

Yasko AW, Lane JM, Fellinger EJ, Rosen V, Wozney JM, Wang EA: The healing of segmental bone defects, induced by recombinant human bone morphogenetic protein (rhBMP-2): A radiographic, histological, and biomechanical study in rats. *J Bone Joint Surg* 1992;74A:659–670.

Biophysical Enhancement

Bassett CA: Fundamental and practical aspects of therapeutic uses of pulsed electromagnetic fields (PEMFs). *Crit Rev Biomed Eng* 1989;17:451–529.

Borsalino G, Bagnacani M, Bettati E, et al: Electrical stimulation of human femoral intertrochanteric osteotomies: Double-blind study. *Clin Orthop* 1988;237:256–263.

Brighton CT: The treatment of non-unions with electricity. *J Bone Joint Surg* 1981;63A:847–851.

Brighton CT, Pollack SR: Treatment of recalcitrant non-union with a capacitively coupled electrical field: A preliminary report. *J Bone Joint Surg* 1985;67A:577–585.

Cochran GV, Pawluk RJ, Bassett CA: Electromechanical characteristics of bone under physiologic moisture conditions. *Clin Orthop* 1968;58:249–270.

Colson DJ, Browett JP, Fiddian NJ, Watson B: Treatment of delayed- and non-union of fractures using pulsed electromagnetic fields. *J Biomed Eng* 1988;10:301–304.

Cook SD, Ryaby JP, McCabe J, Frey JJ, Heckman JD, Kristiansen TK: Acceleration of tibia and distal radius fracture healing in patients who smoke. *Clin Orthop* 1997;337:198–207.

Duarte LR: The stimulation of bone growth by ultrasound. *Arch Orthop Trauma Surg* 1983;101:153–159.

Fukada E, Yasuda I: On the piezoelectric effect of bone. *J Phys Soc Japan* 1957;10:1158–1162.

Heckman JD, Ryaby JP, McCabe J, Frey JJ, Kilcoyne RF: Acceleration of tibial fracture-healing by non-invasive, low-intensity pulsed ultrasound. *J Bone Joint Surg* 1994;76A:26–34.

Kristiansen TK, Ryaby JP, McCabe J, Frey JJ, Roe LR: Accelerated healing of distal radial fractures with the use of specific, low-intensity ultrasound: A multicenter, prospective, randomized, double-blind, placebo-controlled study. *J Bone Joint Surg* 1997;79A:961–973.

McLeod K, Rubin C: Clinical use of electrical stimulation in fracture healing, in Mehta AJ (ed): Rehabilitation of Fractures: Physical Medicine and Rehabilitation: *State of the Art Reviews.* Philadelphia, PA, Hanley & Belfus, 1995, pp 67–76.

McLeod KJ, Rubin CT: The effect of low-frequency electrical fields on osteogenesis. *J Bone Joint Surg* 1992;74A:920–929.

Otter MW, McLeod KJ, Rubin CT: Effects of electromagnetic fields in experimental repair. *Clin Orthop* 1998;335(suppl):S90–S104.

Otter MW, Palmieri VR, Wu DD, Seiz KG, MacGinitie LA, Cochran GV: A comparative analysis of streaming potentials in vivo and in vitro. *J Orthop Res* 1992;10:710–719.

Pilla AA, Mont MA, Nasser PR, et al: Non-invasive low-intensity pulsed ultrasound accelerates bone healing in the rabbit. *J Orthop Trauma* 1990;4:246–253.

Pilla AA, Schmukler RE, Kaufman JJ, Rein G: Electromagnetic modulation of biological processess: Consideration of cell-waveform interactions, in Chiabrera A, Nicolini C, Schwan HP (eds): *Interactions Between Electromagnetic Fields and Cells.* New York, NY, Plenum Press, 1985.

Rubin CT, McLeod KJ, Lanyon LE: Prevention of osteoporosis by pulsed electromagnetic fields. *J Bone Joint Surg* 1989;71A:411–417.

Steinberg ME, Brighton CT, Corces A, et al: Osteonecrosis of the femoral head: Results of core decompression and grafting with and without electrical stimulation. *Clin Orthop* 1989;249:199–208.

Wang S-J, Lewallen DG, Bolander ME, Chao EY, Ilstrup DM, Greenleaf JF: Low intensity ultrasound treatment increases strength in a rat femoral fracture model. *J Orthop Res* 1994;12:40–47.

Ziskin MC: Applications of ultrasound in medicine: Comparison with other modalities, in Repacholi MH, Grandolfo M, Rindi A (eds): *Ultrasound: Medical Applications, Biological Effects, and Hazard Potential.* New York, NY, Plenum Press, 1987, pp 49–59.

Chapter 15

Biologic Response to Orthopaedic Implants

Joshua J. Jacobs, MD

Stuart B. Goodman, MD, PhD

Dale R. Sumner, PhD

Nadim J. Hallab, PhD

This chapter at a glance

This chapter presents current knowledge on the nature of the biologic response to orthopaedic implants and focuses on implants intended for permanent use, particularly joint replacement components.

Introduction

Metal, ceramic, and polymeric materials have a proven track record in the treatment of musculoskeletal disorders. Internal fixation of fractures, spinal stabilization, joint replacement, ligament replacement and augmentation, and the reconstruction of massive bone defects resulting from infectious, congenital, or neoplastic disease have all, to some extent, relied on the use of nonbiologic engineering materials. These materials and their degradation products interact with the surrounding physiologic environment and may elicit a local host response that influences clinical outcomes of surgical reconstruction. Recently, there have been considerable advances in the understanding of both the nature of this host response and of the relationship between local cellular and subcellular events and the clinical performance of the device. As basic information in this area has been gained, new strategies have emerged for the manipulation of the host response and modification of potentially adverse effects. In addition, there is an increasing recognition that there is a potential for orthopaedic implants to have remote and systemic effects as a result of migration of ionic and particulate degradation products from the peri-implant tissues into the lymphatics and bloodstream.

This chapter presents current knowledge on the nature of the biologic response to orthopaedic implants and focuses on implants intended for permanent use, particularly joint replacement components, because much of the concern about long-term adverse biologic effects pertains to these devices. The acute and subacute local response to cemented and cementless joint replacement implants is discussed in detail, given that the initial skeletal fixation may be critical in dictating long-term clinical performance. The chronic local response to these implants in the form of adaptive bone remodeling ("stress-shielding") and osteolysis is also presented. The latter topic has generated intense research activity because it appears to be the major mechanism of long-term failure of joint replacement devices. Finally, the remote and systemic implications of orthopaedic implants are discussed, including the phenomena of hypersensitivity and implant-associated carcinogenesis.

Local Effects

Acute/Subacute Response to Cemented Implants

Polymethylmethacrylate (PMMA) is the material used most often for prosthetic stabilization within bone. It is formed by the polymerization of methylmethacrylate in an exothermic reaction. Sir John Charnley popularized the use of PMMA, borrowing the concept of stabilization of metal and plastic within bone from his dentistry colleagues. Technically, PMMA is a grout, not a glue, because no true adhesive bond occurs between the prosthesis and bone.

Before reviewing the response of bone to a cemented total joint implant, the response of bone to cement alone should be elucidated. In one study, 1 month after doughy Palacos R cement was injected into the canine femora, the endosteum was necrotic and a layer of new periosteal bone was being formed. By 3 to 4 months, the endosteum had revascularized and a thin connective tissue layer had formed at the bone-cement interface. Macrophages and foreign body giant cells were abundant in this tissue layer. The new periosteal bone continued to mature; however, the original cortical bone became less compact, secondary to dilation of the medullary vasculature. These findings were attributed to mechanical trauma during surgery, vascular trauma due to plugging of the nutrient arteries by PMMA, and thermal trauma during polymerization of the cement. In similar experiments, interface temperatures as high as 60°C were observed during cement curing. It was believed that thermal and chemical trauma rather than mechanical and circulatory disturbances were responsible for the extensive cortical necrosis and regeneration. Experiments in rabbits supported these histologic findings.

Cement has also been shown to retard revascularization of the endosteum following reaming of the medullary canal. In another study, the femoral canals of dogs were reamed and then a bolus of bone cement was finger packed into each femur; a Steinman pin was inserted to simulate a femoral prosthesis. The contralateral femur functioned as a reamed but noncemented control. Reaming of the canal compromised the vascularity of the endosteum and caused widespread necrosis, which abated after about 6 months. When cement was implanted, a fibrous tissue membrane formed at the cement-bone interface; revascularization of the endosteum was not complete by 12 months, the time of sacrifice.

Mechanical factors may play a more important role than thermal or chemical trauma in the long-term response to PMMA. Histologic studies comparing tissue response to prepolymerized and doughy PMMA implants in rabbit bones show that both types of implants became encapsulated by fibrous tissue, with occasional macrophages and giant cells. After several months, inflammation was not an important facet of the cellular response. Because prepolymerized PMMA would not result in an exothermic reaction on implantation and would leach less monomer into the surrounding tissue, the formation of a fibrous interface around cemented implants is likely to result, at least in part, from the mechanical and physical mismatch of the cement and the bone bed.

When considering the early effects of cemented implants in humans, results from Charnley's 23 autopsy specimens, harvested up to 7 years after successful total hip replacement, are very enlightening. By 2 to 4 weeks, endosteal necrosis had occurred adjacent to the cement to a depth of

500 μm. A fibrous interfacial membrane then formed, which was fibrocartilaginous in areas of high mechanical load. By 1 year, metaplasia of fibrous tissue to fibrocartilage and bone was more widespread. In other areas, dense fibrous tissue assumed a parallel alignment to the underlying bone. Bony remodeling was very active along the interface. Normal bone marrow was seen adjacent to the cement in some areas. Macrophages and foreign body giant cells were most evident at the interface at 2 to 5 years, and these cells appeared only in the nonweightbearing areas. These findings have been confirmed in similar autopsy retrieval studies of cemented implants.

It has been demonstrated that bone cement adversely affects the complement system, chemotaxis and migration of polymorphonuclear leukocytes, and the phagocytosis and killing of bacteria. The blood lymphocytes are also adversely affected. Furthermore, it has been shown that PMMA was more likely to be associated with infection by a standardized inoculum of bacteria than were conventional metals and plastics without PMMA. Thus, it would appear that cemented implants induce localized, transitory changes in the inflammatory response, beyond those expected of a foreign body alone.

In general terms, whenever a material is implanted in the body, surgical and mechanical trauma evoke an acute inflammatory response. The acute inflammatory cascade results in localized cell necrosis and tissue degeneration. Reparative and regenerative processes then follow in a pre-programmed manner, leading to the next stage of chronic inflammation and fibrosis. In the case of a cemented prosthesis, mechanical, vascular, thermal, and chemical trauma all appear to play a role in disturbing normal bone function. These disturbances take longer to rectify when cement is employed, compared to the use of a cementless implant. Over the ensuing months and years, the endosteal blood supply is reestablished as fibrovascular granulation tissue and cutting cones generate a new interface between the cement and bone. It is quite remarkable that the microinterlock and macrointerlock between cement and bone provide a durable interface and a high level of prosthetic stability during tissue remodeling.

Acute/Subacute Response to Cementless Implants

Basic Biology of Cementless Fixation

Although most cementless joint replacements in North America involve the use of implants with macrotextured surfaces (porous coatings in most cases), there is increasing interest in the use of implants with microtextured surfaces and ceramic coatings. These latter surfaces increase the options for controlling the location of fixation and may eventually represent a less costly but equally effective

means of obtaining cementless fixation than is possible with porous coatings. Although not universally held, it is generally believed that successful cementless fixation depends on establishment and maintenance of a durable connection between the implant and host skeleton. In contrast to cemented fixation, in which interdigitation of cement and the surrounding trabecular bone provides a degree of fixation, with cementless fixation the connection occurs at the implant's surface via newly formed bone tissue.

Certain conditions must exist for bone ingrowth into a porous coating to occur, and it is likely that these conditions are important for cementless fixation in general. Specifically, it is important that there be close contact between the implant surface and host bone, minimal relative motion at the bone-implant interface, and the appropriate surface characteristics (pore size and interconnectedness in the case of macrotextured surfaces, surface roughness in the case of microtextured surfaces, and surface chemistry in the case of ceramic coated surfaces).

Cementless fixation of a joint replacement implant occurs in the context of the surgical trauma created at the time of implantation. The response of the skeleton to trauma has been well studied mechanically and histologically and there is increasing interest in the molecular biology of this phenomenon. The initial skeletal response to the preparation of the bony bed for the implant is hematoma formation and mesenchymal tissue development, leading to the formation of woven bone through the intramembranous pathway (Fig. 1). Lamellar bone forms on the spicules of woven bone and a hematopoietic marrow is established. During this process a mechanically competent connection between the implant's surface and the host bone is established if the conditions outlined above exist.

Injury apparently stimulates mesenchymal stem cells, which reside within the marrow or along the endosteal surface, to divide and differentiate into osteoblasts. Some aspects of the underlying molecular biology of intramembranous bone formation in response to skeletal injury are now being worked out. For instance, following ablation of the rat tibial diaphysis, there is a rapid increase in osteoblast cell density, and expression of the alkaline phosphatase, procollagen $\alpha 1$ (I), and osteopontin genes. This is correlated with production of alkaline phosphatase-enriched matrix vesicles. These extracellular organelles form the nidus for mineral deposits in the matrix. Later, osteocalcin and then collagenase gene expression peak. Matrix vesicles undergo a maturation cascade, culminating in hydroxyapatite crystal formation. The type II collagen gene is not expressed, consistent with the histologic observations that bone formation in this context is intramembranous. Woven bone is present within a few days in rats and within 1 week in canines and humans.

In vitro studies have shown that 3 phases of osteoblast function characterize bone tissue formation: proliferation, extracellular matrix maturation, and mineralization. While

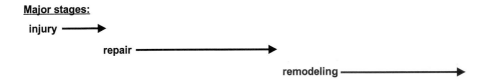

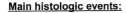

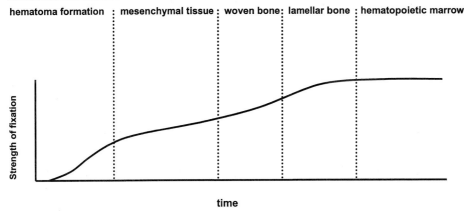

Figure 1

Schematic diagram summarizing the major stages of skeletal response to injury and key histologic events as related to the development of mechanical fixation of cementless implants.

the cells proliferate, genes for type I collagen, fibronectin, and transforming growth factor-β (TGF-β) are maximally expressed and the gene for osteopontin is also expressed to a certain degree. During the second phase, proliferation is downregulated and expression of alkaline phosphatase peaks and then declines. During mineralization, osteocalcin and osteopontin expression increase. The data from the rat tibial ablation model are similar except TGF-β does not increase until later, but insulin-like growth factor-I peaks early. It can be hypothesized that factors that increase proliferation without inhibiting matrix maturation or mineralization may be useful for enhancing bone regeneration around orthopaedic implants.

It is not known if the pattern of gene expression changes at the site of skeletal injury if an implant is placed there, but circumstantial evidence indicates that this may well be the case. For instance, several in vitro studies have shown that osteoblast adhesion to implant surfaces is highly dependent on substrate composition and surface preparation; therefore, it seems reasonable to assume that the presence of an implant must have some effect on the pattern of gene expression. Indeed, it may be possible to control the response by appropriate surface treatment. In addition, several studies examining endosteal bone formation around implant materials using the tibial marrow ablation model described above demonstrate that matrix vesicle production and function are modified not only locally but also in bones distant from the implant. Moreover, both the local and systemic effects depend on the type of material used.

The osteogenic potential of the implantation site is most likely an important factor. It can be anticipated that if the appropriate stem cells are not present, osteogenesis following skeletal trauma would be inhibited. This finding seems consistent with observations of decreased bone formation following revision of an aseptically loosened cemented implant, in which the marrow spaces are filled by granuloma rather than normal marrow tissue. Similarly, because stem cell density is thought by many to decrease with age a diminished response can be expected, but, paradoxically, there is no definitive evidence of decreased osteogenesis in response to skeletal trauma in the mature skeleton.

Following marrow ablation, the newly formed bone will persist indefinitely if it forms in a site where bone is normally present, but will be completely resorbed and replaced by marrow in sites where bone is not normally found (the diaphysis of a long bone). The long-term persistence of the newly formed bone tissue is presumably related to its mechanical function. When a prosthesis is placed in the prepared site, the basic steps in the skeletal wound response ensue. If the implant becomes fixed to the host skeleton, the newly formed bone now has a mechanical role (load transfer) and will persist and adapt to this role. It is possible that the load at the interface could exceed the strength of the connecting bone tissue, in which case failure of fixation is expected. This situation could occur if the area for fixation was insufficient and the interface stresses "overwhelmed" the capacity of the newly formed bone to support the implant.

Under ideal conditions, mechanical fixation strength (bonding strength) plateaus at 2 weeks in canine models and the interface should be protected during this period; it is not absolutely certain what this time period is in humans. However, most clinicians recommend a 6- to 12-week period of protected weightbearing. Initially, the distribution of bone at the interface is relatively homogenous under ideal conditions, but as the newly formed bone tissue adapts to the pattern of implant-to-bone stress transfer, the spatial distribution of bone ingrowth changes accordingly.

However, because it is never certain that ideal conditions for bone ingrowth existed initially, the meaning of anatomic variation in bone ingrowth in implants retrieved from patients must be interpreted with care. Thus, the distribution of bone ingrowth in retrievals could easily reflect the distribution of good initial bone-implant contact and not the pattern of stress transfer that would be expected to develop in an implant with initial uniform contact.

The early studies of bone ingrowth in porous coated implants in humans seemed to indicate that bone ingrowth was a rare occurrence. More recent studies, many of which include a significant number of implants retrieved at autopsy from patients who had excellent function with their implants, indicate that bone ingrowth occurs reproducibly. Some studies have shown comparable mechanical stability of implants fixed by bone ingrowth and cemented implants.

Factors Inhibiting Cementless Fixation

Numerous studies have shown that gaps as small as 0.5 mm can inhibit bone ingrowth. This is a matter of concern because gaps of 1 to 2 mm between the implant and host bone are routinely created in total knee replacement and gaps of at least 3 mm can exist at the acetabular interface, particularly when the bone bed is underreamed to permit a press fit.

Although it is generally agreed that excessive motion is inhibitory to bone ingrowth/ongrowth, the precise amount of interface motion that is tolerable and the mechanism of inhibition are still poorly defined. One study showed bone formation within a porous coated implant in a situation in which 40 µm to 150 µm of interface motion were present, but there was a lack of connecting trabeculae between the implant and host skeleton. Implants with initial motion of 20 µm had bone within the porous coating in continuity with the endosteal bone. These are interesting findings that would suggest that excessive motion causes fibrous tissue formation rather than allowing bone formation. Perhaps bone forms in the presence of some degree of motion, but cannot maintain or establish connectivity with the host skeleton in the presence of "excessive" motion because of the high interface stresses the motion would cause. Interface motion greater than 150 µm normally cannot support bone ingrowth/ongrowth, but application of a ceramic (in this case, hydroxyapatite) to the porous surface permitted bone ingrowth even in the presence of 150 µm of initial interface motion. This is an area in which interpretation of the results is not always obvious, but the ability to ensure fixation in the presence of motion would be of great clinical benefit.

The revision environment represents a severe challenge for bone regeneration because of the presence of gaps, motion, and an inherently diminished osteogenic capacity due to replacement of the normal medullary contents by granulation tissue. There is clinical as well as experimental evidence that these sites still retain some osteogenic potential, but there is great need to develop ways to enhance bone regeneration in this context.

Implant studies and studies of fracture healing have shown that numerous factors can inhibit bone regeneration (Table 1). Of most importance are adjuvant treatments that are sometimes administered to patients receiving cementless joint replacements. For instance, it has been shown that the bisphosphonate ethane hydroxydiphosphate, indomethacin, and certain doses of radiation (prophylactic treatments for heterotopic ossification) can inhibit bone ingrowth. In general, any factor that inhibits fracture healing should be assumed to have a similar effect on implant fixation unless otherwise demonstrated.

Factors Enhancing Cementless Fixation

Various materials (for example, bone graft substitutes) and external modalities (for example, electrical stimulation) have been tested as means to enhance cementless implant fixation (Table 2). In models that replicate ideal conditions for bone ingrowth, enhancement of fixation has been, at best, modest, underscoring the importance of initial fit and stability. However, ideal conditions may be difficult to obtain clinically so there is considerable interest in enhancement, which can mean increasing the rate at which bone forms, without necessarily increasing the amount

Table 1	
Factors Inhibiting Cementless Fixation	
Factor	**Comment**
Excessive interface motion	Still a matter of controversy, but may be as low as 30 µm
Excessive interface gaps	1 to 2 mm gaps can be bridged, but gaps often reduce initial stability causing excessive motion
Inappropriate porosity	This caveat applies to the porous coating and to any gap filling material
Radiation	Dose-dependent, seems to be a therapeutic range for prevention of heterotopic ossification without compromising implant fixation
EHDP (disodium ethane-1-hydroxy-1, 1-diphosphonate)	Once used to prevent heterotopic ossification, but no longer used for that indication
Indomethacin	Short-term, transient inhibition only
Warfarin	Only inhibitory in absence of a calcium phosphate coating on the implant
cis-platinum	
Methotrexate	

formed (acceleration), or increasing the amount of newly formed bone (augmentation) (Fig. 2). Presumably, both would lead to improved long-term rates of successful cementless fixation.

The current strategy for investigating enhancement of fixation is to use a model that impairs bone ingrowth or ongrowth and then to test the usefulness of this model or modality for rescuing the failure. A simple means of impairing bone ingrowth/ongrowth is to create a gap between the implant and host skeleton. In this situation, treatment of the implant with a ceramic (hydroxyapatite, tricalcium phosphate, or a mixture of the two) or treatment of the gap with a graft (such as autogenous bone) enhances bone ingrowth/ongrowth. More recently, certain growth factors (namely recombinant TGF-β and bone morphogenetic protein-2) have been found to be effective (Fig. 3).

Relatively little is known about enhancing fixation in the presence of implant motion, except that a hydroxyapatite coating appears to permit bone ingrowth/ongrowth in the presence of 150 μm of interface motion, an amount of motion that normally does not permit bone ingrowth/ongrowth.

In the context of revision arthroplasty even less is known, although it is clear that autogenous bone grafting works better than the use of a ceramic-based bone graft substitute.

Chronic Local Response

Adaptive Remodeling

One of the chronic responses to an orthopaedic implant involves adaptive bone remodeling. In general, the term adaptive bone remodeling refers to changes in bone mass and geometry in response to an alteration in the bone's mechanical environment. The most familiar examples are increased bone mass with certain kinds of exercise (such as tournament level tennis playing, particularly during growth) and bone loss following space flight-induced disuse. The presence of the implant alters the bone's mechan-

Table 2	
Factors Enhancing Cementless Fixation*	

Factor	Comment
Transforming growth factor-β	Several positive studies (dose-dependent) with effectiveness even in presence of large interface gaps (3 mm)
Bone morphogenetic protein	One positive study (dose-dependent) with effectiveness even in presence of large interface gaps (3 mm)
Autogenous bone graft	Shown to be effective in numerous situations even in presence of large interface gaps (3 mm)
Low amplitude mechanical strains	Very stimulatory in a disuse model
Fresh-frozen allogeneic bone graft	Several positive studies in the presence of interface gaps
Factor XIII	Limited studies, but positive findings with systemic administration
Calcium phosphate coatings	Numerous positive studies, but only if interface gaps less than or equal to 1 mm
Prostaglandin	Limited studies, but positive findings with systemic administration
Electrical stimulation	Some positive findings in the absence of interface gaps (not tested in presence of gaps)
Calcium phosphate granules	Mixed experimental results
Freeze-dried allogeneic bone graft	Mixed experimental results
Fibrin glue	Mixed experimental results
Demineralized bone matrix	No evidence of enhancement

* Listed in the order of apparent effectiveness; permissive factors such as adequate initial implant stability and fit are not included here.

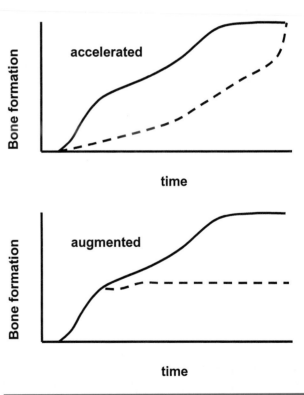

Figure 2

Definitions of enhancement. In both cases, the dashed line depicts the control or normal situation and the solid line depicts the enhanced situation. Acceleration refers to achieving the same level of bone formation, but at a faster rate. Augmentation refers to achieving a higher level of bone formation.

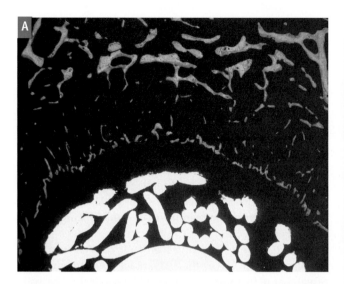

Figure 3

Enhancement with transforming growth factor-β (TGF-β). These back-scatter scanning electron micrographs depict at 4 weeks a control (**A**) and an implant (**B**) treated with TGF-β. In both cases, there was an initial 3-mm gap between the implant and host bone. Note the lack of bone ingrowth in the control implant, whereas the growth factor-treated implant has bone formation across the interface and throughout the depth of the porous coating. The amount of new bone formation was nearly 3 times greater in the treated implants compared to the control implants (original magnification × 15). (Reproduced with permission from Sumner DR, Turner TM, Purchio AF, Gombotz WR, Urban RM, Galante JO: Enhancement of bone ingrowth by transforming growth factor-beta. *J Bone Joint Surg* 1995;77A:1135–1147.)

ical environment and in many areas diminishes the load to the native bone. This phenomenon is called "stress-shielding" and is considered to be an important cause of periprosthetic bone loss (Fig. 4). The general consensus is that there is a negative feedback loop in which implant-induced perturbation of an unidentified mechanical factor causes net bone loss, thereby returning the mechanical set-point to normal (Fig. 5). It is not yet clear that bone loss induced by stress-shielding is a cause of failure, but it is already apparent that loss of bone stock complicates revision surgery.

It is useful to recognize that the term "remodeling" has a special meaning to those who study metabolic bone disease. In that domain, the term refers to coupled bone resorption and formation at discrete anatomic locales. As used here, "remodeling" has a much more general connotation, implying change in mass or geometry without any specific recognition of the underlying tissue mechanisms.

Stress-shielding has been most closely studied in the context of the femoral component in total hip replacement. The severity of stress-shielding is determined by the relative stiffness of the implant and the host skeleton. This relationship depends, then, on the geometry and material properties of both the implant and the host bone and the relative placement of the implant within the bone. Implants made of cobalt-chromium alloy cause more stress-shielding than similarly shaped implants made from titanium alloy because the former alloy has twice the elastic modulus of the latter alloy. Similarly, large diameter implants cause more stress-shielding than small diameter implants. Implants placed eccentrically will tend to cause more

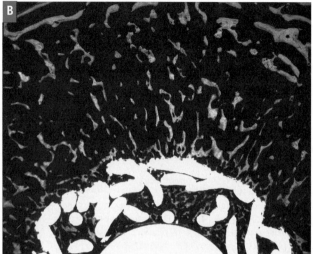

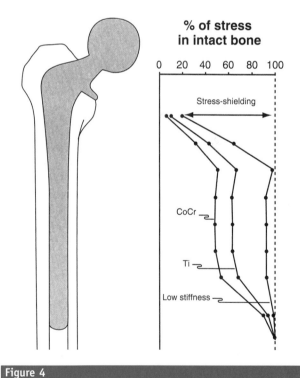

Figure 4

Schematic diagram of stress-shielding. CoCr = Cobalt-chromium; Tr = titanium. (Adapted with permission from Huiskes R, Weinans H, Dalstra M: Adaptive bone remodeling and biomechanical design considerations for noncemented total hip arthroplasty. *Orthopedics* 1989;12:1255–1267.)

stress-shielding than implants placed centrally within the medullary canal. Implant length and extent of porous coating have also been shown in computer models to affect

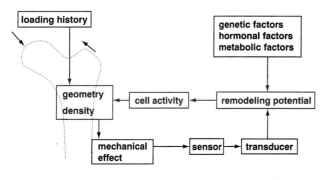

Figure 5

Feedback loop thought to control adaptive remodeling. (Adapted with permission from Huiskes R, Weinans H, Dalstra M: Adaptive bone remodeling and biomechanical design considerations for noncemented total hip arthroplasty. *Orthopedics* 1989;12:1255–1267.)

stress-shielding. Of course, implant design and selection is a compromise between numerous factors such as the need for large, bulky implants to obtain initial mechanical stability to permit bone ingrowth/ongrowth versus the stress-shielding induced bone loss that can be expected to occur with such an implant.

A number of studies have been reported and are currently underway that use dual energy x-ray absorptiometry (DXA or DEXA) to examine bone loss in patients following total joint replacement. This technique was originally developed for osteoporosis, but has been adapted to periprosthetic remodeling. This method is precise (repeatable) and detects much smaller changes in bone mass than can be detected using conventional radiographic techniques.

It is important to understand what these machines measure. Even though the term "density" is often used in conjunction with DXA, these machines do not measure density (mass/volume). Rather, they measure the bone mineral content (BMC)—the mass of mineral in a volume of bone. Unfortunately (and unlike computed tomography), the volume of tissue sampled cannot be determined with DXA. However, to normalize for differences in size, BMC is often divided by the area of interest projected onto a 2-dimensional (2-D) image, and this derived variable is commonly called the bone mineral density (BMD). In a perfectly cylindrical specimen, rotation of the specimen will not affect BMC or BMD, but in a specimen with an elliptical cross-section, BMD can vary significantly while BMC remains constant because the projected area of interest changes as a function of rotation. Most authors report the change in BMD, either compared to the contralateral limb or to a baseline measurement, while some report the change in BMC. The interpretation of the latter is more straightforward in theory, but in practice both are usually highly correlated so it is not too misleading to compare studies that use these different methods of reporting.

The DXA studies to date suggest that most of the bone loss occurs adjacent to the proximal part of the implant within the first 6 to 12 months; the use of extensively porous-coated cobalt chromium alloy stems leads to more bone loss than the use of proximally porous-coated titanium alloy stems; and the use of proximal coatings in cobalt-chromium stems helps to preserve bone stock. These studies cannot yet be considered definitive because of differences in how bone loss was assessed, demographic characteristics of the study populations, and length of follow-up. In addition, most studies are not controlled for limb usage, which can account for a considerable proportion of the apparent periprosthetic bone loss. In general, it is not unusual to find reductions in proximal medial BMC or BMD of 30% to 50% on average, with some individuals experiencing loss of bone of up to 80%.

Adaptive bone remodeling has been studied in animal models, which have the advantage of allowing the researcher to focus on 1 variable at a time (Fig. 6). The average amount of bone loss in many of the animal studies is similar to that observed in human studies; in some individuals, bone loss is severe. These studies indicate that the amount or pattern of bone remodeling is not influenced by the type of porous coating; proximally coated devices do not appear to protect against bone loss compared to fully coated devices; uncoated implants cause as much (if not more) proximal bone loss over time as fully coated implants; and proximal bone loss is reduced with more flexible implants. This latter finding is, perhaps, the clearest support for the stress-shielding mechanism of bone loss following total hip arthroplasty.

In general, the DXA studies and data from computer and animal models are in agreement. However, the animal model data on porous coating location do not support the clinical impression of less bone loss with less extensively coated stems. This difference may be attributed to confounding factors, such as the degree of distal fit and, hence, stress transfer from the implant to the host bone. Thus, from a strictly mechanical point of view, the best method of protection against long-term bone loss in the proximal femur following total hip arthroplasty would be to reduce stress-shielding by reducing the stiffness of the implant. It may eventually be possible to also consider a biologic approach, namely, to reduce stress-shielding by increasing the stiffness of the host bone. Indeed, some DXA studies indicate that the amount of periprosthetic bone loss is highly dependent on the initial bone mass, and, hence, the stiffness of the host femur (Fig. 7). Treatments being developed for osteoporosis or the local use of growth factors might provide a mechanism for increasing the structural stiffness of the femur prior to or at the time of hip replacement. In this way, it may be possible to reduce stress-shielding by altering the bone side of the equation as well as by altering the implant side of the equation.

An alternative biologic approach to inhibit bone loss is to use a drug such as a second- or third-generation bisphosphonate, which suppresses metabolic bone remodeling

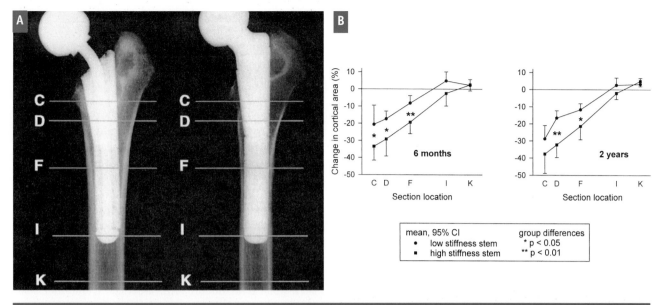

Figure 6

An animal model to examine adaptive remodeling. The contact radiographs in **A** were taken of the treated limbs of 2 animals treated with a unilateral hip replacement, using a low stiffness stem (*left*) or a high stiffness stem (*right*). The graphs in **B** depict the amount of cortical bone loss at 6 months and 2 years and demonstrate that stiffer stems cause more periprosthetic bone loss, presumably because they cause more stress-shielding. The graphs suggest that most of the adaptive process occurred in the first 6 months in this canine model, in general agreement with patient data indicating that most of the bone loss appears to occur within the first 6 to 12 months. CI = confidence interval. (Adapted with permission from Turner TM, Sumner DR, Urban RM, Igloria R, Galante JO: Maintenance of proximal cortical bone with use of a less stiff femoral component in hemiarthroplasty of the hip without cement. *J Bone Joint Surg* 1997;79A:1381–1390.)

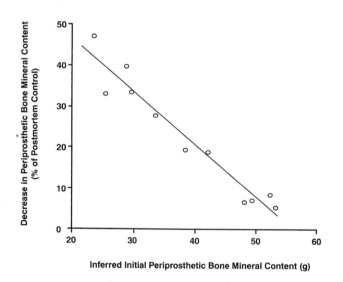

Figure 7

Graph showing that femurs with the most bone mass experienced the least net bone loss. Note that the decrease in periprosthetic bone mineral content was inversely proportional to the inferred initial periprosthetic bone mineral content. (Adapted with permission from Sychterz CJ, Engh CA: The influence of clinical factors on periprosthetic bone remodeling. *Clin Orthop* 1996;322:285–292.)

(coupled bone resorption and formation) by suppressing resorption. The long-term consequences of this approach on the mechanical competence of the tissue are not clearly known, although in the short-term (1 to 2 years) there does not seem to be a worrisome decline in important mechanical properties such as strength and fatigue life.

It can be presumed that many of the principles learned from hip replacement apply to total knee and total shoulder replacement as well. Indeed, there has been considerable interest in how the design of the tibial component in cementless total knee replacement can be altered to minimize the initial motion between the implant and host bone. There is some concern with bone loss in the distal femur, apparently caused by stress-shielding. To date, the best initial fixation with cementless tibial implants occurs with the use of screws, but more recent studies have shown that screw tracts or holes can serve as conduits for particulate debris to gain access to the interface, leading to the development of granuloma formation and possibly osteolysis. This paradox underscores the complexity of implant design; generally, a series of compromises are required to optimize the performance of the device.

There has also been considerable interest in the mechanical consequences of spine instrumentation and fracture fixation plates. Indeed, many of the issues regarding long-term adaptive remodeling currently being studied in the context of total hip replacement were first described with fracture fixation plates. Thus, the effects of implant material and geometry on stress-shielding and the subsequent remodeling of the host skeleton are recurring themes any time an implant is used in orthopaedics.

Chronic Soft-Tissue Response to Orthopaedic Implants

In general, implants placed in an extraosseous environment in the musculoskeletal system are encapsulated by fibrous tissue. However, the precise nature of the tissue is determined by the biologic and mechanical environments to which the implant and surrounding tissues are subjected. For example, spinal rods are frequently covered by fibrous tissue, separating them from the overlying paraspinal musculature. However, in areas adjacent to bone, these same rods are covered by a thick shell of bone, often making extraction difficult. Similarly, plates for internal fixation are often buried in a thick mass of bone, which must be excised, in part, to remove the plate. The plate may also be covered by fibrous tissue having a synovial lining layer and mucinous, viscous fluid within the cavity that surrounds the plate. This inflammatory bursa separates the plate from the surrounding soft tissues. In some cases, a low-grade infection is suspected, but cultures invariably prove to be sterile. Whether the formation of this bursal tissue is caused by interfacial motion, the local biologic environment, or by-products from the implant is unknown. All of these factors are probably contributory.

The response to ligament prostheses follows a series of biologic events similar to that of other artificial implants. These prostheses provide a scaffold onto which immature fibrous tissue and fibrocartilage are produced. Near the attachment areas of these implants where they are anchored to bone, fibrocartilage and bone are formed; the different tissue types probably form in response to the local biomechanical environment.

Long-Term Biologic Response to Nonosseointegrated Implants

Retrieval studies have shown that the interface surrounding mechanically stable implants, whether cemented or cementless, is composed of some areas of direct bone to cement or bone to prosthesis apposition; in other areas, the interface is composed of fibrous tissue, fibrocartilage, granulation tissue, and foreign body reaction. Thus, even in radiographically stable prostheses, the bone-implant interface is heterogeneous.

When a metallic or polymeric implant is placed in an extraosseous location in animals, after several months, the local inflammatory reaction eventually produces a fibrous encapsulation tissue. When an implant is placed in an intraosseous location, the interface tissue is determined primarily by the design, material, topography, and other surface characteristics of the implant, the presence of voids and gaps, the initial implant stability and subsequent parameters of mechanical loading, local biologic stimuli such as coatings and growth factors, the vascularity and viability of the prosthetic bed, and constitutional factors such as the general health and metabolic state of the host. Stress, chronic illnesses, medications, and external stimuli such as electrical stimulation may also have a major impact on the interface. Surgical factors are also important; a poorly prepared prosthetic bed will be less likely to facilitate the local apposition and remodeling of bone.

If an intraosseous implant does not become integrated with the surrounding bone, an intervening fibrous tissue interface forms. Mechanically loose implants undergo displacement with physiologic loads. The subsequent motion usually leads to reactive fibrosis, and in some cases, a synovial-like layer at the bone-implant interface. As loosening progresses and larger prosthetic displacements occur, the fibrous membrane thickens. A thin, bony encapsulation may surround the fibrous tissue layer. Pressure necrosis of bone may occur when an implant subsides or angulates to abut the cortex, and loading becomes more concentrated over a small area. Motion at the articulating and nonarticulating surfaces produces wear debris, which accumulates locally within the tissues and especially within macrophages. This begins a series of cellular and biochemical events that results in the periprosthetic destruction of bone known as osteolysis.

Osteolysis

Osteolysis is characterized by destruction of bone as seen on conventional radiographs. It may present as a focal process or may be more diffusely distributed. Osteolysis has many etiologies, including primary and metastatic bone tumors, infection, rheumatologic diseases, and metabolic abnormalities such as hyperparathyroidism. With respect to joint prostheses, 2 radiographic types of osteolysis have been described. The first type, linear, is associated with slowly progressive, thin radiolucent lines of about 2 mm in thickness surrounding a loose prosthesis. These lines are searched for during radiographic assessment of the stability of a total joint replacement. The more problematic radiolucencies associated with osteolysis are those associated with progressive ballooning and scalloping in the periprosthetic bony bed (Fig. 8). These areas are greater than 2 mm in width, and are often much larger in volume than simple 2-D radiographs might suggest. These radiolucent areas may balloon out from the prosthesis, eroding both cancellous and cortical bone, and in some cases, a pathologic fracture may result. To date, these osteolytic areas have been associated with joint prostheses of all types and at all locations in the body, but are especially prevalent around the knee and hip.

Clinical and basic research have suggested an important role for particulate wear debris and its by-products in the etiology of periprosthetic osteolysis. Wear debris is formed at normal joint articulations (such as at the ball and socket of a normally functioning hip replacement), at modular interfaces (such as the junction of the trunion and ball, or

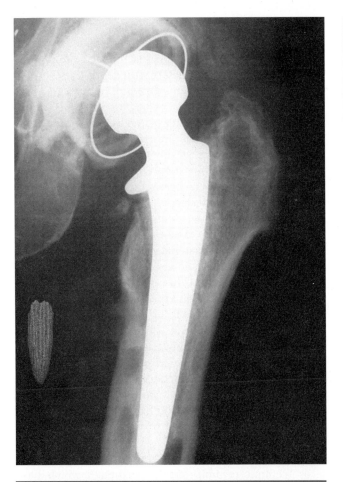

Figure 8

This radiograph of a cemented total hip replacement shows distal femoral osteolysis. Note the large radiolucent areas that have eroded the cortex around the distal aspect of the femoral stem. (Reproduced with permission from Wright TM, Goodman SB (eds): *Implant Wear: The Future of Total Joint Replacement*. Rosemont, IL, American Academy of Orthopaedic Surgeons, 1996.)

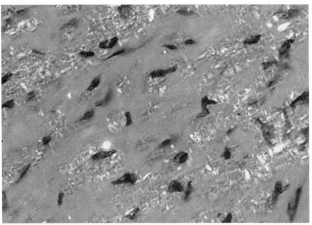

Figure 9

Polarized light photomicrograph of tissue surrounding a loose total hip replacement, showing sheets of macrophages that have phagocytosed numerous, positively birefringent polyethylene wear particles. (Reproduced with permission from Wright TM, Goodman SB (eds): *Implant Wear: The Future of Total Joint Replacement*. Rosemont, IL, American Academy of Orthopaedic Surgeons, 1996. Photomicrograph courtesy of Dr. Pat Campbell, Joint Replacement Institute, Los Angeles.)

polyethylene liner and metallic supporting shell), at areas of impingement (such as when the femoral neck impinges on the rim of the acetabular cup at extremes of motion), and at nonarticulating interfaces due to abrasion with the surrounding bone, cement mantle, or debris. Wear debris formation may be accelerated in the setting of third body wear (when bone particles or debris become interposed within the joint articulation). It has been estimated that tens of thousands of particles are generated with each step during ambulation. Most of the particles are less than 5 μm in diameter and can undergo phagocytosis by macrophages. Particles of a variety of compositions have been implicated in the etiology and pathogenesis of osteolysis around total joint replacements. Metallic, polymeric, and ceramic debris all have been associated with osteolysis. What was originally thought of as "cement disease" has now been recognized as "particle disease." Recent research has especially stressed the importance of polyethylene, because it is almost uniformly used in all joint replace-

ments and its particulate debris tends to be the most abundant in the periprosthetic tissues.

The macrophage is a key cell in the events associated with periprosthetic osteolysis (Fig. 9). Osteolysis appears to result from increased local synthesis of bone-resorbing factors by activated macrophages. These cells phagocytose small particles but are unable to digest them. Through cellular and biochemical signaling mechanisms, phagocytosed particles stimulate increased macrophage accumulation, proliferation, and the synthesis of bone-resorbing factors. It has been shown by in vitro studies that the cellular response is determined by the size, composition, and dose of the particulate. Other factors, such as the shape, surface energy, and nature of the proteins bound to the surface, have not been as well characterized and may also be critical in the cellular response. In conjunction with osteoblasts, fibroblasts, osteoclasts, and other cells, prostanoids (such as prostaglandin E2), cytokines and growth factors (such as interleukin-1, interleukin-6, tumor necrosis factor-α, platelet-derived growth factor, and others), metalloproteinases (such as collagenase and stromelysin), lysosomal enzymes, and other factors are released locally into the interfacial tissues and synovial fluid. The prostanoids, cytokines, and growth factors may act in an autocrine and paracrine manner to stimulate the differentiation, maturation, and activation of osteoclasts and produce localized bone resorption (Fig. 10). Furthermore, recent studies have shown that in addition to their stimulatory effects on bone resorption, particles can inhibit osteoblast function, thus affecting bone formation. The production of autocrine and paracrine regulators by osteoblasts is also affected. Specifically, prostanoid production is increased whereas TGF-β production is decreased. Both of these factors may contribute to increased bone resorption.

This reaction is self-sustaining: the indigestible particles are eventually egested and recirculated. Increased local bone resorption and decreased bone formation undermine the bony support of the prosthesis. The foreign body response due to particulate debris may then begin a vicious cycle: as bone resorption and prosthetic loosening progress, abrasion and fretting at the interface may produce increased amounts of particulate debris. Particles may be circulated throughout the interface, through nonosseo-integrated areas or gaps, into the cancellous bone, and to the joint. The latter factor may lead to increased amounts of articular wear debris generation by a 3-body mechanism, thus increasing the local particulate burden. Furthermore, normal gait cycles produce time periods of increasing and decreasing intra-articular pressure, which may serve as a pumping mechanism for the particles throughout the joint and periprosthetic space.

The primary reaction to particulate debris appears to be a nonspecific foreign body type reaction. In some patients, however, there may be an immune reaction to the particle-protein complex, similar to the type IV hypersensitivity reaction seen in selected patients with implanted devices (see below). This type IV reaction has been shown for patients with either titanium alloy or cobalt-chromium alloy prostheses and presumably occurs with other alloys and materials. One study suggested that severe, progressive osteolysis may be caused by an uncoupling of the events encompassing the foreign body response and reactive fibrosis, resulting in an aggressive granulomatous reaction due to activated fibroblasts and macrophages. The role of individual host responsiveness to wear debris, whether on a specific (antigen/antibody mediated) or nonspecific basis, has been widely suspected but has not been well established. This is currently an area of intense research that may produce useful methods for prospectively screening patients who may be at increased risk of aggressive periprosthetic cellular reactions.

The generation of wear debris from joint prostheses is dependent on mechanical forces, the wear properties of the materials, and surgical technique. Strategies for mitigation of the adverse response to particles include proper choice and manufacturing of materials, optimal prosthesis design and surgical technique, and limits on prosthetic loading to improve the longevity of the prosthesis. Currently, thin polyethylene liners are discouraged, and the processing and storage of materials is being carefully scrutinized. For example, many orthopaedic companies have modified their procedures for sterilizing polyethylene and are storing the polyethylene in a nonoxygen-containing environment. Furthermore, there is considerable activity in the development of extensively cross-linked ultrahigh molecular weight polyethylene (UHMWPE) bearing surfaces, which have demonstrated improved wear performance in joint simulator testing.

Also under consideration are hard-on-hard bearing surfaces (ceramic/ceramic and metal/metal), which have demonstrated very low levels of volumetric wear in joint simulator studies and on implant retrieval. These bearing couples can eliminate or greatly reduce (in the case of those systems that use a polyethylene carrier) the polyethylene particulate burden. Circumferential porous coatings have presently replaced incomplete, partial porous coatings, because particles were shown to migrate along the fibrous, nonporous coated interface. Improved osseointegration of implants has been sought using hydroxyapatite coatings to prevent migration of particles around the prosthesis and improve and accelerate fixation. A resurgence in the use of bone cement has also been suggested as a method to limit particle migration.

There is also an increasing recognition that the corrosion and wear debris generated at modular interfaces (for example, the head/trunion junction of femoral total hip replacement components) can be minimized by appropriate design and manufacturing modifications. Recently, bisphosphonates have been used in preliminary studies to suppress osteoclast-mediated bone resorption in the prosthetic bed. Other pharmacologic strategies directed at intracellular signal transduction pathways are also being investigated. Whether these and other treatments will prove effective remains to be seen. Future improvements in prosthetic design and manufacturing, surgical technique, and pharmacologic treatments may limit the degree of

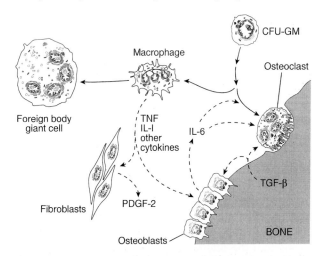

Figure 10

This diagram depicts some of the cells and cytokines thought to participate in the periprosthetic bone resorption associated with wear particles from joint replacements. Interactions between particles and cells lead to the release of cytokines and other substances that modulate osteoclast differentiation and maturation at the bone-implant interface. TNF = tumor necrosis factor; IL-1 = interleukin 1; PDGF-2 = platelet derived growth factor-2; CFU-GM = colony forming unit, granulocyte-monocyte stem cell, TGF-β = transforming growth factor-β. (Diagram courtesy of Dr. Tom Bauer, Department of Pathology, Cleveland Clinic.)

loosening and osteolysis, and the morbidity associated with revision surgery.

Remote and Systemic Effects

In the majority of patients, permanent orthopaedic implants are well tolerated; that is, they are biocompatible. However, there is an increasing recognition that, in the long term, permanent orthopaedic implants may be associated with adverse local and remote tissue responses in some individuals. These adverse effects are mediated by the degradation products of the implant materials that may be present as (1) particulate wear and corrosion debris; (2) colloidal organometallic complexes (specifically or nonspecifically bound); (3) free metallic ions; (4) inorganic metal salts/oxides; and/or (5) substances sequestered in an organic storage form such as hemosiderin.

Much of the focus on the long-term biocompatibility of implant materials has centered on the metallic components because of their tendency to undergo electrochemical corrosion resulting in the formation of, at least transiently, chemically active degradation products. There are 6 reasons why the issue of metal release from implanted devices has taken on an increasing sense of urgency. The first is the recognition in a variety of clinical settings of the deposition of extensive metallic particulate debris within local and remote tissues, in which these particles have enormous specific surface areas available for electrochemical interaction with the surrounding tissue fluids. The second is the reintroduction of metal-on-metal articulating devices in Europe and North America as a consequence of the recognition of the deleterious local effects (periprosthetic osteolysis) of polyethylene wear debris from metal/UHMWPE wear couples. The third is the observation of severe mechanically-assisted crevice corrosion processes in modular and multipart metallic joint replacement components associated with extensive local deposition of corrosion products and elevations in serum metal content. The fourth is the continued popularity of porous-coated cementless devices with high specific surface areas, particularly important in young patients with long life expectancies. The fifth is the concern that metal degradation products can act as a stimulus to osteolysis both directly, by virtue of macrophage activation, and indirectly, by accelerating polyethylene debris generation by a third-body wear mechanism. The sixth reason is the realization that in certain clinical settings the serum transport of metallic degradation products is greater than has been generally appreciated.

Because of the known potential toxicities of the elements (titanium, aluminum, vandadium, cobalt, chromium, and nickel) used in modern orthopaedic implant alloys, concern about the release and distribution of metallic degradation products is justified. Toxicity may be by virtue of several factors: metabolic alterations; alterations in host/parasite interactions; immunologic interactions of metal moieties by virtue of their ability to act as haptens (specific immunologic activation), antichemotactic agents (nonspecific immunologic suppression), or lymphocyte toxins; and chemical carcinogenesis. At this time, the association of metal release from orthopaedic implants with any metabolic, bacteriologic, immunologic, or carcinogenic toxicity remains conjectural because cause and effect have not been established in human subjects. This may be attributable to the difficulty of observation; most symptoms caused by systemic and remote toxicity can be expected to occur in a finite frequency in any population of orthopaedic patients.

Metal Ion Release

Implants or the wear debris they generate may release chemically active metal ions into the surrounding tissues. Although these ions may stay bound to local tissues, metal ions may also bind to protein moieties that are then transported in the bloodstream and/or lymphatics to remote organs. The issue of "metal ion release" can be broken down into 4 basic questions: (1) How much metal is released from the implant? (2) Where is the metal transported and in what quantity? (3) What is the chemical form of the released metal (for example, inorganic precipitate versus soluble organometallic complex)? and (4) What are the pathophysiologic consequences of such metal release? There is a growing body of literature addressing the first 2 issues; however, little is currently known with regard to the other 2 questions.

Broad reviews of the toxicology of the elements used in orthopaedic metal alloys are available and are briefly summarized below. Cobalt, chromium, and possibly nickel and vanadium are essential trace metals in that they are required for certain enzymatic reactions. In excessive amounts, however, these elements may be toxic. Cobalt may lead to polycythemia, hypothyroidism, cardiomyopathy, and carcinogenesis; chromium to nephropathy, hypersensitivity, and carcinogenesis; nickel to eczematous dermatitis, hypersensitivity, and carcinogenesis; and vanadium to cardiac and renal dysfunction, hypertension, and manic depressive psychosis. The nonessential metallic elements also have specific toxicities. Titanium, although generally regarded as biocompatible, has been associated with pulmonary disease in patients with occupational exposure and with platelet suppression in animal models. Aluminum toxicity is well documented in the setting of renal failure and can lead to anemia, osteomalacia, and neurologic dysfunction, possibly including Alzheimer's disease. However, when considering the litany of documented toxicities of these elements, it is important to remember that the toxicities generally apply to soluble forms of the elements and may not apply to the chemical species that result from the degradation of prosthetic implants.

There is a considerable body of literature concerning

serum and urine chromium, cobalt, and nickel levels following total joint replacement, but there are relatively fewer studies examining titanium, aluminum, and vanadium levels. Many investigations have been hampered by technical limitations of the analytic instrumentation, inadequate contamination precautions, and/or suboptimal study designs. Furthermore, it is difficult to compare the results from different laboratories because different techniques and protocols produce different results. Investigations reporting trace metal levels in body fluids and tissues must report precise methodologies and account for metal contamination with prevention protocols. Normal human serum levels of prominent implant metals are approximately 1 to 10 ng/ml for aluminum, 0.15 ng/ml for chromium, <0.01 ng/ml for vanadium, 0.1 to 0.2 ng/ml for cobalt, and <4.1 ng/ml titanium. Following total joint arthroplasty, levels of circulating metal have been shown to increase.

Multiple studies have demonstrated chronic elevations in serum and urine cobalt and chromium following uncomplicated primary total joint replacement. In addition, transient elevations of urine and serum nickel have been noted immediately following surgery. This hypernickelemia/hypernickeluria may be unrelated to the implant itself because there is such a small percentage of nickel within these implant alloys. Rather, this may be related to the use of stainless steel surgical instruments (which contain a relatively higher percentage of nickel in the alloy) or to metabolic changes associated with the surgery itself. Chronic elevations in serum titanium concentrations in subjects with well-functioning total joint replacements with titanium-containing components have also been reported (Fig. 11). These studies have also shown no measurable differences in urine titanium concentrations, serum aluminum concentrations, or urine aluminum concentrations. Serum and urine vanadium concentrations have not been found to be elevated in patients with total joint replacements, partially as a result of the technical difficulty associated with measuring the minute concentrations present in serum and urine.

Metal ion levels within the serum and urine of patients with total joint replacements can be affected by a variety of factors. For example, patients with total knee replacement components containing titanium-based alloy and carbon fiber-reinforced polyethylene wear couples demonstrated tenfold elevations in serum titanium concentration at an average of 4 years after implantation. Substantial serum titanium elevations have also been reported in patients with failed metal-backed patellar components where unintended metal/metal articulation was possible. In the latter example, some individuals with such failed implants had serum titanium levels up to 100 times higher than normal control values (Fig. 12). However, even among these patients, there was no elevation in serum or urine aluminum, serum or urine vanadium, or urine titanium levels. Mechanically-assisted crevice corrosion in patients with

modular femoral total hip replacement components has been correlated with elevations in serum cobalt and urine chromium (Fig. 13). Although it had been previously assumed that extensively porous coated cementless stems would give rise to higher serum and urine chromium concentrations (due to the larger surface area available for passive dissolution), a recent study suggested that fretting corrosion at the modular head/neck junction was the predominant source of disseminated chromium degradation products, giving rise to elevated serum and urine cobalt and chromium levels (Fig. 14).

A limited number of studies have been conducted examining metal levels in remote sites. Metal content analysis of homogenates of remote organs and tissue obtained postmortem from subjects with cobalt-base alloy total joint replacement components has indicated that significant increases in cobalt and chromium concentrations occur in the heart, liver, kidney, spleen, and lymphatic tissue. Similarly, patients with titanium-base alloy implants have demonstrated elevated titanium levels in the spleen. Spleen aluminum and liver titanium levels can also be markedly elevated in selected patients with failed titanium-alloy implants. Spectroscopic analysis of homogenated tissue digests can be a very sensitive method for metal detection; however, this must be supplemented with histologic and ultrastructural studies of the retrieved tissues to gain insight into the tissue localization and pathologic sequelae.

The toxicologic importance of the aforementioned find-

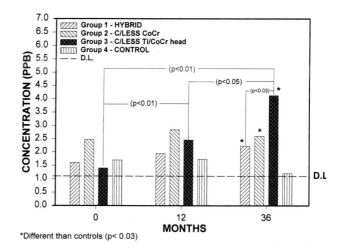

Figure 11

Bar graph showing the concentrations of titanium in the serum, in nanograms per milliliter (parts per billion), as a function of time in 3 groups of subjects with titanium-containing acetabular components (and femoral stems in Group 3) and a group of controls without implants. Note elevations in serum titanium in all three groups at 36 months after surgery. PPB = parts per billion; DL = detection limit; C/LESS = cementless. (Adapted with permission from Jacobs JJ, Skipor AK, Patterson LM, et al: Metal release in patients who have had a primary total hip arthroplasty: A prospective, controlled, longitudinal study. *J Bone Joint Surg* 1998;80A:1447–1458.)

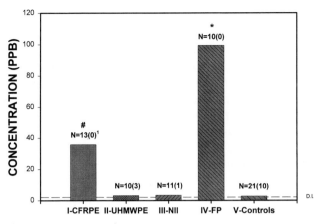

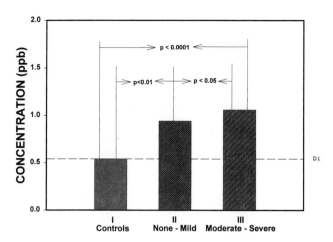

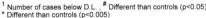

Figure 12

Bar graph of the mean concentrations of titanium in the serum, in nanograms per milliliter (parts per billion) in 4 subject groups with titanium-containing total knee replacement and a group of controls without implants. Note dramatic elevations in serum titanium in patients with failed patellar components (FP). PPB = parts per billion; DL= detection limit; CFRPE = carbon fiber reinforced polyethylene; NII = nitrogen ion-implanted.

Figure 13

Bar graph showing the concentrations of cobalt in the serum, as a function of the degree of corrosion at the femoral head/neck junction seen on retrieved implants. DL = detection limit.

ings is not known. Characterization of the bioavailability and bioreactivity of the metal species that have been released from prosthetic materials is the next step in this line of investigation. Central to this determination is the speciation of the metal moieties present in body fluids and tissue stores that result from implant degradation, because many of the metals used in implants have valence- and ligand-dependent toxicities in mammalian systems. Such studies represent an enormous challenge given the technical complexities of working with concentrations in the parts per billion range. Current technologic tools (graphite furnace Zeeman atomic absorption spectrophotometry and inductively coupled plasma-mass spectrometry) can measure only the concentration of the element, and provide no information on the chemical form or biologic activity. The information in the literature that describes the chemical form of the degradation products of metallic joint replacement prostheses is quite limited. Ultimately, specific toxicologic investigation of relevant chemical species (as identified by bioavailability studies) can be used in animal models and cell cultures to delineate the biologic effects of these degradation products. However, at the present time this information is not available.

Particle Release and Distribution

Particulate debris comprises a substantial portion of metal degradation products generated by joint replacement prostheses. The degradation products of ceramics and polymers

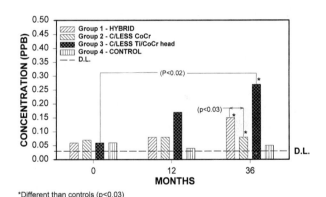

*Different than controls (p<0.03)

Figure 14

Bar graph showing the concentrations of chromium in the serum, in nanograms per milliliter (parts per billion), as a function of time in 3 groups of subjects with chromium-containing total hip replacement components and a group of controls without implants. At 36 months, all groups have elevated levels with respect to controls and cemented Co-Cr stems were associated with higher levels than extensively-coated Co-Cr cementless stems. The high levels in cementless titanium-alloy stems at 36 months is most likely due to corrosion of the Co-Cr modular head. DL = detection limit; C/LESS = cementless. (Adapted with permission from Jacobs JJ, Skipor AK, Patterson LM, et al: Metal release in patients who have had a primary total hip arthroplasty: A prospective, controlled, longitudinal study. J Bone Joint Surg 1998;80A:1447–1458.)

are exclusively in particulate form, as these classes of materials are generally considered insoluble in physiologic environments. Although polyethylene particles are generally recognized as the most prevalent particles in the periprosthetic milieu, metallic and ceramic particulate species are also present in variable amounts and may have important sequelae. When present in sufficient amounts, particulates generated by wear, corrosion, or a combination of these processes induce the formation of an inflammatory, foreign-body granulation tissue with the ability to invade the bone-implant interface. This may result in progressive, periprosthetic bone loss that threatens the fixation of both cemented and cementless devices, limiting the survivorship of total joint replacement prostheses. Consequently, particulate wear debris of polymers, ceramics, and metal alloys used in prosthetic components has been the subject of intense study concerning its role in bone resorption and aseptic loosening.

Less attention has been focused on particles generated by corrosion, perhaps because evidence of macroscopic corrosion in the current generation of single-part components is rare. Recently, however, there have been numerous reports indicating that modular femoral total hip replacement components can undergo severe corrosion at the tapered interface between the head and neck. Several investigators have also observed that, as a result of this process, solid products of corrosion may form. The clinical significance of corrosion at the modular head/neck junction lies, in part, in the effects that solid corrosion products may have at the bone-implant interface. Fragments of these corrosion products increase the particulate burden within the joint and migrate along bone-implant interface membranes to sites remote from their origin (Fig. 15), thereby contributing to periprosthetic bone loss and aseptic loosening. Although there have been numerous investigations concerning the presence of particulate debris within the periprosthetic tissues, relatively little is known about the dissemination of wear debris beyond the local tissues. Indeed, particles thought to be generated by a prosthetic device have been previously reported in distant organs of only a few patients with orthopaedic implants. Identification of implant-generated wear debris in remote tissues can be difficult, even in regional lymph nodes, because of the coexistence of particles from other sources.

In a recent study, wear particles that had disseminated beyond the periprosthetic tissue were primarily in the submicron size range. Metallic wear particles were detected in the para-aortic lymph nodes in up to 70% of patients with total joint replacement components (Fig. 16). In some cases, these particles further disseminated to the liver or spleen where they were found within small aggregates of macrophages or as epithelioid granulomas throughout the organs (Fig. 17). Metallic particles in the liver or spleen were more prevalent in subjects with previously failed arthroplasties (88% of such cases) when compared with cases of well-functioning primary joint replacements (with an average of 17% incidence). Unlike polyethylene debris, metal particles can be characterized by electron microprobe

analysis, which allows identification of the composition of individual particles against a background of particles from environmental or iatrogenic sources other than the prosthetic components. Overall, the smallest particles identified by the microprobe were approximately 0.1 µm in diameter. However, it has been recently suggested that metallic wear debris may extend into the nanometer size range, meaning that alternative methods of specimen preparation and analytic instrumentation may be required to more fully define the burden of metallic wear particles in remote tissues.

Polyethylene particles also make up a substantial fraction of the disseminated wear particles in subjects with joint replacement components. Although the presence of larger (greater than 1 µm) polyethylene particles in lymph nodes, liver, and spleen can be confirmed by Fourier transform infrared spectroscopy microanalyses and/or microraman spectroscopy, finer size particles have so far precluded unequivocal identification. In these sites, differentiation from other birefringent endogenous and exogenous particles is impossible by polarized light microscopy alone. It is evident that dissemination of wear particles to liver, spleen, or abdominal lymph nodes can be considered a common occurrence in patients with a total hip or knee replacement.

Mechanisms of Particle Transport

Variables influencing accumulation of wear debris in remote organs are not clearly identified. When the magnitude of particulate debris generated by a prosthetic device is increased, it seems likely that a corresponding elevation in both the local and systemic burden of particles may be

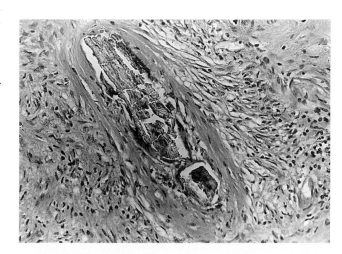

Figure 15

Light micrograph of chromium orthophosphate hydrate-rich corrosion products measuring approximately 350 µm in aggregate in a hip joint pseudocapsule from a patient with corrosion of the modular head-neck couple of the femoral component. The pale, translucent, and nonbirefringent particles are associated with elongated giant cells and macrophages (hematoxylin & eosin, × 250). (Adapted with permission from Jacobs JJ, Gilbert JL, Urban RM (eds): *Advances in Operative Orthopaedics*. St. Louis, MO, Mosby, 1994, Vol 2, p 300.)

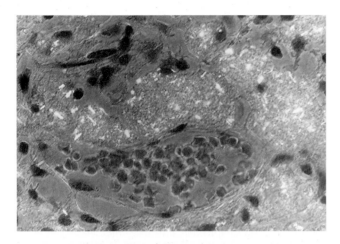

Figure 16

Polarized light micrograph of an abdominal para-aortic lymph node from a patient with total hip arthroplasty with multiple revision procedures for aseptic loosening. An abundance of birefringent polyethylene particles are seen within macrophages (hematoxylin & eosin, × 160).

expected. Thus, component loosening seems an obvious factor for increasing systemic exposure to particles. The duration of implantation is another likely factor important in determining both the cumulative amount of particulate debris generated and dissemination to remote organs. The modular design of contemporary hip and knee replacement prostheses provides the potential for increased generation of metallic and polymeric debris. Modular head/neck junctions, screw/component interfaces, and wire and cable systems used in bony fixation all contribute to the systemic burden of wear and metallic corrosion particles.

Lymphatic transport is thought to be a major route for dissemination of wear debris. Wear particles may migrate via perivascular lymph channels as free or as phagocytosed particles within macrophages. Within the abdominal para-aortic lymph nodes the majority of disseminated particles are submicron in size; however, metallic particles as large as 50 μm and polyethylene particles as large as 30 μm also have been identified. Within the liver and spleen, the maximum size of metallic wear particles is nearly an order of magnitude less than that in lymph nodes, indicating that there may be additional stages of filtration downstream or that there may be alternate routes of particle migration. Hematogenous dissemination of wear debris is also thought to occur. Transport of particles to remote bone marrow by circulating monocytes or by entry of small particles directly into the bloodstream has been hypothesized and may be important in the migration of particles to end organs.

Concurrent disease is another possible factor influencing systemic dissemination of wear particles. Diseases that cause obstruction of lymph flow, such as metastatic tumor, or generalized disturbances of circulation, such as chronic congestive heart failure and diabetes, may be expected to decrease particle migration to remote organs. A clear understanding of the effects of concurrent disease state on the dissemination of particulate debris will require future large-scale investigations.

The clinical significance of orthopaedic wear debris accumulation at remote sites has been understood based for the most part on examination of lymph node biopsy specimens obtained at revision surgery or obtained for cancer staging in patients in whom replacement arthroplasty had been previously performed. Numerous case reports document

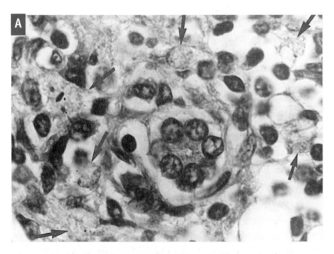

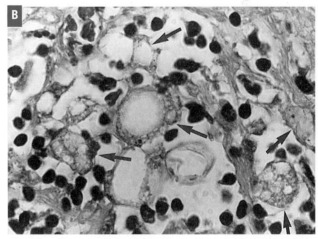

Figure 17

Metal alloy particles within macrophages were found in the portal tracts of the liver of patients with total joint replacement components. **A,** Light micrograph showing several pale staining, vacuolated macrophages (*arrows*) containing minute titanium particles as determined by electron microprobe analysis. The macrophages surround a bile duct in the liver of a patient with revision total hip arthroplasty. In this case, recurrent dislocation had resulted in severe wear of the titanium acetabular shell. The metallic particles were as large as 6 μm, but most were less than 1 μm in size (hematoxylin & eosin, × 1,250). **B,** Light micrograph of macrophages (*arrows*) containing cobalt-chromium-molybdenum-alloy particles (as determined by electron microprobe analysis) in the portal tract of the liver of a patient who had hosted well-functioning, bilateral cemented total knee replacements for 15 years. Nearly all of the metallic particles were submicron in size (hematoxylin & eosin, ×1,250).

the presence of metallic, ceramic, and polymeric wear debris from hip and knee prostheses in regional and pelvic lymph nodes along with the findings of lymphadenopathy, gross pigmentation caused by metallic debris, fibrosis, lymph node necrosis, and histiocytosis, including complete effacement of nodal architecture. The inflammatory response to metallic and polymeric debris in lymph nodes has been demonstrated to include immune activation of macrophages and associated production of cytokines.

In the liver and spleen, as in the lymph nodes, cells of the mononuclear-phagocyte system may accumulate small amounts of a variety of foreign materials without apparent clinical significance. However, it is well established that heavy accumulation of exogenous particles can induce granulomas or granulomatoid lesions in the liver and spleen. Such lesions have been reported in association with inhalation of mineral dusts or agricultural fungicides containing copper sulfate; hematogenous dissemination of silicone from hemodialysis tubing; injection of silicone for cosmetic procedures; gold therapy for rheumatoid arthritis; fragmentation of silicone rubber aortic valve prostheses; the use of radiographic contrast materials; and injection of talc and other materials by intravenous drug abusers. It is likely that the inflammatory reaction to particles in the liver, spleen, and lymph nodes is modulated, as it is in other tissues, by material composition, size, number of particles, their rate of accumulation, duration that they are present, and the biologic reactivity of cells to these particles. Granulomatous lesions in the liver, spleen, and lymph nodes have been reported in response to heavy accumulation of metallic wear particles generated by joint replacement prostheses fabricated from either cobalt or titanium alloys. The implications of remote site accumulation with regard to systemic immune response require further study; however, accumulation of such debris in the spleen and lymph nodes may explain, in part, recent observations suggesting that circulating peripheral blood monocytes from patients with joint replacements are more reactive to particulate wear debris stimulation than monocytes from individuals without implants.

Hypersensitivity

Classification of Immune Response and Clinical Test Methods

Dermal hypersensitivity to metals is fairly common, affecting about 10% to 15% of the population. The term "hypersensitivity" refers to the induction of the immune system by a "sensitizer." This response can be humoral (initiated by antibody or formation of antibody-antigen complexes), taking place within minutes (type I, II, and III reactions), or cell-mediated (a delayed-type hypersensitivity [DTH] response) occurring over days (type IV). Despite the useful-ness of the classification scheme presented below, it is difficult to categorize an allergic response as purely of one type or another because of a large crossover of secondary effects. Although an "allergy" in the strictest sense refers only to immediate immune activation (seen in types I, II, and III), it is commonly used to imply both immediate and delayed types of hypersensitivity reactions.

Type I (immunoglobulin E-[IgE] mediated) humoral response is typified by IgE-induced degranulation of basophils or mast cells and the subsequent release of active pharmacologic agents on the surrounding tissue, causing primarily vasodilatation, increased vascular permeability, and smooth muscle contraction. Typical manifestations include systemic anaphylaxis, localized anaphylaxis, hay fever, asthma, hives, and eczema. Type II (antibody-mediated) hypersensitivity is characterized by antibody-mediated activation of the complement system or cytotoxic cells. Type III (immune complex-mediated) involves locally high concentrations of antibody-antigen complexes resulting in local mast cell degranulation (increasing vascular permeability) and chemotactically-activated neutrophils. This "arthrus" reaction causes local accumulation of fluids (edema) and red blood cells (erythema). A mild reaction is marked by redness and swelling, and more severe reactions are characterized by tissue necrosis, caused by neutrophilic release of lytic enzymes in response to the immune complexes.

Type IV DTH is immune cell-mediated. Hypersensitivity reactions observed with orthopaedic implants (metal sensitivity or metal allergy) are generally associated with this type of response. Antigen-sensitized T lymphocytes release various cytokines, which results in the accumulation and activation of macrophages. Only 5% of the participating cells are antigen-specific T lymphocytes (T-DTH cells) within a fully developed DTH response. The majority of DTH participating cells are macrophages. There are basically 3 phases of a DTH response. The first phase is characterized by at least a 1- to 2-week exposure to the offending antigen. During this phase, there is antigen-induced proliferation of specific T cells. The second, or effector, phase is initiated by contact of sensitized T cells with antigen. In this phase, the antigen-activated T cells are termed T-DTH cells and secrete a variety of cytokines that recruit and activate macrophages, monocytes, neutrophils, and other inflammatory cells. These released cytokines include interleukin-3 (IL-3) and granulocyte/monocyte colony stimulating factor (GM-CSF), which promote hematopoiesis of granulocytes; monocyte chemotactic activating factor, which promotes chemotaxis of monocytes toward areas of DTH activation; interferon-γ and tumor necrosis factor-β (TNF-β), which produce a number of effects on local endothelial cells facilitating cellular extravasation; and migration inhibitory factor (MIF), which inhibits the migration of macrophages away from the site of a DTH reaction. Activation, infiltration, and eventual inhibition of migration of macrophages is the third phase of the DTH response. Activated macrophages, because of their increased ability to present class II major histocompatability complex molecules and IL-1, can trigger the activation of more T-DTH cells, which in turn activate more macrophages, which activate more T-DTH cells, and so on. This DTH self-perpetuation response can create extensive tissue damage.

Delayed (type IV) hypersensitivity reactions may be induced by the ionic degradation products of metal implants, which can function as haptenic moieties in a complex formed with endogenous proteins. This may lead to specific responses, such as severe dermatitis, urticaria, and/or vasculitis. Metals implicated as sensitizers are nickel, cobalt, chromium, and, to a lesser extent, tantalum, vanadium, and beryllium. Although controversial, some case reports have implicated titanium as a sensitizer. The most common sensitizers, in descending order, are nickel, cobalt, and chromium. The amounts of these metals found in medical grade alloys are shown in Table 3.

Dermal contact and ingestion of metals have been widely documented to cause immune reactions. Most typically, these take the form of skin lesions manifesting as hives, eczema, redness, and itching. Furthermore, growing numbers of case reports link immune reactions to adverse performance of metallic cardiovascular, orthopaedic, plastic surgical, and dental implants.

Testing for metal allergy has historically been conducted using either skin testing (patch testing or intradermal testing) and/or in vitro leukocyte migration inhibition testing (termed leukocyte inhibitory factor or MIF testing). Patch testing involves embedding an antigen in an adjuvant and exposing this to the skin by means of an affixed bandage or patch. After 48 to 96 hours of exposure, the skin reaction is graded on a scale of 1 to 4 with 4 being the most severe reaction, characterized by erythema and small, possibly encrusted, weeping blisters with discoloration of the skin. In vitro blood testing for delayed hypersensitivity was first used in 1928 to show tuberculin-induced migration inhibition of white blood cells. Subsequently, many experimental methods have been used to determine migration inhibition

behavior of leukocytes after exposure to a suspected antigen. In the 1960s, capillary tube techniques were used to detect leukocyte migration, which appears as fanlike areas of cells traversing the mouth of the tube. Other techniques developed in the 1970s, such as observing leukocyte migration under agarose gels and across chambers separated by membranes, have remained popular.

Metal Sensitivity in Patients With Surgical Implants

The first apparent association of eczematous dermatitis (skin rash with redness and weeping blisters) with metallic orthopaedic implants was reported in 1966 by Foussereau and Lauggier. In the following years there were a number of case reports linking eczematous reactions of patients with implants to metal sensitivity (particularly to nickel). In these cases, the eczematous reactions abated when the implant was removed. Investigations of orthopaedic implant-related metal sensitivity gained popularity in the 1970s when several "failures" of total hip prostheses with metal-on-metal bearing surfaces were reported to be associated with metal allergy. Among patients with loose implants, most (approximately 64%) tested positive for metal sensitivity (with patch testing), whereas no patients with well-fixed implants were positive. There was a 25% greater incidence of metal sensitivity associated with metal-on-metal bearing surfaces than with metal/UHMWPE bearing couples (Fig. 18). Interest in this association intensified, prompting similar investigations in the late 1970s and early 1980s.

Data from numerous investigations regarding the prevalence of metal sensitivity, albeit with heterogeneous patient populations and testing methodologies, have been compiled (Figs. 19, 20, and 21). The combined results of approximately 50 studies show that the prevalence of metal sensitivity among the general population is about 10% to 15%, with nickel sensitivity the highest (about 14%) (Fig. 19). The cross reactivity of these antigens is high, with cross reactiv-

Table 3

Weight Percent of Different Metals Within 3 Common Alloys

Alloy	%Ni	%Co	%Cr	%Ti	%Mo	%Al	%V
Stainless Steel (F138)*	13–15.5	—	17–19	—	2–4	—	—
CoCrMo (F75)*	1 max	Bal	27–30	—	5–7	—	—
Ti-6Al-4V (F136)*	—	—	—	Bal	—	5.5–6.5	3.5–4.5

* Designation of the American Society for Testing and Materials (ASTM) specification.

(ASTM Annual Book of Standards, Vol 13.01, Medical Devices; Emergency Medical Services. American Society for Testing and Materials, West Conshohocken, PA, 1997). Bal = balance; 1 max = maximum 1%.

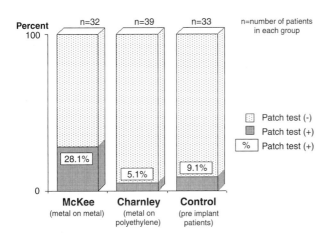

Figure 18

Comparison of metal sensitivity among patients with metal/metal and metal/polyethylene prosthesis. (Data from Benson et al, 1975.)

patients with metal implants. The increased prevalence of metal sensitivity among patients with loose prostheses has prompted the speculation that immunologic processes may be a factor in implant loosening. At this time, however, it is unclear whether metal sensitivity causes the increased prevalence of implant loosening or whether implant loosening results in the development of metal sensitivity. The lack of direct causal evidence implicating cell-mediated immune responses has led some researchers such as Carlsson to conclude "...implantation of cemented metal-to-plastic joint prosthesis is safe, even in the case of a preexisting metal allergy, from both an orthopaedic and a dermatologic point of view."

Other investigations have concluded that metal sensitivity can be a contributing factor to implant failure. Such cases include instances in which clinical immunologic symptoms lead directly to the need for device removal. In these cases, there have been reported reactions of severe dermatitis, urticaria, and/or vasculitis—all presumably linked to what has been reported as metallosis, excessive periprosthetic fibrosis, and muscular necrosis. The clinical observation of apparent immune sensitivity to metallic implants is not limited to orthopaedic surgery. Some case reports have suggested metal sensitivity to pacemakers, heart valves, dental implants, and other reconstructive devices. The temporal and physical evidence associated with such cases leaves little doubt that the phenomenon of metal-induced hypersensitivity does occur. It is currently unclear whether metal sensitivity exists only as an unusual complication in a few susceptible patients, or is more common and plays a

ity between nickel and cobalt being the most common.

The incidence of metal sensitivity among patients with both well and poorly functioning implants is approximately twice as high (about 25%) as that of the general population (Fig. 20). Furthermore, the prevalence of metal sensitivity among patients with a "failed" implant, compiled from 5 investigations (Fig. 21), is 50% to 60%, approximately 5 times the incidence of metal sensitivity found in the general population and more than double that of all

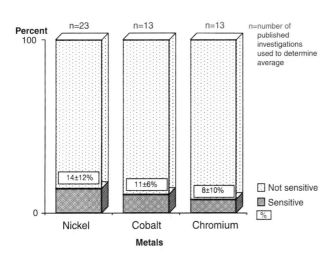

Figure 19

Percentages of metal sensitivity among the general population for nickel, cobalt, and chromium. Data compiled from numerous published reports and listed as the average ± standard deviation. (Data from Basketter et al, 1993.)

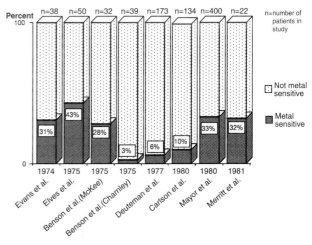

Figure 20

A compilation of 8 investigations in which patients with implants were tested for metal allergy by either patch or lymphocyte migration assay testing. Percentage is of patients with metal sensitivity after receiving a metal implant.

Carcinogenesis

The carcinogenic potential of the metallic elements used in orthopaedic implants continues to be of interest. This is particularly true for the metallic elements comprising joint replacement components. This is because cementless porous coated devices with large surface areas available for metal release are intended for implantation in younger, more active patient populations that may have life expectancies of more than 30 years. Animal studies have documented the carcinogenic potential of orthopaedic implant materials; small increases in rat sarcomas were noted to correlate with metal implants that had high cobalt, chromium, or nickel content. Furthermore, lymphomas with bone involvement were more common in rats with metallic implants. Implant site tumors—primarily osteosarcoma and fibrosarcoma—in dogs and cats have been associated with stainless steel internal fixation devices.

The occurrence of tumors at the site of metallic implants in humans has also been reported. In a review of the literature that included publications up until 1992, 24 cases of malignancies adjacent to a total joint replacement device were cited. The most common lesion was malignant fibrous histiocytoma. Given the large number of joint replacement devices inserted up until that time, this would appear to be a relatively small number of cases and would suggest that the occurrence of peri-implant malignancies may be coin-cidental. However, given that many such cases may go unreported and that these tumors may have relatively long latency periods, additional surveillance and broad-based epidemiologic studies are warranted.

There have been several human epidemiologic studies of systemic and remote cancer incidence in the first and second decades following total hip replacement. In 2 studies, slight increases in the risk of lymphoma and leukemia were found in patients who had a cobalt-alloy total hip replacement, particularly in those patients who had a metal-on-metal device. Larger, more recent studies have found no significant increase in leukemia or lymphoma; however, these studies did not include as large a proportion of subjects with metal-on-metal prostheses. Interestingly, some studies have demonstrated a decreased incidence of certain tumors, including breast carcinoma, in recipients of total joint replacements. Thus, it may be that there are constitutive differences in the populations with and without implants that are independent of the implant itself. This clearly confounds the interpretation of these epidemiologic investigations. The association of metal release from orthopaedic implants with carcinogenesis remains conjectural because causality has not been definitely established in human subjects. Longer-term epidemiologic studies are required to fully address this issue.

Summary

Implants fabricated from nonbiologic engineering materials continue to be crucial tools in the armamentarium of the orthopaedic surgeon. When used for the appropriate indications and when inserted with proper technique, these implants have been quite successful with few serious short- and long-term clinical sequelae. However, as more experience is gained with these devices, it is evident that, in certain situations, adverse biologic effects may occur that may compromise the clinical outcome. As advances in molecular biology and materials science are applied to the study of the host tissue response to implanted devices, it is likely that understanding of the critical determinants of implant biocompatability will increase, providing new opportunities for the development of improved biomaterials, novel diagnostic and screening modalities, and pharmacologic strategies to modify host response. Ultimately, this promises to lead to improved clinical outcomes for patients requiring implanted devices.

Acknowledgments

NIH grants AR16485, AR42862, AR 39310, Rush Arthritis and Orthopaedics Institute.

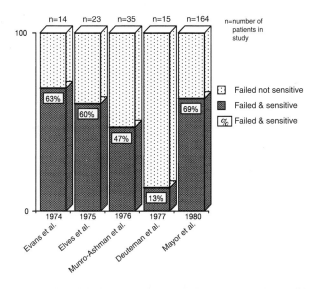

Figure 21

A compilation of investigations showing the percentage of metal sensitivity among patient populations with "failed" or "loose" implants.

Selected Bibliography

Local Effects

Acute/Subacute Response to Cemented Implants

Charnley J (ed): *Low Friction Arthroplasty of the Hip: Therapy and Practice*. Berlin, Germany, Springer-Verlag, 1979.

Jasty M, Maloney WJ, Bragdon CR, Haire T, Harris WH: Histomorphological studies of the long-term skeletal responses to well fixed cemented femoral components. *J Bone Joint Surg* 1990;72A:1220–1229.

Lindwer J, Van Den Hooff A: The influence of acrylic cement on the femur of the dog: A histological study. *Acta Orthop Scand* 1975;46: 657–671.

Petty W: The effect of methylmethacrylate on bacterial phagocytosis and killing by human polymorphonuclear leukocytes. *J Bone Joint Surg* 1978;60A:752–757.

Rhinelander FW, Nelson CL, Stewart RD, Stewart CL: Experimental reaming of the proximal femur and acrylic cement implantation: Vascular and histologic effects. *Clin Orthop* 1979;141:74–89.

Slooff TJ: The influence of acrylic cement. *Acta Orthop Scand* 1971;42:465–481.

Sund G, Rosenquist J: Morphological changes in bone following intramedullary implantation of methyl methacrylate: Effects of medullary occlusion. A morphometrical study. *Acta Orthop Scand* 1983;54:148–156.

Basic Biology of Cementless Fixation

Bilezikian JP, Raisz LG, Rodan GA (eds): *Principles of Bone Biology*. San Diego, CA, Academic Press, 1996.

Braun G, Kohavi D, Amir D, et al: Markers of primary mineralization are correlated with bone-bonding ability of titanium or stainless steel in vivo. *Clin Oral Implants Res* 1995;6:1–13.

Martin JY, Schwartz Z, Hummert TW, et al: Effect of titanium surface roughness on proliferation, differentiation, and protein synthesis of hyman osteoblast-like cells (MG63). *J Biomed Mater Res* 1995;29: 389–401.

Önsten I, Carlsson AS, Ohlin A, Nilsson JA: Migration of acetabular components, inserted with and without cement, in one-stage bilateral hip arthroplasty: A controlled, randomized study using roentgensterero-photogrammetric analysis. *J Bone Joint Surg* 1994;76A: 185–194.

Schwartz Z, Sela J, Ramirez V, Amir D, Boyan BD: Changes in extracellular matrix vesicles during healing of rat tibial bone: A morphometric and biochemical study. *Bone* 1989;10:53–60.

Schwartz Z, Swain L, Sela J, et al: In vivo regulation of matrix vesicle concentration and enzyme activity during primary bone formation. *Bone Miner* 1992;17:134–138.

Schwartz Z, Boyan BD: Underlying mechanism at the bone/biomaterial interface. *J Cell Biochem* 1994;56:340–347.

Sela J, Schwartz Z, Amir D, Swain LD, Boyan BD: The effect of bone injury on extracellular matrix vesicle proliferation and mineral formation. *Bone Miner* 1992;17:163–167.

Sela J, Shani J, Kohavi D, et al: Uptake and biodistribution of 99mtechnetium methylene-[32P] diphosphonate during endosteal healing around titanium, stainless steel and hydroxyapatite implants in rat tibial bone. *Biomaterials* 1995;161:1373–1380.

Shimizu T, Mehdi R, Yoshimura Y, et al: Expression of BMP, TNF, and their receptors in bone forming reaction after femoral marrow ablation. *Bone* 1998;22(suppl 3):19.

Sumner DR, Kienapfel H, Jacobs JJ, Urban RM, Turner TM, Galante JO: Bone ingrowth and wear debris in well-fixed cementless porous-coated tibial components removed from patients. *J Arthroplasty* 1995; 10:157–167.

Sumner DR, Turner TM: Animal models of bone ingrowth and joint replacement, in An YH, Friedman RJ (eds): *Animals Models in Orthopedic Research*. Boca Raton, FL, CRC Press, 1998.

Suva LJ, Seedor JG, Endo N, et al: Pattern of gene expression following rat tibial marrow ablation. *J Bone Miner Res* 1993;8:379–388.

Tanaka H, Barnes J, Liang CT: Effect of age on the expression of insulin-like growth factor-I, interleukin-6, and transforming growth factor-beta mRNAs in rat femurs following marrow ablation. *Bone* 1996;18:473–478.

Urban RM, Jacobs JJ, Sumner DR, Peters CL, Voss FR, Galante JO: The bone-implant interface of femoral stems with non-circumferential porous coating: A study of specimens retrieved at autopsy. *J Bone Joint Surg* 1996;78A:1068–1081.

Factors Inhibiting Cementless Fixation

Bragdon CR, Burke D, Lowenstein JD, et al: Differences in stiffness of the interface between a cementless porous implant and cancellous bone in vivo in dogs due to varying amounts of implant motion. *J Arthroplasty* 1996;11:945–951.

Callaghan JJ: The clinical results and basic science of total hip arthroplasty with porous-coated prostheses. *J Bone Joint Surg* 1993;75A: 299–310.

Callahan BC, Lisecki EJ, Banks RE, Dalton JE, Cook SD, Wolff JD: The effect of warfarin on the attachment of bone to hydroxyapatite-coated and uncoated porous implants. *J Bone Joint Surg* 1995;77A: 225–230.

Hollister SJ, Guldberg RE, Kuelske CL, Caldwell NJ, Richards M, Goldstein SA: Relative effects of wound healing and mechanical stimulus on early bone response to porous-coated implants. *J Orthop Res* 1996;14:654–662.

Qin YX, McLeod KJ, Guilak F, Chiang F-P, Rubin CT: Correlation of bony ingrowth to the distribution of stress and strain parameters surrounding a porous-coated implant. *J Orthop Res* 1996;14:862–870.

Ryd L, Albrektsson BE, Carlsson L, et al: Roentgen stereophotogrammetric analysis as a predictor of mechanical loosening of knee prostheses. *J Bone Joint Surg* 1995;77B:377–383.

Sumner DR, Turner TM, Pierson RH, et al: Effects of radiation on fixation of non-cemented porous-coated implants in a canine model. *J Bone Joint Surg* 1990;72A:1527–1533.

Turner TM, Urban RM, Sumner DR, Galante JO: Revision, without cement, of aseptically loose, cemented total hip prostheses: Quantitative comparison of the effects of four types of medullary treatment on bone ingrowth in a canine model. *J Bone Joint Surg* 1993;75A:845–862.

Factors Enhancing Cementless Fixation

Dalton JE, Cook SD, Thomas KA, Kay JF: The effect of operative fit and hydroxyapatite coating on the mechanical and biological response to porous implants. *J Bone Joint Surg* 1995;77A:97–110.

Kienapfel H, Griss P: Fixation by ingrowth, in Callaghan JJ, Rosenberg AG, Rubash HE (eds): *The Adult Hip*. Philadelphia, PA, Lippincott-Raven, 1998, pp 201–209.

Sumner DR, Turner TM, Purchio AF, Gombotz WR, Urban RM, Galante JO: Enhancement of bone ingrowth by transforming growth factor-beta. *J Bone Joint Surg* 1995;77A:1135–1147.

Chronic Response

Adaptive Remodeling

Chao EY, Aro HT, Lewallen DG, Kelly PJ: The effect of rigidity on fracture healing in external fixation. *Clin Orthop* 1989;241:24–35.

Cheal EJ, Hayes WC, White AA III, Perren SM: Stress analysis of compression plate fixation and its effects on long bone remodeling. *J Biomech* 1985;18:141–150.

Claes L: The mechanical and morphological properties of bone beneath internal fixation plates of differing rigidity. *J Orthop Res* 1989;7:170–177.

Huiskes R: Bone remodeling around implants can be explained as an effect of mechanical adaptation, in Galante JO, Rosenberg AG, Callaghan JJ (eds): *Total Hip Revision Surgery*. New York, NY, Raven Press, 1995, pp 159–171.

McAfee PC, Farey ID, Sutterlin CE, Gurr KR, Warden KE, Cunningham BW: The effect of spinal implant rigidity on vertebral bone density: A canine model. *Spine* 1991;16(suppl 6):S190–S197.

Maloney WJ, Sychterz C, Bragdon C, et al: Skeletal response to well fixed femoral components inserted with and without cement. *Clin Orthop* 1996;333:15–26.

Sumner DR: Bone remodeling of the proximal femur, in Callaghan JJ, Rosenberg AG, Rubash HE (eds): *The Adult Hip*. Philadelphia, PA, Lippincott-Raven, 1998, pp 211–216.

Sumner DR, Turner TM, Igloria R, Urban RM, Galante JO: Functional adaptation and ingrowth of bone vary as a function of hip implant stiffness. *J Biomech* 1998;31:909–917.

Sychterz CJ, Engh CA: The influence of clinical factors on periprosthetic bone remodeling. *Clin Orthop* 1996;322:285–292.

Turner TM, Sumner DR, Urban RM, Igloria R, Galante JO: Maintenance of proximal cortical bone with use of a less stiff femoral component in hemiarthroplasty of the hip without cement: An investigation in a canine model at six months and two years. *J Bone Joint Surg* 1997;79A:1381–1390.

Woo SL, Lothringer KS, Akeson WH, et al: Less rigid internal fixation plates: Historical perspectives and new concepts. *J Orthop Res* 1984;1:431–449.

Long-Term Biologic Response to Nonosseointegrated Cemented and Cementless Implants

Albrektsson T, Albrektsson B: Osseointegration of bone implants: A review of an alternative mode of fixation. *Acta Orthop Scand* 1987;58:567–577.

Goodman SB, Chin RC, Chiou SS, Schurman DJ, Woolson ST, Masada MT: A clinical-pathological-biochemical study of the membrane surrounding loosened and nonloosened total hip arthroplasties. *Clin Orthop* 1989;244:182–187.

Goodman SB, Fornasier VL, Kei J: The effects of bulk versus particulate polymethylmethacrylate on bone. *Clin Orthop* 1988;232:255–262.

Santavirta S, Gristina A, Konttinen YT: Cemented versus cementless hip arthroplasty: A review of prosthetic biocompatibility. *Acta Orthop Scand* 1992;63:225–232.

Osteolysis

Allen MJ, Myer BJ, Millett PJ, Rushton N: The effects of particulate cobalt, chromium and cobalt-chromium alloy on human osteoblast-like cells in vitro. *J Bone Joint Surg* 1997;79B:475–482.

Anthony PP, Gie GA, Howie CR, Ling RS: Localised endosteal bone lysis in relation to the femoral components of cemented total hip arthroplasties. *J Bone Joint Surg* 1990;72B:971–979.

Blaine TA, Pollice PF, Rosier RN, Reynolds PR, Puzas JE, O'Keefe RJ: Modulation of the production of cytokines in titanium-stimulated human peripheral blood monocytes by pharmacological agents: The role of cAMP-mediated signaling mechanisms. *J Bone Joint Surg* 1997;79A:1519–1528.

Chiba J, Rubash HE, Kim KJ, Iwaki Y: The characterization of cytokines in the interface tissue obtained from failed cementless total hip arthroplasty with and without femoral osteolysis. *Clin Orthop* 1994;300:304-312.

Collier JP, Surprenant VA, Jensen RE, Mayor MB, Surprenant HP: Corrosion between the components of modular femoral hip prostheses. *J Bone Joint Surg* 1992;74B:511–517.

Dean DD, Schwartz Z, Blanchard CR, et al: Ultrahigh molecular weight polyethylene (UHMWPE) particles have direct effects on proliferation, differentiation, and local factor production of MG63 osteoblast-like cells. *J Orthop Res* 1999;17:9–17.

Dean DD, Schwartz Z, Liu Y, et al: The Effect of UHMWPE wear debris on MG63 osteosarcoma cells in vitro. *J Bone Joint Surg* 1999;81A:452–461.

Gilbert JL, Buckley CA, Jacobs JJ: In vivo corrosion of modular hip prosthesis components in mixed and similar metal combinations: The effect of crevice, stress, motion, and alloy coupling. *J Biomed Mater Res* 1993;27:1533–1544.

Glant TT, Jacobs JJ, Molnar G, Shanbhag AS, Valyon M, Galante JO: Bone resorption activity of particulate-stimulated macrophages. *J Bone Miner Res* 1993;8:1071–1079.

Glant TT, Jacobs JJ: Response of three murine macrophage populations to particulate debris: Bone resorption in organ cultures. *J Orthop Res* 1994;12:720–731.

Goldring SR, Schiller AL, Roelke M, Rourke CM, O'Neil DA, Harris WH: The synovial-like membrane at the bone-cement interface in loose total hip replacements and its proposed role in bone lysis. *J Bone Joint Surg* 1983;65A:575–584.

Goodman SB: The effects of micromotion and particulate materials on tissue differentiation: Bone chamber studies in rabbits. *Acta Orthop Scand Suppl* 1994;258:1–43.

Goodman SB, Fornasier VL, Lee J, Kei J: The histological effects of the implantation of different sizes of polyethylene particles in the rabbit tibia. *J Biomed Mater Res* 1990;24:517–524.

Goodman SB, Huie P, Song Y, et al: Loosening and osteolysis of cemented joint arthroplasties: A biologic spectrum. *Clin Orthop* 1997;337:149–163.

Goodman SB, Knoblich G, O'Connor M, Song Y, Huie P, Sibley R: The heterogeneity in cellular and cytokine profiles from multiple samples of tissue surrounding revised hip prostheses. *J Biomed Mater Res* 1996;31:421–428.

Goodman S, Wang J-S, Regula D, Aspenberg P: T lymphocytes are not necessary for particulate polyethylene-induced macrophage recruitment: Histologic studies of the rat tibia. *Acta Orthop Scand* 1994;65:157–160.

Horowitz SM, Rapuano BP, Lane JM, Burstein AH: The interaction of the macrophage and the osteoblast in the pathophysiology of aseptic loosening of joint replacements. *Calcif Tissue Int* 1994;54:320–324.

Howie DW, Vernon-Roberts B, Oakeshott R, Manthey B: A rat model of resorption of bone at the cement-bone interface in the presence of polyethylene wear particles. *J Bone Joint Surg* 1988;70A:257–263.

Jacobs JJ, Shanbhag A, Glant TT, Black J, Galante JO: Wear debris in total joint replacements. *J Am Acad Orthop Surg* 1994;2:212–220.

Jiranek W, Jasty M, Wang JT, et al: Tissue response to particulate polymethylmethacrylate in mice with various immune deficiencies. *J Bone Joint Surg* 1995;77A:1650–1661.

Jiranek WA, Machado M, Jasty M, et al: Production of cytokines around loosened cemented acetabular components: Analysis with immunohistochemical techniques and in situ hybridization. *J Bone Joint Surg* 1993;75A:863–879.

Jones LC, Hungerford DS: Cement disease. *Clin Orthop* 1987;225:192–206.

Lee SH, Brennan FR, Jacobs JJ, Urban RM, Ragasa DR, Glant TT: Human monocyte/macrophage response to cobalt-chromium corrosion products and titanium particles in patients with total joint replacements. *J Orthop Res* 1997;15:40–49.

Maloney WJ, Jasty M, Harris WH, Galante JO, Callaghan JJ: Endosteal erosion in association with stable uncemented femoral components. *J Bone Joint Surg* 1990;72A:1025–1034.

Maloney WJ, Jasty M, Rosenberg A, Harris WH: Bone lysis in well-fixed cemented femoral components. *J Bone Joint Surg* 1990;72B:966–970.

Maloney WJ, Peters P, Engh CA, Chandler H: Severe osteolysis of the pelvis in association with acetabular replacement without cement. *J Bone Joint Surg* 1993;75A:1627–1635.

Maloney WJ, Smith RL: Periprosthetic osteolysis in total hip arthroplasty: The role of particulate wear debris. *J Bone Joint Surg* 1995;77A:1448–1461.

Murray DW, Rushton N: Macrophages stimulate bone resorption when they phagocytose particles. *J Bone Joint Surg* 1990;72B:988–992.

Pollice PF, Silverton SF, Horowitz SM: Polymethylmethacrylate-stimulated macrophages increase rat osteoclast precursor recruitment through their effect on osteoblasts in vitro. *J Orthop Res* 1995;13:325–334.

Quinn J, Joyner C, Triffitt JT, Athanasou NA: Polymethylmethacry-late-induced inflammatory macrophages resorb bone. *J Bone Joint Surg* 1992;74B:652–658.

Santavirta S, Konttinen YT, Bergroth V, Eskola A, Tallroth K, Lindholm TS: Aggressive granulomatous lesions associated with hip arthroplasty: Immunopathological studies. *J Bone Joint Surg* 1990;72A: 252–258.

Schmalzried TP, Kwong LM, Jasty M, et al: The mechanism of loosening of cemented acetabular components in total hip arthroplasty: Analysis of specimens retrieved at autopsy. *Clin Orthop* 1992;274: 60–78.

Schmalzried TP, Jasty M, Harris WH: Periprosthetic bone loss in total hip arthroplasty: Polyethylene wear debris and the concept of the effective joint space. *J Bone Joint Surg* 1992;74A:849–863.

Shanbhag AS, Hasselman CT, Rubash HE: Inhibition of wear debris mediated osteolysis in a canine total hip arthroplasty model. *Clin Orthop* 1997;344:33–43.

Shanbhag AS, Jacobs JJ, Black J, Galante JO, Glant TT: Human mono-cyte response to particulate biomaterials generated in vivo and in vitro. *J Orthop Res* 1995;13:792–801.

Shanbhag AS, Jacobs JJ, Black J, Galante JO, Glant TT: Macrophage/particle interactions: Effect of size, composition and surface area. *J Biomed Mater Res* 1994;28:81–90.

Spector M, Shortkroff S, Hsu H-P, Lane N, Sledge CB, Thornhill TS: Tissue changes around loose prostheses: A canine model to investigate the effects of an anti-inflammatory agent *Clin Orthop* 1990;261: 140–152.

Wright TM, Goodman SB (eds): *Implant Wear: The Future of Total Joint Replacement*. Rosemont, IL, American Academy of Orthopaedic Surgeons, 1996.

Yao J, Cs-Szabo G, Jacobs JJ, Kuettner KE, Glant TT: Suppression of osteoblast function by titanium particles. *J Bone Joint Surg* 1997;79A: 107–112.

Yao J, Glant TT, Lark MW, et al: The potential role of fibroblasts in periprosthetic osteolysis: Fibroblast response to titanium particles. *J Bone Miner Res* 1995;10:1417–1427.

Remote and Systemic Effects

Metal Ion Release

Agins HJ, Alcock NW, Bansal M, et al: Metallic wear in failed titanium-alloy total hip replacements: A histological and quantitative analysis. *J Bone Joint Surg* 1988;70A:347–356.

Black J, Sherk H, Bonini J, Rostoker WR, Schajowicz F, Galante JO: Metallosis associated with a stable titanium-alloy femoral component in total hip replacement: A case report. *J Bone Joint Surg* 1990; 72A:126–130.

Brien WW, Salvati EA, Betts F, et al: Metal levels in cemented total hip arthroplasty: A comparison of well-fixed and loose implants. *Clin Orthop* 1992;276:66–74.

Dorr LD, Bloebaum R, Emmanual J, Meldrum R: Histologic, bio-chemical, and ion analysis of tissue and fluids retrieved during total hip arthroplasty. *Clin Orthop* 1990;261:82–95.

Jacobs JJ, Silverton C, Hallab NJ, et al: Metal release and excretion from cementless titanium alloy total knee replacements. *Clin Orthop* 1999;358:173–180.

Jacobs JJ, Skipor AK, Black J, Urban RM, Galante JO: Release and excretion of metal in patients who have a total hip replacement component made of titanium-base alloy. *J Bone Joint Surg* 1991;73A: 1475–1486.

Jacobs JJ, Skipor AK, Patterson LM, et al: Metal release in patients who have had a primary total hip arthroplasty: A prospective, controlled, longitudinal study. *J Bone Joint Surg* 1998;80A:1447–1458.

Jacobs JJ, Urban RM, Gilbert JL, et al: Local and distant products from modularity. *Clin Orthop* 1995;319:94–105.

Michel R, Nolte M, Reich M, Loer F: Systemic effects of implanted prostheses made of cobalt-chromium alloys. *Arch Orthop Trauma Surg* 1991;110:61–74.

Stulberg BN, Merritt K, Bauer TW: Metallic wear debris in metal-backed patellar failure. *J Appl Biomat* 1994;5:9–16.

Sunderman FW Jr, Hopfer SM, Swift T, et al: Cobalt, chromium, and nickel concentrations in body fluids of patients with porous-coated knee or hip prostheses. *J Orthop Res* 1989;7:307–315.

Urban RM, Jacobs JJ, Gilbert JL, Galante JO: Migration of corrosion products from modular hip prostheses: Particle microanalysis and histopathological findings. *J Bone Joint Surg* 1994;76A:1345–1359.

Wang JY, Wicklund BH, Gustilo RB, Tsukayama DT: Prosthetic metals impair murine immune response and cytokine release in vivo and in vitro. *J Orthop Res* 1997;15:688–699.

Particle Release and Distribution

Case CP, Langkamer VG, James C, et al: Widespread dissemination of metal debris from implants. *J Bone Joint Surg* 1994;76B:701–712.

Hicks DG, Judkins AR, Sickel JZ, Rosier RN, Puzas JE, O'Keefe RJ: Granular histiocytosis of pelvic lymph nodes following total hip arthroplasty: The presence of wear debris, cytokine production, and immunologically activated macrophages. *J Bone Joint Surg* 1996;78A: 482–496.

Jacobs JJ, Skipor AK, Urban RM, et al: Systemic distribution of metal degradation products from titanium alloy total hip replacements: An autopsy study. *Trans Orthop Res Soc* 1994;19:838.

Jacobs JJ, Urban RM, Wall J, Black J, Reid JD, Veneman L: Unusual foreign-body reaction to a failed total knee replacement: Simulation of a sarcoma clinically and a sarcoid histologically: A case report. *J Bone Joint Surg* 1995;77A:444–451.

Urban RM, Jacobs JJ, Tomlinson MJ, Gavrilovic J, Black J, Peoc'h, M: Dissemination of wear particles to liver, spleen and abdominal lymph nodes of patients with hip or knee replacement. *J Bone Joint Surg*, in press.

Hypersensitivity

Classification of Immune Response and Test Methods

Black J (ed): *Orthopaedic Biomaterials in Research and Practice.* New York, NY, Churchill Livingstone, 1988.

Kuby J (ed): *Immunology.* New York, NY, WH Freeman, 1992.

Metal Sensitivity in Patients With Surgical Implants

Benson MK, Goodwin PG, Brostoff J: Metal sensitivity in patients with joint replacement arthroplasties. *Br Med J* 1975;4:374–375.

Carlsson AS, Magnusson B, Moller H: Metal sensitivity in patients with metal-to-plastic total hip arthroplasties. *Acta Orthop Scand* 1980;51:57–62.

Deutman R, Mulder TJ, Brian R, Nater JP: Metal sensitivity before and after total hip arthroplasty. *J Bone Joint Surg* 1977;59A:862–865.

Elves MW, Wilson JN, Scales JT, Kemp HB: Incidence of metal sensitivity in patients with total joint replacements. *Br Med J* 1975;4:376–378.

Evans EM, Freeman MAR, Miller AJ, Vernon-Roberts B: Metal sensitivity as a cause of bone necrosis and loosening of the prosthesis in total joint replacement. *J Bone Joint Surg* 1974;56B:626–642.

Fisher AA: Allergic dermatitis presumably due to metallic foreign bodies containing nickel or cobalt. *Cutis* 1977;19:285–286.

Foussereau J, Laugier P: Allergic eczemas from metallic foreign bodies. *Trans St Johns Hosp Dermatol Soc* 1966;52:220–225.

Mayor MB, Merritt K, Brown SA: Metal allergy and the surgical patient. *Am J Surg* 1980;139:477–479.

Merritt K, Brown SA: Metal sensitivity reactions to orthopedic implants. *Int J Dermatol* 1981;20:89–94.

Merritt K, Rodrigo JJ: Immune response to synthetic materials: Sensitization of patients receiving orthopaedic implants. *Clin Orthop* 1996;326:71–79.

Munro-Ashman D, Miller AJ: Rejection of metal to metal prosthesis and skin sensitivity to cobalt. *Contact Dermatitis* 1976;2:65–67.

Carcinogenesis

Gillespie WJ, Frampton CM, Henderson RJ, Ryan PM: The incidence of cancer following total hip replacement. *J Bone Joint Surg* 1988;70B:539–542.

Gillespie WJ, Henry DA, O'Connell DL, et al: Development of hematopoietic cancers after implantation of total joint replacement. *Clin Orthop* 1996;329(suppl):S290–S296.

Jacobs JJ, Rosenbaum DH, Hay RM, Gitelis S, Black J: Early sarcomatous degeneration near a cementless hip replacement: A case report and review. *J Bone Joint Surg* 1992;74B:740–744.

Lewis CG, Sunderman FW Jr: Metal carcinogenesis in total joint arthroplasty: Animal models. *Clin Orthop* 1996;329(suppl):S264–S268.

Nyren O, McLaughlin JK, Gridley G, et al: Cancer risk after hip replacement with metal implants: A population-based cohort study in Sweden. *J Natl Cancer Inst* 1995;87:28–33.

Visuri T, Pukkala E, Paavolainen P, Pulkkinen P, Riska EB: Cancer risk after metal on metal and polyethylene on metal total hip arthroplasty. *Clin Orthop* 1996;329(suppl):S280–S289.

Waalkes MP: Metal carcinogenesis, in Goyer R, Klaassen CD, Waalkes MP (eds): *Metal Toxicology.* San Diego, CA, Academic Press, 1995.

Chapter 16

Growth and Metastasis of Musculoskeletal Tumors

Denis R. Clohisy, MD

This chapter at a glance

This chapter presents an introductory review of oncogenesis and tumor cell metastasis, the cell cycle, oncogenes and tumor suppressor genes, and chromosomal abnormalities and cancer.

Introduction

Techniques for diagnosing cancer are frequently ineffective; in some cases, a diagnosis is made only after a large tumor, which has metastasized, is discovered. With certain types of cancer, treatment is strictly palliative, and the majority of treatments do not provide a cure. Fortunately, potential new anticancer therapies are being developed. Therefore, it is important for clinicians to understand the biochemical and molecular mechanisms of oncogenesis and tumor cell metastasis. This chapter will present an introductory review of oncogenesis and tumor cell metastasis, the cell cycle, oncogenes and tumor suppressor genes, and chromosomal abnormalities and cancer.

The Cell Cycle

Cells progress through the cell cycle in a coordinated and controlled fashion. Their task is monumental, but it is achieved with astonishing speed and accuracy. To complete the cell cycle, 3 billion DNA base pairs must be copied and then sorted into 2 daughter cells.

Because cancer is a disease of the cell cycle, the rationale for many current and future cancer therapies is or will be based on the science of the cell cycle, which can be divided into 4 phases (Fig. 1): DNA synthesis and precise copying of cellular DNA (S phase), mitosis and separation of duplicate sets of DNA into daughter cells (M phase), and the gaps that separate them (G_1 and G_2). The S and M phases are functional phases; that is, changes occur in either the amount or distribution of DNA. During phases G_1 and G_2, cells are prepared for the S and M phases, respectively.

At any given point in time most normal cells are not passing through the cell cycle. These cells are either waiting to enter the cell cycle and are in a temporary noncycling state, G_0, or they are permanently incapable of dividing and have achieved terminal differentiation. In contrast, a significant portion of cancer cells are dividing at all times, and it is this feature that permits cancer cells to grow both at the site of the primary tumor and at distant sites of metastasis.

Genes regulate cell division by controlling the orderly progression of a cell from S phase to M phase. These genes encode specific proteins that assemble the machinery required for successful passage of a cell through the cell cycle.

Cyclins and Cyclin-Dependent Kinases

The key to initiation of cell division is stimulation of progression through G_1. This event is initiated by mitogenic stimuli and is carried out by interactions between distinct families of intracellular proteins. Mitogenic stimulation is typically provided by extracellular growth factors.

The binding of mitogenic growth factors to cell membrane receptors in G_1 cells initiates a cascade of orderly and tightly controlled intracellular events that enable cells to progress through the cell cycle. The key intracellular regulators of progression through the cell cycle are cyclins and cyclin-dependent kinases (CDKs). The G_1 cyclins include 3 D-type cyclins (D1, D2, and D3) and cyclin E. D-type cyclins are produced as long as growth factor stimulation persists. Their production occurs throughout the cell cycle, but peaks near the G_1-S phase transition (Fig. 2). Cyclin E, in contrast, is produced periodically but maximal levels of cyclin E occur at the G_1-S phase transition. The CDKs include CDK2, 4, and 6. Their defining property is that they require a cyclin partner for activation.

Cyclins alone cannot influence progression through G_1; they can only exert influence as activated holoenzymes. Formation of holoenzymes involves cyclins binding to CDKs, and activation requires phosphorylation of CDK within the cyclin/CDK complex (Fig. 3). D-type cyclins and cyclin E form holoenzymes with different CDKs. D-type cyclins form holoenzymes by binding to CDK4 and CDK6, and cyclin E forms a holoenzyme by binding to CDK2 (Fig. 2). Phosphorylation (activation) of CDK is performed by CDK-activating kinase (CAK). This enzyme uses cyclin E-bound CDK2 and cyclin D-bound CDK4 (or 6) as the substrate for phosphorylation. Having recognized the cyclin-bound CDK substrate, CAK directs phosphorylation of a single threonine on CDK. Activated (phosphorylated) CDK then directs a plethora of intracellular events that guide the cell through G_1 phase to S phase.

Activated cyclins direct progression through all phases of the cell cycle. Just as G_1 cyclins (D cyclins and E) direct pro-

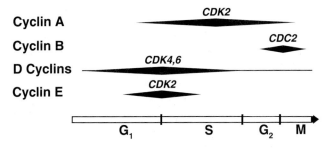

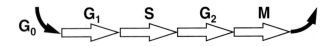

Figure 1

Phases of the cell cycle. G_0 = non-cycling state, G_1 = preparing for S phase, S = DNA replication, G_2 = preparing for M phase, M = segregation of duplicate sets of DNA.

Figure 2

Cyclin expression during the cell cycle and corresponding cyclin-dependent kinases. Cyclins A, B, E, and D type are listed with expression throughout the cell cycle and appropriate matching cyclin-dependent kinases (CDK or CDC) provided.

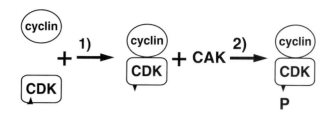

Figure 3

Cyclin/cyclin dependent kinase (CDK) complex activation (phosphorylation). Step 1 — formation of cyclin/CDK complex exposes threonine (t). Step 2 — cyclin-activating kinase (CAK) phosphorylates CDK at a threonine site.

gression through G_1 phase, mitotic cyclins direct progression through the S and G_2 phases. Mitotic cyclins are cyclins A and B. Cyclin A is predominant in S phase, and to a lesser degree, in M phase, and cyclin B is predominant during G_2 (Fig. 2). Both the mitotic cyclins, A and B, are rapidly degraded during S phase. Like the G_1 cyclins, the mitotic cyclins bind protein kinases to form holoenzymes. Cyclin A forms a holoenzyme by binding to CDK2, and cyclin B forms a holoenzyme by binding to the CDK-designated CDC2. Cyclin A-bound CDK4 and cyclin B-bound CDC2 are then activated by CAK-directed phosphorylation (Fig. 3).

Passage of a cell through the cell cycle is dependent on CAK-directed activation (phosphorylation) of CDKs within the cyclin/CDK complex. Activation of CDKs can be influenced at several different points in the cell cycle. Four well-characterized points of regulation are cyclin synthesis/degradation, cyclin/CDK complex formation, CAK activation of CDK, and CDK inhibition by CDK inhibitors.

Protein Targets for Cyclin/CDK Holoenzymes

Activated cyclin/CDK complexes exert their biologic activity by phosphorylating target proteins. Many proteins have been proposed as targets of different cyclin/CDK holoenzymes and they can be separated into proteins that encourage or inhibit progression through the cell cycle. Two of the most widely studied proteins that are targets of cyclin/CDK complexes are pRb and p21.

pRb is the protein encoded by the retinoblastoma tumor suppressor gene. Unphosphorylated pRb is believed to be the active form of this protein, and conversion to the phosphorylated form (pRb-P) occurs in a cell cycle-dependent manner. Phosphorylation (inactivation) of pRb occurs during the G_1/S phase transition, and phosphorylation is performed by activated (phosphorylated) D-type cyclin/CDK complexes (Fig. 4). During late G_1 phase and early S phase these complexes phosphorylate pRb (pRb-P). This phosphorylation renders pRb inactive until late M phase, when pRb-P loses its phosphate and regains the ability to bind to

and inactivate S phase transcription factors. The phosphorylated and unphosphorylated forms of pRb have different properties. Unphosphorylated pRb blocks cells in G_1 phase by binding to a variety of transcription factors. In contrast, pRbP cannot bind such proteins and therefore permits cell passage through the cell cycle.

The most important family of proteins that bind to unphosphorylated pRb is the transcription factors known as E2F. E2F factors are responsible for transcription of a set of genes at the end of G_1 that are required for DNA synthesis. Unphosphorylated pRb prevents E2F-mediated activation of gene transcription by binding to E2F proteins during mid to late G. E2F factors are active, however, after they are released from pRb. Release of E2F from pRb follows phosphorylation of pRb by cyclin/CDK complexes and allows unbound E2F to activate genes that are required for DNA synthesis (Fig. 4).

The absence of pRb has been associated with the malignant phenotype. Because active (unphosphorylated) pRb binds (thus inactivates) transcription factors that are required for DNA synthesis, the retinoblastoma gene is considered to be a tumor suppressor gene. This gene is either absent or inactivated in many different cancers such as retinoblastoma, sarcomas, and small-cell lung carcinomas.

p21 protein is a CDKI and acts as a potent and universal inhibitor of CDK enzyme activity. Inactivation of CDKs by p21 occurs after CDKs have complexed with their corresponding cyclins. Inactivation of a cyclin/CDK complex requires binding of multiple p21 molecules to each cyclin/CDK complex. It is suspected that p21 coordinates the effects of cyclin/CDK complexes on cell cycle progression at the level of DNA replication and/or repair. This is based on the finding that p21-cyclin/CDK complexes bind to subunits of DNA polymerase.

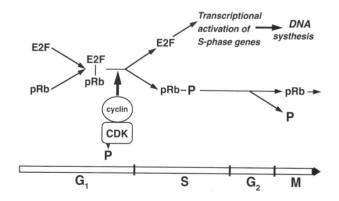

Figure 4

Interaction between the retinoblastoma protein and cyclin/cyclin dependent kinase (CDK) complexes. pRb = inactive retinoblastoma protein; pRb-P-active (phosphorylated) retinoblastoma protein; E2F = transcriptional factors.

Cell Cycle Checkpoints

To prevent genomic abnormalities such as aneuploidy, polyploidy, and chromosomal rearrangements during cell division, normal cells use 4 checkpoints during the cell cycle to survey cellular contents and to establish that progression through the cell cycle is occurring as planned. Two checkpoints survey mitotic spindle function and the duplication of spindle poles (centromere); the other 2 detect defects in DNA replication.

One checkpoint for DNA damage is at the G_1/S phase transition and the other is at the G_2/M phase transition (Fig. 5). The checkpoint controlling entry into S phase prevents the cell from replicating damaged DNA. Although all the details of the cellular mechanisms that block progression at the G_1/S phase checkpoint have not been elucidated, several critical observations have been made. Targets for the G_1/S phase checkpoints are CDKs that are part of cyclin/CDK complexes that formed early in the cell cycle. The components of the cyclin/CDK complexes that are involved include cyclins D, E, and A and CDKs 2, 4, and 6. Cells with DNA damage at the G_1/S phase checkpoint rapidly increase their levels of TP53 protein. When problems at the G_1/S phase checkpoint are detected, the TB53 protein enters the scene and inactivates cyclin/CDK complexes, whose influences are required for progression into S phase. The increase in levels of the TP53 protein occurs through posttranscriptional mechanisms and results in transcriptional activation of several TP53-dependent genes. Transcriptional activation of these genes leads to either cellular arrest in G_1 or to programmed cell death (apoptosis).

Loss of the G_1/S phase checkpoint may lead to malignancy. When functioning properly, the G_1/S phase checkpoint prevents cells with damaged DNA from progressing through the cell cycle and thus functions as a "cancer prevention" tool. Unfortunately, some cells with damaged DNA may progress through the G_1/S phase checkpoint. Progression of such a cell through the G_1/S phase checkpoint can lead to genomic instability, inappropriate surveillance of genetically damaged cells, and evolution of cells to malignancy. The majority of evidence linking loss of the G_1/S phase checkpoint to malignancy is derived from studying cancer and mutations of the TP53 gene. Chromosomal analysis has revealed that the TP53 gene is commonly mutated in human cancers. Aneuploidy is common on TP53 mutant cells and gene products of several DNA cancer viruses alter the function of the TP53 protein. When TP53 is not functioning, then tumor suppression is lost and the G_1/S phase checkpoint is also lost.

The G_2/M phase checkpoint involves surveillance of cells just before entry into M phase (Fig. 5). Transition of G_2 cells into M phase is prevented when DNA damage and incompletely replicated DNA are detected, and this checkpoint prevents chromosomal replication if the chromosome is not intact. One double-strand break in the DNA will activate this checkpoint and prevent progression to mitosis. The mechanism for cellular regulation of the G_2/M phase checkpoint has not been completely identified and is not understood as clearly as the mechanisms controlling the G_1/S phase checkpoint. The feedback loop controlling this checkpoint appears to target the CDC2 kinase in late G_2 and involves keeping the cyclin B/CDC2 complex in an inactive state, thus blocking its permissive effect on entry into M phase. It is generally believed that defects in regulation at

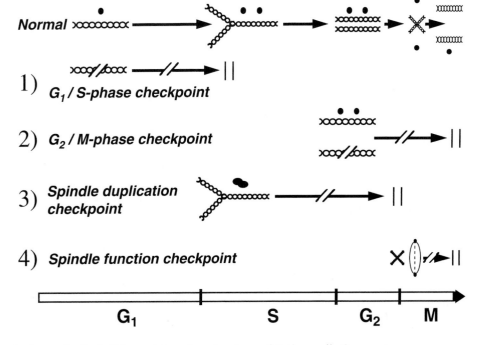

Figure 5

Cell cycle checkpoints. Normal DNA replication, mitotic spindle duplication, and separation into daughter cells are shown in 4 cell cycle checkpoints.

this checkpoint may also contribute to the evolution of malignancy.

The checkpoint that evaluates centromere duplication occurs at the G_2/M phase transition, and detection of defective centromere duplication arrests progression through the cell cycle at this point (Fig. 5). The checkpoint that evaluates the function of the mitotic spindle occurs during mitosis at metaphase. If 1 or more chromosomes are not positioned appropriately at the metaphase plate, then segregation of chromosomes at the metaphase-anaphase transition is prevented (Fig. 5).

DNA Synthesis

Several biochemical events must occur to permit a cell to replicate its DNA efficiently and accurately. These events not only direct synthesis of DNA but also safeguard against the synthesis of inaccurate, injured, or incomplete DNA. The original strands of DNA are used as templates for placement of deoxyribonucleotides. The enzyme that directs deoxyribonucleotide assembly is DNA polymerase. This enzyme requires an RNA primer to begin DNA synthesis and it directs synthesis in a 5´ to 3´ direction. One strand is therefore replicated in a continuous fashion and the other strand is replicated discontinuously with fragment RNA primers. These primers are then reannealed and the open segments, with the exception of the open site at the 3´ end of the DNA template, are filled in with Okazaki fragments.

To protect against failed copy fidelity, the actions of DNA polymerases are linked to proofreading enzymes called exonucleases. Cell-directed DNA repair mechanisms may also be used to remove or repair mismatched DNA bases. To counteract incomplete replication, the open site at the 3´ end of the DNA template must be filled in. This filling-in is accomplished by activity of the telomere-telomerase system, and results in completion of the replication process. Telomeres are specific DNA sequences located on the ends of chromosomes. These sequences solve the end-replication problem by acting as templates for telomerase, an enzyme that lengthens telomeres and thus fills in the replication defect.

Oncogenes and Tumor Suppressor Genes

It is not known which gene alterations cause most cancers. Although many gene alterations are associated with cell transformation, few have been proven to be a direct cause of cancer. Attempts to decipher the role of cancer-associated gene alterations in cell transformation have led to classifying cancer-associated genetic events into those that encourage cell transformation (oncogenes) and those that inhibit cell transformation (tumor suppressor genes).

The identification and study of oncogenes have contributed greatly to the understanding of molecular regulation of both normal and neoplastic cells. Oncogenes were initially detected in experimental systems that studied viral-induced tumorigenesis in animals. Careful analysis of the genome of tumor-inducing viruses led to identification of transforming genes (oncogenes) within viral genomes. Viruses can gain or lose genetic material upon infection of a host cell, and it is believed that viruses copied genetic sequences from infected cells and then incorporated these sequences into their own genome. If the virus had copied a sequence (oncogene) that provided a survival advantage to cells that were subsequently infected, then the virus that had altered its genome with the oncogene had a survival advantage over the parent virus. As these viral oncogenes were discovered, it was predicted and later proved that they would be present in spontaneous human tumors of nonviral etiology.

The molecular biology of events that regulate cell proliferation, genomic stability, cell differentiation, and apoptosis has been largely revealed through the study of oncogenes and tumor suppressor genes. Defining the role of oncogenes and tumor suppression genes in normal cells led to understanding the role of growth factors, receptor tyrosine kinases, transcription factors, and DNA repair mechanisms in normal and cancerous cells.

Oncogenes and tumor suppressor genes play a role in the development of cancer in several primary musculoskeletal malignancies (sarcomas). The oncogene that has received the most attention in this regard is the *MDM2* gene and the tumor suppressor genes that clearly play a role in musculoskeletal oncogenesis are the retinoblastoma (*RB*) and *TB53* genes.

The *MDM2* gene and the protein that it encodes, MDM2, are uniquely expressed in a striking number of bone and soft-tissue sarcomas. Both amplified *MDM2* gene expression and increased levels of the MDM2 protein have been detected in approximately one third of sarcomas analyzed, including liposarcomas, malignant fibrous histiocytomas, and osteosarcomas. MDM2 protein has tumor growth-promoting influences through its effects on the TP53 protein. MDM2 protein binds to TP53 and, by virtue of this binding, prevents *TB53* from exerting its growth inhibitory effects. Therefore, by stopping TP53-mediated growth-inhibition, MDM2 has growth-promoting effects. The fact that *MDM2* gene and protein expression is significantly amplified in a substantial number of sarcomas suggests that this oncogene may contribute to the development of the malignant phenotype in many musculoskeletal cancers.

The tumor suppressor genes that have been closely associated with bone sarcomas are the *RB*, which was the first tumor suppressor gene identified, and the *TB53* gene. The *RB* gene was found to be mutated in the familial cancer retinoblastoma and was later determined to be absent or expressed at low levels in a variety of tumors, including osteosarcoma and carcinomas of the lung, bladder, and breast. The function of the Rb protein has already been described (Fig. 4). In summary, this protein exerts its action at the G_1/S phase checkpoint by inactivating cyclin/CDK complexes that are required for progression into S phase.

The *TB53* gene plays a role in oncogenesis of many malignant musculoskeletal tumors. Interestingly, this tumor suppressor gene is present in over 50% of cancers and is a defining characteristic of a hereditary cancer syndrome called the Li-Fraumeni syndrome. Cancers in which this tumor suppressor gene is absent or expressed at low levels include rhabdomyosarcoma, osteosarcoma, leukemias, melanoma, and carcinomas of the breast, lung, larynx, and colon.

Chromosomal Abnormalities and Cancer

Chromosomal abnormalities are the basis for the malignant phenotype. Some groups of malignancies, such as hematologic malignancies, have established chromosomal abnormalities that are responsible for or always associated with the malignant phenotype. Other groups of malignancies, such as solid tumors, have been shown, in a few specific instances, to have established chromosomal abnormalities. In evaluating and managing patients with hematologic malignancies, cytogenetic analysis of chromosomal abnormalities plays a pivotal role in determining the diagnosis and can provide useful information regarding prognosis. With solid tumors, cytogenetic analysis has not assumed a prominent role in diagnosis or prognosis. This can be attributed to technical difficulties in performing cytogenetic analysis as well as difficulties in interpretation of cytogenetic analysis that are unique to solid tumors. It is likely, however, that cytogenetic data will some day assume a prominent role in the diagnosis and management of solid tumors, including musculoskeletal tumors.

Nomenclature describing normal and pathologic chromosomes involves delineating the arms, region, and bands of chromosomal material. Each chromosome has a numeric assignment. Arms are either short arm (designated p) or long arm (designated q). Regions are subdivisions of each arm and they are designated numerically (1, 2, 3, etc), increasing in number as the region moves away from the centromere. Each region contains bands. These are also assigned numerically and their number increases as they move away from the centromere. An example of such nomenclature is 12q13, which describes the third band in the first region on the long arm of chromosome number 12 (Fig. 6).

Chromosomal abnormalities are described by providing the total chromosome number followed by the sex chromosomes. Gains or losses of whole chromosomes are denoted by + or - before the chromosome number. Gene translocations are designated with t. The genes involved in the translocation are indicated in the first set of brackets and the chromosomal description sites (breakpoints) are in the second set of brackets. A gene translocation between chromosomes 12 and 18 that exchanges chromosomes between the third band within the region closest to the centromere on the long arm of chromosome 12 and the first band within the region closest to the centromere on the short arm of chromosome 16 would be designated t(12;16)(q13;p11). This gene arrangement is seen in myxoid liposarcoma.

In some cancers, the chromosomal abnormalities that cause or are strongly suspected to cause the malignant phenotype have been identified. Identification of nonrandom chromosomal rearrangements in specific tumors has led to the identification of genes that are involved in oncogenesis. These rearrangements have been identified in the form of gene translocations, inversions, and deletions. Deletions simply represent loss of a gene, with the most common example being the loss of a tumor suppressor gene. Translocations and inversions are best described together as translocations.

Chromosomal translocations are the type of gene rearrangement most commonly associated with the malignant phenotype. Chromosomal translocation occurs when there is a break in 2 chromosomes and an exchange of chromosomal sequences between the chromosomes (Fig. 6). The site of breakage is called the breakpoint and the resulting chimeric gene represents fusion of the 2 genes at the site of the breakpoint, which produces a gene rearrangement. The transforming genes involved in chromosomal translocations have been shown to involve protein kinases, cell surface receptors, growth factor receptors, and transcription factors.

The most common chromosomal translocations in cancer cells involve transforming genes that encode transcription factors. Transcription factors are intracellular proteins that direct and/or maintain the differentiation of cells. These proteins are typically located within the nucleus and regulate expression of specific genes by binding to target DNA sequences. This regulation alters gene function either by deregulation of gene expression or by expression of a novel fusion protein. Gene rearrangements that result in deregulation can induce overexpression, underexpression, or inappropriate expression (expression in a cell type or tissue that does not ordinarily express the gene) of affected genes.

Expression of a novel protein, or fusion protein, can result from the positioning of coding sequences from 2 genes that are normally located on different chromosomes in continuous sequence. Fusion proteins can be responsible for the malignant phenotype and are tumor-specific, that is, they do not exist in nonmalignant cells. Thus, detection of the chimeric gene or the resultant fusion protein will establish a diagnosis of malignancy and pinpoint residual or recurrent disease.

Chromosome   # Translocation

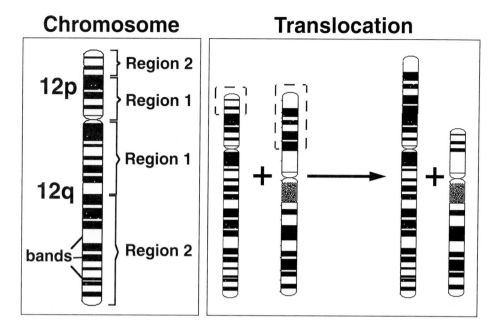

Figure 6

Chromosome nomenclature and gene translocation.

Gene rearrangements have been identified in several primary malignant musculoskeletal malignancies. Both soft-tissue and bone sarcomas have been shown to have highly specific gene translocations (Table 1). Three soft-tissue sarcomas that are known to have specific fusion genes are myxoid liposarcomas, synovial sarcomas, and rhabdomyosarcomas. Myxoid liposarcomas have a (12:16) (q13;p11) translocation. Synovial sarcomas have a (x:18) (p11;q11) translocation and some rhabdomyosarcomas have a (2:13)(q35-37;q14) reciprocal translocation. The one bone sarcoma known to have a specific fusion gene is Ewing's sarcoma. These malignancies are characterized by a (11:22)(q24;q12) translocation.

The chimeric genes identified in myxoid liposarcoma, synovial sarcoma, rhabdomyosarcoma, and Ewing's sarcoma are all suspected to involve transforming genes that encode for fusion-derived transcription factors. The t(12;16)(q13;p11) rearrangement found in many myxoid liposarcomas involves the *CHOP* gene at 12q13, its DNA binding site, and the *FUS* gene at 16p11. *FUS* encodes a transcription factor with a transactivation region. The resultant fusion protein (CHOP/*FUS*) contains the DNA-binding characteristics of *CHOP* and the transactivation region of *FUS*. The t(x:18)(p11;q11) rearrangement in synovial sarcoma involves the *SSX* gene at p11 on the X chromosome and the *SYT* gene at 18q11. The resultant fusion protein (*SSX*/SYT) is believed to be a novel chimeric transcription factor. The t(2:13)(q35-37;q14) rearrangement seen in rhabdomyosarcoma is a reciprocal rearrangement that combines the *PAX3* homeobox gene (2q;35-37) and the *FKHR* gene (13q;14) to create a fusion gene (*PAX3/FKHR*) that encodes a unique fusion transcription factor. The t(11;22)(q24;q12) reciprocal rearrangement in Ewing's sar-

coma produces a fusion protein (EWS/FL11) with similar theoretical characteristics to the fusion protein that results from the gene rearrangements identified in myxoid liposarcomas. With the rearrangements in Ewing's sarcoma, the fusion transcription factor contains the transactivation domain of the *EWS* gene (22q12) and the DNA binding domain of the *FL11* gene (11q24).

Identification of tumor-specific gene translocations and the proteins encoded by these rearrangements will ultimately assist in the design of new cancer therapies. These therapies will underscore the fact that these novel proteins are only present on tumor cells and will deliver treatment targeted only at cells expressing the fusion gene.

Not all tumors that have recurring gene rearrangements are malignant. Recurring chromosomal abnormalities have been identified in benign fatty tumors. Benign tumors of fatty origin (lipomas) are usually karyotypically abnormal and commonly display 12q13-15 abnormalities. This chromosomal change has been shown to be the only genetic anomaly and therefore probably represents a primary genomic alteration.

Table 1
Gene Translocations and Sarcomas

Tumor	Rearrangement
Myxoid liposarcoma	t(12:16) [q13;p11]
Synovial sarcoma	t(x:18) [p11;q11]
Rhabdomyosarcoma	t(2:13) [q35-37;q14]
Ewing's sarcoma	t(11:22) [q24;q12]

Tumor Cell Metastases

Although the genetic basis for tumor development varies greatly between malignancies, the steps required for development of clinically relevant tumor metastases are similar for all tumors. For tumor cells to metastasize to bone and form clinically relevant tumors, malignant cells from the primary tumor must gain access to the vascular system, travel through the circulation, settle within the bone marrow space, induce bone resorption, and grow within bone. Thus, tumor cells must be capable of performing or inducing several basic, reproducible, biologic events: angiogenesis, invasion of soft tissues, and bone resorption.

Angiogenesis

Tumors develop in 2 phases: prevascular and vascular. The prevascular phase can exist for many years and is usually characterized by limited growth and few or no metastases. The vascular phase, in contrast, is characterized by rapid tumor growth, bleeding, and the potential for developing microscopic metastases.

The formation of blood vessels at the site of primary tumor cells is required for tumors to enter the vascular phase of development. In the absence of localized angiogenesis, tumor masses will outgrow their diffusible nutrient supply and will not reach a diameter greater than 2 mm (about 10^6 cells). After formation of vascular access to tumors, a conduit is established that removes toxic molecules, provides tumor cell access to the systemic circulation, and permits delivery of growth factors and matrix proteins to the tumor. These growth factors and matrix proteins are produced by the new capillary endothelium, direct tumor growth, and act in a paracrine fashion (Fig. 7) on tumor cells to direct their growth and invasion.

Physiologic formation of blood vessels involves matrix proteolysis and motility and proliferation of endothelial cells (Fig. 8). Proteolysis is necessary for endothelial cell degradation of and penetration through both the endothelial basement membrane and the perivascular stroma. This extracellular tissue degradation permits capillary sprout penetration into the extracellular matrix and lateral expansion of the capillary sprout within the stroma. Motility is required for endothelial cell chemotaxis away from the parent vessel toward the angiogenic stimulus, for endothelial cell migration through the perivascular stroma, and for endothelial cell alignment within the stroma to form a capillary sprout. Proliferation is needed to produce new endothelial cells to occupy the expanding microvascular network. The completion of these steps results in capillary sprouts that emanate from existing vessels and form in the direction of the source of angiogenic molecules. These capillary sprouts ultimately expand and, through morphogenesis, yield capillaries that provide an expanding blood supply to the area of stimulation.

Although the same triad of matrix proteolysis, endothelial cell motility, and endothelial cell proliferation that characterizes physiologic angiogenesis also characterizes tumor-associated angiogenesis, the difference between physiologic and tumor-associated angiogenesis is the regulation of the process. Normal angiogenesis is tightly regulated by a balance between positive and negative regulators, and

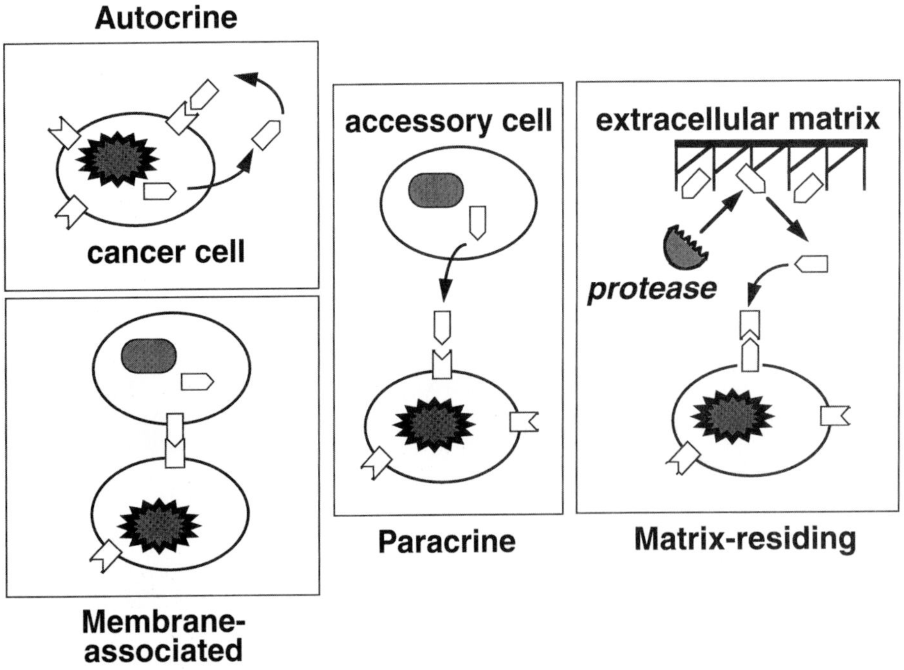

Figure 7

Mechanisms of growth factor or motility factor delivery to cancer cell.

endothelial cells can return to a nonangiogenic state when the angiogenic stimulus is removed. There do not seem to be functional differences between the molecules that influence normal and tumor-associated angiogenesis; that is, the regulators of tumor-induced angiogenesis are normal molecules. They are not molecules that have been modified secondary to a genetic, cancer-inducing mutation. Noncancer-associated endothelial cell proliferation and angiogenesis occur primarily in response to injury; after the response to injury is complete, endothelial cells return to a nonangiogenic state. Tumor-associated angiogenesis, in contrast, is either unregulated or autoregulated and therefore not subject to the checks and balances of physiologic angiogenesis. Endothelial cells in this milieu do not revert back to a nonangiogenic state, and therefore, uncontrolled and unregulated angiogenesis occurs.

The degree of angiogenesis at tumor sites is determined by the net result of factors that stimulate (angiogenic) and those that inhibit (antiangiogenic) the formation of new blood vessels. The balance between angiogenic and antiangiogenic growth factors determines the angiogenic phenotype. Progression to the angiogenic phenotype requires that tumor cells in the prevascular phase be exposed to both an increase in angiogenic factors and a decrease in antiangiogenic factors.

Angiogenic and antiangiogenic factors can originate from several different sources, including tumor cells, accessory cells, or mobilized components of the extracellular matrix. Accessory cells may include the new capillary endothelial cells or normal host cells (such as macrophages) that have been attracted to the tumor. Factors can be presented in soluble, membrane-associated, or matrix-sequestered forms (Fig. 7) and they can influence one or more of the steps in the triad (motility, proteolysis, and growth) of endothelial cell activity during angiogenesis.

Many angiogenic stimuli that influence tumor-associated angiogenesis have been identified. Growth factors produced at sites of tumor-induced angiogenesis and known to stimulate endothelial cell proliferation include glycoproteins from the fibroblast growth factor family, vascular endothelial cell growth factor, vascular permeability factor, angiogenin, epidermal growth factor (EGF), transforming growth factor-alpha (TGF-α), transforming growth factor-beta (TGF-β), and tumor necrosis factor-alpha (TNF-α).

Many antiangiogenic stimuli that influence tumor-associated angiogenesis have been identified. Growth factors that inhibit endothelial cell proliferation include platelet factor 4, angiostatin, and thrombospondin. Platelet factor 4 inhibits endothelial cell proliferation by blocking the mitogenic action of glycoproteins from the fibroblast growth factor family. Thrombospondin and angiostatin are secreted by normal cells and inhibit angiogenesis. Production of thrombospondin and angiostatin is downregulated as "normal" cells assume the transformed phenotype. It is suspected that thrombospondin is under control of the *TP53* tumor-suppressor gene. This suspicion is based on the finding that fibroblasts from patients with Li-Fraumeni syndrome who have a single, mutated copy of the *TP53* gene have decreased production of thrombospondin and increased angiogenic activity.

Proteinases produced at sites of vascular phase tumors can promote or inhibit matrix proteolysis. Proteinases produced at sites of vascular phase tumors and known to stimulate degradation of the endothelial cell basement membrane and/or the extracellular matrix include members of the matrix metalloproteinase family, especially type IV collagenase and several serine proteinases. Proteinases that block degradation of the endothelial basement membrane and/or the extracellular matrix include general metalloproteinase inhibitors, inhibitors of type IV collagenase, and serine proteinase inhibitors. Cartilage-derived growth factor has secondary effects that increase levels of tissue inhibitors of metalloproteinases (TIMPs). This growth factor exerts antiangiogenic activity by inhibiting tumor cell-secreted collagenase activity, which results in inhibition of matrix destruction and blocks endothelial cell motility.

The importance of angiogenesis to the metastatic process is highlighted by the finding that with some cancers, there

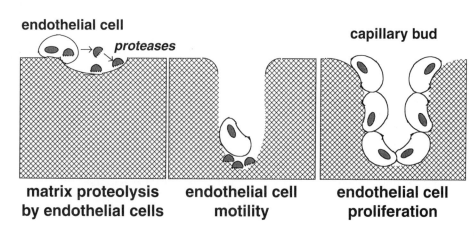

endothelial cell

proteases

capillary bud

matrix proteolysis by endothelial cells

endothelial cell motility

endothelial cell proliferation

Figure 8

Angiogenesis and the 3 phases of proteolysis, motility, and proliferation.

is an inverse relationship between the degree of vascularity and patient survival. This has been shown to be true with breast and prostate cancers, the 2 malignancies that most commonly metastasize to bone. When the degree of vascularity of primary tumors was quantified in patients with nonmetastatic breast cancer, it was determined that this variable was an independent predictor of long-term survival. That is, patients who had tumors with the most vascularity had a higher probability of developing distant metastases and higher probability of dying from their disease than patients who had tumors with lower levels of vascularity.

Invasion of Soft Tissue

Tumor cell invasion of stroma and basement membranes is required at both ends of the metastatic process. Invasion of tissue surrounding the primary tumor and penetration of adjacent blood vessels by tumor cells are both necessary steps to initiate tumor spread. Similarly, following the arrival of tumor cells in distant organs, attachment to target organs/tissues, penetration through blood vessel walls, and movement through the surrounding tissue must occur before a metastatic tumor deposit can be established.

Invasion of soft tissues involves 3 steps: attachment, matrix destruction, and migration. Tissue invasion by cancer cells uses the unique abilities of cancer cells to attach to components of the extracellular matrix, secrete extracellular matrix-degrading enzymes, and move through tissue. Without the ability to alter normal cell motility and to secrete matrix-degrading enzymes, cancer cells could not penetrate adjacent blood vessels or lymphatics and, as a result, cancer cells would not be capable of traveling to distant organs such as bone or lung.

It is attachment of tumor cells to the extracellular matrix that permits sensing, protrusion, burrowing, and traction through tissue at the site of the primary tumor. These attachments are transient and are dependent on rapid expression, turnover, and activation of cell surface proteins (receptors) that recognize and bind to specific elements of the extracellular matrix. One family of cell surface proteins that plays a critical role in tumor cell attachment is the integrin receptor family. These transmembrane receptors are heterodimeric molecules. They are composed of various a and b subunits with numeric designations ($a_{1,2,3,...}$ and $b_{1,2,3,...}$) and they bind the RGD (arginine-glycine-aspartic acid) peptide sequences of a variety of extracellular matrix molecules. The matrix molecules that integrin receptors recognize and bind to are ubiquitous in many tissues and include laminin, fibronectin, vitronectin, and various collagens. Integrins are essential molecules for attachment of metastatic tumor cells to bone and bone marrow. Breast cancer cells use the $\alpha_v\beta_3$ integrin (and surely others) to attach to bone, and experimental models have identified a_4b_1 as an important molecule for attachment of other metastatic cancer cells to bone.

Cancer cell secretion of extracellular matrix-degrading enzymes plays an irreplaceable role in invasion. The basement membrane and the interstitial stroma are the foremost obstacles to cancer cell invasion, and the family of enzymes that has been shown to be vital for matrix destruction during tumor invasion is the matrix metalloproteinases (MMP) enzymes. These enzymes represent a family of zinc-binding enzymes that degrade components of the extracellular matrix. MMPs can be secreted directly by tumors or they can be secreted by normal host cells that are stimulated by tumor-secreted cytokines. Secretion of MMPs has been correlated with tumor invasiveness, and metalloproteinase inhibitors have been shown to inhibit invasiveness of normal and malignant cells.

Secretion of MMPs can be regulated by cytokines, growth factors, and hormones. Production of most MMPs is induced by interleukin-1β (IL-1β), TNF-α, platelet derived-growth factor, EGF, basic fibroblast growth factor, and nerve growth factor. MMP production is repressed by TGF-β.

MMPs are secreted as proenzymes, which require activation after secretion. These enzymes can be divided into 3 classes: interstitial collagenases, stromelysins, and gelatinases. Interstitial collagenases degrade type I, II, III, VII, VIII, and X collagens in their triple helix regions. Stromelysins degrade nonhelical regions of type IV collagen, fibronectin, and proteoglycans. Gelatinases degrade gelatin, intact types IV, V, VII, IX, and X collagen, fibronectin, and elastin.

Matrix destruction at sites of tumor is achieved by an imbalance between MMP enzymes and their endogenous inhibitors, TIMPs. There are 3 TIMP molecules; TIMP-1 and TIMP-2 are soluble proteins and TIMP-3 is a protein that is sequestered in the extracellular matrix. TIMP-1 inhibits activated interstitial collagenase, stromelysin, and gelatinase B. TIMP-2 inhibits type IV collagenase (gelatinase A).

MMP and TIMP play a role in tumor invasion and metastasis. A positive correlation has been found between tumor cell MMP expression and tumor invasion and metastasis, and consistent expression of MMP has been shown in nonneoplastic cells that are adjacent to invasive malignant tumors. The MMP that has received the most support as playing a pathologic role in tumor invasion and metastasis is type IV collagenase. Overexpression of type IV collagenase is associated with genetic induction of the metastatic phenotype, and agents that inhibit type IV collagenase secretion can prevent tumor cell invasion. TIMPs have been shown to act as suppressors of tumor invasion. Specifically, TIMP-1, which inhibits type IV collagenase, has been shown to hold the malignant phenotype in check.

The motility of cancer cells through extracellular matrix is directed by factors that regulate tumor cell adhesion, membrane fluidity, cytoskeletal configuration, and shape. These factors can be separated into 3 types: those secreted by tumor cells (autocrine factors), those secreted by normal host cells (paracrine factors), and those released from the extracellular matrix (Fig. 8).

Three autocrine motility factors have been clearly identified, and many other such factors will most likely be identified in the future. The 3 well-defined tumor-secreted motility factors are hepatocyte growth factor/scatter factor (HGF/SF), insulin-like growth factor II (IGF-II), and autotaxin. The actions of HGF/SF result in phosphorylation of several intracellular proteins including Src, Ras, and mitogen-activated protein kinase. The mechanisms through which IGF-II and autotaxin exert their influence on tumor cell biochemistry are less well understood. Although the intracellular influences provided by IGF-II stimulation are not clearly identified, this growth factor has been shown to act as an autocrine motility factor in human rhabdomyosarcoma.

Three paracrine motility factors, insulin-like growth factor I (IGF-I), interleukin-8 (IL-8), and histamine, have been identified and it is likely that many other paracrine motility factors will be elucidated in the future. These factors are secreted by host cells and they direct tumor cells toward the cells (or organs that contain those cells) that produce them. It is important to appreciate that the biologic role of these factors in cancer cell pathophysiology is probably multifaceted and, as a result, the role of these molecules as motility factors is simply one of their many pathologic influences on cancer cells.

At least 6 motility factors are released from the extracellular matrix: vitronectin, fibronectin, laminin, type I collagen, type IV collagen, and thrombospondin. These factors are released from the matrix by tumor-secreted MMP and, after being cleaved from the extracellular matrix, these proteins stimulate tumor cell motility toward the site of matrix degradation. This important process therefore couples extracellular matrix protein degradation to tumor cell motility. In bone, the most likely motility factors are degradative components of type I collagen, although in the future it is likely that several noncollagenous proteins of bone will prove to serve as motility factors. Two such candidates are osteocalcin and TGF-β.

The effect of motility factors on cancer cells is mediated by the actions of pseudopodia, the cellular tools used for motility and invasion. These structures are cylindrical protrusions of the cell membrane that contain the sensory and motor equipment that cells need for motility. They protrude from cells at regions on the cell surface that bind motility factors and, based on the presence and concentration of these factors, the sensing capacity of these structures provide direction for movement.

Formation of pseudopodia and subsequent cell movement involve a series of well-coordinated events. Proteolysis occurs in the extracellular space adjacent to pseudopodia. This requires that the pseudopodia secrete activated MMP. Cellular detachment and attachment occur at both the advancing tip of the pseudopodia and at the rear of the cell. As cells extend pseudopodia, in response to stimulation for motility, adhesion of the leading edge to the extra-

cellular matrix is required for attachment. Following attachment, MMP are secreted from the pseudopodia, a zone of matrix lyses is created, and the cell moves into this zone by attaching the leading edge of the pseudopodia to the matrix and pulling the cell forward. As the cell moves forward, the rear of the cell detaches and follows the pseudopodia.

Bone Resorption

Invasion of tumor cells at sites of skeletal metastases is very different from invasion at the site of the primary tumor, because bone, unlike the basement membrane or interstitial stroma, is mineralized. To invade bone, tumor cells must penetrate mineralized connective tissue. The components of bone that stand in the way of the invading tumor cell are the mineralized (inorganic) portion and the collagenous (organic) portion. Both of these constituents must be destroyed in order for tumors to invade and grow in bone. Removal of the mineralized portion is a passive process that requires acid pH, and removal of the collagenous portion is an active process that requires the action of collagenolytic enzymes.

Unlike tissue destruction that occurs during tumor cell invasion of soft tissues, tumor-induced bone resorption is not actually performed by tumor cells. The destruction of bone at tumor sites is performed by osteoclasts. Osteoclasts are the body's principal bone-resorbing cells. These cells are multinucleated cells and are derived from fusion of macrophage lineage hematopoietic cells. They are designed for the very specific function of resorbing bone.

Osteoclasts destroy both the inorganic and organic components of bone. These cells are uniquely capable of demineralizing bone by virtue of their ability to create and acidify closed extracellular compartments on bone surfaces. These closed compartments are called resorption bays, and they are positioned at the interface between the bone surface and the osteoclast cell membrane. Resorption bays are actually extracellular compartments that are sealed at the bone-osteoclast surface membrane interface. Osteoclasts treat these resorption bays as if they were lysosomes. They provide the resorption bays with an acidic pH and with proteolytic lysosomal-like enzymes that can destroy the organic portion of bone.

The process of osteoclast-mediated bone resorption is initiated by demineralization and then later by proteolysis of bone. Demineralization requires acidic pH and occurs in the resorption bay because of the acidic pH within this closed compartment. Demineralization exposes the organic portion of bone and results in the unwinding of type I collagen. Degradation of the organic portion of bone follows demineralization. Both the collagenous and noncollagenous proteins of bone are then removed via the lysosomal-like enzymes secreted by osteoclast into the resorption bay.

Regulation of osteoclast-mediated bone resorption can

occur at several different points in the life cycle of the osteoclast and is manifested as either a change in the number of osteoclasts or as a change in the bone-resorbing activity of osteoclasts. The life cycle of the osteoclasts involves formation of osteoclasts from hematopoietic precursor cells, attachment of osteoclasts to bone, stimulation (activation) of osteoclasts to resorb bone, and osteoclast death (Fig. 9). Regulation of osteoclast number can occur through changes in the rate of osteoclast formation or through changes in the rate of osteoclast death. Regulation of osteoclast activity by tumors occurs via direct influences on the osteoclasts. These influences can be delivered in the form of bone matrix proteins released from regions where bone resorption occurs or can be in the form of growth factors secreted by cells that are adjacent to the osteoclasts (Fig. 10).

The influence that a tumor has on bone will reflect the intensity with which the tumor can influence osteoclastic bone resorption. Less aggressive tumors may modestly stimulate osteoclasts at a single site within their life cycle, whereas aggressive tumors will intensely regulate osteoclasts at multiple sites within their life cycle. Most tumors that destroy bone cause an increase in osteoclast number and also stimulate (activate) bone resorption by osteoclasts. The aggressiveness of an individual tumor or a family of tumors will be determined by the number of points of regulation of osteoclast number and osteoclast stimulation as well as by the intensity regulation at each point.

Many tumors destroy bone by increasing osteoclast number. This is true of primary bone malignancies (sarcomas), metastatic bone tumors (breast cancer), and hematologic malignancies (multiple myeloma). The phenomena of increased osteoclast number at sites of invasive tumors

could reflect either an increase in osteoclast formation or a decrease in osteoclast death. Although the impact of tumors on osteoclast death has not been studied, the effect of tumors on osteoclast number has been studied and findings indicate that invasive bone tumors increase osteoclast number by increasing the rate of osteoclast formation.

The increase in osteoclast formation that occurs at sites of invasive bone tumors reflects influences of the tumor on osteoclast precursor cells. These influences, in general, cause an increase in the number of osteoclast precursor cells, which is manifested secondarily as an increase in the number of osteoclasts. Several different osteoclast precursor cells have been identified, and these include pluripotent hematopoietic progenitor cells, lineage committed precursor cells, and lineage committed, differentiated precursor cells (Fig. 9). The pluripotent hematopoietic progenitor cell is capable of forming hematopoietic cells of various lineage, including erythrocytes, eosinophils, granulocytes, macrophages, and ultimately osteoclasts. Because of their high proliferating potential (HPP) and their ability to form colonies of cells from a single colony-forming cell (CFC), these cells are designated HPP-CFC. The lineage committed precursor cell (CFC-gm) is capable of forming granulocytes (g), macrophages (m), and ultimately osteoclasts. These cells can form colonies that contain granulocytic cells, macrophage cells, or both. They are designated CFC-gm or CFC-m based on their ability to form either granulocytes and macrophages or just macrophages. The lineage-committed, differentiated precursor cell is of macrophage lineage, can form osteoclasts, and is incapable of cell division.

The target cell through which invasive tumors exert their osteoclastogenic influences varies with different types of tumors, and different types of tumors vary with respect to

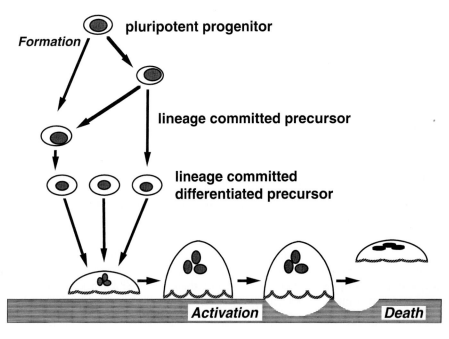

Figure 9

Osteoclast life cycle.

the extent to which they influence target cells. Some tumors target CFC-gm and CFC-ms, and other tumors target the lineage committed, differentiated precursor cell. Some tumors influence cells throughout the body and others influence cells only at sites of bone-residing tumor. Systemic effects of osteolytic tumors on the skeleton are most likely mediated through an increase in the number of CFC-gm cells and effects at localized sites of tumor are most likely mediated through an increase in the number of lineage-committed, differentiated precursor cells.

Several tumor-secreted cytokines stimulate an increase in the number of osteoclasts at sites of tumor. Some of these cytokines have direct effects on osteoclast precursor cells and others have indirect effects, that is, they exert influences by acting on intermediary cells. Tumor-secreted cytokines that are suspected to stimulate osteoclast formation via direct actions toward osteoclast precursor cells are granulocyte/macrophage colony stimulating-factor (GM-CSF), macrophage colony stimulating-factor (M-CSF), IL-1, and IL-6. All of these cytokines can increase the number of osteoclasts by increasing the number of osteoclast precursor cells. GM-CSF, IL-1, and IL-6 primarily target CFC-gm. M-CSF targets both CFC-m and the lineage-committed, differentiated precursor cells. Biologic actions of these factors, however, are very diverse and although these molecules contribute to, and with selected tumors are probably required for, tumor-induced osteoclastogenesis, they probably act in concert with other tumor-secreted factors and/or with components of the extracellular matrix to direct osteoclast formation at sites of bone tumors.

Tumor-secreted cytokines that are suspected to stimulate osteoclast formation via actions on intermediary cells which then stimulate osteoclast formation are parathyroid hormone-related protein (PTH-rp), TGF-α, IL-1, IL-6, and TNF. Among these cytokines, the one that thus far plays the most convincing role in mediating tumor-induced, osteoclast-mediated bone resorption is PTH-rp. It has been determined that the majority of breast cancers that invade bone secrete PTH-rp, whereas breast cancers that metastasize to soft tissue, and not to bone, secrete PTH-rp only rarely. It is suspected that PTH-rp exerts its influence on osteoclasts by stimulating osteoblasts or marrow stromal cells to produce cytokines that will either encourage osteoclast formation or will stimulate osteoclast activation. IL-6 is such a secondary mediator. It is secreted by osteoblasts and marrow stromal cells exposed to PTH-rp and it increases the number of CFC-gm precursors, resulting in an increase in the number of osteoclasts.

Extracellular bone matrix proteins may also play a role in development or progression of tumor invasion into the skeleton. The organic portion of bone contains collagenous and noncollagenous proteins. Although the noncollagenous protein portion of the organic component of bone is only very small, it contains a plethora of potent growth factors with the potential to be involved in the regulation of bone resorption and involved in the growth of bone-residing tumor cells. During tumor-induced bone resorption, these growth factors are released from the organic matrix and they can influence both osteoclasts and the tumor (Fig. 10). Release of osteoclast-directed cytokines from bone during tumor-induced bone resorption can result in increased chemotaxis of osteoclasts and their precursors to sites of tumor, increase in osteoclast precursor cell number (formation) at sites of tumor, and direct stimulation (activation) of osteoclasts at sites of tumor. Release of tumor-directed cytokines from bone during tumor-induced bone

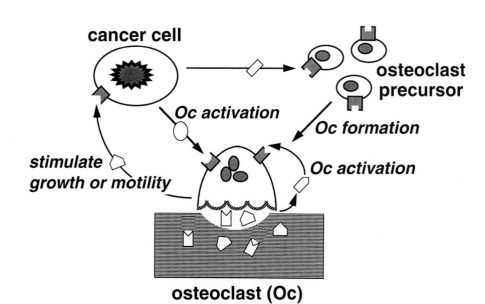

Figure 10

Interactions between cancer cells, osteoclast precursors, and osteoclasts. Open symbols = cytokines, solid symbols = cytokine receptors.

resorption can stimulate tumor cell division and can accelerate tumor growth within bone.

The effect of tumor-induced bone resorption on tumor growth is best illustrated by the effect of breast cancer-induced bone resorption on tumor growth. TGF-β is released from the extracellular bone matrix during tumor-induced, osteoclast-mediated bone resorption. This growth factor influences breast cancer tumor cells to increase production of PTH-rp. This results in an increase in the number of osteoclasts and in an increase in tumor growth. These complex interactions involving osteoclast-mediated bone resorption, tumor cells, and the extracellular bone matrix determine how successful a cluster of bone-residing cancer cells will be at developing into a clinically relevant, invasive bone tumor.

Recent studies have examined the possibility that inhibition of osteoclast-mediated bone resorption decreases tumor osteolysis in experimental animals and decreases the frequency of skeletal complications in cancer patients. Findings in experimental animals have shown that osteoclast-inhibiting bisphosphonates reduce tumor osteolysis and skeletal tumor burden in metastatic breast cancer models, and decrease the number of osteolytic lesion in mice with myeloma. Findings are encouraging in cancer patients who were treated with the bisphosphonates. Patients with skeletal metastases from breast cancer or myeloma who were treated with pamidronate experienced a decrease in the number of skeletal complications, and patients with breast cancer who are at risk for developing skeletal metastases and were treated with the clodronate experienced a decrease in growth and number of breast cancer metastases to bone.

If tumor invasion of bone is so important for successful development of bone cancer, then how can some tumors, such as prostate metastases, seem to primarily form bone? The answer to this question is that no tumor is just bone-forming without having been, at some point in time, bone-resorbing. This notion is supported by 2 findings. First, prostate cancer metastases are predominantly bone-forming neoplasms, but the osteoblastic bone formation within metastases is preceded by osteoclastic activation. This osteoclastic phase leads to focal bone resorption and provides room for deposition of new bone as the new bone associated with blastic prostate metastases actually replaces the old (resorbed) bone. Second, patients with blastic metastases and bone pain improve dramatically following treatment with agents that inhibit osteoclast-mediated bone resorption, such as bisphosphonates.

Selected Bibliography

Cell Cycle

Graña X, Reddy EP: Cell cycle control in mammalian cells: Role of cyclins, cyclin dependent kinases (CDKs), growth suppressor genes and cyclin-dependent kinase inhibitors (CKIs). *Oncogene* 1995;11:211–219.

Hartwell LH, Kastan MB: Cell cycle control and cancer. *Science* 1994;266:1821–1828.

Pines J: Cyclins, CKDs and cancer. *Semin Cancer Biol* 1995;6:63–72.

Sherr CJ, Kato J, Quelle DE, Matsuoka M, Roussel MF: D=type cyclins and their cyclin-dependent kinases: G_1 phase integrators of the mitogenic response, in Stillman B (ed): *Cold Spring Harbor Symposia on Quantitative Biology: Molecular Genetics of Cancer*. Cold Spring Harbor, NY, Cold Spring Harbor Laboratory Press, 1994, vol 59, pp 11–19.

Sherr CJ, Roberts JM: Inhibitors of mammalian G_1 cyclin-dependent kinases. *Genes & Dev* 1995;9:1149–1163.

Sherr CJ: G_1 phase progression: Cycling on cue. *Cell* 1994;79:551–555.

Oncogenes and Tumor Suppressor Genes

Oliner JD, Kinzler KW, Meltzer PS, George DL, Vogelstein B: Amplification of a gene encoding a TP53—associated protein in human sarcomas. *Nature* 1992;358:80–83.

Perkins AS, Stern DF: Molecular biology of cancer: Oncogenes, in DeVita VT Jr, Hellman S, Rosenberg SA (eds): *Cancer: Principles & Practice of Oncology*, ed 5. Philadelphia, PA, Lippincott-Raven, 1997, pp 79–102.

Springfield DS, Bolander ME, Friedlaender GE, Lane N: Molecular and cellular biology of inflammation and neoplasia, in Simon SR (ed): *Orthopaedic Basic Science*. Rosemont, IL, American Academy of Orthopaedic Surgeons, 1994, pp 219–276.

Weinberg RA: Tumor suppressor genes. *Science* 1991;254:1138–1146.

Chromosomal Abnormalities

Douglass EC, Valentine M, Etcubanas E, et al: A specific chromosomal abnormality in rhabdomyosarcoma. *Cytogenet Cell Genet* 1987;45:148–155.

Rabbitts TH: Chromosomal translocations in human cancer. *Nature* 1994;372:143–149.

Solomon E, Borrow J, Goddard AD: Chromosome aberrations and cancer. *Science* 1991;254:1153–1160.

Turc-Carel C, Limon J, Dal Cin P, Rao U, Karakousis C, Sandberg AA: Cytogenetic studies of adipose tissue tumors: II. Recurrent reciprocal translocation t(12;16)(q13;p11) in myxoid liposarcomas. *Cancer Genet Cytogenet* 1986;23:291–299.

Turc-Carel C, Dal Cin P, Limon J, et al: Involvement of chromosome X in primary cytogenetic change in human neoplasia: Nonrandom translocation in synovial sarcoma. *Proc Natl Acad Sci USA* 1987;84: 1981–1985.

Tumor Cell Metastases

Clohisy DR, Palkert D, Ramnaraine ML, Pekurovsky I, Oursler MJ: Human breast cancer induces osteoclast activation and increases the number of osteoclasts at sites of tumor osteolysis. *J Orthop Res* 1996;14:396–402.

Clohisy DR, Ramnaraine ML: Osteoclast formation during tumor osteolysis does not require proliferating osteoclast precursor cells. *J Orthop Res* 1997;15:301–306.

Dallas SL, Garrett IR, Oyajobi BO, et al: Ibandronate reduces osteolytic lesions but not tumor burden in a murine model of myeloma bone disease. *Blood* 1999;93:1697–1706.

Deil IJ, Solomayer EF, Costa SD, et al: Reduction in new metastases in breast cancer with adjuvant clodronate treatment. *N Engl J Med* 1998;339:357–363.

de la Mata J, Uy HL, Guise TA, et al: Interleukin-6 enhances hypercalcemia and bone resorption mediated by parathyroid hormone-related protein in vivo. *J Clin Invest* 1995;95:2846–2852.

El-Badry OM, Minniti C, Kohn EC, Houghton PJ, Daughaday WH, Helman LJ: Insulin-like growth factor II acts as an autocrine growth and motility factor in human rhabdomyosarcoma tumors. *Cell Growth Differ* 1990;1:325–331.

Folkman J: Angiogenesis in cancer, vascular, rheumatoid and other disease. *Nat Med* 1995;1:27–31.

Folkman J: How is blood vessel growth regulated in normal and neoplastic tissue? G.H.A. Clowes Memorial Award Lecture. *Cancer Res* 1986;46:467–473.

Folkman J, Cotran R: Relation of vascular proliferation to tumor growth. *Int Rev Exp Pathol* 1976;16:207–248.

Guise TA, Yin JJ, Taylor SD, et al: Evidence for a causal role of parathyroid hormone-related protein in the pathogenesis of human breast cancer-mediated osteolysis. *J Clin Invest* 1996;98:1544–1549.

Heimann R, Ferguson D, Powers C, Recant WM, Weichselbaum RR, Hellman S: Angiogenesis as a predictor of long-term survival for patients with node-negative breast cancer. *J Natl Cancer Inst* 1996;88:1764–1769.

Horton MA, Davies J: Perspectives: Adhesion receptors in bone. *J Bone Miner Res* 1989;4:803–808.

Hughes DE, Salter DM, Dedhar S, Simpson R: Integrin expression in human bone. *J Bone Miner Res* 1993;8:527–533.

Liotta LA, Steeg PS, Stetler-Stevenson WG: Cancer metastasis and angiogenesis: An imbalance of positive and negative regulation. *Cell* 1991;64:327–336.

Manolagas SC, Jilka RL: Cytokines, hematopoiesis, osteoclastogenesis, and estrogens. *Calcif Tissue Int* 1992;50:199–202.

Matrisian LM: Metalloproteinases and their inhibitors in matrix remodeling. *Trends Genet* 1990;6:121–125.

Mundy GR: Hypercalcemia of malignancy revisited. *J Clin Invest* 1988;82:1–6.

Ray JM, Stetler-Stevenson WG: The role of matrix metalloproteases and their inhibitors in tumour invasion, metastasis and angiogenesis. *Eur Respir J* 1994;7:2062–2072.

Sasaki A, Boyce BF, Story B, et al: Bisphosphonate risedronate reduces metastatic human breast cancer burden in bone in nude mice. *Cancer Res* 1995;55:3551–3557.

Silberman MA, Partin AW, Veltri RW, Epstein JI: Tumor angiogenesis correlates with progression after radical prostatectomy but not with pathologic stage in Gleason sum 5 to 7 adenocarcinoma of the prostate. *Cancer* 1997;79:772–779.

Uy HL, Guise TA, De La Mata J, et al: Effects of parathyroid hormone (PTH)-related protein and PTH on osteoclasts and osteoclast precursors in vivo. *Endocrinology* 1995;136:3207–3212.

Weidner N, Semple JP, Welch WR, Folkman J: Tumor angiogenesis and metastasis: Correlation in invasive breast carcinoma. *N Engl J Med* 1991;324:1–8.

Yamada KM: Adhesive recognition sequences. *J Biol Chem* 1991;266: 12809–12812.

Yoneda T, Sasaki A, Mundy GR: Osteolytic bone metastasis in breast cancer. *Breast Cancer Res Treat* 1994;32:73–84.

Chapter 17

Articular Cartilage Structure, Composition, and Function

Henry J. Mankin, MD

Van C. Mow, PhD

Joseph A. Buckwalter, MD

Joseph P. Iannotti, MD, PhD

Anthony Ratcliffe, PhD

This chapter at a glance

This chapter reviews current understanding of how the unique structure and composition of articular cartilage give the tissue its remarkable mechanical properties and durability.

Introduction

Articular cartilage, the resilient load-bearing tissue that forms the articulating surfaces of diarthrodial joints, provides these surfaces with the low friction, lubrication, and wear characteristics required for repetitive gliding motion. It also absorbs mechanical shock and spreads the applied load onto subchondral bone. In most synovial joints, articular cartilage provides these essential biomechanical functions for 8 decades or more. No synthetic material performs this well as a joint surface. This chapter reviews current understanding of how the unique structure and composition of articular cartilage give the tissue its remarkable mechanical properties and durability.

Structure and Composition

Articular cartilage consists primarily of a large extracellular matrix (ECM) with a sparse population of highly specialized cells (chondrocytes) distributed throughout the tissue. The primary components of the ECM are water, proteoglycans, and collagens, with other proteins and glycoproteins present in lower amounts. These all combine to provide the tissue with its unique and complex structure and mechanical properties.

The structure and composition of the articular cartilage vary throughout its depth (Fig. 1), from the articular surface to the subchondral bone. These differences include cell shape and volume, collagen fibril diameter and orientation, proteoglycan concentration, and water content. The carti-

lage can be divided into 4 zones: the superficial zone, the middle or transitional zone, the deep zone, and the zone of calcified cartilage.

The superficial zone is the uppermost zone of the cartilage and forms the gliding surface. The thin collagen fibrils are arranged parallel to the surface, the chondrocytes are elongated with the long axis parallel to the surface, the proteoglycan content is at its lowest level, and the water content is at its highest level. The middle, or transition, zone contains collagen fibers with a larger diameter and less apparent organization, and the chondrocytes have a more rounded appearance. The deep zone contains the highest concentration of proteoglycans and the lowest water content; the collagen fibers have a large diameter and are organized perpendicular to the joint surface. The chondrocytes are spherical and often are arranged in a columnar fashion. The deepest layer, the zone of calcified cartilage, separates the hyaline cartilage from the subchondral bone. It is characterized by small cells distributed in a cartilaginous matrix encrusted with apatitic salts. Histologic staining with hematoxylin and eosin shows a wavy bluish line, called the tidemark, which separates the deep zone from the calcified zone. The number of tidemarks increases with age as the tissue is remodeled.

In addition to these articular surface-to-bone zonal distinctions, the ECM is divided into pericellular, territorial, or interterritorial regions, depending on its proximity to the chondrocyte (Fig. 2). These regions differ in their content (collagen, proteoglycan, and other matrix components), and in the collagen fibril diameter and organization. The pericellular matrix is a thin layer adjacent to the cell mem-

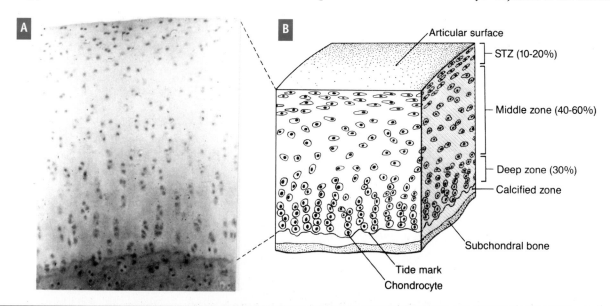

Figure 1

A, Histologic section of normal adult articular cartilage showing even Safranin O staining and distribution of chondrocytes. **B,** Schematic diagram of chondrocyte organization in the 3 major zones of the uncalcified cartilage, the tidemark, and the subchondral bone. STZ = superficial tangential zone. (Reproduced with permission from Mow VC, Proctor CS, Kelly MA: Biomechanics of articular cartilage, in Nordin M, Frankel VH (eds): *Basic Biomechanics of the Musculoskeletal System,* ed 2. Philadelphia, PA, Lea & Febiger, 1989, pp 31–57.)

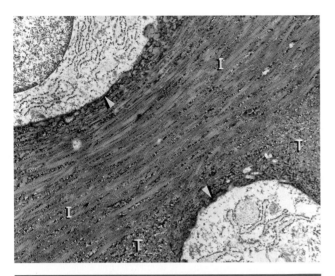

Figure 2

Electron microscopic view (8700 ×) of mature rabbit articular cartilage from the radial zone of the medial femoral condyle. Micrograph shows cytoskeletal elements, and pericellular matrix (arrow), territorial matrix (T), and interterritorial matrix (I). The pericellular matrix lacks cross-striated collagen fibrils, whereas the territorial matrix has a fine fibrillar collagen network. The collagen of the interterritorial matrix has coarser fibers, and they tend to be parallel. (Reproduced with permission from Buckwalter JA, Hunziker EB: Articular cartilage biology and morphology, in Mow VC, Ratcliffe A (eds): *Structure and Function of Articular Cartilage*. Boca Raton, FL, CRC Press, 1993.)

brane and completely surrounds the chondrocyte. It contains primarily proteoglycans and other noncollagenous matrix components; almost no collagen fibrils appear to be present. The territorial matrix surrounds the pericellular matrix, and it is characterized by thin collagen fibrils that, at the boundary of the territorial matrix, appear to form a fibrillar network that is distinct from the surrounding interterritorial matrix. Recent studies have reintroduced the term chondron to describe the chondrocyte and its pericellular and territorial matrices. The interterritorial matrix is the largest of the matrix regions and contributes most of the material properties of the articular cartilage. It encompasses all of the matrix between the territorial matrices of the individual cells or clusters of cells and contains the large collagen fibers and the majority of the proteoglycans.

Chondrocytes

The formation and maintenance of articular cartilage depends on the chondrocytes. They are derived from mesenchymal cells, which differentiate during skeletal morphogenesis and development to form chondrocytes. During skeletal growth, these cells increase the volume of ECM, and in mature tissue, where they occupy less than 10% of the total tissue volume, they are responsible for the maintenance of the ECM. Chondrocytes are metabolically active and are able to respond to a variety of environmental stimuli. These stimuli include soluble mediators, such as

growth factors, interleukins, and pharmaceutical agents; matrix molecules; mechanical loads; and hydrostatic pressure changes. Although the chondrocytes generally maintain a stable matrix, their response to some factors (for example, interleukin-1) may lead to degradation of the ECM. However, the response of articular cartilage chondrocytes to other types of messages commonly used to regulate many body processes is limited. The cartilage has no nerve supply; therefore, neural impulses cannot provide information, and the immune responses (cellular and humoral) are not likely to occur in cartilage because both monocytes and immunoglobulins tend to be excluded from the tissue by steric exclusion.

Matrix Composition

Because the chondrocytes of articular cartilage occupy only a small proportion of the total volume of the tissue, its composition is determined primarily by the matrix. Normal cartilage has water contents ranging from 65% to 80% of its total wet weight (Fig. 3, Table 1). The remaining wet weight of the tissue is accounted for principally by 2 major classes of "structural" macromolecular materials, collagens and proteoglycans. Several other classes of molecules, including lipids, phospholipids, proteins, and glycoproteins, make up the remaining portion of the ECM. Although their precise role in the ECM has not yet been determined, it is impor-

Table 1

Biomechanical Composition of Articular Cartilage

Component	% Wet Weight
Quantitatively Major Components	
Water	65 to 80
Collagen (type II)	10 to 20
Aggrecan	4 to 7
Quantitatively Minor Components (less than 5%)*	
Proteoglycans	
Biglycan	
Decorin	
Fibromodulin	
Collagens	
Type V	
Type VI	
Type IX	
Type X	
Type XI	
Link protein	
Hyaluronate	
Fibronectin	
Lipids	

* Although these components are present in lower overall amounts, they may be present in similar molar amounts compared to type II collagen and aggrecan (for example, link protein), and may have major roles to play in the functionality of the matrix

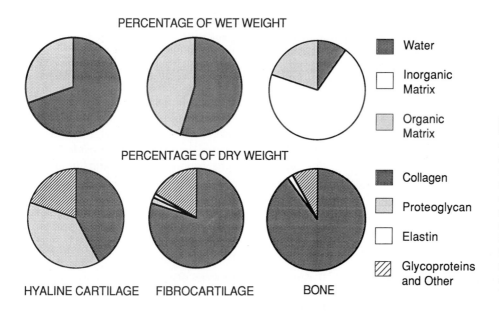

PERCENTAGE OF WET WEIGHT

PERCENTAGE OF DRY WEIGHT

HYALINE CARTILAGE   FIBROCARTILAGE   BONE

Water

Inorganic Matrix

Organic Matrix

Collagen

Proteoglycan

Elastin

Glycoproteins and Other

Figure 3

Composition of 3 classes of skeletal connective tissues: hyaline cartilage, fibrocartilage, and bone. Notice that hyaline cartilage has the highest water content and the highest proteoglycan content. (Reproduced with permission from Buckwalter JA, Cooper RR; Bone structure and function, in Griffin PP (ed): *Instructional Course Lectures XXXVI*. Park Ridge, IL, American Academy of Orthopaedic Surgeons, 1987, pp 27–48.)

tant to recognize that there are other constituents besides collagens and proteoglycans. For example, one type IX collagen is a hybrid; that is, it has regions that consist of collagen and other regions that consist of glycosaminoglycans covalently bound to protein. This molecule may promote interactions between fibrillar collagens and proteoglycans.

Water

Water is the most abundant component of normal articular cartilage, making up from 65% to 80% of the wet weight of the tissue. During the early phases of osteoarthritis, water content may increase to over 90% before disintegration of the tissue occurs. A small percentage of this water is contained in the intracellular space, about 30% is associated with the intrafibrillar space within the collagen, and the remainder is contained in the molecular pore space of the ECM. Inorganic salts, such as sodium, calcium, chloride, and potassium, are dissolved in the tissue water. Water content varies throughout cartilage, decreasing in concentration from approximately 80% at the surface to 65% in the deep zone. Most of the water may be moved through the ECM by applying a pressure gradient across the tissue, or by compressing the solid matrix. Frictional resistance against this flow through the molecular size pores of the ECM is very high, and thus the permeability of the tissue is very low. This frictional resistance and the pressurization of the water within the ECM are the 2 basic mechanisms from which articular cartilage derives its ability to support very high joint loads (please refer to the section on biomechanics of articular cartilage in this chapter). The flow of water through the tissue and across the articular surface also promotes the transport of nutrients and may provide a source of lubricant for the joint. The fluid mechanics of water flow through cartilage is governed by mechanical and physicochemical laws. From these laws, it is possible to show that

very large pressures are required to move water through the ECM. For example, to move water at a rate of 17.5 µm/s (very slow) through normal cartilage, a pressure of 1 MPa (145 psi) is required. Conversely, if water is flowing through cartilage at this rate, a pressure differential of 1 MPa must be developed across the tissue. To appreciate the magnitude of this pressure, note that the pressure in an automobile tire usually is not greater than 30 psi (0.21 MPa).

The affinity of articular cartilage for water derives mostly from the hydrophilic nature of proteoglycans, and less from collagen. Water will wet materials made of pure collagen as a result of capillary or surface tension effects. This is a relatively weak physical mechanism. The ability of proteoglycans to attract water involves 2 physicochemical mechanisms: Donnan osmotic pressure, which is caused by the interstitial freely mobile counterions (for example, Ca^{2+}, Na^+) that are required to neutralize the charges on the proteoglycans, or equivalently, the electrostatic repulsive forces that are developed between the fixed negative charges along the proteoglycan molecules; and the entropic tendency of the proteoglycan to gain volume in solution. For articular cartilage, the degree of hydration is determined by a balance of the total swelling pressure (the sum of these 2 effects) exerted by the proteoglycans, and the constraining forces developed within the strong collagen network surrounding the trapped proteoglycans. Thus, when water is in contact with either of these macromolecules, a cohesive and strong solid matrix is formed, which allows the tissue to hold its water with avidity.

Collagens

Collagens are the major structural macromolecules of the ECM (Table 2). There are at least 15 distinct collagen types composed of at least 29 genetically distinct chains. All members of the collagen family contain a characteristic triple-helical structure that may constitute the majority of the length of the molecule, or may be interrupted by 1 or more nonhelical domains. Over 50% of the dry weight of articular cartilage consists of collagen. The major cartilage collagen, which represents 90% to 95% of the total, is known as type II. However, the articular cartilage matrix also contains types V, VI, IX, X, and XI. Articular cartilage collagens provide the tissue's tensile and shear properties and immobilize the proteoglycans within the ECM. Collagen fibers in cartilage are generally thinner than those seen in tendon or bone, and this may, in part, be a function of their interaction with the relatively large amount of proteoglycan in this tissue. The fibers in articular cartilage vary in width from 10 to 100 nm, although their width may increase with age and disease. Initial studies of their macro-organization suggested that they formed arcades, but recent studies show that the fibers have a less ordered organization, especially in the middle zone of the tissue, where they appear to be randomly distributed (Fig. 4).

Figure 5 shows the stages of collagen fibril formation and the typical dense banding pattern seen under the electron microscope. The triple helix, which is characteristic of all collagens, is composed of 3 polypeptide chains (α chains). The amino acid composition of the chains includes large quantities of glycine (~33% of total residues) and proline (~25% of total residues). Because of their proline content, each of these chains exhibits a characteristic left-handed helical configuration, and in the triple helix, each is wound around a common axis in a right-handed helical configuration to create a structure uniquely designed to resist tensile forces. Collagen also contains hydroxyproline, hydroxylysine, and glycosylated (either galactosyl- or galactosylglucosyl-) hydroxylysine. The amino acid sequence for the triple-helical region of collagen can be represented by $(Gly-Xaa-Yaa)_n$, where Xaa and Yaa can be any amino acid other than glycine, but most are frequently proline and hydroxyproline, respectively. The location of glycine, the

smallest amino acid, is an absolute steric requirement for the triple-helical structure because a functional group of every third residue occupies the interior of the helix. The presence of hydroxyproline is a requirement for the stability of the collagen helix because it allows the formation of intramolecular hydrogen bonds along the length of the molecule. Hydroxylysine participates in the formation of covalent cross-links that principally stabilize collagen fibrillar assemblies; the role of glycosylated hydroxylysine is

Table 2
Types of Collagen

Type	Tissue	Polymeric Form
Class 1 (300-nm triple-helix)		
Type I	Skin, bone, etc	Banded fibril
Type II	Cartilage, disk	Banded fibril
Type III	Skin, blood vessels	Banded fibril
Type V	With type I	Banded fibril
Type XI (1α, 2α, 3α)	With type II	Banded fibril
Class 2 (basement membranes)		
Type IV	Basal lamina	Three-dimensional network
Type VII	Epithelial basement membrane	Anchoring fibril
Type VII	Endothelial basement membrane	Unknown
Class 3 (short-chain)		
Type VI	Widespread	Microfilaments, 110-nm banded aggregates
Type IX	Cartilage (with type II)	Cross-linked to type II
Type X	Hypertrophic cartilage	Unknown
Type XII	Tendon, other?	Unknown
Type XIII	Endothelial cells	Unknown

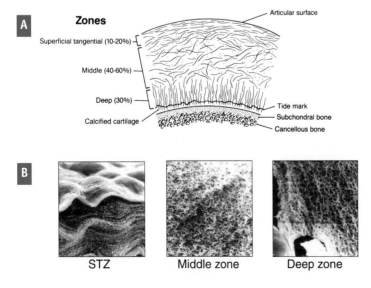

Figure 4

A, Diagram of collagen fiber architecture in a sagittal cross section showing the 3 salient zones of articular cartilage. **B,** Scanning electron micrographs that show actual arrangements of collagen in the 3 zones. STZ = superficial tangential zone. (Reproduced with permission from Mow VC, Proctor CS, Kelly MA: Biomechanics of articular cartilage, in Nordin M, Frankel VH (eds): *Basic Biomechanics of the Musculoskeletal System,* ed 2. Philadelphia, PA, Lea & Febiger, 1989, pp 31–57.)

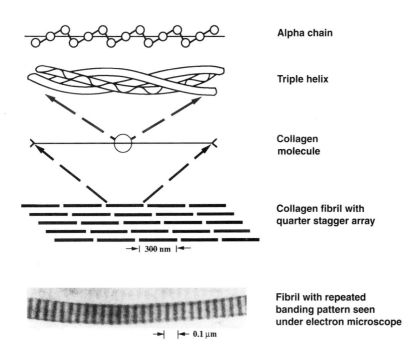

Alpha chain

Triple helix

Collagen molecule

Collagen fibril with quarter stagger array

|← 300 nm →|

Fibril with repeated banding pattern seen under electron microscope

|← 0.1 µm →|

Figure 5

A scheme for the formation of collagen fibrils. The triple helix is made from 3 α chains, forming a procollagen molecule. Outside the cell the N- and C-terminal globular domains of the α chains are cleaved off to allow fibril formation, which occurs in a specific quarter-staggered array that ultimately results in the typical banded fibrils seen under electron microscopy. (Reproduced with permission from Mow VC, Zhu W, Ratcliffe A: Structure and function of articular cartilage and meniscus, in Mow VC, Hayes WC (eds): *Basic Orthopaedic Biomechanics*. New York, NY, Raven Press, 1991, pp 143–198.)

unknown, although it has been postulated to play a role in regulating collagen fibril assemblies and collagen fibril diameters.

Some collagens (for example, type II) appear to be distributed throughout the cartilaginous matrix, whereas others (for example, types VI, IX, and XI) may be localized to specific areas. The prototypical organization of collagen monomers (tropocollagen in the older literature) is shown in Figure 5. In the ECM, monomers containing an uninterrupted triple helix align head-to-tail and side-by-side in a quarter-staggered array such that overlaps and holes are created in the 3-dimensional (3-D) structure. This type of alignment results in the characteristic banding pattern of the fibrillar collagens. In cartilage, this organization is typical of type II collagen. Type XI collagen can also form fibrils, albeit thinner, and currently it is thought that these structures can act as nuclei for the deposition of type II collagen. Type IX collagen, because of interruptions in its triple-helical domains, does not form fibrillar structures on its own, but it associates with the surface of the fibrils. Recent studies have shown that in addition to covalent cross-links between chains of type II collagen, there are links between types II and IX, and between chains of type XI collagen. Such an extensive network of cross-links undoubtedly contributes to the relative insolubility of these cartilage collagens and to the stability and strength of the ECM.

The macromolecular organization of type VI collagen is quite different from those described above because its triple-helical domain represents less than half of the molecular mass and is capped at both the amino and carboxyl termini by noncollagenous domains. These monomers readily aggregate into antiparallel tetramers that align end-to-end to form beaded microfibrils stabilized by disulfide bonds. Thus, type VI collagen can be readily extracted from cartilage using chaotropic (for example, guanidine HCl) and reducing agents. On the other hand, type X collagen appears to exist extracellularly in the form of fine fibrous mats. The roles of collagen types VI and X in articular cartilage are not yet known, but type VI appears to be localized to the pericellular capsule of the chondrons and type X to the deep calcified zone of mature joints. Type VI collagen may be important in tethering the chondrocyte to its pericellular matrix, whereas type X may play a role in the mineralization process that occurs just above the underlying subchondral bone.

Collagen Cross-Links

The collagens of cartilage form a cross-linked network. This intra- and intermolecular cross-linking is thought to add 3-D stability to the fibril network and is likely to contribute to the tensile properties of the tissue. The chemical cross-links prevalent in articular cartilage are the trifunctional hydroxypyridinium cross-links formed by hydroxylysine aldehydes being changed to 3-hydroxypyridinium residues. There are several chemical intermediates in the formation of the final mature cross-links, and their formation in cartilage may take several weeks. Data from recent studies have shown that every type IX collagen molecule in cartilage is cross-linked to type II collagen. Therefore, stabilizing the collagen network by linking the type II collagen fibrils has been proposed to be a function of type IX collagen.

Proteoglycans

Proteoglycans are complex macromolecules that, by definition, consist of a protein core with covalently bound polysaccharide (glycosaminoglycan) chains (Fig. 6). Proteoglycans were formerly called protein-polysaccharides or mucopolysaccharides, and this latter term still is used to describe some inherited storage disorders.

Glycosaminoglycans consist of long-chain, unbranched, repeating disaccharide units. Three major types have been found in cartilage proteoglycans: (1) chondroitin sulfate 4- and 6-isomers; (2) keratan sulfate; and (3) dermatan sulfate (Fig. 7). The chondroitin sulfates are the most prevalent glycosaminoglycans in cartilage. They account for 55% to 90% of the total population, depending principally on the age of the subject or the presence of osteoarthritis. Each chain is composed of 25 to 30 repeating disaccharide units, giving an average chain weight of 15 to 20 kd. The keratan sulfate constituent of articular cartilage, which resides primarily in the large, aggregating proteoglycan, is not as well defined as the chondroitin sulfates. The keratan sulfate composition and degree of sulfation vary in human articular cartilage and may be altered with age. Keratan sulfate chains from human articular cartilage are shorter than chondroitin sulfate chains, with an average molecular weight of 5 to 10 kd. Hyaluronate is also a glycosaminoglycan, but, unlike those described above, it is not sulfated. A further distinguishing feature of hyaluronan is that it is not covalently bound to a protein core, and, therefore, is not part of a proteoglycan. In cartilage it is present as unbranched chains that can be very large (greater than 1×10^6 kd).

All the glycosaminoglycan chains found in cartilage have repeating carboxyl (COOH) and/or sulfate (SO_4) groups (Fig. 7). In solution, these groups become ionized (COO^- and SO_3^-), and in the physiologic environment, they require positive counterions such as Ca^{2+} and Na^+ to maintain overall electroneutrality. These free-floating ions within the interstitial water give rise to the Donnan osmotic pressure effect. Equivalently, because the proteoglycans are packed to within one fifth of their free-solution volume in the tis-

sue, the fixed-charge groups are spaced 10 to 15 Å apart, resulting in a strong charge-to-charge repulsive force. The magnitude of this repulsive force also depends on the concentration of the counterions present in the tissue.

Eighty percent to 90% of all proteoglycans in cartilage are of the large, aggregating type, called aggrecan (Fig. 6). They consist of a long, extended protein core with up to 100 chondroitin sulfate and 50 keratan sulfate glycosaminoglycan chains covalently bound to the protein core. In young individuals the concentration of keratan sulfate is relatively low, and chondroitin 4 sulfate is the predominant form of chondroitin sulfate. With increasing age, the concentration of keratan sulfate increases and chondroitin 6 sulfate becomes the predominant form of chondroitin sulfate. The aggrecan protein core is large (molecular weight 2 kd or larger) and complex, and has several distinct globular and extended domains. One extended domain contains the

Proteoglycan Aggregate

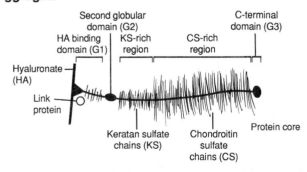

Figure 6 caption references: Hyaluronate (HA), Link protein, HA binding domain (G1), Second globular domain (G2), KS-rich region, CS-rich region, C-terminal domain (G3), Keratan sulfate chains (KS), Chondroitin sulfate chains (CS), Protein core

Chondroitin sulfate:
1,4-glucuronic acid - 1,3- galactosamine

Keratan sulfate:
1,3-galactosamine - 1,4-glucosamine

Hyaluronate:
1,4-glucuronic acid - 1,3-glucosamine

Figure 6

A schematic diagram of the aggrecan molecule and its binding to hyaluronate. The protein core has several globular domains (G1, G2, and G3), with other regions containing the keratan sulfate and chondroitin sulfate glycosaminoglycan chains. The N-terminal G1 domain is able to bind specifically to hyaluronate. This binding is stabilized by link protein.

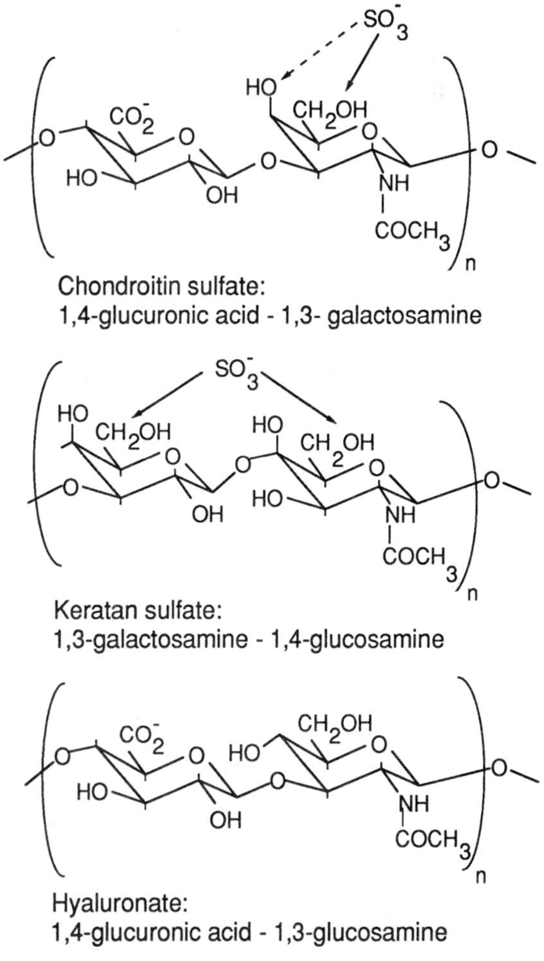

Figure 7

Chemical formula and structure of three primary glycosaminoglycans present in articular cartilage. (Adapted from Wight TN, Heinegård DK, Hascall VC: Proteoglycans: Structure and function, in Hay ED (ed): *Cell Biology of the Extracellular Matrix*, ed 2. New York, NY, Plenum Press, 1991, pp 45–78.)

majority of the keratan sulfate glycosaminoglycan chains, and is adjacent to the longest extended region, which has the chondroitin sulfate chains attached with some interspersed keratan sulfate chains. Small oligosaccharides are also attached along the protein core. At the N-terminal end of the protein core, one of the globular domains (G1) has the specific function of binding to hyaluronan (Fig. 8). The functions of the other globular domains of aggrecan are unknown. A separate, smaller molecule called link protein binds to both the G1 domain of aggrecan and the hyaluronan, stabilizing the bond and, thus, forming the aggrecan-hyaluronate-link protein complexes referred to as proteoglycan aggregates. The interactions forming these complexes are not covalent bonds. However, the noncovalent interactions of this complex are so strong that without proteolytic degradation this binding can be regarded as almost irreversible. Aggregation helps stabilize the aggrecan molecules within the ECM and, because each hyaluronate chain is long and unbranched, many aggrecan molecules can bind to a single hyaluronan chain to form a large proteoglycan aggregate. Aggregate size varies with age and disease state; with increasing age and cartilage degeneration aggregates decrease in size. Aggregates containing more than 300 aggrecans have been identified in fetal cartilages, but most articular cartilage aggregates are a fraction of this size.

The other proteoglycans in cartilage are genetically distinct, containing different core proteins. These include 2 small proteoglycans termed biglycan and decorin, both of which have a protein core of approximately 30 kd. Biglycan contains 2 dermatan sulfate chains, and decorin contains 1. Decorin is located on the surface of collagen fibrils and is thought to be involved with the control of fibrillogenesis and fibril diameter. In addition, type IX collagen usually carries a chondroitin sulfate chain, and thus, is also a proteoglycan. Fibromodulin (50 to 65 kd) is another small proteoglycan present in cartilage and contains keratan sulfate. Despite the relatively minor contribution of small proteoglycan molecules to the mass of proteoglycans, there are nearly as many of these small proteoglycan molecules in cartilage as there are aggrecans. Thus, the small proteoglycans are not minor components of the tissue and they may play important, though not yet defined, roles in providing tissue biomechanical properties.

The proteoglycans of articular cartilage are not homogeneously distributed throughout the depth of the tissue. The surface superficial zone is rich in collagen and relatively poor in proteoglycans. In the transitional zone, the concentration of proteoglycans increases, and they are more homogeneously distributed. In the deep zone, the distribution is more variable. Around each chondrocyte in the pericellular matrix, there is an approximately twofold increase in proteoglycan concentration, compared to that in the matrix distant from the cells.

Figure 9 depicts the composite nature of the porous-permeable, collagen-proteoglycan solid matrix. Undoubtedly, the size of the proteoglycans would arrest or minimize diffusion or hydrodynamic connective transport of these molecules through the ECM because of steric exclusion or intermolecular frictional effects. Thus, within the ECM, the size, structural rigidity, and molecular conformation of the charged proteoglycans trapped in the interfibrillar space will influence the mechanical behavior of articular cartilage. The size and complex organization of the proteoglycans also are known to promote proteoglycan-proteoglycan networking and proteoglycan-collagen interactions. This networking capacity enhances the ability of cartilage to maintain structural rigidity and adds to the stiffness and strength of the ECM. The lack of covalent bonds between the proteoglycan and collagen may be necessary to allow the collagen fibers to slide through the proteoglycan gel. In

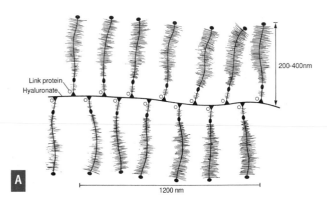

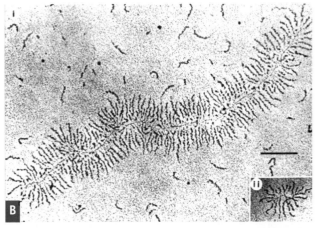

Figure 8

A, A diagram of the aggrecan molecules arranged as a proteoglycan aggregate. Many aggrecan molecules can bind to a chain of hyaluronate, forming macromolecular complexes that effectively are immobilized within the collagen network. **B,** Electron micrographs of bovine articular cartilage proteoglycan aggregates from (i) skeletally immature calf and (ii) skeletally mature steer. These show the aggregates to consist of a central hyaluronic acid filament and multiple attached monomers (bar = 500 μm). (Reproduced with permission from Buckwalter JA, Kuettner KE, Thonar EJ: Age-related changes in articular cartilage proteoglycans: Electron microscopic studies. *J Orthop Res* 1985;3:251–257.)

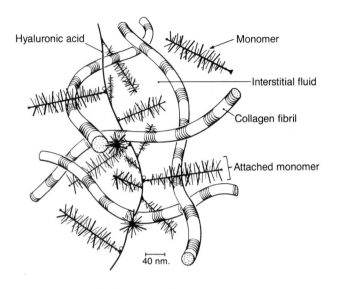

Hyaluronic acid

Monomer

Interstitial fluid

Collagen fibril

Attached monomer

40 nm.

Figure 9

Molecular organization of the solid matrix of articular cartilage as a fiber-reinforced composite solid matrix. The swelling pressure exerted by the proteoglycan keeps the collagen network inflated. (Reproduced with permission from Mow VC, Proctor CS, Kelly MA: Biomechanics of articular cartilage, in Nordin M, Frankel VH (eds): *Basic Biomechanics of the Musculoskeletal System,* ed 2. Philadelphia, PA, Lea & Febiger, 1989, pp 31–57.)

this way the collagen fibrils may resist the tensile stresses developed within the matrix during joint loading and motion. (See Chapter 5.)

Noncollagenous Proteins and Glycoproteins

A variety of noncollagenous proteins and glycoproteins exists within articular cartilage, but thus far only a few of them have been studied. In general, they consist primarily of proteins and have a few attached monosaccharides and oligosaccharides. At least some of these molecules appear to help organize and maintain the macromolecular structure of the ECM. Anchorin CII, a collagen-binding chondrocyte surface protein, may help "anchor" chondrocytes to the matrix collagen fibrils. As yet, the details of these interactions have not been worked out. Cartilage oligomeric protein (COMP), an acidic protein, is concentrated primarily within the chondrocyte territorial matrix. It appears to be present only within cartilage and have the capacity to bind to chondrocytes. This molecule may have value as a marker of cartilage turnover and of the progression of cartilage degeneration in patients with osteoarthritis. Fibronectin and tenascin, noncollagenous matrix proteins that are found in a variety of tissues, have also been identified within cartilage. Their functions in articular cartilage remain poorly understood, but they may have roles in matrix organization, cell-matrix interactions, and in the responses of the tissue in inflammatory arthritis and osteoarthritis.

Lipids

Lipids, which form 1% or less of the wet weight of human adult articular cartilage, are found in both the cells and the matrix. Their exact function is not known, but they vary with age and the presence of osteoarthritis. Phospholipase A_2 is an enzyme that has sparked interest in the past few years. This enzyme may be important both in arachidonic acid metabolism and in the degradative pathway. Pericellular osmiophilic matrix vesicles measure 50 to 250 nm, contain apatitic calcific nodules, and are found in the radial zone. These vesicles appear to increase with age and may play a role in the pathogenesis of osteoarthritis.

Metabolism

Metabolism refers to both synthesis (anabolism) and degradation (catabolism). A surprisingly high level of metabolism exists in articular cartilage. Historically, one of the factors that led to the impression that articular cartilage was inert was the early demonstration that, although articular cartilage had a well-defined glycolytic system, oxygen use was considerably lower in articular cartilage than in other tissues. This difference subsequently was found to be related to the sparse cell population rather than to a lack of metabolic activity per cell. Nevertheless, articular cartilage chondrocytes rely principally on the anaerobic pathway for energy production.

Chondrocytes synthesize and assemble the cartilaginous matrix components and direct their distribution within the tissue. These synthetic and assembly processes are complex, and involve synthesis of proteins, synthesis of glycosaminoglycan chains and their addition to the appropriate protein cores, and secretion of the completed molecules into the ECM. The final incorporation of these components into the matrix also appears to depend on the chondrocyte. All of these actions take place under avascular and, at times, anaerobic conditions, with considerable variation in local pressure and physicochemical states. In addition, the chondrocyte directs internal ECM remodeling by means of an elaborate series of degradative enzymes.

The maintenance of a normal ECM depends on the chondrocytes being able to balance the rates of synthesis of matrix components, the components' appropriate incorporation into the matrix, and the components' degradation and release from the cartilage. The cells do this by responding to their chemical and mechanical environments. Soluble mediators (for example, growth factors, interleukins), matrix composition, mechanical loads, hydrostatic pressure changes, and electric fields can all influence the metabolic activities of the chondrocytes. The response of the chondrocytes usually will maintain a stable matrix. However, in some cases the response of the cells can lead to a change of matrix composition and ultrastructural organization, and eventually to cartilage degeneration.

Nutrition

The source of nutrients for articular cartilage is somewhat of an enigma. Because the tissue is avascular in adult life, most investigators believe that nutrients diffuse through the matrix either from the surrounding synovial fluid or from the underlying bone. Experimental evidence suggests that in skeletally immature animals a portion of the nutrients that enter articular cartilage do so by diffusion from the permeable underlying bony substrate before closure of the physis. In the adult, however, this type of diffusion disappears or becomes severely limited with the appearance of the tidemark and a heavy deposition of apatite in the calcified cartilage zone, leaving the synovial fluid as the most likely source of nutrition. The extremely small pore size (estimated to be 50 Å) of the superficial zone should permit only low molecular weight components of the fluid (less than 20 kd) to diffuse into the tissue. Measured diffusion times range from 10 seconds to 1 hour depending on the molecular weight, structure, size, and charge of the molecules diffusing through the tissue. However, molecules from the synovial fluid (for example, interleukin-1 and the prostaglandins) and some growth factors appear to move freely through the tissue. Further, fragments of proteoglycans and other matrix components, generated by proteolytic activity in normal turnover and in degeneration, are able to leave the tissue rapidly. Normal joints contain very small amounts of synovial fluid. For example, even in a large joint such as the normal knee, there is less than 4 ml of synovial fluid, which forms a coating over the articular surfaces of the joint just 10 to 20 µm thick. Yet, sufficient nutrients and oxygen from the metabolically active synovium reach the chondrocytes, presumably by diffusion through the cartilage matrix via the synovial fluid.

Proteoglycan Synthesis

The chondrocyte is responsible for the synthesis, assembly, and sulfation of the proteoglycan molecule (Fig. 10). At the molecular level, this activity begins with proteoglycan gene expression and the transcription of the messenger RNA (mRNA) from the DNA within the nucleus. In the endoplasmic reticulum, the mRNA is translated and the protein is synthesized at the ribosome. The protein core is then transported to the Golgi complex, where the glycosaminoglycan chains are added. Although the addition appears to be very specific and well coordinated, little is known about how the cell controls these events. Chondroitin/dermatan sulfate chains are attached to specific serine residues in the

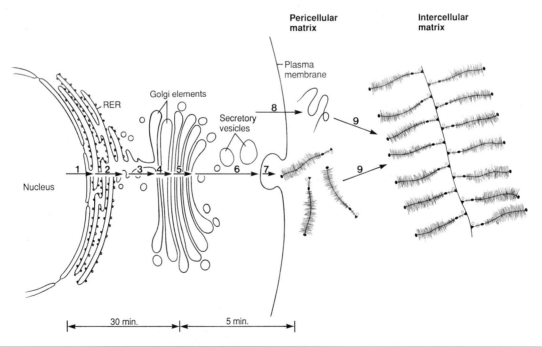

Figure 10

Diagram depicting the various stages involved in the synthesis and secretion of aggrecan and link protein by a chondrocyte. (1) The transcription of the aggrecan and link protein genes to mRNA. (2) The translation of the mRNA in the rough endoplasmic reticulum (RER) to form the protein core of the aggrecan. (3) The newly-formed protein is transported from the RER to (4) the cis and (5) medial-trans Golgi compartments where the glycosaminoglycan chains are added to the protein core. (6) On completion of the glycosylation and sulfation, the molecules are transported via secretory vesicles to the plasma membrane, where (7) they are released into the extracellular matrix. (8) Hyaluronate is synthesized separately at the plasma membrane. (9) Only in the extracellular matrix can aggrecan, link protein, and hyaluronate come together to form proteoglycan aggregates.

sequence Ser-Gly via a unique tetrasaccharide:

-glucuronic acid-galactose-galactose-xylose-ser
|

The repeating disaccharide glucuronic acid-galactosamine is then added to this linkage region; in dermatan sulfate, some of the glucuronic acid residues are subsequently isomerized to iduronic acid. On the other hand, keratan sulfate chains are attached to either serine or threonine by a different sequence:

-galactose-glucosamine
| |
  galactosamine-ser(thr)
| |
sialic acid-galactose

The repeating disaccharide galactose-glucosamine is then added to the linkage region galactose. All of the carbohydrate constituents of glycosaminoglycan chains are added 1 sugar at a time. While the chains are being elongated, hexosamine residues of both chondroitin/dermatan sulfate and keratan sulfate chains are being sulfated. All of the above steps are posttranslational enzymic reactions and, therefore, are not under direct genetic control. For this reason, the glycosaminoglycan chains vary in length. Once glycosylation is complete, the proteoglycan molecules are secreted into the ECM. The protein core may represent as little as 10% of the completed molecule by weight. Thus, the addition of the glycosaminoglycan chains and the other oligosaccharides as posttranslational modifications offers tremendous opportunity for variations in the composition of the completed molecule and can create significant variability of the structure of the molecules synthesized at any particular time. In articular cartilage from young individuals, newly synthesized proteoglycans are relatively uniform, but with aging or development of osteoarthritis, the cells produce aggrecans that vary considerably in size and composition.

Synthesis of some of the proteoglycans by the chondrocyte appears to occur at a rapid rate and is affected by numerous endogenous and exogenous environmental alterations. Studies have shown that such diverse physical and pathologic states as lacerative injury; osteoarthritis; altered interstitial hydrostatic pressure; stresses, strains, and flows in the tissue; varied oxygen tension; pH alteration; calcium concentration; substrate or serum concentration; growth hormones; insulin-like growth factor-I (IGF-I); ascorbate; vitamin E; cortisol; prostaglandins; diphosphonates; salicylates and several other nonsteroidal anti-inflammatory drugs; hyaluronate; uridine diphosphate; xyloside; synovial tissue; and a variety of other factors have significant effects on the rate of synthesis of the proteoglycans. These data suggest that the control mechanisms for proteoglycan synthesis are extraordinarily sensitive to biochemical, mechanical, and physical stimuli. It is also evident that the turnover rate for a small fraction of the proteoglycans is quite rapid. This rapidity seems far in excess of that necessary merely to compensate for any attrition that may occur in cartilage in a joint that operates in an almost frictionless state. These observations strongly suggest the presence of an elaborate internal remodeling system for proteoglycans, which is presumed to be dictated by circumstances other than attrition.

Proteoglycan Catabolism

In normal tissue, in repair processes, and in degradation, proteoglycans of articular cartilage are continually being broken down and released from the cartilage. This activity is a normal event in maintenance of the tissue; it can occur as part of remodeling in repair processes, and in degenerative events it appears to occur at an accelerated rate. The rate of catabolism can be affected by soluble mediators and by various types of joint loading. For example, interleukin-1 will accelerate proteoglycan degradation, and immobilization of a joint will cause loss of proteoglycans from the cartilage matrix.

Current understanding of proteoglycan breakdown in articular cartilage comes from studies of aggrecan and proteoglycan aggregates. The heterogeneity of proteoglycans in articular cartilage is likely to be derived from some limited enzymatic cleavage of the protein core. A major cleavage site of the protein core is between the G1 and G2 domains (Fig. 11), separating the part of the proteoglycan involved in aggregation (binding to hyaluronate and link protein) from the part that contains the glycosaminoglycan chains. The free glycosaminoglycan-containing fragment, although it is large, is able to pass through the matrix and leave the cartilage. This appears to be an efficient mechanism of turnover of the large proteoglycan. The G1 domain and link protein also are susceptible to proteolytic degradation and can thus be released from the cartilage. These fragments can be found in synovial fluid, from which they are taken up through the synovium to the lymphatic system (Fig. 12). The glycosaminoglycan chains can be found further along in this system, in the bloodstream, and even in the urine. The levels of proteoglycan fragments (for example, keratan sulfate) in the body fluids can be quantified and, at least in synovial fluid, it is thought that these levels can be used to measure catabolic activities in the cartilage of that joint. It is hoped that this type of analysis may offer some diagnostic and prognostic help in the clinical evaluation of early degenerative joint disease.

Collagen Synthesis

The collagen network of articular cartilage is much more stable than the proteoglycan components. However, the collagen network is subject to metabolism, and in

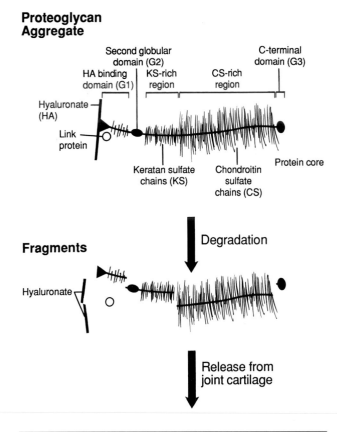

Proteoglycan Aggregate

Fragments

Figure 11

Representation of the mechanism of degradation of proteoglycan aggregates in articular cartilage. The major proteolytic cleavage site is between the G1 and G2 domains, making the glycosaminoglycan-containing portion of the aggrecan molecule nonaggregating. This fragment can now be released from the cartilage. Other proteolytic events can result in G1 domain and link protein also disaggregating and leaving the cartilage.

osteoarthritic cartilage, or cartilage that has undergone lacerative injury, the collagen turnover increases. Most knowledge about collagen synthesis has come from studies of the major fibrillar types (for example, types I to III) (Fig. 13). In a manner identical to that for other secretory proteins, mRNA for the constituent α chains is translated to form a polypeptide containing a signal sequence and noncollagenous propeptide domains on both the amino and carboxy termini flanking the collagenous domain. The nascent chains are extruded into the cisterna of the rough endoplasmic reticulum where the signal peptide is immediately removed and where the posttranslational events of propeptide glycosylation, proline and lysine hydroxylation, lysine glycosylation, and triple helix formation occur. The latter step, which is propagated in a carboxy to amino terminal direction, is obligatory for the procollagen molecule to enter the secretory apparatus. It is useful to note that the hydroxylation reactions require vitamin C as a cofactor and that deficiencies (for example, scurvy) can result in alterations in collagen synthesis. After secretion, the propep-

tides are cleaved from both ends of the triple-helical domain, and the resultant collagen molecules can self-assemble into the fibrillar arrays discussed previously. The final step in this process is covalent cross-link formation, which is catalyzed by the enzyme lysyl oxidase.

In cartilage, the above steps are generally followed for types II and XI collagen. For each of the other cartilage collagen types, there are variations on this process. Types VI, IX, and X collagen, for example, retain their noncollagenous terminal domains after secretion, and these unprocessed forms are used in subsequent matrix interaction. In addition, type IX collagen has a single site that usually contains a chondroitin sulfate chain, which probably is added intracellularly in the Golgi compartment. Finally, recent evidence has uncovered another level of complexity in cartilage collagen synthesis at the transcription level where collagen types II and IX can be alternatively spliced to yield slightly different products in different tissues.

Collagen Catabolism

As yet, little is known about the mechanisms of collagen breakdown. In normal cartilage it occurs at a slow rate, although in degenerative cartilage and in cartilage undergoing repair and remodeling (for example, during skeletal growth), there is evidence of accelerated breakdown of the collagen network. The mechanism of breakdown may be enzymatic, with the metalloproteinase collagenase able to specifically cleave the triple helix of collagen.

Growth Factors

Recent work shows that polypeptide growth factors play a role in the regulation of the synthetic processes of normal cartilage. In addition, it has been speculated that these growth factors may even have a greater role in osteoarthritis. The methods by which these agents act on the chondrocyte have not been elucidated fully but appear to be related principally to interaction with cell surface receptor sites on the responsive cells. In the case of at least 2 of these agents (IGF-1 and insulin), competitive binding is present, which may alter the end result. For most of the factors, however, the cell receptor is highly specific and the response is dictated by the concentration of the growth factor and the number of receptors on the cell. The various growth factors are discussed below.

Platelet-Derived Growth Factor (PDGF)

PDGF is a 30-kd glycoprotein that consists of a dimer of disulfide-bonded A and B polypeptide chains. Various isoforms have been identified and seem to have different activities. Although several studies have suggested that PDGF has a mitogenic effect on chondrocytes, the method of action is not clear nor does it seem likely that this material is active in the joint under normal conditions. In osteoarthritis, and especially in lacerative injury, a greater likelihood exists for the role of these peptides in healing.

Basic Fibroblast Growth Factor (bFGF)

This material, like many of the other factors, comes from multiple sources. In the past, the peptide coming from the pituitary was referred to as cartilage growth factor, and that generated by the cartilage was called cartilage-derived growth factor. It is now evident that these are identical to bFGF, which acts in connective tissues principally as a very powerful mitogen. Studies have shown that bFGF alone is a powerful stimulator of DNA synthesis in adult articular chondrocytes in culture. This material, although contributory to matrix production, seems less active unless it is

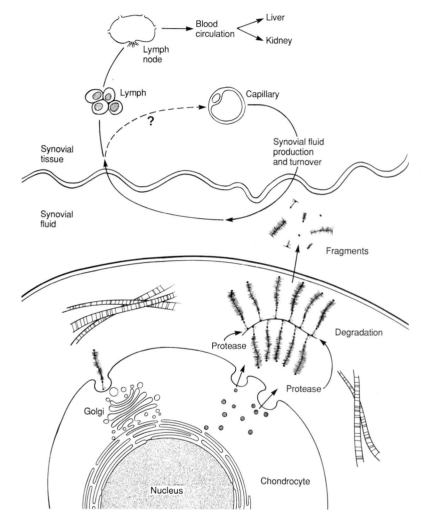

Figure 12

Schematic representation of the metabolic events controlling the proteoglycans in cartilage. The chondrocytes synthesize and secrete aggrecan, link protein, and hyaluronate, and they become incorporated into functional aggregates. Enzymes released by the cells break down the proteoglycan aggregates. The fragments are released from the matrix into the synovial fluid, and from there the fragments are taken up by the lymphatics and moved into the circulating blood.

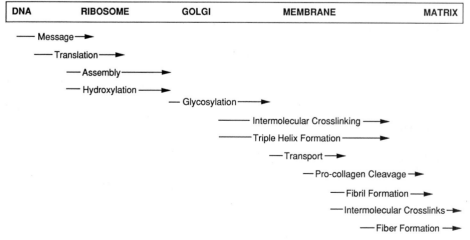

Figure 13

The events involved in the synthesis of collagen, showing the intracellular sites that are used for each procedure. (Reproduced with permission from Mankin HJ, Brandt KD: Biochemistry and metabolism of articular cartilage in osteoarthritis, in Moskowitz RW, Howell DS, Goldberg VM, et al (eds): *Osteoarthritis: Diagnosis and Medical/Surgical Management,* ed 2. Philadelphia, PA, WB Saunders, 1992, pp 109–154.)

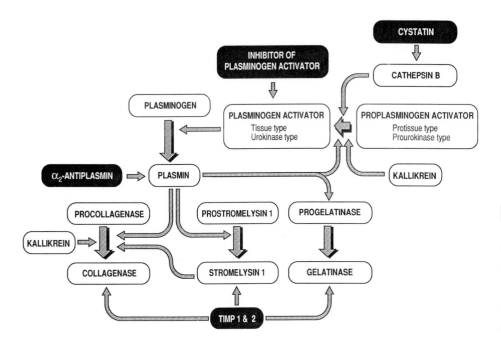

Figure 14

The proteolytic enzymes, their activators and inhibitors involved in the catabolism of articular cartilage matrix. (Reproduced with permission from Mow VC, Ratcliffe A, Poole AR: Cartilage and diarthrodial joints as paradigms for hierarchical structures. *Biomaterials* 1992;13:67–97.)

introduced with other materials, such as insulin. Recent studies have shown that bFGF markedly stimulates repair of cartilage slices in an in vivo rabbit model.

Insulin and Insulin-Like Growth Factors (IGF-I and IGF-II)

Perhaps the best studied of the growth factors, insulin, IGF-I, and IGF-II are 3 homologous peptides that bind with varying affinity to 3 distinct receptors on the cells. IGF-I and IGF-II are structurally homologous to proinsulin, almost the same size (70 and 67 amino acids), and share about 65% homology. IGF-I, formerly known as somatomedin-C, has been found to stimulate DNA and matrix synthesis in growth plate, in immature cartilage, and, more recently, in adult articular cartilage. There is little evidence to suggest that these growth factors are synthesized by articular cartilage, and it is unknown whether IGF is produced locally or in the liver. IGF-I is more effective when coadministered with other factors, including bFGF, but not insulin. Recent evidence suggests that IGF-I maintains a steady state for proteoglycan synthesis in adult tissue.

Transforming Growth Factor-Beta (TGF-β)

TGF-β is a 25-kd protein composed of 2 identical polypeptides linked by disulfide bonds. It shares its receptor with no other factors and is known to exist in at least 5 isoforms. Numerous cellular activities have been attributed to this material in relation to bone and more recently cartilage, and not all of these are stimulatory. The material seems to potentiate the stimulation of DNA synthesis by bFGF, epidermal growth factor, and IGF-I rather than initiating it de novo. Recent studies have shown that TGF-β is synthesized locally by the chondrocytes and appears to stimulate proteoglycan synthesis and, at the same time, suppress type II

collagen synthesis. There is now evidence to suggest that, in addition to its other functions, TGF-β is responsible for stimulating the formation of tissue inhibitor of metalloproteinase (TIMP) and plasminogen activator inhibitor-1, 2 materials believed to prevent the degradative action of stromelysin and plasmin.

Degradative Enzymes

The breakdown of the cartilage matrix in normal turnover, and in articular cartilage degeneration, appears to be by the action of proteolytic enzymes (proteinases) that are synthesized by the chondrocytes. This is part of the complex orchestration of events performed by the chondrocytes to maintain the normal cartilage matrix. It is likely that the overactivity of some of these enzymes is ultimately responsible for cartilage degradation in osteoarthritis and rheumatoid arthritis. The most important proteinases thought to be involved in cartilage turnover are shown in Figure 14. The major groups are metalloproteinases (collagenase, gelatinase, and stromelysin) and the cathepsins (cathepsins B and D).

The metalloproteinases derive their name from the fact that their activity depends on the presence of zinc in the active site. Collagenase is highly specific in its action on collagen, because it is the only enzyme that can cleave the triple-helical part of the molecule, at a single site three fourths of the way along the molecule from the amino terminus. Gelatinase cleaves the denatured α chains generated by prior collagenase activity. Stromelysin can act on type II collagen within the nonhelical domain and can also act on type IX collagen. Breakdown of the protein core of aggrecan has been thought to be a major activity of stromelysin. Although it cleaves the protein core between the G1 and G2 domains (as occurs in normal aggrecan breakdown), the specific cleavage products identified in vivo and in vitro cannot be assigned to stromelysin. The possibility therefore remains that another enzyme, yet to be defined, is responsible for the cleavage of aggrecan, or that stromelysin acts together with another enzyme.

The activities of these metalloproteinases appear to be controlled by 2 mechanisms, their activation and their inhibition. Collagenase, stromelysin, and gelatinase are all synthesized as latent enyzmes (proenzymes), and they require activation outside of the cell by enzymatic modification. Plasmin, produced from plasminogen by the activity of a plasminogen activator, can activate collagenase. Stromelysin can superactivate collagenase to produce maximal activity. The mechanisms of activation for prostromelysin and progelatinase remain to be determined. The active enzymes can be inhibited irreversibly by TIMP, which also is secreted by the chondrocyte. The molar ratios of metalloproteinases and TIMP will determine whether there is net metalloproteinase activity.

The cathepsins are a second group of articular cartilage enzymes that have the capacity to degrade aggrecan. These have been identified as cathepsins D and B, and both are known to occur in articular cartilage. Of some concern, however, has been the low pH optima at which these acid cathepsins act (pH 5.5), because it may exclude them from having a major role in the degradation of proteoglycan in the interterritorial matrix. However, there is some evidence that low pH can be achieved in the cartilage, possibly in the pericellular matrix; therefore, the ability of acid pH optimum enzymes to participate in cartilage metabolism cannot be excluded.

Development and Aging

Unlike many other tissues, immature articular cartilage differs considerably from adult articular cartilage. On gross inspection, the cartilage from a skeletally immature animal appears blue-white in color, presumably because of the reflection of the vascular structures in the underlying immature bone, and is relatively thick. The thickness appears to be primarily a function of the dual nature of the cartilage mass, which serves not only as a cartilaginous articular surface for the joint but also as a microepiphyseal plate for endochondral ossification of the underlying bony nucleus of the epiphysis.

On histologic examination, it is apparent that immature articular cartilage is considerably more cellular than the adult tissue, and numerous studies have corroborated the high number of cells per unit volume or mass in immature articular cartilage (Fig. 15, A). The high level of cellularity appears fairly uniform throughout immature cartilage. The structural organization of the tissue also differs from that of adult cartilage in that the zonal characteristics show major variation, particularly in the lower zones. The gliding or tangential layer is evident in immature articular cartilage, although the surface cells are somewhat larger and less discoid than those seen in adult cartilage. The midzone is wider and contains a larger number of randomly arranged cells. In the lower zones, however, the orientation differs markedly; at about the halfway mark in the distance from the surface to the underlying bone, the chondrocytes are arranged in irregular columns and, at further depth, the columnation becomes more evident. With further distance from the surface, the cells are increased in size and show

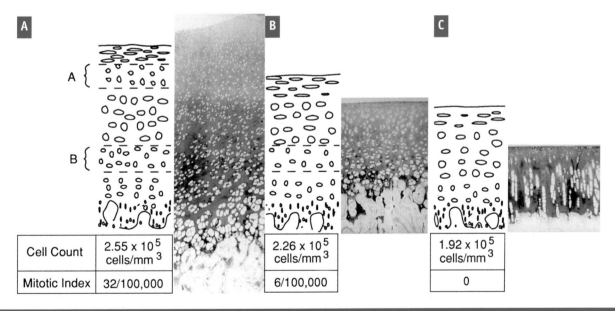

	Cell Count	Mitotic Index
A	2.55×10^5 cells/mm^3	32/100,000
B	2.26×10^5 cells/mm^3	6/100,000
C	1.92×10^5 cells/mm^3	0

Figure 15

Estimates of number density of chondrocytes and histologic sections of articular cartilage, showing changes in thickness and cellular population. **A,** immature. **B,** maturing. **C,** adult. (Photomicrographs provided by EB Hunziker, MD, 1990, Bern, Switzerland.)

shrunken pyknotic nuclei and large intracytoplasmic vacuoles that have been demonstrated to contain glycogen. Vascular buds from the underlying bone invade the cartilage columns in a pattern resembling the zone of provisional calcification of the epiphyseal plate.

When immature articular cartilage is examined by light microscopy, mitotic figures are readily noted, and all stages of mitosis can be seen. Cell replication is not uniformly present throughout the tissue. In the very young animal, the mitotic activity occurs in 2 distinct zones. One lies subjacent to the surface and presumably accounts for the growth of the cellular complement of the articular portion of the cartilage mass; the second lies below this region and consists of a narrow band of cells that morphologically resemble the proliferative zone of the microepiphyseal plate of the subjacent bony nucleus. Figure 15 shows the changes observed in rabbit articular cartilage. It should be noted that a 2-month-old rabbit is immature; a 6-month old rabbit, pubertal; and an 18-month-old rabbit, a young adult. As the animal ages and approaches maturity, the pattern of cell replication changes. The mitotic activity is confined to the area just above the zone of vascular invasion in the lowermost portion of the cartilage, which now demonstrates a diffuse calcification. No evidence for cell replication can be found in the more superficial regions.

In the adult animal, mitotic activity ceases with the development of a well-defined calcified zone, the tidemark, and, in some species, with closure of the epiphyseal plate. Careful search of normal articular cartilage from adult animals of numerous species has failed to demonstrate mitotic figures, and ^{3}H-thymidine studies have not demonstrated grains over the nucleus to indicate DNA replication. Although it has been suggested that the chondrocyte may divide by amitotic division, there is only limited evidence for such an activity, and cytophotometry and cytofluorometry have failed to demonstrate evidence of nuclear polyploidy in the adult tissue (Fig. 15, C).

In recent years, investigations have demonstrated significant variation in the chemistry of articular cartilage with advancing age. Water content appears to be relatively high in immature animals and slowly diminishes during skeletal growth to a level that remains relatively constant throughout most of adulthood. The collagen content of fetal articular cartilage is considerably lower than that of mature animals. The collagen concentration climbs to adult levels shortly after birth, and it is maintained throughout the life of the animal. The principal chemical changes that occur in articular cartilage matrix with advancing age appear to be in the proteoglycans. Proteoglycan content in articular cartilage is highest at birth and diminishes slowly through the period of skeletal growth. The protein core and the glycosaminoglycan chains are longer in immature animals. As the animal approaches adolescence and maturity, the average length of the proteoglycan protein core becomes less, probably because of enzymatic cleavage of the resident proteoglycan population, near the C-terminal end of the protein core, and the lengths of the glycosaminoglycan chains, particularly those of chondroitin sulfate, diminish. Although an extraordinarily high concentration of chondroitin 4-sulfate has been noted in immature animals, a fairly rapid diminution in the value is noted with aging accompanied by an increase in the concentration of chondroitin 6-sulfate. Furthermore, with advancing age, the total chondroitin sulfate concentration falls and that of keratan sulfate increases until at approximately age 30 in humans, keratan sulfate represents 25% to 50% of the total glycosaminoglycans. This value then remains constant through old age. It should be noted that aggregation appears to diminish with advancing age, possibly on the basis of an alteration in the core protein or link protein, but this does not appear to be a result of any change in the concentration of hyaluronate. Synthesis of proteoglycans in vitro is diminished for rabbit and bovine articular chondrocytes from mature animals, which is consistent with a maintenance process of the ECM after its remodeling during growth, development, and maturation. In addition, with increasing age, chondrocytes may become less responsive to anabolic cytokines.

Biomechanics

Chapter 5, Biomechanics, and the glossary will be helpful to the reader who is not familiar with the terminology and the constructs of biomechanics.

The Biphasic Nature of Articular Cartilage

The articular cartilage of diarthrodial joints is subject to high loads applied statically, cyclically, and repetitively for many decades. Thus, the structural molecules, that is, collagens, proteoglycans, and other molecules, must be organized into a strong, fatigue-resistant, and tough, solid matrix capable of sustaining the high stresses and strains developed within the tissue from these loads. In terms of material behavior, this solid matrix is described as being porous and permeable, and very soft. Water, 65% to 80% of the total weight of normal articular cartilage, resides in the microscopic pores, and this water may be caused to flow through the porous-permeable solid matrix by a pressure gradient or by matrix compaction. Thus, the biomechanical properties of articular cartilage are understood best when the tissue is viewed as a biphasic material, composed of a solid phase and a fluid phase (including the dissolved ions). Because of technical difficulties, early studies on cartilage biomechanics have generally ignored the water component of the tissue. Over the past 2 decades, however, a theory has been developed, which is capable of describing the biphasic deformational behaviors of hydrated soft tissues such as cartilage. This theory has been used to describe the experimentally measured behaviors of articular cartilage, as well as to calculate interstitial fluid flow and stresses and strains in the collagen-proteoglycan solid matrix. The material coefficients can be calculated from the experimental data by using the biphasic theory, and these define the intrinsic behavior of the collagen-proteoglycan solid matrix and its frictional resistance against interstitial fluid flow. Within this theoretical framework, the structure-function relationships of the collagen-proteoglycan solid matrix of normal cartilage, and changes of these intrinsic material properties in osteoarthritic cartilage are determined.

Permeability

A series of studies have shown that water is capable of flowing through the cartilage when a pressure gradient is imposed. In these experiments, a tissue sample of thickness h is subjected to an applied pressure gradient ($\Delta P/h$) across the specimen. The rate of volume discharge Q across the permeation area A is related to the hydraulic permeability coefficient k by Darcy's law, which expresses a direct linear proportionality between Q and ($\Delta P/h$), $Q = kA(\Delta P/h)$. The permeation speed V is related to Q by the expression $V = Q/A\phi^f$ where ϕ^f, the porosity of the tissue (65% to 80%), is defined as the ratio of the interstitial fluid volume V^f to the total tissue volume V^T. Results from this permeation experiment show that for normal cartilage and meniscus, the permeability coefficient k ranges from 10^{-15} to 10^{-16} m^4/Ns. The diffusive drag coefficient K is inversely related to the permeability coefficient k and is given by the following simple equation: $K = (\phi^f)^2/k$. Because the porosity ϕ^f for cartilage ranges from 0.65 to 0.80, K ranges from 10^{14} to 10^{15} Ns/m^4. This very large frictional drag coefficient indicates that any interstitial fluid flow will cause large drag forces to be generated within the tissue. In turn, very high pressures are required to move the water through cartilage; a flow speed of 17.5 µm/s requires a pressure gradient of 1 MPa (or 145 psi).

Water also will flow through the porous-permeable solid matrix as the tissue is compressed. In this case, the compressive stress causes the solid matrix to be compacted, raising the pressure in the interstitium and forcing the fluid out of the tissue. The rate of efflux is controlled by the drag force generated during flow. In general, the manner with which an applied load is shared between the fluid phase (hydrodynamic pressure) and the solid phase (stress in the solid matrix) is determined, among other things, by the volumetric ratios within the tissue, that is, the porosity ϕ^f and solidity ϕ^s (= V^s/V^T, where V^s is the volume of the solid matrix), the loading rates, and the type of loading (tension, compression, and shear). The load-carrying capacity of each phase is determined by balancing the frictional drag forces against the elastic forces at each point within the tissue. For example, flow of fluid through a highly permeable,

stiff solid matrix would cause little frictional drag force or fluid pressurization. A compressive stress acting on such a material would be supported predominantly by the stress developed within the solid matrix (for example, a highly porous rigid steel filter). Conversely, flow of fluid through a soft solid matrix with very low permeability would cause high frictional drag forces and require high hydrodynamic pressures to maintain a significant flow. In this case, fluid pressure provides a significant component of total load support, thus minimizing the stress acting on the solid matrix. Such is the case for normal articular cartilage. This phenomonon is referred to as stress shielding of the solid matrix.

Articular cartilage permeability, as calculated using Darcy's law, is based on data obtained from permeation experiments. This permeability decreases nonlinearly with compression ε_c (Fig. 16). This strain-dependent permeability effect serves to regulate the response of cartilage to compression by preventing rapid and excessive fluid exudation from the tissue with compressive loading, and by promoting interstitial fluid pressurization for load support. It also regulates the ability of cartilage to dissipate energy during cyclic loading. There are 2 reasons for this nonlinear effect: (1) as the tissue is compressed, the water content or porosity is reduced; and (2) as the tissue is compressed, the density of the negative charges on the proteoglycan (COO^- and SO_3^-) in the interstitium is increased (see below for a discussion on swelling pressure). Because proteoglycan is the main reason why water is held so tightly within the interstitium of cartilage, an increase in its concentration would act to decrease permeability. These observations have been verified experimentally by correlating the permeabilities of different osteoarthritic cartilages with tissue water and proteoglycan contents. Indeed, there is a direct relationship between permeability and water content, and an inverse relationship between permeability and proteoglycan content.

Flow-Dependent Viscoelasticity in Compression

Articular cartilage is viscoelastic; it will exhibit a time-dependent behavior when subjected to a constant load or constant deformation. When a constant compressive stress (load/area) is applied to the tissue, its deformation will increase with time; it will creep until an equilibrium value is reached (Fig. 17, *top*). Similarly, when the tissue is deformed and held at a constant strain, the stress will rise to a peak, followed by a slow stress-relaxation process until an equilibrium value is reached (Fig. 17, *bottom*). In polymeric materials, these viscoelastic behaviors arise from the frictional force generated by the sliding motion of long-chain molecules within the material, resulting in internal energy dissipation. In articular cartilage, however, there are 2 mechanisms responsible for viscoelasticity: a flow-independent and a flow-dependent mechanism. The flow-independent viscoelastic behavior of the collagen-proteoglycan matrix of cartilage derives from intermolecular friction, and this is measured with a pure shear experiment in which no fluid flow occurs within the tissue. The flow-dependent mechanism depends on interstitial fluid flow and pressurization, as discussed above. It is now known that the drag resulting from interstitial fluid flow is the main contributor to the compressive viscoelastic behavior of cartilage (Fig. 18).

Interstitial fluid pressure is generated in cartilage during loading (compression), and it combines with matrix compression in supporting the applied load. However, under constant load, as creep continues, the load support is gradually transferred from the fluid phase (as the fluid pressure dissipates) to the solid phase. Typically, for normal cartilage, this equilibration process takes 2.5 to 6.0 hours to achieve. At equilibrium the fluid pressure vanishes, and load support is provided entirely by the compressed collagen-proteoglycan solid matrix. It has been experimentally determined that this equilibrium compressive strain is related linearly to the applied compressive stress. The proportionality constant of this linear relationship defines the equilibrium compressive modulus. Typically, this compressive modulus of the solid matrix of normal articular cartilage ranges from 0.4 to 1.5 MPa. Table 3 provides Poisson's ratio, compressive aggregate modulus, and permeability coefficients for articular cartilage from the lateral condyle and patellar groove of young normal humans, steers, beagles, greyhounds, cynomolgus monkeys, and New Zealand white rabbits.

Because of the long equilibration time, articular cartilage is almost always dynamically loaded under physiologic conditions, that is, no equilibrium state occurs because the joints are always moving, even during sleep. Thus, fluid pressurization almost always will occur within the tissue. It is likely, then, that in normal articular cartilage, fluid pressurization is the dominant physiologic load-support mechanism in diarthrodial joints. This unique behavior of cartilage occurs only because the solid matrix is very soft and has a very low permeability. The known values of normal articular cartilage permeability and compressive modulus have been used in calculations to determine that fluid pressure supports, by far, the larger part of the applied load. In fact, the ratio of load supported by the fluid pressure to that supported by the solid matrix stress is greater than 20 to 1 in normal articular cartilage.

The most apparent early changes in human osteoarthritic cartilage are increased water content and decreased proteoglycan content. These changes increase tissue permeability. Increased permeability diminishes the fluid pressurization mechanism of load support in cartilage and, thus, requires the collagen-proteoglycan solid matrix to bear more of the load. Increased loading of the solid matrix is detrimental for the long-term survival of cartilage, and may be an important factor in the development and progression of cartilage degeneration in patients with osteoarthritis.

Flow-Independent Viscoelastic Shear Properties

The random organization of the collagen architecture through the middle zones of the tissue contributes significantly to the shear properties of articular cartilage. Stretching of these randomly dispersed collagen fibrils and shear-

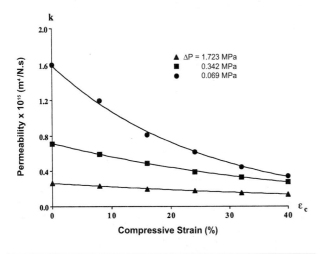

Figure 16

Permeability of normal bovine articular cartilage showing nonlinear strain dependence and pressure dependence. The decrease of permeability with compression acts to retard rapid loss of interstitial fluid during high joint loadings. (Reproduced with permission from Mow VC, Zhu W, Ratcliffe A: Structure and function of articular cartilage and meniscus, in Mow VC, Hayes WC (eds): *Basic Orthopaedic Biomechanics.* New York, NY, Raven Press, 1991, pp 143–198.)

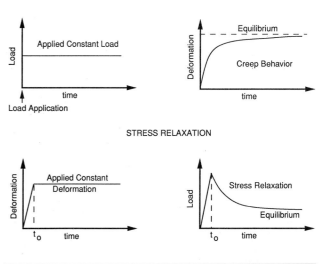

Figure 17

Top, Creep of a viscoelastic material under constant loading. **Bottom,** Stress rise during a ramp-displacement compression of a viscoelastic material and stress relaxation under constant compression. (Reproduced with permission from Mow VC, Ratcliffe A, Poole AR: Cartilage and diarthrodial joints as paradigms for hierarchical structures. *Biomaterials* 1992;13: 67–97.)

ing of the entrapped proteoglycan molecules provide cartilage with its shear stress-strain response (Figs. 4 and 19). No interstitial fluid flow occurs under pure shear because no pressure gradients or volume changes are developed within the tissue. Thus, the pure shear experiment provides a direct method to determine the flow-independent viscoelastic properties of articular cartilage. For normal human and bovine articular cartilage, the equilibrium shear moduli have been determined to range from 0.05 to 0.30 MPa.

To assess the flow-independent viscoelastic properties, a dynamic (sinusoidal) pure shear experiment must be performed. In these experiments, the magnitude of the dynamic shear modulus $|G^*(\omega)|$ and $\tan\delta$ are measured.

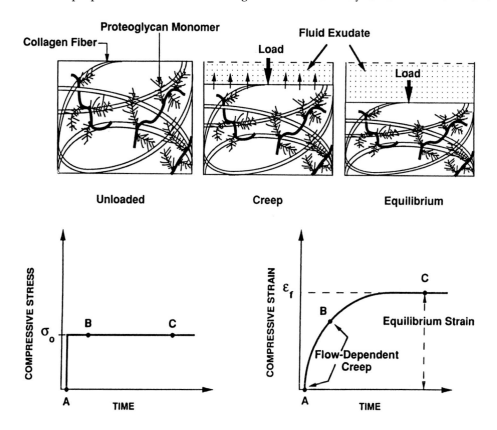

Figure 18

Biphasic creep behavior of a hydrated soft tissue such as articular cartilage during compression. Rate of creep is governed by the rate at which fluid may be forced out from the tissue, which, in turn, is governed by the permeability and stiffness of the porous-permeable, collagen-proteoglycan solid matrix.

Table 3

Average Poisson's Ratio, Compressive Aggregate Modulus and Permeability Coefficient of Lateral Condyle Cartilage and Patellar Groove Cartilage

	Human*	Bovine*	Canine*	Monkey*	Rabbit*
Poisson's Ratio (ϑ)					
Lateral condyle	0.10	0.40	0.30	0.24	0.34
Patellar groove	0.00	0.25	0.09	0.20	0.21
Compressive Aggregate Modulus (MPa)					
Lateral condyle	0.70	0.89	0.60	0.78	0.54
Patellar groove	0.53	0.47	0.55	0.52	0.51
Permeability Coefficient ($10^{-15}m^4/N{\cdot}s$)					
Lateral condyle	1.18	0.43	0.77	4.19	1.81
Patellar groove	2.17	1.42	0.93	4.74	3.84

*   Animals are young normal humans; 18 months to 2-year-old steers; mature beagles and greyhounds; mature cynomolgus monkeys; and mature New Zealand white rabbits

The dynamic shear modulus is a measure of the intrinsic shear stiffness of the solid matrix at any given frequency ω, and tan δ is a measure of the viscoelastic energy dissipation in the tissue during a cycle of shear. A value of $\delta = 0°$ represents a purely elastic material with no energy dissipation, whereas a value of $\delta = 90°$ represents a purely viscous material that is highly dissipative. The value of $|G^* (\omega)|$ depends on the frequency of oscillation, and it has been measured to vary from 0.2 to 2.5 MPa with increasing frequency from 0.01 to 20 Hz; the corresponding values of δ range from 20° to 9° in an inverse manner with increasing frequency. The effects of compression on cartilage are to stiffen the tissue in shear and make it less dissipative. Again, this nonlinear effect is important in that the resistance of cartilage to shear stress increases with compression.

How does shear stress arise in cartilage when the articular surface is nearly frictionless? Consider the simple act of compressing a strip of cartilage. The tissue not only would be compressed in the direction of the applied load, but also would expand in the transverse direction; this is known as the Poisson's ratio effect. If a surface of the strip is firmly attached to a rigid surface, such as the deep zone cartilage is attached to the tidemark in situ, then the cartilage cannot expand freely at this interface. To prevent its expansion, a shear stress must be imparted onto the articular cartilage at the interface by the hard, bony substrate. Indeed, it has been shown that by compressing articular cartilage on bone, the shear stress attains a maximum value at the tidemark. Also, it is well known that high compressive loads, such as those that occur during blunt impact, will cause articular cartilage to be sheared off of the bone. The fact that any materials with a Poisson's ratio other than zero will spread in the transverse direction during compression means that tensile stresses and strains will also be developed within the material. For cartilage, these tensile stresses and strains may be sufficiently large to cause collagen fiber and network damage at the articular surface.

The low values of δ (9° to 20°) for articular cartilage as compared with ~150° for solutions of pure concentrated proteoglycan networks indicate that the collagen-proteoglycan solid matrix of articular cartilage is more elastic and less dissipative than the pure concentrated proteoglycan solutions. The collagen-proteoglycan matrix is, however, considerably more viscoelastic and dissipative than is collagen alone, with $\delta \sim 4.0°$ for a highly collagenous tissue such as canine medial collateral ligament. Figure 20 provides a comparison of energy dissipation for collateral ligament, articular cartilage, and proteoglycan solutions. In addition, the dynamic shear modulus $|G^* (\omega)|$ of pure proteoglycan solutions indicates that the proteoglycan-collagen matrix is approximately 10^5 times stiffer than pure solutions of proteoglycan-proteoglycan networks alone. These differences lead to the conclusion that proteoglycan-proteoglycan networks in solution add little to the observed stiffness and elasticity of articular cartilage in shear. Furthermore, these

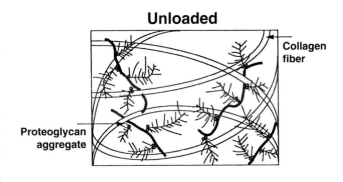

Unloaded

Collagen fiber

Proteoglycan aggregate

Pure shear

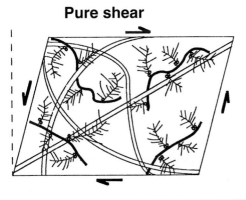

Figure 19

Schematic depiction of how the collagen-proteoglycan solid matrix may act under shear. The randomly dispersed fibers are stretched during shear (bottom) to provide the shear rigidity to the tissue. (Reproduced with permission from Buckwalter JA, Mow VC: Cartilage repair in osteoarthritis, in Moskowitz RW, Howell DS, Goldberg VM, et al (eds): *Osteoarthritis: Diagnosis and Medical/Surgical Management,* ed 2. Philadelphia, PA, WB Saunders, 1992, pp 71–107.)

results indicate that the stiffness and energy dissipation properties of cartilage in shear are provided by the proteoglycan-collagen structure present in the tissue, not by the proteoglycan-proteoglycan network. Thus, it is most likely that the networking capacity of proteoglycans functions to maintain the inflated spatial form of the collagen network in the ECM, and not to provide any appreciable stiffness in shear (Figs. 9 and 19).

Tensile Properties

A change of volume always occurs when a piece of material is stretched (increase) or compressed (decrease). Thus, in any tensile experiment, both flow-dependent and flow-independent viscoelastic mechanisms contribute to the response of cartilage in tension. If specimens are stretched at extremely slow rates, or if the force response to stretch is obtained at equilibrium, both mechanisms of viscoelasticity will be defeated. The intrinsic tensile response of the collagen-proteoglycan solid matrix has been measured in such slow strain-rate or equilibrium experiments. Figure 21 shows a typical tensile stress-strain curve for articular cartilage, with a toe region followed by a linear response. The

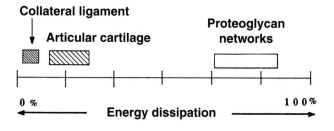

Figure 20

Diagram providing comparison of energy dissipation in a material composed predominantly of collagen (collateral ligament), a material composed of a collagen and proteoglycan mix (articular cartilage), and pure proteoglycans. (Reproduced with permission from Buckwalter JA, Mow VC: Cartilage repair in osteoarthritis, in Moskowitz RW, Howell DS, Goldberg VM, et al (eds): *Osteoarthritis: Diagnosis and Medical/Surgical Management,* ed 2. Philadelphia, PA, WB Saunders, 1992, pp 71–107.)

proportionality constant in the linear portion of the stress-strain curve is called the tensile modulus, and it reflects the stiffness of the collagen network in tension. The tensile modulus of articular cartilage may vary from 5 to 50 MPa, depending on the location, depth, and orientation of the test specimen relative to the split line direction, surface fibrillation, or compositional changes. From numerous studies, it is known that samples from the superficial zone of articular cartilage are stiffer than middle and deep zone samples because of the high concentration and high degree of orientation of collagen fibrils in this zone. Tensile stiffness decreases as mild fibrillation moves toward end-stage osteoarthritic degenerative changes (Fig. 22). The tensile moduli of normal and mildly fibrillated human articular cartilage correlate well with collagen content and ratio of

collagen to proteoglycan present in the tissue. Figure 23 provides a comparison of the tensile, compressive, and shear properties of some important hydrated connective soft tissues.

Physicochemical Forces Responsible for Cartilage Swelling

Swelling is defined as the ability of a material to gain (or to lose) in size or weight when soaked in a solution. This swelling occurs as a result of the chemical or physical nature of the material. For articular cartilage, the reason for the swelling often is referred to as physicochemical because it is derived mainly from the charged nature of the proteoglycan component of the tissue. In cartilage, the proteoglycans contain 1 or 2 negative charge group(s) on each dimeric hexosamine (for example, SO_3^- and COO^-; Fig. 8), and these groups are spaced 10 to 15 Å apart. For normal articular cartilage, the total fixed charge density ranges from 0.1 to 0.5 mEq/ml at physiologic pH; for osteoarthritic cartilage, it drops dramatically as a result of proteoglycan loss from the tissue. Because each of these negative charges requires an opposite (positive) charge to maintain electroneutrality, the total ion concentration inside the tissue must be greater than the ion concentration in the external bathing solution. The maximum difference occurs when the tissue is equilibrated in a very dilute external electrolyte solution. This imbalance of ion concentrations gives rise to

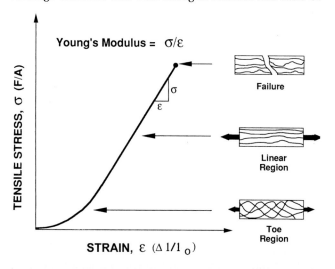

Figure 21

Representation of how the collagen network in a fibrous composite material such as articular cartilage might function during tension. (Reproduced with permission from Buckwalter JA, Mow VC: Cartilage repair in osteoarthritis, in Moskowitz RW, Howell DS, Goldberg VM, et al (eds): *Osteoarthritis: Diagnosis and Medical/Surgical Management,* ed 2. Philadelphia, PA, WB Saunders, 1992, pp 71–107.)

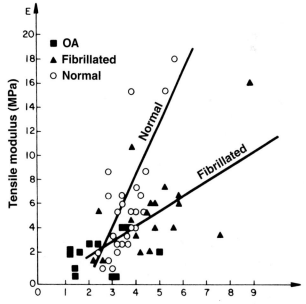

Figure 22

Variation of human knee joint cartilage tensile stiffness for normal, mildly fibrillated, and osteoarthritic (OA) tissue (from a site adjacent to frank OA lesions). (Reproduced with permission from Akizuki S, Mow VC, Muller F, et al: The tensile properties of human knee joint cartilage I: Influence of ionic conditions, weight bearing, and fibrillation on the tensile modulus. *J Orthop Res* 1986;4:379–392.)

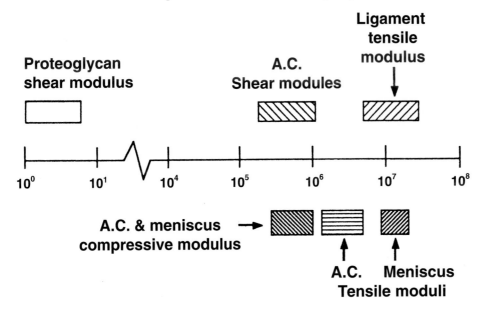

Comparison of moduli (Pa)

Figure 23

Comparison of tensile, compressive and shear properties for common connective tissues. (Reproduced with permission from Buckwalter JA, Mow VC: Cartilage repair in osteoarthritis, in Moskowitz RW, Howell DS, Goldberg VM, et al (eds): *Osteoarthritis: Diagnosis and Medical/Surgical Management*, ed 2. Philadelphia, PA, WB Saunders, 1992, pp 71–107.)

an internal swelling pressure greater than the pressure in the external bath. The extent of swelling is limited by the stress generated in the solid matrix to resist its expansion. The swelling pressure caused by the counterions in association with the fixed charge density is known as the Donnan osmotic pressure, and it usually is denoted by the symbol π.

The swelling pressure can be modulated by changing the external electrolyte (for example, NaCl) concentration. The ideal osmotic pressure law is given by $\pi = RT\Delta c$, where R is the universal gas constant, T is the absolute temperature, and Δc is the difference of ion concentrations between the interstitium and the external bathing solution. This difference of ion concentrations is determined by the fixed charge density c^F of proteoglycans within the interstitium, and the electrolyte concentration c^* in the external bathing solution. First, according to the Donnan equilibrium ion distribution law, for a tissue equilibrated in a monovalent salt (NaCl) solution under ideal conditions, the concentration c of Na^+ in the interstitium is given by the simple quadratic equation $c(c + c^F) = (c^*)^2$. The difference Δc between the total ion concentration of NaCl in the interstitium and the external solution is $\Delta c = (2c + c^F) - 2c^*$, and it may be calculated from the Donnan equilibrium ion distribution law. The Donnan osmotic pressure π may be determined from the idealized law for osmotic pressure. From this analysis, a bit of reflection will show that as c^* becomes large, Δc will vanish, and π will become zero. In other words, when cartilage is bathed in a high-concentration salt solution (hypertonic), the Donnan osmotic pressure becomes negligible, causing the tissue to shrink and lose water. Conversely, when cartilage is bathed in a low concentration salt solution (hypotonic), Δc will become large, causing the tissue to swell and gain water.

For normal cartilage equilibrated in physiologic saline (0.15M NaCl), the swelling pressure π has been calculated to range from 0.1 to 0.25 MPa. The contribution of the swelling pressure toward load support, when normal cartilage is at a compressed equilibrium state, depends on the applied load. For a lightly loaded tissue, the swelling pressure may contribute significantly to the load support. But for highly loaded tissues (that is, physiologic loading conditions), and certainly for dynamically loaded tissues in which interstitial fluid pressurization dominates, the contribution of this swelling pressure to load support is difficult to assess.

Equilibrium Swelling Behavior of Articular Cartilage

The physicochemical forces along an aggrecan would cause the molecule to assume a stiff, fully-extended configuration in an infinitely dilute solution. Under these circumstances, the free-solution volume of the aggrecan is limited only because the stiffness of the molecule itself resists the swelling forces. In cartilage, however, the proteoglycans are trapped and entangled within the interfibrillar space, and compacted to within a volume that is one fifth of the free-solution volume. As a result of interactions between collagen fibrils, such as cross-linking, and interactions between collagen, proteoglycans, and other molecules, the solid matrix of articular cartilage is strong and cohesive. Thus, in the tissue, the swelling pressure is resisted by the stresses developed in the solid matrix where both collagen and proteoglycan share the load. It is likely that, in situ, collagen provides most of the resistance to the swelling pressure. This heuristic description is suggested in the schematic depiction of the collagen-proteoglycan composite matrix for cartilage (Fig. 9).

Recently, it has been shown that at free-swelling equilibrium, the stress tensor σ^s acting in the solid matrix has 3 equal normal stress components given by $\sigma^s = P_s$. For an elastic solid matrix, the dilatation $\Delta V/V_0$ (volumetric change per unit volume) produced by the swelling pressure is given by $P_s=B(\Delta V/V_0)$, where B is the elastic bulk modulus of the solid matrix, which may be measured by material testing methods described above and in Chapter 5. This simple equation may be used to calculate $\Delta V/V_0$ at every point within the tissue as well as for the tissue as a whole. Determination of $\Delta V/V_0$ results in some important conclusions: (1) A swelling pressure will exist within the articular cartilage, and this swelling pressure will cause the porous-permeable, collagen-proteoglycan solid matrix to expand and imbibe water. (2) The elastic stiffness, more specifically the bulk modulus B of the solid matrix, resists the swelling pressure. If the collagen network is damaged in any manner, swelling (gain in volume or water) will occur. (3) Loss of proteoglycans resulting in a decrease of P_s will not necessarily mean a loss of water because more space is available within the interstitium for water, and the loss of proteoglycans will alter the elastic bulk modulus of the porous-permeable solid matrix to allow greater expansion. However, an increase of tissue hydration in early osteoarthritic cartilage is a universal experimental finding. Clearly, then, from the dilatation law $\Delta V/V_0 = P_s/B$, the bulk modulus B of the solid matrix must be decreasing faster than the swelling pressure P_s during the early stages of osteoarthritis. In other words, during early osteoarthritic cartilage changes, the loss of swelling pressure is less severe than the compromise in mechanical properties of the solid matrix. Each molecular, compositional, and ultrastructural change of collagen, proteoglycan, and quantitatively minor glycoproteins, which compose and organize the solid matrix, has a specific influence on solid matrix properties. Thus, in recent decades, the biochemistry and molecular structure of major components of normal and diseased articular cartilages have been studied intensely. Concomitantly, changes of cartilage material properties during early

osteoarthritis in animal models of the disease and in human cartilage specimens obtained at necropsy also have been the object of much investigation. Table 4 provides the mechanoelectrochemical swelling properties of articular cartilage.

Reponse to Loading

Mechanosignal Transduction

Articular cartilage is an aneural tissue. Thus, the nerve impulses that regulate many of the body processes cannot provide information to chondrocytes. Cellular and humoral immune responses also are not likely to occur in cartilage, because both monocytes and immunoglobulins tend to be excluded from the tissue by virtue of their size. Thus, if transport of such messages does occur, it may be considerably slower than in more vascular tissue. In theory at least, chondrocytes receive only limited information regarding the rest of the body state via the standard neural, lymphatic, or humoral pathways. On the other hand, the available evidence strongly suggests that the cells are pressure- or deformation-sensitive; therefore, they may derive considerable information from alterations in the stresses and strains that act on the cell membranes as a result of alteration of the physical forces acting on the tissue. A large number of recent studies have resulted in reports on the effects of pressure, stresses, and strains on chondrocyte metabolism in vitro and the effects of joint instability and joint immobilization on cartilage degeneration and chondrocyte metabolism. These reports indicate that articular cartilage remodels following alterations of mechanical stimuli to the tissue in vivo, and can change its metabolic activities in vitro. Thus, acts such as loading, unloading, or movement of the joint appear to serve as a principal stimuli to biochemical alterations in the cartilage and, ultimately, to its biomechanical properties. How the chondrocytes sense their mechanical environment and convert the information received to changes in specific gene expression in the

Table 4

Summary of Mechanoelectrochemical Properties of Articular Cartilage

Fixed Charge Density (c^F in mEq/ml)	Osmotic Pressure (π in MPa)	Electric Conductivity (κ in S/m)	Na+ Diffusion (D^+ in $m^2/s \times 10^{-9}$)	Cl- diffusion (D^-) (D^- in $m2/s \times 10^{-9}$)
0.01–0.5	0–0.25	0.5–1.5	0.25–1.0	0.5–1.5

Articular Cartilage Streaming Potential per Applied Pressure ($\Delta\Psi/\Delta p$): 30–50 mV/MPa

N = Newtons; s = seconds; m = meters; Eq = number of equivalent monovalent charges; mV = millivolt; Pa = N/m^2 (pascal); Mpa = 145 lb/in^2; S = Seimans = m/s

Note: D^- is always greater than D^+; diffusion coefficients are measured in 0.15M NaCl

nucleus is unknown, although it is thought that integrins, which are molecules that span the plasma membrane and are connected to the intracellular cytoplasm, are likely to be involved. Eventually, the mechanical signals are transmitted to the nucleus resulting in mRNA expression that directs synthesis of proteins.

Effects of Joint Motion and Loading

Joint loading and motion are required to maintain normal adult articular cartilage composition, structure, and mechanical properties. The type, intensity, and frequency of loadings necessary to maintain normal articular cartilage vary over a broad range. When the intensity or frequency of loading exceeds or falls below these necessary levels, the balance between synthesis and degradation processes will be altered, and changes in the composition and microstructure of cartilage follow.

Reduced joint loading, in the form of rigid immobilization or casting, leads to atrophy or degeneration of the cartilage. The effects can be separated into those occurring in contact areas and those occurring in noncontact areas. The use of external fixation to effect continuous and static compression of 2 opposing cartilage surfaces in the absence of normal joint motion may produce severe degenerative lesions and chondrocyte death in the area of contact. The severity of damage depends on the magnitude and duration of loading. Changes in the noncontact areas resulting from rigid immobilization include fibrillation, decreased proteoglycan content and synthesis, and altered proteoglycan conformation, such as a decrease in the size of aggregates and amount of aggregate. These changes result, in part, because normal nutritive transport to cartilage from the synovial fluid by means of diffusion and convection has been diminished. With immobilization by casting or strapping, a limited range of joint motion is maintained and the changes are less severe than in cases of rigid immobilization. In addition to the alterations in articular cartilage composition, the mechanical properties of articular cartilage will be compromised with immobilization. Fluid flux and deformation in response to compression will increase, although these changes are minimal in areas where some level of joint contact is maintained. Normal tensile properties are maintained, reflecting the biochemical finding that proteoglycan rather than collagen is affected primarily by reduced joint motion and loading. All of these biochemical and biomechanical changes are, at least in part, reversible on remobilization of the joint, although the extent of this recovery decreases with increasing periods of joint immobilization and increasing rigidity of the immobilization.

Increased joint loading, either through excessive use, increased magnitudes of loading, or impact, also may affect articular cartilage. Catabolic effects can be induced by a single-impact or repetitive trauma, and may serve as the initiating factor for progressive degenerative changes. Moderate running exercise may increase the articular cartilage proteoglycan content and compressive stiffness, decrease the rate of fluid flux during loading, and increase the articular cartilage thickness in skeletally immature animals. However, no significant changes in articular cartilage mechanical properties were observed in dogs in response to lifelong increased activity that did not include high impact or torsional loading of their joints.

Disruption of the intra-articular structures, such as menisci or ligaments, will alter the forces acting on the articular surface in both magnitude and areas of loading. The resulting joint instability is associated with profound and progressive changes in the biochemical composition and mechanical properties of articular cartilage. In experimental animal models, responses to transection of the anterior cruciate ligament or meniscectomy have included fibrillation of the cartilage surface, increased hydration, changes in the proteoglycan content, reduced number and size of proteoglycan aggregates, joint capsule thickening, and osteophyte formation. It seems likely that some of these changes result from the activities of the chondrocytes, because their rates of synthesis of matrix components, breakdown of matrix components, and secretion of proteolytic enzymes are all increased. Changes in the mechanical properties also have been observed together with these histologic and biochemical composition changes. Significant and progressive decreases in the tensile and shear modulus have been observed in response to transection of the anterior cruciate ligament. Furthermore, decreases in the compressive modulus and increases in the hydraulic permeability occur in response to joint instability, which will produce increased matrix deformation, elevated fluid flux under physiologic loading, and diminution of the fluid pressurization and stress shielding effects of load carriage. There is evidence of increased chondrocyte mitotic and anabolic activity in joint instability, although these elevated chondrocyte responses are insufficient to repair early damage and to inhibit progression of cartilage degeneration. Rather, it appears that the increased anabolism is outpaced by an elevated catabolism, which is activated in models of altered joint loading.

The specific mechanisms by which joint loading influences chondrocyte function remain unknown, although various mechanical, physicochemical, and electrical transduction mechanisms have been proposed. Matrix deformation will produce fluid and ion flow, which may facilitate chondrocyte nutrition and chemical transduction signals, and chondrocyte deformation, which may directly control the metabolic activity. Deformation and fluid flow will lead to changes in the local charge density within the matrix, resulting in an electric potential that may serve as an electric transduction mechanism. In vitro studies have shown that loading of the cartilage matrix can cause all of these mechanical, electric, and physicochemical events, but thus far it has not been shown clearly which signals are most important in stimulating the anabolic and catabolic activity of the chondrocytes.

Summary

The unique mechanical properties of articular cartilage make possible normal synovial joint function. These properties depend on the structure and composition of the tissue. Articular cartilage consists of isolated cells, chondrocytes, embedded in an abundant extracellular matrix consisting of a macromolecular framework filled with water. Chondrocytes are highly differentiated cells that rely primarily on anaerobic metabolism. They form the matrix macromolecular framework from 3 classes of molecules: collagens, proteoglycans, and noncollagenous proteins. Types II, IX, and XI collagens form a fibrillar meshwork that gives the tissue its form and tensile stiffness and strength. Type VI collagen forms part of the matrix immediately surrounding chondrocytes and may help them attach to the matrix macromolecular framework. Large aggregating proteoglycans, aggrecans, give the tissue its stiffness to compression, resilience, and contribute to its durability. Small proteoglycans, including decorin, biglycan, and fibromodulin, bind to other matrix macromolecules and thereby help stabilize the matrix. Noncollagenous proteins including tenascin and fibronectin can influence chondrocyte matrix interactions. The structural molecules, primarily the collagens and proteoglycans, form a strong, fatigue-resistant, solid matrix capable of sustaining the high stresses and strains developed within the tissue during joint use. This solid matrix is porous, permeable, and very soft. Water, 65% to 80% of the total weight of normal articular cartilage, resides in the microscopic pores. A pressure gradient or matrix compaction causes the water to flow through the porous-permeable solid matrix. Significant flow of fluid through the solid matrix requires high hydrodynamic pressures because the very low permeability of the solid matrix causes high frictional drag forces. Thus, fluid pressure provides a significant component of total load support for articular cartilage, minimizing the stress acting on the solid matrix. In fact, the ratio of load supported by the fluid pressure to that supported by the solid matrix stress is greater than 20:1 in normal articular cartilage. For these reasons, the biomechanical properties of articular cartilage are understood best when the tissue is viewed as a biphasic material, composed of a solid phase and a fluid phase. Throughout life the tissue undergoes continual internal remodeling as the cells replace matrix macromolecules lost through degradation. Loading of the tissue caused by joint use creates mechanical, electrical, and physicochemical signals that help direct chondrocyte synthetic and degradative activity. Prolonged, severely decreased joint use leads to alterations in matrix composition and eventually loss of tissue structure and mechanical properties, whereas joint use stimulates chondrocyte synthetic activity and possibly internal tissue remodeling.

Selected Bibliography

General Reference Texts

Hay ED (ed): *Cell Biology of Extracellular Matrix*, ed 2. New York, NY, Plenum Press, 1991.

Mayne R, Irwin MH: Collagen types in cartilage, in Kuettner KE, Schleyerbach R, Hascall VC (eds): *Articular Cartilage Biochemistry*. New York, NY, Raven Press, 1986, pp 23–38.

Mow VC, Hayes WC (eds): *Basic Orthopaedic Biomechanics*, ed 2. Philadelphia, PA, Lippincott-Raven, 1997.

Structure

Buckwalter JA, Mankin HJ: Articular cartilage I: Tissue design and chondrocyte-matrix interactions. *J Bone Joint Surg* 1997;79A: 600–611.

Clarke IC: Articular cartilage: A review and scanning electron microscope study: 1. The interterritorial fibrillar architecture. *J Bone Joint Surg* 1971;53B:732–750.

Clark JM: The organization of collagen in cryofractured rabbit articular cartilage: A scanning electron microscopic study. *J Orthop Res* 1985;3:17–29.

Schenk RK, Eggli PS, Hunziker EB: Articular cartilage morphology, in Kuettner KE, Schleyerbach R, Hascall VC (eds): *Articular Cartilage Biochemistry*. New York, NY, Raven Press, 1986, pp 3–22.

Scott JE: Proteoglycan: Collagen interactions in connective tissues. Ultrastructural, biochemical, functional and evolutionary aspects. *Int J Biol Macromol* 1991;13:157–161.

Physicochemistry

Maroudas A: Tissue composition and organization, in Maroudas A, Kuettner KE (eds): *Methods in Cartilage Research*. London, England, Academic Press, 1990, pp 209–239.

Mow VC, Ratcliffe A, Poole AR: Cartilage and diarthrodial joints as paradigms for hierarchical materials and structures. *Biomaterials* 1992;13:67–97.

Biomechanics

Anderson DD, Brown TD, Radin EL: The influence of basal cartilage calcification on dynamic juxtaarticular stress transmission. *Clin Orthop* 1993;286:298–307.

Brown TD, Radin EL, Martin RB, Burr DB: Finite element studies of some juxtaarticular stress changes due to localized subchondral stiffening. *J Biomech* 1984;17:11–24.

Froimson MI, Ratcliffe A, Gardner TR, Mow VC: Differences in patellofemoral joint cartilage material properties and their significance to the etiology of cartilage surface fibrillation. *Osteoarthritis Cartilage* 1997;5:377–386.

Grodzinsky AJ: Mechanical and electrical properties and their relevance to physiological processes, in Maroudas A, Kuettner KE (eds): *Methods in Cartilage Research.* London, England, Academic Press, 1990, pp 275–311.

Mow VC, Ratcliffe A: Structure and function of articular cartilage and meniscus, in Mow VC, Hayes WC (eds): *Basic Orthopaedic Biomechanics,* ed 2. Philadelphia, PA, Lippincott-Raven, 1997, pp 113–177.

Newton PM, Mow VC, Gardner TR, Buckwalter JA, Albright JP: The effect of lifelong exercise on canine articular cartilage. *Am J Sports Med* 1997;25:282–287.

Biology

Bachrach NM, Valhmu WB, Stazzone E, Ratcliffe A, Lai WM, Mow VC: Changes in proteoglycan synthesis of chondrocytes in articular cartilage are associated with the time-dependent changes in their mechanical environment. *J Biomech* 1995;28:1561–1569.

Buckwalter JA, Mankin HJ: Articular cartilage I: Tissue design and chondrocyte-matrix interactions. *J Bone Joint Surg* 1997;79A:600–611.

Buschmann MD, Hunziker EB, Kim YJ, Grodzinsky AJ: Altered aggrecan synthesis correlates with cell and nucleus structure in statically compressed cartilage. *J Cell Sci* 1996;109:499–508.

Guilak F: Compression-induced changes in the shape and volume of the chondrocyte nucleus. *J Biomech* 1995;28:1529–1541.

Helminen HJ, Kiviranta I, Saamanen AM, Tammi M, Paukkonen K, Jurvelin J (eds): *Joint Loading: Biology and Health of Articular Structures.* Bristol, England, Wright, 1987.

Kim YJ, Sah RL, Grodzinsky AJ, Plaas AH, Sandy JD: Mechanical regulation of cartilage biosynthetic behavior: Physical stimuli. *Arch Biochem Biophys* 1994;311:1–12.

Palmoski MJ, Brandt KD: Running inhibits the reversal of atrophic changes in canine knee cartilage after removal of a leg cast. *Arthritis Rheum* 1981;24:1329–1337.

Palmoski MJ, Brandt KD: Effects of static and cyclic compressive loading on articular cartilage plugs in vitro. *Arthritis Rheum* 1984; 27:675–681.

Stockwell RA (ed): *Biology of Cartilage Cells.* Cambridge, England, Cambridge University Press, 1979, pp 7–31.

Stockwell RA: Structure and function of the chondrocyte under mechanical stress, in Helminen HJ, Kiviranta I, Tammi M, Saamanen AM, Paukkonen K, Jurvelin J (eds): *Joint Loading: Biology and Health of Articular Structures.* Bristol, England, Wright, 1987, pp 126–148.

Water

Armstrong CG, Mow VC: Variations in the intrinsic mechanical properties of human articular cartilage with age, degeneration, and water content. *J Bone Joint Surg* 1982;64A:88–94.

Mankin HJ, Thrasher AZ: Water content and binding in normal and osteoarthritic human cartilage. *J Bone Joint Surg* 1975;57A:76–80.

Maroudas A: Physicochemical properties of articular cartilage, in Freeman MAR (ed): *Adult Articular Cartilage.* Kent, England, Pitman Medical Publishing, 1979, pp 215–290.

Maroudas A, Bayliss MT, Venn MF: Further studies on the composition of human femoral head cartilage. *Ann Rheum Dis* 1980; 39:514–523.

Proteoglycans

Hardingham TE, Fosang AJ: Proteoglycans: Many forms and many functions. *FASEB J* 1992;6:861–870.

Lohmander S: Proteoglycans of joint cartilage: Structure, function, turnover and role as markers of joint disease. *Baillieres Clin Rheumatol* 1988;2:37–62.

Mow VC, Zhu W, Lai WM, Hardingham TE, Hughes C, Muir H: The influence of link protein stabilization on the viscometric properties of proteoglycan aggregate solutions. *Biochim Biophys Acta* 1989; 992:201–208.

Muir H: Proteoglycans as organizers of the intercellular matrix. *Biochem Soc Trans* 1983;11:613–622.

Rosenberg LC, Buckwalter JA: Cartilage proteoglycans, in Kuettner KE, Schleyerbach R, Hascall VC (eds): *Articular Cartilage Biochemistry.* New York, NY, Raven Press, 1986, pp 39–57.

Roughley PJ: Structural changes in the proteoglycans of human articular cartilage during aging. *J Rheumatol* 1987;14:14–15.

Link Protein

Baker JR, Caterson B: The isolation of "link proteins" from bovine nasal cartilage. *Biochim Biophys Acta* 1978;532:249–258.

Buckwalter JA, Rosenberg LC, Tang L-H: The effect of link protein on proteoglycan aggregate structure: An electron microscopic study of the molecular architecture and dimensions of proteoglycan aggregates reassembled from the proteoglycan monomers and link proteins of bovine fetal epiphyseal cartilage. *J Biol Chem* 1984; 259:5361–5363.

Hardingham TE: The role of link-protein in the structure of cartilage proteoglycan aggregates. *Biochem J* 1979;177:237–247.

Tang LH, Buckwalter JA, Rosenberg LC: Effect of link protein concentration on articular cartilage proteoglycan aggregation. *J Orthop Res* 1996;14:334–339.

Collagens

Bruckner P, Vaughan L, Winterhalter KH: Type IX collagen from sternal cartilage of chicken embryo contains covalently bound glycosaminoglycans. *Proc Natl Acad Sci USA* 1985;82:2608–2612.

Eyre DR, Wu JJ, Apone S: A growing family of collagens in articular cartilage: Identification of 5 genetically distinct types. *J Rheumatol* 1987;14:25–27.

Mayne R, Irwin MH: Collagen types in cartilage, in Kuettner KE, Schleyerbach R, Hascall VC (eds): *Articular Cartilage Biochemistry.* New York, NY, Raven Press, 1986, pp 23–38.

Nimni ME, Harkness RD: Molecular structures and functions of collagen, in Nimni ME (ed): *Collagen, Vol 1: Biochemistry.* Boca Raton, FL, CRC Press, 1988, pp 1–78.

Fibronectin

Brown RA, Jones KL: The synthesis and accumulation of fibronectin by human articular cartilage. *J Rheumatol* 1990;17:65–72.

Burton-Wurster N, Horn VJ, Lust G: Immunohisto-chemical localization of fibronectin and chondronectin in canine articular cartilage. *J Histochem Cytochem* 1988;36:581–588.

Lipids

Bonner WM, Jonsson H, Malanos C, Bryant M: Changes in the lipids of human articular cartilage with age. *Arthritis Rheum* 1975;18:461–473.

Ohira T, Ishikawa K, Masuda I, Yokoyama M, Honda I: Histologic localization of lipid in the articular tissues in calcium pyrophosphate dihydrate crystal deposition disease. *Arthritis Rheum* 1988;31: 1057–1062.

Scotchford CA, Ali SY: Association of magnesium whitlockite crystals with lipid components of the extracellular matrix in human articular cartilage. *Osteoarthritis Cartilage* 1997;5:107–119.

Vignon E, Mathieu P, Louisot P, Vilamitjana J, Harmand MF, Richard M: Phospholipase A2 activity in human osteoarthritic cartilage. *J Rheumatol Suppl* 1989;18:35–38.

Noncollagenous Proteins

Fife RS, Palmoski MJ, Brandt KD: Metabolism of a cartilage matrix glycoprotein in normal and osteoarthritic canine articular cartilage. *Arthritis Rheum* 1986;29:1256–1262.

Heinegard D, Lorenzo P, Sommarin Y: Articular cartilage matrix proteins, in Kuettner KE, Goldberg VM (eds): *Osteoarthritic Disorders.* Rosemont, IL, American Academy of Orthopaedic Surgeons, 1995, pp 229–237.

Metabolism

Guilak F, Sah R, Setton LA: Physical regulation of cartilage metabolism, in Mow VC, Hayes WC (eds): *Basic Orthopaedic Biomechanics,* ed 2. Philadelphia, PA, Lippincott-Raven, 1997, pp 179–207.

Mankin HJ, Brandt KD: Biochemistry and metabolism of articular cartilage in osteoarthritis, in Moskowitz RW, Howell DS, Goldberg VM, Mankin HJ (eds): *Osteoarthritis: Diagnosis and Medical/ Surgical Management,* ed 2. Philadelphia, PA, WB Saunders, 1992, pp 109–154.

Mankin HJ, Johnson ME, Lippiello L: Biochemical and metabolic abnormalities in articular cartilage from osteoarthritic human hips: III. Distribution and metabolism of amino sugar-containing macromolecules. *J Bone Joint Surg* 1981;63A:131–139.

Oegema TR Jr, Thompson RC Jr: Metabolism of chondrocytes derived from normal and osteoarthritic human cartilage, in Kuettner KE, Schleyerbach R, Hascall VC (eds): *Articular Cartilage Biochemistry.* New York, NY, Raven Press, 1986, pp 257–271.

Osborn KD, Trippel SB, Mankin HJ: Growth factor stimulation of adult articular cartilage. *J Orthop Res* 1989;7:35–42.

Treadwell BV, Mankin HJ: The synthetic processes of articular cartilage. *Clin Orthop* 1986;213:50–61.

Enzymes

Campbell IK, Piccoli DS, Butler DM, Singleton DK, Hamilton JA: Recombinant human interleukin-1 stimulates human articular cartilage to undergo resorption and human chondrocytes to produce both tissue- and urokinase-type plasminogen activator. *Biochim Biophys Acta* 1988;967:183–194.

Gunja-Smith Z, Nagase H, Woessner JF Jr: Purification of the neutral proteoglycan-degrading metalloproteinase from human articular cartilage tissue and its identification as stromelysin matrix metalloproteinase-3. *Biochem J* 1989;258:115–119.

Nguyen Q, Murphy G, Roughley PJ, Mort JS: Degradation of proteoglycan aggregate by a cartilage metalloproteinase: Evidence for the involvement of stromelysin in the generation of link protein heterogeneity in situ. *Biochem J* 1989;259:61–67.

Sandy JD, Brown HL, Lowther DA: Degradation of proteoglycan in articular cartilage. *Biochim Biophys Acta* 1978;543:536–544.

Yamada H, Stephens RW, Nakagawa T, McNicol D: Human articular cartilage contains an inhibitor of plasminogen activator. *J Rheumatol* 1988;15:1138–1143.

Aging

Bayliss MT: Age-related changes in the stoichiometry of human articular cartilage proteoglycan aggregates, in Maroudas A, Kuettner KE (eds): *Methods in Cartilage Research*. London, England, Academic Press, 1990, pp 220–222.

Buckwalter JA, Roughley PJ, Rosenberg LC: Age-related changes in cartilage proteoglycans: Quantitative electron microscopic studies. *Microsc Res Tech* 1994;28:398–408.

Buckwalter JA, Kuettner KE, Thonar EJ: Age-related changes in articular cartilage proteoglycans: Electron microscopic studies. *J Orthop Res* 1985;3:251–257.

Front P, Aprile F, Mitrovic DR, Swann DA: Age-related changes in the synthesis of matrix macromolecules by bovine articular cartilage. *Connect Tissue Res* 1989;19:121–133.

Martel-Pelletier J, Pelletier JP: Neutral metalloproteases and age related changes in human articular cartilage. *Ann Rheum Dis* 1987;46:363–369.

Martin JA, Ellerbroek SM, Buckwalter JA: Age-related decline in chondrocyte response to insulin-like growth factor-I: The role of growth factor binding proteins. *J Orthop Res* 1997;15:491–498.

Chapter 18

Articular Cartilage Repair and Osteoarthritis

Henry J. Mankin, MD

Van C. Mow, PhD

Joseph A. Buckwalter, MD

This chapter at a glance

This chapter provides a review of the current understanding of the processes involved during articular cartilage injury and repair and osteoarthritis.

Introduction

Articular cartilage has remarkable durability. Under normal physiologic situations, naked-eye examinations of necroscopy specimens show that this tissue may appear pristine even after 8 or 9 decades of use, without any signs of wear and tear. However, this tissue may be damaged by trauma or inflammatory disease processes, or it may undergo progressive degeneration causing the clinical syndrome of osteoarthritis (OA). Although articular cartilage is metabolically active, it has a limited capacity for repair. Because of this limitation, damaged articular cartilage is not restored to a normal condition. Often, once damage is done, it accumulates, leading to a complete loss of the articular surface exposing the underlying bone. Concomitant with these cartilage changes, osteophyte formation occurs, severely altering joint form and congruency. These changes are almost always associated with a severely impaired joint function, with clinical symptoms of redness, swelling, and pain. At that point, prosthetic joint replacements offer the best hope of restoring pain-free mobility. Although joint replacement procedures have revolutionized orthopaedic surgery, they are appropriate only for the treatment of end-stage degenerative joint disease, often after prolonged suffering by the patient; in a small percentage of cases (< 10%), these total joint replacements lack the durability of normal diarthrodial joints. New research on articular cartilage biology and biomechanics, with advances in the understanding of the etiology of OA and the processes of limited articular cartilage repair, offers hope for the development of biologically based alternatives to end-stage total prosthetic joint replacements. The aim of this chapter is to offer a review of the current understanding of the processes involved during articular cartilage injury and repair and OA.

Articular Cartilage Repair

Repair refers to the replacement of damaged or lost cells and matrix of a tissue with new cells and matrix. Unfortunately, repair tissue restores neither the original structure nor function of normal articular cartilage. For vascularized tissues, the most common form of repair tissue, referred to as scar tissue, consists of densely packed collagen fibrils and scattered fibroblasts. Scar tissue can often be remodeled over a prolonged period of time with cells and matrix macromolecules being replaced and reorganized, and with the composition of the extracellular matrix (ECM) modified. In most tissues, type I collagen is the predominant matrix macromolecule of the mature scar. Under most circumstances, vascularized fibrous tissues such as ligaments, tendon, and joint capsule, and repair of lost or injured tissues, and repair of defects filled with new cells and ECM, if formed, closely resembles the original tissue. These repaired tissues can restore normal or near-normal function. Repair of significant defects in articular cartilage, however, is rarely, if ever, this successful. Factors that limit the response of articular cartilage to injury include a lack of blood vessels and a lack of cells in the tissue that can migrate to the injured site; also, endogenous cells at these sites cannot repair defects of any significant size.

Lack of Blood Supply

Because adult cartilage lacks blood vessels, disruption of the tissue does not cause fibrin clot formation or migration of inflammatory cells and undifferentiated cells from blood vessels to the site of tissue damage. Repair of injuries to vascularized tissues, including bone, tendon, and ligament, joint capsules, and the peripheral third of knee meniscus begins with hemorrhage and fibrin clot formation. These events are followed by migration of inflammatory cells and then undifferentiated cells from blood vessels to the injury site. The undifferentiated cells proliferate, differentiate, and synthesize a new matrix. Injured cells and platelets release mediators that can promote the vascular response to injury and stimulate cell migration and proliferation. The inflammatory cells may help remove necrotic tissue and, as they do so, release mediators that stimulate migration of mesenchymal cells capable of invading a fibrin clot, proliferating, differentiating into a wide range of connective tissue cells, and synthesizing a new ECM. For these reasons the repair response of vascularized tissues is more effective than the repair response of nonvascularized tissues.

Lack of Undifferentiated Cells

In addition to lacking blood vessels, cartilage lacks undifferentiated cells within the tissue that can migrate, proliferate, and participate in the repair response. The only cell type found in articular cartilage, the highly differentiated chondrocyte, has limited capacity for proliferation or migration because they are encased within the dense collagen-proteoglycan ECM of the tissue. During cartilage growth, chondrocytes proliferate rapidly, depositing the ECM along the way. For normal articular cartilage, this ECM is composed mainly of type II collagen (10% to 20%), aggregating proteoglycans (5% to 10%), and water (70% to 85%). However, the rate of cell division declines with increasing age until, in normal mature articular cartilage, few if any chondrocytes show signs of mitotic activity. Following cartilage injury or in OA some chondrocytes do proliferate, but this response is very limited, and there is no evidence that these cells can migrate through the dense collagen-proteoglycan ECM to the site of tissue damage or deterioration.

Chondrocytes in the tissue also may have a limited capacity for increasing matrix synthesis. In normal mature cartilage, chondrocytes synthesize sufficient matrix macromolecules to maintain the ECM, and they can increase their rate of matrix synthesis in response to injury or osteoarthritic changes. However, chondrocytes do not synthesize sufficient amounts of proteoglycans or collagen to repair significant tissue defects. Moreover, the matrix macromolecules that they do synthesize appear to change with age. For example, the size of cartilage aggrecan and proteoglycan aggregates declines with increasing fetal age, and, with skeletal maturity and increasing age, the size of the cartilage proteoglycans further decreases and these molecules become more variable in size. These age-related changes in matrix proteoglycans may adversely affect the cartilage, and it is not known if mature chondrocytes can be stimulated to produce the larger, more uniform proteoglycans. Other factors that may limit the ability of mature cartilage to repair tissue defects are that the number of chondrocytes declines during aging and the responsiveness of chondrocytes to anabolic growth factors may also decline, thus reducing the capacity of the tissue to repair itself.

When cartilage injury or disease extends to the blood vessels in the subchondral region, cells that can repair tissue defects enter the injury site. These cells, however, do not consistently repair the injury with a tissue that has the unique composition, structure, and material properties of normal articular cartilage matrix. Cartilage alone among the primary musculoskeletal tissues (bone, dense fibrous tissue, and articular cartilage) has an ECM macromolecular framework consisting primarily of type II fibrillar collagen, large, elaborately structured cartilage proteoglycans, and cartilage-specific noncollagenous proteins. Following most injuries, the cells responsible for repair do not produce these cartilage macromolecules in amounts sufficient to create a cohesive and strong extracellular matrix, and they fail to organize the molecules into a layered, anisotropic structure like that of articular cartilage. Because of the unique characteristics of articular cartilage, the repair responses to superficial lacerations, blunt trauma, and injuries that damage subchondral bone as well as articular cartilage differ considerably.

Response of Articular Cartilage to Superficial Lacerations

The earliest visible articular cartilage degeneration begins as a fraying of the superficial zone (top 10% to 15% of the tissue). Fraying is commonly seen under the scanning electron microscope, with short tufts and sheets of collagen fibers being peeled off the surface. With time, as damage progresses into the tissue, vertical clefts and fissures appear and become progressively deeper, giving the affected tissue an irregular, matted, dull, and fibrillated appearance—even to the naked eye. In the most superficial regions, proteoglycan is lost from the matrix as evidenced by a diminished safranin O staining. Perhaps in response to the loss of matrix proteoglycan, chondrocytes proliferate, forming clusters or clones, and begin to synthesize increased

amounts of various matrix macromolecules, particularly proteoglycans. However, the chondrocytes do not migrate into the areas of the defects nor does the matrix they synthesize fill the defects. The newly synthesized proteoglycans are localized in the immediate neighborhood of clusters of chondrocyte clones. As the deterioration of the matrix progresses, fragments of cartilage may tear loose and be released into the joint, leaving deeper regions exposed. Eventually, more tissue is lost, exposing subchondral bone and resulting in bony eburnation. The inability of the chondrocytes to repair the damaged tissue or to prevent further damage allows the disintegration of the articular surface to progress until only a hard, dense eburnated bone remains.

Superficial laceration injuries to articular cartilage that do not cross the tidemark, the boundary between the uncalcified cartilage and the calcified cartilage, generally do not heal. Despite some suggestions to the contrary, performing intracartilaginous lacerative surgery through the arthroscope does not stimulate cartilage healing any more than surgery done in an open procedure, and using a shaver, laser, or cautery doesn't change the results either. If the injury to mature cartilage is superficial, it will not heal. Conversely, lacerations of mature cartilage perpendicular to the surface only kill chondrocytes at the site of the injury, and the matrix defects remain, apparently without any further progression. Thus, presumably these lesions could remain at the joint surface unaltered, presumably for the life of the joint (Fig. 1).

Why do superficial lacerations behave this way? First, these lesions do not cause hemorrhage or initiate an inflammatory response. Also, fibrin clots rarely form on

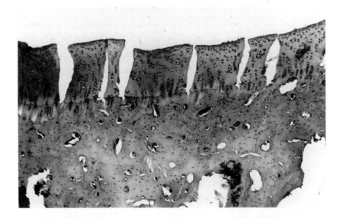

Figure 1

Light micrograph showing multiple laceration defects in rabbit articular cartilage 6 months after injury. These defects did not penetrate the subchondral bone. The chondrocytes have not migrated into the defects or formed a new matrix. (Reproduced with permission from Buckwalter JA, Mow VC: Cartilage repair in osteoarthritis, in Moskowitz RW, Howell DS, Goldberg VM, Mankin HJ (eds): *Osteoarthritis: Diagnosis and Medical/Surgical Management*, ed 2. Philadelphia, PA, WB Saunders, 1992, pp 71–107.)

exposed surfaces of normal cartilage. Platelets do not bind to the damaged cartilage and a fibrin clot does not appear; nor do inflammatory cells, invading capillaries, or undifferentiated mesenchymal cells. Chondrocytes near the injury may proliferate and form clusters or clones and synthesize new matrix, but the chondrocytes do not migrate into the lesion, the new matrix they produce remains in the immediate region of the chondrocytes, and their proliferative and synthetic activity fails to provide new tissue to repair the damage. This repair phase is initially brisk. It is, however, limited in scope and duration, disappearing within a matter of weeks.

Superficial lacerations made tangential or parallel to the articular surface follow a similar course. Some cells directly adjacent to the lacerations die, whereas others show evidence of proliferation and increased matrix synthesis. A thin layer of new matrix may form over the surface, but there is no evidence of significant repair, although the remaining tissue does not degenerate.

Results from experimental studies of injuries limited to cartilage clearly demonstrate the inability of chondrocytes to repair cartilage defects. However, they also show that limited experimental injuries to normal articular surfaces in normal synovial joints generally do not progress to full-thickness loss of cartilage. Thus, it appears that the existence of the superficial cartilage lesions alone will not cause OA in otherwise normal joints and that the progression of superficial osteoarthritic lesions results either from an abnormality of the cartilage in the osteoarthritic joint or from other factors associated with the disease.

Response of Articular Cartilage to Blunt Impact

Articular cartilage can withstand single or multiple moderate- and, occasionally, high-impact loads. However, a number of studies have addressed the effects of either a single excessive high-impact force causing injury to the cartilage without a break in the surface, or repetitive below-trauma threshold loads causing an accumulation of damage to the cartilage by a repeated application of the load. From animal models of subfracture impact studies, 600 N of peak impact force on the mature rabbit patellofemoral joint, and 6 kN of peak impact force on the porcine patellofemoral joint, are sufficient to cause a biomechanical weakening of the articular cartilage. From these and other studies, it is evident that cartilage can be damaged by either loading process, and that the damage caused may be significant. Chondrocyte death, matrix damage, fissuring of the surface, injury to the underlying bone, and thickening of the tidemark region can occur. At a certain threshold of impact loading, the cartilage may be sheared off of the subchondral bone. For the porcine model, 6 kN of peak impact load is required to cause a shear fracture of the cartilage-bone interface (that is, at the tidemark).

Perhaps the most provocative aspect of these studies is the suggestion that impact, especially in repetitive multiple injuries, leads to thickening or progressing of the tidemark, increasing the thickness of the calcified zone, and, ultimately, to an advance and even reduplication of the tidemark at the expense of uncalcified articular cartilage thickness. These changes also may stiffen the cartilage-bone junction. Alterations in these parameters (thinning of the uncalcified cartilage and stiffening of the subchondral bone) have been hypothesized to lead to changes in the stresses and strains acting within the thinner cartilage layer during normal function and, with time, to osteoarthritic changes. According to this hypothesis, these changes in the calcified and subchondral tissues on which the articular cartilage rests are critical and necessary for the progression of articular cartilage damage observed in OA.

Repair of Articular Cartilage and Subchondral Bone Injuries

Repair of cartilage defects that penetrate the subchondral bone (that is, osteochondral defects) may depend to some extent on the severity of injury as measured by the volume of tissue or surface area injured, and on the location of the injury in the joint (that is, high or low load bearing areas). Experimental studies indicate that repair of larger osteochondral defects generally is less predictable and less complete than repair of smaller defects.

Another factor that may influence osteochondral repair is the age of the individual. Although possible age-related differences in healing of synovial joint injuries have not been investigated thoroughly, it is known that fractures heal more rapidly in children, and chondrocytes from skeletally immature animals proliferate and synthesize larger cartilage proteoglycans than those from mature animals. Thus, it is possible that osteochondral injuries and perhaps chondral injuries in very young people have the potential to heal more effectively than similar injuries in skeletally mature or elderly individuals. It is known, though not very well publicized, that immature cartilage does have a blood supply, albeit very limited.

Mechanical injury that disrupts bone as well as articular cartilage causes hemorrhage, fibrin clot formation, and inflammation. Soon after creation of the defect, a fibrin clot fills the injury site and inflammatory cells migrate into the clot. In addition to these visible differences between injuries limited to cartilage and injuries that penetrate subchondral bone, there is another important difference. Injury to bone and the subsequent clot formation cause the release of growth factors, proteins that influence multiple cell functions including migration, proliferation, differentiation, and matrix synthesis from bone. Bone matrix contains a number of growth factors, and platelets release multiple growth factors, including platelet-derived growth factor and transforming growth factor-β.

At present, the role of growth factors in cartilage repair has not been defined clearly. It is likely that the growth factors stimulate migration of undifferentiated mesenchymal cells or fibroblast-like cells into the clot and that the local concentrations and types of growth factors in the tissue defect influence the proliferative and synthetic activity of these cells. Within as little as 2 weeks after osteochondral injury, some of these mesenchymal cells have assumed the rounded form of chondrocytes and have begun to produce a matrix that contains type II collagen and a relatively high concentration of proteoglycans. Six to 8 weeks after injury, the tissue within the chondral portion of the defect contains a relatively high proportion of chondrocyte-like cells and a matrix consisting of type II collagen, proteoglycans, and some type I collagen. Simultaneously, cells within the bone portion of the defect form immature bone, fibrous tissue, and cartilage with a hyaline matrix. The bone formation restores the original level of subchondral bone but rarely, if ever, progresses into the chondral portion of the defect. In general, by 6 months after injury the subchondral bone defect has been repaired with a tissue that consists primarily of bone but also contains some regions of fibrous tissue and hyaline cartilage.

In contrast, the chondral defect rarely is repaired completely, and although it contains a higher proportion of hyaline-appearing cartilage than the bony portion of the defect, it also contains substantial amounts of fibrous tissue. In many instances the composition and structure of the chondral repair tissue are intermediate between those of hyaline cartilage and fibrocartilage, the repair tissue does not bond to the surrounding cartilaginous tissue, and the subchondral bone does not form an impermeable barrier. Thus, the repair tissue does not restore the normal structure, composition, or mechanical properties of an articular surface.

In most injuries the chondral repair tissue begins to show evidence of fibrillation, loss of cells with the appearance of chondrocytes, and loss of the hyaline-appearing matrix in less than 1 year. The remaining cells usually have the appearance of fibroblasts, and the surrounding matrix consists of densely packed collagen fibrils. However, the fate of cartilage repair tissue is not always progressive deterioration. Occasionally, the repair tissue persists and appears to function satisfactorily as an articular surface for a prolonged period of time. It may even remodel until it more closely resembles normal articular cartilage. The reasons why some repair tissue persists for a prolonged period while most repair tissue deteriorates remain unknown. Because of the potential for repair tissue to provide a functional articular surface in some instances, many orthopaedic surgeons continue to drill or abrade joint surfaces into the bleeding bone in their attempt to restore an articular surface.

The striking difference in the differentiation of the repair tissue in the chondral and bony parts of the same defect suggests that the different environments in the 2 regions of the defect cause the same type of repair cells to produce different types of tissue. It is not clear whether the differences in the environment in the 2 regions of the same defect are mechanical, biologic, humoral, or related to unknown factors. However, the differentiation of the repair tissue in the chondral defect suggests that there is potential for directing the cartilage repair response toward restoration of an articular surface.

Figure 2, A, shows a light micrograph of a well-formed repair tissue filling an osteochondral defect in a rabbit knee 8 weeks after surgery. No graft material has been used in this defect to promote repair. The repair tissue stained well with safranin O, indicating that a significant component of the extracellular matrix is proteoglycan, although the cellular organization is quite different from that of normal articular cartilage. Figure 2, B, is a higher magnification of the same healed defect, showing a lack of safranin O staining near the surface. Figure 2, C, is a photomicrograph of repair tissue 6 months after surgery. Note the well-formed tidemark in this repair tissue. However, in this section, safranin O staining is streaked and the extracellular matrix now appears fibrillar. Typical surface defects have begun to appear. Figure 2, D, is a photomicrograph at a higher magnification, showing fragmentation of rabbit cartilage repair 1 year after the injury. Clinically, in the majority of cases, repair tissue in large osteochondral defects (those that cause mechanical joint dysfunction or synovitis) goes on to degeneration.

Material Properties of Cartilage Repair Tissue

The material properties of fibrocartilaginous repair tissue have not been extensively studied, but clinical experience suggests that in most patients the long-term performance of this tissue is inferior to that of normal articular cartilage. Studies have been performed on rabbits in which the compressive viscoelastic properties of normal joint cartilage were compared with those of repair tissues obtained from arthroplasties. The arthroplasty repair tissue always deformed more easily than normal cartilage, and this result correlated with the lower proteoglycan concentration of the repair tissues. In several studies on larger animals (pigs), the fibrocartilage repair tissue in osteochondral defects did not possess the same biomechanical properties as normal cartilage, and this repair tissue swelled excessively when bathed in physiologic Ringer's solution. A recent report of a detailed study indicates that osteochondral healing at a high weightbearing area of a primate knee joint does not produce a repair tissue with material properties similar to those of normal articular cartilage. More specifically, repair tissues have a solid matrix with lower elastic modulus and higher permeability than those of normal tissues. Both of these qualities act to negate the fluid-pressure load-

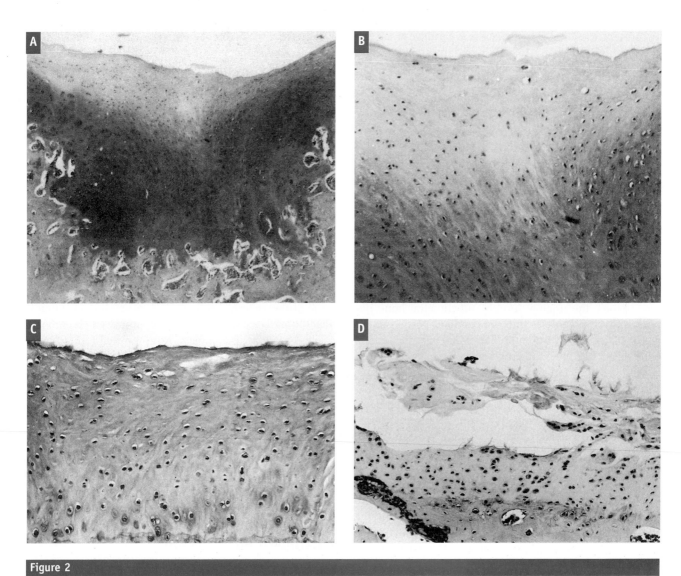

Figure 2

A, Light micrograph of a well-formed repair tissue filling an osteochondral defect (3.2 mm) in a mature rabbit, 8 weeks after surgery. The dark staining by safranin O indicates the presence of glycosaminoglycans. **B,** Same defect. Mild fibrillation of the surface is seen at higher magnification. **C,** A well-formed defect after 6 months, with irregular safranin O staining in the interterritorial matrix. **D,** Fragmentation of rabbit repair tissue 1 year after surgery. (Reproduced with permission from Buckwalter JA, Mow VC: Cartilage repair in osteoarthritis, in Moskowitz RW, Howell DS, Goldberg VM, Mankin HJ (eds): *Osteoarthritis: Diagnosis and Medical/Surgical Management,* ed 2. Philadelphia, PA, WB Saunders, 1992, pp 71–107.)

carrying capacity of the tissue.

The differences in material properties between repair cartilage and normal cartilage may help explain the frequent deterioration of repair cartilage over time. Presumably, these differences can be explained as well by examination of the repair cartilage matrix, composition, and organization. In normal cartilage, the collagen meshwork gives the tissue its form and tensile strength and restrains the swelling of proteoglycans. The increased swelling of repair cartilage may reflect a lack of organization of the collagen fibrillar network. Inspection of repair cartilage shows that the orientation of the collagen fibrils does not follow the pattern seen in normal articular cartilage. Specifically, in most regions of repair cartilage the interterritorial matrix

collagen fibrils appear to have a random orientation relative to the articular surface throughout the tissue, rather than having different orientations in the superficial, middle, and deep zones.

Another possible explanation of the increased swelling of repair cartilage is that the repair tissue may fail to establish the normal relationships between proteoglycans and the collagen network. This might occur because of formation of a different type of collagen (type I), a lack of organization of the collagen network, insufficient concentrations of necessary adhesive molecules (for example, type IX collagen), or the presence of molecules that interfere with assembly of a normal articular cartilage matrix. Either a lack of organization of the collagen network or a failure to establish the normal relationships between the collagen and proteoglycans might make the repair tissue less durable. In addition, the inferior material properties of repair cartilage, including decreased stiffness, will subject the tissue to increased strain fields during joint use, thereby causing progressive structural damage. Finally, the repair tissues do not integrate well with the surrounding tissue, leaving gaps that permit abnormally easy fluid exudation, thus adversely affecting the mechanical properties of the tissue.

Improving Articular Cartilage Repair

The poor quality of most articular cartilage repair tissue has led surgeons to develop procedures intended to improve articular cartilage repair and thereby improve joint function and decrease joint pain for patients with damaged articular cartilage or OA. Surgeons frequently penetrate subchondral bone using a variety of techniques, including abrasion with a burr, drilling, and microfracture with an awl, with the intent of restoring a functional articular surface and decreasing symptoms. Although some patients notice at least a temporary decrease in pain and these procedures can promote formation of fibrocartilaginous repair tissue, the results vary considerably among patients.

Altering the loading of osteoarthritic joints by osteotomy or joint distraction can also stimulate formation of fibrocartilaginous repair tissue. Unfortunately, the relationships between joint loading and formation and maturation of cartilage repair tissue are poorly understood, and osteotomies and joint distraction have not been shown to produce consistent long-term results. Advances in understanding of the effects of joint loading and motion on articular cartilage repair should help improve the results of these procedures. Experimental studies show that chondrocyte and mesenchymal stem cell transplantation, periosteal and perichondrial grafting, insertion of synthetic matrices, application of growth factors, and other methods have the potential to stimulate formation of a new articular surface. Limited clinical studies suggest that periosteal and perichondrial grafts and chondrocyte transplants may help promote restoration of a damaged articular surface in humans.

However, none of these methods has been shown to restore a durable articular surface in an osteoarthritic joint on a predictable basis, and it is unlikely that any one of them will be uniformly successful in the restoration of articular surfaces. Instead, the available clinical and experimental evidence indicates that future methods of improving articular cartilage repair will begin with a detailed analysis of the structural and functional abnormalities of the involved joint and the patient's expectations for future joint use. Based on this analysis the surgeon will develop a treatment plan that potentially combines correction of mechanical abnormalities (including malalignment, instability, and intra-articular causes of mechanical dysfunction), debridement of degenerated articular cartilage and possibly limit-

ed penetration of subchondral bone, and applications of growth factors or implants that may consist of a synthetic matrix that incorporates cells or growth factors. These treatments will need to be followed by a postoperative course of controlled joint loading and motion to ensure the formation and maturation of the cartilage repair tissue.

Osteoarthritis

Definition and Pathology

OA, also referred to as degenerative joint disease, degenerative arthritis, osteoarthrosis, or hypertrophic arthritis, is the most prevalent clinical entity within the domain of the orthopaedist. The clinical picture is well documented, is easily recognized on the basis of physical examination and radiographic imaging, and, if necessary, can be confirmed by arthroscopy. OA consists of a generally progressive loss of articular cartilage accompanied by attempted repair of articular cartilage, remodeling, and sclerosis of subchondral bone, and in many instances the formation of subchondral bone cysts and marginal osteophytes. In addition to the changes in the synovial joint, diagnosis of the clinical syndrome of OA requires the presence of symptoms and signs that may include joint pain, restriction of motion, crepitus with motion, joint effusions, and deformity. Pathologically, the disease is characterized by fissuring and focal erosive cartilage lesions (Fig. 3), cartilage loss and destruction (Fig. 4), subchondral bone sclerosis (Fig. 5), and cyst and large osteophyte formation at the margins of the joint (Fig. 6). OA appears to originate in the cartilage, and the virtually pathognomonic changes in that tissue are progressively more severe as the disease advances. It is always associated with structural aberrations in the underlying bone.

Unlike the joint destruction seen in joint diseases with a major inflammatory component, OA consists of a retrogressive sequence of cell and matrix changes that result in loss of articular cartilage structure and function accompanied by cartilage repair and bone remodeling reactions. Because of the repair and remodeling reactions, the degeneration of the articular surface in OA is not uniformly progressive, and the rate of joint degeneration varies among individuals and among joints. Occasionally it occurs rapidly, but in most joints it progresses slowly over many years, although it may stabilize or even improve spontaneously with at least partial restoration of the articular surface and a decrease in symptoms.

The changes in joint tissues that occur with development and progression of OA include articular cartilage fibrillation and ulceration, thickening of joint capsule and synovium, bone remodeling and eburnation, osteophyte formation, and bone cyst formation.

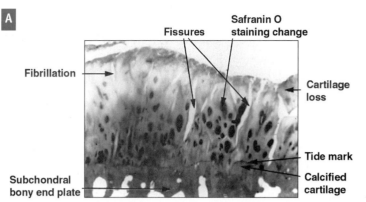

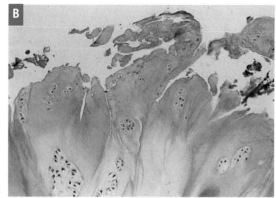

Figure 3

A, Low power magnification of a section of a glenohumeral head of osteoarthritic cartilage removed at surgery for total shoulder replacement. Note the significant fibrillation, vertical cleft formation, the tidemark, and the subchondral bony end plate. **B,** A higher power magnification of surface fibrillation showing vertical cleft formation and widespread large necrotic regions of the tissue devoid of cells. Clusters of cells, common in osteoarthritic tissues, are also seen.

Articular Cartilage Fibrillation and Ulceration

The gross appearance of hyaline articular cartilage in an osteoarthritic joint shows a highly variable pattern (Fig. 3). In some areas, the cartilage shows softening and a yellowish or brownish discoloration, whereas in other areas the normally smooth glistening surface appears as a soft, velvety, felt work. Remnants of old, irregularly scarred, or ulcerated cartilage may lie adjacent to a pebble-grained newly formed material, which is dull white in color and lacks the smooth surface characteristic of ordinary hyaline cartilage. Ulcerations, fissures, and cracks appear on the surface and, at times, are extensively focally denuded as to reveal the underlying sclerotic and eburnated subchondral bone (Fig. 4).

Histologic changes in osteoarthritic articular cartilage are a striking feature of the disease. The earliest alterations include surface erosion and irregularities, deep fissures, and alterations in the staining of the matrix (Fig. 3, *A*). The tidemark, when identifiable, often shows irregularities, duplication, and discontinuities, and often is perforated with blood vessels. As the disorder progresses, the surface layer becomes more fragmented, and short vertical clefts often descend through the gliding zone of the cartilage into the transitional zone (Fig. 3). Deep horizontal clefts can sometimes be identified. A usual pattern is extension of the vertical clefts deep into the cartilage with horizontal components. The matrix shows greater irregularity in staining even with hematoxylin and eosin. With metachromatic stains, such as toluidine blue or alcian blue, or an orthochromatic stain, such as safranin O, a patchy, progressive depletion of color can be detected (Fig. 3, *B*). At first confined to the surface areas, it later extends to the deeper layers. Initially in the interterritorial areas and subsequently in the

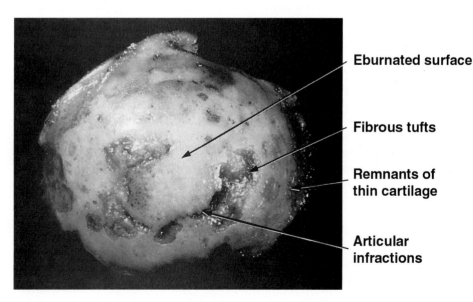

Figure 4

Macrophotograph showing total loss of articular cartilage on a human humeral head. The bone is eburnated and pitted. Regions showing remnants of cartilage are also present.

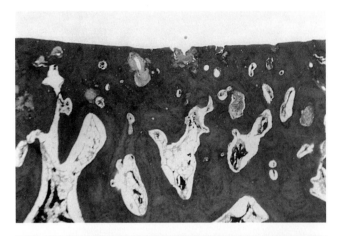

Figure 5

A histologic section of an eburnated section of bone with a dense sclerotic appearance.

territorial regions, a staining alteration occurs, which closely parallels the progressive depletion of proteoglycan. As the disease advances, the focal fragmentation of the joint surface becomes greater, the clefts deeper (descending as far as the calcified zone), and the matrix staining even more irregular and depleted. Finally, at end stage, only wisps of cartilage are left clinging to the denuded eburnated sclerotic subchondral bone (Fig. 4).

Thickening of Joint Capsule and Synovium

Gross examination of an osteoarthritic joint demonstrates that other structures are also affected. The joint capsule is usually thickened and occasionally adheres to the deformed underlying bone. This condition probably accounts for the limitation of movement. Histologic examination of the capsule, particularly in advanced disease, also demonstrates focal areas of inflammatory infiltrate, neovascularity, and, in some areas, a hyalinization, amyloid deposition, and sparse cellularity. The synovial lining in an osteoarthritic joint may show mild to moderate inflammatory changes that are thought to be secondary when compared with those of rheumatoid arthritis. The surface of the affected synovium is generally hypervascular and hemorrhagic. During OA, the synovium shows a pattern ranging from nearly normal tissues with only slight thickening of the subsynovial tissues and duplication of the synovial layer to tissues with marked thickening, villous formation, inflammatory change, and neovascularity. These, however, normally occur at a later stage of the disease.

Bone Remodeling

From etymology, the Greek root "osteo-" in the name of the disease, the bones in osteoarthritic joints often show remarkable changes (Fig. 6). Although considerable remod-

eling of the underlying bone is evident from alterations in gross structure, thickening of the cortices, and changes in trabecular bone pattern (often considered to parallel the principal stress lines from loading), the bone of the joint itself shows the most striking changes. The most severe changes are found at the point of maximum pressure against the opposing articulating surface. After total denudation of the cartilage has occurred, a dense sclerosis with fibrous and fibrocartilage tufts at the surface and evidence for new bone formation may be seen (Figs. 4 through 6). Despite the OA subchondral hypervascularity, strongly supported by angiography and bone scans of this region, small islands and, sometimes, large segments of osteonecrotic bone are often encountered.

Osteophyte Formation

These bony and cartilaginous structures, a cardinal feature of OA, arise from the bony margins of the osseous components of the joint, surround it, and significantly alter its bony contours (Fig. 6). The majority of articular osteophytes are covered with apparently normal hyaline cartilage. This has been thought of as a biologic way to resurface the diseased joint. Careful examination of the bone often shows extensive thickening of the cortex, bony sclerosis frequently having prominent cement lines, and dilated vascular spaces that may penetrate the lower layers of the cartilage.

Bone Cyst Formation

Osteoarthritic cysts (Fig. 6), another cardinal feature of OA, frequently develop within the subchondral bone. The cysts usually are located quite close to the joint surface, although

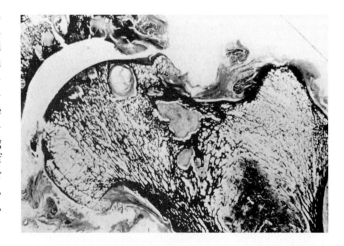

Figure 6

A macrosection of an osteoarthritic human femoral head demonstrating a large cyst subjacent to the superior aspect of the head, sclerotic bone formation, and a large osteophyte at the inferior border. The acetabulum also shows similar bony reactions.

they occasionally appear at a considerable distance from the cartilage, even extending into the metaphyseal areas. The margins of the cysts are sclerotic, which helps to distinguish them from the cysts seen in patients with rheumatoid arthritis. The cysts on cut surfaces contain homogeneous, clear or cloudy gelatinous material with a consistency resembling that found within ganglions adjacent to tendon sheaths. Microscopically, they appear as loose, sparsely cellular amorphous regions surrounded by thickened bone that stain poorly with hematoxylin and eosin.

Etiology of OA

OA has no single cause, but by a variety of means reaches a common end stage. Considerable speculation exists concerning various factors that may contribute to the initiation, perpetuation, and pathogenesis of the disorder. OA develops most commonly in the absence of a known cause, a condition referred to as primary or idiopathic OA. Less frequently it develops as a result of joint injuries, infections, or a variety of hereditary, developmental, metabolic, and neurologic disorders, a group of conditions referred to as secondary OA (Table 1). The age of onset of secondary OA depends on the underlying cause; therefore, it may develop in young adults and even children as well as the elderly. In contrast, a strong association exists between primary OA and age. The percentage of people with evidence of OA in 1 or more joints increases from less than 5% of people between 15 and 44 years of age, to 25% to 30% of the people 45 to 64 years of age, to more than 60%, and as high as 90% in some populations, of the people 65 years of age and older. Despite this strong association, and the widespread view that OA results from "wear and tear," the relationships between joint use, aging, and joint degeneration remain uncertain. Furthermore, the changes observed in articular cartilage of older individuals differ from those observed in OA (Table 2), and normal lifelong joint use has not been shown to cause degeneration. Thus, OA is not simply the result of mechanical wear from joint use. The available evidence suggests that the following factors contribute to the development of OA.

Aging

There is little doubt that OA is more common in the elderly and is, in fact, virtually nonexistent in children. But the disease is not an inevitable consequence of aging. Furthermore, as noted above, the changes in articular cartilage brought about by aging differ from the changes seen in OA (Table 2), and the occurrence of posttraumatic OA in young adults precludes the possibility that age-related changes in cartilage are prerequisite in the development of the disease. Thus, it seems most likely that age-related changes in articular cartilage increase the risk of developing OA, but do not in themselves cause the disease.

Table 1

Causes of Joint Degeneration (Secondary Osteoarthritis)

Cause	Presumed Mechanism
Intra-articular fractures	Damage to articular cartilage and/or joint incongruity
High-intensity impact joint loading	Damage to articular cartilage and/or subchondral bone
Ligament injuries	Joint instability
Joint dysplasias (developmental and hereditary joint and cartilage dysplasias)	Abnormal joint shape and/or abnormal articular cartilage
Aseptic necrosis	Bone necrosis leads to collapse of the articular surface and joint incongruity
Acromegaly	Overgrowth of articular cartilage produces joint incongruity and/or abnormal cartilage
Paget's disease	Distortion or incongruity of joints caused by bone remodeling
Ehlers-Danlos syndrome	Joint instability
Gaucher's disease (hereditary deficiency of the enzyme glucocerebrosidase, leading to accumulation of glucocerebroside)	Bone necrosis or pathologic bone fracture leading to joint incongruity
Stickler's syndrome (progressive hereditary arthro-ophthalmopathy)	Abnormal joint and/or articular cartilage development
Joint infection (inflammation)	Destruction of articular cartilage
Hemophilia	Multiple joint hemorrhages
Hemochromatosis (excess iron deposition in multiple tissues)	Mechanism unknown
Ochronosis (hereditary deficiency of enzyme, homogentisic acid oxidase articular cartilage homogentisic acid)	Deposition of homogentisic acid polymers in leading to accumulation of
Calcium pyrophosphate deposition disease	Accumulation of calcium pyrophosphate crystals in articular cartilage
Neuropathic arthropathy (Charcot joints, syphilis, diabetes mellitus, syringomyelia, meningomyelocele, leprosy, congenital insensitivity to pain, amyloidosis)	Loss of proprioception and joint sensation results in increased impact loading and torsion, joint instability and intra-articular fractures

(Reproduced with permission from Buckwalter JA, Mankin HJ: Articular cartilage: Degeneration and osteoarthritis, repair, regeneration and transplantation, in Cannon WD Jr (ed): *Instructional Course Lectures 47.* Rosemont, IL, American Academy of Orthopaedic Surgeons, 1998, pp 487–504.)

Alterations in Matrix Structure

Although secondary changes occur in matrix structure during the progress of OA, little support is offered for the concept that such changes are primary and lead to the eventual development of the disease. A recent observation of an alteration in the genetic structure of type II collagen in certain families provides some evidence for an inherited basis of OA in a small number of people.

Alterations in Cellular Activity

There is no doubt that the metabolic activity of the OA chondrocyte is abnormal, and that its differences are phenotypic and dependent on the environment. The question arises, however, as to whether these changes are primary or merely alterations (presumably permanent) that occur when the cells are stimulated either acutely or chronically by some initiating factors for the disease. A large body of data indicates that altered stresses and strains in the solid matrix, osmotic pressure, streaming potential, and a whole host of other physical factors may play a role in modulating chondrocyte activities. The specific nature of the signal (that is, mechanical, physicochemical, and/or electrical) in the ECM, and the specific nature of the signal transduction mechanism at the cellular level is unknown.

Alterations in Mediators

Humoral, synovial, and cartilage-derived chemical mediators and mechanoelectrochemical stimuli play a major role in the regulation of synthetic processes. Ample evidence exists to demonstrate that such factors may have a significant effect on the cell. Biochemical and mechanoelectrochemical factors may indeed interact and reinforce each other. Factors such as interleukin-1 can produce profound, specific alterations in the metabolism of chondrocytes, severely diminishing anabolism while enhancing catabolism, and can facilitate the disassembly of the large proteoglycan aggregates by its action on the link protein and thereby enhance proteoglycan migration through the ECM. The relative contribution of these factors in the progression of OA is not yet clear.

Table 2

Differences Between Articular Cartilage Aging and Osteoarthritis

	Structural	Cells	Matrix
Aging	Stable localized superficial fibrillation	Decreased chondrocyte density with skeletal growth	Decreased water concentration
		Alternation in synthetic activity (smaller, more variable aggrecans)	Loss of large proteoglycan aggregates (decreased aggregate stability?)
		Decreased response to growth factors	Increased decorin concentration
		Decreased synthetic activity	Accumulation of degraded molecules (aggrecan and link protein fragments)
			Increased collagen cross-linking
			Increased collagen fibril diameter and variability in fibril diameter
			Decreased tensile strength and stiffness in superficial layers
Osteoarthritis	Progressive superficial fibrillation	Initial increase in synthetic and proliferative activity	Initial increase in water content and in some instances proteoglycan concentration
	Fibrillation and fragmentation extending to subchondral bone	Loss of chondrocytes	Disruption of collagenous macromolecular organization
	Loss of tissue (decreased cartilage thickness and complete loss of cartilage in some regions)	Eventual decreased synthetic activity	Progressive degradation and loss of proteoglycans and hyaluronan
	Formation of fibrocartilaginous repair tissue	Increased degradative enzyme activity	Progressive degradation and loss of collagens
		Appearance of fibroblast-like cells in regions of fibrocartilaginous repair tissue	Increased permeability and loss of tensile and compressive stiffness and strength

(Reproduced with permission from Buckwalter JA, Mankin HJ: Articular cartilage: Degeneration and osteoarthritis, repair, regeneration and transplantation, in Cannon WD Jr (ed): *Instructional Course Lectures 47*. Rosemont, IL, American Academy of Orthopaedic Surgeons, 1998, pp 487–504.)

Altered Joint Mechanics

An ankle fracture that is not reduced and leaves the joint incongruent will, in a short time, lead to OA. Chronic states, such as recurrent dislocation of the patella, developmental dislocation of the hip, and joint incongruency as a result of osteonecrotic collapse, also will frequently lead to OA. The disease also may result from a single severe mechanical insult, but usually the evolution of the process is so slow that it is manifested only in later years, or OA may result from repetitive low-intensity insults. Excessive joint laxity caused by traumatic ligamentous injury or excessive joint tightness secondary to diseased or unintentional surgical overshortened ligaments can lead to chronic asymmetric cartilage loading and result in OA. A large number of animal studies and much clinical experience indicate that loss of the anterior cruciate ligament and meniscectomy will result in cartilage degeneration as well.

Immune Responses

Recent evidence suggests that some cartilaginous matrix proteins are not recognized by the immune system as autogenous. When they escape from the cartilage into the synovial fluid, the local lymphocytic elements identify them as antigens. This may explain why a minor injury to the cartilage may initiate or perpetuate a local autoimmune synovial inflammation. But such minor injuries are not associated with any chronic processes, nor do these joints develop OA.

Biochemical Alterations in Osteoarthritic Cartilage

DNA Content

Cell counts and measurements of the quantity of DNA per unit tissue show considerable variation in OA, depending on the site tested and extent of the disease. Usually, however, DNA concentrations are near normal or slightly increased in OA. This supports the concept that, despite a reduction in tissue volume, the cell count is reasonably well maintained. Some of the chondrocyte clones show intense activity when studied autoradiographically using 3H-cytidine, whereas others may show little or no evidence of RNA metabolism and are probably dead or dying. As the disease worsens, large regions of the tissues become hypocellular and, eventually, all cellular substance is lost over large areas of the diseased tissue.

Water

The water content of articular cartilage has been the subject of numerous studies over several decades. These have demonstrated that one of the earliest detectable changes is an increase in water content of osteoarthritic cartilage that is statistically significant, although it is only a few percentage points over that of normal tissues. At first, this finding seemed inconsistent with the fact that the concentration of proteoglycans, which constitute approximately 4% to 7% of the wet weight of normal cartilage, is significantly reduced in later stages of OA. Several hypotheses put forth to explain this observation have been discussed. Several other possible explanations, along the ultrastructural line, also have been offered for the observed increase of hydration. One possibility is that removal of the proteoglycans opens up water-binding sites on the collagen that were otherwise obscured, and that these sites hold water better than the collagen-proteoglycan solid matrix. A second possibility is that removal of some of the proteoglycans present in the interstitium allows the remainder to uncoil, thereby increasing both its negatively charged domain and its hydrophilic character. Alternatively, disruption of the collagen network may allow the proteoglycans to expand, thereby decreasing their concentration and increasing the water concentration. Recent scientific evidence suggests that collagen network stiffness and strength in resisting proteoglycan swelling may be the dominant mechanism in controlling tissue hydration. Specimens derived from enzymatically treated normal cartilage to exhaustively extract the proteoglycan content, without affecting collagen network organization and stiffness, do not gain water. No matter how the phenomenon is explained, osteoarthritic tissue always swells (gains water or size) relative to normal tissue.

Proteoglycan

The proteoglycans of osteoarthritic articular cartilage also have been studied intensely. It has been established that the proteoglycan content of osteoarthritic cartilage is diminished and that this decrease appears to be directly proportional to the severity of the disease. Since these initial studies, additional investigations have been undertaken in an attempt to define the nature of the proteoglycan macromolecules present in osteoarthritic articular cartilage, particularly in relation to aggregation, glycosaminoglycan chain length, and distribution of the glycosaminoglycans. Evidence exists for a marked increase in chondroitin sulfate concentration, especially chondroitin 4-sulfate, with a diminution in the concentration of keratan sulfate. One explanation for this alteration is that the articular chondrocytes in osteoarthritic cartilage synthesize proteoglycans similar to those found in immature cartilage. Another explanation is the possibility of an asymmetric degradation of the proteoglycan moiety that could selectively attack the hyaluronate-binding region of the macromolecule or possibly the keratan sulfate-containing region. A third possible explanation is supported by the finding of 2 populations of proteoglycans in cartilage: a larger one, rich in chondroitin sulfate, and a smaller one, with increased concentrations of keratan sulfate. Keratan sulfate has been shown to be reduced in OA, perhaps reinforcing the concept that during the early stages of the disease, cartilage more closely resembles immature than adult cartilage.

In normal cartilage, aggrecans, which consist of a core

protein and glycosaminoglycan side chains, usually exist in the form of very large aggregates that are linked at specific binding sites to a long-chain, single filament of hyaluronic acid in the presence of link proteins. Results from many studies have shown that: (1) proteoglycans appear to be considerably more extractable from osteoarthritic articular cartilage than from normal cartilage; (2) a higher percentage of the cartilage proteoglycan exists in the nonaggregating form; and (3) conversely, a smaller proportion of the proteoglycans are aggregated. These changes suggest that increased proteolytic activity attacks both the free terminal end of the aggrecan and the protein-rich portion, thus reducing the chain length and damaging the hyaluronate-binding region of the core protein to the extent that, when more hyaluronate is added, no additional aggregation occurs. Link proteins appear to be normal in character, but are quickly lost from osteoarthritic cartilage, whereas hyaluronate is only moderately reduced.

Collagen

The collagen of osteoarthritic cartilage may show some marked variations in the size and ultrastructural arrangement of the fibers, usually demonstrating a much less orderly network. This variation allows for swelling of the surface with increased water content and loss of its tensile stiffness and weakening of its tensile strength, even at the earliest stages of the disease process. Nevertheless, no change in the concentration of collagen in early osteoarthritic cartilage has been demonstrated. In severe OA, when the cartilage is almost totally destroyed, the collagen content must fall along with that of other constituents, but the relative concentration of collagen in relation to total mass (net weight, dry weight, or per microgram of DNA) is increased appreciably, reflecting a rapid loss of proteoglycan relative to collagen during the progression of the disease. This loss is reflected in the dramatic reduction of collagen network tensile stiffness and strength in the advanced stages of the human OA process.

It is not clear if the primary fibrillar collagen of osteoarthritic cartilage remains as type II. Conflicting evidence exists, but the consensus suggests that the newly formed cartilage collagen, which attempts to repair the damage in the diseased tissue, is mostly type II rather than type I. Type I collagen may be increased slightly, particularly in osteophytes. Investigators are just beginning to assess the variation in types IV, V, IX, and X collagen in OA. Such alterations may explain some of the characteristics of the disease and, perhaps, how these characteristics might influence the water content and proteoglycan distribution within the tissue.

Other Molecules

Severe OA-like changes occur in patients with alkaptonuric ochronosis or hemachromatosis. These disorders seem to occur in relation to a tanning of the collagen fiber present

as a result of the deposition in the cartilage substance of molecules of homogentisic acid or hemosiderin. A more subtle form of chemical disorder has been suggested by recent studies that note the increased frequency of joint cartilage calcification (chondrocalcinosis articularis) in OA. A considerable body of data has evolved that demonstrates increased calcium pyrophosphate in the joint, increased numbers of membrane-bound, calcium-containing vesicles, and increased alkaline phosphatase concentration in cartilage from some patients with OA. The relationship of these alterations to the pathogenesis of the disease is obscure, but one theory suggests that the midzones of the tissue are stiffened and perhaps more brittle, and therefore more prone to mechanical injury.

Material Property Changes During OA

Alterations in cartilage composition, molecular structure, and ultrastructural organization are known to produce significant degradation of the material properties of cartilage that is dictated by the tissue's water content. The swelling theory states that $\Delta V/V = \pi/B$, where ΔV is the volume gained by the tissue during swelling, that is increased water content; V is the original volume of the tissue, π is the Donnan osmotic pressure, that is, swelling pressure; and B is the bulk modulus of the collagen-proteoglycan solid matrix. The coefficient B is analogous to the Young's modulus or shear modulus of any material. Clearly from this simple relationship, the volume gained is a balance between the Donnan osmotic pressure and the bulk modulus of the tissue.

Over many decades, the hydration data from normal and OA tissues shows that there is generally a gain in water content, always by a few percentage points, from normal tissues to OA tissues. It can be concluded, therefore, that the compositional and structural changes of OA cartilage always affect the mechanical properties of the solid matrix (bulk modulus) to a greater extent than they do the swelling pressure. The tensile stiffness and strength of the solid matrix have been measured and correlated with the collagen/proteoglycan ratio. There is a significant drop of cartilage tensile stiffness with increasing severity of the lesion, although much more collagen than proteoglycan is present. This change probably reflects damage to the collagen network. This information on the cause for the increase in water content is consistent with that obtained from the enzymatic treatment studies referred to above.

In recent studies on a canine OA model based on transection of the anterior cruciate ligament, it was found that the tensile stiffness may be reduced by 50% at 3 to 4 months after surgery, water content increased by 7.5%, collagen content decreased by 25%, and collagen cross-link density decreased by 11%. These results show that, as early as 3 months after surgical transection of the anterior cruciate ligament, there are dramatic, and possibly irreversible changes in cartilage collagen composition and tensile properties. In a similar series of studies, it was found that the equilibrium shear modulus in the experimental knee joint cartilage was reduced by 65% at 6 weeks, with a slight bit of progression at 12 weeks. The dynamic modulus |G*| of cartilage in this canine OA model was reduced by 62%, with a slight recovery at 12 weeks. The energy dissipation factor (δ) was significantly increased at 6 and 12 weeks. These results indicate a general loosening and weakening of collagen-proteoglycan solid matrix in early osteoarthritic cartilage.

Typically, the increase in water content in early osteoarthritic cartilage is associated with the loss of proteoglycan and an increase in the collagen/proteoglycan ratio. From the biphasic nature of cartilage, it can be anticipated that water content of the tissue is a major factor in determining its compression properties and load support. Figure 7 shows the effects of increased water content and decreased total glycosaminoglycan content in human knee joint cartilage. The loss of the equilibrium compressive modulus results from an increase in porosity (that is, water content) and a decrease in fixed charge density (swelling pressure). Also associated with these changes is an increased permeability (Fig. 8). An interesting finding from these studies is that the permeability does not increase linearly with porosity ϕ^f, but increases quadratically. This functional dependence clearly shows how important it is for the tissue to maintain normal levels of hydration because of its accentuated effect on permeability.

Changes in the Load Support Mechanism in Cartilage During OA

In normal articular cartilage, the permeability is extremely low, in the range of 1 to 5×10^{-15} m^4/Ns (a unit of perme-

ability). Because of this extremely low permeability, it is very difficult to force the interstitial water to flow through the tissue by compression. However, it is important to realize that the interstitial water will always flow through the ECM during compression, albeit very slowly. Because of this, when normal cartilage is compressed, 90% to 95% of the load support is provided by the interstitial water. This mechanism effectively shields the collagen-proteoglycan solid matrix from heavy load bearing. However, for osteoarthritic tissues, namely those tissues with increasing water content and permeability (Fig. 8), resistance to interstitial water flow through the tissue is greatly reduced, and consequently the hydraulic pressure is proportionally reduced as well. Hence, load support must shift from the interstitial water to the collagen-proteoglycan solid matrix, defeating the highly effective stress-shielding mechanism that exists in normal cartilage. This no doubt will exacerbate the ongoing degenerative processes in osteoarthritic tissues.

All of these findings support the hypothesis that, compositionally and structurally altered cartilage from OA degenerative processes will have inferior material properties, causing it to lose its ability to effectively support the loads of joint articulation by interstitial fluid pressurization. More specifically, the altered cartilage will lose its fluid pressurization stress-shielding mechanism, which is important for it to maintain a normal functioning collagen-proteoglycan solid matrix in cartilage. Eventually, failure of this load-bearing material occurs as OA develops. Thus, it is seen that the amount of water in cartilage plays a pivotal role in the biomechanical properties and function of the tissue.

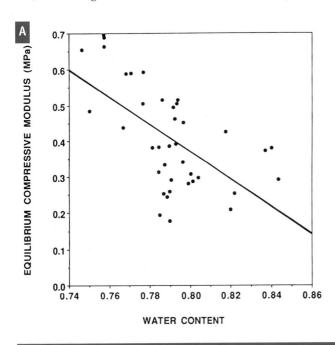
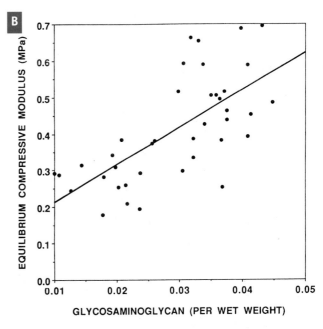

Figure 7

A, Decrease of equilibrium compressive modulus with increasing water content for human knee joint cartilage. **B,** Increase of equilibrium compressive modulus with increasing glycosaminoglycan content.

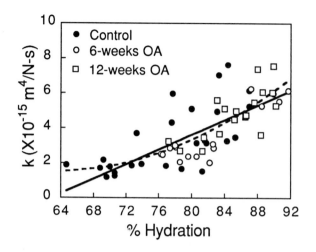

Change of canine knee joint cartilage water content and permeability 6 and 12 weeks after the anterior cruciate ligament has been transected. Note the statistical data follow the trend predicted by theory, indicating that permeability varies with the square of the hydration.

The Metabolism of Osteoarthritic Cartilage

Perhaps the most controversial issue in the biochemical study of osteoarthritic cartilage has been the assessment of the metabolic rate of the tissue as compared with that of normal tissue. The early hypotheses suggested that the process consisted of a passive mechanical erosion by wear and tear of a relatively inert tissue. Therefore, it would seem logical that the cells would show no signs of degeneration and decreased synthetic activity as the disease progressed. In fact, chondrocytes from osteoarthritic human joints are considerably more active metabolically than those from normal articular cartilage. Furthermore, regardless of the material used to trace proteoglycan synthesis (radioactive sulfate or glucosamine), the rates of incorporation are not only higher in diseased than in normal tissue, but appear to parallel the severity of the disease process. In a recent study, hyaluronate synthesis was found to be markedly increased in OA, which seems unusual in view of the decreased aggregation and the diminished concentration of hyaluronate. Considering the data, it seems reasonable that: (1) the hyaluronate that is synthesized is abnormal and, hence, does not allow aggregation; or (2) the excess synthesis is a response to a rapid degradation of the synthesized product.

Collagen Synthesis and Breakdown

Several metabolic studies have shown that collagen synthesis varies with the severity of the disease. The rate of collagen synthesis is increased, but it is not established whether all of the collagen synthesized can be incorporated into the collagenous network in a manner that will maintain the integrity of the solid matrix. Information on the catabolism of the collagen network in OA is limited. The network is dis-

rupted, but overall loss appears to be limited, until end-stage cartilage degeneration occurs. Further studies have shown, at least in several animal models, that the material synthesized is type II rather than type I collagen, supporting the concept that the repair tissue in OA is hyaline cartilage rather than fibrocartilage.

Another minor constituent protein of cartilage, fibronectin, has been found to show significant increments in both concentration and rate of synthesis in OA. The significance of this finding is currently unknown.

Proteoglycan Synthesis and Breakdown

Proteoglycan synthesis has been found to be elevated in osteoarthritic cartilage. This elevation generally is regarded as a mechanism used by the chondrocytes for matrix repair—a repair process that ultimately is doomed to failure for those patients developing OA. Animal studies have shown this synthesis to be one of the first biochemical events to occur in the early development of OA. The proteoglycans synthesized are similar to those in normal cartilage, but they appear to have slightly longer chondroitin sulfate chains, which suggests that there are some fundamental changes in the synthesis mechanisms in osteoarthritic chondrocytes. This observation is supported by recent data obtained using a monoclonal antibody to chondroitin sulfate, which shows that the chondroitin sulfate chains in osteoarthritic cartilage have subtle but potentially important structural differences.

However, the decrease in the overall proteoglycan content in osteoarthritic tissue leads to the conclusion that the proteoglycan breakdown rate and migration rate through the ECM have increased. This is indeed the case, and the increased rate of proteoglycan breakdown is a major metabolic change in osteoarthritic cartilage, particularly at the early stages of development of the joint disease. However, no difference has been shown between the molecular mechanisms involved in proteoglycan breakdown in normal tissues, and those in accelerated degradation. It therefore seems that the increased rate of catabolism is caused by increased activities of enzymes already present and active in normal tissue. The proteolytic fragments are released from the cartilage into the synovial fluid, and then are cleared by the lymphatics. Recent studies indicate that the detection of significantly elevated levels of proteoglycan in synovial fluids, particularly at early stages of OA, may represent a means for detection and monitoring of the disease. The maintenance of the cartilage matrix is, therefore, a balance between the rates of synthesis and breakdown and loss; cartilage degeneration appears to be an imbalance of these events.

DNA Synthesis

Studies of DNA synthesis in osteoarthritic cartilage have shown both mitotic activity and increased ^{3}H-thymidine incorporation, particularly in the cells of the chondrocyte clones. This finding is supported by electron microscopic studies of osteoarthritic cartilage. All of these data indicate that the articular chondrocyte in OA "turns on the switch" for DNA synthesis and makes new cells that presumably become metabolically active. The rate of DNA synthesis appears to vary directly with the morphologic severity of the process up to a point of failure, after which the rate falls.

Degradative Enzymes in Osteoarthritic Articular Cartilage

Despite the findings that the rates for synthesis of proteoglycan, collagen, and DNA are all increased, OA is a disorder that produces inexorable and sometimes rapid cartilage degeneration. The catabolic activity of the tissue, therefore, can be extraordinarily high and can ultimately dominate the picture. The degradation of articular cartilage by enzymes has been the subject of many studies. Much of the work has been directed at determining which enzymes are present in the cartilage, and what are their in vitro activities. The determination of which specific enzyme is responsible for a specific degradative event has been elusive, partly because there has been a lack of enzyme inhibitors with the specificity to provide this information.

The enzymes found in articular cartilage include the metalloproteinases collagenase, gelatinase, and stromelysin; the serine proteases, including tissue plasminogen activator, elastase, and cathepsin G; and the cathepsins B and D. The activities of the metalloproteinases are controlled by the presence of their specific inhibitor, TIMP.

Levels of metalloproteinases and the cathepsins B and D are increased in osteoarthritic cartilage. The increase in collagenase and gelatinase activities appears to correspond to the observed disruption of the collagenous network. The increased activity of stromelysin, which is likely to use the proteoglycans as a major substrate, corresponds to the increased release of proteoglycan from the articular cartilage. This enzyme also has recently been shown to degrade type IX collagen in cartilage, and thus may play an important role in the disruption of the collagen network. The level of TIMP is not increased, and it even may be decreased in osteoarthritic cartilage. This phenomenon provides support for the hypothesis that the balance of the levels of enzyme and inhibitor dictates the rate of matrix degradation, and that in OA degradation of the matrix is the result of an imbalance of these enzymes. Good evidence for the involvement of the cathepsins B and D in cartilage matrix degradation is lacking.

An important mediator of cartilage degradation, particularly in inflammatory events, is interleukin-1. Although this material may originate in the monocytes of inflamed joints, it also has been found to be synthesized by chondrocytes as a paracrine activity. Interleukin-1 enhances enzyme synthesis and activation of a number of enzyme systems in the cartilage including latent collagenase, stromelysin, and gelatinase, and a tissue plasminogen activator (Fig. 9). Plasminogen is presumed to be synthesized by the chondrocytes or passes across the synovial cell membrane to enter the matrix. The stimulation of collagenase and stromelysin production by interleukin-1 is thought to be important in elevating the catabolic events in cartilage.

Summary

Although the articular cartilage of most joints performs well for the lifetime of the individual, it may be damaged by trauma or inflammatory diseases, or it may undergo progressive degeneration leading to the clinical syndrome of

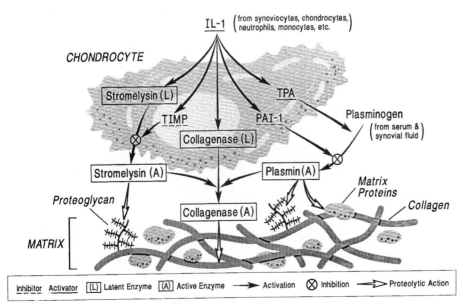

Figure 9

The cascade of enzymes, their activators and inhibitors involved in interleukin-1–stimulated degradation of articular cartilage.

OA. Because articular cartilage has a limited capacity for repair, the response to functionally significant tissue damage caused by injury or disease rarely, if ever, restores a normal articular surface. Mechanical disruption of articular cartilage stimulates chondrocyte synthetic activity, but this increased matrix synthesis does not repair injuries in skeletally mature individuals. Disruption of articular cartilage and subchondral bone stimulates chondral and bony repair, but it does not restore an articular surface that duplicates the biologic and mechanical properties of normal articular cartilage. However, in some instances the repair tissue could provide a functional joint surface for many years.

Degeneration of articular cartilage as part of the clinical syndrome of OA is one of the most common causes of pain and disability in middle-aged and older people. The strong correlation between increasing age and the prevalence of OA suggests that age-related changes in articular cartilage can contribute to the development and progression of OA. Although the mechanisms responsible for OA remain poorly understood, lifelong moderate use of normal joints does not increase the risk of OA. Thus, degeneration of normal articular cartilage is not simply the result of mechanical wear. A number of methods of restoring articular cartilage are being investigated, including altering joint loading, periosteal and perichondrial grafts, chondrocyte and mesenchymal stem cell transplants, artificial matrices, and growth factors. None of these methods has been shown to restore normal articular cartilage, but the results demonstrate that the potential for restoring a biologic articular surface exists.

Selected Bibliography

General Reference Texts

Buckwalter JA, Einhorn TA, Bolander ME, Cruess RL: Healing of the musculoskeletal tissues, in Rockwood CA Jr, Green DP, Bucholz RW, Heckman JD (eds): *Fractures in Adults*, ed 4. Philadelphia, PA, Lippincott-Raven, 1996, pp 261–304.

Kuettner KE, Goldberg VM (eds): *Osteoarthritic Disorders*. Rosemont, IL, American Academy of Orthopaedic Surgeons, 1995.

Mow VC, Hayes WC (eds): *Basic Orthopaedic Biomechanics*, ed 2. Philadelphia, PA, Lippincott-Raven, 1997.

Woo SL-Y, Buckwalter JA (eds): *Injury and Repair of the Musculoskeletal Soft Tissues*. Park Ridge, IL, American Academy of Orthopaedic Surgeons, 1988.

Cartilage Injury and Repair

Buckwalter JA: Mechanical injuries of articular cartilage, in Finerman GAM, Noyes FR (eds): *Biology and Biomechanics of the Traumatized Synovial Joint: The Knee as a Model*. Rosemont, IL, American Academy of Orthopaedic Surgeons, 1992, pp 83–96.

Buckwalter JA, Mow VC: Cartilage repair in osteoarthritis, in Moskowitz RW, Howell DS, Goldberg VM, Mankin HJ (eds): *Osteoarthritis: Diagnosis and Medical/Surgical Management*, ed 2. Philadelphia, PA, WB Saunders, 1992, pp 71–107.

Buckwalter JA, Mow VC, Ratcliffe A: Restoration of injured or degenerated articular cartilage. *J Am Acad Orthop Surg* 1994;2:192–201.

Donohue JM, Buss D, Oegema TR Jr, Thompson RC Jr: The effects of indirect blunt trauma on adult canine articular cartilage. *J Bone Joint Surg* 1983;65A:948–957.

Mankin HJ: The response of articular cartilage to mechanical injury. *J Bone Joint Surg* 1982;64A:460–466.

Mitchell N, Shepard N: Effect of patellar shaving in the rabbit. *J Orthop Res* 1987;5:388–392.

Mow VC, Ratcliffe A, Rosenwasser MP, Buckwalter JA: Experimental studies on repair of large osteochondral defects at a high weight bearing area of the knee joint: A tissue engineering study. *J Biomech Eng* 1991;113:198–207.

Newberry WN, Zukosky DK, Haut RC: Subfracture insult to a knee joint causes alterations in the bone and in the functional stiffness of overlying cartilage. *J Orthop Res* 1997;15:450–455.

O'Driscoll SW, Keeley FW, Salter RB: Durability of regenerated articular cartilage produced by free autogenous periosteal grafts in major full-thickness defects in joint surfaces under the influence of continuous passive motion: A follow-up report at one year. *J Bone Joint Surg* 1988;70A:595–606.

Salter RB, Simmonds DF, Malcolm BW, Rumble EJ, MacMichael D, Clements ND: The biological effect of continuous passive motion on the healing of full-thickness defects in articular cartilage: An experimental investigation in the rabbit. *J Bone Joint Surg* 1980;62A:1232–1251.

Setton LA, Mow VC, Muller FJ, Pita JC, Howell DS: Mechanical properties of canine articular cartilage are significantly altered following transection of the anterior cruciate ligament. *J Orthop Res* 1994;12:451–463.

Setton LA, Elliott DM, Mow VC: Altered mechanics of cartilage with osteoarthritis: Human osteoarthritis and an experimental model of joint degeneration. *Osteoarthritis Cartilage* 1999;7:2–14.

Thompson RC, Oegema TR, Lewis JL, Wallace L: Osteoarthrotic changes after acute transarticular load: An animal model. *J Bone Joint Surg* 1991;73B:990–1001.

Wakitani S, Kimura T, Hirooka A, et al: Repair of rabbit articular surfaces with allograft chondrocytes embedded in collagen gel. *J Bone Joint Surg* 1989;71B:74–80.

Osteoarthritis

Akizuki S, Mow VC, Muller F, Pita JC, Howell DS, Manicourt DH: Tensile properties of human knee joint cartilage: I. Influence of ionic conditions, weight bearing, and fibrillation on the tensile modulus. *J Orthop Res* 1986;4:379–392.

Buckwalter JA: Osteoarthritis and articular cartilage use, disuse, and abuse: Experimental studies. *J Rheumatol* 1995;43(suppl):13–15.

Buckwalter JA, Lane NE: Athletics and osteoarthritis. *Am J Sports Med* 1997;25:873–881.

Buckwalter JA, Mankin HJ: Articular cartilage: Degeneration and osteoarthritis, repair, regeneration, and transplantation, in Cannon WD Jr (ed): *Instructional Course Lectures 47.* Rosemont, IL, American Academy of Orthopaedic Surgeons, 1998, pp 487–504.

Dean DD, Martel-Pelletier J, Pelletier JP, Howell DS, Woessner JF Jr: Evidence for metalloproteinase and metalloproteinase inhibitor imbalance in human osteoarthritic cartilage. *J Clin Invest* 1989;84: 678–685.

Ehrlich MG, Armstrong AL, Treadwell BV, Mankin HJ: The role of proteases in the pathogenesis of osteoarthritis. *J Rheumatol* 1987;14: 30–32.

Froimson MI, Ratcliffe A, Gardner TR, Mow VC: Differences in patellofemoral joint cartilage material properties and their significance in the etiology of cartilage surface fibrillation. *Osteoarthritis Cartilage* 1997;5:377–386.

Hunziker EB: Articular cartilage repair: Are the intrinsic biological constraints undermining this process insuperable? *Osteoarthritis Cartilage* 1999;7:15–28.

Kuettner KE, Schleyerbach R, Peyron JG, Hascall VC (eds): *Articular Cartilage and Osteoarthritis.* New York, NY, Raven Press, 1992.

Mankin HJ, Dorfman H, Lippiello L, Zarins A: Biochemical and metabolic abnormalities in articular cartilage from osteo-arthritic human hips: II: Correlation of morphology with biochemical and metabolic data. *J Bone Joint Surg* 1971;53A:523–537.

Moskowitz RW, Howell DS, Goldberg VM, Mankin HJ (eds): *Osteoarthritis: Diagnosis and Medical/Surgical Management,* ed 2. Philadelphia, PA, WB Saunders, 1992.

Mow VC, Setton LA: Mechanical properties of normal and osteoarthritic cartilage, in Brandt KD, Doherty M, Lohmander LS (eds): *Osteoarthritis.* Oxford, UK, Oxford University Press, 1998, pp 108–122.

Radin EL: Factors influencing the progression of osteoarthrosis, in Ewing JW (ed): *Articular Cartilage and Knee Joint Function: Basic Science and Arthroscopy.* New York, NY, Raven Press, 1990, pp 301–309.

Ryu J, Treadwell BV, Mankin HJ: Biochemical and metabolic abnormalities in normal and osteoarthritic human articular cartilage. *Arthritis Rheum* 1984;27:49–57.

Setton LA, Mow VC, Pita JC, Muller F, Howell DS: Altered structure-function relationships for articular cartilage in human osteoarthritis and an experimental canine model, in van den Berg WB, van der Kraan PM, van Lent PLEM (eds): *Joint Destruction in Arthritis and Osteoarthritis.* Basel, Switzerland, Birkhauser Verlag, 1993, pp 27–48.

Telhag H: Nucleic acids in human normal and osteoarthritic articular cartilage. *Acta Orthop Scand* 1976;47:585–587.

Chapter Outline

Chapter 19

Pathophysiologic Aspects of Inflammation in Diarthrodial Joints

Anneliese D. Recklies, PhD

A. Robin Poole, PhD, DSc

Subhashis Banerjee, MD

Earl Bogoch, MD, PhD

John DiBattista, PhD

C.H. Evans, PhD, DSc

Gary S. Firestein, MD

Cyril B. Frank, MD, FRCSC

David R. Karp, MD, PhD

John S. Mort, PhD

Nancy Oppenheimer-Marks, PhD

John Varga, MD

Wim van den Berg, PhD

Yiping Zhang, MD

This chapter at a glance

This chapter reviews the pathologic changes that occur in the various joint tissues as well as the cellular and molecular processes involved in the etiology of inflammatory joint diseases.

Introduction

Loss of diarthrodial joint function is commonly observed in all populations and is a major cause of disability in all societies. Pathologic changes in the joint environment are triggered by a combination of local and systemic factors. Localized traumatic or degenerative events, exacerbated by abnormal loading, lead to degradation of cartilage matrix components of individual joints. Alterations in the homeostasis of the underlying bone may also be involved in the development of pathology. The term osteoarthritis (OA) is generally used to describe this group of degenerative joint diseases, which usually affects the large, weightbearing joints. Although not commonly associated with OA, inflammatory events driven by matrix components and wear particles may contribute to the disease in later stages.

Inflammatory joint diseases, of which rheumatoid arthritis (RA) presents the most common form, generally involve many joints because of the systemic nature of the disease. Both weightbearing and nonweightbearing joints are affected. One major aspect of RA is the chronic and progressive nature of the disease. The inflammatory processes lead to dramatic changes in all the tissues and structures of the joint. The final outcome is usually total destruction of the joint and loss of joint function. This chapter will review the pathologic changes that occur in the various joint tissues as well as the cellular and molecular processes involved in the etiology of inflammatory joint diseases.

Structure and Function of Diarthrodial Joints

To appreciate the cellular and molecular processes that lead to pathologic changes in inflammatory joint diseases, it is necessary to review the components of a diarthrodial joint. The function of the diarthrodial joint is to allow free and painless movement of 2 juxtaposed bone surfaces. The components of such a joint have evolved based on the primary requirements for this function, namely to provide smooth articulation within the required range of motion for a particular joint, to allow for adequate distribution of load, and to provide stability.

The basic components of a diarthrodial joint, using the knee as an example, are illustrated in Figure 1. The articular cartilage covering the opposing bone surfaces provides the main interface for articulation. The matrix composition of this tissue and its associated mechanical properties are crucial for its role as a protective buffer, absorbing and distributing mechanical loads applied across the joint during movement. It is thus self evident that any disturbance in the homeostasis of the cartilage matrix will result in impaired function. The structure and composition of the cartilage matrix are reviewed elsewhere in this book.

The joint cavity is filled with synovial fluid, which provides nutrients to the articular cartilage and, because of its viscous

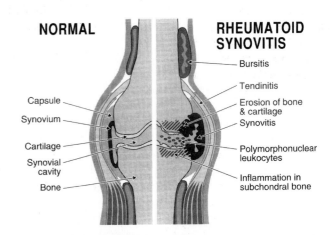

Figure 1

Schematic illustration of a diarthrodial joint and tissues affected by inflammatory processes, using the knee joint as an example. The left side shows structures in the healthy joint; the right side illustrates the widespread involvement of all joint tissues.

nature, allows almost frictionless articulation of the juxtaposed surfaces. This space is delimited laterally by the synovial membrane. Many of the inflammatory processes associated with RA are centered in the synovial tissue, and will be addressed in detail in this chapter. The joint is stabilized by the joint capsule and ligaments. In the knee joint, further stabilization is provided by the cruciate ligaments. The integrity and tone of the muscles and their tendons as well as the nerve supply involved in the movements of a particular joint are also important aspects of maintaining the joint in a proper functional state, because disuse can lead to imbalances in the homeostasis of the joint tissues and initiate pathologic changes.

Pathophysiology of Articular Cartilage

Although all joint tissues are affected by the inflammatory processes of RA, the loss of joint function is caused primarily by the progressive erosion of the articular cartilage, ligaments, and subchondral bone. The final outcome is usually total loss of articular cartilage followed by ankylosis of the joint, resulting from the formation of granulomatous tissue or from bony fusion. Because of the avascular nature of the articular cartilage, matrix breakdown is mediated by agents, mainly proteolytic enzymes, secreted by the chondrocytes or by the cells of the surrounding tissues in response to proinflammatory agents, such as the cytokines interleukin-1 (IL-1) or tumor necrosis factor-α (TNF-α).

Cartilage Erosion

In contrast to OA, in which prominent pathologic features, such as surface fibrillation, formation of fissures, and cloning of chondrocytes, have been described and are used in the histologic determination of the extent of cartilage damage, relatively little is known about early pathologic changes in the articular cartilage of involved joints in patients with RA. Cartilage erosion, the mechanisms of which are discussed in greater detail later in this chapter, occurs at 2 fronts. Cartilage erosion in inflammatory joint diseases occurs predominantly from the lateral aspects of the joint at the junction between the invading synovium (the pannus) and the cartilage. The pathophysiologic processes in this region are mediated and regulated by a complex network of inflammatory cytokines and chemokines, which stimulate the production of proteolytic enzymes from the pannus and neighboring chondrocytes (Fig. 2).

The propensity of human rheumatoid synovial cells to invade and erode articular cartilage has been demonstrated by cotransplantation of these tissues into the SCID (severe combined immunodeficient) mouse. In addition to the erosion at the invading edge, mediated by proteolytic enzymes released from the synovial cells, lysis of cartilage matrix is also observed around the chondrocytes in the near vicinity. These cells are activated by cytokines and other inflammatory mediators released from the pannus.

More recent work, in which molecular markers were used for degradation of individual matrix components, most notably type II collagen (as discussed in more detail below), has demonstrated that degradation also occurs in the interior of the cartilage of the affected joints, particularly adjacent to the subchondral bone. This degradation appears to be the result of a poorly studied inflammatory process originating in the underlying bone, leading to the release of cytokines and activation of chondrocytes in this region.

Studies involving cartilage from patients with inflammatory joint diseases have been restricted to late stages, where there is often very little cartilage left; however, some understanding of the mechanisms of destruction has been obtained from studies using animal models. Similar to observations with osteoarthritic cartilage, an early loss

of aggrecan has been reported. In vitro studies indicate that degradation of collagen fibrils occurs at a later stage, after loss of a significant proportion of the cartilage proteoglycan, aggrecan. Presumably the destruction of the large aggrecan complexes allows proteinases to access the collagen fibrils.

In addition to an increase in degradation of matrix components, inhibition of synthesis of new matrix is also observed, and, in fact, the overall loss of matrix is a result of both increased catabolism and decreased anabolism. While the same molecular mediators influence both processes (that is, IL-1 increases synthesis and secretion of matrix metalloproteinases [MMPs] while it inhibits the synthesis of many of the matrix components, most notably aggrecan and type II collagen), inhibition of synthesis of matrix molecules is observed at concentrations at least 10-fold lower than those necessary to induce synthesis and secretion of MMPs. The progressive loss of articular cartilage has been demonstrated both in the human and in many different animal models, but there is no evidence for any attempts at repair, as is observed in the osteoarthritic joint. This lack of repair may be a result of the suppression of matrix synthesis by inflammatory mediators.

Erosion of the cartilage matrix leads to deterioration and eventually complete loss of joint function. At the molecular level this process has a more immediate effect in supplying cartilage antigens that are thought to drive the autoimmune aspect of the disease. The agents initiating RA in humans are as yet unknown; however, it is widely believed that the chronic aspects are caused by the establishment of an autoimmune response to cartilage matrix components released into the synovial fluid. Because of the avascular nature of articular cartilage, many of the components, particularly those whose expression is restricted to this tissue, probably evade recognition as self antigens during the maturation of the immune system. Although direct proof of an involvement of autoantigens in human disease is still

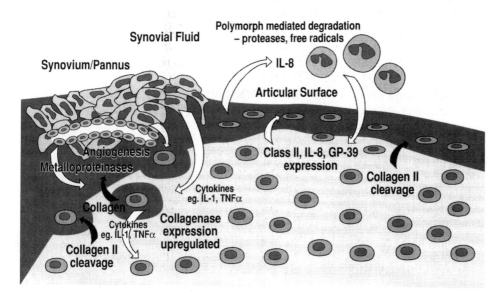

Figure 2

An extensive cytokine network is involved in the establishment of joint inflammation, leading to erosion of articular cartilage at the pannus/cartilage junction, as well as to chondrocyte-mediated matrix loss.

lacking, various animal models have demonstrated that type II collagen, the G1 domain of the aggrecan molecule, and other molecules present in cartilage matrix (cartilage oligomeric matrix protein [COMP] and cartilage gylcoprotein-39 [HCgp-30]) can elicit an erosive inflammatory arthritis. The common clinical observation that the inflammatory processes usually diminish once the cartilage is completely eroded or resected at arthroplasty, thus removing the source for autoantigens, supports this hypothesis.

Mediators of Cartilage Degradation

Degradation of the components of extracellular matrix (ECM) is caused mainly by the action of proteolytic enzymes, although nonenzymatic mechanisms may contribute to this process. The family of MMPs has received the greatest attention with respect to cartilage matrix degradation. Currently 23 members of this proteinase family have been described, and the list is still growing. They function in the normal remodeling of ECM, which takes place during embryologic development and skeletal growth as well as in physiologic turnover and resorption of tissues, such as cervical ripening and involution of the uterus preceding and following parturition, respectively, or the involution of mammary gland tissue upon cessation of lactation.

The MMPs are secreted as inactive proforms. Activation is achieved by proteolytic cleavage of the propeptide, which blocks access of substrate to the active site in the proform. The exact mechanism operating in vivo is not clearly understood. The plasminogen activator/plasmin system has been implicated, but this may not be the case for all MMPs or in all tissues. The common structural feature of all MMPs is the presence of a zinc ion in the active site, which is essential for the catalytic activity of the enzymes.

Of major importance with respect to cartilage degradation are the collagenases, MMP-1 (collagenases-1 or interstitial collagenase), MMP-8 (collagenase-2 or neutrophil collagenase), and MMP-13 (collagenase-3). Although a number of different proteinases cleave collagen fibrils in the telopeptide region, the collagenases are the only proteinases (other than cathepsin K) that cleave collagen fibers in the triple helical domain as illustrated in Figure 3. Binding to the triple helical region of collagen is mediated by the C-terminal hemopexin domain of the collagenases. Other members of the MMP family cleave denatured collagen (gelatinase A and B) or show a broad substrate specificity (MMP-1 or stromelysin).

Although all 3 collagenases cleave type I, II and II collagen fibrils, MMP-13 shows an increased activity toward type II collagen and is currently thought to be the major enzyme involved in type II collagen cleavage in the physis of the growth plate. Both MMP-1 and MMP-13 are involved in collagen degradation in RA. MMP-8, the major source of which is the neutrophil, has recently been shown to be synthesized also by articular chondrocytes and may contribute to the degradative process in inflammation.

In addition to the secreted MMPs several recently described members of this proteinase family are associated with the plasma membrane of the cell (the membrane-type or MT-MMPs). MT-MMP-1 appears to be involved in the activation of MMP-2 (gelatinase A or 72 kd gelatinase).

There is now good evidence that proteinases other than the MMPs are also involved in the cleavage of matrix molecules. The lysosomal cysteine proteinase, cathepsin B, has been shown to be involved in the cascade of events leading to matrix degradation stimulated by IL-1. It may play a role in the activation of pro-MMPs or MMP activators. Another member of the cysteine proteinase family, cathepsin K, is produced almost exclusively by the multinucleated osteoclast and may be involved in the erosion of cartilage from the aspect of the subchondral bone. Cells of the macrophage/monocyte lineage are also present in this region and have been implicated in the erosion of subchondral bone and adjacent articular cartilage. These cells are rich in cathepsin L, which is also a cysteine proteinase with a predominantly lysosomal distribution.

The cysteine proteinases are synthesized as inactive precursor molecules. Activation usually occurs in the acidic environment of the lysosome. A unique feature of the mature enzymes is their instability at physiologic pH, whereas the proforms are generally stable, allowing processing and transport from the endoplasmic reticulum to their final destination, the lysosome. Under some circumstances, the proforms of both cathepsins B and L can be secreted and accumulate in the extracellular milieu, thus providing a pool of potential degradative activity.

Nonenzymatic mechanisms can also contribute to the degradation of matrix components. Generation of free radicals is an important aspect of the immune defense repertoire of neutrophils and macrophages, and they may therefore play a role in acute inflammation. The short-lived

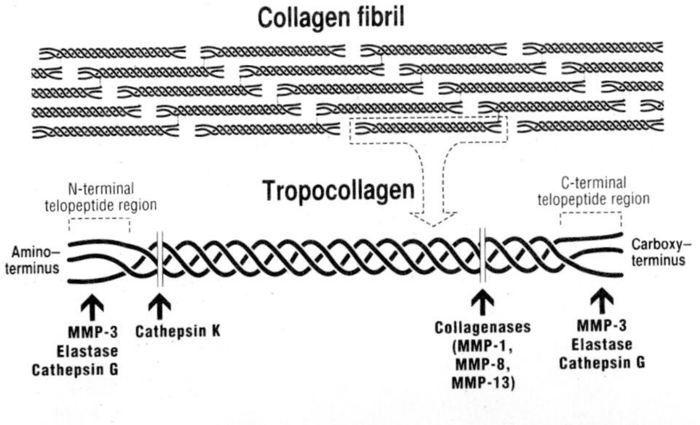

Figure 3

Proteolytic degradation of fibrillar collagen, illustrating regions susceptible to proteolytic attack by proteases present in the joint environment. Tropocollagen is the repeating unit of collagen fiber. Cleavage in the non-helical telopeptide domain by proteinases such as MMP-3 can lead to the loss of the triple helical segments. The collagenases and cathepsin K cleave fibrillar collagens at unique sites in the triple-helical domain.

hydroxyl and superoxide radicals have been implicated in the breakdown of cartilage matrix molecules. Free radicals are capable of inducing cleavage of aggrecan, collagen, and hyaluronic acid.

Stimulation of Cartilage Degradation

The MMPs involved in cartilage degradation are secreted by cells resident in many of the joint tissues, given an appropriate stimulatory environment. Although there is some difference in the set of MMPs elaborated by a particular cell type, the synthesis and secretion of many MMPs (with the exception of MMP-2) are regulated in a similar fashion in most connective tissue cells. The most well-characterized regulators of MMP-production are the proinflammatory cytokines IL-1α and β (collectively referred to as IL-1) and TNF-α. Because of their pivotal role in inflammation, their effects and mechanism of action will be discussed in more detail later in this chapter. Adding IL-1β or TNF-α to articular cartilage in vitro induces loss of aggrecan and, after an initial delay, degradation of collagen. Degradation of cartilage matrix is decreased by transforming growth factor-β (TGF-β), which limits the amount of extracellular proteolytic activity by inhibiting transcription of the MMP genes and by stimulating the production of inhibitors of MMPs (tissue inhibitors of matrix metalloproteinases or TIMPs) and of other proteinases, such as plasminogen activator inhibitor (PAI).

Turnover of matrix components is a normal physiologic process in articular cartilage; thus, it is not surprising that degradative events should be regulated by the interactions of the cells with their surrounding matrix. Fragments of the ubiquitous extracellular matrix component, fibronectin, induce synthesis of several MMPs in a variety of connective tissue cells, including chondrocytes and synovial cells, and induce loss of aggrecan in intact articular cartilage in vitro. This effect is mediated by $\alpha_5\beta_1$ integrin, the cellular receptor for fibronectin which binds to the well-characterized RGD motif (an internal sequence of the 3 amino acids arginine [R], glycine [G], and aspartic acid [D]) of the fibronectin molecule. The sequence of events downstream of the receptor engagement, which leads to increased MMP gene expression, is not clearly understood at present. In articular chondrocytes, fibronectin fragments are thought to stimulate increased production of IL-1, which in turn acts on MMP gene expression.

Hyaluronan (hyaluronic acid, HA) fragments of a molecular size less than 300 kd activate monocytes, stimulating increased production of inflammatory cytokines (IL-1, TNF-α) and chemokines (IL-8). This process is partially mediated by binding to the cellular HA-receptor, CD44. HA fragments also stimulate loss of aggrecan from cartilage explants, which may be mediated by induction of IL-1 synthesis in articular chondrocytes.

In addition to molecular messengers, biomechanical factors may also regulate matrix homeostasis. Chondrocytes are very sensitive to mechanical loading. Cyclic compressive loading, which mimics the normal biomechanical environment of the cell, enhances matrix synthesis relative to unloaded tissue. Continuous or static loading, on the other hand, inhibits synthesis and accelerates degradation of both proteoglycan and collagen. The mechanisms of transmission of biomechanical signals to the cells is not clearly understood but it has recently been shown that cyclic pressure induces hyperpolarization of articular chondrocytes and that the $\alpha_5\beta_1$ integrin is involved in the signaling pathway. It is thus possible that biomechanical parameters affect the interaction of chondrocytes with matrix components, forming an integral part of the regulation of normal tissue turnover in the joint.

Mechanisms of Degradation of Matrix Molecules

The understanding of the degradative events in articular cartilage has been aided greatly by 2 relatively recent developments. The identification of the various MMPs and the production of recombinant forms have provided the quantities of enzyme necessary for in vitro studies and allowed the precise identification of the cleavage sites in a number of matrix molecules. Proteolytic cleavage of matrix molecules generates new N- and C-terminals, which are specific for cleavage by a given proteinase. These new terminal sequences are referred to as neoepitopes because the charged terminal residues are not normally present on the parent protein (Fig. 4). Hence, antibodies specific for these neoepitopes can be generated and used to study the recent proteolytic history of a tissue, giving some indication about the identity of the proteinases involved.

Cartilage erosion either in OA or in RA involves the proteolytic attack on all the major matrix components by a variety of MMPs and other matrix degrading proteinases, as illustrated in Figure 5. However, these events do not necessarily occur simultaneously. One of the earliest events is the degradation and loss of aggrecan. This molecule is particularly susceptible to proteolysis in the interglobular domain between the G1 and G2 domains. Because the G1 domain is responsible for binding to HA and, hence, the retaining of aggrecan within the matrix, this cleavage results in the loss of the part of the molecule bearing the chondroitin sulfate- and keratan sulfate-rich domains. These fragments of the aggrecan molecule can be readily detected in synovial fluids using antibodies to either the chondroitin sulfate or keratan sulfate side chains.

There are 2 main cleavage sites in the interglobular domain. One is the site at which numerous metalloproteinases, such as MMP-3, cleave. Cleavage at the second site, which is closer to the G2 domain and referred to as the "aggrecanase cleavage site," has been shown to occur in vitro on stimulation of cartilage with IL-1. This proteolytic event also occurs in vivo; aggrecan fragments bearing the

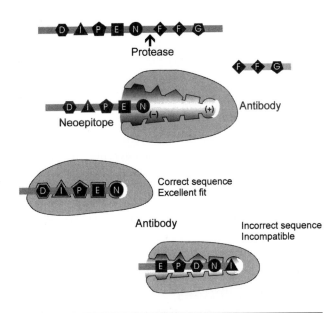

Figure 4

The use of antineoepitope antibodies to demonstrate the action of specific proteinases. Prototypic cleavage of a matrix protein at a specific site (the matrix metalloproteinase-3 cleavage site of aggrecan is illustrated here) generates fragments with new amino and carboxy-termini, referred to as neoepitopes. They are not present in their charged form in the parent molecule, and can be used to generate specific antibodies. Charge-charge interactions of subsites in the antibody binding region of the immunoglobulin molecule with the amino or, in the case illustrated here, carboxy-terminal residue, contribute greatly to the specificity and affinity of neoepitope antibodies.

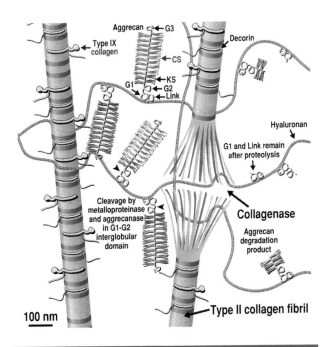

Figure 5

Diagrammatic representation of the organization of the proteoglycan aggrecan and type II collagen fibrils in cartilage matrix. Sites of attack on collagen and aggrecan by collagenases and other proteinases, respectively, are shown.

aggrecanase neoepitope can be found in articular cartilage and synovial fluids from patients with RA and OA. The existence of a specific "aggrecanase" was thus postulated. Two proteases belonging to the ADAMs (a disintegrin and metalloprotease) family have recently been identified, which generate the specific cleavage fragments of aggrecan. The control of their expression and activity is currently being studied intensively in the hope of designing effective inhibitors for the control of cartilage erosion.

In experimental models of arthritis, both the MMP-3 and aggrecanase cleavage sites are present, suggesting that both are involved in the proteolysis of aggrecan. However, mice bearing a null mutation for MMP-3 still develop an antigen-induced arthritis, providing further evidence that other proteinases are involved in the cleavage of aggrecan, both in normal tissue remodeling during endochondral ossification and in pathologic situations.

Degradation of type II collagen follows the initial loss of proteoglycan. The triple helix of this collagen is primarily cleaved by collagenases that have the capacity to cleave at a single site within the triple helix between residues 775–776, approximately three fourths of the way from the amino terminus of the mature collagen molecule. This cleavage leads to denaturation of the triple helix at physiologic temperature followed by further cleavage of the denatured α-chains by collagenases, particularly collagenase-3 (MMP-13), as well as by the gelatinases A (MMP-2) and MMP-9 and stromelysin-1 (MMP-3). Antibodies to the neoepitopes of the collagenase cleavage site as well as to "hidden epitopes," which are exposed on denaturation of the cleaved triple helix, have been used to detect cleavage of cartilage collagen in situ, demonstrating that collagen degradation occurs not only at the cartilage-pannus junction in RA, but also in remote areas and adjacent to the subchondral bone. In OA, cleavage of collagen occurs both in the superficial and deep zones of the cartilage, depending on the state of the disease.

Measurement of Cartilage Degradation In Vivo

The present knowledge of cartilage-specific components and the degradative events that take place in this tissue under inflammatory or degenerative conditions has led to the development of new immunoassays that can be used to monitor cartilage erosion. Degradation products, including markers for aggrecan and type II collagen, can be detected in synovial fluid, serum, and urine. COMP and HC-gp39, can be detected in serum and synovial fluid.

Increased biosynthesis of matrix components can be followed using a similar approach. Assembly of new type II collagen fibrils is preceded by the extracellular cleavage of the C-terminal peptide from the newly synthesized and secreted proform. The C-propeptide is released from the cartilage and, hence, its presence in body fluids is indicative of the level of new matrix synthesis. A chondroitin sulfate epitope specific for newly synthesized aggrecan has also been identified and can be used to monitor aggrecan synthesis. This aspect is important if biologic repair of damaged cartilage by therapeutic intervention is to be achieved and evaluated.

The Synovium

Normal Synovium

The normal adult synovium provides nutrients to articular cartilage and produces lubricants that allow the joint surfaces to glide smoothly across each other. It is generally divided into 2 distinct layers, the intimal lining and the sublining. The intimal lining is in direct contact with the intra-articular cavity and is responsible for the production of synovial fluid components such as HA. It is a loosely organized, avascular layer that is usually 1 or 2 cells deep. Ultrastructural studies show that this region comprises 2 main cell types, called type A and type B cells. Type A cells are derived from the bone marrow and have many features of tissue macrophages, including a prominent Golgi apparatus, abundant digestive vacuoles, and expression of surface Fc receptors. Type B cells originate from mesenchyme and have a fibroblast-like morphology. Production of the enzyme uridine diphosphoglucose dehydrogenase by type B synoviocytes is a unique feature of this type of fibroblast. The intimal lining acts as a porous barrier of loosely associated type A and B cells and lacks a true basement membrane or tight junctions.

The synovial sublining lies directly below the intimal lining. Normally, this region is relatively acellular and contains scattered blood vessels, fat cells, and fibroblasts. A network of small capillaries and venules is found immediately below the sublining, and larger vessels penetrate the deep sublining tissues. Occasional mononuclear cells, including lymphocytes and macrophages, infiltrate the sublining space. The acellular ECM contains a variety of macromolecules, including types I and III collagen, fibronectin, and proteoglycans.

The Synovium in Rheumatoid Arthritis and Other Arthritides

In RA, synovial tissue becomes hyperplastic, with redundant folds, and villae (Outline 1). In very early disease, blood vessel growth (angiogenesis) and endothelial cell damage predominate and are soon accompanied by increased cellularity in the intimal lining. Over the ensuing months, intimal lining hyperplasia becomes prominent, attaining a depth of up to 10 to 20 cell layers. Local proliferation of the fibroblast-like type B synoviocytes and migration of new macrophage-like type A synoviocytes from bone marrow contribute to cell accumulation in the intima.

An abnormally low rate of cell death (apoptosis) probably also contributes to this process.

Chronic inflammatory cells, including T cells, B cells, macrophages, and plasma cells, accumulate in the sublining region in long-standing disease. Lymphocytes, mostly CD4$^+$ memory T cells, organize into discrete aggregates, although diffuse mononuclear cell infiltrates or relatively acellular fibrous tissue can also be present. The lymphocytes express many distinct surface macromolecules, suggesting prior activation. These macromolecules include the major histocompatibility complex (MHC) class II proteins, HLA-DR, and a variety of adhesion molecules. Proliferation of blood vessels remains prominent in the chronic phase of RA. Capillary morphometry studies suggest that the vascular tree is more disorganized in arthritis compared to normal tissue and that relative ischemia of synovial tissue occurs despite the presence of more blood vessels.

These histopathologic findings are not unique to RA. Most inflammatory arthritides display similar characteristics, although usually to a lesser degree. Even "noninflammatory" forms of arthritis, such as OA, are often marked by mild synovial lining hyperplasia and sublining mononuclear cell infiltration. For this reason, synovial biopsy has little use as a diagnostic tool in inflammatory synovitis unless infectious etiologies are being considered.

Pannus and Bone Destruction

The invasive region of rheumatoid synovium that erodes into cartilage, bone, and ligament is called "pannus." It contains macrophages and primitive mesenchymal cells, but very few lymphocytes. The mesenchymal cells in the pannus might be related to type B synoviocytes or derived from a separate lineage. Morphologic and functional studies suggest that the pannus-derived fibroblasts, which have been called "pannocytes," have distinctive characteristics, such as very high expression of vascular cell adhesion molecule-1.

Outline 1

Histologic Features of Chronically Inflamed Synovium

Intimal lining hyperplasia

Lymphocyte accumulation

CD4+ T cells

Perivascular lymphoid aggregates

Blood vessel proliferation

Rare neutrophils

Pannus formation (rheumatoid arthritis only)

Damage to bone and cartilage caused by synovial tissue and pannus is mediated by degradive enzymes, including members of the serine-, cysteine-, and metalloproteinase families. MMP-1, -2, and -3 have all been detected in synovial tissue and synovial fluid in RA, as have the cysteine proteinases cathepsin B and L. The primary sources of metalloproteinases in inflammatory synovitis are fibroblast-like synoviocytes in the intimal lining. The same genes are expressed by the synovial lining in OA, albeit at lower levels. Enzyme production is regulated by cytokines, and IL-1 and TNF-α are the most potent inducers. Protease inhibitors like the TIMPs are also expressed by the rheumatoid synovial lining, although the balance between proteinases and inhibitors favors increased proteolytic activity in inflammatory arthritis.

Synovial Inflammation and the Pathogenesis of Rheumatoid Arthitis

The pathogenesis of RA has been the subject of intense study over the last few decades. Early studies focused on the acute inflammatory response mediated by autoantibodies such as rheumatoid factor, complement, and small molecular mediators like the leukotrienes. Subsequent observations suggested that T cells are intimately involved in the disease and coordinate an antigen-specific process directed against 1 or more antigens derived from the articular cartilage. More recently, studies of cytokines, macrophages, and fibroblasts have suggested that a more complex disease process accounts for the chronic, destructive nature of RA (Fig. 6).

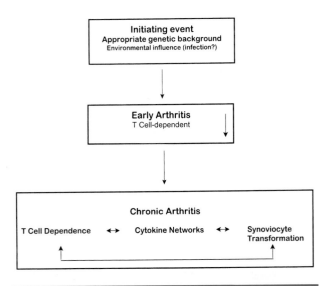

Figure 6

Pathogenesis of rheumatoid arthritis is a complex process involving immune processes driven by T cells, leading to autoimmune responses, cytokine-driven events (responsible for most of the erosive events), and synovial transformation, resulting in pannus formation and hyperplasia.

The Role of T Cells in Rheumatoid Arthritis

The most widely accepted model to explain the pathogenesis of RA invokes antigen-specific T cells that orchestrate chronic synovial inflammation. This notion is partially based on the observation that the synovium in RA is extensively infiltrated with CD4+ T cells. Second, many animal models of arthritis involve T-cell-mediated responses, such as collagen-induced arthritis and adjuvant arthritis in rodents. Third, specific HLA-DR haplotypes are associated with the susceptibility to RA. These major histocompatibility molecules are known to present peptides to T cells, and the association could be a result of the ability of unique disease-associated DR molecules to bind to arthritogenic peptides.

Immunosuppressive agents have some clinical efficacy in severe rheumatoid synovitis, suggesting that T lymphocytes contribute to arthritic symptoms. Despite the enthusiasm for T-cell-suppressive therapy, however, the results in controlled clinical trials have been generally disappointing. Monoclonal antibodies that bind to T-cell surface receptors, including anti-CD4, -CD5, and -CD52, offer minimal or no therapeutic benefit even though T cells are removed from the blood, and, in some cases, synovial tissue.

The T-cell hypothesis suggests that lymphocytes mediate synovitis through the generation of immunoregulatory proteins known as cytokines. However, protein and messenger RNA studies in RA suggest that T-cell products are relatively deficient in the rheumatoid joint, possibly as a result of the production of endogenous suppressive agents like TGF-β or IL-10. Notably, some animal models suggest that the presence of membrane-bound cytokine factors on T cells can also cause arthritis, although this has not been studied extensively in human disease.

The population of T helper (Th) cells can be divided into functional subsets based on their pattern of cytokine production. Th1 cells produce IL-2 and interferon γ (IFN-γ), but not IL-4 or IL-10, whereas Th2 cells secrete the converse. Th1 cytokines are involved in the inflammatory phase of many animal models of autoimmunity, whereas Th2 cytokines suppress disease. For instance, IFN-γ and Th1 cells are important in murine collagen-induced arthritis. In contrast, IL-10 and IL-4 gene expression correlate with disease remission. These findings have some relevance to RA. Although the amount of T-cell cytokines in the rheumatoid joint is low, the products that can be detected are primarily produced by Th1 cells while Th2-cytokines are essentially absent. This has led many investigators to propose the use of Th2 cytokines to treat RA.

Autocrine/Paracrine Cytokine Networks

In contrast to T-cell cytokines, those produced mainly by macrophages and fibroblasts of the intimal lining are abundant in rheumatoid synovium and synovial fluid. IL-1 and

TNF-α are present in high concentrations in the joint and can enhance production of prostaglandins, metalloproteinases, and complement, as well as increase cell recruitment into the inflamed joint. These cytokines can establish paracrine or autocrine loops that, in turn, increase the local production of other cytokines. An alternative explanation for the perpetuation of RA involves these complex, intertwined cytokine networks. If the synovium lacks sufficient amounts of suppressive cytokines (like those derived from Th2 cells), this process can become self-perpetuating.

The clinical importance of cytokine networks has recently been demonstrated in studies using specific anticytokine therapy. For instance, inhibition of TNF-α leads to dramatic improvement in RA and demonstrates the importance of this proinflammatory factor. Blockade of IL-1 and IL-6 using either biologic or small molecular inhibitors is also promising. It is not known whether anticytokine therapy will alter the progression of joint destruction in addition to improving subjective measures of disease activity.

Partial Transformation of Synoviocytes

One intriguing hypothesis suggests that RA synoviocytes achieve a degree of autonomy in chronic disease and continue to invade cartilage independent of the inflammatory process. For example, cultured RA synoviocytes exhibit some features of cellular transformation, including growth under anchorage-independent conditions and loss of contact inhibition. Therefore, RA synoviocytes appear to be permanently altered by their articular environment. This was best demonstrated when synoviocytes were implanted along with cartilage explants into SCID mice. RA synoviocytes migrated into cartilage matrix over the ensuing 1 to 2 months, while synoviocytes derived from osteoarthritic or normal tissue did not.

Investigations of the molecular mechanism of RA synoviocyte transformation led to studies on the *p53* tumor suppressor gene. Immunohistochemistry and Western blot analysis showed that the p53 protein is overexpressed in the synovial lining of patients with destructive synovitis as well as in cultured synoviocytes. More important, somatic mutations were identified in the *p53* gene in rheumatoid synovium and in cultured synoviocytes. The specific synovial mutations localized to regions of the gene that had been associated with cell transformation, suggesting that the mutations have functional importance. Other genes might also be altered in arthritis, and mutations in the H-*ras* oncogene have been recently identified in RA and OA synovium.

The mutations identified in rheumatoid synovial tissue probably do not cause arthritis. Instead, the genotoxic environment of the inflamed joint probably leads to mutations that accumulate over time. Proinflammatory mediators such as nitric oxide and reactive oxygen species can damage DNA in synovium, ultimately altering key genes.

Changes in the *p53* gene or other cell cycle regulators can subsequently increase synoviocyte autonomy and destructive potential.

Each of these pathways for the pathogenesis of RA has strengths and weaknesses that still must be addressed. Also, it is important to recognize that they are not mutually exclusive. For instance, RA might be initiated by a T-cell-specific process. Later, cytokine networks involving macrophages and fibroblasts might become more important but still require intermittent T-cell input. In chronic disease, partially transformed synoviocytes might arise as a result of the production of local oxygen radicals. The recognition that arthritis is a complex process involving multiple overlapping mechanisms suggests a need for therapeutic intervention at multiple levels.

Bone

Inflammation within bone may occur as a result of various etiologies, some of which are discussed elsewhere in this book. Osteitis (inflammation of bone) is a historic term for numerous conditions not now considered to be truly inflammatory, such as osteitis fibrosa cystica (hyperparathyroidism) and osteitis deformans (Paget's disease). The term still is used occasionally for infection in bone. The term osteomyelitis refers to inflammation of bone and bone marrow associated with infection and is discussed elsewhere in this book. In addition to the above conditions, inflammation in bone may occur as a foreign body reaction (such as reaction to wear debris from prosthetic implants) or in association with inflammatory arthritides, which is the focus of this chapter.

Inflammation within bone is modified by the specific anatomy of bone, which varies according to site (trabecular cancellous bone versus cortical bone), and by the calcified matrix, which limits cellular invasion and diffusion of molecules. Inflammation can alter the physiology and structure of bone by modifying the normal pattern of remodeling and stimulating increased bone resorption and formation.

Bone turnover is the result of an ordered, well-controlled sequence of events. Bone is resorbed by osteoclasts. They are succeeded by transitional cells, which then give way to osteoblasts producing osteoid. Osteoblasts surrounded by osteoid become osteocytes, while at the bone surface active osteoblasts are replaced by resting cells. Each packet of such cells and/or the succession of cells at the bone surface make up 1 bone multicellular unit or BMU, and the activity of multiple BMUs results in bone turnover.

The specialized cells within bone that affect bone structure and respond to disease-induced stress are the osteoblasts and osteoclasts. Osteoblasts synthesize bone. They are mononucleated cells that arise from mesenchymal stem cells of the bone marrow stroma, as do chondrocytes, adipocytes, and fibroblasts. Osteoclasts resorb bone.

They are multinucleated cells of a monocytic lineage; that is, they are derived from hematopoietic precursor cells. In addition to multinuclearity, distinguishing morphologic features of osteoclasts are the presence of a ruffled border, which is the resorptive portion of the cell membrane, and a "clear zone" thought to be the site of attachment to matrix. At the molecular level, osteoclasts are characterized by the presence of large quantities of the lysosomal enzyme, tartrate-resistant acid phosphatase, which is involved in the resorption of hydroxyapatite; the cysteine proteinase, cathespin K, which is responsible for a major proportion of the degradative events of bone resorption; and the membrane receptors for calcitonin.

A key cellular event occurring in bone as a result of inflammation is the activation of osteoclasts by inflammatory cytokines, resulting in increased bone remodeling and loss, with important clinical implications. RA is the paradigm of these effects of inflammation on bone. Although bone loss is detectable by radiography only after 30% or more of bone mass has been lost, osteopenia is a very common and predictable radiographic feature of severe rheumatoid disease. The clinician performing joint arthroplasty or internal fixation in the rheumatoid patient must consider osteopenia to be an important component of the patient morbidity. Preoperative planning and special intraoperative methods are indicated to avoid fracture and loss of fixation. Current noninvasive techniques for identifying and quantifying osteopenia, including imaging (x-ray absorptiometry, quantitative computed tomography) and serologic techniques (osteocalcin and alkaline phosphatase are bone turnover markers indicative of osteoblast activity, and deoxypyridinoline crosslinks, an end-product of collagen degradation, are diagnostic for the level of bone resorption) have led to a better understanding of bone loss associated with inflammatory arthritides.

Data obtained from human tissues are limited and much of the knowledge acquired in this field has been obtained from animal models of inflammatory arthritis, induced by systemic or intra-articular injection of irritants or immunogens. Osteopenia is a primary feature of these experimental models. Modified bone structure resulting from abnormal remodeling associated with joint inflammation is observed remote from the inflamed joint, in the network of subchondral cancellous bone adjacent to the articular surface, and also in bone marrow between the subchondral bone spaces. In hard tissues the primary pathologic event is bone loss but more recently, soft-tissue changes in the subchondral bone marrow have also been documented.

The diaphyses and metaphyses of long bones of patients who have severe, long-standing polyarticular RA usually appear radiolucent and demonstrate cortical thinning resulting from endosteal resorption. Histologic descriptions of the anatomic pathology that results in radiolucency of the cortex are few, and are usually confined to a description of endosteal bone loss. Rheumatoid cortical bone may show haversian canals containing increased numbers of osteoclasts, osteoblasts, and high endothelial vessels (HEV). HEV are associated with leukocyte extravasation to inflamed tissues, where activated endothelial cells facilitate their recruitment to the site of inflammation.

Radiographic lucency, decreased bone mineral density, and cortical thinning are well documented in animal models. A significant loss of cortical bone strength has been correlated to the appearance of large (-800-1,200 mμ) foci of bone resorption in the femoral cortex in carrageenan-induced inflammatory arthritis of the rabbit tibiofemoral joint. Suppression of osteoclast activity through administration of bisphosphonate prevented not only the appearance of the defects in bone but also the associated loss in bone strength.

Subchondral bone, which separates articular cartilage from underlying trabecular bone and marrow spaces, provides mechanical support for the cartilage. Mechanical failure of subchondral bone in chronic inflammatory arthritis (RA) may occur at joint surfaces of the femoral head (collapse), the medial wall of the pelvis (acetabular protrusion), and the weight-bearing tibial surfaces in the knee (deformity, collapse), and plays a role in the destruction of the joint and loss of articular cartilage. Proximal tibial and femoral bone specimens collected from patients undergoing joint replacement for RA are weaker than osteoarthritic or normal bone. Inflammation-induced abnormalities of subchondral bone are readily identifiable in radiographs of patients who have chronic, severe RA. Typical findings are erosions (circumscribed radiolucencies resulting from focal bone resorption) and diffuse cancellous osteopenia adjacent to joints.

Early histologic observations suggested increased evidence of resorptive activity and increased osteoid, indicating bone formation. Profound acceleration of bone remodeling driven by active bone resorption takes place adjacent to inflamed joints. The rate of bone formation and osteoblast function associated with increased bone resorption appears to vary. Reports of increased or decreased bone formation may result from differences in study methodology. Variation in bone remodeling rates may also be caused by differences in the stage (early or late), location (such as hip or finger joints), and type of disease (erosive or nonerosive; juvenile or adult-onset; RA or seronegative inflammatory arthritides), as well as gender (women appear to have more severe bone loss than men).

Origin and Activation of Osteoclasts

Inflammation-induced bone loss is mediated by increased numbers of osteoclasts as well as by increased resorptive activity of these cells. Inflammatory processes can affect the recruitment of osteoclast precursors from the circulation, their rate of maturation, and their level of activity. These processes are mediated by osteoblasts and bone marrow stromal cells and by the cytokine profile in this environment.

Osteoclast precursors are derived from peripheral blood monocytes that migrate into the bone and are induced to mature by the bone microenvironment. Their differentiating and maturation is influenced by hematopoietic and other growth and differentiation factors as well as systemic hormones. The most important hematopoietic growth factors for osteoclasts are granulocyte macrophage colony stimulating factor (M-CSF) and IL-6. M-CSF is obligatory for osteoclast proliferation and differentiation. Its role is demonstrated in studies of osteopetrotic animals in which abnormal bone remodeling is traced to a defect in the synthesis of M-CSF by bone marrow stromal cells. TGF-β depresses differentiation and maturation of hematopoietic cells, including osteoclast precursors, while the cytokines IL-1α, IL-1β, IL-6, IL-11, leukemia inhibitory factor, and TNF-α all promote osteoclast precursor formation. The systemic hormones, parathyroid hormone (PTH), PTH-related peptide (PTHrp), calcitonin, and vitamin D_3, as well as prostaglandins, are all involved in osteoclast ontogeny and fusion of cells to form mature multinucleated cells. Most of these factors affect osteoblasts and/or bone marrow stromal cells, so that the osteoblast is now considered to play a significant role in the normal ontogeny, fusion, and activation of the osteoclast through the release of paracrine factors and through cell-cell interaction. One direct link between osteoblast and osteoclast is via osteoclast differentiation factor (ODF), also known as TNF-related activation-induced cytokine or receptor activator of nuclear factor kappa B ligand. ODF located on the cell surface of the osteoblast interacts with a receptor on osteoclast precursors known as receptor activator of nuclear factor kappa B to promote osteoclastogenesis and resorptive activity. This interaction is sufficient for this process and does not require any other factor.

The Role of Inflammation in Osteoclast Ontogeny and Activation

Many of the cytokines that normally promote osteoclast formation and activation are synthesized excessively by inflammatory cells at sites of inflammation. The major mediators of inflammation that are substantially increased in the synovial fluid, synovial tissue, or serum of RA patients and that have been shown to act in experimental models are IL-1, IL-6, TNF-α, and M-CSF. These are the same cytokines that profoundly influence osteoclast differentiation and maturation. The cytokine network and cellular interactions which may lead to osteopenia in RA are shown in Figure 7. A similar biosynthetic cytokine profile is found in monocytes recruited in significant numbers to sites of bone injury and remodeling, and many of the processes involved in this aspect of bone turnover are identical, albeit more tightly controlled. Thus, upregulation of the inflammatory process implies activation of the osteoclast, and osteopenia is a reflection of intense inflammation.

Tendons and Ligaments

Despite the long history of clinical and basic scientific investigations of inflammatory processes within joints, there have been very few investigations of tendons and ligaments in these conditions, per se. This section will briefly review what has been published about pathophysiologic processes in human tendons and ligaments. These processes have been investigated during noninvasive diagnostic means (such as magnetic resonance imaging or by ultrasound), or using postsurgical or postmortem analysis of

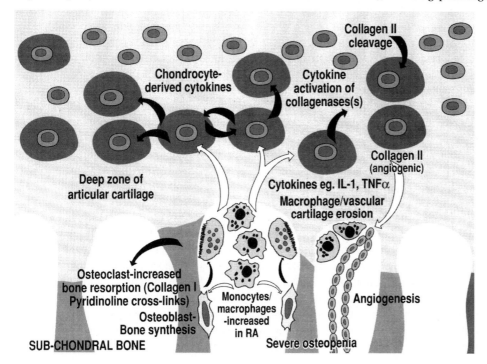

American Academy of Orthopaedic Surgeons | Orthopaedic Basic Science

Figure 7

Inflammatory processes in cartilage and subchondral bone and the pathologic consequences on bone structure. The cytokine network operating in this scenario is similar to that active in the synovium/cartilage compartment.

selected specimens. Unfortunately, these clinical reports have been neither controlled nor comprehensive, making it impossible to make broad or definitive statements concerning pathophysiologic mechanisms from these samples alone. Further, although there are numerous basic studies on ligament and tendon injury, repair, and transplantation that have documented alterations of tissue properties in a healing environment, animal models of inflammatory joint disease have not yet been used to study associated tendon or ligament pathology alone. This deficiency results in an inability to use the same detail used for other joint tissues to define the mechanisms by which tendons and ligaments may be altered by joint inflammation. With these qualifications, what follows is a synthesis of current knowledge in this area.

Tendons

Normal Tendons

Normal tendons are anatomically and functionally discrete, very complex dense collagenous structures, which, by definition, connect muscles to bones. Tendons cross diarthrodial joints and carry the muscle forces required to move those joints. Along the course from their parent muscle to their bony attachment site, normal tendons have several important features that contribute to the understanding of how tendons can be altered by inflammatory processes.

First, all tendons consist of highly oriented fibers of dense connective tissue that contains a relatively poor blood supply and few cells, making the tissue relatively hypometabolic. They contain a small number of nociceptive and proprioceptive nerves, particularly near their attachment sites. These cellular and physiologic features are thought to endow tendons with a relatively slow and poor repair capacity.

Second, tendons have long been classified into 2 types based on their surface anatomy. One type of tendon has a synovial surface layer and slides through a connective tissue sheath that also is lined with synovium. Despite these tendons being extra-articular, this synovial surface anatomy appears to make them unique, allowing them to move and glide over relatively great distances while being partially nourished within a type of "synovial environment." As with other intrasynovial tissues, this synovial environment likely has unique pathophysiologic implications. The second type of tendon, which does not have such a synovial sheath, is simply referred to as being an "extrasynovial" tendon.

Third, although some tendons do not pass directly through synovial sheaths or have synovium on their surfaces, many of them probably come in contact with synovially-lined bursae as they pass around bony contours on their way to their insertions. Others are in very close proximity to joint capsules, which are lined by synovium. This proximity to either bursae or capsular tissues with synovial linings can provide some potential for these tendons to be altered by inflammatory components or inflammatory breakdown products that likely originate in the inflamed synovium.

Although it has been shown that there are subtle differences between the synovial tissues themselves in these various locations, which contribute to the many varied patterns of synovial diseases that affect different joints and different tendons, it appears that the proximity of synovium to a tendon is key to the development of tendinopathy in many forms of arthritis.

Tendinopathy From Synovial Inflammation

Clinical observations suggest that there are at least 3 ways that tendons can be altered and damaged by synovial inflammation that exists around the tendons themselves, in immediately adjacent synovial bursae, or in nearby synovial joints. Two ways are "direct effects" of the inflammatory mediators or synovial cells themselves; the third is what would be called an "indirect" effect on a tendon, the effect of inflammatory-mediated changes to adjacent bone. According to empirical clinical observations, all 3 of these mechanisms appear to be preventable, by excising the peritendinous synovium early in the disease process, clearly suggesting that chronicity of synovial inflammation in the peritendinous area is a critical factor in the pathologic changes that occur in the tendons over time. This is distinct from nonsynovial inflammatory effects on tendons themselves (reviewed in a separate subsection below).

The first and apparently most common pathology noted in tendon samples taken from the extremities of patients with chronic synovial inflammatory types of arthritis is a direct attack on the tendon matrix by some component of the inflammatory process. This attack results in matrix disorganization of the normally dense tendon and replacement of the tendon matrix by relatively disorganized, immature, "scar-like" tissue. Ultrastructural studies have shown the replacement tissue to consist of interfibrillar dysplastic collagen fibrils, variable collagen fibril sizes, but mainly small diameter collagen fibrils that are either broken-down, large, original collagen fibrils or newly synthesized small fibrils; and intracellular collagen fibrils that are either newly synthesized or broken down. Inflammatory processes of synovium have somehow promoted these changes, either by a secondary effect on the tendon cells themselves, by infiltration of the tendon with extrinsic inflammatory cells, or by matrix destruction secondary to diffusion into the tendon of destructive enzymes secreted from peritendinous inflammatory cells. Recent evidence suggests that tension on the tendon affects its infiltration and destruction by enzymes, if not by cells. Less tensile force on a tendon exposed to a degradative enzyme such as collagenase appears to allow more rapid and perhaps more extensive enzymatic tendon destruction. Regardless of the source of change, the matrix changes must clearly be interpreted as being degradative because of the high incidence of tendon ruptures in patients with these types of inflammatory diseases.

The second means by which inflamed synovium appears to damage tendons may be by the pathologic, hypervascular, inflamed synovium itself directly growing into the tendon surfaces, thus replacing their dense matrix with synovial tissue. This phenomenon has been observed in tendons taken from patients with RA but it has not yet been verified through any type of cell marker studies. Thus, it remains to be proven that the hypervascular tissues seen within inflamed tendons are actually synovial, as opposed to these areas simply representing altered tendon or scar tissue. Regardless of the actual source of abnormal cells seen within tendons, these processes do result in a net degradation and weakening of the tendon matrix. Further work to resolve the cell types, sources, and mechanisms of tendinous infiltration is still required.

The third and fourth means by which an inflamed joint can alter an adjacent tendon are by causing bone spurring along the path of the tendon, or by joint destruction leading to tendon subluxations; both potentially cause secondary tendon abrasion on bone and subsequent tendon breakdown. This secondary mechanical damage to a periarticular tendon has only been described clinically as an infrequent consequence of bony change, but it must be considered as a potential source of tendinopathy around inflamed joints as well.

Direct Inflammatory Tendinopathy or Mechanical Tendinopathy

There are at least 2 other means by which tendons can become damaged as a result of joint inflammation. Both are direct effects on the tendons themselves; although they do not involve any synovial effect, they nonetheless result in similar intratendinous cellular changes and matrix alterations.

The direct attack of inflammatory cells that are either resident in the tissues or have migrated from the vasculature within tendon tissue as a result of neurogenic inflammation has been hypothesized. This type of intrinsic (nonsynovially mediated) inflammatory change within a tendon as a primary event seems possible depending on the physiology of its vasculature, but this has not yet been established for tendons in vivo.

A much better defined cause of tendinopathy is that of "tendon overuse"—mechanical damage to tendon matrix causing a peritendinous or intratendinous inflammatory cascade, which may lead to ongoing tendon matrix turnover, intratendinous hypervascularity, potential cyst formation, and possible tendon replacement by inappropriate materials. Although these mechanisms have been described and studied mainly in athletic populations and in attempted models of muscle-induced tendon overuse, the concept also is relevant to the understanding of tendinopathy of chronic joint inflammation in which muscle and joint forces are being dramatically altered by pain, by the pathologic processes themselves, and by therapeutic interventions (surgery, physiotherapy, and so forth). Presumably, mechanical damage occurs more readily in already weak-ened tendons (secondary to inflammatory processes), potentially causing an ongoing cycle of damage and intratendinous injury even with "normal loading." Thus, tendinitis during rehabilitation of either inflammatory or degenerative joint disease may be induced by mechanical effects.

The best studied effects of inflammation on tendons can be found in the surgical literature on tendon transfers and transplantation in which bleeding and inflammation accompany the processes of tendon healing. These effects are very similar to those noted in ligament surgery in which inflammation has been shown to have dramatic effects on the vascularity, cellularity, cellular metabolism, matrix production, and matrix organization (including integration of scarring into the tendon or ligament) of the original tissue. In these circumstances, peritendinous inflammation causes scar formation and adherence, scar infiltration, and partial replacement of the dense connective tissue matrix by scar-like matrix (less organized, altered collagen types, small fibril sizes, altered proteoglycan types, and so forth), resulting in relative weakening, increasing compliance, and increased relative viscosity of the viscoelastic structure of the original. These changes have been documented extensively by investigators in the tendon transfer/transplant literature and have been shown to be different for intrasynovial and extrasynovial tendons.

Ligaments

There is even less scientific information about the effects of synovial or joint inflammation, per se, on ligaments than on tendons. There are only a few case reports of inflammatory changes within ligaments as a direct result of the inflammatory disease process itself and no studies of inflammatory joint disease have been reported that have looked specifically at the ligaments.

Inflammatory Joint Disease

What is known about inflammatory effects on ligaments is that, as with tendons, synovium may be critical to either ligament destruction or protection. One clinical report has suggested that there is more significant destruction of the anterior cruciate ligament than the posterior cruciate ligament in the rheumatoid knee, perhaps as a result of its relatively smaller mass or perhaps because of its relative lack of protection from synovial fluid. This has not been proven and is far from being resolved.

Direct Effects of Inflammation on Ligaments

As noted above with tendons, the best evidence for the effects of inflammation on ligaments has come from the surgical transplant literature in which it has been shown that inflammation induced by injury causes dramatic biologic effects on both ligament structures and functions. The major effect appears to be a semidestructive infiltration and replacement of ligament tissue by hypervascular scar tissue, producing a scar-ligament composite that has altered mechanical qualities (weaker, less stiff, more compliant, more viscous). These changes, if similar in nonsurgically induced joint inflammation, could result in permanent elongation and possibly in ligament failure, even under loading conditions that would be normal for that joint. Unfortunately, it has never been proven that the inflammatory processes associated with either immune-mediated or degenerative joint diseases are the same as these following injury. It may be speculated that the former would be more destructive to the inflamed ligament because of the suppression of a reparative scar response; however, this has not yet been investigated. A great deal of investigation still is required to understand all of the pathophysiologic mechanisms and implications of joint inflammation on ligaments.

Cellular Mechanisms of Inflammation

Chronic inflammation is the defining feature of RA. Its establishment requires multiple cellular interactions that are evident throughout the etiology of the disease. There is a constant traffic of cells into the inflamed synovium and the joint space. Large numbers of neutrophils from the circulatory system move through the synovial tissue into the synovial fluid during active phases of the disease. Other immune system cells invade the synovium; cellular invasion is also evident at the pannus-cartilage junction. This section provides an overview of the cellular interactions involved in various aspects of the development of joint inflammation and synovial hypertrophy.

Cytokine Networks in Inflammatory Joint Disease

The establishment and perpetuation of inflammatory processes in general, including those characteristic of RA, require the interaction of many different cells, leading to the generation of autoimmune processes and to the destruction of cartilage and bone. An increasingly extensive network of cytokines acting in autocrine or paracrine fashions regulates both immune and nonimmune processes in the arthritic joint. Table 1 summarizes the proinflammatory cytokines and their major biologic effects. These cytokines are secreted from a variety of cells, although activated monocytes, macrophages, and synovial cells are often a major source. In addition, many different cells respond to the proinflammatory cytokines with the response pattern often dependent on the cell type responding.

A second group of cytokines, also sometimes referred to as lymphokines, is secreted predominantly by T cells at various stages of activation. These cytokines are summarized in Table 2. Their primary role is the controlled amplification of an activating event. Several cytokines in this group enhance the proliferation and function of specific T and B cells, whereas others inhibit these responses. IFN-γ is a hallmark of the Th1 response, as is IL-2. IFN-γ stimulates MHC class II expression on monocytes and connective tissue cells, increasing the capacity for antigen presentation and thereby further augmenting the activation of T cells.

An interface between the immune cells and the inflammatory compartment is provided by factors that control synthesis of proinflammatory cytokines. Thus, IL-17 is produced by activated memory T cells and stimulates connective tissue cells to produce IL-6, the chemotactic cytokines (chemokines) IL-8 and monocyte chemotactic protein and granulocyte colony-stimulating factor. IL-10 is produced by a subset of activated T cells, referred to as Th2 cells. Its main effect is the suppression of proinflammatory cytokine synthesis by activated monocytes and macrophages. IL-15, on the other hand, is produced by macrophages (whether or not synovial cells or chondrocytes can also secrete IL-15 is currently not known) and, similar to IL-2, promotes T-cell proliferation. These cytokines thus provide for a large amount of cross talk between the different compartments of the immune and nonimmune responses. The following discussion will concentrate on those cytokines that may play a major role in the pathogenesis of RA, particularly with respect to the chronic nature of the disease.

Tumor Necrosis Factor-α and Interleukin-1

The most extensively-studied cytokines with respect to the pathogenesis of RA are TNF-α and IL-1. The terms mononuclear cell factor, lymphocyte-activating factor, and catabolin were originally used for the molecule now known as IL-1, and they aptly describe the major source and biologic effects of this cytokine, namely the augmentation of cellular immune response and the destruction of ECM, particularly in articular cartilage. As its name implies, TNF-α was originally studied as a factor that induces tumor cell death and cachexia (thus the alternate term, cachexin). However, studies with pure preparations of TNF-α revealed that it had many other biologic effects that overlapped to some degree with those of IL-1, although quantitative differences with respect to both dose and response were often observed. Because IL-1 and TNF-α are produced generally by the same cells, stimulate each other's synthesis, and, in many cases, act synergistically, it is often difficult to assign specific effects to one particular cytokine. However, most evidence currently supports the thesis that both cytokines play a crucial role in the development of RA, but that TNF-α affects inflammatory and immune events in the synovium predominantly, whereas the erosive processes in articular cartilage (and bone) are the result of IL-1 action. This concept is illustrated in Figure 8.

Table 1

Proinflammatory Cytokines and Their Role in the Pathogenesis of Arthritis*

Cytokine	Major Cellular Source	Major Targets and Biologic Effects
TNF-α	Monocytes Macrophages T lymphocytes	Monocytes, synovial macrophages, fibroblasts, chondrocytes, endothelial cells Stimulation of proinflammatory cytokine and chemokine synthesis Activation of granulocytes Increased MHC class II expression Secretion of MMPs leading to cartilage matrix degradation
IL-1	Monocytes, Macrophages (many other cells)	Monocytes, synovial macrophages, fibroblasts, chondrocytes, endothelial cells Inhibition of matrix synthesis in chondrocytes Secretion of MMPs leading to matrix degradation Stimulation of proinflammatory cytokine and chemokine synthesis Fibroblast proliferation T cell proliferation
IL-6	Activated T cells (Th2) Many cell types (induced by IL-1 or TNF-α)	Stimulation of acute phase protein synthesis in liver B cell proliferation and differentiation T cell proliferation Differentiation of hematopoietic precursor cells Differentiation and maturation of osteoclasts (induction of MMP-inhibitor, TIMP-1)
TGF-β	Many cell types	Immune suppression (inhibition of B and T cell proliferation) Monocyte chemotaxis Differentiation of mesenchymal and epithelial cells (chondrogenesis) Anabolic for cartilage – stimulation of matrix synthesis – reduced production of MMPs – increased production of proteinase inhibitors

*   TNF-α, tumor necrosis factor-α; IL, interleukin; TGF-β, transforming growth factor-β; MHC, major histocompatibility complex; MMP, matrix metalloproteinases; TIMP, tissue inhibitors of matrix metalloproteinases

Table 2

Major Cytokines Involved in Immune Regulation*

Cytokine	Cellular Source	Biologic Effects
IL-2	Activated T cells (Th1)	Clonal proliferation of T cells Proliferation of B cells
IFN-γ	Activated T cells (Th1)	Induction of MHC class II expression on monocytes, connective tissue cells (fibroblasts, chondrocytes) and endothelial cells Increased expression of MHC class I molecules
IL-4	Activated T cells (Th2)	B cell proliferation and class switching of immunoglobulin synthesis Inhibition of production of proinflammatory cytokines by monocytes
IL-5	Activated T cells (Th2)	Growth and differentiation of eosinophils
IL-12	Activated macrophages	Development of the Th1 response
IL-10	Activated T cells (Th2) Macrophages	Inhibition of synthesis of proinflammatory cytokines by T cells and macrophages
IL-15	Activated macrophages Connective tissue cells?	T cell proliferation (similar to IL-2)

IL-17	Activated memory T cells	Proinflammatory; stimulation of cytokine secretion (IL-6, IL-8, MCP1, granulocyte-
		  stimulating factor) and prostaglandin E_2 in epithelial, endothelial, and fibroblastic
		  cells

*   IL, interleukin; IFN-α, interferon-α; MHC, major histocompatibility complex; MCP1, monocyte chemotactic protein 1

Studies in a range of animal models of arthritis, including joint inflammation induced by bacterial cell wall fragments, immune complexes, or T-cell reaction to cartilage autoantigens, confirmed that TNF-α is important both at the onset and during acute exacerbations of arthritis. Treatment with neutralizing anti-TNF-α antibodies leads to rapid improvement of collagen-induced arthritis in mice and to a pronounced reduction of inflammation in RA patients. A reduced influx of leukocytes into the joints and expression of vascular adhesion molecules have been observed. TNF-α affects both immune-cell driven events and nonimmune, inflammatory events. Increased production of chemokines and changes in the expression of cellular adhesion molecules result in increased recruitment of lymphocytes as well mononuclear cells. TNF-α stimulates expression of MHC class II receptors on antigen-presenting cells, thus augmenting responses to autoantigens and activation of T cells. Induction of prostaglandin E2 and MMPs (collagenases, stromelysin) is the major response of connective tissue cells, including synovial fibroblasts and chondrocytes.

Although IL-1 may not be the dominant cytokine in the onset of arthritis, it appears to be the pivotal cytokine in amplification of late cellular infiltration in the synovium and progression of cartilage damage. Uncoupling between TNF-α dependent joint swelling and late IL-1 dependent cartilage destruction was clearly noted. Studies using transgenic mice confirmed that overexpression of TNF-α leads to chronic erosive arthritis, yet the arthritis was fully abolished with antibodies to the IL-1 receptor, suggesting

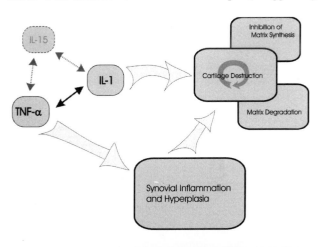

Figure 8

Although a plethora of cytokines is found in the inflamed joint environment, some of these occupy a pivotal role, initiating and perpetuating many different inflammatory processes. Current evidence supports the suggestion that tumor necrosis factor-alpha (TNF-α) and interleukin-1 (IL-1) occupy such a role. While TNF-α may control many of the processes attributed to the monocytes/synoviocytes in the inflamed joint, IL-1 plays a prominent role in the orchestration of events taking place within the articular cartilage, which lead to joint erosion. The position of IL-15 in this hierarchy is currently hypothetical, but existing data suggest that IL-15 may act to initiate the T-cell driven autoimmune process.

TNF-α-induced IL-1 production as a major pathway in this model. In human arthritides, it is not clear whether most IL-1 production is indeed controlled by TNF-α. This is of crucial therapeutic importance because IL-1 is by far the most destructive cytokine for articular cartilage because of enhanced release of destructive enzymes and profound inhibition of the synthetic function of the chondrocyte.

Control of TNF-α and IL-1 Action

The cellular response to TNF-α and IL-1 is mediated via specific receptors for these molecules on the cell surface, namely the type I and type II receptors for TNF-α and the IL-1 receptor, respectively. Activation of cellular pathways stimulated by these inflammatory cytokines is thus dependent on their local concentration. Various mechanisms exist to control the levels of bioavailability (that is, free) cytokines. Release of the extracellular portion of the TNF-α receptors (referred to as receptor shedding) leads to a soluble form of these receptors that will bind to free TNF-α and thus prevent its interaction with the cellular receptors. IL-1 action on its cellular targets is modulated in a different fashion. Many cells secrete an IL-1 analog, that competes with IL-1 for binding to the IL-1 receptor, but does not elicit a cellular response. This molecule is known as IL-1 receptor antagonist (IL-1ra or IRAP).

Treatment of experimentally-induced arthritis with IL-1ra results in only limited improvement of inflammatory symptoms and cartilage erosion. Because of its rapid clearance from the circulatory system, a thousandfold excess of IL-1ra over IL-1 is needed to block IL-1 interaction with the IL-1 receptor. IL-1ra expression is abundant in the inflamed synovium, with a tendency toward higher levels in OA as compared to RA. Localization is mainly in the synovial lining cells. Nevertheless, the increased levels of IL-1ra in the inflamed synovium appear to be insufficient to control IL-1 action effectively.

Interleukin-6

IL-6 is found in very high concentrations in the synovial fluid of the inflamed joints. Both TNF-α and IL-1 can induce IL-6 production in synovial macrophages, fibroblasts, and chondrocytes. One of the major functions of this cytokine is the induction of acute phase protein synthesis by the liver. However, many other effects on a variety of cell types have been reported. IL-6 is a potent B-cell growth factor. With respect to cartilage destruction, IL-6 can increase TIMP-1 synthesis as well as IL-1ra and TNF-α soluble receptors, thus counteracting the effects of IL-1 and TNF-α in the cartilage-erosion compartment. This suggestion is supported by the observation in a nonimmune inflammation model in IL-6-deficient mice that the cellular infiltrate was reduced, yet cartilage destruction was higher in the arthritic joints.

IL-6 may have a proinflammatory function as well, contributing to autoantibody production in RA. The observation that IL-6-deficient mice are protected against collagen-induced arthritis, a disease model that depends on both T- and B-cell driven processes, suggests a role for IL-6 in the autoimmune aspects of the disease. Because lack of IL-6 does not affect the development and severity of the polyarthritis observed in mice overexpressing TNF-α (by breeding the IL-6$^{-/-}$ genotype into mice transgenic for human TNF-α), the role of IL-6 in nonimmune inflammatory processes may be minimal.

Finally, IL-6 may promote bone resorption, because it is produced locally by osteoblasts and activating osteoclasts. Turning again to the IL-6 deficient mouse, it has become apparent that although IL-6 is not required for normal bone development, which involves extensive remodeling and hence osteoclast activity, it may mediate the increased bone turnover in mature females caused by reduced estrogen levels. This may be important because a majority of patients with RA are postmenopausal women.

Parathyroid Hormone-Related Peptide

A hormone-cytokine acting distal to the TNF-α-IL-1 axis, but proximal to IL-6, is PTHrp. This peptide plays a pivotal role in skeletal development and bone turnover. It has recently been shown to be produced by RA and OA synoviocytes both in vivo and in vitro. Normal synoviocytes increase production of PTHrp in response to TNF-α and IL-1, suggesting that PTHrp is part of the proinflammatory repertoire elicited by these factors. PTHrp, in turn, can stimulate IL-6 production, which may contribute to the increased levels of the latter both in experimental models of RA and in the human disease. Receptors for PTHrp are present on both chondrocytes and synoviocytes. The catabolic effects of this hormone on bone metabolism are well established, as is its role in the differentiation and maturation of hypertrophic chondrocytes. Because PTHrp has been shown to inhibit collagen synthesis in articular chondrocytes, it may be another factor affecting cartilage matrix loss.

Interleukin-4 and Interleukin-10

Apart from the control by specific soluble receptors, antibodies, or antagonists, the actions of TNF-α and IL-1 are modulated by additional regulatory cytokines. These include IL-4, IL-10, and IL-13. IL-4 has many activities in common with IL-13, and the latter will not be addressed in detail. This set of cytokines is produced by Th2 cells, whereas macrophages are an additional source of IL-10 and TNF-α. At the local level in the inflamed joint, the macrophage derived mediators probably contribute to a greater extent to the regulation of arthritis compared to Th2 cells. Th2 cells are virtually absent in RA synovia as is IL-4.

IL-4 and IL-10 act on a variety of target cells, suppressing proinflammatory events. They inhibit the maturation of Th1 cells, the major immune cell component in RA. The major effect on nonimmune cells is the reduction of TNF-α and IL-1 synthesis by synovial macrophages. Increased shedding of TNF-α receptors can be induced by IL-10, whereas IL-4 has been reported to increase the synthesis of IL-1ra.

IL-10 is abundant in inflamed synovial tissue. Neutralization of IL-10 increases TNF-α and IL-1 production in cultures of inflamed synovia. Moreover, treatment of animals with experimental arthritis using neutralizing anti-IL-10 antibodies enhances both the severity and chronicity of the arthritis. However, the control by endogenous IL-10 is not maximal; addition of recombinant IL-10 further inhibits TNF-α-IL-1 production in the synovial cultures and in vivo treatment in arthritis models reduces the disease severity. Sensitivity to IL-10 regulation depends on the maturation state of the synovial cells, and the impact might therefore be different at various stages of arthritis.

Although IL-4-IL-10 treatment may seem a promising option as compared to plain inhibition of TNF-α-IL-1, because of additional upregulation of inhibitors, there are potential side effects. IL-10 is a potent B-cell stimulator and may be involved in rheumatoid factor production in RA synovia. IL-4 is an effective fibroblast growth factor and might thus increase synovial proliferation.

Transforming Growth Factor-Beta

TGF-β is a strong immunosuppressor, but also has marked chemotactic activity for inflammatory cells. TGF-β also stimulates chondrocyte proliferation and matrix synthesis. When given systemically, it reduces the severity of arthritis in experimental models. However, injection of TGF-β into a naïve joint increases recruitment of leukocytes and stimulates local fibroblast proliferation. In an inflamed joint, additional TGF-β exacerbates the inflammation, increasing the cell mass in the synovial tissue. Yet it counteracts the proteoglycan depletion in the articular cartilage by stimulation of chondrocyte proteoglycan synthesis, inhibition of metalloproteinase production, and induction of TIMP-1. Because of its activation of periosteal cells and its cartilage inductive potential, TGF-β induces characteristic osteophytes at the joint margins, although these are not found in RA joints, in spite of the high levels of TGF-β in synovial fluid. Because numerous physiologic processes are affected by TGF-β, it is difficult to assess which of the many actions of this growth factor-cytokine contribute to the pathogenesis of chronic arthritis.

Interleukin-12

IL-12 is a heterodimeric cytokine, which mainly is produced by activated macrophages. It promotes the development of naïve T cells into Th1 cells and stimulates IFN-γ secretion by such cells. IL-12 is considered to be a principal protective factor in bacterial infections, stimulating antigen-specific immunity. However, IL-12 may unmask Th1-dependent autoimmune reactions by skewing the Th1-Th2 balances, and it is a likely intermediate in the often suggested link between nonspecific bacterial infections and expression of autoimmune arthritis. Moreover, IL-12 is a potent inducer of nitric oxide (NO) and displays proinflammatory activity in early stages of nonimmune arthritis. Elimination with neutralizing anti-IL-12 antibodies reduces arthritis severity. However, in established arthritis, IL-12 induces IL-10 production in macrophages and T cells, thus playing a protective role. This bimodal activity will seriously complicate IL-12 directed therapy.

Interleukin-15

IL-15 is an IL-2 homolog present in inflamed synovia of RA patients. Many cell types, including macrophages and fibroblasts (with the notable exception of normal T cells), can produce IL-15 but the inducing stimulus is as yet unknown. Its potent T-cell activity and subsequent triggering of macrophage TNF-α production by these IL-15-activated T cells makes it a pivotal candidate in the RA process. IL-15 attracts memory T cells and accounts for much of the T-cell chemotactic activity in arthritis synovial fluid. The induction of macrophage TNF-α production is dependent on cell-cell contact, with a critical role for CD69 expression. Interestingly, CD69 is also pivotal in cell-cell interaction between T cells and synoviocytes, resulting in release of cartilage degrading proteases. Studies with antibodies to IL-15 in models or patients are needed to evaluate its contribution to the pathogenesis of RA.

Chemokines

Although much of the destructive process in an arthritic joint is linked to proliferation of synovial macrophages and fibroblasts, the influx of leukocytes may amplify this process. The cellular composition of the infiltrate depends on the local generation of particular chemotactic factors (chemokines).

Chemokines can be divided into 2 groups, the -CXC-group and the -CC-group, based on a cysteine motif in their amino acid sequence near the amino terminus of the peptide. The CXC cytokines contain 2 cysteine residues separated by 1 amino acid, the identity of which is variable, depending on the individual member of this group. In the CC cytokines, the 2 cysteine residues are adjacent to each other. These motifs are critical for the secondary structure of the molecules and determine which chemokine receptor group the molecules interact with. Chemokines act on responsive leukocyte subsets through G-protein-coupled transmembrane receptors; a number of receptors have been identified for each group. IL-8, a member of the -CXC-group, is a major chemoattractant of granulocytes. It is one of the most abundant proteins synthesized and secreted by both synoviocytes and chondrocytes on stimulation with IL-1, and it may be responsible for the accumulation of granulocytes in synovial fluid. IL-8 also stimulates angiogenesis, and the presence of receptors for -CXC-chemokines on endothelial cells suggests that IL-8 acts directly on the endothelial cells. Other members of this family (gro-β, ip-10, and PF-4) inhibit angiogenesis. Monocyte chemotactic protein and macrophage inflammatory protein are members of the -CC-family. Various closely related forms of these factors exist. They are mainly involved in monocyte-macrophage infiltration, although specific lymphocyte targets have also been described.

In addition to local production of subsets of chemokines, the infiltrate at a particular site is dependent on the expression of selectin receptors on the cell surface. Th1 cells can accumulate in inflamed synovia, whereas Th2 cells have great difficulty reaching this site. It is now clear that these T-cell subsets have different chemokine receptors. IL-5, a major product of Th2 cells, is a potent chemoattractant for eosinophils. The relative lack of Th2 cells in inflamed RA synovia is in line with the paucity of eosinophils in such inflammatory synovial infiltrates.

The synovial lining macrophages provide an important source of chemokines. TNF-α-IL-1 can induce cell influx and generation of chemotactic activity in normal joints, but lose this capacity in experimentally induced synovial lining cell-depleted joints. In addition to blocking the action of TNF-α-IL-1, the propagation of the arthritic process can be inhibited by elimination of the relevant chemokines.

In general, the destructive character of an arthritis depends more on the balance of proinflammatory and modulatory cytokines than on their absolute levels. Some forms of arthritis are more destructive than others, and this difference may be linked to different cytokine balances, related to different underlying processes, with emphasis on either T-cell or macrophage-fibroblast driven pathogenesis. Variations in the genetic regulation of proinflammatory and modulatory cytokines could also contribute to the final cytokine balance and, thus, the disease progression.

The Role of Immune Cells in Inflammatory Joint Disease

Specificity is a fundamental feature of immune recognition for distinguishing between foreign and self antigens. The specific immune responses are classified into 2 categories, depending on which type of cells, T or B lymphocytes, are involved in the process. Humoral immunity is mediated by B lymphocytes, which produce antibodies responsible for the recognition of soluble foreign antigens and their elimination with the help of complement. Cellular immunity is mediated by T lymphocytes, which recognize and eliminate intracellular antigens. This process requires the help of antigen presenting cells (APC).

Specific recognition and destruction of self-antigen(s) by the immune system is observed in humans in autoimmune diseases, such as myasthenia gravis, multiple sclerosis, systemic lupus erythematosus, and RA, and in animal models of these diseases. Autoantibodies and auto-reactive T lymphocytes, however, are also present in normal healthy individuals, suggesting that autoimmunity may not necessarily lead to destructive autoimmune diseases. Moreover, self-reactivity mediated by certain T-cell subsets, such as Th2 cells, may provide suppressive signals to ongoing immune responses. The exact extent to which cellular and humoral autoimmunity contribute to the pathogenesis of RA is still unresolved.

Specific Immune Response Mediated by T Lymphocytes

Three essential elements are involved in specific T-cell recognition: the T cell receptor (TCR), MHC molecules, and antigen. Because a specific immune response is regulated by T cells, the TCR-MHC-antigen peptide complex can be considered a control switch for the immune system.

T cells are derived from bone marrow stem cells that are committed to the T lymphocyte lineage. They differentiate into mature T cells in the thymus and then enter the circulatory system. The TCR is expressed in mature T cells in combination with either CD4 or CD8 glycoproteins on the cell surface that serve as accessory molecules to define and help T-cell recognition. The major function of CD4 T cells is the secretion of cytokines (lymphokines) to regulate cellular and humoral immune responses; the principal function of CD8-expressing T cells, also referred to as cytotoxic T lymphocytes (CTLs), is to kill the antigen-bearing target cells by releasing perforin, lymphotoxin, and other cytokines.

The TCR is the recognition unit of the T cells. It is a disulfide-linked heterodimer consisting of 2 polypeptide chains, each of approximately 45,000 daltons.

There are 2 types of TCRs, designated α/β and γ/δ. The majority of mature T cells express the α/β TCR, whereas the γ/δ TCR is found only on a small subset of T cells. The genes for the TCRα and TCRβ chains are located on chromosomes 14 and 7, respectively. A functional TCRα gene is assembled from 3 of the discontinuous gene segments, called Vα (variable), Jα (joining), and Cα (constant). In a similar fashion, the TCRβ gene is assembled from discontinuous gene segments with 1 additional diversity segment (Dβ) inserted between Vβ and Jβ. There are up to 100 Vα, and approximately 50 Jα, 70 Vβ, 2Db, 13 Jβ, and 2 Cβ gene segments to choose from. Thus, a high degree of TCR diversity is generated through combinatorial rearrangement.

T cells cannot recognize antigen directly. The TCR binds a peptide antigen only when the latter is associated with a single allelic form of a MHC molecule expressed on an APC. Conventional APCs are dendritic cells, cells of the monocyte-macrophage lineage, and memory B cells. Two cellular properties are an absolute requirement for the function of APCs, namely the expression of MHC molecules at the cell surface and the ability to process antigen, ie, to convert a native protein to an MHC-associated peptide fragment (a T-cell epitope). Moreover, APCs also provide pivotal costimulatory factors to promote the T-cell response (Fig. 9).

The MHC is a region of highly polymorphic genes involved in immune recognition. The human MHC, also named HLA, is located on the short arm of chromosome 6. Two different groups of MHC gene products, called MHC class I and class II molecules, participate in T-cell recognition. CD8 T cells are class I restricted, while all CD4 T cells are restricted by class II MHC molecules. The HLA class I complex consists of a membrane-associated heavy chain glycoprotein of 44,000 d, and a noncovalently attached light chain (12,000 d) called β2-microglobulin. The latter is encoded outside the MHC locus. In humans, 3 loci, termed HLA-A, B, and C, encode the principal HLA class I molecules, which are expressed on all nucleated cells. All 3 loci are highly polymorphic, with more than 80 alleles described for HLA-A and B.

The class II molecule is a heterodimer consisting of 2 membrane-associated chains, α and β, of similar size (about 30,000 d) that express on cells, such as monocyte-macrophages, dendritic cells, and B cells, that are known to present antigen to T cells. The α and β subunits are coded for by 3 sets of genes, designated DR, DP, and DQ. Thus DRA and DRB code for the α and β subunits of the DR group, and a similar nomenclature is used for the other 2 groups.

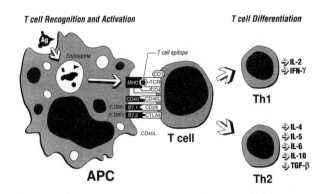

Figure 9

The mechanism of T-cell activation and differentiation. In addition to antigen-specific engagement of the T-cell receptor, costimulatory interactions between cell-surface receptors on the antigen-presenting cells (APC) and the T cell are required to stimulate T-cell differentiation. The end-stage of the T-cell activation process is defined by the panel of cytokines synthesized by the cells. Which factors determine whether the T cells follow a Th1 or Th2 differentiation path is currently not clear.

Although there is limited variation in the genes encoding the α chains, those coding for the β chains are extremely polymorphic. All 3 sets of genes are used in humans and expressed in a concomitant fashion, which implies that antigen-presenting cells display 6 different HLA class II complexes on their cell surfaces. Both HLA class I and class II complexes were originally defined serologically, and class II genes were further classified by mixed lymphocyte culture, which accounts for the terminology used for the members of this gene family. Now, individual polymorphisms are defined precisely by the nucleic acid sequence.

The principal function of MHC molecules is to present peptide antigen to T cells. These antigens are derived from foreign proteins by intracellular proteolytic processing. They are also referred to as T-cell epitopes, although this is a functional definition, implying recognition and activation of a particular set of T cells. A typical T-cell epitope is a peptide consisting of 9 or 10 amino acid residues that fit the peptide-binding site of the MHC molecule. Class II molecules present peptide fragments derived from extracellular proteins to T cells of the CD4 phenotype, whereas class I molecules present peptides derived from endogenously synthesized proteins, for example viral proteins, to T cells with the CD8 phenotype. The requirement for binding of the peptide fragments to the particular MHC molecules expressed by a given cell imparts a controlling role to the MHC phenotype in the generation of immune responses, because only those peptide fragments that can bind to the MHC will be presented to the T-cell population for further selection. This phenomenon is called MHC restriction. The high degree of polymorphism of the MHC genes generates functional molecules with different affinities for peptide fragments, allowing the presentation of a wide variety of peptide motifs.

The recognition of a peptide-MHC complex by a T cell initiates a sequence of events that culminates in cell proliferation and cytokine secretion. In addition to the binding of antigen to the TCR, T-cell activation requires the engagement of costimulatory factors. One important aspect is the B7-CD28/CTLA4 interaction. It consists of 2 costimulatory ligands on the APC, B7-1 (CD80) and B7-2 (CD86), which bind to their respective receptors on T cells, called CD28 and CTLA4. Both resting and activated T cells express CD28, whereas only activated T cells express CTLA4 after TCR engagement. Why the immune system needs 2 pairs of costimulatory ligands and receptors is still unknown. The role of CTLA4 as a negative signal in T-cell activation has drawn attention recently.

Activated CD4$^+$T cells can be divided into 2 subsets, based on the set of lymphokines elaborated following antigen stimulation; Th1 cells mainly synthesize IL-2 and IFN-γ, and Th2 cells principally secrete IL-4, IL-5, and IL-10. Th1 cells mediate delayed hypersensitivity, activate macrophages, and are involved in many autoimmune diseases. In contrast, Th2 cells mainly provide help for B cells by promoting an immunoglobulin (Ig) class switch from IgM to IgG1 and IgE and suppressing cellular autoimmunity.

T Lymphocytes and Rheumatoid Arthritis

In RA, the synovial histopathology in oligoarthritis is not distinguishable from that seen in polyarthritis; both involve an inflammatory reaction in the joint mediated by T cells, B cells, and macrophages. These features favor the local intra-articular expression of immunity. Most studies have focused on the pathogenetic roles of CD4$^+$ T cells; less is known on whether and how CD8$^+$ T cells act in RA.

The TCR repertoire in RA patients has been intensively studied. Analyses of TCR repertoire expression, mostly Vβ genes, in RA synovial fluid and membrane indicate both selected (Vβ, 3, 17) and multiple Vβ gene usage. Studies of TCR antigen binding sites (complementary-determining region, CDR3) have also shown both oligoclonal and polyclonal T-cell expansion in RA tissues, indicating the involvement of an antigen-driven and nonantigen-specific T-cell responses. Polyclonality may be more pronounced in long-standing chronic disease or in an active phase. Hence studies of patients with early disease, ideally up to 2 years from onset, would be desirable. This is more often possible in juvenile RA. In active RA lesions, autoreactive T cells may be only a small component (less than 1%) of the total T-cell infiltrate. However, a few antigen-specific clones might play a critical role in the up- or downregulation of a vast population of nonspecific T-cell responses in the inflammatory tissue.

Synovial T lymphocytes commonly express markers of T-cell activation, such as the IL-2 receptor, HLA class II molecules, and CD45RO$^+$, compared with peripheral blood in which there is no correlation with disease subtype. These T cells preferentially secrete IL-2 and IFN-γ, a cytokine profile indicative of the presence of a Th1 subset in RA. It is not known whether these cells are activated elsewhere and then migrate into joints or enter the synovium first and then are activated locally. There are, however, reports indicating that T-cell activation occurs in joints of RA patients. The latter is associated with induction of synovial hyperplasia when such T cells are transferred to SCID mice. They also produce cytokines, such as IL-1 and TNF-α, that initiate and perpetuate the degradation of cartilage matrix. The release of putative cartilage autoantigens is a result of this process.

In RA, the inflamed synovial tissue is enriched in monocytes and macrophages, dendritic cells, and B cells; these are 'professional' APCs for T-cell activation. Moreover, local secretion of proinflammatory cytokines by Th1 cells (IFN-γ) or monocytes (TNF-α) induces the expression of HLA class II molecules on the cell surface of fibroblasts, chondrocytes, or endothelial cells. These cell types can then serve as APCs and secrete T-cell growth factors other than IL-2, such as IL-15, to upregulate the inflammatory T-cell responses.

The role of metalloproteinases, especially the MMPs, in the destruction of cartilage and bone in RA is well established.

MMPs are also used by T cells during extravasation and homing to various target organs, which require migration through basement membranes and the ECM of connective tissues. Activated T cells produce a signaling protein, gp39 (also called CD40L), which binds to CD40 receptors on B cells. This receptor-ligand engagement stimulates the expression and secretion of MMPs, predominantly the gelatinases MMP-2 and -9, and proinflammatory cytokines. Specific MMP inhibitors can significantly decrease edema and inflammatory tissue damage, suggesting possible therapeutic benefits.

Specific subtypes of the HLA class II molecules have been associated with RA; HLA DR4 and DR1 are frequently found in patients with RA and are related to the severity of the disease as well. Both genes are located in the HLA-DRB1 gene complex. The association between the individual DR subtypes and RA is listed in Table 3.

In addition to subtypes that clearly are associated with RA, there are those that clearly are not associated with the disease. Because all these subtypes are now defined by the amino acid sequence of the β chain they code for, certain patterns can be recognized. Differences in amino acid sequence (the basis for the observed polymorphism) are most prominent in the region of the molecule that forms the binding groove for the peptide to be presented. Thus the amino acid sequence in this region will determine what kind of peptide will bind to the HLA molecule (eg, a peptide with acid or basic residues in certain positions) and be presented to the T cells. Comparisons of all the DR subtypes in different ethnic groups that have been associated with RA show that the amino acid residues in the peptide binding groove that interact with the peptide antigen are conserved, although this is not the case in the nonassociated subtypes. This conserved sequence motif is sometimes referred to as a "shared epitope." The implication of this observation is that the disease-associated HLA molecules will present similar peptide fragments to the cell-mediated immune system.

Autoantigen(s)

It is generally accepted that immune responses to autoantigens play a key role in the induction of RA. However, the causative antigen(s) is still unknown. Articular cartilage contains a number of molecules primarily concentrated in this tissue that can induce an experimental arthritis resembling RA in mice. These include types II, IX, and XI collagen, the proteoglycan aggrecan, and link protein. Type II collagen was the first autoantigen to be identified as being capable of inducing a polyarticular disease with erosive joint inflammation in mice, rats, and primates. In addition to an erosive polyarthritis, aggrecan also induces a spondylitis and ankylosis of the spine that are not seen in type II collagen-induced arthritis.

Thus, as observed for other organ-specific autoimmune diseases, a number of antigens may be involved in the pathogenesis of RA. It is very difficult to identify the initiating antigen, because after the initial immune response there is a series of T- and B-cell responses to other epitopes on the same or other antigens at the site of inflammation. This phenomenon is called epitope spreading. It is seen in virtually all autoimmune diseases. Although the identification of an initiating antigen in RA may be of little practical value with respect to treatment, analysis of antigens involved in the later, chronic stages of the disease may lead to the identification of treatment modalities to block their specific effects.

Specific Immune Response Mediated by B Lymphocytes

In humans, naive B lymphocytes (B cells) are generated within the bone marrow and migrate into the secondary lymphoid organs, including tonsils, lymph nodes, spleen, and mucosal-associated lymphoid tissues. The B cell recognizes an antigen via its membrane-bound Ig receptor (B-cell receptor, BCR) and initiates the B-cell response. In contrast to T cells, BCRs are able to bind cell-bound as well as free soluble antigens. In general, B-cell recognition does not require the presence of APCs and MHC molecules. Two major types of B-cell response are distinguished: thymus-dependent and thymus-independent B-cell responses. Thymus-independent antigens make up a small minority of the antigenic universe; most antigens are thymus-dependent, which means that they can only stimulate B cells with the help of T cells. Activated T cells express gp39 (CD40L) that binds to CD40 on APCs and mediates helper functions for B cells.

Upon encountering an antigen within a secondary lymphoid organ, the rapid expansion of a few founder cells leads to the establishment of a new structure called the ger-

Table 3		
Members of the HLA Family Associated with Arthritis		
Antibodies	**Nomenclature Defined by Mixed Lymphocyte Culture**	**Nucleotide Sequences**
HLA Class II		
DR1	DR1. Dw1	DRB1*0101
DR4	DR4, Dw4	DRB1*0401
DR4	DR4, Dw14, 14.1	DRB1*0404
DR4	DR4, Dw15	DRB1*0405
HLA Class I		
B27	B*2702	
B27	B*2704	
B27	B*27052	
B27	B*27053	
B27	B*2707	

minal center (GC). Within the GC dark zone, B cells bearing specific BCR undergo somatic hypermutation. This is followed by selection for specificity and affinity by antigens on follicular dendritic cells and molecules expressed by GC-T cells within the GC light zone. B cells with low affinity are eliminated through apoptosis (negative selection), while B cells with high affinity survive under the influence of T cell help and differentiate into either memory B cells or plasma cells. The memory B cells express high affinity antigen-specific BCRs, while the plasma cells secrete large amounts of Igs, with a specificity identical to that of the BCR.

B Lymphocytes and Rheumatoid Arthritis

Currently most studies are focused on the role of T cells in the pathogenesis of RA. The involvement of autoreactive B cells and antibodies is much less well defined. The first evidence for the autoimmune nature of RA and a role for B-cell mediated immunity stems from the observation that the majority of RA patients have autoreactive antibodies called rheumatoid factors, which are directed against the Fc-region of human IgG. In addition to rheumatoid factors, antinuclear antibodies and antibodies against the cartilage matrix proteins, type II collagen and aggrecan, have been reported. However, autoreactive antibodies are also produced in other diseases as well as in normal subjects. In animal models of autoimmune inflammatory arthritis, the disease cannot be transferred to healthy animals by injection of autoantibodies or B cells, suggesting a subordinate role for B lymphocytes.

A T-cell mediated autoimmune disease can, by definition, be transferred passively to nonimmunized animals using T-cell lines reactive against the putative autoantigen. This has been demonstrated for experimental autoimmune encephalomyelitis, a model for multiple sclerosis in which the autoantigen is derived from myeline basic protein. The situation in RA appears to be more complex. Both T and B cells are required for the passive transfer of either type II collagen or aggrecan-induced arthritis from arthritic to naïve mice; neither T cells nor B cells alone are sufficient. Moreover, the development of disease in animal models is directly related to humoral immunity against type II collagen or aggrecan. Thus, these data suggest that both T and B cells are involved in the pathogenesis of RA.

B-cell infiltrates and structures reminiscent of GC are found in tissues normally devoid of this cell population in a number of autoimmune diseases. The thymus is a primary lymphoid organ for the differentiation and maturation of T cells; it contains virtually no B cells. GC-like structures have been described in the thymus of patients with myasthenia gravis (a well characterized autoimmune disease directed against the acetylcholine receptor), as well as in thyroid tissue of patients with Hashimoto's disease and in the salivary glands of patients with Sjögren's syndrome. These diseases also are believed to be mediated by tissue-specific autoantibodies. In RA, GC-like structures have been observed in synovial tissue and in the subchondral bone, and large aggregates appear to consist mainly of B cells. Somatic hypermutation and clonal expansion have been documented for B cells derived from RA synovium. Together these findings suggest that B cells play an important role in the pathogenesis of RA. If B-cell infiltration into arthritic lesions is an antigen-dependent process, the question arises whether or not these antigens are tissue specific.

Specific Immunotherapy in the Treatment of Rheumatoid Arthritis

Removal of circulating lymphocytes by thoracic lymphatic duct drainage can produce marked clinical improvement in RA patients. Therapeutic studies with anti-CD4 antibodies have produced mixed results with evidence of clinical improvement in some cases. Whether such immunotherapies are effective may depend on the rates of T-cell migration in different patients and access of antibody to T-cells in extravascular sites. In summary, there is clear evidence in support of T cell-dependent mechanisms, but T-cell independent mechanisms may also be important. This may vary from patient to patient and with disease duration.

Endothelial Interactions and Angiogenesis

Chronic inflammation is established after the migration of leukocytes from the blood stream into the affected joint tissue. This section focuses on mechanisms of cell adhesion used by leukocytes during their migration into tissue. In particular, the role of cell surface adhesion receptor molecules, which mediate cell attachment to each other and to ECM components, and the capacity of soluble mediators to regulate the activity of many of these receptors are discussed. This section also deals with angiogenesis, which is the process of new blood vessel development in tissues. Angiogenesis is especially prominent during wound healing and tissue repair, but also is important for tumor growth and metastasis and the development of immunologically mediated chronic inflammation. The most important features of each of these processes are highlighted; more extensive reviews are available for additional information.

Established rheumatoid synovitis is characterized by unremitting immunologic activity resulting from cellular interactions and the release and activity of a number of proinflammatory cytokines. The predominant cell found in inflamed synovium is the T cell, although B cells, APCs, and synovial cells are also present and are critically involved in the pathogenesis of RA. To enter synovial tissue, T cells must migrate through the endothelial cell lining of postcapillary venules. The cells, therefore, have to pass through a barrier that is 1 endothelial cell layer thick and then must penetrate the basement membrane composed of extracellular molecules and present underneath the endothelial cell layer, supporting the structure of the blood vessel. The cells then either migrate to areas in the tissue where they remain as a result of specific interactions with antigen and APCs, or they migrate to areas where they are involved in nonspecific, antigen-independent interactions. Alternatively, the T cells may percolate through the tissue and exit into the synovial fluid where they are removed by draining lymphatics.

Mechanisms of Cell Adhesion and Transendothelial Migration

The adhesion and transendothelial migration of T cells are essential to a number of physiologic and pathologic processes involving the perivascular accumulation of T cells in lymphoid and nonlymphoid tissues. Which tissue T cells migrate into depends, in part, on the differentiation state of the T cell. For example, naive T cells that have not previously encountered their specific antigen outside the thymus predominantly recirculate from the blood into secondary lymphoid tissues, such as the lymph nodes and Peyer's patches. Memory T cells, which develop as a result of binding their specific antigen, are recruited to migrate into nonlymphoid tissues, such as the rheumatoid synovial membrane. As part of their immune surveillance function, memory T cells will also enter lymph nodes, but they appear to do so through the afferent lymphatics draining the tissues. Regardless of whether they migrate into lymphoid tissue, T cells always appear to use similar mechanisms of adhesion and transendothelial migration, involving the concerted activities of specific cell surface adhesions receptors expressed by both T cells and endothelial cells. In addition, T-cell motility is critical for migration into tissue, as is the action of certain cytokines.

Essential to the process of transendothelial migration of T cells are the activities of members of the selection, integrin, and Ig superfamilies of adhesion receptors. An extensive review of all members of these adhesion receptor families is beyond the scope of this chapter. In general, the initial interaction of all leukocytes with endothelial cells is relatively weak. It is sensitive to shear stress imparted by blood flow and is mediated by adhesion receptors on leukocytes such as L-selectin (CD62L) (Table 4) that are always ready and able to bind their ligand (Fig. 7). This particular adhesion receptor binds specialized complex carbohydrates containing sialic acid and fucose, which are found on a number of different endothelial cell receptors, including mucosal addressin cell adhesion molecule, peripheral node addressin, E-selectin (CD62E), and P-selectin (CD62P).

As a result of L-selectin binding to its specific receptor, changes occur in the bound T cells. Prominent is the alter-

ation of another set of T-cell adhesion receptors that are members of the integrin family of adhesion receptors, lymphocyte function-associated antigen (LFA)-1 (CD11a/CD18) and very late antigen (VLA)-4 (CD49d/CD29), which normally are not able to bind their ligand. When L-selectin binds to its ligand, chemical messages are generated in the bound T cells that cause the integrin receptors to change their structure and become capable of binding their specific receptors, intercellular adhesion (ICAM)-1 (CD54) and vascular cell adhesion molecule (VCAM)-1 (CD106), respectively, which are present on endothelial cells at sites of inflammation. This integrin-mediated binding of T cells to endothelial cells is relatively stable and resistant to the shear stress of blood flow (Fig. 10).

Many bound T cells will subsequently migrate through the endothelial cell layer and underlying basement membrane to reach the tissue. Other bound T cells will detach from the endothelial cell and return to the circulation. Similar to T cell-endothelial cell binding, transendothelial migration also is mediated by specific adhesion receptors, mainly LFA-1 on T cells and ICAM-1 on endothelial cells. Adhesion receptors, therefore, may be involved in both the binding of T cells to endothelial cells and transendothelial migration. Alternatively, they may promote only 1 step of the process. For example, VLA-4 and VCAM-1 mediate T-cell binding to endothelial cells but they do not play a role in transendothelial migration.

Transendothelial migration additionally requires the development of motility in T cells so that they can move through the endothelial cell layer and within the tissue. The mechanisms involved in this are not completely understood. A number of reports have indicated that the binding of chemokines and IL-15 to their specific receptors on T cells induces additional chemical signals to facilitate activation of adhesion receptors and cause alterations in the shape of the bound T cells (Fig. 10). Chemokines are low molecular weight cytokines produced by a variety of cell types, including leukocytes, epithelial cells, and endothelial cells. They mediate the chemotaxis, or directed migration, of leukocytes. IL-15 is a cytokine produced by a number of nonhematopoietic cell types, including endothelial cells. It shares many biologic activities with IL-2, including the ability to promote T-cell proliferation. In addition, it activates LFA-1 to bind ICAM-1, induces T-cell shape changes, and increases T-cell migration.

The Vascular Endothelium at Sites of Chronic Inflammation

The vascular endothelium is essential for the maintenance of hemostasis, inflammatory responses, and immune function. Endothelial activity mediated by cytokine secretion and cellular interactions is necessary for the control of vasomotor tone, vascular permeability, regulation of platelet adhesion and activation, modulation of the complement cascade, activation of procoagulant and fibrinolytic pathways, and immune modulation. Poised at the interface between the blood and extravascular tissue, it is continuously influenced by both environments.

Endothelial cells are able to alter their morphologic and biologic phenotypes in response to environmental stimuli. T cells migrate into lymph nodes through the endothelium of specialized postcapillary venules, known as high endothelial venules. These blood vessels are distinguished from others based on their characteristic cuboidal or columnar morphology. At sites of chronic inflammation, endothelial cells assume morphologic and cytochemical characteristics of high endothelial venules. The development of these types of vessels has been examined in sites of delayed type sensitivity reaction in the skin of baboons and was found to depend on the exposure of the tissue to proinflammatory cytokines. Thus, concomitant stimulation with TNF-α and IFN-γ induced the appearance of high endothelial venules as well as the adhesion and extravasation of inflammatory cells.

Exposure to multiple cytokines in chronically inflamed human tissue is likely to induce high endothelial venules in a similar manner. The high endothelial venule-like blood vessels in synovial tissue of patients with RA, like those of lymphoid tissue, have been shown to be sites of adhesion of lymphocytes; thus infiltration of mononuclear cells into the inflamed tissue is likely to occur here. In rheumatoid synovium, high endothelial venules are found in areas containing aggregates of CD4+ T cells, suggesting that they play a role in the extravasation of specific subsets of T cells.

In addition to these phenotypic changes, endothelial cells undergo functional changes to adapt their activity to the inflammatory environment. For example, in response to actions of proinflammatory cytokines such as TNF-α, IFN-γ, or IL-1β, endothelial cells produce adhesion receptors, including ICAM-1 (CD54), VCAM-1 (CD106), E-selectin (CD62E), P-selectin (CD62P), and the β7 integrin. They also elaborate factors and cytokines, such as those involved in procoagulation and chemotaxis, with the net result being enhancement of leukocyte trafficking into the tissue.

Angiogenesis

At sites of chronic inflammation, angiogenesis (growth of new blood vessels) is a prominent response of endothelial cells to the actions of growth factors. Several features of angiogenesis, or neovascularization, have been reported, involving the dissolution of basement membrane connec-

Table 4

Adhesion Receptors Mediating T-cell Interactions with Endothelial Cells at Sites of Chronic Inflammation

T-Cell Receptor	Superfamily	Counterreceptor on Endothelial Cells*
Receptors mediating T-cell arrest[†]		
CD2	Immunoglobulin	LFA-3
PECAM-1 (CD31)	Immunoglobulin	PECAM-1αVβ3, heparin
CD44	?	Hyaluronic acid, ?
L-selectin (CD62L)	Selectin	MadCAM-1, PNAd, sialylated oligosaccharides
CLA	?	E-selectin
Others[§]	?	
Receptors mediating stable T-cell binding to endothelial cells[†]		
LFA-1 F(CD1 1a/CD18)	Integrin	ICAM-1 (CD54), ICAM-2 (CD102)
VLA-4 (α4β1, CD49d/CD29)	Integrin	VCAM-1 (CD106), MadCAM-1, Fibronectin
α4β7 (CD49d/β7)	Integrin	MadCAM-1, VCAM-1
Receptors mediating transendothelial migration[†]		
LFA-1	Integrin	ICAM-1
CD44	?	?
Others[§]	?	

*   LFA-3, leukocyte function associated antigen-3; PECAM-1, platelet endothelial cell adhesion molecule-1; MadCAM-1, mucosal addressin cell adhesion molecule-1; PNAd, peripheral node addressin-1; ICAM-1, -2, intercellular adhesion molecule-1, -2; VCAM-1, vascular cell adhesion molecule-1.

†   Receptors are listed because either they have been shown to mediate T-cell arrest to endothelial cells under shear stress of blood flow (CD44, CD62L) in functional assays, or they do not require a chemical signal to be able to bind to their receptor ligand (CD2, CD31).

§   It is anticipated that other adhesion receptors will be identified that mediate T-cell arrest on endothelial cell surfaces, stable T-cell binding to endothelial cells, and transendothelial migration.

tive tissue, separation of endothelial cells from the vessel walls, endothelial cell migration, endothelial cell adhesion to ECM molecules, endothelial cell proliferation, and subsequent endothelial cell tube formation (Fig. 10). A family of angiogenic factors known as vascular endothelial growth factors (VEGF) and a vascular permeability factor, vasculotropin, have recently been identified. Other growth factors, such as a basic fibroblast growth factor, also stimulate endothelial cell proliferation, but they are not specific for this cell type. VEGF, on the other hand, targets endothelial cells specifically.

VEGF is produced by several cell types during tumorigenesis, wound healing, and chronic inflammatory disorders, including RA. In rheumatoid synovium, VEGF mRNA is largely associated with cells associated with the synovial lining. Endothelial cells express 2 specific receptors for VEGF, namely, kinase-insert domain receptor, VEGFR-2 and fms-like tyrosine kinase (flt-1) VEGFR-1, which are members of the immunoglobulin superfamily of molecules. Ligation of these receptors stimulates endothelial cell proliferation and alters endothelial expression of integrin adhesion receptors, including $\alpha V\beta5$, $\alpha1\beta1$, and $\alpha2\beta1$, which mediate binding to ECM molecules. In addition, VEGF stimulates the release of ECM degrading enzymes. Thus, the activity of growth factors such as VEGF, elaborated at sites of chronic inflammation, results in the degradation of the connective tissue, facilitating migration of endothelial cells, as well as their proliferation. In RA, the process of angiogenesis may partly account for the numerous small blood vessels that develop in rheumatoid synovium connective tissue, particularly around the developing pannus.

Summary

Transendothelial migration is an intrinsic property of certain T-cell populations. The activities of a variety of adhesion receptors are critical for T-lymphocyte infiltration into sites of chronic inflammation. Adhesion receptor activity is an essential feature of transendothelial migration of T cells as well as angiogenesis. It is the persistence of these endothelial-cell and T-cell mediated mechanisms that may be pivotal in the perpetuation of chronic inflammatory joint disorders.

Fibrosis

Definition of and Clinical Spectrum of Fibrosis

Fibrosis is characterized by excessive accumulation of connective tissue macromolecules in an affected organ. Connective tissue formation is an essential component of the physiologic processes of development, growth, and tissue repair. Under certain conditions, however, the orderly physiologic process of connective tissue synthesis and deposition escapes its normal controls, resulting in the development of pathologic fibrosis. Connective tissue is composed of ECM, a complex superstructure of collagens, fibronectin, proteoglycans, and other self-aggregating macromolecules, which are attached via $\alpha1\beta$ and $\alpha2\beta1$ integrin receptors to stromal cells such fibroblasts, myofibroblasts, osteoblasts, and mesangial cells. Previously regarded

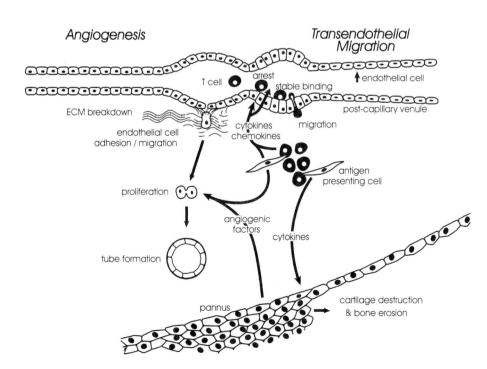

Figure 10

Model of events involved in angiogenesis and transendothelial migration.

simplistically as an inert structural "scaffold" for maintaining tissue integrity, the ECM in fact is in a dynamic and carefully balanced equilibrium with cellular components of connective tissue. These cells are responsible for the synthesis, as well as the degradation, of ECM under a process that is normally carefully regulated. In turn, the ECM communicates with cellular components, regulating their migration, differentiation, proliferation, metabolism, contractility, and survival. Perturbation of the dynamic equilibrium between the cellular and extracellular components of connective tissue results in fibrosis on the one hand, and pathologic matrix degradation on the other.

Fibrosis is a prominent feature of a diverse group of acquired human diseases (Outline 2). Although some of these are uncommon, others are prevalent and account for substantial morbidity and mortality. The fibrosing diseases can be classified as systemic, characterized by fibrosis of virtually every organ, and organ-limited, characterized by fibrosis confined predominantly to a single organ. These include fibrosis of the lung, the liver, the eye, the thyroid glands, the penis, the bone marrow, and the skin. In a broader sense, atherosclerosis may also be properly viewed as a form of vascular fibrosis. In each of these forms of fibrosis, dysregulated local production and accumulation of connective tissue leads to disruption of the normal architecture of the affected organ, resulting in its progressive failure.

Pathogenesis of Fibrosis

Collagens and Their Degradation

The collagens are the major structural proteins of the ECM, accounting for up to 70% of the dry weight of the dermis and 90% of the organic matrix of bone. They represent a large family of genetically distinct proline- and hydroxyproline-rich proteins. All collagens have a unique triple helical structure that requires a glycine in every third position of the amino acid sequence The fiber-forming collagens (types I, III, and V) are widely distributed, most abundant in the skin and tendons, and in cartilage (type II collagen). In addition, types VI and XII collagens are important in the skin, whereas types IX, X, and XI collagens are found in cartilage, and types IV and VII collagens in basement membrane. The genes for the interstitial collagens are unusually large and have complex exon-intron structures.

The procollagen precursors have large nonhelical terminal domains that control fibril formation and macromolecular organization. Following hydroxylation of lysine and proline residues, procollagens are secreted, and undergo extracellular cleavage of the terminal propeptides, followed by fibril formation, and assembly and stabilization of mature collagens. Tissue deposition of collagen can be decreased through its intracellular degradation, its phagocytosis by fibroblasts, or its extracellular degradation by collagenase. Abnormally regulated expression of collagenase and other matrix-degrading enzymes is a hallmark of

arthritis, periodontal disease, skin disorders such as dystrophic epidermolysis bullosa, and cancer tissue invasion.

Fibroblast Activation

Although the fibrosing diseases listed in Outline 2 display distinct clinical and pathologic features depending on the structure and cellular composition of the affected organs, the overlap in the pathogenetic pathways resulting in these different entities is striking. An initial injury—such as a physical, chemical, or immunologic insult; ionizing radiation; viral (especially retroviral) infection; or "idiopathic" injury—results in activation of fibroblasts and related connective tissue-synthesizing stromal cells. Several mechanisms of fibroblast activation that are not mutually exclusive have been implicated in the development of fibrosis (Fig. 11). First, injury may lead to proliferation and/or recruitment of connective tissue-synthesizing cells in affected tissue, resulting in net overproduction and subsequent deposition of connective tissue macromolecules. Induction of genetic programs for the synthesis of connec-

---

Outline 2

Selected Human Diseases Characterized by Prominent Tissue Fibrosis

Primarily cutaneous fibrosis
Localized scleroderma (morphea)
Sclerodema; scleromyxedema
Eosinophila-myagia syndrome; Spanish toxic oil syndrome
Keloids
Dupuytren's contractures

Systemic fibrosis
Systemic sclerosis
Retroperitoneal fibrosis
Chronic graft versus host disease
Metastatic carcinoid
Postsurgical adhesions
Radiation-induced fibrosis

Organ-specific fibrosis
Idiopathic pulmonary fibrosis
Bleomycin-induced pulmonary fibrosis
Cryptogenic cirrhosis
Veno-occlusive disease
Biliary cirrhosis
Sclerosing cholangitis
Retro-orbital fibrosis
Riedel's struma
Diabetic nephropathy
Chronic renal allograft rejection
Human immunodeficiency virus nephropathy
Mesangial fibrosis
Vascular restenosis
Atherosclerosis (?)
Peyronie's disease
Cystic fibrosis-associated colonopathy

tive tissue macromolecules may result from inappropriate and sustained activation of fibroblasts by cytokines or hormones. Alternatively, failure to appropriately downregulate and thus limit fibroblast activation following a physiologic stimulus for repair may also result in deregulated synthesis of collagen and related macromolecules. Finally, impaired production of matrix-degrading enzymes, or increased synthesis of their inhibitors, such as TIMP and PAI-1 may lead to defective turn-over of connective tissue, resulting in fibrosis.

Although each of these 3 mechanisms of fibroblast activation may be operative in pathologic fibrogenesis, current evidence suggests that constitutive activation of fibroblast connective tissue synthesis may be the most important. Various cytokines and extracellular signals with a role in tissue repair have been implicated in the development of pathologic fibrosis. Platelet-derived growth factor, fibroblast growth factor, IL-1, TNF-α, connective tissue growth factor, TGF-β, and hypoxia positively influence connective tissue accumulation, whereas prostaglandin E_2, relaxin, and IFN-γ inhibit this process.

Transforming Growth Factor-β

The best studied of the fibroblast-activating signaling molecules is TGF-β. This pleiotropic cytokine has 3 mammalian isoforms of nearly identical biologic activity. TGF-β is secreted by activated lymphocytes and monocytes in a latent form that undergoes extracellular cleavage to yield a biologically active 25 kd homodimer. Fully mature TGF-β binds to 3 distinct and ubiquitously distributed serine-

theronine kinase transmembrane receptors. On ligand binding, TGF-β receptor type II phosphorylates receptor type I, resulting in the formation of activated heterodimeric receptor complexes, which then phosphorylate additional intracellular proteins. Several targets of TGF-β receptor type I phosphorylation have been identified, although their functional role in propagating TGF-β signal to the nucleus are still unknown. In contrast, the newly discovered SMAD proteins clearly appear to be essential for TGF-β signal transduction.

The SMAD family consists of 7 members related by the high degree of similarity in their amino acid sequence, particularly in the N- and C-terminal domains of the molecules. Some of these family members are involved in signal transduction from the ligand-occupied TGF-β receptor to the final target in the nucleus, namely specific genes whose expression is controlled by this growth factor. This process involves phosphorylation of SMADs associated with the TGF-β receptor, which initiates events leading to their translocation to the nucleus and binding to specific regulatory elements of the genome. Other members of the SMAD family act as intracellular negative regulators of TGF-β signaling. Their role may be to prevent constitutive or inappropriate receptor signaling.

TGF-β in Tissue Repair and Pathologic Fibrogenesis

Several lines of evidence implicate TGF-β in fibrosis of the liver, kidney, lung, and other organs. First, exogenous TGF-β in animals not only promotes tissue repair, but can also cause pathologic fibrosis. Thus, intraperitoneal injections of TGF-β cause generalized tissue fibrosis, and overexpression of biologically active TGF-β by gene transfer or gene targeting results in fibrosis of the target organs. Second, elevated expression of TGF-β is associated with tissue fibrosis. In liver biopsy specimens from patients with active liver diseases, for instance, TGF-β mRNA levels are elevated in areas of fibrosis and correlate closely with levels of type I collagen mRNA. In patients undergoing autologous bone marrow transplantation, elevated plasma TGF-β predicts the rapid onset of liver and lung fibrosis. Third, no other cytokine has such generalized effects on connective tissue accumulation via stimulation of fibroblast chemotaxis and connective tissue production, inhibition of matrix-degrading enzyme synthesis, and stimulation of protease inhibitor synthesis, as TGF-β.

In vitro, TGF-β stimulates the transcription of the genes for both chains of type I collagen. Transient transfection analysis using chimeric DNA constructs, which were carrying the regulatory regions of these genes fused to a reporter, identified elements targeted by TGF-β-induced intracellular signaling cascades. In the gene coding for the α2 chain of type I collagen, a 300-base pair segment of the proximal promoter is necessary and sufficient for activation of transcription by TGF-β. This region harbors multiple binding sites for members of the Sp1 family of transcription factors.

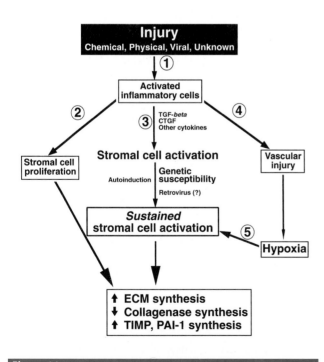

Figure 11

Mechanisms in the development of pathologic fibrosis.

It has been suggested that TGF-β signaling results in post-transcriptional modification of Sp1, resulting in its enhanced DNA-binding. In the gene coding for the α1 chain of type I collagen, a different proximal promoter element appears to mediate the response to TGF-β. Work from different investigators has implicated different sequences of the type I collagen genes as "TGF-β response elements," highlighting the inherent limitations of in vitro transient transfection analysis.

Finally, the sequestration of active TGF-β in the kidney or the lung by neutralizing antibodies, soluble TGF-β receptors, or the TGF-β binding protoglycan decorin effectively abrogates the subsequent development of fibrosis of these tissues in animal models. The causal relation between secretion of TGF-β and the pathologic accumulation of ECM in animal models of fibrosis and human fibrotic diseases appears to be well established. Following acute injury, normally only a transient increase in TGF-β and limited connective tissue accumulation, resulting in tissue repair, occur. This is because both the production of TGF-β and the intracellular signaling cascades it triggers are promptly terminated. Whether pathologic fibrogenesis is the result of sustained production of TGF-β as a result of repeated injury or sustained autoinduction, enhanced fibroblast responsiveness to TGF-β resulting from upregulation of TGF-β receptors, or a failure to terminate TGF-β-induced intracellular signaling is currently unknown.

Approaches to Treatment of Fibrosis

Traditional, empirically-based antifibrotic treatments are generally ineffective and are frequently associated with significant side effects. For instance, inhibition of collagen production by glucocorticoids is associated with skin atrophy, increased tendon fragility, and osteoporosis, but provides little benefit in preventing or reversing fibrosis. Current and future treatment strategies are summarized in Table 5. A detailed understanding of the molecular basis of tissue fibrosis has resulted in the identification of several molecules with essential roles in pathologic fibrogenesis. This, in turn, is likely to facilitate the development of antifibrotic treatment strategies aimed at selectively interfering with signaling through these molecules. Particularly promising are various antagonists of TGF-β that inhibit production, extracellular activation, receptor binding, or signaling by these fibrogenic cytokines.

Summary

Fibrosis resulting from excessive accumulation of connective tissue in various organs is a prominent feature of many prevalent and currently incurable human diseases. Fibrosis represents a pathologic excess of the physiologic process of tissue repair. Overproduction of collagen and other connective tissue macromolecules is due to activation of stromal cells. TGF-β is a key molecular mediator in both normal tissue repair and in pathologic fibrosis. In the former, it is self-limited, whereas in the latter, signaling by TGF-β to stromal cells becomes constitutive. Therapeutic strategies targeted at specific steps in stromal cell activation and ECM biosynthesis offer promising future approaches for the amelioration and treatment of pathologic fibrosis.

Apoptosis

Apoptosis is an evolutionarily conserved form of programmed cell death in which a cell actively contributes to its own destruction. The term was first used in 1972 by Wyllie and others, and comes from a Greek word denoting the dropping of a leaf from a tree in the autumn or the falling of a petal from a flower. It is characterized morphologically by shrinkage of the cell, condensation of nuclear chromatin, nuclear fragmentation, and bleeding of the cell membrane to form vesicles called apoptotic bodies. These processes occur without disruption of the plasma membrane until late in the process. The apoptotic cell expresses novel surface phospholipids and glycoproteins that are recognized by specific receptors on a neighboring macrophage, leading to rapid engulfment of the dead cell without stimulation of the phagocyte. The process thus leads to the 'dropping off' of unwanted cells from tissues without leading to inflammation (Fig. 12). This is to be contrasted with the other form of cell death called necrosis, where the cell, after exposure to severe environmental insults, enlarges in size and ruptures, spilling the proinflammatory cellular contents into the extracellular milieu.

Apoptotic processes are important in embryogenesis and in the maintenance of homeostasis of various tissues in the body. Processes during development, such as formation of the brain, pharyngeal clefts, and interdigital web spaces, are critically dependent on apoptosis. The induction of immune tolerance to self-antigens and immune-mediated killing of infected cells and tumors is also mediated by apoptosis. Resolution of acute inflammatory processes is accompanied by apoptosis of infiltrating neutrophils. Apoptosis also appears to be important in the death of hypertrophic chondrocytes during the normal ossification process in the growth plates, as well as removal of osteoclasts in late stages of bone remodeling. Abnormalities in the apoptotic processes can lead to pathologic states such as neoplasias, autoimmunity, neurodegenerative diseases, and acquired immune deficiency syndrome (AIDS) as described later in this section.

Induction of Apoptosis

Apoptotic cells have been described in almost every organ in the body in pathologic conditions. Events that can induce apoptosis include withdrawal of growth factors, infection with viruses, stimulation through specific death receptors on the membrane, and exposure to stressful environmental stimuli such as DNA-damaging (genotoxic) agents.

Molecular and Biochemical Characterization

On a molecular level, apoptosis is an irreversible process characterized by disruption of the cytoskeletal architecture and ordered cleavage of the chromosomal DNA leading to a characteristic "ladder" pattern on agarose gel electrophoresis. New protein synthesis is not required, thereby suggesting that the players in this process preexist in the cell, waiting to be triggered on initiaion of apoptosis. The elucidation of the biochemical steps involved in apoptosis is an area of active research. Regardless of the initial stimulus, there appears to be a final common pathway of cell damage in most, if not all, cases of apoptosis. This process involves proteolytic degradation of cytoskeletal elements by a family of proteases called caspases and ordered degradation of nuclear DNA by specific nucleases. Enzymes involved in DNA repair are also cleaved during the process, thus ensuring that the nuclear damage is irreversible. The mitochondria appear to be actively involved in at least some forms of apoptotsis. Other intracellular mediators that may be involved in apoptosis include ceramide and protein kinases called stress-activated protein kinases. The apoptotic process is tightly regulated by the requirement for sequential activation of caspases, which are present as inactive zymogens in normal cells, as well as by antiapoptotic proteins such as members of the Bcl-2 family and other apoptosis inhibitory proteins in the cytosol. The delicate balance between the apoptotic mediators and antiapoptotic proteins governs the final fate of the cell.

Caspases

Caspases (cysteine aspartate specific proteases) are members of a family of cysteine proteases that cleave their substrates after aspartate (D) residues. Ten members of the

Table 5
Selected Approaches to the Treatment of Fibrosis

Mechanism of Action	Representative Agent/ Intervention
Decrease inflammation	Cyclophosphamide Glucocorticoids Cyclosporine A* Photophoresis*
Inhibit collagen production	Interferon-γ* Glucocorticoids Relaxin* Antisense oligonucleotide Lysyl oxidase inhibitors Prolyl 4-hydroxylase inhibitors
Inhibit collagen fiber formation	D-penicillamine
Enhance collagen degradation	Interferon-α* Relaxin*
Inhibit transforming growth factor-β (TGF-β)	Decorin Anti TGF-β antibody[†] Soluble receptor[†] Angiotensin II blockade[†] Dietary protein restriction[†] Certain retinoids and estrogens[†] Mannose-6-phosphate[†] Antisense gene therapy[†]
Inhibit other "fibrogenic" cytokine signaling	Receptor tyrosine kinase inhibitors[†]

* Experimental intervention

† Potential treatment strategy

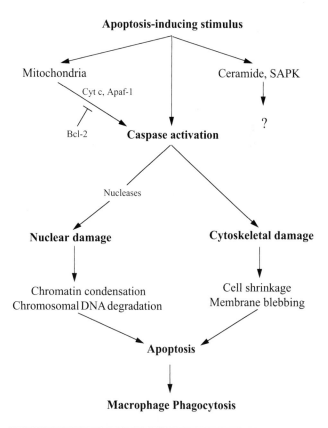

Figure 12

A generic scheme of mediators and processes involved in apoptosis. Because not all the intermediary steps induced by different apoptotic stimuli have yet been characterized, it is possible that other mediators not shown may be critically involved in certain pathways.

family have been described so far, and they appear to belong to various subfamilies depending on their preferred substrate specificities in vitro and possibly in vivo. Caspases 8 and 10 activate caspases 3, 6, and 7, which are thought to be involved in the final 'execution' stage of cell death. Numerous intracellular protein substrates have been described for caspases 3, 6, and 7; however, it is not clear at present whether any of these is absolutely essential for cell survival. The role of caspases in the apoptotic process has been studied extensively in those pathways initiated by activation of Fas and tumor necrosis factor receptor 1 (TNFR1) (p55TNF receptor) belonging to the TNFR family.

Fas-Mediated Apoptosis

The Fas antigen (APO-1, CD95) is expressed ubiquitously on cells. It has an extracellular domain which binds to the Fas ligand (FasL) and a cytoplasmic region containing a death domain (DD). This domain is present on a number of proteins involved in apoptotic processes; hence, its name. It mediates interaction with other proteins, leading to heterodimer formation, an important aspect in many activation processes. Cross-linking of Fas on the surface of cells by the FasL or agonistic antibodies leads to the recruitment and activation of caspase 8 by adapter proteins. This eventually leads to activation of downstream caspases, such as caspases 3 and 7, and finally to cell death. The Fas pathway can be antagonized in cells by a natural protein called FLIP (Fas-inhibitory protein). FasL usually is expressed only on CD8+ cytotoxic T lymphocytes, cytotoxic CD4+ T helper-1 (Th1) lymphocytes, natural killer cells, in the eye, and in the testis. Expression of FasL in the normal eye and the testis leads to these sites being 'immune privileged,' because infiltrating leukocytes are killed by Fas-mediated apoptosis at these sites. The Fas antigen has been shown to be important in the dampening of the immune response after antigenic stimulation. A defect in this process leads to massive lymphadenopathy and autoimmunity in mice with a mutation in the Fas gene (lpr mutation) or the FasL gene (gld mutation).

Tumor Necrosis Factor Receptor

The TNFR1 has some homology with the Fas antigen and has a DD in the cytoplasmic domain similar to the Fas antigen. However, signaling through the TNFR1 is somewhat more complex and can initiate both an apoptotic pathway similar to Fas and a usually dominant survival pathway through activation of the proinflammatory transcription factor NF-kB. Other members of the TNFR family that can transduce apoptotic symbols have been recently described including DR3 (death receptor 3), DR4, and DR5, all of which contain cytoplasmic DDs. Two surface decoy receptors (DcR1 and DcR2) lacking DD, or with mutated DD, have been recently described that can antagonize the proapoptotic actions of the DR ligand called TRAIL (TNF-related apoptosis inducing ligand).

Mitochondria and Bcl-2

It has been known for some time that a loss in the transmembrane potential in mitochondrial membranes caused by formation of large channels in these membranes accompanies almost all forms of apoptosis. This loss allows the diffusion of large molecules such as cytochrome c and apoptosis inducing factors from the mitochondria to the cytosol after induction of apoptosis. Cytochrome c appears to complex with another mitochondrially derived protein called apaf-1 (apoptosis activating factor-1) and recruits and activates caspase-9. Caspase-9 can then cleave and activate caspase-3, leading eventually to nuclear degradation and cell death. Bcl-2 and other members of the family are present on mitochondrial membranes and can regulate this process. Bcl-2 itself or another antiapoptotic family member such as Bcl-xL may inhibit the mitochondrial release of cytochrome c and thereby suppress apoptosis, whereas other proapoptotic Bcl-2 family members such as Bax and Bad can enhance the apoptotic process by complexing with and inactivating the antiapoptotic members of the family.

Apoptosis in Disease Processes

Intracellular proteins such as p53 and retinoblastoma protein have been shown to be important in inducing apoptosis in cells arrested in the cell cycle after events such as DNA damage. Mutations in these proteins are thought to be important in the induction of neoplasia. Increased Bcl-2 expression may play a role in the pathogenesis of B-cell lymphomas.

Hepatocytes are exquisitely sensitive to Fas-induced cytotoxicity and fulminant hepatitis, and hepatic failure can result from unchecked Fas-mediated killing by cytotoxic T lymphocytes and natural killer cells. There is some evidence that the death of uninfected T lymphocytes in AIDS may be secondary to Fas-mediated apoptosis. Recent findings suggest that at least some tumors of hepatic, breast, and other origins may express FasL and may kill immune cells by Fas-mediated apoptosis before the latter cells can kill the tumor. The tumors can thereby escape immune surveillance. The rare disorder called autoimmune lymphoproliferative syndrome, or the Canale-Smith syndrome, is caused by Fas mutations, and the phenotype has similarities with mice with the lpr mutation.

The synovial hyperplasia in the pannus seen in RA could be partly due to decreased apoptosis of the synovial cells. Mutations in the p53 gene leading to defects in apoptosis in vitro have been detected in synovial tissues of RA patients with long-standing disease. There is evidence to suggest that increased neuronal apoptosis plays an important role in neurodegenerative disorders such as Alzheimer's disease and Parkinson's disease, in myopathies, and after ischemic injury following acute myocardial infarction and stroke. Indeed, there is increasing evidence of abnormal apoptosis in diseases in almost any organ in the body. The contribution of abnormal apoptotic processes to these disease processes is an area of ongoing investigation.

Efforts to suppress apoptosis in a tissue-specific manner in conditions such as Alzheimer's disease and AIDS and following ischemia may alleviate these conditions, whereas methods to increase apoptosis in neoplasias would induce regression of the tumors.

Nitric Oxide, Other Free Radicals, and Related Species

Free radicals are atoms or molecules that contain 1 or more unpaired electrons. Chemical species with this property tend to be highly reactive and therefore short-lived under physiologic conditions. Although a large number of free radicals are generated in biologic systems, those that are thought to contribute most prominently to orthopaedic disorders are nitric oxide ($\cdot$NO) and superoxide ($\cdot O_2^-$). Discussion of these 2 molecules cannot proceed without consideration of the related, nonradical species, hydrogen peroxide (H_2O_2) and peroxynitrite ($ONOO^-$). Collectively, these molecules are likely to be involved in several key pathophysiologic aspects of RA and OA, as well as in the healing and repair of orthopaedic tissues.

Nitric Oxide

Nitric oxide is synthesized by a family of enzymes known as NO synthases, which use arginine and molecular oxygen as substrates (Fig. 13).

Three distinct isoforms of NO synthase (NOS) have been identified, purified, and cloned (Table 6). It is not known whether further isoforms of NOS await identification. Two of the NOS isoforms are expressed constitutively by many cells and are known as constitutive cNOS. One of these isoforms was first identified in neural tissue and is often referred to as neural nNOS or brain bNOS. The other isoform of cNOS was first identified in endothelial cells and is often referred to as eNOS. In addition to these 2 isoforms of cNOS, there is a so-called inducible species of NOS often referred to as iNOS, which is not normally present in cells but it is induced in response to specific stimuli. Ambiguities accompanying the nomenclature nNOS, iNOS and eNOS have led many authors to revise these to NOS-1, NOS-2, and NOS-3, respectively (Table 6). Both nomenclatures are found in the literature.

Constitutive isoforms of NOS require exogenous Ca^{2+} for activity. Cells expressing cNOS usually synthesize small amounts of $\cdot$NO transiently in response to stimuli that increase intracellular concentrations of Ca^{2+}. These are important in the maintenance of homeostasis in the cardiovascular and nervous systems. The role of $\cdot$NO in the regulation of blood pressure has been particularly well investigated in this regard. Such studies have shown convincingly that $\cdot$NO, produced constitutively by the endothelial lining of blood vessels, relaxes the surrounding smooth muscle, thereby acting as a vasodilator. Inhibitors of NOS are undergoing phase III clinical trials as a means of maintaining blood pressure in patients with septic shock.

Unlike cNOS, iNOS plays no known role in homeostatic physiology although it may be important in nonspecific immunity. Its expression is associated with a number of inflammatory and degenerative conditions. Once expressed, iNOS produces large amounts of $\cdot$NO for extended periods in the absence of exogenous Ca^{2+}. Because the sustained production of large quantities of $\cdot$NO is thought to be associated with a number of diseases, there has been a considerable effort by the pharmaceutical industry to develop specific inhibitors of iNOS for therapeutic purposes. None, however, are yet in clinical use.

A variety of musculoskeletal tissues express 1 or more of the various isoforms of NOS (Table 6). Under normal conditions, cNOS is expressed in skeletal muscle and bone. Cartilage synovium, meniscus, tendons, ligaments, and intervertebral disk do not appear to generate $\cdot$NO spontaneously, suggesting that cNOS is absent. Cytokine stimulation of rodent articular cartilage, meniscus, synovium, ligaments, and tendons, as well as bovine disk, results in the production of large amounts of $\cdot$NO. In the case of articular cartilage this has been formally shown to result from iNOS induction. Cells obtained from laboratory animals generally tend to be more enthusiastic in the production of iNOS than human cells. In this regard, human articular chondrocytes are notable for the high levels of $\cdot$NO synthesis following exposure to IL-1.

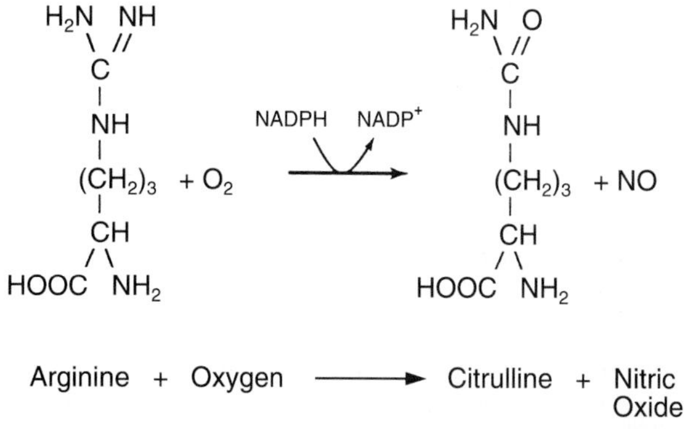

Figure 13

Nitric oxide synthase reaction. (Reproduced with permission from Evans CH, Stefanovic-Racic M, Lancaster J: Nitric oxide and its role in orthopaedic disease. *Clin Orthop* 1995;312:275–294.)

Superoxide, Peroxynitrite, and Others

Unlike ·NO, ·O_2^- can be synthesized biologically in a number of different ways. Polymorphonuclear leukocytes use the enzyme NADPH (reduced form of nicotinamide-adenine oxidase dinucleotide phosphate) to generate large amounts of ·O_2^- which, like ·NO, has antimicrobial properties. Patients lacking this enzyme are prone to infections. A number of metabolic reactions and mitochondrial respiration also generate ·O_2^-. These 2 free radicals are the substrates for a number of enzymatic and spontaneous chemical reactions leading to the generation of various reactive molecules as shown in Figure 14. The enzyme superoxide dismutase (SOD) protects cells from the toxic effects of ·O_2^-, forming hydrogen peroxide (H_2O_2) by reaction with water. H_2O_2 is itself a reactive and potentially toxic molecule that is converted to water and oxygen by catalase. As shown in Figure 13, H_2O_2 can undergo the Harber-Weiss reaction with ·O_2^- to form the highly reactive hydroxyradical (·OH). In the presence of transition metals, such as Fe^{3+}, H_2O_2 can also generate ·OH via the Fenton reaction. Polymorphonuclear leukocytes generate hypochlorous acid, an antimicrobial agent, from H_2O_2 and chloride using the enzyme myeloperoxidase.

There is presently much interest in the reaction between ·O_2^- and ·NO to form peroxynitrite ($ONOO^-$). This is a very rapid reaction which dominates the chemistry of these 2 radicals where they are coproduced. Increasingly, $ONOO^-$ is seen as an agent of the pathophysiologic properties that were formerly ascribed to ·NO. One way in which $ONOO^-$ may damage biologic systems is by rearranging to form the highly toxic hydroxyl radical ·OH and the nitrogen dioxide radical (·NO_2). Alternatively it may rearrange to form the harmless products, water and nitrite. Peroxynitrite also nitrosylates aromatic amino acids and the presence of nitro-tyrosine is taken as evidence of $ONOO^-$ reduction. To add further complexity, there is evidence that ·NO inhibits catalase and SOD, as well as NOS. Determining the biologic conditions under which each of these possible outcomes occurs is an area of active research.

Biologic Properties of Free Radicals and Related Molecules

In general, free radicals are powerful oxidants that damage proteins, nucleic acids, sugars, and lipids. They consequently interfere with most facets of cellular activity, including energy metabolism and protein synthesis, as well as produce mutations and damage cell membranes. Their potency is enhanced by their high rates of diffusion and their ability to cross cell membranes.

Many biologic responses, to ·NO reflect the affinity of this molecule for Fe, sulfhydryl groups (-SH) and, as shown in Figure 14, oxygen and its derivatives. A number of iron-containing enzymes are inhibited by ·NO, including ribonucleotide reductase, aconitase, and prolyl hydroxylase. Guanyl cyclase, in contrast, is activated by ·NO. The consequent increase in intracellular cGMP (cyclic guanosine 3,5´-monophosphate) underlies a variety of cellular responses to ·NO including the relaxation in vascular smooth muscle that leads to vasodilation.

Because these radicals are so reactive, there are a number of biologic defense mechanisms that limit their activities. Probably all cells possess catalase, SOD, and an enzyme called glutathione reductase. Glutathione reductase contains a sulfhydryl group and is an important antioxidant. Other naturally occurring antioxidants are α-tocopherol (vitamin E), ascorbic acid (vitamin C,) β-carotene, bilirubin, uric acid, pyruvate, flavinoids, ubiquinol, and a variety of molecules rich in thiol groups. Biologic mechanisms are also in place to limit the availability of free iron and copper ions, as these are powerful catalysts of the Fenton reaction (Fig. 14) and other reactions that generate free radicals.

Free Radicals in Orthopaedic Conditions

Inflammation

Large amounts of ·NO are synthesized at sites of inflammation in experimental animals. There is also evidence for the production of ·O_2^-, H_2O_2 and $ONOO^-$. In rodents, much of

Table 6		
Nitric Oxide Synthases		
Isoform	**Human Chromosomal Location**	**Presence in Musculoskeletal System**
nNOS=NOS-1	12	Skeletal muscle
iNOS=NOS-2	17	Cartilage, bone, intervertebral disk, synovium (?), meniscus (?)*
eNOS=NOS-3	7	Bone

* NOS-2 is only observed in these tissues after induction by cytokines or endotoxin.

the $\cdot$NO is produced by macrophages. In many, but not all animal models, including models of RA and lupus, inhibitors of iNOS prevent disease onset. As a result, there is considerable interest in developing inhibitors of this nature as antirheumatic and anti-inflammatory drugs. This enthusiasm needs to be tempered by several considerations, including the observations that not all NOS inhibitors are effective in all models; indeed, exacerbation is sometimes seen. In addition, human macrophages do not generate the large amounts of NO that rodent macrophages produce. SOD has proven to be a poor anti-inflammatory agent when administered to patients in human trials.

Osteoarthritis and Cartilage Repair

Articular chondrocytes do not synthesize NO constitutively, but become enthusiastic producers of this molecule after activation by cytokines such as IL-1. Moreover, cartilage recovered from arthritic joints spontaneously synthesizes elevated amounts of $\cdot$NO. Great interest was aroused by the recent observation that the NOS present in osteoarthritic cartilage was abnormal, and possibly a dysregulated form of nNOS. Until this enzyme is better characterized, it is being referred to as OA-NOS.

The role of $\cdot$NO in the metabolism of cartilage is better understood than in the metabolism of other musculoskeletal tissues. There is general agreement that $\cdot$NO inhibits the synthesis of the cartilaginous matrix, but the mechanism through which it does this is unknown. Whether $\cdot$NO also mediates matrix catabolism is presently controversial. Superoxide and H_2O_2 also inhibit matrix synthesis, possibly by lowering cellular levels of adenosine triphosphate. There is evidence that they activate latent matrix metalloproteinases and inactivate certain proteinase inhibitors. They may further damage matrix macromolecules directly.

Evidence also exists to suggest that $\cdot$NO causes apoptosis in chondrocytes. Interestingly, other free radicals such as $\cdot O_2^-$

may protect chondrocytes from this fate, by reacting with $\cdot$NO to form less harmful products (Fig. 14). When these same free radicals are produced in large excess over $\cdot$NO, they are no longer protective but produce necrotic cell death. This is a good example of why it is difficult to ascribe protective or destructive roles to individual free radicals under in vivo conditions. The complexity of the chemistry and biology of these substances defies such simplistic assertions.

The ability of these radicals to kill chondrocytes and reduce matrix synthesis suggests a role for them in OA, as well as indicates how they may impair cartilage repair. One problem with this hypothesis is the observation that matrix synthesis is increased in the cartilage of early and midstage disease.

Bone Metabolism and Aseptic Loosening

Osteoblasts, osteocytes, and osteoclasts possess cNOS and can be stimulated to express iNOS. The former enzyme produces small amounts of NO within bone in response to mechanical stress and is thought to be involved in the adaptive responses of bone to loading. The high levels of $\cdot$NO resulting from iNOS induction in bone inhibit osteoblast proliferation and differentiation, and may also induce apoptosis in these cells. High concentrations of $\cdot$NO have also been reported to inhibit osteoclastic activities. It is thus likely that $\cdot$NO is involved both in the normal, homeostatic physiology of bone, as well as in fracture healing and pathologic conditions such as osteoporosis. Recent data indicate the presence of iNOS in the pseudosynovium that surrounds aseptically loosened joint prostheses.

Summary

Free radicals posses highly complex biologies because their properties are highly dependent on concentration and the local biomechanical milieu. Unlike the other species discussed in this section, the regulated production of low

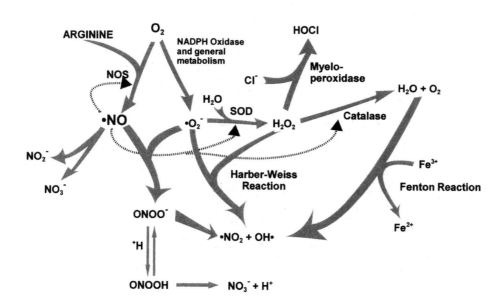

Figure 14

Free radical synthesis and interactions. Dashed lines indicate negative regulation by NO. SOD = Superoxide dismutase; NOS = Nitric oxide synthase; ONOO = Peroxynitrite; ONOOH = Peroxynitrous acid; HOCl = Hypochlorous acid.

levels of ·NO is of great importance to normal, homeostatic physiology. The large amounts of ·NO generated by iNOS, in contrast, appear to be related to disease but the details await definition. The chemical and biomechanical interactions between different radicals and their products are still being elucidated and will determine their ultimate biologic and pathophysiologic properties.

Cyclooxygenases and Inflammation

The analgesic, antipyretic and anti-inflammatory properties of certain nonsteroidal anti-inflammatory drugs were recognized as early as the middle of the nineteenth century but it was not until 1971 that a plausible mechanism of action was elucidated. It was discovered that these drugs blocked the synthesis and release of prostaglandins, such as prostaglandin E_2 (PGE_2) by inhibiting the activity of a rate-limiting enzyme called prostaglandin endoperoxide synthase or, as it is now referred to, cyclooxygenase (COX). As such, the discovery provided a unifying explanation for the therapeutic efficacy of this class of drugs but also firmly established PGs as important mediators of inflammatory diseases such as RA.

Two Isoforms of Cyclooxygenase

Cellular activation by proinflammatory stimuli results in, among other responses, increased PG synthesis, which may be important in the pathogenesis of many immune and inflammatory diseases. Acting locally in a paracrine or autocrine fashion, PGE_2 can initiate and modulate cell and tissue responses involved in many physiologic processes affecting essentially all organ systems. The formation of prostanoids results from the phospholipase-induced release of phospholipid-derived arachidonic acid (AA) and conversion of AA to prostaglandin H_2 (PGH_2) by the peroxidase activity of COX. PGH_2 is then converted to PGE_2 by the cyclooxygenase activity that has been determined to be rate-limiting. Two forms of COX have been identified to date: the constitutive COX-1 and the inducible COX-2. They are both integral, monotopic, endoplasmic-reticulum associated, homodimeric enzymes that posses heme-dependent peroxidase and COX activity. Structurally speaking, these bifunctional enzymes are composed of 3 independent folding units: an epidermal growth factor-like domain, a membrane-binding motif, and an enzymatic domain. Although the sites for the peroxidase and COX activities are adjacent, they have been shown to be spatially distinct as judged by x-ray crystallography. The COX-1 active site forms a long hydrophobic channel with critical tyrosine (385) and serine (530) amino acid residues at the apex of the channel. Aspirin and aspirin-like drugs (ibuprofen) act by excluding AA from the enzyme's active site although they do so by chemically distinct mechanisms. Aspirin irreversibly acetylates serine 530 (covalent modification) whereas ibuprofen excludes AA by steric hindrance.

Physiology of COX-1 and COX-2

COX-1 is constitutively expressed and, as such, is generally accepted to be involved in physiologically protective functions. Its activation leads, for instance, to the production of prostacyclin, which is antithrombogenic and cytoprotective when released by the endothelium and gastric mucosa, respectively. Current theory suggests that gastric ulceration caused by nonsteroidal anti-inflammatory drugs is a result of their inhibition of COX-1 catalysed PG synthesis. By extrapolation, elimination of COX-1 should result in spontaneous gastric ulceration. However, recent studies with COX-1 knockout mice (COX-1, –/–) indicate that the animals show no signs of gastric pathology or inflammation. Although the PG levels in the stomach of COX-1 (–/–) mice were the same as in indomethacin-treated wild-type animals, the latter had far higher incidences of gastric ulceration. Thus, PGs may not be required for gastric protection, and gastritis associated with nonsteroidal anti-inflammatory drug use may not be the result of COX-1 inhibition.

COX-2 is induced by inflammatory cytokines, tumor-promoting phorbol esters, and mitogenic factors; it is thus associated with pathophysiologic conditions, notably inflammation. COX-2 mRNA and enzyme levels are elevated in animal models of inflammation and in human articular synovial membranes and cartilage derived from patients suffering from OA and RA. Taken together, the data strongly implicated COX-2 in the pathogenesis of inflammatory disorders and resulted in heightened interest for developing COX-2 selective inhibitors that would be more efficacious and less toxic. However, the COX-2 knockout mouse model (COX-2, –/–) revealed some surprising results and led to a reevaluation of the role of COX-2 in inflammation. Using various model systems designed to elicit a local inflammatory response (leading to recruitment of monocytes and neutrophils and edema), no difference was observed between COX-2 (–/–) and their wild type counterparts, suggesting a certain redundancy in the pathways controlling inflammatory responses. COX-1 may be mediating the inflammatory response in the COX-2-deficient mice. Alternatively, leukotrienes produced from AA via the 5-lipoxygenase pathway could also be involved. The contribution of this latter pathway to the inflammatory response is evident in the 5-lipoxygenase knockout mouse in which ear inflammation produced by AA is substantially reduced.

Notwithstanding the traditional biologic functions associated with COX-2 expression, the COX-2-deficient mouse model has revealed the essential role of COX-2 in normal kidney development, vasoprotection, colon cancer, and fertility and ovulation. Rationalization of the role of COX-2 in the latter processes awaits further studies but the rather narrow view of PGs as merely inflammatory mediators must be reevaluated to include the notion that they are pleiotropic feedback bioregulators of tissue homeostasis.

Induction and Activation of the *COX-2* Gene

The *COX-2* gene (mRNA 4.1 kb) is rapidly induced by tumor promoters, growth factors, cytokines, and mitogens in many cell model systems. Regulation of COX-2 expression has been shown to occur at both transcriptional and post-transcriptional levels. The COX-2 message has an extensive 3' untranslated region with at least 2 distinct polyadenylation sites and 22 Shaw-Kamen 5' $AUUU_n$-A-3' motifs. The latter sequences are believed to be associated with message instability and rapid turnover. Sequence analysis of the 5'-flanking region has revealed the presence of several potential transcription regulatory sequences, as shown in Figure 15. These sites allow binding of specific nuclear factors whose translocation to the nucleus is the end result of signaling cascades initiated by specific growth factors, cytokines or other mediators. For example, binding of nuclear factor kappa B (NF-κB) or nuclear factor IL-6 (NF-IL-6) to their respective sites in the promoter region has been shown to mediate the induction of COX-2 by TNF-α, while lipopolysaccharide stimulation involves binding of NF-IL-6 and cAMP-responsive element. Despite this wealth of structural information, it is still unclear how the COX-2 gene is regulated by external stimuli in terms of signaling pathways.

In human synovial fibroblasts and chondrocytes, COX-2 gene expression is controlled to a large extent by serine/threonine phosphatase activity (such as PP-1, PP-2A). These enzymes regulate the level of phosphorylation and thus transcriptional activity of a number of nuclear factors that control COX-2 promoter activity. Signaling pathways probably include the protein kinase A and the Ras/MEKK-1/JNK cascades. It is likely, however, that COX-2 gene transcription induced by various classes of agonists is mediated by multiple, complex, and interacting pathways, dependent on cellular context.

Role of COX-2 in the Pathogenesis of Rheumatoid Arthritis

Synovial tissues of patients with RA display characteristics that are strikingly similar to malignancies, including cell proliferation, angiogenesis, and invasion of surrounding tissues. This aggressively transformed phenotype appears to be the result of locally produced factors that include cytokines, growth factors, and eicosanoids. Complex cell-cell and cell-biologic effector interactions appear to be fundamental to the maintenance of this aggressive phenotype. The principal source of cytokines and other chemical factors

is likely to be infiltrating macrophages and lymphocytes, particularly natural killer cells.

Large increases in COX-2 mRNA expression, protein synthesis, and PGE_2 production have been observed in RA synovia and cartilage. It is known that PGE_2 is antiapoptotic in human connective tissue cells, based on the observation that exogenously added PGE_2 prevents actinomycin D-induced apoptosis in synovial fibroblasts in culture. Furthermore, PGE_2 prevented nonsteroidal anti-inflammatory drug-induced apoptosis in these same cells, strongly supporting the notion that the eicosanoid is cytoprotective and/or antiapoptotic in an autocrine/paracrine context. Perhaps as a result of this action, PGE_2 can stimulate cell proliferation of type B human synovial fibroblasts and may contribute to pannus formation in patients with RA. In support of this notion is the observation that the proinflammatory cytokines can increase COX-2 expression and proliferation of human vascular endothelial cells, thereby contributing to angiogenesis.

Although COX-1 is also increased in RA synovia as a result of increased cellularity, COX-2 is the only isoform capable of producing the levels of PGE_2 necessary to stimulate proliferation and inhibit apoptosis. The role played by PGs in the development and perpetuation of chronic inflammatory rheumatic diseases is likely to be quite complex, and there is now evidence that eicosanoids can elicit effects that are clearly proinflammatory but also homeostatic.

Selective Inhibition of COX-2

Anti-inflammatory glucocorticoids (eg, prednisone) are by far the most potent inhibitors of COX-2 and display some selectivity to the extent that COX-1 expression is not affected to any significant degree. However, virtually every tissue is a glucocorticoid target and the untoward side effects, eg, immunosuppression, of using this type of medication for protracted periods of time make their use questionable. On the other hand, since nonsteroidal anti-inflammatory drug gastropathy is the second most deadly rheumatic disease, the need to develop more selective COX inhibitors is even more urgent. Several classes of COX-2 inhibitors have now been tested and have been shown to have a far more favorable side effects profile than the nonselective nonsteroidal anti-inflammatory drug currently in use. Selective COX-2 inhibitors decrease PG production in situations where COX-2 activity is increased (inflammatory episodes), but do not alter basal production due to COX-1 activity. As such, in tissues, such as the kidney, endothelium, and gastrointestinal tract, where PGs mediate important homeostatic functions, there is a decreased likelihood of tissue pathologies. Furthermore, selective COX-2 inhibitors block the local production of PGs by inflamed joint tissues far more effectively and are thus indicated for the treatment of inflamma-

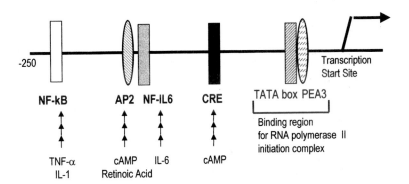

Figure 15

Schematic representation of the cyclooxygenase-2 (COX-2) promotor region and possible pathways of activation. This region contains various sequence motifs which bind nuclear activation factors, such as nuclear factor κB (NF-κB), activator protein 2 (AP-2), and cAMP responsive element (CRE). These factors regulate the expression of numerous other genes activated during inflammatory conditions. The transcription start site is indicated by the arrow. The TATA sequence (TATA box) is commonly found upstream but in close proximity to the transcription start site. The RNA polymerase II initiation complex, consisting of the TATA box binding protein (TBP) and 8 or more other subunits (TAFs, transcription activating factors), assembles around the TATA box, allowing RNA polymerase II to bind and start the transcription process. Binding of PEA3 (polyoma virus enhancer A3) further enhances transcription, as might occupation of sites further upstream by their appropriate nuclear binding proteins. Multiple arrow sequences indicate signaling cascades initiated by binding of cytokines or growth factors to their respective receptors and that lead to binding of regulatory proteins to specific sequences in the promoter region, resulting in increased transcription.

tory rheumatic diseases. However, it remains to be determined what the role of COX-2 and PGs is in terms of the progression of erosive joint disease.

Proteases

The agents ultimately responsible for damage to articular joint tissues are the proteases. The function of a protease is to cleave peptide bonds between contiguous amino acid residues. This is accomplished by nucleophilic attack on the peptide bond, resulting in the addition of a water molecule and thus the generation of new C- and N-terminal amino acid residues. The catalytic efficiency of this process depends on the protein substrate being positioned in the enzyme molecule in such a way that the residue serving as a nucleophile is in close proximity to the peptide bond to be cleaved. A bewildering array of proteases is present in all compartments of cells and tissues, and many of them are involved in inflammatory processes (Table 7). However, while they represent a diverse group of enzymes, proteases all use similar mechanisms for substrate binding and catalysis.

The substrate binding site of a typical protease consists of an extended cleft containing, in addition to the catalytic residues, subsites termed S_3 to S_1 and S_1' to S_3' that interact with residues of the protein substrate upstream and downstream of the peptide bond to be cleaved (Fig. 16). These subsites confer differing degrees of specificity to the enzyme, determining where the protein molecule will be cleaved. In the extreme case, the caspases, discussed earlier in this section, cleave uniquely after an aspartyl residue. However, protease selectively is usually much more general in nature; for example, the lysosomal cysteine proteases,

such as cathepsin L, prefer large aromatic residues such as phenylalanine at the S_2 subsite, and exhibit little selectivity at other positions, whereas the MMPs show their major preference in the type of residue occupying the S_1' subsite. Although all proteases consist of a catalytic unit, many also contain additional domains that aid in substrate recognition and binding. The collagenases, for example, consist of a typical MMP catalytic domain that is connected by a flexible linker to a so-called hemopexin domain, which provides this group of enzymes with the ability to bind to and cleave triple helical collagen.

Protease Classification

The original protease classification system, based on the catalytic group in the active site, was proposed in 1960 and is still widely used, although it requires slight refinement based on recent findings. Four classes are commonly recognized; the aspartic-, serine-, cysteine-, and metalloproteinases (Table 8).

The catalytic activity of the aspartic proteases is based on the presence of 2 active site aspartic residues that account for the acidic pH optimum of these enzymes. Although the lysosomal aspartic protease, cathepsin D, is probably responsible for a considerable proportion of the proteolysis of endocytosed matrix components, it is unlikely that enzymes in this class play any role in ECM degradation of cartilage matrix. The absence of inhibitors for this family of enzymes reinforces this proposal.

Serine proteases in which the active serine residue is responsible for nucleophilic attack on the peptide bond represent the most abundant class. These enzymes are active at neutral pH and mediate many normal extracellu-

Table 7
Proteases Mediating Inflammation and Joint Erosion

Site of Action		Protease	Function
Intracellular	Cytosol	Caspases (cysteine)	Apoptosis; IL-1 activation
		Proteasome (threonine)	Antigen processing (MHC class I); inactivation of I-κB
	Lysosome	Cathepsin D (aspartic)	General proteolysis
		Cathepsin B, L (cysteine)	General proteolysis
		Cathepsin K (cysteine)	Bone resorption
	Endosome	Cathepsins L, S, etc (cysteine)	Antigen processing (MHC class II)
	Specialized granules	Cathepsin G, Elastase (serine)*	Neutrophils — removal of cellular debris and degradation of extracellular matrix
		Chymases, tryptases (serine)*	Mast cells — degradation of extracellular matrix following IGE-mediated degranulation
Cell Surface		MT-MMPs (metallo)	Gelatinase activation
		ADAMs (metallo)	TNF-α activation (TACE)
Extracellular	Tissue	MMPs (metallo)	Matrix degradation
		ADAMTS (metallo)	
		Plasminogen activators (serine)	Removal of fibrin deposits
	Plasma	Plasmin (serine)	Removal of fibrin deposits

* These proteases are active in the extracellular environment following secretion. ADAM = A disintegrin and metalloprotease; ADAMTS = ADAM containing a thrombospondin motif; MT-MMP = Membrane-type matrix metalloprotease; I-κ B = Inhibitor of nuclear factor κ B; TNF-α = Tumor necrosis factor α; TACE = TNF-α converting enzyme; IL-1 = Interleukin-1

lar events such as blood coagulation and clot lysis. Other examples of serine proteases that may play a role in the degradation of cartilage matrix components are the polymorphonuclear leukocyte products, elastase and cathepsin G, and the mast cell chymases and tryptases. A member of the serine protease family that has been studied extensively with respect to inflammatory processes is plasminogen activator. Its main function, as the name implies, is the activation of plasminogen to yield active plasmin, the main mediator of clot lysis. A role for plasmin has been proposed in the activation of some members of the metalloprotease family, particularly the collagenases and stromelysin; however, the relative importance of this activation pathway is not clear.

The catalytic feature of the serine residue is its hydroxyl group. Recently it has been shown that the hydroxyl group of threonine can also play a catalytic role in proteolysis, indicating the existence of an additional protease class. The proteasome, a complex intracellular multisubunit complex responsible for turnover of cytoplasmic proteins, including the processing of antigenic peptides for presentation by the MHC class I system, is composed of a series of threonine protease subunits.

The catalytic nucleophile in the active site of cysteine proteases is a cysteine residue. The pH optimum of most of these enzymes is on the acidic side and some (cathepsins B and L) are inactivated at elevated pH, due to structural instability. This process limits their extracellular activity. In addition, like many other proteases, the cysteine proteases are synthesized as inactive proforms. Many cysteine pro-

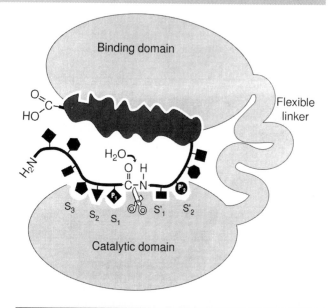

Figure 16

Diagrammatic representation of a multidomain protease consisting of a catalytic domain where peptide bond cleavage occurs (arrow) connected by a flexible linker to a second domain which binds to regions of the protein substrate (black) remote to that under attack. The active site cleft contains a series of subsites (S_3 to S_3') that accept, with different degrees of selectivity, amino acid residues of the substrate. Proteases generally contain subsites for the binding of 5 or more residues. Although many proteases consist of a simple catalytic unit, the multidomain approach shown here allows the enzyme to bind more tightly to its protein substrate or to facilitate access of the catalytic domain to the region to be cleaved. For example, collagenases use a binding domain, referred to as the hemopexin domain, to locally unwind the collagen triple helix, permitting cleavage in this area.

teases are located in the lysosomes; however, there is a remarkably varied distribution between different cell types. Cathepsins B and L are elevated in cells of the monocytic lineage present in areas with increased erosive activity in bone and cartilage. High cathepsin B content characterizes the septoclast, a cell present in the vicinity of blood vessels invading the growth plate during resorption of the calcified matrix. Cathepsin K is almost uniquely restricted to the osteoclast and is thought to be responsible for the majority of proteolysis occurring in osteoclast-mediated bone resorption. In addition, a series of novel cysteine proteases (cathepsins L2, W, and Z) has been discovered recently, and it is becoming clear that these enzymes, together with cathepsins S and L, are important players in antigen presentation through the class II pathway. The activity of the lysosomal cysteine proteases is generally restricted to this intracellular organelle, but evidence for an extracellular role is accumulating. Increased secretion of the precursor forms of cathepsins B and L has been observed under some pathologic conditions. In contrast to their active counterparts, the precursor forms are stable at physiologic pH and thus can accumulate in the extracellular milieu until conditions are favorable for their activation.

A large and still increasing subfamily of the cysteine proteases are the caspases, which are evolutionarily unrelated to the lysosomal cysteine proteases. They are of particular importance in inflammatory processes, because activation of IL-1 is carried out by caspase 1 (IL-1 converting enzyme, ICE), which was the first member of this family to be characterized. The other caspases are mediators of apoptosis, and their properties and mechanism of action are described in more detail in the section dealing with cell death.

The metalloproteinases, in particular the MMPs, are currently believed to be the major mediators of ECM degradation. In this protease class, a metal ion, almost exclusively Zn^{2+}, is chelated into the active site and activates the water molecule that will add to the substrate peptide bond under attack. The MMPs represent a large family of structurally related metalloproteinases that are active at neutral pH. Most are multidomain proteins allowing the enzyme to bind large substrate molecules, such as type II collagen fibers in the case of the collagenases. MMPs degrade aggrecan and other matrix components present in articular cartilage. These enzymes are secreted as inactive precursors, and thus require activation. Whereas several proteases can achieve this important step in vitro, the processes operative under physiologic and pathologic conditions in vivo are still unclear. The plasminogen activator/plasmin system may be operative under some pathologic conditions; however, the essentially normal growth and skeletal development in mice deficient in either one or both forms of plasminogen activator suggests that other mechanisms are responsible for the activation of MMPs. A subfamily of membrane-type (MT) MMPs has been described recently. These enzymes are associated with the cell membrane as a result of the presence of a membrane-spanning domain. They appear to play a role in the activation of other MMPs, in particular gelatinase A.

Another newly described group of metalloproteases is the ADAMs, mentioned earlier. These enzymes also consist of several domains with different functions. In addition to the Zn^{2+}-dependent protease domain, the ADAMs proteases contain an integrin-binding domain as well as the membrane spanning region localizing the enzyme to the cell surface. This functional combination results in a protease that is able to bind to and disrupt molecules close to the cell surface in a very directed fashion. Generation of TNF-α from its membrane-bound proform is mediated by TNF-α-converting enzyme or TACE (ADAM 17), which belongs to this protease family.

A branch of the ADAMs family that lacks the membrane-spanning domain, but contains several copies of a domain similar to the C-terminal portion of thrombospondin (TS

Table 8

Protease Inhibitors

Protease Class	Inhibitors	Representative Proteases
Aspartic	—	Cathepsin D
Serine	Serpins (α_1PI, α_1AP)	Elastase, Plasmin
Cysteine	Cystatins IAPs	Cathepsin B, Cathepsin L, etc Caspases
Metalloproteinase	TIMPs	Collagenase, Stromelysin, ADAMs
General	α_2-macroglobulin	Most proteases

To date, no specific inhibitor of aspartic proteases has been described in mammals.
α_1PI, α_1-protease inhibitor α_1 antitrypsin; α_1AP, α_1-plasmin inhibitor; IAP, inhibitor of apoptosis; TIMP, tissue inhibitor of metalloproteinases; ADAM, a disintegrin and metalloprotease.

domain) has recently been identified. Of particular significance are ADAMTS2, the protease responsible for cleavage of the N-terminal propeptide of fibrillar collagens, and ADAMTS4 and 11, which cleave aggrecan at the aggrecanase cleavage site.

Control of Proteolysis

Control of proteolysis is of paramount importance for the survival of cells and organisms and is achieved in several ways. Rates of synthesis of proteolytic enzymes can be regulated at the transcriptional level. This control mechanism has been well characterized for the MMPs collagenase-1, collagenase-3, and stromelysin, where their synthesis is greatly increased in response to IL-1 and, to a somewhat lesser extent, TNF-α, while constitutive synthesis is usually very low. Other proteases, most notably the cysteine proteases, are produced at relatively constant rates, although often in a cell-specific manner, and the mechanisms regulating the transcriptional activity of their genes are not well understood at present.

As noted above, most proteases are synthesized as inactive precursors, preventing their activity in the biosynthetic and secretory compartments of the cell. Activation, as a result of proteolytic removal of the N-terminal proregion, generally occurs once these enzymes have reached their final destination, as is the case for the lysosomal enzymes in which activation occurs when the proenzyme encounters an acidic environment. Alternatively, activation is only permitted when the need for increased proteolytic activity arises, as in the well-characterized blood coagulation and clot lysis pathways. Activation of the MMPs is less-well understood but is an important aspect of their biology since these protease are released into the extracellular environment as their proforms. In addition to increased synthesis of MMPs, their activation may well be an important control point in the matrix degradation as a result of the action of inflammatory cytokines.

Protease inhibitors represent a final control mechanism. A large variety of inhibitors is present in all organisms, in the cytoplasmic as well as in the extracellular milieu. Table 8 summarizes some of these class-specific inhibitors. Plasma is probably the most well-known source of protease inhibitors for all classes of proteases, with a heavy bias towards the serine proteinases, because these are the most abundant proteases found in this environment. Noteworthy in plasma is the multifunctional protease inhibitor, $\alpha2$-macroglobulin, which acts as a trap, because it contains a bait region presenting substrates for most proteases. Following cleavage of this bait region, the inhibitor covalently captures the protease for subsequent clearance from the circulation.

As indicated above, the MMPs represent a potent source of degradative potential in the ECM but this is normally offset by the presence of a series of family specific inhibitors termed TIMPs. It is only when the balance between active enzyme and inhibitor is overwhelmed that matrix degradation can take place. The elucidation of the 3-dimensional structures of many proteases has provided detailed understanding of the interactions underlying substrate binding and as a result has allowed the design of inhibitors with high affinity for specific proteases—a process referred to as rational drug design. Several inhibitors have been developed for the inactivation of specific metalloproteinases, such as gelatinase A, which is a target for tumor growth and metastasis, and collagenase-3, which is a target for arthritis. Some MMP inhibitors are currently being used therapeutically and others are undergoing clinical trials.

Selected Bibliography

Articular Cartilage

Billinghurst RC, Dahlberg L, Ionescu M, et al: Enhanced cleavage of type II collagen by collagenases in osteoarthritic articular cartilage. *J Clin Invest* 1997;99:1534–1545.

Docherty AJ, O'Connell J, Crabbe T, Angal S, Murphy G: The matrix metalloproteinases and their natural inhibitors: Prospects for treating degenerative tissue diseases. *Trends Biotechnol* 1992;10:200–207.

Poole AR: Cartilage in health and disease, in Koopman WJ (ed): Arthritis and Allied Conditions: *A Textbook of Rheumatology*. Baltimore, MD, Williams & Wilkins, 1997, pp 255–308.

Poole AR: Skeletal and inflammation markers in aging and osteoarthritis: Implications for early diagnosis and monitoring of the effects of therapy, in Hamerman D (ed): *Osteoarthritis: Public Health Implications for an Aging Population*. Baltimore, MD, Johns Hopkins University Press, 1997, pp 187–214.

Poole AR, Alini M, Hollander AP: Cellular biology of cartilage degradation, in Henderson B, Edwards JCW, Pettipher ER (eds): *Mechanisms and Models in Rheumatoid Arthritis*. London, England, Academic Press, 1995, pp 163–204.

Woessner JF Jr: Matrix metalloproteinases and their inhibitors in connective tissue remodeling. *FASEB J* 1991;5:2145–2154.

The Synovium

Arend WP, Dayer JM: Inhibition of the production and effects of interleukin-1 and tumor necrosis factor alpha in rheumatoid arthritis. *Arthritis Rheum* 1995;38:151-160.

Firestein GS, Echeverri F, Yeo M, Zvaifler NJ, Green DR: Somatic mutations in the p53 tumor suppressor gene in rheumatoid arthritis synovium. *Proc Natl Acad Sci USA* 1997;94:10895–10900.

Firestein GS, Zvaifler NJ: How important are T cells in chronic rheumatoid synovitis? *Arthritis Rheum* 1990;33:768–773.

Liblau RS, Singer SM, McDevitt HO: Th1 and Th2 CD4$^+$ T cells in the pathogenesis of organ-specific autoimmune diseases. *Immunol Today* 1995;16:34–38.

Müller-Ladner U, Kriegsmann J, Franklin BN, et al: Synovial fibroblasts of patients with rheumatoid arthritis attach to and invade normal human cartilage when engrafted into SCID mice. *Am J Pathol* 1996;149:1607–1615.

Penzotti JE, Nepom GT, Lybrand TP: Use of T cell receptor/HLA-DRB1*04 molecular modeling to predict site-specific interactions for the DR shared epitope associated with rheumatoid arthritis. *Arthritis Rheum* 1997;40:1316–1326.

Pitsillides AA, Wilkinson LS, Mehdizadeh S, Bayliss MT, Edwards JC: Uridine diphosphoglucose dehydrogenase activity in normal and rheumatoid synovium: The description of a specialized synovial lining cell. *Int J Exp Pathol* 1993;74:27–34.

Roivainen A, Jalava J, Pirala L, Yli-Jama T, Tiusanen H, Toivanen P: H-ras oncogene point mutations in arthritic synovium. *Arthritis Rheum* 1997;40:1636–1643.

Zvaifler NJ, Firestein GS: Pannus and pannocytes: Alternative models of joint destruction in rheumatoid arthritis. *Arthritis Rheum* 1994;37:783–789.

Bone

Athanasou NA: Cellular biology of bone-resorbing cells. *J Bone Joint Surg* 1996;78A:1096–1112.

Bogoch E, Gschwend N, Bogoch B, Rahn B, Perren S: Changes in the metaphysis and diaphysis of the femur proximal to the knee in rabbits with experimentally induced inflammatory arthritis. *Arthritis Rheum* 1989;32:617–624.

Collin-Osdoby P: Role of vascular endotheliel cells in bone biology. *J Cell Biochem* 1994;55:304-309.

Eriksen EF, Axelrod DW, Melson F: *Bone Histomorphometry*. New York, NY, Raven Press, 1994.

Hayashida K, Ochi T, Fujimoto M, et al: Bone marrow changes in adjuvant-induced and collagen-induced arthritis: Interleukin-1 and interleukin-6 activity and abnormal myelopoiesis. *Arthritis Rheum* 1992;35:241–245.

Suzuki Y, Tanihara M, Ichikawa Y, et al: Periarticular osteopenia in adjuvant induced arthritis: Role of interleukin-1 in decreased osteogenic and increased resorptive potential of bone marrow cells. *Ann Rheum Dis* 1995;54:484–490.

van Soesbergen RM, Lips P, van den Ende A, vander Korst JK: Bone metabolism in rheumatoid arthritis compared with postmenopausal osteoporosis. *Ann Rheum Dis* 1986;45:149–155.

Zhang J, Weichman BM, Lewis AJ: Role of animal models in the study of rheumatoid arthritis: An overview, in Henderson B, Edwards JCW, Pettipher ER (eds): *Mechanisms and Models in Rheumatoid Arthritis*. Toronto, Canada, Academic Press Limited, 1995, pp 363–371.

Tendons and Ligaments

Frank C: The biology of ligament reconstruction, in Niwa S, Yoshino S, Kurosaka M, et al (eds): *Reconstruction of the Knee Joint*. Tokyo, Japan, Springer, 1997, pp 7–27.

Gelberman R, Goldberg V, An K-N, Banes A: Tendon, in Woo SL-Y, Buckwalter JA (eds): *Injury and Repair of Musculoskeletal Soft Tissues*. Park Ridge, IL, American Academy of Orthopaedic Surgeons, 1988, pp 5–40.

Nabeshima Y, Grood ES, Sakurai A, Herman JH: Uniaxial tension inhibits tendon collagen degradation by collagenase in vitro. *J Orthop Res* 1996;14:123–130.

Schumacher HR Jr: Morphology and physiology of normal synovium and the effects of mechanical stimulation, in Gordon SL, Blair SJ, Fine LJ (eds): *Repetitive Motion Disorders of the Upper Extremity*. Rosemont, IL, American Academy of Orthopaedic Surgeons, 1995, pp 263–276.

Simmen BR, Gschwend N: Tendon diseases in chronic rheumatoid arthritis. [German] *Orthopade* 1995;24:224–236.

Cytokines and Inflammation

Baggiolini M: Chemokines and leukocyte traffic. *Nature* 1998;392:565–568.

Feldmann M, Brennan FM, Maini RN: Role of cytokines in rheumatoid arthritis. *Annu Rev Immunol* 1996;14:397–440.

Kronenberg HM, Lee K, Lanske B, Segre GV: Parathyroid hormone-related protein and Indian hedgehog control the pace of cartilage differentiation. *J Endocrinol* 1997;154(suppl):S39–S45.

van den Berg WB: Lessons for joint destruction from animal models. *Corr Opin Rheumatol* 1997;9:221–228.

Weckmann AL, Alcocer-Varela J: Cytokine inhibitors in autoimmune disease. *Semin Arthritis Rheum* 1996;26:539–557.

The Role of Immune Cells in Inflammatory Joint Disease

Fox DA: The role of T cells in the immunopathogenesis of rheumatoid arthritis: New perspectives. *Arthritis Rheum* 1997;40:598–609.

Harris ED Jr: Rheumatoid arthritis: Pathophysiology and implications for therapy. *N Engl J Med* 1990;322:1277–1289.

Lanchbury JS, Pitzalis C: Cellular immune mechanisms in rheumatoid arthritis and other inflammatory arthritides. *Curr Opin Immunol* 1993;5:918–924.

Steinman L: A few autoreactive cells in an autoimmune infiltrate control a vast population of nonspecific cells: A tale of smart bombs and the infantry. *Proc Natl Acad Sci USA* 1996;93:2253–2256.

Wucherpfennig KW, Strominger JL: Selective binding of self peptides to disease-associated major histocompatibility complex (MHC) molecules: A mechanism for MHC-linked susceptibility to human autoimmune diseases. *J Exp Med* 1995;181:1597–1601.

Endothelial Cell Interactions and Angiogenesis

Beck L Jr, D'Amore PA: Vascular development: Cellular and molecular regulation. *FASEB J* 1997;11:365–373.

Kavanaugh A, Oppenheimer-Marks N: The role of the vascular endothelium in the pathogenesis of vascultitis, in LeRoy EC (ed): *Systemic Vasculitis: The Biological Basis.* New York, NY, Marcel Dekker, 1992, pp 27–48.

Munro JM, Pober JS, Cotran RS: Tumor necrosis factor and interferon-gamma induce distinct patterns of endothelial activation and associated leukocyte accumulation in skin of Papio anubis. *Am J Pathol* 1989;135:121–133.

Oppenheimer-Marks N, Lipsky PE: Adhesion molecules and the regulation of the migration of lymphocytes, in Hamann A (ed): *Adhesion Molecules and Chemokines in Lymphocyte Trafficking.* Amsterdam, The Netherlands, Harwood Academic Publishers, 1997, pp 55–87.

Picker LJ, Siegelman MH: Lymphoid tissues and organs, in Paul WE (ed): *Fundamental Immunology,* ed 3. New York, NY, Raven Press, 1993, pp 145–197.

Thomas KA: Vascular endothelial growth factor: A potent and selective angiogenic agent. *J Biol Chem* 1996;271:603–606.

Fibrosis

Border WA, Noble NA: Transforming growth factor-beta in tissue fibrosis. *N Engl J Med* 1994;331:1286–1292.

Kovacs EJ, DiPietro LA: Fibrogenic cytokines and connective tissue production. *FASEB J* 1994;8:854–861.

Massague J: TGF-beta signaling: Receptors, transducers, and Mad proteins. *Cell* 1996;85:947–950.

Roberts AB, Sporn MB, Assoian RK, et al: Transforming growth factor type beta: Rapid induction of fibrosis and angiogenesis in vivo and stimulation of collagen formation in vitro. *Proc Natl Acad Sci USA* 1986;83:4167–4171.

Varga J, Jimenez SA: Modulation of collagen gene expression: Its relation to fibrosis in systemic sclerosis and other disorders. *Ann Intern Med* 1995;122:60–62.

Apoptosis

Nagata S: Apoptosis by death factor. *Cell* 1997;88:355–365.

Nicholson DW, Thornberry NA: Caspases: Killer proteases. *Trends Biochem Sci* 1997;22:299–306.

Rudin CM, Thompson CB: Apoptosis and disease: Regulation and clinical relevance of programmed cell death. *Annu Rev Med* 1997;48:267–281.

Hughes DE, Boyce BF: Apoptosis in bone physiology and disease. *Mol Pathol* 1997;50:132–137.

Thornberry NA, Lazebnik Y: Caspases: Enemies within. *Science* 1998;281:1312–1316.

Nitric Oxide, Other Free Radicals, and Related Species

Caderas E: Biochemistry of oxygen toxicity. *Ann Rev Biochem* 1989;58:79–110.

Evans CH, Stefanovic-Racic M, Lancaster J: Nitric oxide and its role in orthopaedic disease. *Clin Orthop* 1995;312:275–294.

Evans C, Watkins SC, Stefanovic-Racic M: Nitric oxide and cartilage metabolism. *Meth Enzymol* 1996;269B:75–88.

Farrell AJ, Blake DR: Nitric oxide. *Ann Rheum Dis* 1996;55:7–20.

Halliwell B: Oxygen radicals, nitric oxide and human inflammatory joint disease. *Ann Rheum Dis* 1995;54:505–510.

Murrell GAC, Dolan MM, Jan D, Szabo C, Warren RF, Hannifin JA: Nitric oxide: An important articular free radical. *J Bone Joint Surg* 1996;78A:265–274.

Nathan C, Xie Q-W: Nitric oxide synthases: Roles, tolls and controls. *Cell* 1994;78:915–918.

Cyclooxygenases and Inflammation

Vane JR: Inhibition of prostaglandin synthesis as a mechanism of action for aspirin-like drugs. *Nature* 1971;231:232–235.

Vane JR, Botting RM: New insights into the mode of action of antiinflammatory drugs. *Inflamm Res* 1995;44:1–10.

Herschman HR: Prostaglandin synthase-2. *Biochim Biophys Acta* 1996;1299:125–140.

Bazan N, Botting J, Van J (eds): *New Targets in Inflammatory Inhibitors of COX-2 or Adhesion Molecules.* Boston, MA, William Harvey Press, 1996.

Proteases

Chapman HA, et al: Emerging roles for cysteine proteases in human biology. *Ann Rev Physiol* 1997;59:63–88.

Birkedal-Hansen H: Proteolytic remodeling of extracellular matrix. *Curr Opin Cell Biol* 1995;7:728–735.

Chapter 20

The Meniscus: Structure, Function, Repair, and Replacement

Steven P. Arnoczky, DVM

Cahir A. McDevitt, PhD

This chapter at a glance

This chapter describes some of the basic science aspects of the human meniscus.

Introduction

The menisci are C-shaped disks of fibrocartilage interposed between the condyles of the femur and tibia. Once described as the functionless remains of leg muscle, the menisci are now realized to be integral components in the complex biomechanics of the knee joint. This realization has resulted in a renewed interest in the basic science of the meniscus in terms of its structure, function, and physiology. This chapter will describe some of these basic science aspects of the human meniscus.

Gross Anatomy

The menisci of the knee joint are soft-tissue extensions of the tibia that serve to deepen the articular surfaces of the tibial plateau to better accommodate the condyles of the femur. The peripheral border of each meniscus is thick, convex, and attached to the inside capsule of the joint; the opposite border tapers to a thin free edge. The proximal surfaces of the menisci are concave and in contact with the condyles of the femur; their distal surfaces are flat and rest on the head of the tibia (Fig. 1).

The medial meniscus is semicircular in form. It is approximately 3.5 cm in length and considerably wider posteriorly than it is anteriorly (Fig. 2). The anterior horn of the medial meniscus is attached to the tibial plateau in the area of the anterior intercondylar fossa in front of the anterior cruciate ligament (ACL). The posterior fibers of the anterior horn attachment merge with the transverse ligament, which connects the anterior horns of the medial and lateral menisci. The posterior horn of the medial meniscus is firmly attached to the posterior intercondylar fossa of the tibia between the attachments of the lateral meniscus and the posterior cruciate ligament. The periphery of the medial meniscus is attached to the joint capsule throughout its length. The tibial portion of the capsular attachment is often referred to as the coronary ligament. At its midpoint, the medial meniscus is almost firmly attached to the femur and tibia through a condensation in the joint capsule known as the deep medial collateral ligament.

The lateral meniscus is almost circular and covers a larger portion of the tibial articular surface than the medial meniscus (Fig. 2). It is approximately the same width from front to back. The anterior horn of the lateral meniscus is attached to the tibia in front of the intercondylar eminence and behind the attachment of the ACL, with which it partially blends. The posterior horn of the lateral meniscus is attached behind the intercondylar eminence of the tibia in front of the posterior end of the medial meniscus. Although there is no attachment of the lateral meniscus to the lateral collateral ligament, there is a loose peripheral attachment to the joint capsule.

Several ligaments run from the posterior horn of the lateral meniscus to the medial femoral condyle, either just in front of or behind the origin of the posterior cruciate ligament; these are known as the anterior meniscofemoral ligament (ligament of Humphrey) and the posterior meniscofemoral ligament (ligament of Wrisberg) (Fig. 3).

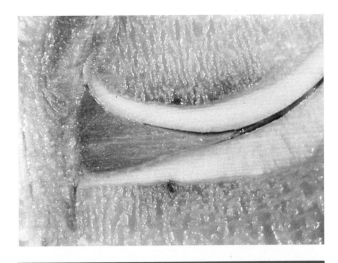

Figure 1

Frontal section of the medial compartment of a human knee illustrating the articulation of the menisci with the condyles of the femur and tibia. (Reproduced with permission from Warren RF, Arnoczky SP, Wickiewicz TL: Anatomy of the knee, in Nicholas JA, Hershman EB (eds): *The Lower Extremity and Spine in Sports Medicine*. St. Louis, MO, CV Mosby, 1986, pp 657–694.)

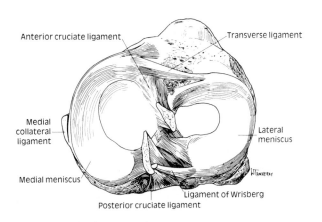

Figure 2

Drawing of a tibial plateau showing the shape and attachments of the medial and lateral menisci. (Reproduced with permission from Warren RF, Arnoczky SP, Wickiewicz TL: Anatomy of the knee, in Nicholas JA, Hershman EB (eds): *The Lower Extremity and Spine in Sports Medicine*. St. Louis, MO, CV Mosby, 1986, pp 657–694.)

Meniscal Function

Meniscal Motion

As the knee passes through the range of motion, the menisci move with respect to the tibial articular surface. A classic study demonstrated that from 0 to 120° of knee flexion, the mean meniscal excursion (defined as the average antero-posterior displacement of the anterior and posterior meniscal horns along the tibial plateau in the midcondylar, parasagittal plane) of the medial meniscus was 5.1 ± 0.96 mm, whereas that of the lateral meniscus was 11.2 ± 3.27 mm (Fig. 7). The lack of bony opposition (that is, convex femoral condyle and tibial plateau), an unconstrained peripheral margin, and the close approximation of its central tibial attachment appear to allow the lateral meniscus a greater degree of movement.

Rotation of the knee joint also has an effect on meniscal motion with a greater effect being observed in the lateral meniscus. The posterior oblique fibers of the medial collateral ligament appear to limit the movement of the medial meniscus in rotation, which may increase its risk of tear injury.

In addition to their anteroposterior translation, the menisci deform to remain in constant congruity to the tibial and femoral articular surfaces throughout the full range of joint motion. This deformation allows the meniscus to provide additional joint stability. The anterior horn segments of the medial and lateral menisci demonstrate differing mobility compared with posterior horn segments. This differential allows the menisci to assume a decreasing radius with flexion that correlates with a decreasing radius of curvature of the posterior femoral condyle. The change in radius enables the menisci to maintain congruity with the articulating surfaces throughout flexion. The greatest deformation appears to occur at the anterior medial horn as it moves onto the tibial plateau with flexion and is manifested as an increase in the concavity of the superior articulating meniscal surface. This is probably caused by the increasing load resulting from femoral flexion.

Material Properties

The functional behavior of the meniscus can best be understood when it is viewed as a biphasic medium comprising a fluid phase (the interstitial water with the inorganic salts dissolved in it) and a solid phase (the collagen-proteoglycan organic solid matrix composing the fluid-filled porous-permeable medium). This biphasic nature can explain the fundamental mechanism by which the interstitial fluid flow and the porous solid matrix deformation contribute to the overall mechanical behavior of the meniscus. Like articular cartilage, the mechanical behavior of meniscal tissue is viscoelastic when subjected to loading. This viscoelastic response is probably dependent on 2 fundamental physical

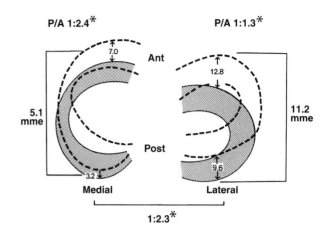

Figure 7

Diagram of mean meniscal excursion (mme) along the tibial plateau. The ratio of posterior to anterior translation (P/A) was significant (* $p < 0.05$). (Reproduced with permission from Thompson WO, Thaete FL, Fu FH, Dye SF: Tibial meniscal dynamics using three-dimensional reconstruction of magnetic resonance images. *Am J Sports Med* 1991;19:210–215.)

mechanisms: the intrinsic viscoelastic properties of the macromolecules (collagen, proteoglycan, and other structural macromolecules) comprising the organic solid matrix, and the frictional drag exerted by the interstitial fluid as it flows through the porous-permeable solid matrix.

Experimental studies have shown that in compression the meniscus has approximately half the intrinsic elastic modulus and one sixth to one tenth the permeability of articular cartilage. This would suggest that the compressive viscoelastic creep behavior of the meniscus is governed, to a large degree, by the interstitial fluid flowing through the tissue during compression. The combination of low compressive stiffness and low permeability suggests that the menisci, as structures, should function as highly efficient shock absorbers. Because the combined mass of the menisci is much greater than that of the articular cartilage-bearing load across the femoromeniscotibial articulation, it is likely that most of the mechanical shocks generated in the knee joint by loading are absorbed by the meniscus. The deformable nature of the menisci with this low compressive (and shear) stiffness and permeability allows them to distribute load well in the knee.

The tensile properties of the meniscus have been shown to be nonlinear, anisotropic, and nonhomogeneous. There appears to be direct correlation between the tensile properties of meniscal tissue and its collagen fiber architecture, although the tensile properties of the meniscus reveal significant regional and directional variations in stiffness and strength (Fig. 8). This would suggest that variations in tensile stiffness and strength appear to be related to local differences in the collagen fiber ultrastructure and fiber bundle direction. Indeed, polarized light studies have

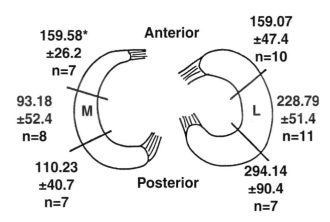

Figure 8

Drawing of the medial (M) and lateral (L) menisci showing the regional variation of the mean tensile modulus. (Reproduced with permission from Fithian DC, Kelly MA, Mow VC: Material properties and structure-function relationships in the menisci. *Clin Orthop* 1990;252:19–31.)

revealed a greater degree of fiber bundle orientation in areas of the meniscus that demonstrate superior tensile strength and stiffness. This suggests that collagen ultrastructure, and perhaps intermolecular interactions (such as collagen cross-linking), are the important factors influencing the inhomogeneity in the tensile responses of the menisci.

Because the meniscus is subjected to significant levels of shear stress and strain during load, it is extremely important to understand the response of the tissue to shear. Experimental studies have shown that the meniscus exhibited anisotropic shear properties that were dependent on the applied compressive strain. The meniscus was shown to exhibit a complex shear modulus approximately one tenth that of articular cartilage. It is thought that this low shear modulus is important in the physiologic function of the tissue, allowing the meniscus to easily distort its shape to conform to the anatomic form of the articulating surfaces of the femur and tibia. Although the anisotropic shear behavior of the meniscus may be accounted for by the collagen fiber ultrastructure (the location of the weakest shear planes corresponded to the frequently observed clinical patterns of horizontal cleavage lesions and longitudinal bucket-handle tears), it is likely that the collagen fiber-proteoglycan and other matrix protein interactions may be responsible for the observed compressive strain dependence of the shear properties. The latter would suggest that the rapidity of stress application to the meniscus is important in the development of tears.

Functional Roles of the Meniscus

Load Bearing

The meniscus has been shown to play a vital role in load transmission across the knee joint. Biomechanical studies

have demonstrated that at least 50% of the compressive load of the knee joint is transmitted through the meniscus in extension, whereas approximately 85% of the load is transmitted in 90° of flexion. In the meniscectomized knee the contact area is reduced approximately 50% (Fig. 9). This significantly increases the load per unit area and results in articular cartilage damage and degeneration. This evidence explains the osteophyte formation, joint space narrowing, and flattening of the femoral condyle that have been observed following total meniscectomy.

Partial meniscectomy has also been shown to significantly increase contact pressures. It has been shown that resection of as little as 15% to 34% of the meniscus increased contact pressures by more than 350%. Thus, even a partial meniscectomy can affect the ability of the meniscus to function in load transmission across the knee.

Shock Absorption

Another proposed function of the meniscus is that of shock absorption. It has been suggested that the viscoelastic menisci may function to dampen the load generated during walking. Experimental studies have shown that the normal knee has a shock-absorbing capacity about 20% higher than knees that have undergone meniscectomy. Because the inability of a joint system to absorb shock has been

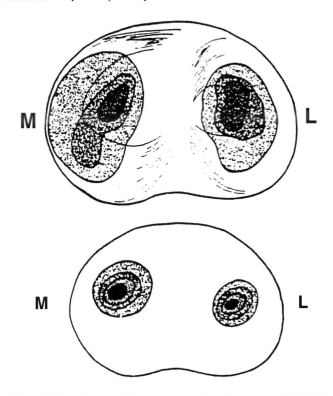

Figure 9

Drawing of a tibial plateau showing contact area and contact stress in the intact knee (**top**) and meniscectomized knee (**bottom**). M = medial; L = lateral. (Reproduced with permission from Fukubayashi T, Kurosawa H: The contact area and pressure distribution pattern of the knee: A study of normal and osteoarthrotic knee joints. *Acta Orthop Scand* 1980;51:871–879.)

strongly implicated in the development of osteoarthritis, the meniscus appears to play an important role in maintaining the health of the knee.

Joint Stability

The menisci are also thought to contribute to knee joint stability. Although medial meniscectomy alone does not cause a significant increase in anterior-posterior joint translation, it has been demonstrated that medial meniscectomy in association with ACL insufficiency signifiantly increases the anterior laxity of the knee (Figs. 10 and 11). However, lateral meniscectomy, alone or in association with ACL insufficiency, has not been shown to increase knee joint laxity.

Joint Lubrication

Because the menisci serve to increase the congruity between the condyles of the femur and tibia they contribute significantly to overall joint conformity. It has been suggested that this conformity promotes the viscous hydrodynamic action required for full fluid-film lubrication and this function assists in the overall lubrication of the articular surfaces of the knee joint. However, the exact contribution of the meniscus to joint lubrication has yet to be elucidated.

Proprioception

Finally, the menisci may serve as proprioceptive structures providing a feedback mechanism for joint position sense. This role has been inferred from the presence of type I and type II nerve endings observed in the anterior and posterior horns of the meniscus (see section on neuroanatomy). As with similar structures identified on and within the cruciate ligaments, these neural elements are thought to be part of a proprioceptive reflex arc that may contribute to the functional stability of the knee.

Vascular Anatomy

The menisci of the knee are relatively avascular structures whose limited peripheral blood supply originates predominantly from the lateral and medial genicular arteries (both inferior and superior). Branches from these vessels give rise to a perimeniscal capillary plexus within the synovial and capsular tissues of the knee joint. This plexus is an arborizing network of vessels that supplies the peripheral border of the meniscus throughout its attachment to the joint capsule (Figs. 12 and 13). These perimeniscal vessels are oriented in a predominantly circumferential pattern with radial branches directed toward the center of the joint. Anatomic studies have shown that the degree of vascular penetration is 10% to 30% of the width of the medial meniscus and 10% to 25% of the width of the lateral meniscus.

The middle genicular artery, along with a few terminal branches of the medial and lateral genicular arteries, also

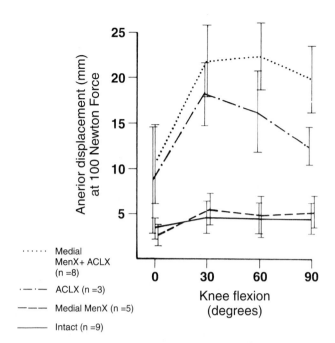

Figure 10

A graph illustrating the effect of anterior cruciate ligament insufficiency (ACLX), medial meniscectomy (Medial MenX), and combined anterior cruciate ligament deficiency and medial meniscectomy (Medial MenX + ACLX) on anterior translation of the tibia resulting from a 100-N anteriorly directed force as a function of flexion angle. (Reroduced with permission from Levy IM, Torzilli PA, Warren RF: The effect of medial meniscectomy on anterior-posterior motion of the knee. *J Bone Joint Surg* 1982;64A:883–888.)

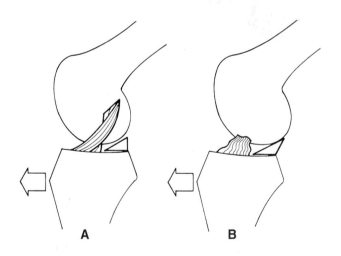

Figure 11

A, When the tibia translates anteriorly as a result of an applied force, the intact anterior cruciate ligament (ACL) stops the translation short of contact with the body of the medial meniscus. B, After disruption of the ACL, the medial meniscus helps to limit the continued anterior translation of the tibia. (Reproduced with permission from Levy IM, Torzilli PA, Warren RF: The effect of medial meniscectomy on anterior-posterior motion of the knee. *J Bone Joint Surg* 1982;64A:883–888.)

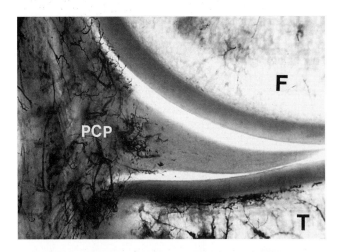

Figure 12

A 5-mm thick frontal section of the medial compartment of the knee is shown after vascular perfusion with India ink and tissue clearing with a modified Spalteholz technique. Branching radial vessels from the perimeniscal capillary plexus (PCP) can be seen penetrating the peripheral border of the medial meniscus. (F) Femur, (T) Tibia. (Reproduced with permission from Arnoczky SP, Warren RF: Microvasculature of the human meniscus. *Am J Sports Med* 1982;10:90–95.)

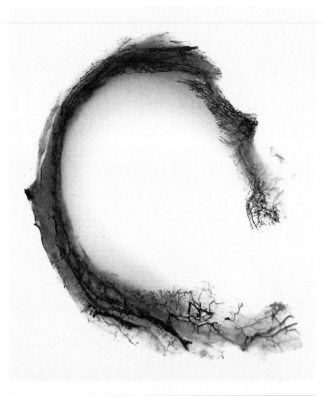

Figure 13

Superior aspect of a medial meniscus after vascular perfusion with India ink and tissue clearing with a modified Spalteholz technique. Note the vascularity at the periphery of the meniscus as well as the anterior and posterior horn attachments. (Reproduced with permission from Arnoczky SP, Warren RF: Microvasculature of the human meniscus. *Am J Sports Med* 1982;10:90–95.)

supplies vessels to the meniscus through the vascular synovial covering of the anterior and posterior horn attachments. These synovial vessels penetrate the horn attachments and give rise to endoligamentous vessels that enter the meniscal horns for a short distance and end in terminal capillary loops. A small reflection of vascular synovial tissue is also present throughout the peripheral attachment of the medial and lateral menisci on both the femoral and tibial articular surfaces. (An exception is the posterolateral portion of the lateral meniscus adjacent to the area of the popliteal tendon.) This "synovial fringe" extends for a short distance (1 to 3 mm) over the articular surfaces of the menisci and contains small, terminally looped vessels. Although this vascular synovial tissue adheres intimately to the articular surfaces of the menisci, it does not contribute vessels into the meniscal tissue.

Whereas the peripheral aspects of the menisci are vascular, the vast majority of the meniscus is avascular and must therefore derive its nutrition through either diffusion or mechanical pumping; the latter mechanism derives from intermittent compression of the tissue during function. Clinical and experimental observations have suggested that because of its dense, fibrous, extracellular matrix, diffusion into the central core of the meniscus may be marginal; thus, mechanical pumping (that is, joint motion) may be essential for continued tissue nutrition. An interesting study recently showed the presence of openings on the articular surfaces of human and animal menisci. These openings (approximately 10 to 200 μm in diameter) are believed to be connected with a system of canals within the substance of the menisci. It was theorized that these canals may represent spaces between collagen bundles through which a transudate of serum could pass, thus supplying nutrients to cells throughout the meniscus. Further study is needed to elucidate the exact mechanism of meniscal nutrition to its avascular portion.

Neuroanatomy

Histologic studies of human and animal menisci have identified the presence of neural elements within the meniscal tissue. Although the anterior and posterior horns of the menisci appear to be the most richly innervated, myelinated and unmyelinated nerve fibers have been identified within the peripheral body of the meniscus. These nerve fibers originate in the highly innervated perimeniscal tissue and radiate into the peripheral third of the meniscus. Many of these fibers accompany the vascular network of the meniscus; however, some neural elements were not exclusively paravascular in position, suggesting a function other than vasomotor or vasosensory.

Studies of human specimens have identified 3 morphologically distinct mechanoreceptors within the medial meniscus: Ruffini endings, Golgi tendon organs, and pacinian corpuscles. These neural elements were found in greater concentration in the horns of the meniscus, particularly the posterior horn. The presence of these neuroreceptors in the meniscus has led to the hypothesis that the menisci may serve an important afferent role in the sensory feedback mechanism of the knee. During extremes of knee flexion and extension, the horns of the menisci become more taut. This increase in tension would activate the mechanoreceptors located in the meniscal horns and provide the central nervous system with information regarding joint position. This may, in turn, contribute to a reflex arc that stimulates protective or postural muscular reflexes. It is theorized that the greater concentration of neural elements found in the anterior and posterior horns of the meniscus reflects the need for afferent feedback at the extremes of flexion and extension.

Meniscal Pathology

Joint Instability

Studies in animals have demonstrated that following ACL transection the menisci undergo alterations in their extracellular matrices, including an increase in water content. This increase in water content presumably represents a defect in the collagenous fibrillar system resulting in a decreased ability of this meshwork to withstand the swelling pressures of the proteoglycans. This results in the imbibition of more water in the tissue. Following ACL transection an initial decrease in the concentration of GAGs has also been observed. A 30% decrease in chondroitin sulfate and a 70% decrease in keratan sulfate has been reported in animals. However, in the more chronic joints the concentration of GAGs was found to increase substantially. This reflects a remarkable ability on the part of the fibrochondrocytes to replenish the lost proteoglycans.

Degenerative areas of the menisci have also been shown to have a higher content of noncollagenous protein as compared to normal menisci. It is not known whether this represents imbibition of exogenous proteins by fibrillated tissue or by neosynthesis and accumulation of endogenous proteins.

Age-Related Meniscal Changes

With age, the menisci undergo discoloration and an increase in the deposition of calcium pyrophosphate dihydrate crystals. The water content of menisci has not been shown to change with age. However, GAG content is altered and an increase in the ratio of chondroitin-6 sulfate to chondroitin-4 sulfate is observed. Similar changes have been reported in articular cartilage as a function of age. Collagen content of normal menisci has been found to increase until 30 years of age, where it remains steady until the eighth decade and then declines. Noncollagenous protein

concentration declines from about 20% in neonatal human menisci to approximately 10% in adults aged 50 to 70 years.

Meniscal Healing

In 1885, Thomas Annandale was credited with the first surgical repair of a torn meniscus, but it was not until 1936, when King published his classic experiment on meniscus healing in dogs, that the actual biologic limitations of meniscus healing were set forth. King demonstrated that, for meniscus lesions to heal, the lesion must communicate with the peripheral blood supply. Although the vascular supply of the meniscus is an essential element in determining its potential for repair, of equal importance is the ability of this blood supply to support the inflammatory response characteristic of wound repair. Clinical and experimental observations have demonstrated that the peripheral blood supply is capable of producing a reparative response similar to that observed in other connective tissues.

After injury within the peripheral vascular zone, a fibrin clot forms that is rich in inflammatory cells. Vessels from the perimeniscal capillary plexus proliferate through this fibrin scaffold, accompanied by the proliferation of undifferentiated mesenchymal cells. Eventually, the lesion is filled with a cellular, fibrovascular scar tissue that bonds the wound edges together and appears continuous with the adjacent normal meniscal fibrocartilage. Vessels from the perimeniscal capillary plexus, as well as the proliferative vascular pannus from the "synovial fringe," penetrate the fibrous scar to provide a marked inflammatory response.

Experimental studies have shown that radial lesions of the meniscus extending to the synovium are completely healed with fibrovascular scar tissue by 10 weeks (Fig. 14). Modula-

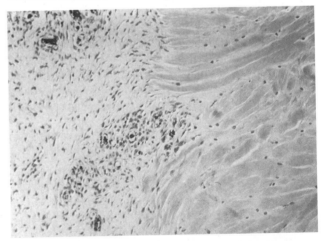

Figure 14

Photomicrograph of healing meniscus at the junction of the fibrovascular scar and the normal adjacent meniscal tissue. (Hematoxylin and eosin, magnification × 75.) (Reproduced with permission from Arnoczky SP, Warren RF: The microvasculature of the meniscus and its response to injury: An experimental study in the dog. *Am J Sports Med* 1983;11:131–141.)

tion of this scar into normal-appearing fibrocartilage, however, can require several months. The initial strength of this repair tissue as compared to the normal meniscus has not been thoroughly evaluated; 1 study suggests it is approximately 33% at 8 weeks, 52% at 4 months, and 62% at 6 months. Although the absolute strength values may be debated, the relative increase over time parallels the histologic maturation of the repair tissue.

The ability of meniscal lesions to heal has provided the rationale for the repair of peripheral meniscal injuries, and numerous clinical reports have demonstrated excellent results after primary repair of peripheral meniscal injuries. Postoperative examinations of these peripheral repairs have revealed a process of repair similar to that noted in the experimental models.

When examining injured menisci for potential repair, lesions are often classified by the location of the tear relative to the blood supply of the meniscus and the "vascular appearance" of the peripheral and central surfaces of the tear. The so-called red-red tear (peripheral capsular detachment) has a functional blood supply on the capsular and meniscal side of the lesion and, obviously, has the best prognosis for healing. The red-white tears (meniscus rim tears through the peripheral vascular zone) has an active peripheral blood supply, whereas the central (inner) surface of the lesion is devoid of functioning vessels. Theoretically, these lesions should have sufficient vascularity to heal by the aforementioned fibrovascular proliferation. The white-white tears (meniscus lesion completely in the avascular zone) are without blood supply, and theoretically cannot heal.

Meniscus repair has generally been limited to the peripheral vascular area of the meniscus (red-red, red-white tears), but a significant number of lesions occur in the central, avascular portion of the meniscus (white-white tears). Experimental and clinical observations have shown that these lesions are incapable of healing and have thereby provided the rationale for partial meniscectomy. In an effort to "extend" the level of repair into these avascular areas, techniques have been developed that provide vascularity to these white-white tears. These techniques include vascular access channel and synovial abrasion.

Initial attempts to extend the peripheral vascular response of the meniscus into the avascular zone used the creation of vascular access channels. This concept was based on the observation that when avascular lesions were extended into the peripheral blood supply of the meniscus, vessels would migrate into those lesions and heal them by the aforementioned process.

In an experimental study in dogs, a longitudinal lesion in the avascular portion of the medial meniscus was connected, at its midportion, to the peripheral vasculature of the meniscus by a full-thickness vascular access channel. Vessels from the peripheral tissues migrated into the channel and healed the meniscal lesion by the proliferation of fibrovascular scar tissue. This same mechanism was successful in healing lesions in the avascular portion of rabbit menisci. When using the vascular access technique it is imperative to remember that the function of the meniscus can be destroyed through the destruction of the peripheral rim. However, because the vascularity extends into the meniscus at least 25% of its width, a vascular access channel can be created without completely disrupting the integrity of the peripheral rim of the meniscus.

Another technique of "manipulating" the vascular supply of the meniscus that is being used more frequently is synovial abrasion. In this technique, the synovial fringe is abraded in an effort to incite a more robust vascular response near the site of the meniscal lesion. As noted previously, the meniscal synovial fringe is a vascular synovial tissue that extends over the femoral and tibial articular surfaces of the meniscus. Although it does not contribute vessels to the meniscal stroma under normal circumstances, it plays a major role in the healing of meniscal lesions in contact with the peripheral vasculature of the meniscus. It has been theorized that by stimulating (through rasping or abrading) the synovial fringe, a proliferative vascular response could be extended over the meniscal surface to previously avascular areas of the meniscus. Although clinical results have suggested an improved healing rate when synovial abrasion is used, the exact extent and character of the repair tissue has yet to be determined.

Finally, the use of an exogenous fibrin clot has been shown to heal avascular lesions without benefit of a blood supply in a canine model. Previous work had suggested that white-white tears in the meniscus were incapable of repair. This was based on the belief that the meniscal cells were incapable of mounting a repair response and that a blood supply was a prerequisite for wound repair. However, in an experimental study, Webber and associates demonstrated that meniscal fibrochondrocytes are capable of proliferation and matrix synthesis when exposed to chemotactic and mitogenic factors normally present in the wound hematoma. Using cell cultures, they demonstrated that meniscal cells exposed to PDGF were able to proliferate and synthesize an extracellular matrix.

In normal wound repair, hemorrhage from vascular injury gives rise to a fibrin clot that provides a scaffolding to support a reparative response. In addition, the clot provides substances such as PDGF and fibronectin, which act as chemotactic and mitogenic stimuli of reparative cells. Clinical use of the fibrin clot techniques has suggested that it can improve the healing rate in meniscal tears at or near the limit of vascularity.

Meniscal Regeneration

Controversy exists within the orthopaedic literature regarding the ability of a meniscus or a meniscus-like tissue to regenerate after meniscectomy. This dichotomy may have resulted from confusion as to the extent of meniscectomy, partial versus total, and/or the fact that much of the data regarding meniscal regeneration has been limited to investigations in animals.

Experiments in rabbits and dogs have demonstrated that after total meniscectomy there is regrowth of a structure that is similar in shape and texture to the removed meniscus. It is thought that after removal of the meniscus, bleeding from the incised perimeniscal vessels results in an organized clot within the peripheral joint space. Cells, believed to be from the synovium and capsule, then migrate onto this fibrin scaffold. The cells proliferate and synthesize a fibrous connective tissue. In time, joint motion and the resultant hydrostatic pressure provide the proper environment for the transformation of this fibrous tissue into fibrocartilage. Studies have shown that by 7 months this tissue has the histologic appearance of fibrocartilage and grossly resembles a meniscus. For this meniscus-like tissue to regenerate, however, the entire meniscus must be resected to expose the vascular synovial tissue or, in the case of subtotal meniscectomy, the excision must extend into the peripheral vasculature of the meniscus. The importance of the peripheral synovial tissues in meniscal regeneration has been shown in experimental studies in rabbits. In animals in which total meniscectomy was accompanied by synovectomy, there was no evidence of tissue regrowth at 12 weeks. However, total meniscectomy alone was followed by regrowth of a meniscus-like structure in 83% of the animals studied.

Smillie has observed that, in humans, the most perfect replica of a regenerated meniscus follows total meniscectomy. Evidence that the fibrous joint capsule may also be instrumental in the regeneration of fibrocartilaginous tissue within the joint space has been demonstrated by the presence of regenerated fibrocartilaginous rims in patients after total knee implantation. These regenerated tissues grossly resembled normal menisci, and histologic examination revealed a fibrocartilage-like tissue consisting of chondrocytes in a dense connective tissue matrix.

Although the frequency and degree of meniscal regeneration have not been precisely determined, it has been theorized that, after total meniscectomy, only the peripheral rim of the meniscus regenerates. A clinical study evaluating 22 cases of total meniscectomy 10 years after surgery revealed that regeneration of a meniscus-like structure that had a radius of at least a third of that of the normal meniscus was observed in all cases. It should be noted, however, that although a more consistent, albeit limited, regeneration of a meniscus-like tissue occurs after total meniscectomy, the functional role of this replacement tissue is, at best, unknown. Because of this it is generally believed that the degenerative changes associated with the initial absence of a peripheral meniscal rim make partial meniscectomy a more desirable procedure.

Meniscal Replacement

The significance of the menisci to the overall well-being of the knee has underscored the importance of maintaining these structures whenever possible. Although techniques of meniscal repair and partial meniscectomy have limited the cases of total meniscectomy there are instances in which total resection of the tissue is the only option. Because of the deleterious consequences to the joint as a result of meniscal loss, replacement of the meniscus through allografting or synthetic scaffold is being explored.

Allografts

As with any tissue, successful transplantation is dependent on several factors, including tissue preservation, the immunologic compatability of the donor and host, and the long-term biologic and biomechanical integrity of the transplant. Because several studies have shown that viable articular cartilage allografts are biomechanically superior to nonviable grafts, the effect of cryopreservation on meniscal tissue was examined. Using a technique of cryopreservation originally developed for articular cartilage, meniscal tissue was controlled-rate frozen to −100°C using dimethylsulfoxide (DMSO) as a cryopreservative. The results of the study demonstrated that while the preservation technique had no untoward effects on the overall structure or tensile properties of the menisci, only 10% of the cells survived the preservation process and remained viable at 1 week. Although other studies demonstrated varying amounts of cell viability using other preservation techniques, the role of viable cells in the success or failure of transplanted menisci is still a matter of debate. One study has shown that 4 weeks following transplantation of a totally viable meniscus, no donor DNA could be found in the tissue. This would suggest that cell viability at the time of transplant is a moot point. Indeed, experimental studies examining meniscal transplantation using fresh, cryopreserved, and deep-frozen allografts have shown a similar biologic incorporation of the graft. In all cases, cells (presumably from the peripheral synovial and capsular tissues) migrate into the transplant and ultimately repopulate the tissue with cells resembling meniscofibrochondrocytes. Histologic and vascular studies have shown a normal vascular and cellular pattern at 6 months following transplant. Limited mechanical and biochemical evaluations have shown that while the transplant has normal tensile properties at 6 months there is a decrease in the proteoglycan content and an increase in the water content. The long-term effect of these findings has not been examined. The use of a synthetic scaffold is currently being investigated as a way to accomplish effective meniscal regeneration.

The meniscus, like articular cartilage, has long been considered an immunologically privileged tissue and while histologic evaluation of fresh, cryopreserved, and deep-frozen meniscal transplants used in experimental studies have not identified evidence of an immune response, a recent clinical case challenged that concept. An acute, noninfectious, inflammatory reaction comprised of lymphocytes and plasma cells has been reported in a patient receiving a cryopreserved meniscal allograft.

Finally, a recent experimental study has shown that meniscal tissue is capable of transmitting a retrovirus, even after deep-freezing. Although gamma irradiation has been used to "sterilize" meniscal allografts, the exact dose of radiation required for viricidal action and its ultimate effect on the structural and mechanical properties of the tissue is still a matter of debate.

Tissue Engineered Meniscus

Creating a tissue-engineered meniscus requires that specific biologic considerations such as cell type, matrix scaffold, bioreactor design, and environmental conditions be addressed. Meniscal cells, fibroblasts, and mesenchymal stem cells have been proposed as potential cell sources and have been grown (both in vivo and in vitro) on various cell matrices including collagen-based scaffolds, biodegradable polymers, and small intestine submucosa. Although these tissue engineering paradigms have produced a meniscus-like construct, the long-term functional capabilities of this engineered tissue have yet to be proven.

Gene Therapy

Several investigators have demonstrated the ability to transfer specific genes into meniscal fibrochondrocytes using retroviral recombinant adenoviral vectors. It has been postulated that such genetic manipulation could promote secretion of therapeutic cytokines which could improve meniscal healing and regeneration. Although it is not yet clear what genes should be selected for transfer, the possibilities that these biologic interventions offer for meniscal repair and regeneration are both realistic and exciting.

Selected Bibliography

General

Annandale T: An operation for displaced semilunar cartilage. *Br Med J* 1885;1:779.

Arnoczky S, Adams M, DeHaven K, Eyre D, Mow V: Meniscus, in Woo SL-Y, Buckwalter JA (eds): *Injury and Repair of the Musculoskeletal Soft Tissues*. Park Ridge, IL, American Academy of Orthopaedic Surgeons, 1988, pp 487–537.

Bullough PG, Vosburgh F, Arnoczky SP, Levy IM: The menisci of the knee, in Insall JN (ed): *Surgery of the Knee*. New York, NY, Churchill Livingstone, 1984, pp 135–146.

Mow VC, Arnoczky SP, Jackson DW (eds): *Knee Meniscus: Basic and Clinical Foundations*. New York, NY, Raven Press, 1992.

Anatomy

Arnoczky SP: Gross and vascular anatomy of the meniscus and its role in meniscal healing, regeneration, and remodeling, in Mow VC, Arnoczky SP, Jackson DW (eds): *Knee Meniscus: Basic and Clinical Foundations*. New York, NY, Raven Press, 1992, pp 1–14.

Arnoczky SP, Warren RF: Microvasculature of the human meniscus. *Am J Sports Med* 1982;10:90–95.

Aspden RM, Yarker YE, Hukins DW: Collagen orientations in the meniscus of the knee joint. *J Anat* 1985;140:371–380.

Bullough PG, Munuera L, Murphy J, Weinstein AM: The strength of the menisci of the knee as it relates to their fine structure. *J Bone Joint Surg* 1970;52B:564–567.

Gardner E: The innervation of the knee joint. *Anat Rec* 1948;101:109–130.

Ghadially FN (ed): *Fine Structure of Synovial Joints: A Text and Atlas of the Ultrastructure of Normal and Pathological Articular Tissues*. London, England, Butterworths, 1983, pp 103–144.

Heller L, Langman J: The menisco-femoral ligaments of the human knee. *J Bone Joint Surg* 1964;46B:307–313.

Kennedy JC, Alexander IJ, Hayes KC: Nerve supply of the human knee and its functional importance. *Am J Sports Med* 1982;10:329–335.

O'Connor BL: The histological structure of dog knee menisci with comments on its possible significance. *Am J Anat* 1976;147:407–417.

O'Connor BL: The mechanoreceptor innervation of the posterior attachments of the lateral meniscus of the dog knee joint. *J Anat* 1984;138:15–26.

O'Connor BL, McConnaughey JS: The structure and innervation of cat knee menisci, and their relation to a "sensory hypothesis" of meniscal function. *Am J Anat* 1978;153:431–442.

Warren R, Arnoczky SP, Wickiewicz TL: Anatomy of the knee, in Nicholas JA, Hershman EB, (eds): *The Lower Extremity and Spine in Sports Medicine.* St. Louis, MO, CV Mosby, 1986, pp 657–694.

Wilson AS, Legg PG, McNeur JC: Studies on the innervation of the medial meniscus in the human knee joint. *Anat Rec* 1969;165:485–491.

Zimny ML, Albright DJ, Dabezies E: Mechanoreceptors in the human medial meniscus. *Acta Anat (Basel)* 1988;133:35–40.

Biochemistry

Adams ME, Hukins DWL: The extracellular matrix of the meniscus, in Mow VC, Arnoczky SP, Jackson DW (eds): *Knee Meniscus: Basic and Clinical Foundations.* New York, NY, Raven Press, 1992, pp 15–28.

Ghosh P, Taylor TK: The knee joint meniscus: A fibrocartilage of some distinction. *Clin Orthop* 1987;224:52–63.

Herwig J, Egner E, Buddecke E: Chemical changes of human knee joint menisci in various stages of degeneration. *Ann Rheum Dis* 1984;43:635–640.

McDevitt CA, Marcelino J: Composition of articular cartilage. *Sports Med Arthroscopy Rev* 1994;2:1–12.

McDevitt CA, Miller RR, Spindler KP: The cells and cell matrix interactions of the meniscus, in Mow VC, Arnoczky SP, Jackson DW (eds): *Knee Meniscus: Basic and Clinical Foundations.* New York, NY, Raven Press, 1992, pp 29–36.

McDevitt CA, Webber RJ: The ultrastructure and biochemistry of meniscal cartilage. *Clin Orthop* 1990;252:8–18.

Miller RR, McDevitt C.: Thrombospondin in ligament, meniscus, and intervertebral disc. *Biochim Biophys Acta* 1991;1115:85–88.

Peters TJ, Smillie IS: Studies on the chemical composition of the menisci of the knee joint with special reference to the horizontal cleavage lesion. *Clin Orthop* 1972;86:245–252.

Proctor CS, Schmidt MB, Whipple RR, Kelly MA, Mow VC: Material properties of the normal medial bovine meniscus. *J Orthop Res* 1989;7:771–782.

Roughley PJ, McNicol D, Santer V, Buckwalter J: The presence of a cartilage-like proteoglycan in the adult human meniscus. *Biochem J* 1981;197:77–83.

Function

Ahmed AM: The load-bearing role of the knee menisci, in Mow VC, Arnoczky SP, Jackson DW (eds): *Knee Meniscus: Basic and Clinical Foundations.* New York, NY, Raven Press, 1992, pp 59–73.

Ahmed AM, Burke DL: In-vitro measurements of static pressure distribution in synovial joints: Part I. Tibial surface of the knee. *J Biomech Eng* 1983;105:216–225.

Aspden RM, Hukins DWL: Structure, function, and mechanical failure of the meniscus, in Yettram AL (ed): *Material Properties and Stress Analysis in Biomechanics.* Manchester, England, Manchester University Press, 1989, pp 109–122.

Burr DB, Radin EL: Meniscal function and the importance of meniscal regeneration in preventing late medial compartment osteoarthrosis. *Clin Orthop* 1982;171:121–126.

Fairbank TJ: Knee joint changes after meniscectomy. *J Bone Joint Surg* 1948;30B:664–670.

Fithian DC, Zhu W, Ratcliffe A, Kelly MA, Malinin TI, Mow VC: Exponential law representation of tensile properties of human meniscus. *Proc Inst Mech Engng Bioengn* 1989;85–90.

Fithian DC, Kelly MA, Mow VC: Material properties and structure-function relationships in the menisci. *Clin Orthop* 1990;252:19–31.

Fukubayashi T, Kurosawa H: The contact area and pressure distribution pattern of the knee: A study of normal and osteoarthrotic knee joints. *Acta Orthop Scand* 1980;51:871–879.

Kettelkamp DB, Jacobs AW: Tibiofemoral contact area: Determination and implications. *J Bone Joint Surg* 1972;54A:349–356.

Krause WR, Pope MH, Johnson RJ, Wilder DG: Mechanical changes in the knee after meniscectomy. *J Bone Joint Surg* 1976;58A:599–604.

Levy IM, Torzilli PA, Fisch ID: The contribution of the menisci to the stability of the knee, in Mow VC, Arnoczky SP, Jackson DW (eds): *Knee Meniscus: Basic and Clinical Foundations.* New York, NY, Raven Press, 1992, pp 107–115.

Levy IM, Torzilli PA, Warren RF: The effect of medial meniscectomy on anterior-posterior motion of the knee. *J Bone Joint Surg* 1982;64A:883–888.

Mow VC, Fithian DC, Kelly MA: Fundamentals of articular cartilage and meniscus biomechanics, in Ewing JW (ed): *Articular Cartilage and Knee Joint Function: Basic Science and Arthroscopy.* New York, NY, Raven Press, 1990, pp 1–18.

Mow VC, Ratcliffe A, Chern KY, Kelly MA: Structure and function relationships of the menisci of the knee, in Mow VC, Arnoczky SP, Jackson DW (eds): *Knee Meniscus: Basic and Clinical Foundations.* New York, NY, Raven Press, 1992, pp 37–57.

Myers ER, Zhu W, Mow VC: Viscoelastic properties of articular cartilage and meniscus, in Nimni ME (ed): *Collagen: Biochemistry and Biomechanics.* Boca Raton, FL, CRC Press, 1988, vol 2, pp 267–288.

Shrive NG, O'Connor JJ, Goodfellow JW: Load-bearing in the knee joint. *Clin Orthop* 1978;131:279–287.

Spilker RL, Donzelli PS: A biphasic finite element model of the meniscus for stress-strain analysis, in Mow VC, Arnoczky SP, Jackson DW (eds): *Knee Meniscus: Basic and Clinical Foundations.* New York, NY, Raven Press, 1992, pp 91–106.

Thompson WO, Thaete FL, Fu FH, Dye SF: Tibial meniscal dynamics using three-dimensional reconstruction of magnetic resonance images. *Am J Sports Med* 1991;19:210–215.

Voloshin AS. Wosk J: Shock absorption of meniscectomized and painful knees: A comparative in vivo study. *J Biomed Eng* 1983; 5:157–161.

Walker PS, Erkman MJ: The role of the menisci in force transmission across the knee. *Clin Orthop* 1975;109:184–192.

Injury, Repair, Regeneration, and Replacement

Arnoczky SP, McDevitt CA, Schmidt M, Mow VC, Warren RF: The effect of cryopreservation on canine menisci: A biochemical, morphologic, and biomechanical evaluation. *J Orthop Res* 1988;6:1–12.

Arnoczky SP, Warren RF: The microvasculature of the meniscus and its response to injury: An experimental study in the dog. *Am J Sports Med* 1983;11:131–141.

Arnoczky SP, Warren RF, McDevitt CA: Meniscal replacement using a cryopreserved allograft: An experimental study in the dog. *Clin Orthop* 1990;252:121–128.

Arnoczky SP, Warren RF, Spivak JM: Meniscal repair using an exogenous fibrin clot: An experimental study in dogs. *J Bone Joint Surg* 1988;70A:1209–1217.

Cabaud HE, Rodkey WG, Fitzwater JE: Medial meniscus repairs: An experimental and morphologic study. *Am J Sports Med* 1981;9: 129–314.

Cox JS, Cordell LD: The degenerative effects of medial meniscus tears in dogs' knees. *Clin Orthop* 1977;125:236–242.

Cox JS, Nye CE, Schaefer WW, Woodstein IJ: The degenerative effects of partial and total resection of the medial meniscus in dogs' knees. *Clin Orthop* 1975;109:178–183.

DeYoung DJ, Flo GL, Tvedten H: Experimental medial meniscectomy in dogs undergoing cranial cruciate ligament repair. *J Am Anim Hosp Assoc* 1980;16:639–645.

DiCarlo EF: Pathology of the meniscus, in Mow VC, Arnoczky SP, Jackson DW (eds): *Knee Meniscus: Basic and Clinical Foundations.* New York, NY, Raven Press, 1992, pp 117–130.

Doyle JR, Eisenberg JH, Orth MW: Regeneration of knee menisci: A preliminary report. *J Trauma* 1966;6:50–55.

Elmer RM, Moskowitz RW, Frankel VH: Meniscal regeneration and postmeniscectomy degenerative joint disease. *Clin Orthop* 1977;124: 304–310.

Evans DK: Repeated regeneration of a meniscus in the knee. *J Bone Joint Surg* 1963;45B:748–749.

Hamlet W, Liu SH, Yang R: Destruction of a cryopreserved meniscal allograft: A case for acute rejection. *Arthroscopy* 1997;13:517–521.

Heatley FW: The meniscus: Can it be repaired? An experimental investigation in rabbits. *J Bone Joint Surg* 1980;62B:397–402.

Henning CE, Lynch MA, Clark JR: Vascularity for healing of meniscus repairs. *Arthroscopy* 1987;3:13–18.

Jackson DW, McDevitt CA, Simon TM, Arnoczky SP, Atwell EA, Silvino NJ: Meniscal transplantation using fresh and cryopreserved allografts: An experimental study in goats. *Am J Sports Med* 1992;20: 644–656.

Jackson DW, Simon TM: Biology of meniscal allograft, in Mow VC, Arnoczky SP, Jackson DW (eds): *Knee Meniscus: Basic and Clinical Foundations.* New York, NY, Raven Press, 1992, pp 141–152.

Jackson DW, Whelan J, Simon TM: Cell survival after transplantation of fresh meniscal allografts: DNA probe analysis in a goat model. *Am J Sports Med* 1993;21:540–550.

Kim JM, Moon MS: Effect of synovectomy upon regeneration of meniscus in rabbits. *Clin Orthop* 1979;141:287–294.

King D: Regeneration of the semilunar cartilage. *Surg Gynecol Obstet* 1936;62:167–170.

King D: The healing of semilunar cartilages. *J Bone Joint Surg* 1936; 18:333–342.

Nemzek JA, Arnoczky SP, Swenson CL: Retroviral transmission by the transplantation of connective-tissue allografts: An experimental study. *J Bone Joint Surg* 1994;76A:1036–1041.

Noble J, Hamblen DL: The pathology of the degenerate meniscus lesion. *J Bone Joint Surg* 1975;57B:180–186.

Roeddecker K, Muennich U, Nagelschmidt M: Meniscal healing: A biomechanical study. *J Surg Res* 1994;56:20–27.

Smillie IS: Observations on the regeneration of the semilunar cartilages in man. *Br J Surg* 1944;31:398–401.

Stone KR, Rodkey WG, Webber RJ, McKinney LA, Steadman JR: Development of a prosthetic meniscal replacement, in Mow VC, Arnoczky SP, Jackson DW (eds): *Knee Meniscus: Basic and Clinical Foundations.* New York, NY, Raven Press, 1992, pp 165–173.

Veth RP, den Heeten GJ, Jansen HW, Nielsen HK: Repair of the meniscus: An experimental investigation in rabbits. *Clin Orthop* 1983;175: 258–262.

Webber RJ, Harris MG, Hough AJ Jr: Cell culture of rabbit meniscal fibrochondrocytes: Proliferative and synthetic response to growth factors and ascorbate. *J Orthop Res* 1985;3:36–42.

Webber RJ, York L, Vander Schilden JL, Hough AJ Jr: Fibrin clot invasion by rabbit meniscal fibrochondrocytes in organ culture. *Trans Orthop Res Soc* 1987;12:470.

Chapter 21

Intervertebral Disk Structure, Composition, and Mechanical Function

Joseph A. Buckwalter, MS, MD

Van C. Mow, PhD

Scott D. Boden, MD

David R. Eyre, PhD

Mark Weidenbaum, MD

This chapter at a glance

This chapter discusses the unique structure and biologic and mechanical behavior of the intervertebral disk.

One or more of the authors or the department with which they are affiliated has received something of value from a commercial or other party related directly or indirectly to the subject of this chapter.

Introduction

Normal function of the axial skeleton is made possible by the intervertebral disks. They stabilize the spine and maintain its alignment by anchoring adjacent vertebral bodies to each other (Fig. 1). The intervertebral disks allow the movement between vertebrae that gives the spine its flexibility, and they absorb energy and distribute loads applied to the spine. These multiple functions are made possible by the structure of disks, which consist of a firm fibrous ring, called the anulus fibrosus, which surrounds a softer gelatinous mass called the nucleus pulposus (Fig. 2). Although both are components of the intervertebral disk, the anulus fibrosus and nucleus pulposus each has a distinct composition and mechanical properties. Recent investigations have dramatically advanced understanding of the unique structure-function relationships of the anulus fibrosus and nucleus pulposus and thereby help clarify the biologic and mechanical behavior of intervertebral disks.

Structure and Composition

The 23 intervertebral disks of the human spine increase in height and diameter from the cervical to the lumbar spine (Fig. 1); even though they vary considerably in size, all intervertebral disks have the same basic structure and biochemical composition. Like other connective tissues, they consist of a sparse population of cells (Fig. 3) and an abundant extracellular matrix formed by an elaborate framework of macromolecules filled with water. The cells synthesize these biomacromolecules and then maintain the framework created from these molecules. The structural integrity and mechanical properties of the disk depend on the macromolecules and their interactions with water. Because a blood supply is found solely in the periphery of the normal disk, the nutrition of disk cells is derived from diffusional and convective transport of nutrients and wastes through the porous-permeable solid matrix. Movement of these nutrient and waste molecules through the matrix depends on the composition and organization of the macromolecular framework (that is, pore size and pore torturosity) and the interstitial water content, which in turn is largely determined by the charged proteoglycan concentration (that is, Donnan osmotic pressure, which is the colligative physical properties associated with the excess ionic concentration in the interstitium).

Three concentrically arranged component tissues form the normal human intervertebral disk: (1) the outer anulus fibrosus, a ring of highly oriented, densely packed type I collagen fibrous lamellae including collagen fibrils that

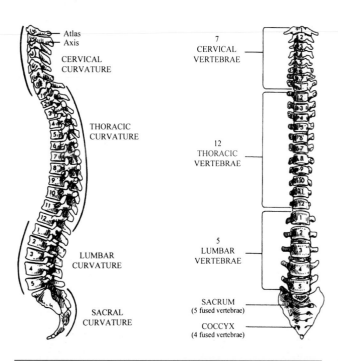

Figure 1

Drawing of the human spine that shows how the 23 intevertebral disks unite the 24 vertebral bodies to form the 4 regions (cervical, thoracic, lumbar, and sacral) of the central column of the axial skeleton. The differences in the sizes of the vertebral bodies and intervertebral disks are shown. (Reproduced with permission from Ashton-Miller JA, Schultz AB: Biomechanics of the human spine, in Mow VC, Hayes WC (eds): *Basic Orthopaedic Biomechanics*. Philadelphia, PA, Lippincott-Raven, 1997, pp 353–393.)

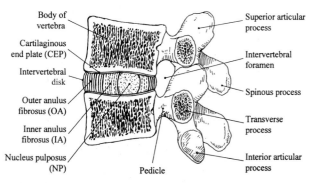

Figure 2

Sagittal section view of a motion segment comprising two vertebral bodies and an intervertebral disk forming a strong connection between the 2 bones. The 4 regions of the disk are shown: cartilaginous end plate (CEP), outer anulus fibrosus (OA), inner anulus fibrosus (IA), and nucleus pulposus (NP). The posterior articular and spinous processes and the articular surface of a facet joint are also shown. (Reproduced with permission from Ashton-Miller JA, Schultz AB: Biomechanics of the human spine, in Mow VC, Hayes WC (eds): *Basic Orthopaedic Biomechanics*. Philadelphia, PA, Lippincott-Raven, 1997, pp 353–393.)

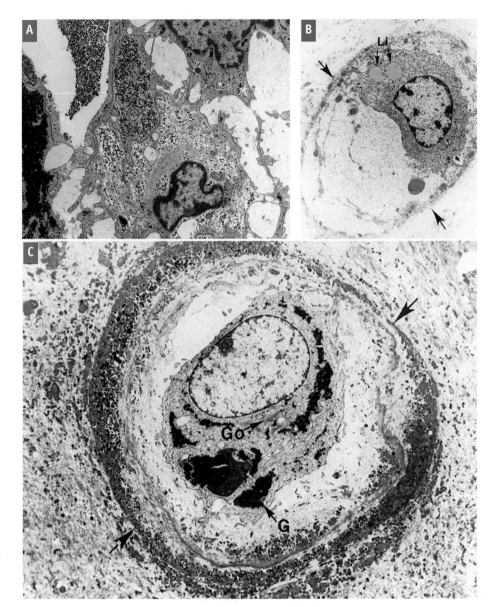

Figure 3

Electron micrographs showing viable cells from human nucleus pulposus. **A,** Notochordal cells from a newborn. Note the interdigitation of the cell membranes and the regions of extracellular matrix surrounded by cell membranes. **B,** Chondrocyte-like cell from a 14-month-old infant. Li indicates lipid deposits and the arrows mark the edges of accumulated granular pericellular material. **C,** Chondrocyte-like cell from a 91-year-old. Go indicates Golgi membranes, G indicates glycogen, and arrows mark the edges of the accumulated granular pericellular material. Note the increased density of the granular material in the tissue matrix. (Reproduced with permission from Buckwalter JA, Woo SL, Goldberg VM, et al: Soft-tissue aging and musculoskeletal function. *J Bone Joint Surg* 1993;75A:1533–1548.)

insert into the vertebral bodies; (2) the larger fibrocartilaginous inner anulus fibrosus, which consists of a less dense type II collagenous matrix that lacks the clearly distinct lamellar organization of the outer anulus; and (3) the central nucleus pulposus (Fig. 2). Vertebral end plates in children and young adults consisting of hyaline cartilage and in the aged consisting of calcified cartilage and bone, form the superior and inferior boundaries of the intervertebral disks. The cells of the cartilage end plates resemble chondrocytes found in other hyaline cartilages. The outer anulus contains fibroblast- or fibrocyte-like cells, whereas the cells of the inner anulus more closely resemble chondrocytes. At birth the nucleus pulposus contains a mass of interconnected notochordal cells (Fig. 3, *A*). During growth and development notochordal cells appear to separate from the mass of interconnected notochordal cells and then disappear completely by early adult life, leaving scattered chondrocyte-like cells in their place (Fig. 3, *B* and *C*). The mechanisms

responsible for the disappearance of the notochordal cells and the appearance of the chondrocyte-like cells in the nucleus have not yet been defined.

Collagens and proteoglycans are the primary structural components of the intervertebral disk macromolecular framework. Collagens give the disk tissues their form and tensile strength (Fig. 4). Proteoglycans, through their interactions with water, give the tissues stiffness, resistance to compression, and viscoelasticity. The relative amounts of collagen and proteoglycan differ significantly in the matrices of disk components. Collagens account for as much as 70% of the dry weight of the outer anulus, but less than 20% of the dry weight of the central nucleus of younger individuals. In contrast, proteoglycans account for only a few percent of the dry weight of the outer anulus, but as much as 50% of the dry weight of the nucleus from a child.

The profile of collagen types changes across the disk. Fibrillar collagens, primarily type I and type II, make up most

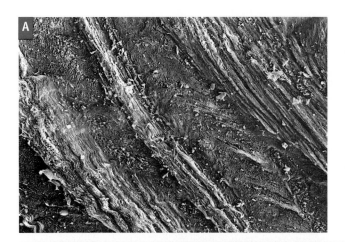
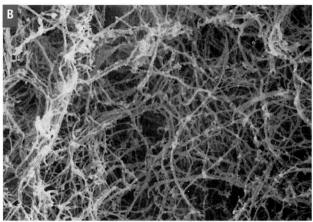

Figure 4

Scanning electron micrographs showing the arrangement of the collagen fibrils in the outer anulus (**A**) and the central nucleus pulposus (**B**). Note the tightly packed, highly oriented lamellae of collagen fibrils in the outer anulus and the loose, almost random pattern of collagen fibrils in the nucleus. (Reproduced with permission from Buckwalter JA: The fine structure of human intervertebral disc, in White AA III, Gordon SL (eds): *American Academy of Orthopaedic Surgeons Symposium on Idiopathic Low Back Pain*. St. Louis, MO, CV Mosby, 1982, pp 108–143.)

of the total disk collagen, but short helix collagens that do not form fibrils are also present (Table 1). The dense fibrous matrix of the outer anulus consists primarily of type I collagen. The concentration of type II collagen relative to type I collagen increases going from the outer edge to the interior of the anulus. On average, the human anulus in young adults contains a ratio of approximately 60% type II collagen to 40% type I collagen. Proteoglycan concentration increases with type II collagen concentration. In the nucleus, the concentration of type II collagen reaches 80% of the total collagen and type I collagen is absent. Both type V and type XI collagens are present in small amounts in the disk, about 3% of the total collagen. Their concentrations vary across the disk: type V is present in higher concentrations when type I collagen is the predominant collagen, and type XI is present in higher concentrations when type II collagen is the predominant collagen. Other quantitatively minor collagens also form part of the disk matrix (Table 1).

Disks also contain remarkably high concentrations of type VI collagen, as much as 10% of the total collagen in the anulus and 15% or more in the nucleus. This collagen does not form fibrils; instead, it consists of fine filaments connected to dense transverse bands with central lucent areas or as a network of fine filaments. Its unusually high concentration in the disk, when compared with other connective tissues, suggests that it contributes to the unique properties of the disk matrix. In the anulus and nucleus, both type I and type II collagens are heavily cross-linked with pyridinoline residues. These mature trivalent cross-links are found in the collagens of many tissues, but they reach their highest levels in the intervertebral disk. There is some evidence that this form of cross-linking is most pronounced in tissues that bear high mechanical loads, as they are needed for maintaining tissue cohesiveness.

Proteoglycan aggregates consisting of central hyaluronan filaments and multiple attached aggrecan molecules exist in all the component tissues of disks of newborns and infants (Fig. 5). Link proteins, small proteins that bind to aggrecan molecules and hyaluronan, stabilize these large aggregates. The anulus and cartilage end plate contain aggregates that closely resemble those found in articular cartilage; but even in disks from infants, nucleus pulposus aggregates are smaller, and their concentration declines rapidly with increasing age. In addition, with increasing age the proportion of nonaggregated proteoglycans progressively increases and the size of the aggrecan molecules decreases, especially in the nucleus pulposus. These extensive alterations in proteoglycan structure begin early in life, years before the appearance of age-related changes in disk morphology.

Table 1
Intervertebral Disk Collagens

Type	Predominant Location	Percent of Total Collagen (%)
Fibril-Forming Collagens		
I	Anulus	0-80
II	Anulus & Nucleus	0-80
III	Anulus	< 5
V	Anulus & Nucleus	1-2
XI	Anulus & Nucleus	1-2
Short Helix Collagens		
VI	Anulus & Nucleus	5-20
IX	Anulus & Nucleus	1-2
XII	Anulus	< 1

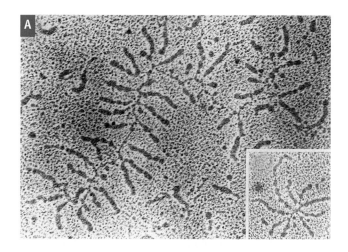

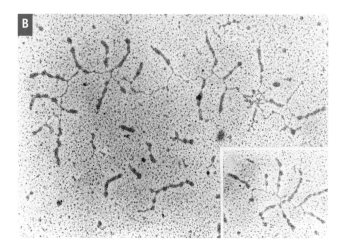

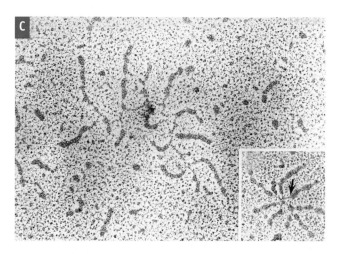

Figure 5

Electron micrographs showing aggregating proteoglycans from human infant intervertebral disks. The central filament consists of hyaluronan and the projecting arms are aggrecans. **A,** Large and small (inset) aggregates from cartilage end plate. **B,** Large and small (inset) aggregates from anulus fibrosus. **C,** Large and small (inset) aggregates from nucleus pulposus. (Reproduced with permission from Buckwalter JA, Pedrini A, Tudisco C, Pedrini V: Proteoglycans of human infant intervertebral disc: Electron microscopic and biochemical studies. *J Bone Joint Surg* 1985;67A:284–294.)

A variety of noncollagenous proteins and small amounts of elastin exist throughout the disk tissues. Although the noncollagenous proteins have not been extensively studied, they appear to contribute significantly to the organization and stability of the matrix. The contribution of elastin to the mechanical properties of the disk remains uncertain, but its low concentration suggests that it does not have a major role.

Blood Supply and Innervation

In normal disks of skeletally mature individuals, vascular supply and innervation are limited. Blood vessels lie on the surface of the anulus and may penetrate a short distance into the outer layers of the anulus. The blood vessels of the vertebral bodies lie directly against the end plates as well, but do not enter the central regions of the disk. Simple and plexiform unmyelinated nerve endings and encapsulated nerve endings have been found on the surface of the anulus and small nerves with simple free nerve endings enter the outer layers of the anulus, but nerves have not been identified within the central regions of normal human disks. Facet joint capsules and spinal ligaments have free and encapsulated nerve endings.

Mechanical Function

The unique structure and composition of the intervertebral disk make possible its specialized mechanical functions. The anulus fibrosus contains the nucleus pulposus between the vertebral end plates and the inner anulus fibrosus (Fig. 2). Collagen fibers of the anulus pass into the bone of the vertebral bodies binding adjacent vertebrae together, contributing to the stability of the spine and joining the anulus fibrosus to the vertebral bodies. The dense collagenous cross-ply, circumferential lamellae of the outer anulus fibrosus (Figures 2 and 4) resist the large tensile stresses, minimize intervertebral disk bulging, and reduce the strains that are developed during axial compressive and torsional loading, sagittal and transvere bending, or axial torsional loading of the spine. When the disks are subjected to prolonged high levels of axial loading, such as during long periods of upright posture (standing), tissue consolidation will squeeze the intersitial water out of the disks; thus, their height will decrease and bulging will occur (Fig. 6, *A*). When the load is removed from the disks, or decreased, such as during sleep in a recumbent position, water will flow back into the disks and their volume is restored. The propensity to regain the water is mainly because of the Donnan osmotic pressure of the charges on the proteoglycans, and the elasticity of the porous-permeable, collagen-proteoglycan solid matrix (see Chapter 17 for a fuller explanation of this phenomenon). Thus, it can be seen that each component of the intervertebral disk has a structure and a function, and taken together, they provide the entire spine with a supple mobility and stability, while absorbing and distributing the high loads of biomechanical function.

The anulus fibrosus and nucleus pulposus have different roles in disk biomechanical function. The outer anulus fibrosus resists tensile loads and contains the inner anulus fibrosus, and the (physiologically normal) nucleus pulposus provides a hydrostatic barrier that limits their deformations. Because of the cartilaginous nature of the inner anulus fibrosus and nucleus pulposus (that is, characterized by a high proteoglycan content), and their high degree of hydration (70% to 80%), they also contribute to the viscoelastic behavior of the entire disk, including maintaining or restoring disk height and absorbing loads applied to the spine. This viscoelastic behavior is biphasic in nature and is largely caused by the frictional drag associated with the extrusion and imbibition of the interstitial fluid (see Chapter 17). In other words, in the inner anulus and nucleus pulposus, the less dense collagenous matrix permits larger deformations in response to loads, and thus volumetric changes, that in turn create interstitial fluid flows within the disk that dissipate energy and viscoelastic creep. Torques on the vertebra-disk-vertebra motion segments distort the shapes of the anulus fibrosus (with no volume change) while bending and compression causes disk bulging, volumetric changes, and end plate deformation (Fig. 6).

Mechanical responses resulting from the applied loads will be altered with excision, say, of a posterolateral portion of the anulus or of the nucleus pulposus. Selective removal of the nucleus pulposus will result in increased motion at the level of injury, decreased disk height and stiffness, and increased deformations of the anulus. Injection of physiologic saline into the nucleus increases intradiskal pressure and decreases segmental motion, at least temporarily. These results demonstrate that loss of fluid pressure occurs in response to denucleation or isolated anulus fibrosus injury, with subsequent effects on load-deformational responses of the entire disk. Clearly, disturbance of any one component of the disk will affect the mechanical behavior of that component and the disk as a whole.

Biomechanical behavior of the intervertebral disk is determined by many factors. Detailed information regarding disk biomechanics requires analysis of its stress/strain behavior within the disk, as determined by Newton's laws that express a balance between applied loads and restraining forces generated within the disk. Knowledge of material properties of the disk and its components is crucial for understanding these interactions. Correctly formulated material properties, such as swelling pressure, hydraulic permeability, and compressive, tensile, and shear moduli, describe the intrinsic mechanical behavior of given materials regardless of loading conditions and geometric form of

the structure. These properties can be characterized using the biphasic theory developed for soft-hydrated biologic tissues. This theory attributes viscoelastic behavior to frictional drag of interstitial fluid movement within the porous-permeated, solid matrix of the tissue as a result of tissue volumetric change. These intrinsic material properties depend on microstructural organization and compositional factors that define the tissue under consideration (articular cartilage, meniscus, disk, ligament, and tendon).

Swelling pressure in the intervertebral disk arises from osmotic pressure differences between the disk's interstitial fluid and bathing fluid external to the disk. These differences are created by the difference in ion concentration between the 2 fluids that results from the electroneutrality law that dictates that the negative charges on the proteoglycans can be maintained in neutral state; this necessitates an additional counterion concentration (Na+) to be dissolved in the interstitial fluid, thus giving rise to the osmotic pressure. The Donnan osmotic pressure is equivalent to the charge-to-charge repulsive forces arising from fixed charges on the proteoglycans. Deformations caused by this swelling pressure are physically restrained by the stresses created in the fibrillar collagen network, primarily located in the anulus fibrosus. Thus, net swelling depends on the interaction between swelling pressure, the integrity of the restraining collagen network, and the magnitude and directions of the applied mechanical loading.

Osmotic pressure measurements using polyethylene glycol have been used to assess swelling pressure in addition to direct pressure measurements using pressure transducers in the intervertebral disk. Anulus fibrosus and nucleus pulposus swelling pressures are fairly similar, ranging from 0.05 to 0.3 MPa. The nucleus pulposus has an enormous swelling propensity, capable of causing the tissue to imbibe large amounts of water, and swelling up to 200% of its initial volume. The high water and proteoglycan contents of the normal nucleus pulposus enable it to function predominantly as a viscous fluid under normal physiologic conditions, thus capable of providing a high degree of hydrostatic load support. When degenerative disk materials are tested under the same loading conditions, they tend to exhibit a solid-like behavior. The Donnan osmotic swelling pressure resulting from the high proteoglycan concentration also helps maintain disk height and contributes to load support and distribution. The nucleus pulposus resists axial compressive load and its biomechanical behavior is highly dependent on rate of loading such as under dynamic conditions. In continuous or dynamic loading, it behaves more like a viscoelastic solid. Thus, there are 3 mechanisms of load support in the disk: (1) hydrostatic pressure in the interstitial fluid; (2) Donnan osmotic pressure, and (3) stresses developed in the collagen-proteoglycan solid matrix.

Clearly, then, how much each of these mechanisms contributes to the total load-carrying capacity of the disk depends on the physiologic state of the materials (and

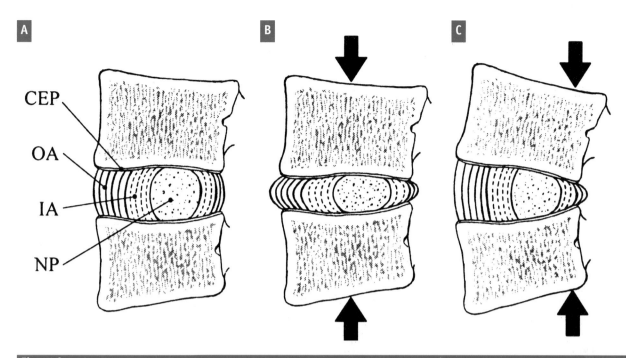

Figure 6

A, Schematic diagram showing a cross-section of a motion segment. The motion segment under axial load showing compression and bulging of the disk is seen in **B.** Under this condition, tensile stresses will be generated in the outer anulus and compressive stresses in the nucleus. High fluid pressures (see text) are generated in the proteoglycan and water components of the nucleus pulposus that help to support the axial load. This fluid pressure has 2 components: osmotic and hydrostatic. After cessation of axial loading, the osmotic pressure causes the extruded fluid to flow back into the disk thus restoring its height (**A**). How bending of the spine (flexion or extension, and lateral bending) would cause an eccentric deformation of the disk is shown in **C,** with a cyclically alternating suction-extrusion action on the interstitial fluids, into and out of the disk. Large shear strains are induced in the disk during bending. Excessive shear stress may be the cause for anulus delamination as commonly found in degenerated disks.

hence their intrinsic material properties) comprising the disk. Analyses of the detailed changes of the structure-function relationship within the disk must be preceded by a detailed determination of the intrinsic biomechanical properties of the components of the disk for normal and pathologic tissues. Only after this has been done, meaningful finite element analyses can be undertaken to determine the details of the biomechanical and pathophysiologic processes occurring within the disk during disk degeneration.

Because compression is a dominant mode of loading for the disk, mechanisms of disk response to compressive load are of great interest. In the spine, very large compressive loads (many times body weight) exist because of muscular action. To resist these loads, the 3 load-carrying mechanisms just described must act in concert. Hydrostatic pressurization of the interstitial fluid has long been considered important for providing load support and energy dissipation in compression. When tested in confined compression, compressive modulus (stiffness), hydraulic permeability, and isometric swelling pressure of nondegenerate anulus fibrosus samples are inhomogeneous, with regional, radial, and circumferential variations. This tissue is highly nonlinear in that the compressive modulus increases with compressive strain. Interestingly, anulus fibrosus also has a

nonlinear permeability function. Its permeability is low compared with that of articular cartilage, but the increase in permeability with compressive strain is relatively low as well. It appears that nonlinear effects may be more important for compressive stiffness than for effects related to fluid movement through the tissue.

Determination of properties of anulus fibrosus in tension is important because the anulus fibrosus experiences large tensile stresses in situ. The intrinsic biomechanical properties of the anulus fibrosus in tension have been shown to be dependent on the pathologic state of the tissue. Tensile stiffness, energy dissipation, and elongation to failure depend on fiber orientation and sample thickness. Single anulus fibrosus layers do not exhibit differences between layers, but multiple-layer samples appear to be weaker than the sum of the layers. This suggests that the interlamellar ground substance between the anulus layers are weaker than the layers themselves. This may explain why delamination of the anulus fibrosus is commonly observed during disk degeneration. In general, when tested in response to uniaxial deformations, the anulus fibrosus exhibits a nonlinear "toe" region, or region of low force for small tensile strains, followed by a near-linear region at higher strains, followed by an abrupt failure. This behavior is characteristic of many collagenous tissues, including articular cartilage, ligament, meniscus, and tendon. The viscoelastic behavior, anisotropy, and inhomogeneous nature of the anulus fibrosus in tension have recently been characterized. The highly oriented and layered structure of the anulus fibrosus suggests that it behaves anisotropically. Such anisotropy in tension has been confirmed for both single layer and multilayer samples of anulus fibrosus tested in tension. In general, tensile modulus and failure stress are greatest when disk tissues are tested along the predominant collagen fibril direction.

Inhomogeneities in anulus fibrosus composition have been documented with variations in water, amount and type of collagen, proteoglycan composition from inner to outer anulus fibrosus (in the radial direction) and from anterior to posterior anulus fibrosus (in the circumferential direction). These inhomogeneities suggest that a variation in the material behavior of the anulus fibrosus may exist in the radial and circumferential directions. Tensile properties of individual layers of anulus fibrosus from differing locations vary, with specimens from anterior/outer locations being stiffer than posterolateral/inner ones. These findings support the conclusion that the stiffer outer layers create a state of uniform hoop stress during compression, while the inner layers deform and act as "shock absorbers" (the biphasic phenomenon). The circumferential direction of loading is important because this is the direction of large tensile hoop stresses generated to resist swelling pressure from the nucleus pulposus. Anulus fibrosus axial compressive strains coupled with large swelling forces in the nucleus pulposus suggest that compressive deformations may be present in the radial direction as well.

The circumferential variation in anulus fibrosus material properties, including a larger tensile modulus and failure stress in the anterior regions as compared to posterolateral regions, is intriguing given the higher proportion of disk herniations in the posterolateral region. Furthermore, this basic science finding is consistent with the conclusions of some investigators that posterior disk injury may be influenced by the regional variation in organization of laminate layers. The combination of incomplete layers, increased fiber-interlacing angle, and "loose" interconnections of fibers of the posterior outer anulus fibrosus may be associated with the decreased tensile stiffness as measured in that region. These findings support the concept that regional differences in material properties of the disk may be related to variations of the structural organization of the intervertebral disk, and that they may predispose the intervertebral disk to damage.

Disk mechanical function depends not only on the anulus fibrosus and nucleus pulposus, but also on the cartilage end plate. Little is known of the compressive behavior of cartilage end plate, but motion segment studies suggest that it undergoes significant compressive deformation.

Although morphologically distinct from anulus fibrosus and nucleus pulposus, the cartilaginous end plate functions in conjunction with the 2 structures to maintain uniform stress distribution across the boundary between the vertebral body and the disk. Because of this, compressive deformation of cartilage end plate is significantly prolonged and more rapid upon initial load as compared with that of articular cartilage. Prolonged cartilage end plate deformation in compressive creep is attributed to the interstitial fluid flow, as well as to intrinsic viscoelastic effects for the solid matrix of the cartilage end plate. Because of its much higher permeability (less fluid frictional drag), the intrinsic viscoelastic behavior of the collagen-proteoglycan solid matrix plays a much more pronounced role than articular cartilage. The high cartilage end plate hydraulic permeability causes rapid fluid transport and less pressurization in response to loading. Thus, the permeability of the cartilage end plates provides a conduit for water to flow from and into the disk, and thereby helps transfer loads in a uniform manner across the inner anulus fibrosus and nucleus pulposus. As important, this also provides an access channel for nutient and waste transport deep into and from the anulus fibrosus and nucleus pulposus, thus augmenting the diffusional transport mechanism.

The charged matrix molecules and fluid flows through the matrix give the disk another important property, the streaming potential. When a fluid passes through a charged hydrated tissue such as the anulus fibrosus, an electrical potential (difference) will occur when the electric current is limited. This electrical potential difference at zero current is called the streaming potential. This potential is a mechanical-to-electrical transduction, a phenomenon that occurs in any charged porous material. The pattern of fiber organization in normal anulus fibrosus suggests that the mechanoelectrical properties are likely to be anisotropic.

The mechanical function of the normal intervertebral disk can be summarized as follows. The nucleus pulposus acts predominantly as a fluid under static loading conditions, generating large hydrostatic pressures. The swelling pressure mechanism, arising in part from a high concentration of negatively charged proteoglycans in the nucleus pulposus, maintains disk height and contributes to the pressurization mechanism of load support and transfer. The relatively high hydraulic permeability of the cartilage end plates allows load transfer in a uniform manner across the anulus fibrosus and nucleus pulposus. The high values for tensile modulus, stiffness, and failure stress of anulus fibrosus indicate that the anulus fibrosus is well suited to resisting large tensile stresses. In particular, the outer anulus fibrosus, with the highest tensile modulus, is ideally suited for minimizing intervertebral disk bulging and anulus fibrosus strains generated during compression, bending, or torsional loading. In contrast, the lower modulus of the anulus fibrosus allows viscoelastic dissipation through a biphasic flow-dependent mechanism. This fluid-flow generated frictional dissipation mechanism in the anulus fibrosus, along with an independent dissipation resulting from nucleus pulposus deformation, are likely to be dominant mechanisms for energy dissipation and "shock absorption" for the entire intervertebral disk.

This current understanding of disk mechanical function has limitations, and further work is needed. Mathematical and numerical modeling is a technique that can be used to study the mechanical behavior of the intervertebral disk and motion segment. Such computational modeling may be used to study loading conditions or material behavior that may not be easily achieved experimentally. Clearly, model predictions will necessarily depend on the assumed geometry, the nature of the stress-strain laws used to describe the components of the disk, and the accuracy of the data for material coefficients associated with these laws. Therefore, the full usefulness of the finite element models will not be completely realized until realistic material models and geometries are used along with experimentally determined material properties. It is hoped that understanding these behaviors will make it possible to accurately model the disk and predict behavior under both normal and pathologic situations.

Selected Bibliography

Structure and Composition

Buckwalter JA: The fine structure of human intervertebral disc, in White AA III, Gordon SL (eds): American Academy of Orthopaedic Surgeons *Symposium on Idiopathic Low Back Pain.* St. Louis, MO, CV Mosby, 1982, pp 108–143.

Eyre D, Benya P, Buckwalter J, et al: The intervertebral disk: Basic science perspectives, in Frymoyer JW, Gordon SL (eds): *New Perspectives on Low Back Pain.* Park Ridge, IL, American Academy of Orthopaedic Surgeons, 1989, pp 147–207.

Eyre DR: Biochemistry of the intervertebral disc. *Int Rev Connect Tissue Res* 1979;8:227–291.

Cells

Trout JJ, Buckwalter JA, Moore KC: Ultrastructure of the human intervertebral disc: II. Cells of the nucleus pulposus. *Anat Rec* 1982; 204:307–314.

Trout JJ, Buckwalter JA, Moore KC, Landas SK: Ultrastructure of the human intervertebral disc: I. Changes in notochordal cells with age. *Tissue Cell* 1982;14:359–369.

Urban JPG: The effect of physical factors on disk cell metabolism, in Buckwalter JA, Goldberg VM, Woo SL-Y (eds): *Musculoskeletal Soft-Tissue Aging: Impact on Mobility.* Rosemont, IL, American Academy of Orthopaedic Surgeons, 1993, pp 391–412.

Proteoglycans

Buckwalter JA, Pedrini-Mille A, Pedrini V, Tudisco C: Proteoglycans of human infant intervertebral disc: Electron microscopic and biochemical studies. *J Bone Joint Surg* 1985;67A:284–294.

Buckwalter JA, Roughley PJ, Rosenberg LC: Age-related changes in cartilage proteoglycans: Quantitative electron microscopic studies. *Microsc Res Tech* 1994;28:398–408.

Buckwalter JA, Smith KC, Kazarien LE, Rosenberg LC, Ungar R: Articular cartilage and intervertebral disc proteoglycans differ in structure: An electron microscopic study. *J Orthop Res* 1989;7:146–151.

Johnstone B, Bayliss MT: Proteoglycans of the intervertebral disk, in Weinstein JN, Gordon SL (eds*): Low Back Pain: A Scientific and Clinical Overview.* Rosemont, IL, American Academy of Orthopaedic Surgeons, 1996, pp 493–509.

Collagens

Ayad S, Sandell LJ: Collagens of the intervertebral disk: Structure, function, and changes during aging and disease, in Weinstein JN, Gordon SL (eds): *Low Back Pain: A Scientific and Clinical Overview.* Rosemont, IL, American Academy of Orthopaedic Surgeons, 1996, pp 539–556.

Buckwalter JA, Maynard JA, Cooper RR: Banded structures in human nucleus pulposus. *Clin Orthop* 1979;139:259–266.

Eyre DR, Muir H: Quantitative analysis of types I and II collagens in human intervertebral discs at various ages. *Biochim Biophys Acta* 1977;492:29–42.

Biomechanics

Acaroglu ER, Iatridis JC, Setton LA, Foster RJ, Mow VC, Weidenbaum M: Degeneration and aging affect the tensile behavior of human lumbar anulus fibrosus. *Spine* 1995;20:2690–2701.

Andersson GB, Schultz AB: Effects of fluid injection on mechanical properties of intervertebral discs. *J Biomech* 1979;12:453–458.

Best BA, Guilak F, Setton LA, et al: Compressive mechanical properties of the human anulus fibrosus and their relationship to biochemical composition. *Spine* 1994;19:212–221.

Ebara S, Iatridis JC, Setton LA, Foster RJ, Mow VC, Weidenbaum M: Tensile properties of nondegenerate human lumbar anulus fibrosus. *Spine* 1996;21:452–461.

Goel VK, Nishiyama K, Weinstein JN, Liu YK: Mechanical properties of lumbar spinal motion segments as affected by partial disc removal. *Spine* 1986;11:1008–1012.

Iatridis JC, Weidenbaum M, Setton LA, Mow VC: Is the nucleus pulposus a solid or a fluid? Mechanical behaviors of the nucleus pulposus of the human intervertebral disc. *Spine* 1996;21:1174–1184.

Setton LA, Zhu W, Weidenbaum M, Ratcliffe A, Mow VC: Compressive properties of the cartilaginous end-plate of the baboon lumbar spine. *J Orthop Res* 1993;11:228–239.

Skaggs DL, Weidenbaum M, Iatridis JC, Ratcliffe A, Mow VC: Regional variation in tensile properties and biochemical composition of the human lumbar anulus fibrosus. *Spine* 1994;19:1310–1319.

Urban JP, Maroudas A: Swelling of the intervertebral disc in vitro. *Connect Tissue Res* 1981;9:1–10.

Weidenbaum M, Iatridis JC, Setton LA, Foster RJ, Mow VC: Mechanical behavior of the intervertebral disk and the effects of degeneration, in Weinstein JN, Gordon SL (eds): *Low Back Pain: A Scientific and Clinical Overview*. Rosemont, IL, American Academy of Orthopaedic Surgeons, 1996, pp 557–582.

Chapter 22

Intervertebral Disk Aging, Degeneration, and Herniation

Joseph A. Buckwalter, MS, MD

Scott D. Boden, MD

David R. Eyre, PhD

Van C. Mow, PhD

Mark Weidenbaum, MD

This chapter at a glance

This chapter discusses age-related deterioration, degenerative disease, and herniation of the intervertebral disk.

One or more of the authors or the department with which they are affiliated has received something of value from a commercial or other party related directly or indirectly to the subject of this chapter.

Introduction

No component of the musculoskeletal system changes more with age than the intervertebral disk. Age-related deterioration of disk structure, composition, and function contribute to the 2 most common clinical disorders of the axial skeleton: degenerative disease of the spine and intervertebral disk herniation.

Once skeletal maturity is achieved, all intervertebral disks undergo progressive alterations in biomechanical properties, volume, shape, microstructure, and composition that can decrease motion of and adversely affect the mechanical properties of the spine. In addition, some intervertebral disks undergo a severe age-related loss of structure and function that is best considered a form of degeneration, leaving only a thin layer of fibrous tissue separating the vertebral bodies. Motion between adjacent vertebral bodies is restricted, and degenerative changes in the facet joints may occur or worsen. In addition to restricted motion, degenerative disease of the spine can cause pain; neurologic deficits may occur when osteophytes compress the spinal cord or spinal nerves. The disk tissue is weakened and there is an increased risk of herniation, which also can cause pain and neurologic deficits.

Disk Aging

The changes in disk volume and shape (including loss of disk height, protrusion of the central disk into the vertebral body with a decrease in the height of the anulus, and buckling or bulging of the anulus) and the rate at which these changes occur following skeletal maturity vary among individuals and among disks. Unfortunately, these changes have not been well defined or correlated with those in disk tissue structure and composition.

Changes in disk tissue microstructure and composition precede and accompany the alterations in gross morphology. The changes in disk size, vascular supply, and composition (especially proteoglycan organization and proteoglycan and water concentrations) begin during growth and development, well before evidence of disk degeneration appears. These early changes may form the basis for the changes that occur following skeletal maturity, including degeneration. In this sense, the age-related disk changes begin soon after birth. The most extensive changes occur, after age 20, in the nucleus pulposus, where there is a decline in the number of viable cells and the concentrations of proteoglycans and water. These changes are accompanied by fragmentation of the aggregating proteoglycans and increases in the concentrations of collagens and noncollagenous proteins.

Newborn

At birth, distinct hyaline cartilage end plates separate the disk tissues from the vertebral bodies. The outer anulus fibrosus consists of dense circumferential layers of collagen fibrils (Fig. 1) that penetrate the cartilage plates of the vertebrae. Occasional elastic fibers lie parallel to the collagen fibrils. Small blood vessels may be found between the outer lamellae of the anulus fibrosus, especially in the posterolateral regions of the disk and adjacent to the cartilage end plates, and occasional blood vessels penetrate the inner anulus. Numerous perivascular and free nerve endings lie on and among the most peripheral layers of the anulus. The nucleus pulposus fills almost half the disk and at birth consists primarily of notochordal tissue: a soft, gelatinous, clear matrix surrounding syncytial cords and clusters of notochordal cells. The matrix of the nucleus contains few collagen fibrils and even fewer sheets of elastin embedded in an abundant network of highly hydrated proteoglycans. In disk tissues of the newborn, collagen fibers have a nearly uniform small diameter (Fig. 1). Proteoglycan aggregates from newborn and infant intervertebral disk anulus fibrosus and cartilage end plate have the same structure as aggregates from hyaline cartilages; only about one third of nucleus pulposus proteoglycan aggregates resemble these large aggregates, and the other two thirds consist of aggrecan clusters that frequently lack a visible central hyaluronan filament.

Childhood and Adolescence

During skeletal growth, disk volume and diameter increase several fold, thereby increasing the distance between the central regions of the disk and the peripheral blood vessels. At the same time the blood vessels of the anulus and the cartilage end plate become smaller and less numerous. The fibrocartilaginous component of the anulus increases in size, but during early adolescence the nucleus pulposus still comprises nearly half the disk and can easily be distinguished from the fibrocartilage of the inner anulus. The number of notochordal cells decreases, and chondrocyte-like cells appear in the central regions of the disk. More collagen fibrils appear in the nucleus, and the collagen fibrils of all disk components increase in mean diameter and variability in diameter (Fig. 1). The proportion of proteoglycans that form aggregates and proteoglycan aggrecan size both decrease, and large proteoglycan aggregates similar to those found in articular cartilage disappear. By adolescence, the proteoglycan population of the nucleus pulposus consists almost entirely of clusters of short aggrecan molecules and nonaggregated proteoglycans. A decline in the concentration of functional link protein may cause at least some of the change in proteoglycan aggregates.

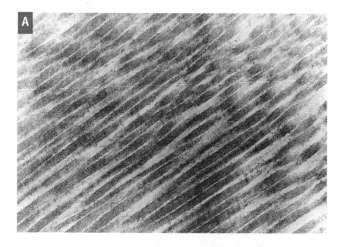

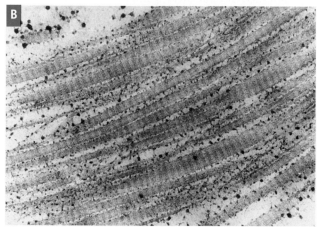

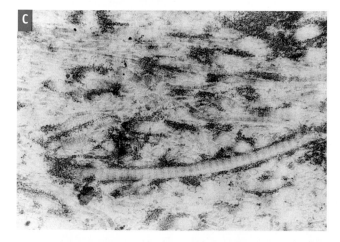

Figure 1

Electron micrographs showing collagen fibrils from the anulus fibrosus. **A,** Newborn. **B,** Young adult. **C,** Older adult. Note that the mean collagen fibril diameter and the variability in collagen fibril diameter increase between birth and skeletal maturity and that with age, electron-dense granular material accumulates in the matrix. (Reproduced with permission from Buckwalter JA: The fine structure of human intervertebral disk, in White AA III, Gordon SL (eds): American Academy of Orthopaedic Surgeons *Symposium on Idiopathic Low Back Pain*. St. Louis, MO, CV Mosby, 1982, pp 108–143.)

Adult

With skeletal maturity, many of the remaining peripheral blood vessels disappear. The size of the outer anulus fibrosus stays about the same, but the apparent size of the fibrocartilaginous inner anulus expands at the expense of the nucleus pulposus as the latter becomes progressively more fibrotic. In portions of the anulus, myxomatous degeneration develops with loss of the normal collagen fiber organization. Fissures and cracks appear in the disk, often between the lamellae, and extend from the periphery to the central regions. The nucleus pulposus becomes firm and white rather than soft and translucent. In all regions of the disk inside the outer anulus, but especially in the most central regions, the concentration of viable cells declines sharply. Few if any notochordal cells remain, but the central regions of the nucleus contain scattered viable chondrocyte-like cells. Proteoglycan and water concentrations decrease and collagen and noncollagenous protein concentrations increase as dense granular material accumulates throughout the matrix (Fig. 1). Although this material appears throughout the matrix, it appears especially concentrated in the regions immediately surrounding the cells and forms thick sheaths around some collagen fibers. Its composition remains unknown, but it may contain degraded matrix molecules or noncollagenous matrix proteins including fibronectin, and its deposition in the matrix may be at least partially responsible for the age-related increase in the concentration of noncollagenous protein. Taken together, the age-related alterations in disk tissue following skeletal maturity appear to decrease the structural integrity of the disk and thereby contribute to the changes in disk volume and shape and the increased probability of mechanical failure of the matrix leading to disk herniation.

Elderly

In the elderly, the entire disk inside the outer lamellae of the anulus fibrosus usually becomes a stiff fibrocartilage. It may be difficult if not impossible to distinguish the inner anulus fibrosus from the nucleus pulposus by gross examination, although the region of the nucleus may still have less densely packed collagen fibrils of smaller diameter, as demonstrated by electron microscopy. In the central regions of the disk, few viable cells remain (Fig. 2). The height of the disk may decline further and prominent fissures and clefts may form in the center. The loss of disk height and alterations in disk composition can affect spine mobility and alter the alignment and loads (vector) applied to the facet joints, spinal ligaments, and paraspinous muscles.

Degeneration

Although all disks undergo aging changes, not all of them degenerate. Disks that have almost disappeared, leaving only a thin layer of fibrotic tissue separating adjacent vertebral bodies, represent the end stage of the degenerative process (Fig. 3). In many instances advanced disk degeneration is associated with vertebral body osteophytes, increased bone density or sclerosis of the vertebral bodies adjacent to the disk, and facet joint osteoarthritis (Fig. 4). Small blood vessels proliferate in the end plates and vertebral bodies and grow into the peripheral regions of degenerated disks. Extension of nerves into the inner regions of the disk may accompany this vascular proliferation and ingrowth, and several investigators have found evidence that these changes are associated with back pain. The loss of disk tissue results from the action of degradative enzymes within the disk and the inability of disk cells to maintain or restore their extracellular matrix. This last stage of disk degeneration leads to a loss of spinal mobility and abnormal loading of the facet joints, spinal ligaments, and muscles. The relationships between disk degeneration and clinical disorders of the spine are complex. Advanced disk degeneration is commonly found in middle-aged and older people with no symptoms, but in others it can lead to spinal stenosis and neurogenic claudication as well as back pain.

Although the end stage of intervertebral disk degeneration can be identified by imaging studies and gross examination, widely accepted criteria for the diagnosis of disk degeneration and for distinguishing between disk aging and degeneration have not been established. Correlation of changes in disk size, shape, composition, and mechanical properties with alterations in spine function may make it possible to develop these criteria. These types of studies have recently been reported in the literature, and may eventually show that disk degeneration differs from the normal aging of the disk, much like osteoarthritis or degenerative joint disease differs from normal aging of synovial joints. In both synovial joints and the joints formed by

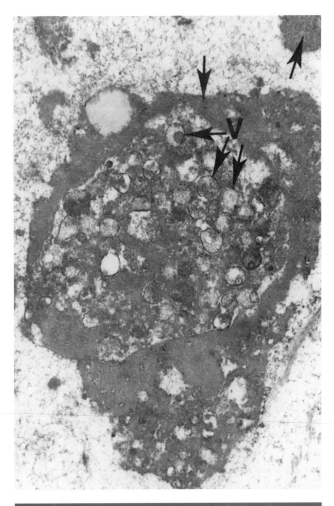

Figure 2

Electron micrograph showing the remains of a necrotic nucleus pulposus cell. V indicates membrane-bound vacuoles and the arrows mark dense cell debris. (Reproduced with permission from Buckwalter JA, Martin J: Intervertebral disk degeneration and back pain, in Weinstein JN, Gordon SL (eds): *Low Back Pain: A Scientific and Clinical Overview.* Rosemont, IL, American Academy of Orthopaedic Surgeons, 1996, pp 607–623.)

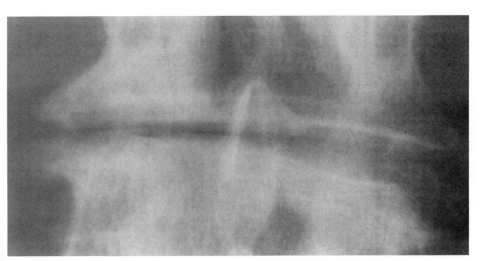

Figure 3

Radiograph showing advanced degeneration of an intervertebral disk. Note the almost complete loss of disk height and the formation of vertebral osteophytes. (Reproduced with permission from Buckwalter JA, Martin J: Intervertebral disk degeneration and back pain, in Weinstein JN, Gordon SL (eds): *Low Back Pain: A Scientific and Clinical Overview.* Rosemont, IL, American Academy of Orthopaedic Surgeons, 1996, pp 607–623.)

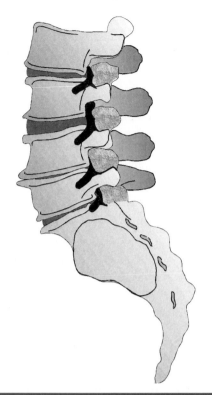

Figure 4

Drawing showing degenerative changes of the spine. Notice the advanced degeneration of the L4-5 and L5-S1 intervertebral disks, the formation of vertebral and facet joint osteophytes, and the narrowing of the intervertebral foramina by the osteophytes.

vertebral bodies and intervertebral disks, degenerative changes may or may not be associated with pain. Articular cartilage and intervertebral disks change with age, and degeneration of both these tissues is closely correlated with increasing age, but despite aging changes these tissues continue to function well throughout life in many individuals. Thus, disk degeneration may result from either an acceleration or exacerbation of normal aging or a distinct process that is superimposed on normal aging; at present a distinction between these 2 alternatives cannot be made.

Mechanisms of Intervertebral Disk Degeneration

A variety of mechanisms, including declining nutrient and waste product transport mechanisms (for example, loss of the cartilage end plate and decreased tissue hydration) decreasing concentration of viable cells, cell senescence, apoptotic debris, loss of aggregating proteoglycans, modification of matrix proteins, degradative enzyme activity, accumulation of degraded matrix macromolecules, and fatigue failure of the matrix, may contribute to disk degeneration. Although each of these mechanisms may alter disk composition and microstructure, their relative importance and the interactions among them have not been established.

Declining nutritional transport appears to be the most critical event responsible for the changes in central disk cells and their matrices. The disk cells rely on diffusion and convection of nutrient waste products through the matrix from blood vessels on the periphery of the anulus fibrosus and within the vertebral bodies. The increase in disk volume during growth, combined with the progressive age-related decline in the number of arteries supplying the periphery of the disk (and possibly calcification of the cartilage end plates), impair delivery of nutrients and removal of waste products. At the same time the blood supply to the periphery of the disk declines, the accumulation of degraded matrix macromolecules and decreasing matrix water concentration within the central disk may interfere with diffusion and convection through the matrix, further compromising cell nutrition.

Not only does the supply of nutrients decline, but the pH is decreased. This decrease is caused by a rise in lactate concentration due to an increase in its production as a result of low oxygen tension and decreased rate of lactate removal. A lower pH compromises cell metabolism and biosynthetic functions and can cause cell death. Factors that may increase the rate and severity of age-related changes in the intervertebral disk by indirectly altering nutrition transport include increased disk loading due to demanding physical activities, immobilization, vibration (such as while driving), or spinal deformity. Factors that directly compromise the vascular supply include smoking, vascular disease, and diabetes.

The age-related decline in nutrition and waste transport to and from the central disk region and the accompanying decline in pH would be expected to have an adverse effect on cell viability. Indeed, electron microscopic studies show that the proportion of necrotic cells and apoptotic debris increases with age. In fetal and infant intervertebral disks, no more than 2% of the nucleus pulposus cells showed morphologic signs of necrosis. In disks of some adolescents and young adults, more than 50% of the nucleus cells were necrotic, and in samples from elderly people, more than 80% were necrotic.

Although age-related changes in disk cell function have not been extensively studied, in other tissues declining cell function contributes to age-related degeneration. Even without decreased cell nutrition, many normal differentiated cells become senescent with age. The cells remain viable, but lose their capacity to replicate DNA and possibly some or all of their synthetic capacity and other specialized functions. Experimental evidence suggests that these alterations in cell capacity result from changes in gene expression, and that these age-related changes are controlled by transcription factors, proteins that bind to specific sequences of DNA and direct gene expression.

Mature intervertebral disks lack large proteoglycan aggregates and aggrecans similar to those found in articular cartilage. The available evidence suggests that a population of articular cartilage-like proteoglycan aggregates exists in the disks of newborns, but disappears during maturation and that the aggrecans become shorter. Other work shows that a decline in proteoglycan concentration precedes and accompanies disk degeneration. The loss of proteoglycan aggregates and large aggrecans and decreased proteoglycan concentration affect the ability of the disk to maintain a high water concentration (see Chapter 21). These changes, combined with the increasing collagen concentration and a decline in water concentration, make the central disk fibrotic and stiff, and decrease its ability to maintain its height and distribute loads.

With increasing age, connective tissue matrices, including those of the intervertebral disk tissues, tend to lose elasticity and strength. These changes may result from modifications of the various matrix collagen molecular form and ultrastructural organization. These alterations, including increased collagen cross-linking, impaired collagen fibril formation, and denaturation of collagen, contribute to disk degeneration. Increasing collagen cross-links through nonenzymatic glycation or lipid peroxidation may cause an increase in brown pigmentation with age, and, more importantly, alter disk mechanical properties. In addition to their potential effects on tissue biomechanical properties, glycation products also can stimulate cells, including chondrocytes, to release cytokines and proteases that contribute to tissue degeneration. Examination of adult human intervertebral disks has shown greater denaturation of type II collagen (loss of triple helical configuration) in the anulus fibrosus and nucleus pulposus than in articular cartilage from the same individuals. This difference may result from accumulation of degraded molecules in the intervertebral disk and could alter the biomechanical properties of the collagen fibrillar framework and the interaction of type II collagen fibrils with other matrix molecules.

Throughout life newly synthesized matrix molecules replace older molecules that are enzymatically degraded. An imbalance between synthesis and degradation leads to a loss of disk tissue. The cause of the imbalance between synthetic and degradative activity in degenerating disks remains unknown.

With aging, accumulation of partially degraded molecules may alter the properties of the disk, including the biomechanical behavior of the tissue and the ability of nutrients and metabolites to diffuse and convect through the matrix. Increasing concentrations of degraded molecules, and possibly noncollagenous proteins, may inhibit or interfere with the ability of cells to synthesize new molecules. Accumulation of degraded molecules may also interfere with the transport and assembly of newly synthesized molecules in the matrix. For example, accumulation of hyaluronan binding fragments of proteoglycan aggrecan core proteins may interfere with assembly of proteoglycan aggregates.

Normal spine movement requires loading and deformation of disks followed by recovery of disk shape. In addition,

maintaining an upright posture decreases disk height by driving water out of the disk matrix. Prolonged recumbency then restores the original disk shape and volume as water returns to the matrix. These repetitive deformations of the disk may lead to fatigue failure of the collagen fibers, and anulus delamination. These failures may appear as macroscopically observable fissures, cracks, or myxoid degeneration (appearance and accumulation of myxoid material within dense fibrous tissue), or as more subtle changes in the macromolecular framework of the matrix including fragmentation of proteoglycans, and disruption of collagen fibrils and the relationships between the collagen network and other matrix macromolecules. These alterations of the matrix may expose cells to increased stresses and strains that compromise their function.

Age-related changes in the disk may lessen the ability of the tissue to recover from deformation, either from a loss of intrinsic elasticity of the solid matrix or from a decrease of the Donnan osmotic pressure resulting from the loss of proteoglycans, and make it more vulnerable to progressive microdamage of the matrix. Loss of proteoglycans and water from the central disk regions (that is, decreased fluid pressure load support from loss of hydrostatic or osmotic pressures, or both) would therefore necessarily increase the loads that the collagen-proteoglycan solid matrix must carry. Modifications of the collagens, decreased water concentration, and accumulation of degraded matrix molecules may make the collagen framework more vulnerable to further mechanical failures, either fatigue or rupture. Also, the decline in cell nutrition, decreased concentration of viable cells, and cell senescence, combined with the accumulation of disorganized molecular debris in the extracellular matrix, could further compromise the ability of the cells to repair the altered organization of the degenerated matrix. This repair process must necessarily depend on the transport of these matrix molecules once the cells have made and extruded them into the interterritorial space. Any hindrance of this transport process clearly will affect extracellular matrix repair.

Alterations in Disk Mechanical Properties

The changes in composition and structure that occur with aging and degeneration alter the mechanical properties of the disk. The most apparent changes include increased deformability, decreased intradiskal hydrostatic and osmotic pressure, reduced fatigue life and failure strength, altered manner of load support Chydrostatic pressure versus osmotic pressure versus matrix stresses, and changes in their biphasic viscoelastic properties. The normal nucleus pulposus behaves in a manner similar to a viscous fluid; with degeneration, it shows an increase in shear modulus (becomes stiffer) and becomes more elastic. This undoubtedly is the result of a shift of composition of the nucleus with increasing collagen content. This shift in composition has been shown to increase tissue stiffness, decrease dissipation, and result in more elastic solid-like behavior. This transition from fluid-like to more solid-like behavior is associated with a decrease in hydrostatic pressurization, resulting in reduced energy dissipation in the disk. This may lead to significantly altered states of stress in the disk, with focal areas of abnormally high stresses and strains in both the nucleus pulposus and anulus fibrosus. The loss of a fluid-like nature suggests a loss of the isotropic stress state in the nucleus pulposus. The maintenance of a fluid-like nature is critical to the ability of the tissue to distribute loads. This mechanical change is likely to result in an increase in the anisotropic and nonuniform deformational behaviors of the entire disk and may be partly responsible for the induction of focal or site-specific damage in the disk. This modified stress-strain environment may have deleterious effects on the entire disk and may contribute to commonly observed degenerative changes such as tearing of the anulus fibrosus.

Anulus fibrosus samples with degenerative changes do not exhibit the same degree of anisotropy in compression as in tension. Significant effects of degeneration or specimen orientation on permeability have not been noted in anulus fibrosus samples with degenerative changes, although significant effects on stress and compressive stiffness have been identified. This implies that the highly organized anulus fibrosus collagen network does not play the major role in compression that it does in tension. Normally, fluid pressurization and osmotic swelling pressure shield the solid matrix from large stress and strains. With degeneration there is a loss of fluid content and thus fluid pressurization. This means that more of the load must now be carried by nonhydrostatic (and nonuniform) mechanisms. This diminution of stress shielding of the collagen-proteoglycan solid matrix is thought to be a major determining factor in disk degeneration.

Permeability is orientation-dependent (anisotropic) for anulus fibrosus specimens without degenerative changes, but not for those with degenerative changes. In anulus fibrosus samples without degenerative changes, permeability is greatest in the radial direction (important in diffusion and convective fluid transport of nutrients). With degeneration, radial permeability decreases (due to decreased water content or clogging of the pores with molecular debris) while axial and circumferential permeability increase (due to structural changes such as fissuring between the lamellae), leading to more isotropic permeability. This pattern is consistent with streaming potential behavior as well. Reduction of steady-state streaming potentials with degeneration may be caused by a decrease in proteoglycan content (that is, decrease of the fixed change density) with disk degeneration.

Degeneration not only affects the nucleus pulposus and anulus fibrosus, but it affects the end plate as well. Thinning, microfracture, or damage to the end plate with degeneration may significantly increase its hydraulic permeability, allowing rapid fluid exudation from the cartilage end plate on loading. Although beneficial for nutrient transport, this rapid fluid exudation would defeat any hydrostatic pressure load-support mechanism provided by the end plate, leading to a more nonuniform load distribution across the entire disk and higher shear stresses, thus contributing to site-specific damage in the disk.

With this understanding of disk mechanics, it is clear that changes with degeneration in the material behaviors of disk components may predispose the disk to mechanical failure. This can occur in the absence of any change in the type, frequency, or magnitude of loading. Degeneration is the natural consequence of either of 2 scenarios: (1) application of normal loads to disk components with abnormal material properties; and (2) application of abnormal loads to components with normal material properties. In traumatic situations, the latter scenario would prevail.

It appears that the degenerative process affects the nucleus pulposus and cartilage end plate more significantly than the anulus fibrosus, at least with respect to changes in material properties. A scenario is therefore suggested in which loss of hydrostatic pressurization and osmotic pressure in both the nucleus pulposus and cartilage end plate with degeneration has a deleterious effect on the entire disk. The loss of the mechanism for uniform load transfer and the loss of the isotropic pressure load support in the nucleus pulposus and cartilage end plate seem to lead to states of nonuniform stress within the anulus fibrosus, resulting in the development of focal stress concentrations and high shear stresses, and thus material failures.

Reduction of steady-state streaming potential with degeneration is due to the decrease in proteoglycan content (fixed charge density) with degeneration along with changes in other material properties (such as stiffness or permeability). These results may provide insight into such phenomenon as signal transduction to cells to modulate their metabolic activities. Changes in the streaming potential response of the disk suggest the possibility of developing sensitive methods for detecting early disk degeneration using electromechanically instrumented arthroscopic probes.

Intervertebral Disk Degeneration and Pain

The relationships between disk degeneration and pain remain poorly understood. Some individuals with minimal morphologic evidence of disk degeneration have chronic back pain and stiffness, while others with advanced disk degeneration have minimal symptoms. Yet, the available information suggests that intervertebral disk degeneration may contribute to back pain through 3 possible mechanisms: loss of disk structure and biomechanical properties, release of mediators that may sensitize nerve endings, and nerve and blood vessel ingrowth into degenerated disks. The loss of disk structure and biomechanical properties alters loading and alignment of vertebral bodies, facet joints, spinal ligaments, and muscles, and decreases the ability of the disks to absorb and distribute loads applied to the spine (Fig. 4). These changes may increase stimulation of nerve endings in bone, spinal ligaments, facet joint capsules, and muscles. By altering the biomechanical function of the spine and the alignment of the facet joints, long-standing advanced disk degeneration may initiate or accelerate development of osteoarthritis of the facet joints.

In addition to these structural and loading changes, the cell and matrix changes associated with disk degeneration, including cell necrosis, may be associated with release of cytokines, free radicals, and other molecular debris from matrix degradation. Some of these substances can sensitize nociceptive nerve endings and thereby contribute to the development of back pain. Although normal intervertebral disks rarely have nerve fibers or blood vessels that penetrate further than the first lamellae of the outer anulus, nerves and blood vessels have been identified in the inner anulus and even in the nucleus pulposus of degenerated disks, and these changes have been correlated with back pain.

Herniation

Intervertebral disk herniation refers to protrusion of tissue from the nucleus pulposus through a defect in the anulus fibrosus (Fig. 5). The herniated tissue may remain attached to the disk or become a free fragment. This material may frequently impinge on the spinal nerves, causing back pain.

Mechanisms of Intervertebral Disk Herniation

Fissures that extend through the full thickness of the anulus fibrosus create a defect that will allow herniation of nucleus pulposus tissue. Experimentally, compressive loads applied to flexed, twisted, fully saturated disks cause propagation of annular fissures, most often starting at the junction of the posterior anulus and the vertebral body. The causes of annular fissures in vivo remain poorly understood, but the fissures are presumed to result from localized degeneration of the anulus fibrosus or from excessive loading of normal annular tissue. It is also not clear how often full-thickness fissures lead to disk herniation; however, once the fissures form, the risk of herniation exists. Because prolonged recumbence allows fluid to flow into the central disk, increasing hydrostatic pressure and in some instances disk volume, many disk herniations occur in the morning, soon after the patients increase disk loading by assuming an upright posture. The most common site of annular disruption and symptomatic disk herniation is at the insertion of the outer anulus into the vertebral body. Hence, herniated tissue commonly tracks from the posterior surface of the anulus near its bony insertion into the space between the anterior surface of the posterior longitudinal ligament and the posterior surfaces of the anulus and vertebral body and then cephalad or caudad into the spinal canal.

Intervertebral Disk Herniation and Pain

Clinical studies show that the relationships between intervertebral disk herniation and pain are complicated. In some patients, back pain precedes a disk herniation, and

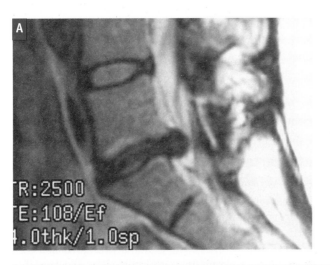
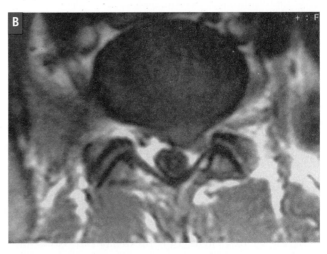

Figure 5

Magnetic resonance images showing herniated intervertebral disks. **A,** Sagittal view showing posterior herniation of the L5-S1 intervertebral disk. Note that the L4-5 intervertebral disk has a well-defined nucleus pulposus, but the L5-S1 disk has a poorly defined nucleus pulposus and reactive changes in the vertebral end plates suggesting the presence of degenerative changes. **B,** Transverse view showing a posterior lateral herniation of the L5-S1 intervertebral disk.

Chapter 23

Transplantation of Musculoskeletal Tissues

Sharon Stevenson, DVM, PhD

Steven P. Arnoczky, DVM

This chapter at a glance

This chapter discusses general principles of musculoskeletal transplantation, including terminology, graft function, incorporation, and evaluation, and bone and cartilage grafts.

General Principles of Musculoskeletal Transplantation

Terminology

The terminology of transplantation is quite exact and, in the case of bone, is complicated by the various histologic types of bone grafts. The first level of description refers to the origin of the graft. A graft moved from 1 site to another within the same individual is an autograft; the corresponding adjective is autologous or autogenous. An allograft (that is, allogeneic tissue) is tissue transferred between 2 genetically different individuals of the same species. A xenograft (xenogeneic) is tissue from 1 species implanted into a member of a different species. Two special situations of grafting exist. When tissue from 1 twin is implanted into an identical (monozygotic) twin, an isograft (isogeneic) occurs. Artificially inbred strains of mice provide the second special situation. These animals are virtually identical genetically, and tissues transferred between them are also termed isografts (syngeneic). Graft placement is either orthotopic (anatomically appropriate) or heterotopic (anatomically inappropriate). Musculoskeletal grafts can be further described as fresh or preserved. Fresh grafts are either transferred directly from the donor to the recipient site in the case of autografts, or held for a relatively short time in culture or storage medium in the case of allografts. Musculoskeletal tissue for transplantation may be preserved by freezing, freeze-drying, irradiation, or chemical means. Maintenance of sterility is a primary concern whether a graft is fresh or preserved.

Graft Function

Musculoskeletal tissue grafts often serve both a mechanical and biologic function. In certain applications one of these functions may be more important to clinical outcome than the other. For example, a massive proximal femoral graft used in a revision total hip arthroplasty provides mechanical support almost entirely, whereas allogeneic demineralized bone matrix used in a posterolateral spinal fusion provides only a stimulus for bone formation and no short-term mechanical support. Most of the time, both functions are intimately intertwined; therefore, the surgeon needs to understand how methods of preparation, processing, storage, and handling affect graft properties. Also, the surgeon needs to understand the local environment into which the graft will be placed. The net biologic activity of a graft is the sum of its inherent biologic activity (living cells and their products); its capacity to activate surrounding host tissues to relevant biologic activity (mediated by bioactive factors within the matrix); and its ability to support the ingrowth of host tissue (if necessary). The graft cannot exert its biologic activity in isolation; it is dependent on the surrounding environment for cells to respond to its signals and, in some cases, for blood supply. The mechanical environment of the graft site is also very important: bone and soft-tissue grafts are remodeled in response to mechanical load. Excessive, inadequate, and inappropriate loads may be deleterious. Thus, the environment into which a graft is placed is a very influential factor in the ultimate success or failure of that graft.

Musculoskeletal graft incorporation is a complex, multi-faceted process, and several variables influence its rate, pattern, and completeness. Although the graft and the perigraft environment each make separate contributions to the process, it is the sum of their interactions that determines the success or failure of the graft. In general, a minimal sum of biologic and environmental processes is necessary for a graft to incorporate successfully: the less biologically active and more dependent on the perigraft environment the graft, the better the environment must be. Conversely, the more biologically active and autonomous the graft, the more an attenuated perigraft environment will be tolerated.

Special Issues With Allogeneic Tissue

Processing, Preservation, and Sterilization

All methods of processing, preservation, and storage must be carefully evaluated in terms of their effects on the biologic and material properties of the tissue. Certain processes such as autoclaving are technically successful; that is, the pathogens are killed, but these processes are not functionally useful because they also denature the graft and reduce its biologic potential. For instance, sterilization by ethylene oxide under certain conditions and 2.5 mrad of gamma irradiation both substantially reduce osteoinductivity of demineralized bone matrix. Other processes adversely affect the material properties of the graft; for example, high levels of irradiation have been shown to reduce soft-tissue graft strength and stiffness. The purposes of processing are to remove as much superfluous protein, cells, and tissue as possible, and thereby to reduce the potential for immune sensitization of the recipient to donor antigens and disease transmission (see below). Modern processing methods usually include the following steps: an optional low dose irradiation step (< 20 kGy) to destroy nonpathogenic surface bacteria; physical debridement to remove unwanted tissue and reduce cellular load; ultrasonic and/or pulsatile water washes to remove most of the remaining cells and blood; ethanol treatment to denature cellular proteins and kill some viruses and bacteria; and an antibiotic soak to kill other bacteria. Soft-tissue allografts are not generally subjected to the ethanol soak because it will affect the material properties of the graft. Some allogeneic bone is demineralized during processing.

The most common methods of preservation of musculoskeletal tissue are freezing, usually to -70°C, and freeze-drying. Freezing has a minimal effect on the material properties of most grafts, but freeze-drying can change the material properties substantially and, at the very least, requires careful rehydration of the tissue. If the tissue has been collected and processed aseptically, no further treatment is necessary. If the tissue is contaminated or has not been processed sterilely, a terminal sterilization step may be performed before or after preservation.

Two methods of sterilization, ethylene oxide and irradiation, have been used for musculoskeletal tissue. Although instruments are well sterilized with ethylene oxide, this method can cause inflammation and, therefore, it cannot be recommended for musculoskeletal tissue. Irradiation is effective, killing bacteria at relatively low doses (< 20 kGy). However, it is difficult to determine the virucidal dose, which depends on the viral load and radiosensitivity of the virus. Doses that are considered potentially virucidal (> 30 kGy) affect the material properties of the graft.

Risk of Disease Transmission

Approximately 150,000 musculoskeletal allografts, including bone, tendon, and cartilage allografts, are used annually by orthopaedic surgeons in the United States. With human allografts, the transmission of disease from the donor to the recipient is a concern. The aggregate risk of disease transmission with allogeneic tissue is a reflection of the rigor of the screening and testing of potential donors and the kind of allogeneic tissue that is transplanted. At this time, the pathogens of principal concern are the human immunodeficiency virus (HIV) and the viruses responsible for hepatitis B and C. Although there are documented cases of the transmission of these diseases by musculoskeletal tissue, it is important to examine the data within the context of the time and circumstances of the occurrence. Most incidents of viral transmission via allogeneic musculoskeletal tissue occurred when the pathogen had not yet been identified or then-current technology did not identify its presence in a potential donor. One of the difficulties encountered in the detection of viral disease in potential tissue donors is that there is an initial period of viremia in which the donor may have infectious disease but have levels of the virus, or antibody in response to the virus, that are not high enough to be detected by blood tests. For example, antibody to the hepatitis B virus or HIV may not be detectable for as long as 4 weeks after exposure to the virus. There are constant improvements in the technology of serologic viral detection, both for antibody and antigen. Current tests are much more sensitive than those used only a few years ago. The most notable advance in the testing of donors for viral diseases is the use of polymerase chain reaction assays. With this method, a single infected cell can be reliably detected in a population of 10^6 uninfected cells.

All grafts should be obtained from tissue banks that follow the standards of the American Association of Tissue Banks (AATB). These tissue banks perform extensive donor screening, including a detailed social and medical history as well as serologic testing for hepatitis B surface antigen, hepatitis B core antibody, hepatitis C antibody, syphilis, human T-lymphotrophic virus-1 antibody, HIV I and II antibodies, and HIV P24 antigen. Some banks perform polymerase chain reaction testing for HIV; this is not required by the AATB.

A review of disease transmission via musculoskeletal allografts has found that the only documented incidents of disease transmission have involved frozen, unprocessed grafts such as patellar tendons or femoral heads (which are particularly at risk because of the presence of marrow contents). In one case, recipients of all organs (both kidneys, the liver, and the heart) and 3 of 4 recipients of frozen, unprocessed musculoskeletal allografts (both femoral heads and a patella-patellar ligament-tibial tubercle complex) became infected with the donor's virus. However, other grafts from this donor, including processed freeze-dried bone chips and freeze-dried segments of fascia lata, tendon, and ligament, did not transmit the disease. None of the approximately 25 recipients of freeze-dried bone chips tested positive for HIV antibody more than 5 years after the transplantation. Also worth noting is that 1 of the 4 frozen, unprocessed bone allografts from this donor did not transmit the virus. This proximal femoral graft was modified by reaming the medullary canal before using it to reconstruct the proximal femur in a revision total hip arthroplasty using a cemented prothesis. It may be that marrow removal by reaming and heating of any residual marrow by cement polymerization were sufficient to remove or kill any virus contained therein.

Processing is thought to be effective because blood, bone marrow, and soft tissue are removed. However, certain grafts such as menisci and bone-tendon-bone complexes may not be processed as mentioned previously. An experimental study using a feline retrovirus model showed that following routine tissue processing and deep-freezing, infected menisci, tendon, and cortical bone transmitted the virus to the allograft recipients in 100% of the cases. Theoretically, a method of sterilization such as gamma irradiation could be used to clear the graft of pathogens. The dose required can be calculated by knowing the bioburden and radiosensitivity of the infectious agent. Doses of gamma irradiation in the range of 30 to 40 kGy have been required before viral DNA of HIV could no longer be detected in musculoskeletal tissues. If irradiation were harmless to the tissue, the solution would be simply to irradiate the tissue with doses that kill the highest potential bioburden. However, irradiation can be harmful to the tissue. As noted elsewhere, doses of around 20 kGy do not seem to affect the mechanical properties of either bone or soft tissue, but doses equal to or greater than 30 kGy have been reported to compromise both bone and soft tissue.

Several authors have attempted to assess the degree of

risk of the transmission of HIV through transplantation of a musculoskeletal allograft. Assuming that the tissue has been obtained from a tissue bank operating under AATB guidelines, the risk of viral transmission through transplantation of processed, freeze-dried bone chips is practically zero, whereas the risk of transmission through transplantation of a frozen, unprocessed femoral head is somewhat less than that of transmission of a disease through transfusion of a unit of blood. Because of the combination of donor-screening and blood-testing it is believed that the risk of viral transmission by unprocessed musculoskeletal grafts is low: about 1 in 1 million.

Immunogenicity

The specific effects of immunogenicity on grafts of individual musculoskeletal tissues will be discussed below, but several important principles must be mentioned. The response of the host to any allograft is predominantly a cell-mediated response to cell surface antigens carried by cells in the allograft. Class I and II antigens, encoded by the genes of the major histocompatibility complex (MHC), are the major alloantigens recognized by the responding T lymphocytes. The cells of all musculoskeletal tissues display class I MHC antigens and, frequently, a subset of cells will display class II MHC antigens. Furthermore, the expression by cells within musculoskeletal tissue of class I and II MHC antigens can be induced by gamma interferon and other inflammatory mediators. Minor histocompatibility antigens are also present on the surface of cells and can be important in the late rejection of parenchymal organs. Their precise role in the host response to musculoskeletal tissue is not known. The mechanisms of rejection of any allogeneic material may include cell-mediated cytotoxicity, antibody-mediated cytotoxicity, and antibody-dependent cell-mediated cytotoxicity. All of these responses have been documented in vivo after the implantation of musculoskeletal tissue allografts.

Musculoskeletal tissue allografts and parenchymal organ allografts appear to sensitize their hosts in a similar manner; however, there are important differences in the mechanisms and outcomes of rejection. Nonvascularized musculoskeletal allografts do not contain a graft-derived vascular tree nor do they often contain living cells, which are the usual targets of rejection in parenchymal organs. Rejection is more difficult to identify and to quantify in transplants of musculoskeletal tissue than in transplants of parenchymal organs (such as kidneys) for which there are readily identifiable markers of function—for example, levels of serum creatinine. Biopsy is difficult in musculoskeletal transplants because a cellular infiltrate is generally not uniform, and it is difficult to obtain an expendable biopsy specimen. Thus, rejection has been inferred from resorption of a bone graft or the premature mechanical failure of a ligament or tendon graft. In almost all studies, experimental or clinical, allogeneic tissue has not performed as well as analogous autologous tissue, but the exact mechanisms and the singular importance of the allogeneic response in the process remain unclear. The incorporation of musculoskeletal tissue transplants is a complex process, dependent not only on the biologic properties of the graft and the responsiveness of the host bed, but also on the stability of the fixation and the mechanical loading of the graft. Many musculoskeletal tissue allografts achieve adequate clinical function.

Graft Incorporation and Evaluation

When any graft is implanted surgically, there is a stereotypic sequence of events at the site of the graft: hemorrhage, inflammation, revascularization of the tissue, and substitution and remodeling of the graft with locally derived tissue (the extent may be variable). Successful graft incorporation is defined as the ability of the transplanted tissue to function as well as the original tissue; that is, to maintain its mechanical integrity and function during and after the process of incorporation. Mechanical function depends not only on the biology of the transplanted tissue but also on surgical technique, stability of fixation, postoperative rehabilitation, the general health of the patient, and a myriad of other factors. Thus, it becomes very difficult to identify the key factors intrinsic to the tissue that affect outcome. It is important when reading the literature to evaluate the functional relevance of the models used and of the methods of assessment.

Bone Grafts

Functions

Osteogenesis refers to bone formation with no indication of cellular origin. When new bone is formed on or about a graft it may be either of graft origin (that is, from cells that survive the transfer and are capable of forming bone) or from cells of host origin. Surface cells on cortical and cancellous grafts that are properly handled can survive and produce new bone. This early bone formed by viable graft cells is often critical in callus formation during the first 4 to 8 weeks after surgery. Cancellous bone, with its very large surface area covered by quiescent lining cells or active osteoblasts, obviously has the potential for more graft origin-new bone formation than does cortical bone. Another way in which a bone graft may function as a source of osteogenesis is by being osteoinductive. Osteoinduction is the recruitment from the surrounding bed of mesenchymal-type cells, which then differentiate into cartilage-forming and bone-forming cells. Osteoinduction is mediated by graft-derived factors. The osteoinductivity of mineralized grafts is thought to be minimal except as living graft cells may be producing osteoinductive factors, but the osteoinductivity of demineralized bone matrix has been repeatedly shown. Bone matrix contains several bone morphogenetic proteins, transforming growth factor-beta, insulin-like growth factors I and II, acidic and basic fibroblast growth factors, platelet-derived growth factors, interleukins, granulocyte colony-stimulating factors, and granulocyte-macrophage colony-stimulating factors.

These moieties induce or influence the differentiation of mesenchymal cells into bone-forming cells. It is important to note that osteogenesis of graft origin occurs independently of the host bed except that diffusion is required for the survival of graft surface cells. For instance, if abundant fresh cancellous autograft is transferred to a densely fibrotic, previously irradiated bed, that graft may still survive, produce new bone, and incorporate successfully because it is capable of forming bone relatively independently of the host bed. On the other hand, the condition of the host bed is critical in the process of osteoinduction, because new osteoprogenitor cells are recruited by induction of residual mesenchymal cells in marrow reticulum, endosteum, periosteum, and connective tissue.

When placed in large defects resulting from trauma or debridement, bone grafts can act as weight-bearing space fillers. Also, cortical bone struts may be used to both stabilize and support fractures in special situations, as in periprosthetic proximal femoral fractures. These grafts are always cortical or corticocancellous bone. In addition to providing mechanical support, they function as a trellis or scaffold for the ingrowth of new host bone. The 3-dimensional process of ingrowth of sprouting capillaries, perivascular tissue, and osteoprogenitor cells from the recipient bed into the structure of a graft is termed osteoconduction. Osteoconduction may result from active bone formation and osteoinduction (for example, in a fresh corticocancellous autograft) or it may occur passively, without the active participation of the graft, as would be the case with most cortical allografts. It is important to note that osteoconduction is not random; indeed, it follows an ordered, predictable, spatial pattern, determined by the structure of the graft, the vascular supply from the surrounding soft tissue, and the mechanical environment of the graft and surrounding structures. Comparative properties of bone grafts are presented in Table 1.

Types of Bone Grafts and the Host Response

Autogenous cancellous bone, properly handled, is robustly osteogenic, easily revascularized, and quickly integrated into the recipient site. It does not provide structural support, but the rapidity with which autogenous cancellous bone both produces and stimulates new bone formation often contributes to the early stabilization of a fracture site. The major source of autogenous cancellous bone is the iliac crest. Although the graft material is extremely useful, significant morbidity accompanies the harvest procedure. The biologic activity of autogenous cancellous bone results from its histocompatibility, large surface area covered with

Table 1
Comparative Properties of Bone Grafts*

Graft Material	Inflammation/ Immunogenicity	Mechanical Properties	Osteogenesis Inductiveness	Osteogenesis Graft-Derived	Biological Dependence on Host Bed
Fresh autogenous cancellous	—	+	+++	++	+
Fresh vascularized autogenous cortical	—	+++	+	+	+
Fresh nonvascularized autogenous cortical	—	+++	+	—/+	++
Processed allogeneic cancellous chips	+	—/+	—	—	+++
Processed allogeneic cortical	+	+++	—	—	+++
Allogeneic demineralized bone matrix	+	—	++	—	+++
Allogenic inductive proteins (BMP-like)	—	—	+++	—	++

*— = not present; + = degree to which each property is represented; BMP = bone morphogenetic protein

(Reproduced with permission from Stevenson S, Goldberg VM: Bone transplantation, in Evarts CE (ed): *Surgery of the Musculoskeletal System*, ed 2. New York, NY, Churchill Livingstone, 1989, pp 115–150.)

osteoblasts and their precursors, and trabecular architecture. Clinicians should be aware that minced or morcellized autogenous cortical bone does NOT have the same robust biologic activity as cancellous bone, although it may be helpful in extending the volume of graft material.

The host response to cancellous autograft is described in 5 stages, which overlap and form a continuum. Hemorrhage and inflammation, the first 2 stages, occur rapidly after the surgical procedure. Many of the grafted cells die, particularly osteocytes in trabecular lacunae, but surface osteoblasts do survive and produce early new bone. Because cancellous bone is quite porous, host vessels, osteoblasts, and osteoblast precursors can infiltrate the graft from the periphery toward the center as early as 2 days after surgery. Osteoclast precursors are blood-borne; therefore, the ingrowth of vessels marks the beginning of graft resorption. As the third stage, vascular invasion of the cancellous graft proceeds, and osteoblasts line the edges of dead trabeculae and deposit a seam of osteoid, which eventually surrounds the central core of dead bone. Subsequently, the graft is remodeled; that is, the new host bone and entrapped cores of necrotic bone are gradually resorbed by osteoclasts and replaced with new bone synthesized by host osteoblasts (the fourth stage). The period of osteoconduction and early remodeling may last for several months in cancellous autografts. The final stage is the integration of the graft into a streamlined mechanical supporting structure. This process is well underway by 6 months and is usually complete by 1 year after surgery.

Nonvascularized cortical autografts, properly handled, provide structural support, are somewhat osteogenic, and revascularize slowly. The delay in revascularization may be attributed to the structure of cortical bone, because the vascular penetration of the graft is primarily the result of peripheral osteoclastic resorption and vascular invasion of Volkmann's and haversian canals. In contrast to cancellous grafts, which initially appear more radiodense because of the deposition of new host bone on dead, grafted trabeculae, cortical bone becomes more radiolucent because osteoclasts spearhead the invasion of vessels from the surrounding host bed. The graft becomes significantly weaker than normal bone, and the weakness persists for months to years depending on the size of the graft. The mechanical phase of incorporation is much more predominant in cortical bone than in cancellous grafts. Large portions of the dead cortical autograft may remain for significant periods of time. The major source of nonvascularized cortical autograft is the fibula, although the use of the anteromedial aspect of the tibia has also been described. The ilium will provide corticocancellous bone, but the mass and strength of the cortex is less than that of the fibula.

A successful vascularized cortical autograft provides limited structural support (if stable, there is rapid healing at the host-graft interface) and functions relatively independently of the host bed. Its turnover and remodeling resemble that of normal bone, and the ingrowth of vascular buds from the host bed is not necessary for its incorporation. Because vascularized cortical autografts are implanted with a functional blood supply, their incorporation differs markedly from that of nonvascularized cortical autografts. When anastomosis of the vessels is a success and the graft suffers only transient intraoperative ischemia, over 90% of osteocytes survive the transplantation procedure. Graft-host union occurs quickly, and resorption followed by osteoconduction and remodeling, as consistently observed in nonvascularized cortical grafts, is not seen. The 3 sources for free vascularized bone autografts are the fibula, iliac crest, and rib. The fibula may be isolated on its peroneal vessels. The iliac crest graft uses the deep circumflex iliac artery and vein, and the rib graft uses the posterior intercostal artery and vein. Although the graft will not be weakened by marked resorption, it must be supported with appropriate internal or external fixation until it can hypertrophy in response to the mechanical loading of its new site. Grafts are remodeled in response to the same local mechanical stimuli (that is, Wolff's law) as normal skeletal bone.

Allogeneic demineralized bone matrix (DBM) is quickly revascularized, provides no structural support, and may be moderately osteoinductive. Implantation of allogeneic DBM is followed by platelet aggregation, hematoma formation, and inflammation characterized by migration of polymorphonuclear leukocytes into implants within 18 hours. Thereafter, fibroblast-like mesenchymal cells are attracted to and establish close contact with the implanted matrix. Interactions between the DBM and mesenchymal cells result in cellular differentiation into chondrocytes around day 5 after implantation. Chondrocytes produce cartilage matrix, which is then mineralized. By days 10 to 12, vascular invasion accompanied by osteoblastic cells is observed, multinuclear cells appear, and chondrocytes begin to degenerate. New bone is formed apposed to the surface of the mineralized cartilage. Remodeling and replacement of these composite structures with new host bone ensues. With time and continued remodeling, all of the implanted DBM will be resorbed and replaced with host bone suitable for the environment in which it finds itself. Adequate cross-linking of collagen in DBM as well as the presence of osteoinductive proteins in a proper amount and proportion are necessary for sustained osteogenesis.

The source and processing of DBM has a direct effect on its osteoinductive capacity. For instance, storage of bone at room temperature for more than 24 hours prior to processing causes the recovered DBM to be biologically inactive. Sterilization by ethylene oxide under certain conditions and 2.5 mrad of gamma irradiation both substantially reduce osteoinductivity. The AATB and the Food and Drug Administration require that each batch of DBM be made from a single human donor so the characteristics of the individual donor will also influence the biologic activity of that batch. A variety of putties, pastes, gels, and sheets based on DBM are commercially available. Each will be made from a single donor. The DBM may be shredded or ground, and may be from cortical or cancellous bone. The carrier may be water soluble (such as glycerol) or non-watersoluble (such as gelatin). In general, commercial vendors attempt to differentiate products based more on their handling, or physical characteristics, than on their biologic activity. However, in assessing commercially available information, orthopaedists should be mindful that passive remineralization of demineralized bone is not biologically equivalent to new, active bone formation, although it will appear as mineral density on radiographs.

Morcellized and cancellous allogeneic bone grafts provide limited mechanical support (mostly resistance to compression) and are osteoconductive only. Morcellized grafts may be derived from either cancellous or cortical bone. Mineralized cancellous or cortical bone may be processed to yield chips ranging from 0.5 to 3 mm in diameter or shapes up to 1 cm in diameter. Morcellized allografts usually are preserved by freeze-drying. Morcellized and cancellous allografts are characterized by an open, porous, almost lattice-like physical structure so there is no physical impairment to the ingrowth of vessels. The same stages of incorporation occur in morcellized/cancellous allografts as in autografts, but the allografts are osteoconductive only, as they have no living cells. They are not osteoinductive because the matrix is mineralized. However, because they are mineralized, the allografts have some inherent mechanical strength; that is, resistance to compression. Thus, allografts may serve as weightbearing structures during the process of graft incorporation. Because resorption is not necessary in order that they be revascularized, allografts do not suffer the transient loss in mechanical strength that is generally seen during the incorporation of mineralized cortical bone.

Corticocancellous and cortical allografts provide structural support and are osteoconductive to a limited degree. Corticocancellous grafts may be prepared from the ilium, distal femur, and proximal tibia. Cortical bone may be cut longitudinally to yield struts that are generally used to buttress preexisting bone or constructs. Full-thickness fibulas may also be used as struts. Full-thickness cortical bone grafts, ranging from short ring-like structures to entire diaphyses, are available and are generally used to fill defects and to buttress constructs. Following processing, cortical bone may be preserved by deep-freezing, usually at -70°C, or by freeze-drying. Freezing has minimal effects on processed bone allografts, because the cells and proteins have already been removed by processing. Deep frozen bone retains its material properties and can be implanted immediately after thawing.

Freeze-drying alters the material properties of mineralized cortical bone and necessitates reconstitution (rehydration) of the graft prior to implantation. Even with reconstitution, freeze-dried cortical bone can be somewhat friable and remains weak in torsion and bending. The early phase of inflammation following implantation of a cortical allograft is similar to that following the implantation of all grafts. Vascular invasion begins, and inflammatory cells migrate into the area. It is during this time that the host encounters graft-derived cellular antigens, if present, and becomes sensitized to them. Cortical bone that has been processed by modern processing techniques generally contains very little protein and few, if any, intact cells. When this bone is implanted, the initial trauma-induced, nonspecific postoperative inflammation subsides within a few days after surgery. Massive cortical allografts are penetrated by vessels and are substituted with host bone very slowly, superficially, and to a limited degree. This may account for the incidence of fracture in these grafts, which is reported to range from 16% to 50%. When biopsies of the fracture site were obtained at the time of surgical treatment of the fracture, a lack of revascularization and soft-tissue attachments was noted. These massive grafts likely sustain fatigue microdamage as cyclic loading occurs over time. Necrotic bone cannot repair itself in response to that damage, which ultimately results in failure of the matrix.

Cortical allografts remain significantly weaker for a considerable time after surgery than cortical autografts. Given enough time and a weightbearing, stable construct, most segmental cortical allografts will eventually resemble autografts biomechanically and structurally, although significantly more unremodeled necrotic bone will be present in allografts. The above comments refer to cortical grafts processed by modern processing techniques, whether frozen or freeze-dried. Cortical grafts that are denatured by harsh alkylating agents or by autoclaving may be slowly revascularized, if they are revascularized at all. There have been several clinical reports of sensitization of recipients to graft-specific histocompatibility antigens. Studies in animals have documented a correlation between a graft-specific immune response and a reduction of revascularization and remodeling of cortical grafts. Bone allografts can induce secretion of graft-specific antibodies, as documented by the previously mentioned clinical case studies as well as animal models. Additionally, cell-mediated immune responses have been documented in response to allogeneic bone. It is important to note that all of these studies have used either fresh bone or bone that has been frozen without complete debridement and cleansing.

In general, 2 physical factors determine the incidence and speed of union between bone grafts and the adjacent host bone more than the characteristics of the grafts themselves: stability of the construct and contact between host-bone and the graft. In animal models, when the host-graft interfaces were intimately apposed and were stably fixed with compression plates, all interfaces healed, whether the grafts were autogenous or allogeneic, or fresh or frozen. Under stable conditions, but without intimate host bone-graft contact, all interfaces did not heal, but the biologic characteristics of the graft did not have a discernible effect. When the grafted site was less stable, almost no unions were seen. Furthermore, a decreasing incidence and maturity of union were noted with decreasing stability of the graft site in that model. The importance of stability of the graft on the parameters of graft incorporation has been noted experimentally and clinically and cannot be overemphasized.

Cartilage Grafts

Types of Cartilage Grafts and the Host Response

The treatment of defects of articular cartilage with an injection of culture-expanded autologous chondrocytes under a periosteal flap has been described in recent clinical and experimental studies. Although clinical reports and early rabbit data appear to be promising, a quantitative histomorphometric examination of long-term reconstitution of femoral trochlear groove articular cartilage in dogs comparing untreated empty defects, empty defects with a periosteal flap, and defects filled with autologous chondrocytes with a periosteal flap showed no significant differences among groups at 12 and 18 months after surgery. Furthermore, in the 2 groups that received a periosteal flap, articular cartilage surrounding the defect showed degenerative changes appearing to be related to the suturing of the flap.

In evaluating all experimental models of articular cartilage repair, the site of the defect, the species of the animal, and the duration of the study must be considered. Defects in full weightbearing sites, such as the femoral condyle, repair differently (and frequently more completely) than those in minimal weightbearing sites such as the trochlear groove. The species of animal is important in drawing conclusions for clinical practice, because the articular cartilage of most experimental animals is substantially thinner (0.7 to 1.2 mm) than that in similar sites of humans (3 mm). The relatively lighter body weight of most experimental species, as well as difficulties in postoperative management (limitation of range of motion and weightbearing immediately after surgery and a progressive rehabilitation regimen are both difficult), and sometimes lack of postoperative use (cage housing) make correlations between animal studies and the expected clinical outcome even more tenuous. It is also very important to examine long-term outcome, both experimentally and clinically. Many treatments that looked promising at 3 or 6 months after surgery do not maintain their advantage when examined at 12 or 24 months after surgery.

The use of multiple autologous osteochondral fragments to repair articular cartilage defects has also been reported clinically. The technique involves taking small osteochondral plugs from an uninvolved area of the injured knee that bears minimal weight and transferring these plugs to the defect site. No fixation is used exclusive of the press-fit. While there have been multiple clinical reports of this technique, at the time of this writing, no experimental studies with histologic or functional evaluation of the long-term integration and maintenance of these plugs have been published.

Fresh allogeneic osteochondral grafts (shell grafts) are articular cartilage with a thin shell of underlying bone, which are held at 4°C prior to transplantation. The rationale for this storage method is that the chondrocytes will survive for up to 4 days while the bone cells will die under these conditions. The intent is to implant living, intact cartilage that can maintain itself after transplantation and dead bone that will remain structurally intact during replacement by host bone. The presence of the cartilaginous matrix is believed to shield the MHC antigen-bearing chondrocytes from recognition by the host. It is also hypothesized that the bone component will be less immunogenic because the cells are dead. The grafts are most often used for traumatic defects in younger, higher-demand patients in whom implants are not desirable and arthrodesis is not acceptable. There is strong correlation between experimental and clinical observations—both types of studies agree that mechanical conditions seem more important to successful results than immunologic factors. Appropriate sizing of the graft, fixation of the graft, realignment of the limb, and a controlled postoperative rehabilitation regimen are critical to a successful outcome. The clinical success rate was reported to be 76%. Long-term (up to 10 years) survival of the chondrocytes has been documented both clinically and experimentally. Histologically, the dead graft bone appeared to have been replaced by host bone. Chronic synovitis, fibrosis of the subsynovial tissue, and mild chronic inflammatory infiltrates have been observed in transplanted joints. The extent to which these reactions reflect a specific immunologic response to donor antigens is not known.

Massive allogeneic osteochondral grafts are used to reconstruct joints in limb-sparing procedures following tumor resection. These grafts comprise cortical bone, metaphyseal cancellous bone, and articular cartilage. The previous comments regarding the incorporation of frozen cortical allografts are relevant to massive osteochondral grafts. The cortical bone is revascularized and replaced to a minimal extent as has been previously described. A retrieval study demonstrated that soft tissue, such as fascia, ligaments, and tendons, became firmly attached to the surface of the allograft through a seam of appositional bone that had been laid on the surface of the allograft. A common complication is nonunion at the host-graft interface. Achieving a stable host-graft interface and robust surgical construct is particularly important because only 1 end of these grafts may be stabilized with internal fixation devices. Unique to this graft type is the entire metaphyseal, epiphyseal, and articular cartilage portion of the graft, which will be bearing weight almost immediately and which can have only minimal protection with internal or external fixation devices.

These grafts are generally stored at -80°C after the cartilage has undergone cryopreservation with dimethylsulfoxide (DMSO). Only the superficial chondrocytes survive cryopreservation and thawing in intact articular cartilage, so the viability of the implanted cartilage is quite limited. Histologic examination of both experimental and clinical cryopreserved osteochondral allografts has shown that no graft chondrocytes survived. The necrotic cartilage functioned well for as long as 5 years, and as it degenerated, it was covered by a pannus of fibrovascular reparative tissue. Good anatomic fit of the graft and satisfactory stability of the joint, mediated by adequate soft-tissue repair, were correlated with maintenance of necrotic articular cartilage architecture. The radiographic appearance was the same whether there was necrotic articular cartilage or fibrovascular pannus.

When massive osteochondral grafts were studied in a dog model at 11 months after surgery, the subchondral trabeculae of fresh autografts were revascularized and well remodeled, resembling sham-operated bones. The subchondral trabeculae of all allografts (both MHC matched and mismatched and fresh and cryopreserved) were thickened because new bone formed on their surfaces without much remodeling. Fibrous connective tissue filled the intertrabecular spaces. In some allografts, focal bone resorption had resulted in distortion of the bony architecture and even breaks in the subchondral plate. These findings are similar to those reported from a clinical study of retrieved osteochondral allografts. In some of those grafts the subchondral plate and adjacent trabeculae remained necrotic and unrepaired. In other grafts, revascularization and trabecular resorption had occurred beneath the articular surface, resulting in major architectural changes. Degenerative changes about the joint and joint instability can be late complications of the surgery.

Meniscal Allografts

Unlike ligament replacement where other allograft tissues (such as Achilles tendon, fascia lata, and patellar tendon) can be used to replace the lost structure, the meniscus requires an exact replacement. As with any tissue, successful transplantation of the meniscus depends on several factors, including tissue preservation, the immunologic compatibility of the donor and host, and the long-term biologic and biomechanical integrity of the transplant.

Several preservation techniques have been proposed for the meniscus, including glutaraldehyde fixation, deep-freezing, cryopreservation, and freeze-drying. Because several studies have shown that viable articular cartilage allografts are biomechanically superior to nonviable grafts, cryopreservation was initially thought to be the method of

choice. In this technique, meniscal tissue is controlled-rate frozen to -100°C using DMSO or glycerol as a cryopreservative. An experimental study has demonstrated that while this technique had no untoward effects on the overall structure or tensile properties of the menisci, only 10% of the cells survived the preservation process and remained viable at 1 week. Although other studies demonstrated varying amounts of cell viability using other preservation techniques, the role of viable cells in the success or failure of transplanted menisci is still a matter of debate. One study has shown that 4 weeks after transplantation of a totally viable meniscus, no donor DNA could be found in the tissue. This would suggest that cell viability at the time of transplantation is a moot point. Indeed, experimental studies examining meniscal transplantation using fresh, cryopreserved, and deep-frozen allografts have shown a similar biologic incorporation of the graft. In all cases, cells (presumably from the peripheral synovial and capsular tissues) migrate into the transplant and ultimately repopulate the tissue with cells resembling meniscofibrochondrocytes. Histologic and vascular studies have shown a normal vascular and cellular pattern at 6 months following transplantation. Limited mechanical and biochemical evaluations have shown that although the transplant has normal tensile properties at 6 months, there is a decrease in the proteoglycan content and an increase in the water content. The long-term effect of these findings has not been examined.

Gamma irradiation with ^{60}Co has been used as a method of secondary sterilization of deep-frozen and freeze-dried menisci. However, precise dose recommendations to achieve complete bactericidal and virucidal activity as well as the effect of such levels on the biomaterial properties of the meniscus have not been determined.

Histologic evaluations of fresh, cryopreserved, and deep-frozen meniscal transplants used in experimental studies have not identified evidence of an immune response. The clinical experience with meniscal allografts has yielded mixed results. Variations in surgical technique, patient selection, and postoperative management have made it difficult to draw any conclusion on the long-term efficacy of meniscal allografts.

Ligament Allografts

The success of autogenous tissues as cruciate ligament substitutes and the fact that these grafts are avascular at the time of transplantation have led to the concept of using allograft tissues for cruciate ligament replacement. Several tissues, including bone-patellar tendon-bone, Achilles tendon, hamstring tendons, iliotibial band, fascia lata, and bone-cruciate ligament-bone have been used as allograft replacements of the cruciate ligaments. Although tissue harvest is usually done under aseptic conditions, several methods of secondary sterilization have been proposed, including the use of ethylene oxide and gamma irradiation. Ethylene oxide has been routinely used in association with freeze-drying of the tissue, allowing it to be stored at room temperature. However, clinical reports have documented sterile reactions to ethylene oxide-sterilized tissue used for cruciate ligament replacement. One study was able to document by-products of ethylene oxide in these grafts several months after transplantation. It was thought that inadequate aeration following sterilization of these grafts was responsible for these reactions.

Gamma irradiation with ^{60}Co has also been used to sterilize these ligament allografts. Although 25 kGy of irradiation has been considered to provide adequate sterilization, many bacteria and viruses have been shown to require higher doses to render these organisms inactive. One study has demonstrated that a dose of at least 30 kGy of irradiation was required to sterilize HIV-infected bone-patellar tendon-bone grafts. However, this dose of irradiation has also been shown to adversely affect the material properties of patellar tendon allografts. These changes range from a slight decrease in tensile modulus to a significant decrease in ultimate stress.

Preservation of allograft tissues used to reconstruct the cruciate ligaments is currently limited to deep-freezing and freeze-drying. Studies have shown that the structural properties of deep-frozen (-80°C) or freeze-dried tissues were not significantly different from those of fresh specimens. The immunogenicity of allografts used to replace the cruciate ligaments remains a matter of debate. Experimental and clinical studies have shown evidence of donor-specific antibodies in the synovial fluid, as well as in the serum of individuals receiving fresh-frozen bone-patellar tendon-bone allografts. However, these findings were not associated with any clinical abnormalities or obvious alterations in graft incorporation.

Numerous studies have examined the biologic incorporation of allografts used for cruciate ligament replacement. As with autogenous tissues, allografts used to reconstruct the cruciate ligaments must be revascularized and revitalized if they are to remain functional within the joint. The vascular tissues of the infrapatellar fat pad and synovium, as well as vessels from the tibial and femoral bone tunnel, contribute to a vascular synovial envelope that surrounds the graft within the first 6 weeks. This extrinsic vascular supply provides the origin for the intrinsic revascularization and cellular proliferation within the allograft. Although experimental studies in animals have shown that allografts and autograft patellar tendons undergo a similar remodeling process, it appears that the allograft tissues remodel at a slower rate. This may be because of the initial lack of cells in the allograft or a result of a localized immune response.

Clinical experience with allograft reconstruction of the cruciate ligaments has produced mixed results. Although most clinicians agree that allografts provide an acceptable level of function, overall results have not been as good as those achieved with autografts because of an increased incidence of effusions and increased long-term laxity. In addition, a clinical study has shown that freeze-dried tissues produced less satisfactory results when compared to fresh-frozen tissue.

Summary

It seems a rather simple act to remove a single segment of diseased or injured bone, cartilage, or soft tissue and to replace it with tissue transferred from another site or with tissue transferred from another person. Certainly, such surgeries are technically feasible—in fact, they are performed frequently in modern medical practice. However, what begins as a technical exercise ends as a journey through the intricacies of immunology, biochemistry, physiology, biomechanics, molecular biology, and pathology. The goal of the clinician who performs a grafting procedure is to choose the right graft or combination of grafts for the biologic and mechanical environment into which the graft will be placed.

Portions of this chapter are reproduced with permission from Stevenson S: Enhancement of fracture healing with autogenous and allogenic bone grafts. *Clin Orthop* 1998; 355(suppl):S236–S246.

Selected Bibliography

Graft Function

Stevenson S, Emery SE, Goldberg VM: Factors affecting bone graft incorporation. *Clin Orthop* 1996;324:66–74.

Processing, Preservation, and Sterilization

Hamer AJ, Strachan JR, Black MM, Ibbotson CJ, Stockley I, Elson RA: Biomechanical properties of cortical allograft bone using a new method of bone strength measurement: A comparison of fresh, fresh-frozen and irradiated bone. *J Bone Joint Surg* 1996;78B: 363–368.

Jackson DW, Windler GE, Simon TM: Intraarticular reaction associated with the use of freeze-dried, ethylene oxide-sterilized bone-patella tendon-bone allografts in the reconstruction of the anterior cruciate ligament. *Am J Sports Med* 1990:18:1–11.

Pelker RR, Friedlaender GE: Biomechanical aspects of bone autografts and allografts. *Orthop Clin North Am* 1987;18:235–239.

Simonian PT, Conrad EU, Chapman JR, Harrington RM, Chansky HA: Effect of sterilization and storage treatments on screw pullout strength in human allograft bone. *Clin Orthop* 1994;302:290–296.

Risk of Disease Transmission

Conrad EU, Gretch DR, Obermeyer KR, et al: Transmission of the hepatitis-C virus by tissue transplantation. *J Bone Joint Surg* 1995; 77A:214–224.

Nemzek JA, Arnoczky SP, Swenson CL: Retroviral transmission by the transplantation of connective-tissue allografts: An experimental study. *J Bone Joint Surg* 1994;76A:1036–1041.

Tomford, WW: Transmission of disease through transplantation of musculoskeletal allografts. *J Bone Joint Surg* 1995;77A:1742–1754.

Immunogenicity

Horowitz MC, Friedlaender GE: Induction of specific T-cell responsiveness to allogeneic bone. *J Bone Joint Surg* 1991;73A:1157–1168.

Khoury MA, Goldberg VM, Stevenson S: Demonstration of HLA and ABH antigens in fresh and frozen human menisci by immunohistochemistry. *J Orthop Res* 1994;12:751–757.

Muscolo DL, Caletti E, Schajowicz F, Araujo ES, Makino A: Tissue-typing in human massive allografts of frozen bone. *J Bone Joint Surg* 1987;69A:583–595.

Muscolo DL, Ayerza MA, Calabrese ME, Redal MA, Santini Araujo E: Human leukocyte antigen matching, radiographic score, and histologic findings in massive frozen bone allografts. *Clin Orthop* 1996; 326:115–126.

Shigetomi M, Kawai S, Fukumoto T: Studies of allotransplantation of bone using immunohistochemistry and radioimmunoassay in rats. *Clin Orthop* 1993;292:345–351.

Skjodt H, Hughes DE, Dobson PR, Russell RG: Constitutive and inducible expression of HLA class II determinants by human osteoblast-like cells in vitro. *J Clin Invest* 1990;85:1421–1426.

Skjodt H, Moller T, Freiesleben SF: Human osteoblast-like cells expressing MHC class II determinants stimulate allogeneic and autologous peripheral blood mononuclear cells and function as antigen-presenting cells. *Immunology* 1989;68:416–420.

Stevenson S: The immune response to osteochondral allografts in dogs. *J Bone Joint Surg* 1987;69A:573–582.

Stevenson S, Horowitz M: The response to bone allografts. *J Bone Joint Surg* 1992:74A:939–950.

Strong DM, Friedlaender GE, Tomford WW, et al: Immunologic responses in human recipients of osseous and osteochondral allografts. *Clin Orthop* 1996;326:107–114.

Bone Graft Functions

Buckwalter JA, Glimcher MJ, Cooper RR, Recker R: Bone biology: Part I. Structure, blood supply, cells, matrix, and mineralization. *J Bone Joint Surg* 1995;77A:1256–1275.

Buckwalter JA, Glimcher MJ, Cooper RR, Recker R: Bone biology: Part II. Formation, form, modeling, remodeling, and regulation of cell function. *J Bone Joint Surg* 1995;77A:1276–1289.

Burchardt H: The biology of bone graft repair. *Clin Orthop* 1983; 174:28–42.

Burwell RG: The fate of bone grafts, in Apley AG (ed): *Recent Advances in Orthopaedics*. Edinburgh, Scotland, Churchill Livingstone, 1969, pp 115–207.

Friedlaender GE: Bone grafts: The basic science rationale for clinical applications. *J Bone Joint Surg* 1987;69A:786–790.

Heiple KG, Chase SW, Herndon CH: A comparative study of the healing process following different types of bone transplantation. *J Bone Joint Surg* 1963;45A:1593–1616.

Vander Griend RA: The effect of internal fixation on the healing of large allografts. *J Bone Joint Surg* 1994;76A:657–663.

Types of Bone Grafts and the Host Response

Berrey BH Jr, Lord CF, Gebhardt MC, Mankin HJ: Fractures of allografts: Frequency, treatment, and end-results. *J Bone Joint Surg* 1990;72A:825–833.

Dell PC, Burchardt H, Glowczewskie FP Jr: A roentgenographic, biomechanical, and histological evaluation of vascularized and non-vascularized segmental fibular canine autografts. *J Bone Joint Surg* 1985;67A:105–112.

Enneking WF, Mindell ER: Observations on massive retrieved human allografts. *J Bone Joint Surg* 1991;73A:1123–1142.

Feighan JE, Davy D, Prewett AB, Stevenson S: Induction of bone by a demineralized bone matrix gel: A study in a rat femoral model. *J Orthop Res* 1995;13:881–891.

Goldberg VM, Shaffer JW, Field G, Davy DT: Biology of vascularized bone grafts. *Orthop Clin North Am* 1987;18:197–205.

Goldberg VM, Stevenson S, Shaffer JW, et al: Biological and physical properties of autogenous vascularized fibular grafts in dogs. *J Bone Joint Surg* 1990;72A:801–810.

Kale AA, Di Cesare PE: Osteoinductive agents: Basic science and clinical applications. *Am J Orthop* 1995;24:752–761.

Leunig M, Yuan F, Berk DA, Gerweck LE, Jain RK: Angiogenesis and growth of isografted bone: Quantitative in vivo assay in nude mice. *Lab Invest* 1994;71:300–307.

Mankin HJ, Gebhardt MC, Jennings LC, Springfield DS, Tomford WW: Long-term results of allograft replacement in the management of bone tumors. *Clin Orthop* 1996;324:86–97.

Schwartz Z, Mellonig JT, Carnes DL Jr, et al: Ability of commercial demineralized freeze-dried bone allograft to induce new bone formation. *J Periodontol* 1996;67:918–926.

Stevenson S, Li XQ, Davy DT, Klein L, Goldberg VM: Critical biological determinants of incorporation of nonvascularized cortical bone grafts: Quantification of a complex process and structure. *J Bone Joint Surg* 1997;79A:1–16.

Stevenson S, Li XQ, Martin B: The fate of cancellous and cortical bone after transplantation of fresh and frozen tissue-antigen-matched and mismatched osteochondral allografts in dogs. *J Bone Joint Surg* 1991;73A:1143–1156.

Cartilage Grafts

Breinan HA, Minas T, Hsu H-P, Nehrer S, Sledge CB, Spector M: Effect of cultured autologous chondrocytes on repair of chondral defects in a canine model. *J Bone Joint Surg* 1997;79A:1439–1451.

Brittberg M, Lindahl A, Nilsson A, Ohlsson C, Isaksson O, Peterson L: Treatment of deep cartilage defects in the knee with autologous chondrocyte transplantation. *N Engl J Med* 1994;331:889–895.

Brittberg M, Nilsson A, Lindahl A, Ohlsson C, Peterson L: Rabbit articular cartilage defects treated with autologous cultured chondrocytes. *Clin Orthop* 1996;326:270–283.

Gross, AE: Use of fresh osteochondral allografts to replace traumatic joint defects, in Czitrom AA, Gross AE (eds): *Allografts in Orthopaedic Practice*. Baltimore, MD, Williams & Wilkins, 1992; pp 67–82.

Lance EM, Kimura LH, Manibog CN: The expression of major histocompatibility antigens on human articular chondrocytes. *Clin Orthop* 1993;291:266–282.

Mankin HJ, Gebhardt MC, Jennings LC, Springfield DS, Tomford WW: Long-term results of allograft replacement in the management of bone tumors. *Clin Orthop* 1996;324:86–97.

Matsusue Y, Yamamuro T, Hama H: Arthroscopic multiple osteochondral transplantation to the chondral defect in the knee associated with anterior cruciate ligament disruption. *Arthroscopy* 1993; 9:318–321.

Oates KM, Chen AC, Young EP, Kwan MK, Amiel D, Convery FR: Effect of tissue culture storage on the in vivo survival of canine osteochondral allografts. *J Orthop Res* 1995;13:562–569.

Ohlendorf C, Tomford WW, Mankin HJ: Chondrocyte survival in cryopreserved osteochondral articular cartilage. *J Orthop Res* 1996;14: 413–416.

Sams AE, Nixon AJ: Chondrocyte-laden collagen scaffolds for resurfacing extensive articular cartilage defects. *Osteoarthritis Cartilage* 1995;3:47–59.

Sellers RS, Peluso D, Morris EA: The effect of recombinant human bone morphogenetic protein-2 (rhBMP-2) on the healing of full-thickness defects of articular cartilage. *J Bone Joint Surg* 1997;79A: 1452–1463.

Shortkroff S, Barone L, Hsu HP, et al: Healing of chondral and osteochondral defects in a canine model: The role of cultured chondrocytes in regeneration of articular cartilage. *Biomaterials* 1996;17:147–154.

Stevenson S, Dannucci GA, Sharkey NA , Pool RR: The fate of articular cartilage after transplantation of fresh and cryopreserved tissue-antigen-matched and mismatched osteochondral allografts in dogs. *J Bone Joint Surg* 1989;71A:1297–1307.

Meniscal Allografts

Arnoczky SP, McDevitt CA, Schmidt MB, Mow VC, Warren RF: The effect of cryopreservation on canine menisci: A biochemical, morphologic, and biomechanical evaluation. *J Orthop Res* 1988;6:1–12.

Arnoczky SP, Warren RF, McDevitt CA: Meniscal replacement using a cryopreserved allograft: An experimental study in the dog. *Clin Orthop* 1990;252:121–128.

Jackson DW, McDevitt CA, Simon TM, Arnoczky SP, Atwell EA, Silvino NJ: Meniscal transplantation using fresh and cryopreserved allografts: An experimental study in goats. *Am J Sports Med* 1992; 20:644–656.

Jackson DW, Simon TM: Biology of meniscal allograft, in Mow VC, Arnoczky SP, Jackson DW (eds): *Knee Meniscus: Basic and Clinical Foundations*, New York, NY, Raven Press, 1992, pp141–152.

Jackson DW, Whelan J, Simon TM: Cell survival after transplantation of fresh meniscal allografts: DNA probe analysis in a goat model. *Am J Sports Med* 1993;21:540–550.

Ligament Allografts

Arnoczky SP, Warren RF, Ashlock, MA: Replacement of the anterior cruciate ligament using a patellar tendon allograft: An experimental study. *J Bone Joint Surg* 1986;68A:376–385.

Bechtold JE, Eastlund DT, Butts MK, Lagerborg DF, Kyle RF: The effects of freeze-drying and ethylene oxide sterilization on the mechanical properties of human patellar tendon. *Am J Sports Med* 1994;22:562–566.

Fideler BM, Vangsness CT Jr, Lu B, Orlando C, Moore T: Gamma irradiation: Effects on biomechanical properties of human bone-patellar tendon-bone allografts. *Am J Sports Med* 1995;23:643–646.

Jackson DW, Corsetti J, Simon TM: Biologic incorporation of allograft anterior cruciate ligament replacements. *Clin Orthop* 1996;324: 126–133.

Jackson DW, Simon TM, Kurzweil PR, Rosen MA: Survival of cells after intra-articular transplantation of fresh allografts of the patellar and anterior cruciate ligaments: DNA-probe analysis in a goat model. *J Bone Joint Surg* 1992;74A:112–118.

Shino K, Kimura T, Hirose H, Inoue M, Ono K: Reconstruction of the anterior cruciate ligament by allogeneic tendon graft: An operation for chronic ligamentous insufficiency. *J Bone Joint Surg* 1986;68B: 739–746.

Vasseur PB, Rodrigo JJ, Stevenson S, Clark G, Sharkey N: Replacement of the anterior cruciate ligament with a bone-ligament-bone anterior cruciate ligament allograft in dogs. *Clin Orthop* 1987;219: 268–277.

Chapter Outline

Chapter 24

Anatomy, Biology, and Biomechanics of Tendon and Ligament

Savio L-Y. Woo, PhD

Kai-Nan An, PhD

Cyril B. Frank, MD

Glen A. Livesay, PhD

C. Benjamin Ma, MD

Jennifer Zeminski, BS

Jennifer S. Wayne, PhD

Barry S. Myers, MD, PhD

This chapter at a glance

This chapter focuses on the basic science of the structure and function of tendons and ligaments, and discusses anatomy, biochemical composition, biomechanical properties, and healing processes.

Introduction

The injury and repair of soft tissues in and about the diarthrodial joints of the human body continue to be significant problems in orthopaedic surgery. With the increased interest in athletic activities and the increased use of high-speed transportation, severe soft-tissue injuries are becoming more common in people of all ages. Proper treatment and management of these injuries play an increasingly important role in clinical practice. Such injuries produce both acute and chronic disability and, although once thought to be of minor consequence, have been shown to lead to premature joint degeneration with significant morbidity. Given the increasing life span of humans, together with the increase in frequency of such soft-tissue injuries, prevention of their sequelae and consequent chronic disability is becoming more significant.

Tendons and ligaments are important structures that govern motion as well as share load in diarthrodial joints. Injury or loss of these structures can lead to marked changes in joint motion and to significant morbidity for patients. This chapter focuses on these important aspects, with the first section focusing on the basic science of the structure and function of tendons, and the second section covering the basic science of ligaments. Each section begins with a review of the anatomy and biochemical composition of tendon and/or ligament. The biomechanical properties as well as the various factors that could affect these properties are then discussed, followed by the healing processes in these structures. At the end of each section, the biomechanics are then related to a clinical application, with examples such as tendon transfer and ligament reconstruction. In order to obtain a true understanding of the behavior of tendons and ligaments, it is necessary to examine the structural hierarchy from the smallest constituents to their biomechanical behavior.

Tendon

Anatomy

Morphologically, tendon is a complex composite material consisting of collagen fibrils embedded in a matrix of proteoglycans, associated with a relative paucity of cells. Fibroblasts, the predominant cell type within tendons, are arranged in the spaces between the parallel collagen bundles. The cell bodies are rod- or spindle-shaped and oriented in rows when seen microscopically in a longitudinally derived section (Fig. 1). When viewed in cross section, the cell's outlines appear as dark, star-shaped structures between the collagen bundles (Fig. 2). The cytoplasm of the fibroblasts stains darkly with basic dyes and contains a clear centrosome adjacent to the single round nucleus.

Although the borders between successive cells in a row are distinct, the lateral borders of the cells are indistinct as a result of thin cytoplasmic processes that extend between collagen bundles (Fig. 3).

The major constituent of tendon is type I collagen (86% fat-free dry weight). Collagen contains a high concentration of glycine (33%), proline (15%), and hydroxyproline (15%). Thus, almost two thirds of the primary structure of the collagen chain consists of these 3 amino acids. Hydroxyproline, a derivative of the incorporated proline, is unique to collagen. Hydroxylysine makes up 1.3% of collagen dry weight and is also unique to the molecule.

The secondary structure of collagen relates to the arrangement of each chain in a left-handed configuration, and in its tertiary structure 3 collagen chains are combined into a collagen molecule. In type I collagen, there are 2

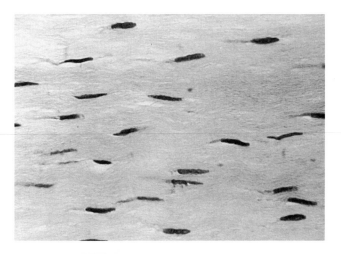

Figure 1

Photomicrograph of a longitudinal section of a human flexor tendon showing the spindle-shaped fibroblasts (hematoxylin and eosin, × 250).

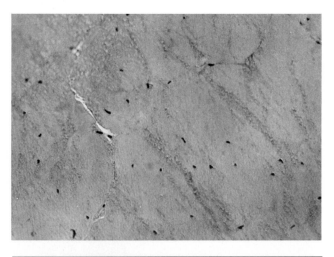

Figure 2

Photomicrograph of a cross section of a human flexor tendon showing the star-shaped fibroblasts with cytoplasmic processes extending between collagen bundles (hematoxylin and eosin, × 250).

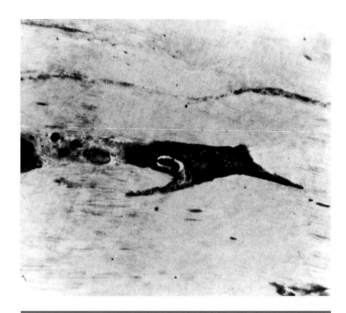

Figure 3

Electron micrograph of fibroblast (× 4000).

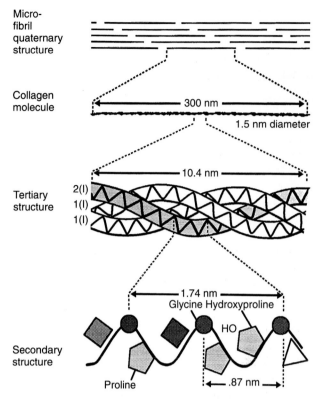

Figure 4

Schematic drawing of structural organization of collagen into the microfibril.

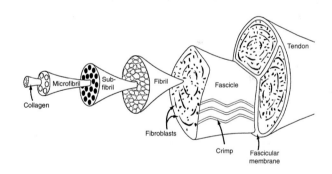

Figure 5

Schematic representation of the microarchitecture of a tendon. (Adapted with permission from Kastelic J, Baer E: Deformation in tendon collagen, in Vincent JFV, Currey JD (eds): *The Mechanical Properties of Biologic Materials.* Cambridge, England, Cambridge University Press, 1980, pp 397–435.)

identical polypeptide chains called α1(I) and a slightly different chain called α2(I) or simply α2. The 3 chains are coiled together in a right-handed triple helix held together by hydrogen and covalent bonds (Fig. 4).

The quaternary structure of collagen relates to the organization of collagen molecules into a stable, low energy biologic unit based on a regular association of adjacent molecules' basic and acidic amino acids. By arranging adjacent collagen molecules in a quarter-stagger, oppositely charged amino acids are aligned. The fact that a great deal of energy and, therefore, force is required to separate these molecules accounts in part for the strength of the structure. In this way, collagen molecules combine to form ordered units of microfibrils (5 collagen molecules), subfibrils, and fibrils (Fig. 5). These units are arranged in closely packed, highly ordered parallel bundles that are oriented in a distinct longitudinal pattern, with proteoglycans and glycoproteins in association with water incorporated in a matrix, binding the fibrils together to form fascicles (Fig. 6).

Proteoglycans make up 1% to 5% of the tendons' dry weight. They are extremely hydrophilic and thus can trap and bind water. Proteoglycans are important for their role in the interaction with collagen fibers. One of the small proteoglycans, decorin, is widely distributed and is thought to play a fundamental role in regulating collagen fiber formation in vivo. It has been suggested that uncontrolled lateral fusion of collagen fibrils in a decorin-deficient tendon would reduce tensile strength of the tendon. On the other hand, it also has been shown that decorin incorporation can increase the ultimate tensile strength of fibers that are not cross-linked. It has been speculated that decorin can prevent fibrillar slippage during deformation, thereby improving the tensile properties of collagen fibers. The distribution

of various proteoglycans changes in response to the in vivo mechanical environment. Analysis of the human posterior tibialis tendon from age 1.5 months to 24 months shows that decorin is the predominant proteoglycan in the proximal (tension-bearing) region of the tendon. In contrast, 2 types of small proteoglycans (decorin and biglycan) and large proteoglycans are present in the region that experiences localized compression where the tendon passes behind the medial malleolus. The same distribution of proteoglycans

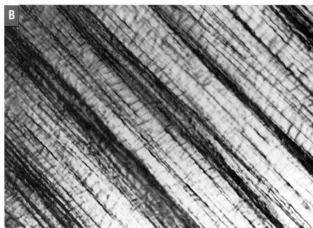

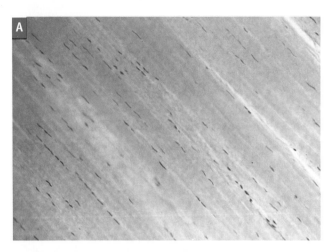

Figure 6

A, Photomicrograph of a longitudinal section of a human flexor tendon. Note the parallel rows of fibroblasts lying between the collagen bundles. **B,** Photomicrograph of the same section under polarized light microscopy, illustrating the parallel, longitudinally arranged collagen bundles (hematoxylin and eosin, × 100).

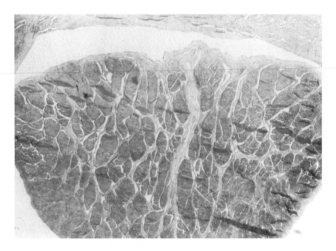

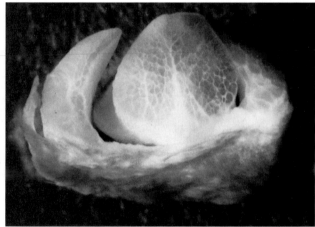

Figure 7

Photomicrograph of a cross section of a human flexor tendon showing the connective tissue (endotenon) that surrounds the fascicles of the tendon (hematoxylin and eosin, × 25).

Figure 8

Cross section of a human flexor tendon (flexor digitorum superficialis, flexor digitorum profundus) at the midportion of the proximal phalanx of the third digit. The endotenon tissue of the profundus is clearly visible.

for tissues under tension alone has also been documented in the human patellar tendon. This distribution showed no distinctive trends related to age after puberty.

The fascicles within the tendon are bound together by loose connective tissue, the endotenon, which permits longitudinal movement of collagen fascicles and supports blood vessels, lymphatics, and nerves (Fig. 7). Tendons typically carry tensile forces (tractions). However, at regions where tendons wrap around an articular surface, large compressive stresses are produced. Tendons in these regions assume a cartilage-like appearance. Tendons that bend sharply, such as the flexor tendons of the hand, are enclosed by a tendon sheath that acts as a pulley and

directs the path of the tendon (Fig. 8). A bifoliate mesotenon originates on the side of the bend opposite from the pulley friction surface and joins the epitenon that covers the surface of the tendon. The sliding of this type of tendon is assisted by synovial fluid, which is extruded from the parietal synovial membrane and from the visceral synovial membrane or epitenon (Fig. 9). Tendons not enclosed within a sheath move in a straight line and are surrounded by a loose areolar connective tissue called the paratenon, which is continuous with the tendon.

Tendons receive their blood supply from vessels in the perimysium, the periosteal insertion, and the surrounding tissue via vessels in the paratenon or mesotenon. In ten-

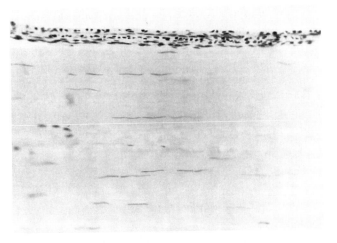

Figure 9

Longitudinal section of a human flexor tendon illustrating the epitenon on the surface of the tendon (hematoxylin and eosin, × 125).

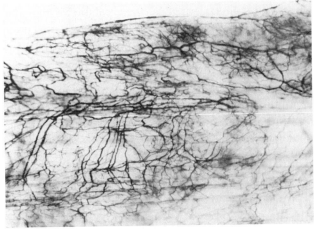

Figure 10

India ink injected (Spalteholz technique) calcaneal tendon of a rabbit, illustrating the vasculature of a paratenon-covered tendon. Vessels enter from many points on the periphery and anastomose with a longitudinal system of capillaries.

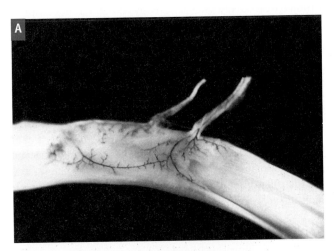
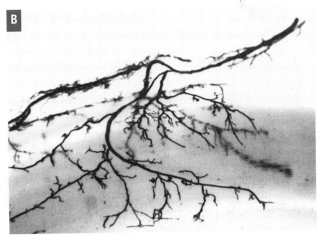

Figure 11

A, India ink injected specimen illustrating the vascular supply of the flexor digitorum profundus in a human through the vinculum longus. **B,** Close-up of specimen (Spalteholz technique) showing the extent of the blood supply from the vinculum longus. The vessels in the vinculum divide into the dorsal, proximal, and distal branches, giving off vertical vascular loops into the tendon substance.

dons surrounded by a paratenon, vessels enter from many points on the periphery and anastomose with a longitudinal system of capillaries (Fig. 10). The vascular pattern of a flexor tendon within a tendon sheath is quite different. Here, blood is supplied by the proximal mesotenons and is reduced to the long and short vinculae (Fig. 11). These tendons also receive their blood supply from their osseous insertions. Despite a large number of vessels supplying these tendons, injection studies have identified consistent areas of avascularity. These avascular regions have led several investigators to propose a dual pathway for tendon nutrition: a vascular pathway and, for the avascular regions, a synovial (diffusion) pathway. The concept of diffusional nutrition is of primary clinical significance in that it implies that tendon healing and repair can occur in the absence of adhesions (that is, a blood supply).

Biomechanics

Tensile Properties

Tendon possesses one of the highest tensile strengths of any soft tissue in the body, both because its main constituent is collagen, one of the strongest fibrous proteins, and because these collagen fibers are arranged parallel to the direction of tensile force. The tensile properties of tendon can be characterized by the mechanical (material) properties of the tendon itself as well as the structural properties of the bone-tendon-muscle structure. The mechanical properties (stress-strain relationship) of the collagen depend primarily on the architecture of the collagen fibers, and the interaction of the collagen with the extracellular matrix and proteoglycans. The structural properties (load-elongation relationship) of the bone-tendon-muscle structure depend on the mechanical properties of the tendon substance as well as its bony insertion site and the myotendinous junction. A more detailed description of the method to determine these biomechanical properties can be found in the section on biomechanics of ligaments.

Briefly, the structural properties of the bone-tendon-muscle structure can be represented by a load-elongation curve (Fig. 12) obtained during a uniaxial tensile test. The load-elongation curve begins with a toe region, in which the tendon stretches easily, without much force. This behavior has been attributed to the straightening of the crimped fibrils and the orienting of the fibers in the direction of loading. The toe region is generally smaller in tendon than in ligament because the collagen fibers are oriented more nearly parallel with the long axis of the tendon, and less realignment is required during loading. From this curve, the stiffness (slope of the curve in N/mm), ultimate load (load at failure in N), and the energy absorbed to failure (area under the curve in N•mm) can be obtained.

The mechanical properties of tendon, represented by the stress-strain relationship, can be obtained if the cross-sectional area of the tendon and the elongation of the tissue substance are known. Stress in N/mm^2 is defined as the load per cross-sectional area of the tendon substance. Strain is obtained by marking out a gauge length within the central region of the tendon and is defined as the change in length divided by the gauge length. The stress-strain curve shows similar nonlinearity as the load-elongation curve (Fig. 13). From the stress-strain curve, parameters such as the modulus (E, slope of the curve in MPa), tensile strength (σ, ultimate tensile strength in MPa), ultimate strain (ϵ), and the strain energy density (ω in MPa) can be determined.

Similar to the load-elongation curve, with increasing strain, the toe region leads into a linear region in which the slope of the curve represents the elastic modulus of the tendon. Following the linear region, the stress-strain curve at larger strains can end abruptly or curve downward as a result of irreversible changes (failure) or permanent stretching in the tendon. Thus, to fully describe the stress-strain curve, the elastic modulus, the ultimate tensile strength, and the ultimate strain, as well as the strain energy density, are required.

It has been shown in animals that the elastic modulus of tendon ranges from 500 to 1,200 MPa, whereas the ultimate tensile strength ranges from 45 to 125 MPa. In humans, the elastic modulus ranges from 1,200 to 1,800 MPa, the ultimate tensile strength of tendon ranges from 50 to 105 MPa, and ultimate strain ranges from 9% to 35%. Structural properties of bone-tendon-muscle complexes have also been studied extensively, but vary greatly with different complexes from various anatomic locations.

Time- and History-Dependent Behavior of Tendons

Tendons, like many soft tissues, exhibit time-dependent and history-dependent viscoelastic properties. In other words, their elongation depends not only on the amount of force but also on the time and history of force application. This viscoelastic behavior reflects the inherent properties of collagen as well as the interactions between collagen and ground substance. The time dependence is best illustrated by the phenomena of creep and stress relaxation. Creep is defined as the time-dependent elongation of a tissue when subjected to a constant load (Fig. 14). Stress-relaxation, on the other hand, is defined as the time-dependent decrease

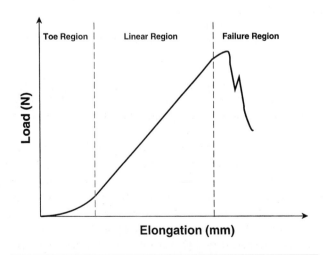

Figure 12

A schematic load-elongation curve for tendon, indicating 3 distinct regions of response to tensile loading.

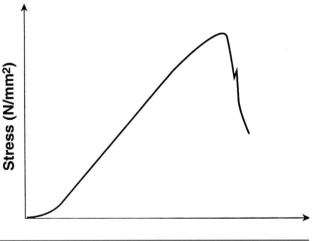

Figure 13

Schematic stress-strain curve resulting from tensile testing of a ligament.

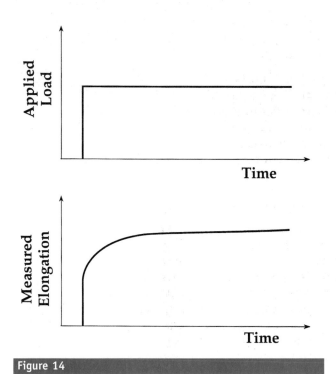

Figure 14

Schematic representation of creep under a constant load.

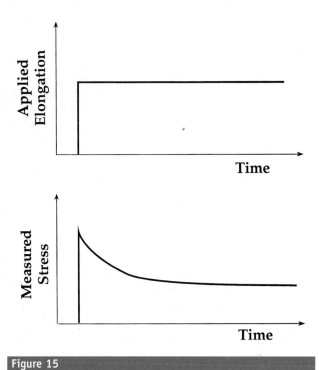

Figure 15

Typical curves demonstrating the stress-relaxation behavior of soft tissue.

in load when the tissue is subjected to constant elongation (Fig. 15). The history-dependent behavior of tendons means that the shape of the load-elongation curve will vary depending on the previous loading. For example, during cyclic loading and unloading of a tendon between 2 limits of elongation, the loading (top) and unloading (bottom) curves from a single cycle follow different paths, forming hysteresis loops (Fig. 16). With increasing numbers of cycles, the peak force decreases. Eventually, after many cycles, the loading and unloading curves become similar to those in the previous cycle. The viscoelastic response will regulate not only tension, but also elongation. For example, in an isometric contraction, the length of the muscle-tendon unit remains constant; however, because of creep, the tendon elongates, allowing the muscle to shorten. Physiologically, the change in length of the muscle decreases the rate of muscle fatigue. Thus, tendon creep increases muscle performance in an isometric contraction.

An additional viscoelastic effect in tendon and ligaments is preconditioning. The first few cycles of elongation following inactivity reveal larger areas of hysteresis (energy loss) than subsequent cycles. Following this conditioning (similar to warm-up exercise), the behavior of the tissues (load-elongation curve) becomes more repeatable. This preconditioning step is important and should be included in biomechanical test protocols to avoid experimental errors caused by the viscoelastic properties of the tissue. For example, after preconditioning, the recovered elastic strain energy of a tendon is 90% to 96% per cycle when loaded in the physiologic range, indicating that tendons do not waste

much energy during repetitive activity.

Like many other soft connective tissues, the properties of tendon are somewhat strain-rate dependent: an increased elongation rate (and therefore a higher strain rate) will make the tendon appear stiffer. However, its strain-rate dependency, like that of ligaments, is not nearly as

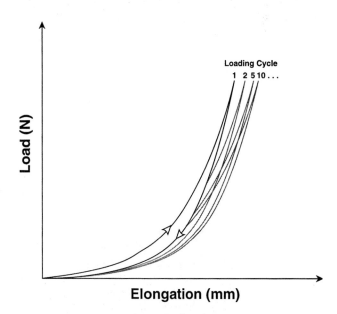

Figure 16

Typical loading (top) and unloading (bottom) curves from cyclic tensile testing of soft tissue. The area between the curves, called the area of hysteresis, represents the energy losses within the tissue.

pronounced as that demonstrated for bone. Although a comprehensive study of tendon has not yet been done, the effects of strain rate have been demonstrated on a specialized tendon, such as the rat tail tendon.

Factors Affecting the Mechanical Properties of Tendons

Many factors have been identified that influence the tensile properties of tendons. In addition to the viscoelastic effects discussed above, anatomic location, the level of activity, age, and heat treatment will also affect the mechanical properties of the tendons.

Anatomic Location Tendons from different anatomic locations experience different biomechanical and biochemical environments; their biomechanical properties also vary. The ultimate tensile strength of the digital flexor tendons of adult miniature swine is about twice as large as those of the digital extensor tendons. Biochemical analysis also reveals that the digital flexors have a much higher collagen concentration than the digital extensors. Further, the hysteresis of extensor tendons is twice as large as that of the flexor tendons. These differences increase with age and maturation (Fig. 17). At birth, the digital flexor and extensor tendons have similar mechanical properties. The reason for the change in tendon properties with anatomic location is probably multifactorial. One hypothesis is that the cross-link stabilization that occurs in collagen during growth and aging, which results in increased modulus and strength, takes place more rapidly in the flexor tendons than in the extensor tendons. This difference may be influenced by the level of stress experienced in vivo.

Exercise and Immobilization Exercise has a positive long-term effect on the structural and mechanical properties of tendons. For example, the modulus and ultimate load of swine digital extensor tendons increase as a result of long-term exercise training. The crimp angle and crimp length have been found to be influenced significantly by exercise. Exercise may also enhance collagen synthesis; this possibility is confirmed by results of biochemical studies of collagen metabolism after physical stress. Furthermore, tendons subjected to exercise have a higher percentage of large diameter collagen fibrils. The large diameter fibrils can be expected to withstand greater tensile forces than small diameter fibrils because they contain a higher number of intrafibrillar covalent cross-links.

The effects of stress shielding on the mechanical properties of the patellar tendon have been examined using a rabbit model. The tensile strength in the completely stress-shielded group was significantly less than that in the partially stress-shielded group at 1, 2, 3, and 6 weeks. However, the cross-sectional area of the completely stress-shielded tendon was significantly larger than that of the partially stress-shielded tendon at 1, 2, and 3 weeks.

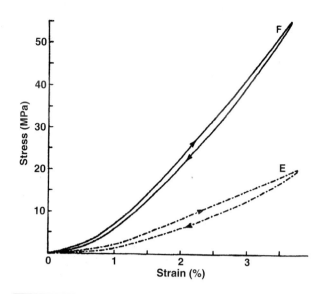

Figure 17

Examples of stress-strain curves obtained from digital flexor (F) and extensor (E) tendons of adult pigs. Arrows show loading and unloading directions. Elastic modulus values at peak stress are 1.8 and 0.7 GPa, and hysteresis values are 7% and 19%, respectively. (Reproduced with permission from Shadwick RE: Elastic energy storage in tendons: Mechanical differences related to function and age. *J Appl Physiol* 1990;68:1036.)

The effect of stress deprivation and cyclic tensile loading on the mechanical properties of the canine flexor digitorum profundus tendon was examined in vitro. Stress deprivation resulted in a progressive and significant decrease in the elastic modulus over an 8-week period. Conversely, in vitro cyclic tensile loading of tendons over a 4-week period resulted in a significant increase in the elastic modulus compared with that of the stress-deprived tendons.

Age Age has a great influence on the mechanical properties of tendons. An age-related decrease in crimp angle contributes to the decrease in the toe region of the stress-strain curve. The modulus increases with age (up to skeletal maturity) and then remains relatively constant. Before maturity, the linear region is followed by a single yield region in which irreversible elongation and structural damage take place (Fig. 18). A near-zero modulus is observed in this yield region. After maturity, this single yield plateau is not as obvious and is replaced by 2 distinct yield regions. The ultimate tensile strength and ultimate strain also increase with maturation. In one study, the age-related changes in the mechanical properties of rabbit Achilles tendon were examined using immature (age 3 weeks), young adult (age 8 to 10 months), and old (age 4 to 5 years) rabbits. The cross-sectional area of the tendon increased with growth. The ultimate tensile strength of the young adult and old tendon was significantly higher than that of the immature tendon. However, there was no significant difference in tensile strength between mature and old tendons. The modulus of the mature tendon was higher than those of the immature

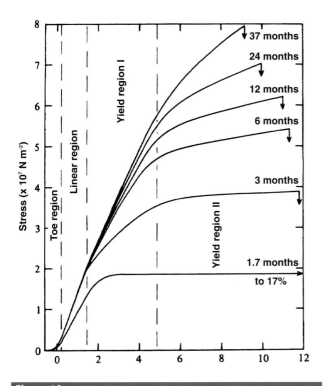

Figure 18

Stress-strain behavior of rat tail tendon as a function of age. (Adapted with permission from Kastelic J, Baer E: Deformation in tendon collagen, in Vincent JFV, Currey JD (eds): *The Mechanical Properties of Biologic Materials.* Cambridge, England, Cambridge University Press, 1980, pp 397–435.)

and old tendons, although the difference was not statistically significant.

The ultrastructural appearance of the proteoglycan filaments and their relationships with the collagen fibrils was investigated in mature and immature tendons. Proteoglycan filaments were seen to be orthogonally arranged in a repeating pattern in mature tendons. In immature tendons, proteoglycan filaments took up more varied orientations, but were mainly orthogonal or axially arranged with respect to the collagen fibrils. Young tendons ruptured at lower tensile strength than mature tendons. It is suggested that proteoglycan bridges between collagen fibrils play a role in tensile stress transmission in tendons and thus contribute to the strength of the tissue.

Laser/Heat Treatment Laser or heat shrinkage of soft tissue is a treatment regimen that is gaining popularity in orthopaedics. The effect of laser energy on the length, stiffness, and structure of connective tissues has been examined using the rabbit patellar tendon. The results indicated significant tendon shrinkage after laser treatment. A sharp increase in shrinkage to approximately 70% of resting length was noted around 70°C. Tensile testing of the tendons shortened 10% of their resting length showed a decrease in load to failure to approximately one third compared with that of control specimens. It should also be

noted that in vivo, the length of the treated tendon had increased significantly beyond immediate post-laser length at 4 weeks and even beyond its original length by 8 weeks. At 8 weeks, the laser-treated tendons had a significantly lower stiffness as well as a significantly larger cross-sectional area than the contralateral controls. Because of the relatively unknown effect of laser treatment, more scientifically based evaluations are needed to better understand the long-term consequences of laser or heat treatment on soft tissue both in vitro and in vivo.

Experimental Considerations in Tensile Testing of Tendons

There are a number of technical considerations associated with the experimental measurement of tensile properties of tendons. The readers should be made aware of and appreciate the potential errors in results obtained when reviewing results reported in the literature.

Testing Environment The environment in which tendons are tested, including specimen hydration and temperature, can affect their mechanical properties. Collagenous tissue swells minimally in water and physiologic saline, but markedly in acid solution with an associated decrease in tendon stiffness. On the other hand, dehydration of the tendon causes it to stiffen and increases the stress at failure, but with a significant decrease in strain at failure. Temperature also influences the mechanical properties and the creep rate of tendons. The stiffness of canine Achilles and patellar tendon decreased significantly with an increase in temperature from 23°C to 49°C. A quantitative relationship has also been demonstrated between temperature and the viscoelastic properties of the canine medial collateral ligament.

Gripping the Tendon Slipping of the tendon in the test grips has been a significant problem in experimental determination of tensile properties of soft tissue. This slippage produces falsely large elongation measurements and may result in failure at erroneously low loads. Also, at the grips, there is a significant stress concentration that can alter the stress-strain curve. For small tendons such as rat tails, methods in which 2 looped ends are jammed into a hole or methods that involve wrapping the ends around a cylindrical surface give satisfactory results with minimal slippage or tearing of the tendon in the grips. For larger tendons, special treatment of the ends is required. Methods in which the tendon ends are bound with wire, suture, or adhesive material have been used. Freezing the tendon ends into a fluid medium has been another successful method for securing test specimens with minimal structural damage.

Tensile tests should be done on longer specimens with a higher length versus width ratio (called the aspect ratio); this will minimize the error due to slippage and stress concentration at the test grips. Also, this testing condition will result in a more uniform stress distribution in the midsubstance of the tendon where the tensile stress is being measured. A uniform stress distribution is important for measuring the stress-strain relationship and, thus, the structural properties. A twisted specimen, which has a nonuniform cross-section, does not produce a proper stress-strain relationship.

Percent Elongation Versus Strain In some experimental studies, the movement between the tissue clamps has been used to represent the amount of elongation, or strain, of a specimen. Unfortunately, this assumption introduces errors as slippage occurs and can lead to erroneous measurements of tendon elongation. When this method is used to determine the mechanical properties (stress-strain relationship) of the tendon, the strain in the tendon is assumed to be uniform along its length; however, a number of studies have demonstrated that the distribution of strain along the tendon substance during tensile testing is not uniform. Usually, the strain near the clamps is much higher (over twice as much in some instances) than that for the midsubstance. It is, therefore, preferable to use an extensometer, which can provide measurements of elongation in a selected portion of the tendon midsubstance during testing to determine strain. Noncontact (optical) methods that depend on either surface markers or markers inserted into the tendon can also be adapted for strain measurements.

Initial Length The definition of the initial length used in strain calculations (the gauge length) has a considerable effect on the reported mechanical properties. This gauge length can be difficult to determine because during the initial portion of the test, small forces produce large changes in length as a result of the low elastic modulus within the toe region. Initial length affects the determination not only of strain but also of the modulus. To help standardize testing, the gauge length is usually determined by the application of a small initial load (or tare load) to the specimen before measurements.

Test Specimen Geometry The ultimate tensile strength of the whole tendon is usually lower than that of single fibers or fiber bundles. Two reasons for this phenomenon have been suggested. First, the stress in thicker tendons is distributed unevenly among the tendon fibers, leading to the sequential failure of fiber bundles. It is therefore extremely important to align specimens in the appropriate orientation to avoid experimental errors when determining tensile properties. Second, a whole tendon consists of both tendon fibers and interfibular noncollagenous protein and glycosaminoglycan. The addition of this material leads to an increase in cross-sectional area and therefore a decrease in ultimate tensile strength.

Cross-Sectional Area Measurement Because stress is defined as the tensile load per cross-sectional area, an accurate measure of cross-sectional area is of great importance. In the earliest studies in biomechanics, gravimetric methods were used in which the volume of water displaced by the specimen of interest could be related to cross-sectional area once a simple cross-sectional shape was assumed. In other studies, histologic sections were used to measure cross-sectional area; however, these methods are destructive (preventing subsequent tensile testing of the same specimen) and may suffer from experimental artifact, such as shrinkage, in the sectioning process. Purely mechanical methods using devices such as calipers have also been used to measure the width and thickness of a specimen, with the cross-sectional area obtained by assuming a simple cross-sectional shape (such as a rectangle or ellipse). These methods are adequate for geometrically simple structures, but may introduce large errors for tendons with more complex geometries.

Noncontact methods have also been developed with the intent of avoiding possible tissue deformation during the measurement of cross-sectional area. These methods involve an optical system (either visible or laser light) for measurement, or an image reconstruction technique to determine the cross-sectional area and/or shape. Examples of noncontact approaches include the shadow amplitude method, the profile method, the laser micrometer method, and more recently the laser reflectance system that can account for concavities in the tissue. As might be expected, these methods will perform much better than some contact methods for more complex geometries; however, the equipment involved is generally more expensive.

In summary, when determining the tensile properties of tendon, it is important to consider the various experimental factors that will affect the results. Preliminary studies should routinely be performed to assess the significance of each of these factors before testing experimental specimens. As noted above, a number of biologic factors can also influence the mechanical properties of tendon, and these factors should be taken into account during experimental design and considered when analyzing and reporting experimental results.

Biomechanical Modeling of Tendons

Characterization and prediction of the behavior of soft tissues is the primary function of biomechanical modeling. If a relatively simple mathematical expression can be used to describe the behavior of a single component (such as a tendon or ligament), this usage enables the construction of a much larger model to describe the function of an entire joint. The relevance of this type of research to orthopaedics can be seen in the prospective use of biomechanical models to evaluate the effects of a particular therapeutic intervention, or as an aid in the design of prosthetics and/or instrumentation. The inputs to these models to describe the behavior of soft tissues will be in the form of data on either load-elongation or stress-strain relationships, with the latter representing a constitutive relationship for the tendon or ligament. A variety of mathematical functions have been used to represent the empirically obtained data. The simplest relationships relate tensile stress, σ, to strain, ε, using a power law,

$$s = ae^b \qquad \text{(Eq. 1)}$$

or a logarithmic function,

$$\sigma = a + b \log \varepsilon \qquad \text{(Eq. 2)}$$

where a and b are constants.

Both of these descriptions are able to account for 2 important characteristics of tendons and ligaments: (1) they can be considered effective elastic materials for most modeling efforts—the current stress depends only on the current strain and not on time; and (2) they also display nonlinear behavior under tensile loading. However, it is important to consider the reasons a particular model has been developed, and the specific questions it will be used to investigate; a model cannot be used to describe behavior that it was not designed to address.

It has been well documented that tendons and ligaments are viscoelastic, meaning the stress in the material depends on the current strain as well as the history of strain. For developing models of viscoelastic behavior, cyclic loading, stress-relaxation, and creep tests are routinely performed. The rate at which the stress (or load) in a tendon or ligament decreases when the structure is held at a constant strain (length) can be determined in a stress-relaxation test. The reduced relaxation function for the structure can then be calculated by determining the current stress as a percentage of the initial stress and plotting it versus time. When the tendon or ligament is stretched and held at a new length, the stress-relaxation test begins, and the current stress is the initial stress (100%). This percentage will fall as the tendon or ligament is held at a stretched state, and the rate at which it falls is used to represent the viscoelastic properties of the structure. Similarly, a creep function can be determined by the rate at which the current strain in the tendon or ligament increases as the structure supports a constant stress. Together, these functions represent the most common approaches for describing the way in which the stress and strain in tendons and ligaments change with time.

One of the most common models developed for describing the viscoelastic response of tendons and ligaments is the quasilinear viscoelasticity, or QLV, theory. This approach combines the elastic stress and strain relationship (as might be described in equation 1 or 2) with the reduced relaxation function used to relate stress and time. In this way, the current stress in the tendon or ligament can be determined mathematically, given that the elastic relationship between stress and strain and the strain history for the structure are known. The QLV theory has found broad application within orthopaedic research and has been widely used to characterize the viscoelastic behavior of not only tendons and ligaments, but also smooth and cardiac muscle, and other soft tissues.

Tendon Injury, Healing, and Repair

Tendon injury occurs as a result of direct trauma with laceration or contusion, or indirect trauma with tensile overload. Direct trauma frequently involves injury with sharp tools. Although direct injury can involve any tendon, it is of special importance to the hand and upper extremity surgeon because of the frequent incidence of injury and the critical role of hand function. The healing process following direct injury to the paratenon covered tendon and sheathed tendon has been studied extensively and will be discussed in detail below.

Indirect injury mechanisms are multifactorial and depend heavily on anatomic location, vascularity, and skeletal maturity, as well as the magnitude of the applied forces. When the force in the muscle-tendon-bone complex exceeds the tolerance of this structure, failure occurs at the weakest link. Most tendons can withstand tensile forces larger than those exerted by the muscles or sustained by the bones. As a result, avulsion fractures and tendon ruptures at the musculotendinous junction occur much more frequently than midsubstance tendon ruptures. In the flexor tendons of the hand, for example, avulsion of the bony insertion of the tendon occurs mainly in young adults during athletic events, and those in the ring finger are injured most often (75%). Although the risk for injury depends on the forces applied and the strength of the tendon, it is interesting to note that the flexor digitorum profundus of the ring finger is significantly weaker than that of the long and index fingers.

Indirect injury to the tendon midsubstance requires the presence of preexisting pathology before the mechanical overload. This requirement is supported by the study of a number of different tendon injuries. Achilles tendon rupture typically occurs in middle-aged individuals who engage in strenuous activity. The rupture is abrupt and is frequently accompanied by a popping sensation, and many patients have no history of injury or discomfort. Histologic study of these injuries reveals tendon pathology described as angiofibrotic hyperplasia, suggesting an ongoing degenerative process or a failure of remodeling in a normal tendon prior to rupture. For midsubstance tendon ruptures, relative avascularity, inflammatory disease, and other local factors are involved. For example, extensor pollicis longus midsubstance rupture occurs in rheumatoid arthritis patients as a result of attrition of the tendon against a bony prominence. Tendon attrition in the absence of inflammation also is cited frequently as a factor in midsubstance rup-

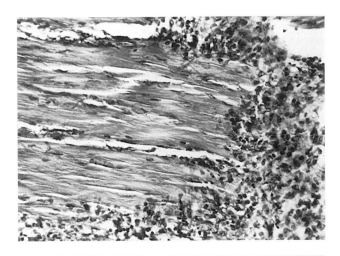

Figure 19

Longitudinal section of a rat calcaneal tendon 3 days after surgical transection and suture reapposition. Note the predominance of inflammatory cells in the wound. Some fibroblasts may be noted (hematoxylin and eosin, × 125; Courtesy of Dr. Scott Wolfe, New York).

ture. For example, attrition of the rotator cuff and biceps brachii against the anteroinferior aspect of the acromion has been thought to contribute to rupture of these tendons.

Healing Process in a Paratenon-Covered Tendon

The rabbit and rat calcaneal tendons have been studied extensively to characterize healing in a paratenon-covered tendon. After the paratenon and tendon are incised, the wound fills with inflammatory products, blood cells, nuclear debris, and fibrin (Fig. 19). This tissue has no tensile strength. During the first week, proliferating tissue from the paratenon penetrates the gap between the tendon stumps and fills it with undifferentiated and disorganized fibro-

blasts. Capillary buds invade the area and together with the fibroblasts compose the granulation tissue between the tendon ends (Fig. 20).

Collagen synthesis can be detected as early as the third day. The process begins with an increased concentration in the protein mucopolysaccharides, which aids in the polymerization of the monomeric collagen. The endoplasmic reticulum of the fibroblasts synthesizes a precursor of collagen. This triple chain helix depends on heat-sensitive hydrogen bonds to connect the hydroxyl groups of hydroxyproline to the ketoimide groups of other amino acids. In this milieu, the collagen molecules begin to polymerize into fibrils. These fibrils progressively accumulate more collagen molecules until they have increased in size to become histologically visible, thin wavy forms.

After 2 weeks, the tendon stumps appear to be fused by a fibrous bridge. Dramatic fibroblast proliferation and collagen production in the granulation tissue continue. The growth and migration of the collagen fibers between the tendon stumps are oriented perpendicular to the long axis of the tendon (Fig. 21). In an animal model, type I collagen production in the wound, documented by radiolabeled proline uptake, increases to 15 to 22 times normal. This rate of synthesis decreases slowly over a period of several months.

Histologically, the tendon stumps show a marked increase in fibroblast and vascular proliferation and a decrease in other cellular reactions. Fibroblasts and collagen fibers bridge the gap and physically unite the tendon ends. The fibrovascular tissue migrating from the paratendinous tissue blends with the epitenon to form the tendon callus (Fig. 22). Between the third and fourth weeks, fibroblasts and collagen fibers near the tendon begin to orient themselves along the long axis of the tendon as a result of stress

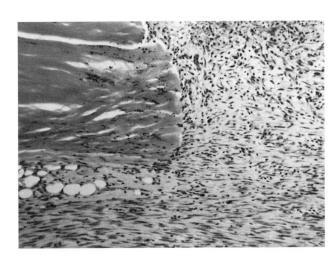

Figure 20

Longitudinal section of a rabbit tendon 1 week after surgical transection and suture reapposition. Note the increase of fibroblasts from the paratenon migrating into the wound (hematoxylin and eosin, × 100; Courtesy of Dr. Larry Stein, University of Illinois).

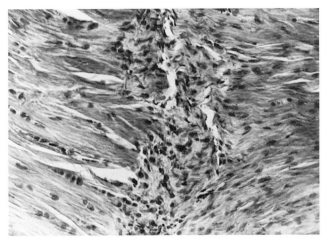

Figure 21

Longitudinal section of a rat calcaneal tendon 2 weeks after surgical transection and suture reapposition. Collagen fibers continue to migrate into the wound and are oriented perpendicular to the long axis of the tendon (hematoxylin and eosin, × 125; Courtesy of Dr. Scott Wolfe, New York).

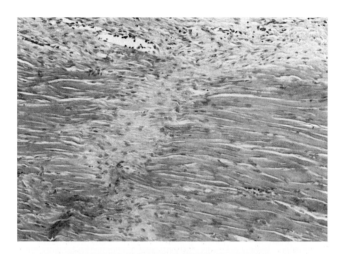

Figure 22

Longitudinal section of a rat calcaneal tendon 21 days after surgical transection and suture reapposition. The collagen within the wound neotendon begins to show evidence of longitudinal orientation.

(Fig. 23). Only the collagen near the tendon reorganizes; the more distant scar-like tissue remains unorganized.

The 2 important factors of this remodeling process are that the increase in the biomechanical properties and the reduction in the mass of the scar-like tissue continue for many months. Tensile properties increase as a result of both the increasing degree of organization of the collagen fibers along the lines of tensile loading and an increase in the number of intermolecular bonds between collagen fibers. The ultimate load of the healing tendon increases despite the decrease in total mass. Such a reduction of cross-sectional area to resist larger tensile load means the ultimate tensile strength (or the quality of tissue) is increasing rapidly. As healing proceeds, remodeling continues until by

the 20th week there is minimal histologic difference in vascularity and cellularity between the healed tendon and the normal tendon. Monomeric collagen production, fibril reorientation, and cross-linking all depend on the presence of applied loads in the tendon. In the absence of loading, collagen production decreases and the remodeling to increase the quality of the healing tendon slows.

Healing Process in a Sheathed Tendon

As mentioned before, tendons that bend sharply, such as the flexor tendons of the hand, are enclosed by a tendon sheath. The healing of these tendons has been a controversial topic for many years. Data from early investigations suggested that healing was affected by granulation from the tendon sheath. It was believed that the lacerated digital flexor tendons from the front paw of the dog healed by means of fibroblasts derived from the tendon sheath and surrounding tissues. The tendon cells themselves played no active role in this repair. However, results of recent experimental investigations have demonstrated that tenocytes appear to have intrinsic capabilities of repair. Flexor tendons in cell culture are able to participate in the repair process; a tissue cap forms on the lacerated tendon ends by means of proliferation and migration of cells from the epitenon and endotenon (Fig. 24).

The flexor tendons of rabbits were transected through 90% of their thickness and placed in cell culture. At 3 weeks, cells from the epitenon migrated into the wound site and differentiated into phagocytes or macrophages. These chains of migrating epitenon cells were frequently joined together via desmosomes. Within the endotenon there was an increase in the number of cells. The cells looked like metabolically active fibroblasts that had well-formed granular endoplasmic reticulum with dilated cisternae contain-

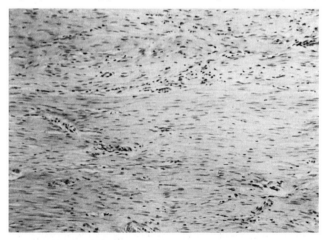

Figure 23

Longitudinal section of a rabbit tendon 28 days after transection and suture reapposition. Note the increased cellularity and vascularity within the repair neotendon and the longitudinal orientation of the collagen bundles (hematoxylin and eosin, × 100; Courtesy of Dr. Larry Stein, University of Illinois).

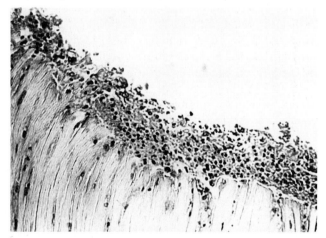

Figure 24

Photomicrograph of monkey flexor tendon after 6 weeks on culture, showing focal area of cellular proliferation. Note the apparent cellular migration from within the endotenon matrix at the tendon end (Courtesy of Dr. P. R. Manske, St. Louis).

ing electron-dense material, indicative of protein synthesis. By 6 weeks, the number of phagocytes within the repair site had increased. By 9 weeks, cellular activity at the repair site continued, and cells migrating from the epitenon retained a phagocytic appearance. The fibroblasts within the endotenon also continued to show evidence of metabolic activity, and an extracellular matrix of collagen fibrils in various stages of polymerization was evident. Thus, a remodeling process is apparent with both active phagocytosis and collagen synthesis.

Therefore, it appears that in the proper environment, the sheathed tendon is capable of repair. In repaired tendons treated with controlled passive motion, this intrinsic response originating from the epitenon predominates. In the immobilized tendon, however, healing occurs through the ingrowth of connective tissue from the digital sheath and cellular proliferation of the endotenon (Fig. 25).

Tendon Repair

Issues regarding tendon repair are numerous, and a detailed discussion is beyond the scope of this chapter. Suture material, the type of suture repair, knotting of sutures, continuous passive motion, weightbearing, and, of course, the nature and location of the injury all impact on the quality of the tendon repair.

There are numerous suture techniques that take advantage of the mechanical strength of the tendon. For example, sutures passed between fascicles are easily pulled out. Sutures placed parallel to the tendon also pull out of the tendon at low forces. This observation has led to the development of current techniques in which a suture is passed perpendicular to the tendon before passing it across the injury; that is, parallel to the tendon (Fig. 26). In vitro evaluations have shown that perpendicularly passed sutures result in stronger tendon-suture-tendon constructs. Instead of pulling through the tendon, these constructs tend to fail by suture ruptures. This indicates that the strength of the suture-tendon interface exceeds the strength of the suture. In view of this observation, new suture techniques have been developed in which multistrand, multigrasp sutures are used for tendon repair to increase the mechanical strength of the repair.

Besides providing adequate mechanical strength, suture repair must also minimize gap formation between the tendon stumps, because even small gaps have been shown to adversely affect outcome. The ability of a construct to resist gap formation depends on the geometry of the construct, the amount of tension placed on the suture, and the viscoelastic creep that occurs not only in the tendon, but also in many suture materials. The resistance to gap formation as a mechanical parameter has led to modification of repair techniques. It is now common practice to have peripheral epitendinous sutures to increase the repair strength and prevent gap formation.

Mechanical strength of the repair alone, however, is an

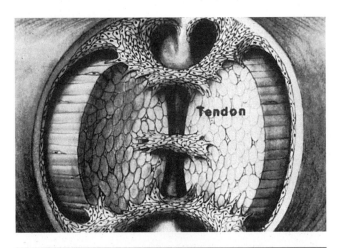

Figure 25

Schematic drawing of an immobilized tendon illustrating extrinsic and intrinsic repair (Courtesy of Dr. R.H. Gelberman, Boston).

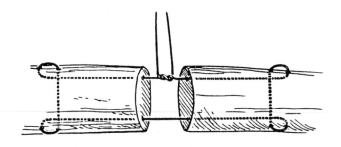

Figure 26

Schematic drawing of a tendon repair. The perpendicular portion of the suture increases the strength of the repair without compromising tendon vascularity. (Adapted with permission from Kleinert HE, Schepel S, Gill T: Flexor tendon injuries. *Surg Clin North Am* 1981;61:267–286.)

insufficient measure of the likelihood of success, because mechanical strength at the expense of tissue viability will compromise repair. For example, the placement of sutures in the volar aspect of the tendon has been advocated to avoid injury to the dorsally located intrinsic longitudinal vessels (Fig. 27). The other important criteria for predicting the success of tendon repair is the gliding function of the sheathed tendon after injury. A tendon repair construct with large scar or adhesion formation, in spite of mechanical strength, would be detrimental to the gliding function of the healed tendon. It is therefore recommended that low profile suturing techniques, in which the suture knots are buried within the lacerated site, should be used for tendon repair.

Animal studies have provided valuable insight into variables such as the gliding function of the healed tendon. These studies also allow for histologic and biochemical evaluation of the repair process. Early weightbearing or aggressive early active mobilization of repaired tendon has been shown to result in rupture and gap formation. However, carefully controlled early passive mobilization stimulates the repair and improves the strength of the tendon in the first few months after repair. Additionally, small

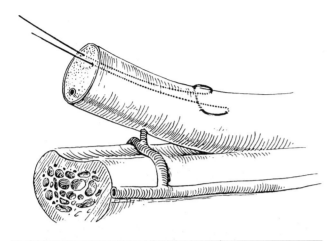

Figure 27

Schematic drawing of a suture placed in the volar surface of the tendon to avoid injury to the longitudinal vessels. (Reproduced with permission from Kleinert HE, Stilwell JH, Netscher DT: Complications of tendon surgery in the hand, in Sandzen SC Jr (ed): *Current Management of Complications in Orthopaedics: The Hand and Wrist.* Baltimore, MD, Williams & Wilkins, 1985, pp 206–227.)

motions applied early have been shown to reduce the number of adhesions associated with tendon healing. Thus, an optimum level of stress and motion exists that promotes healing without resulting in additional damage to the repairing tendon. Limitations in animal studies include the variations in the healing potential of the animal, the expense of long-term follow-up, and the difficulty in controlling the rehabilitation process. Determination of the optimal rehabilitation regimen remains a challenge in tendon repair.

Tendon Transfer

Tendon transfers require considerable clinical experience and acumen. Indications for tendon transfers are numerous and include peripheral nerve injury and replacement of ruptured tendons in rheumatoid patients and patients with central nervous system disorders such as cerebral palsy. Considerations for transfer include absence of inflammation and edema, mobility of the joints, adequacy of the tissue bed, adequacy of skin coverage, and potential for an effective line of action of the transferred tendon.

While these and many other factors contribute to the selection and staging of tendon transfers, the primary considerations include the expendability, excursion, and strength of the muscle being transferred. The expendability of a muscle depends on the particular clinical condition of the patient. Tendon excursion is proportional to the number of sarcomeres connected in series in the muscle; that is, it is proportional to the length of the muscle. Effective tendon excursion includes the sum of the contraction length from rest plus the traction length from rest plus the effect of intercalary joints (tenodesis effect). The tenodesis effect refers to the effective increase in excursion of a tendon that can occur when it crosses 2 joints.

The relationship between the excursion and force of the muscle must be coupled with the needs of the recipient joint, including adequate joint torque generation and adequate range of motion. These relationships depend both on the properties of the muscle and on the insertion site of the tendon. Insertion of the muscle away from the axis of rotation of the joint increases the joint torque that the muscle can produce (torque = force × perpendicular distance). However, the range of motion decreases as the angular rotation is approximately equal to the total excursion/distance to the joint axis of rotation. Thus, for a given muscle, joint torque and range of motion have an inverse relationship governed by the insertion site of the tendon.

Success of tendon transfers is a complex issue that depends on the donor tendon, biomechanics, and rehabilitation. Postoperatively, patients have to undergo long and rigorous rehabilitation to acquire the desired joint motion.

Ligament

Ligaments, like tendons, are classified as dense connective tissue. Ligaments and tendons are similar in structural composition as well as mechanical behavior; however, they differ in a number of ways. Physically, ligaments are load-bearing structures that are shorter and wider tissues that connect between bones, whereas tendons are longer and narrower structures that connect muscle to bone. Biochemically, ligaments contain a lower percentage of collagen and a higher percentage of ground substance than tendons. Biomechanically, the collagen fibers in tendons are more longitudinally organized than those in ligaments, as ligaments experience a more varied loading because of their role in joint stability and, therefore, display a broader distribution of fiber directions.

Ligaments have been studied extensively because of their prevalent role in sports injuries as well as their importance in joint stability. Most studies have concentrated on the ligaments of the knee as well as the capsular ligaments of the shoulder. This section will focus on the knowledge gained from studies of knee ligaments.

Anatomy

Ligaments are short bands of tough, flexible fibrous connective tissue that connect bones and support viscera. Grossly, ligaments appear as band- or cable-like structures with few distinguishing landmarks. Microscopic examination reveals a high level of hierarchical organization, quite similar to that found in tendons. Ligaments contain rows of fibroblasts within parallel bundles of extracellular matrix composed primarily of type I collagen fibers (70% fat-free dry weight). Elastin, a fibrillar protein that affects the mechanical properties, is also present in both tendon and ligament in very small amounts (less than 1% dry weight). In some ligaments, such as the flaval and nuchal ligaments of the spine in particular, elastin forms the primary structural component, resulting in considerably different mechanical properties from nonelastin-dominated ligaments. As with tendons, the mechanical properties of ligaments are influenced by the collagen composition, as well as by the crimping and biochemical bonding between the structural subcomponents.

Ligament insertion into bone represents a transition from one material to the other and can be quite complex. Insertions of ligaments are usually classified as either direct or indirect, the latter being more common. Direct insertions contain 4 morphologically distinct zones, namely ligament, fibrocartilage, mineralized fibrocartilage, and bone (Fig. 28). For indirect insertions, the superficial layer connects directly with periosteum while the deeper layers anchor to bone via Sharpey fibers (Fig. 29). An example of a ligament that exhibits both types of insertion is the medial collateral ligament (MCL) of the knee. Its femoral insertion is direct while its tibial insertion is indirect.

Compared with surrounding tissues, ligaments appear to be hypovascular. However, histologic study reveals that throughout the ligament substance there is uniform microvascularity, which originates from the insertion sites. Despite the small size of the vascular system and its limited blood flow, it is of primary importance in the maintenance of the ligament. Specifically, by providing nutrition for the cellular population, this vascular system maintains the continued process of matrix synthesis and repair.

Ligaments were also once thought to be without innervation; however, a number of human and animal studies have documented a variety of specialized nerve endings. Evidence of pain fibers in spinal facet capsular ligaments has been further demonstrated in histochemical studies. Innervation of a variety of ligaments including the MCL and anterior cruciate ligament (ACL) of the knee, which play a role in proprioception and nociception, has been identified.

Biomechanics

Tensile Properties

Tensile properties of ligaments are expressed in terms of the structural properties of the bone-ligament-bone complex, as well as the mechanical properties of the ligament substance itself. As with tendon, the structural properties characterize the behavior of the overall bone-ligament-bone complex (load-elongation relationship) whereas the mechanical properties characterize the behavior of the ligament substance itself under tensile loading (stress-strain relationship). The mechanical properties of ligaments are influenced by collagen composition, fiber orientation, and the interaction between the collagen and surrounding ground substance. In contrast, the structural properties of the bone-ligament-bone complex are governed by the mechanical properties and the geometry of the ligament, as well as by the properties of the insertion sites. With the correct preparation, both types of data (structural and mechanical properties) can be obtained from a single uniaxial test of the bone-ligament-bone complex.

Structural Properties of a Bone-Ligament-Bone Complex

The structural properties of a bone-ligament-bone complex can be derived from the load-elongation curve

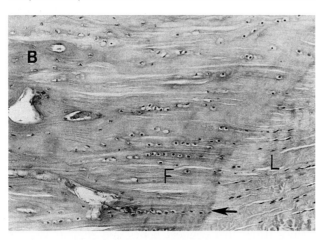

Figure 28

Femoral insertion of a rabbit MCL is typical direct insertion. The deep fibers of the ligament (L) pass into the bone (B) through a well-defined zone of uncalcified and calcified fibrocartilage (F). (Reproduced with permission from Woo SL-Y, Gomez MA, Sites TJ, et al: The biomechanical and morphological changes in the medial collateral ligament of the rabbit after immobilization and remobilization. *J Bone Joint Surg* 1987;69A:1200–1211.)

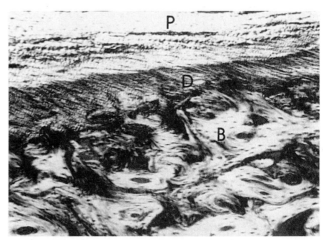

Figure 29

Indirect insertion of a rabbit MCL into the tibia showing superficial fibers (P) inserting into periosteum, and the deep fibers (D) inserting obliquely into bone (B). (hematoxylin and eosin, × 50; Reproduced with permission from Woo SL-Y, Gomez MA, Sites TJ, et al: The biomechanical and morphological changes in the medial collateral ligament of the rabbit after immobilization and remobilization. *J Bone Joint Surg* 1987;69A:1200–1211.)

obtained from uniaxial tensile tests. Similar to tendon, the load-elongation curve can be divided into an initial low stiffness region, the toe region, followed by a linear region with higher stiffness. Thus, ligament has a nonlinear, strain-stiffening structural response. This behavior has been attributed to the undulating pattern (crimp) of the collagen fibrils and to the nonuniform recruitment of the individual fibers. During stretch, small initial forces produce large elongation because the crimp is easily straightened, after which much larger forces are needed for further stretch to cause the fibrils themselves to begin to elongate. Because of the varying degrees of crimping and the different orientations among the fibrils, each fibril uncrimps and begins to resist stretch at a different elongation of the ligament. As elongation is increased, more fiber bundles become uncrimped and oriented in the direction of loading. This recruitment of fibers produces a gradual increase in ligament stiffness.

Stiffness in N/mm, defined as the slope of the load-elongation curve, therefore, increases at the toe region and reaches a relatively constant value at the linear region. The curve then reaches the ultimate load (N) of the bone-ligament-bone complex where failure occurs. The slope of the curve can end abruptly at the ultimate load or decrease slowly as the ligament approaches its ultimate load. The decrease in stiffness reflects the failure of individual fibers before failure of the whole complex. The area under the entire load-elongation curve constitutes the energy absorbed to failure of the structure (N•mm) (Fig. 30).

Mechanical Properties

The mechanical properties (stress-strain relationship) of the ligament substance can also be obtained from the same uniaxial tensile test. From the stress-strain curve, parameters such as the modulus (E, slope of the curve, in MPa), tensile strength (σ_u, ultimate tensile strength, in MPa), ultimate strain (ε_u) as well as the strain energy density (ω, in MPa) can be obtained.

Because of their frequent involvement in knee injuries and different healing responses, extensive research has been devoted to contrasting the MCL and ACL. The two differ anatomically; the MCL is an extra-articular ligament that is relatively flat with rather uniform fiber alignment. The ACL, on the other hand, has fibers that are nonparallel as well as cross-sectional areas that vary greatly from the midsubstance of the ligament to its insertions. There are also cellular, histologic, ultrastructural, and biochemical differences. The mechanical properties of the medial and lateral portions of the rabbit ACL are different from those of the MCL. The elastic modulus (between 4% and 7% strain) is approximately twice as much for the MCL as for the ACL. The tensile strength of the rabbit MCL, 110 ± 19 MPa, is over 70% higher than that of the medial portion of the ACL.

The higher modulus and tensile strength of the MCL when compared to those for the ACL can be attributed, in part, to

their morphologic differences. Rabbit MCL consists of more densely packed fiber bundles that have a lower frequency crimp pattern than the ACL. The subfascicular area fraction of collagen is significantly greater for the MCL than the ACL. Thus, the MCL has more force-bearing collagen fibrils per unit area than the ACL. The mean fibril diameter is also greater for the MCL than the ACL, and larger diameter fibrils are believed to provide greater resistance to elongation.

The mechanical properties of the anterolateral and posteromedial bundles of the human posterior cruciate ligament (PCL) as well as the meniscofemoral ligaments have also been studied. The meniscofemoral ligaments possess a slightly higher elastic modulus (355 ± 234 MPa) than the anterolateral bundle of the PCL (294 ± 115 MPa), while both are higher than that of the posteromedial bundle of the PCL (150 ± 69 MPa).

Time- and History-Dependent Behavior

Ligaments, like tendons, display time- and history-dependent viscoelastic behavior that reflects the interactions of the collagen and ground substance. The characterization of the basic viscoelastic parameters of soft tissue such as creep, stress-relaxation, and hysteresis have been described in more detail in the earlier section on tendons.

Viscoelastic properties of ligaments have a number of clinical implications. During ACL reconstruction, the initial force applied to tension the graft decreases over time as a result of stress relaxation. This has also been demonstrated in the primate patellar tendon in which the stress could be reduced by up to 69.8% of its initial value within 30 minutes. Thus, the amount of tension remaining in the graft postoperatively depends on the viscoelastic characteristics of the graft. It has been shown that preconditioning a ligament can reduce the amount of stress relaxation by approximately 50% when compared to a ligament with no precon-

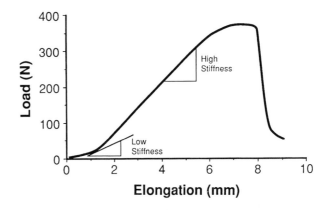

Figure 30

Typical load-elongation curve from tensile testing of a ligament, showing a region of low stiffness (toe region) and a region of high stiffness (linear region).

ditioning. These viscoelastic properties are also used to the clinician's advantage during intraoperative spinal distraction. By applying the distraction in small steps separated by a few minutes, the peak forces applied to the instrumentation and its insertions on the vertebra can be reduced over 50% because of vertebral soft-tissue creep. The importance of creep can also be demonstrated in the reduction of joint dislocation. Shoulder dislocations can sometimes be treated with a hanging weight at the forearm. With the creep behavior of the shoulder capsular ligaments as well as surrounding soft tissue, these lengthened structures help to make subsequent joint relocation easier.

Factors Influencing the Properties of Ligaments

There also is profound variation in the properties of ligaments, based on biologic factors such as species, biochemistry, immobilization, skeletal maturation, and age. To further complicate the issue, different experimental methods have contributed to the differences reported in mechanical properties of ligaments. Difficulties are similar to those encountered in the study of tendon, and include gripping of ligaments, strain measurement, definition of the initial length, and determination of the cross-sectional area. Additional in vitro factors include temperature, freezing, and sterilization techniques. The following section discusses many of these factors.

Biologic Factors Influencing Tensile Properties of Ligaments

Skeletal Maturity Data from rabbit studies show a significant increase in the structural properties of the rabbit femur-MCL-tibia complex (FMTC) and mechanical properties of ligament substance with skeletal maturation. Twofold, fourfold, and tenfold increases in linear stiffness, ultimate load, and energy absorbed at failure, respectively, are observed as the animals age from 3 to 12 months; physeal closure for rabbits occurs at 7 to 8 months. The modulus of the ligament substance also increases between 5% and 15% during skeletal maturation (Fig. 31).

The modes of failure, that is, types of injury, also change with skeletal maturation. With uniaxial tensile load, FMTCs from rabbits with open epiphyses fail by tibial avulsion, while those from skeletally mature rabbits tear in the ligament substance. Thus, the tibial insertion is the weaker link before physeal closure, and the ligament substance is the weaker link after closure. Histologic examination has shown active remodeling of the tibial insertions and incomplete insertion of the deep ligamentous fibers before maturation. Because the ligament crosses the physis and must lengthen and grow with the bone, the insertion is weak and causes the avulsions. Stress relaxation is also more prominent in immature ligaments. Immobilization interferes with the normal increase of ligament structural properties with skeletal maturity. Thus, the structural properties of

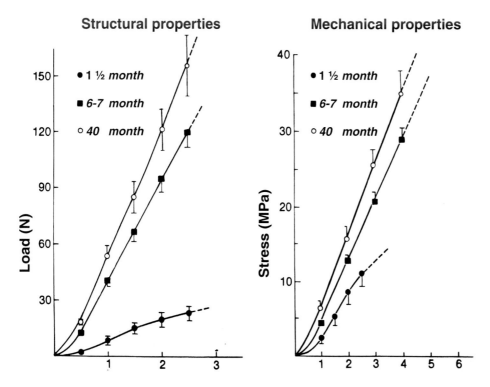

Figure 31

The structural properties (load-deformation curves) of the femur-MCL-tibia complex and the mechanical properties of the ligament substance (stress-strain curves) for 3 age groups: 1-1/2 months (open epiphysis), 6 to 7 months (closed epiphysis), and 40 months (closed epiphysis). (Reproduced with permission from Woo SL-Y, Young EP, Kwan MK: Fundamental studies in knee ligament mechanics, in Daniel D, Akeson WH, O'Connor JJ (eds): *Knee Ligaments: Structure, Function, Injury, and Repair.* New York, Raven Press, 1990, pp 115–134.)

Anatomic orientation

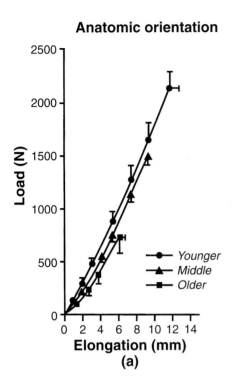

Tibial orientation

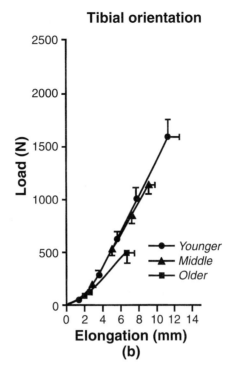

Figure 32

The structural properties (load-elongation curves) for femur-ACL-tibia complexes tested at 30° of flexion in the (a) anatomic orientation and (b) tibial orientation for younger, middle-aged, and older human donors. (Reproduced with permission from Woo SL-Y, Hollis JM, Adams DJ, Lyon RM, Takai S: Tensile properties of the human femur-anterior cruciate ligament-tibia complex: The effects of specimen age and orientation. *Am J Sports Med* 1991;19:217–225.)

immobilized, skeletally immature rabbit FMTC decrease as the animal ages, unlike those of normal MCL, in which strength increases with age until maturation.

Age The significance of aging has been investigated in the rabbit FMTC at 3, 5, 6, 12, 36, and 48 months of age. The elastic modulus of the rabbit FMTC increased with maturity until 12 months when skeletal maturity is reached, and then gradually declined until 48 months. The tensile properties remained relatively constant after 12 months of age with a slight decline at 48 months. However, investigations of human femur-ACL-tibia complex (FATC) reveal a different trend. Values of structural properties of FATCs from young human donors have been found to be significantly higher than those from older donors. The stiffness and ultimate load for the ACLs from young donors (ages 22 to 35 years) are reported as 242 ± 28 N/mm and 2160 ± 157 N, respectively, which are greater than the properties of specimens from older donors by more than threefold (Fig. 32). The values obtained for FATCs from younger donors should be used as a guideline for the strength requirements of ACL replacements. These studies demonstrate that although the tensile properties of ligaments decline with aging, the rate of decline may not be the same for different ligaments.

Immobilization, Remobilization, and Exercise Rehabilitation regimens after musculoskeletal injuries often include immobilization to protect the afflicted tissues from further damage during the early healing phases. However, the side effects of immobilization can be quite detrimental. Increases in joint stiffness caused by synovial adhesions and proliferation of fibrofatty connective tissues have been observed

both clinically and experimentally after immobilization. Joint contracture also has been hypothesized to be the result of new collagen fibrils forming interfibrillar contacts that restrict normal parallel sliding of fibers in ligaments. Quantitative assessment of joint stiffness in animals, following 9 weeks of immobilization of the rabbit knee, demonstrated that large increases in torque and energy were required to extend the joints.

Ligament properties are also compromised by immobilization. Drastic decreases in the structural properties of

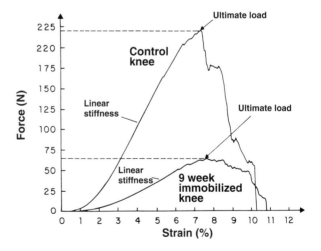

Figure 33

Force-strain curves of rabbit femur-MCL-tibia complex from control and immobilized limbs. (Reproduced with permission from Woo SL-Y, Gomez MA, Woo YK, et al: Mechanical properties of tendons and ligaments: II. The relationship of immobilization and exercise on tissue remodeling. *Biorheology* 1982;19:397–408.)

rabbit FMTC are observed after 9 weeks of knee joint immobilization. The tensile load required for failure (ultimate load) of the FMTC is about 33%, and the energy absorbed at failure is only 16% of the contralateral, nonimmobilized control (Fig. 33). Both elastic modulus and ultimate tensile strength of the MCL also are decreased with immobilization.

The decreases in structural properties of the bone-ligament-bone complex in rabbits are caused by a combination of changes to the insertions and to the ligament substance itself. Histologic evaluation of the MCL tibial insertions following immobilization reveals marked disruption of the deep fibers inserting into bone. Osteoclastic activity results in subperiosteal bone resorption for the tibial insertion but little change to the femoral insertion. This resorption correlates with an increasing occurrence of failure by tibial avulsion for the FMTC from the immobilized knees. Similar decreases in the properties of the ACL and FATC occur in primates. Investigators have observed subperiosteal resorption at both the femoral and tibial insertions.

The resumption of joint motion leads to a rather slow reversal in the effects of immobilization on the structural properties of the FMTC and FATC. The ultimate load and energy absorbed at failure of these 2 complexes reach 80% to 90% of control at 1 year. Histologic evidence of new bone formation at the ligament insertion reveals that the time required to return to normal is much longer than the immobilization period. In contrast, the mechanical properties of the MCL substance return to normal after 9 weeks of remobilization. These data illustrate a delayed recovery of the insertion compared to the ligament substance. Based on these data, the remobilization period should be on the order of months, following only a few weeks of immobilization.

The properties of the ligament substance and the insertion are also affected by exercise. Short-term exercise regimens, ranging from treadmill walking to running and swimming, have been studied using various animal models and tend to show an increase in mechanical and structural properties. Following 12 months of exercise, the structural properties of the FMTC from swine increased when compared to controls; the exercised animals had a 38% increase in ultimate load and a 14% increase in stiffness. The tensile strength and ultimate strain increased 20% and 10%, respectively.

The effects of lifelong exercise were tested on a beagle with an 11-kg backpack running on a treadmill. Surprisingly, there were no changes in the structural properties of its FMTC. Load-elongation curves for exercised and nonexercised, age-matched complexes were similar. The linear stiffness, ultimate load, ultimate elongation, and energy absorbed at failure were unaffected by the exercise, and only minimal changes in the mechanical properties were observed. Although surprising, the lack of improvement in the structural and mechanical properties might be attributed to the processes of aging, which could have masked any positive effects of exercise.

Thus, a relationship between different levels of stress and ligament properties can be derived from the results of the various studies (Fig. 34). Immobilization significantly compromises both the structural properties of the bone-ligament-bone complex and the mechanical properties of the ligament, with more pronounced weakening at the insertion sites. The mechanical properties of ligament substance return to control levels after a relatively short period of remobilization, but the insertions require a much longer period of recovery to regain their previous stiffness and strength. Therefore, the complex remains weak, and avulsion injuries are more likely during this interval. On the contrary, the changes in these properties resulting from exercise or increased stress are not analogous to the marked decrease following immobilization; only moderate improvements are seen. Thus, a highly nonlinear relationship is depicted.

Experimental Factors Influencing the Properties of Ligaments

Strain Rate The tensile properties of ligament increase minimally with increasing rates of elongation (strain rates). This behavior is similar to that of most soft biologic tissues. In a study using skeletally mature rabbit MCL as a model, elongation rates of 0.008 to 113 mm/s corresponding to strain rates of the MCL midsubstance of 0.01% to over 200%/s, a range over 4 decades, were used. The structural properties of the FMTC differed minimally between the lowest and highest rates of elongation (Fig. 35). The ultimate load increased from 311.5 ± 12.1 at 0.008 mm/s to 403.7 ± 7.5 at 113 mm/s. The mechanical properties of the MCL followed similar trends, but the increases were much

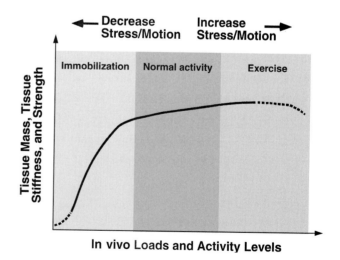

Figure 34

Schematic diagram depicting ligament homeostasis secondary to stress and motion. (Reproduced with permission from Woo SL-Y, Chan SS, Yamaji T: Biomechanics of knee ligament healing, repair and reconstruction. *J Biomechanics* 1997;30:431–439.)

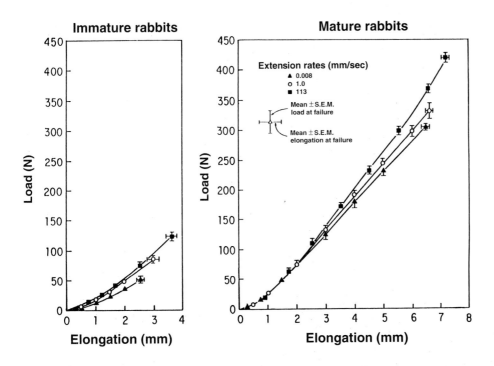

Immature rabbits

Mature rabbits

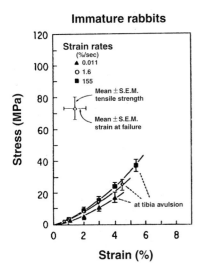

Figure 35

The structural properties (load-elongation curves) of the FMTC of skeletally immature (**left**) and mature (**right**) rabbits as a function of extension rate. (Reproduced with permission from Woo SL-Y, Peterson RH, Ohland KJ, et al: The effects of strain rate on the properties of the MCL in skeletally immature and mature rabbits: A biomechanical and histological study. *J Orthop Res* 1990;8:712–721.)

less marked. The ultimate tensile strength of the MCL increased only 40% from the 0.01% to 200%/s strain (Fig. 36). Studies of the ACL at slow (0.003 mm/s), medium (0.3 mm/s), and fast (113 mm/s) rates of elongation showed similar effects. Small differences were observed in the modulus between the slow and medium strain rates, but the modulus at the fast extension rate was only 30% higher.

The influence of strain rate on injury has caused significant debate. Although clinical injuries to ligaments usually occur at high strain rates, many experimental studies use low to medium rates because of the limitation of the testing as well as data-collecting systems. Some authors have attributed the difference in results to the use of lower strain rates. However, data from recent studies suggest that the effects of strain rate are overstated—especially when comparing strain rates such as 1%/s versus 100%/s. In fact, the status of the insertions, not the strain rate, may be the primary determinant that dictates the type of injury to the bone-ligament-bone complex.

Specimen Orientation Because some bone-ligament-bone complexes are nonuniform in geometry and shape, the direction of applied force and the initial position of the ligament are important for its load-elongation behavior. This is especially true for the ACL with its complex geometry and nonuniform arrangement of the fiber bundles, which makes uniform loading of the entire ligament impossible. Applying the force in the direction of the ACL allows a greater proportion of the fiber bundles to be loaded. This would not be the case if the force were applied in an arbi-

Immature rabbits

Mature rabbits

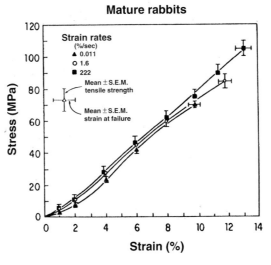

Figure 36

The mechanical properties (stress-strain curves) of the MCL substance from skeletally immature (**left**) and mature (**right**) rabbits, and the influence of the rate of stretching of the ligament (strain rate) on the mechanical properties. (Reproduced with permission from Woo SL-Y, Peterson RH, Ohland KJ, et al: The effects of strain rate on the properties of the MCL in skeletally immature and mature rabbits: A biomechanical and histological study. *J Orthop Res* 1990;8:712–721.)

trary direction. In a study on young human cadaveric FATC, paired specimens were studied with one knee tested along the anatomic axis of the ACL and the other along the tibial axis (Fig. 37). The stiffness and strength of the FATC were greater when tested in the anatomic orientation than when tested in the tibial orientation. The linear stiffness was approximately 242 and 218 N/mm, respectively, while the ultimate load was 2,160 N for specimens tested in the anatomic orientation and only 1,602 N when tested in the tibial orientation.

Data from rabbit knees show that ultimate load for the FATC decreases with increasing knee flexion when load is applied in the tibial orientation. In contrast, flexion angle does not affect the ultimate load of the FATC when the force is applied along the anatomic axis of the ACL. Similar results were also observed in canine studies.

Proper Specimen Storage The effect of freezing on ligaments is of interest because freezing is necessary for many biomechanical experiments as well as for preserving tissue allografts. One method used for knee specimen storage is to freeze the knees with muscle and other tissues left intact to prevent dehydration. Each knee is double-wrapped in

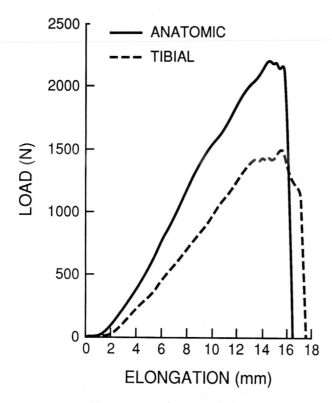

Figure 37

Typical load-elongation curves for paired femur-ACL-tibia complex from a younger donor demonstrating the differences in results between testing in the anatomic versus the tibial orientation. (Reproduced with permission from Woo SL-Y, Hollis M, Adams DJ, Lyon RM, Takai S: Tensile properties of the human femur-anterior cruciate ligament-tibia complex: The effects of specimen age and orientation. *Am J Sports Med* 1991;19:217–225.)

saline-soaked gauze, sealed in an airtight plastic bag, and frozen to -20°C. No significant differences in the structural properties of the FMTC or the mechanical properties of the MCL were noted between fresh rabbit knees and those stored using this method. The single exception, which occurs during the first few cycles of loading and unloading, is a decrease in the area of hysteresis that becomes insignificant with further cycling. Similar results have been reported for other soft tissues.

Appropriate Testing Environment The in vitro environment also has profound effects on ligament behavior. Maintenance of specimen hydration is of primary importance to the study of soft tissues. Temperature has also been shown to be important, although to a lesser degree than hydration. Increases in temperature from 2°C to 37°C resulted in a decrease in stiffness and a decrease in areas of hysteresis. These factors have led many investigators to immerse their specimens in a physiologic saline bath in which pH and temperature are closely controlled.

Consideration of Multiple Degrees of Freedom Joint Motion Besides characterizing the tensile properties of ligaments, studies have also been performed to identify the contribution of each ligament to joint stability. The orientation and tensile properties of the ligaments in combination with the geometry of the joint govern the kinematics or motion of that particular joint. Each joint has 6 degrees of freedom (DOF): 3 translations and 3 rotations. In the human knee joint, there are 3 axes: the femoral shaft axis, the epicondylar axis, and the floating axis. The floating axis is perpendicular to the other 2 axes, and is also known as the anterior-posterior axis. Translation along these 3 axes will lead to distraction-compression, medial-lateral translation, and anterior-posterior translation, respectively; rotation about these 3 axes will lead to internal-external tibial rotation, flexion-extension, and varus-valgus rotation, respectively (Fig. 38).

Early studies on the function of knee ligaments have simplified the complex motion of the joint by limiting the joint to a single DOF, whereas the change in kinematics in response to an applied load was measured before and after transection of the ligament. For example, the amount of anterior tibial translation in response to an anterior tibial load was measured before and after transection of the ACL while the remaining DOF, like medial-lateral translation and internal-external tibial rotation, were artificially constrained. Constraining the translations and rotations in other DOF introduced errors in knee kinematics because coupled motion occurs naturally in the knee joint. When an anterior tibial load is applied, the knee responds with both an anterior tibial displacement as well as a 'coupled' internal tibial rotation at all flexion angles of the knee (Fig. 39). This coupled motion is a result of the joint anatomy as well as the contribution from the various ligaments. Constrain-

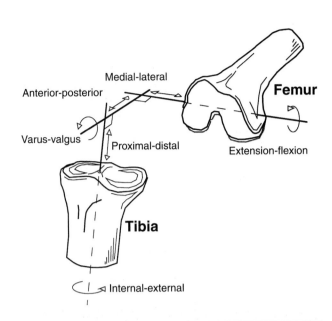

Figure 38

Schematic diagram illustrating the 6 degrees of motion of the human knee joint. (Reproduced with permission from Woo SL-Y, Livesay GA, Smith BA: Kinematics, in Fu FH, Harner CD, Vince KG (eds): *Knee Surgery*. Baltimore, MD, Williams & Wilkins, 1994, pp 155–173.)

ing this motion will limit the normal response of the joint to externally applied loads. The concept of allowing the joint to have multiple DOF of motion is important to study the function of ligaments as well as to understand the complexity of knee motion.

In the laboratory, biomechanical tests are usually performed with 5 DOF, for example, constraining the sixth DOF, the flexion angle. When evaluating the knee, the 5 DOF tests enable investigators to simulate the effect of clinical examinations, such as the anterior drawer test or Lachman test for the ACL, at a chosen flexion angle of the knee.

Healing of Ligaments

Clinical Classification

The clinical classification of ligament injuries is based on the relative degree of injury to the ligament. Generally speaking, ligament damage can be classified as being either partial or complete. Surprisingly, partial tears of ligaments tend to be more painful than complete tears, presumably because they remain partially intact and innervated. In practice, ligament injuries have been classified into 3 grades or degrees (grades I, II, or III). Grade I injuries correspond to the clinical diagnosis of a mild sprain. The injured ligament will be tender to palpation and pain will be induced when stress is applied to the ligament. No laxity of the joint can be detected during a manual stress test of any grade I injury. At the tissue level, the ligament has presum-

ably suffered a minimal rupture of some of its soft-tissue fibers. There will likely be some signal changes seen on magnetic resonance imaging (MRI), but they will be relatively mild. The clinical prognosis of a grade I injury is therefore relatively good. Grade II injuries are more severe and are considered moderate sprains. In such cases, injuries will be more severe, with more acute pain and swelling. As with grade I injuries, there will be pain when the injured ligament is stressed. Unlike the grade I injury, a grade II injury will have some detectable joint laxity. Histopathologically, a grade II injury will involve disruption of some but not all ligament fibers within the structure of the ligament. This partial integrity may also be noted on MRI. A grade II injury can be classified as intermediate; most do well clinically, but some are prone to ongoing instability problems and reinjury. Grade III ligament injuries correspond to the most severe, complete ligament tears, called severe sprains, in which ligament fibers are completely disrupted. Clinically, there will be some pain, swelling, and tenderness in the specific anatomic area of the disruption but, as noted above, stressing the joint to reveal its instability will often be surprisingly nonpainful. At the tissue level, the ligament will be completely disrupted; none of its fibers will be in continuity. Torn ends of the ligament with a fluid-filled gap will be seen on MRI. There will be significant local hemorrhage, inflammation, scar tissue formation, and remodeling over a period of weeks to months. The prognosis of grade III ligament injuries is the most guarded and is more ligament-specific.

Finally, special note should be made of ligament injuries that involve avulsions of bony insertions. These injuries are unique in that they involve bone injury in addition to soft-tissue injury (though not rupture). They can thus be detected on radiographs rather than through physical examina-

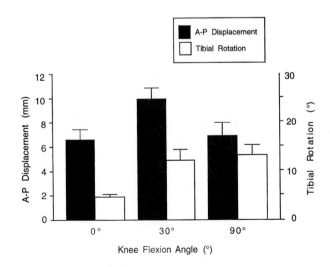

Figure 39

Anterior-posterior displacement and coupled axial tibial rotation in response to ± 100 N of anterior- tibial load.

tion alone, and their prognosis for repair is better if the bony anatomy can be restored surgically. It should be noted that these avulsions disrupt not only bone but also the soft-tissue components of the ligament itself. The clinical prognosis of repaired bony avulsions, however, is reportedly better than that of a pure soft-tissue grade III injury.

Inflammation and Healing of Ligaments

The healing of extra-articular ligaments is analogous to the repair process of other vascular tissues. Following injury there is exudation of blood and associated blood products from disrupted vessels, organization of a fibrin clot, vascularization of this fibrin scaffold, proliferation of cells, synthesis of an extracellular matrix, and, finally, remodeling of the repair tissue. Although this repair process occurs as a continuum, it has been divided into individual phases based on the morphologic and biochemical events that occur.

Phase I: Inflammation Following complete ligament disruption, the torn ends of the ligament retract and usually have an irregular mop-end appearance. In the extra-articular environment, damaged capillaries within the ligament and adjacent tissues produce a hematoma that fills the gap created by the retraction of the ligament ends. In response to the injury and their exposure to the fibrin clot, potent vasodilators, histamine, serotonin, bradykinins, and prostaglandins, are released. Bradykinins, in addition to vasodilation, increase capillary permeability, allowing transudation of fluid and movement of inflammatory cells into the extracellular space. The inflammatory mediators, in combination with the injured tissue and the forming coagulum, initiate the healing process. These events usually occur during the first 72 hours after injury.

Histologically, inflammatory cells and erythrocytes fill the injured area. Leukocytes (polymorphonuclear cells and lymphocytes) migrate through capillary walls and disrupted blood vessels. This migration is followed by the gradual appearance of monocytic cells that, along with macrophages, begin phagocytosis of necrotic tissue. Capillary endothelial buds proliferate in the wound in response to an angiogenic factor secreted by the macrophage.

Toward the end of the inflammatory stage, fibroblast proliferation begins to occur. Thought to arise from undifferentiated mesenchymal cells, these fibroblasts produce a matrix of proteoglycan and collagen, forming a rudimentary scar. Considerable remodeling of the collagen takes place in this phase, with synthesis slightly exceeding degradation. Although most of the newly synthesized collagen scar is type III, a small amount of type I is produced. Type III collagen is thought to be responsible for early stabilization of the collagen meshwork, and type I collagen is more important to the long-term matrix properties.

Phase II: Matrix and Cellular Proliferation Matrix and cellular proliferation occurs over the next 6 weeks and is accompanied by increasing organization of the fibrin clot. The gap between the torn ligament ends is filled with a friable, vascular granulation tissue, and the fibroblast is the predominant cell type. At this stage, the scar is highly cellular and contains macrophage and mast cells in addition to fibroblasts. Vascular endothelial capillary buds communicate with adjacent capillaries in a diffuse network. Active collagen synthesis occurs during this phase in both the proliferating scar and the adjacent normal tissue. However, collagen concentration remains low because of the less dense, woven organization of the collagen framework. Spaces in this framework are thought to be filled with water and other extracellular components. Type I collagen is now the predominant matrix component, and the concentration of glycosaminoglycans also increases. These biochemical changes correlate with an increase in the mechanical strength of the scar.

Phases III and IV: Remodeling and Maturation After several weeks, a gradual transition takes place between the proliferative and remodeling phases. There is a relative decrease in the cellularity and vascularity at the previously ruptured site and an increase in collagen density. In addition, polarized light microscopy of the healing ligament reveals a more organized collagen arrangement, with the collagen becoming aligned along the axis of the ligament.

Biochemically, there is a decrease in active matrix synthesis during this phase, and the biochemical profile of the matrix shifts toward that of normal ligament. While the collagen content of the healing ligament plateaus, the tensile strength of the ligament continues to increase. This increase is thought to reflect collagen reorganization, cross-linking, and other changes in the matrix. In an animal model, the ligament appears to have normal histologic appearance at 6 weeks, and many have proclaimed complete healing on that basis. It should be noted, however, that while the ligament ends may appear to be united, several months are required for the ligament to remodel to achieve complete morphologic normalcy.

The healed ligament remains slightly disorganized and hypercellular. It is thought that as much as 12 months or more may be required to complete remodeling. Numerous factors influence healing and repair, including both host factors (biology) and biomechanics.

The above description of ligament healing relates predominantly to the collateral ligaments as an example of extra-articular ligament healing. Their anatomic location affords them direct access to the vascular supply of the adjacent soft tissue. In addition, the anatomy confines the scar to the gap between the torn ligament ends, effectively closing the gap and facilitating healing. In the intra-articular environment, the cruciate ligaments do not have this advantage. Results of experimental studies have shown that while the ACL has a profuse vascular response following injury, spontaneous repair does not occur. One of the proposed reasons could be the dilution of the hematoma by the synovial fluid, preventing the formation of a fibrin clot and, thus, the initiation of the healing mechanism. Some physicians have suggested that the synovial fluid is hostile to soft-tissue healing, while others have speculated that the high stress carried by the intact ACL prevents effective healing from taking place.

Clinical and Biomechanical Aspects of Extra-Articular Ligament Healing and Repair

Clinical Relevance There are numerous extra-articular ligaments in the body, virtually any of which can be injured. Before implying that all extra-articular ligaments undergo exactly the same "natural history of healing," it is important to recognize that clinical evidence supports the possibility that ligament healing may be not only specific to the severity of the injury (grade), but also may be, to some extent, anatomically-specific and patient-specific (age, gender, etc).

Among the extra-articular ligaments, the MCL of the knee (stifle joint of animals) has been studied most extensively in both the clinical setting and the laboratory. The general consensus of clinical investigations is that virtually all partial MCL injuries (grade I and grade II) heal without surgical treatment, allowing the majority of patients to return to competitive team sports fairly quickly with a very good clinical prognosis. In a review of college football injuries, it was found that 42 of the 51 patients who received nonsurgical treatment for grade I or grade II MCL injuries returned to sports uneventfully within about 3 weeks after injury. In the 9 injuries in which conservative treatment and rehabilitation was unsuccessful, other pathology involving the ACL or damage to the menisci was found. In a prospective review of 38 recreational athletes in Sweden who had nonsurgically treated grade I or grade II injuries of the MCL, 75% returned to sports by 3 months, with 5 patients having objective valgus laxity remaining at that interval. At 4 years, 87% of those patients who returned to sports still had nor-mal knee function during strenuous activities. However, at 10 years, 13% of the patients returning to sports had early radiographic signs of osteoarthritis.

The optimum treatment of grade III, or complete, MCL injuries has been more controversial because, as expected, clinical results have been inferior to those of the 2 milder grades. Between 10% to 25% of patients studied continue to have ongoing clinical problems, regardless of whether they have surgical repair or not. Although it is not entirely clear whether some of those patients may have had other subtle injuries in combination with their MCL damage, it would appear that this "success rate" of 75% to 90% does represent the outcome of treatment of isolated, severe MCL injuries.

In defining the optimal treatment of grade III MCL injuries, early clinical studies advocated surgical repair followed by several weeks of immobilization. Subsequent studies, however, suggested that these reports had compared mixed populations of injuries (the vast majority included ACL and MCL injuries combined), without appropriate controls. Eliminating combined injuries demonstrated that surgical repairs of grade III MCL injuries were probably no better than nonsurgical treatment. In fact, data in several clinical studies demonstrated that the repair and/or the postoperative immobilization protocols actually interfered with the rate of rehabilitation, without any apparent benefits. For example, a recent prospective clinical trial of 33 patients divided between repair or nonsurgical treatment showed a slower rehabilitation period for the subgroup treated with surgery (14.9 weeks versus 11.3 weeks) with otherwise equal clinical outcomes over 2 years after injury.

Biomechanical Aspects: Isolated MCL Injuries—Repair Versus Nonrepair Animal studies using the canine model have been used to evaluate the significance of primary MCL repair with immobilization following transection of the MCL. Results of these studies showed that the valgus rotations of the knee with a nonrepaired and repaired MCL were significantly higher than those of the control at 6

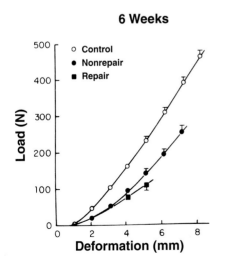

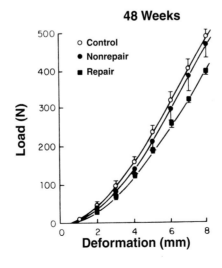

Figure 40

Structural properties of the repaired and nonrepaired canine femur-MCL-tibia complex at 6 and 48 weeks postoperatively. The controls are shown for comparison. (Reproduced with permission from Woo SL-Y, Horibe S, Ohland KJ, et al: The response of ligaments to injury: Healing of the collateral ligaments, in Daniel D, Akeson WH, O'Connor JJ (eds): *Knee Ligaments: Structure, Function, Injury, and Repair.* New York, NY, Raven Press, 1990, pp 351–364.)

weeks. However, the nonrepaired group had near-normal valgus rotation at 12 weeks, while that of the surgical group was larger than normal. The structural properties of the FMTC from the nonrepaired ligaments were also closer to the control than those of the surgically repaired ligaments throughout the 48-week study period. Their values approached those of the controls at 48 weeks (Fig. 40). Despite the normal structural properties of the FMTCs from the nonrepaired group, the mechanical properties of both the repaired and nonrepaired MCL were considerably different from those of the control. Tensile strength reached only 60% of control at 48 weeks. Histologically, this correlates with a more irregular orientation of the collagen fibers.

A rabbit model of MCL healing in which a gap injury was created showed that apposition of ligament ends did provide a small improvement to the early structural properties of the FMTC when compared with healing of a gap early after the injury. The stiffness and ultimate load of the FMTC for the sutured group were about 25% greater than for the gap group up to 14 weeks postoperatively. At 40 weeks, the repaired group reached 85% of normal ultimate load to failure, and only 55% in ultimate tensile strength, whereas gaps reached about 70% and 35%, respectively. These data therefore collectively suggest that gap sizes between ligament ends can cause some detectable weakness of healed ligament as a result of subtle differences in tissue remodeling.

Whether there are significant gaps between torn ligament ends in the clinical situation remains unknown, but as noted above, recent clinical experience suggests that suture repairs of isolated grade III MCL injuries are unnecessary. This may be because the gap between the torn ends is small and the structural properties of the healing MCL are suffi-

cient to allow function. These studies have shown that even though the mechanical properties (ultimate tensile strength) of the healed ligaments are inadequate when compared with the intact ligament, the larger cross-sectional area of the healed ligament accounts for structural properties (ultimate tensile load) that are closer to those of intact ligaments.

An alternative model has been used to evaluate the effects of primary repair versus nonsurgical treatment on the histologic and biomechanical properties of the rabbit MCL. In this model, the MCL of a rabbit hindlimb was ruptured by placing a rod beneath it and causing a mop-end tear of the ligament substance with simultaneous injury to the insertion sites. Primary repair of the MCL initially decreased the varus-valgus rotation; however, after 12 weeks there was no difference between surgically treated and nonsurgically treated MCL. There was no significant effect of repair on in situ force or tensile properties of the MCL (Fig. 41). Failure modes of the FMTC and histologic sections of the ligament insertion sites indicate that after injury the insertion sites recover more slowly than the ligament substance.

Combined ACL and MCL Injuries The management of MCL injury in the presence of ACL injury is more complicated. Of primary importance to this problem is the role of the ACL in stabilizing the MCL-deficient knee. Experimental studies have demonstrated that the MCL is the main stabilizer in valgus rotation when the knee is constrained to 3 DOF; that is, internal-external tibial rotation and anterior-posterior translation are restricted. In nonconstrained knee motion, as would occur during normal activities, valgus instability caused by a torn MCL increased only minimally because of

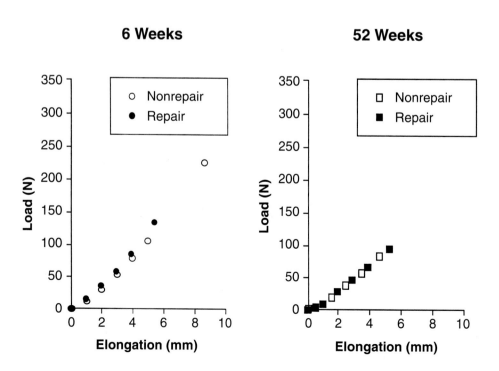

6 Weeks

52 Weeks

Figure 41

Load-elongation curves comparing nonrepaired and repaired rabbit femur-MCL-tibia complex at 6 and 52 weeks postoperatively.

the contributions of the remaining soft-tissue structures, the ACL in particular. Therefore, the effects of transection of the ACL on MCL healing were investigated using both the canine and rabbit knee models. Although all MCLs healed, the valgus rotation and mechanical properties of the healing MCL in the combined ACL/MCL injury failed to recover to normal levels. Thus, ACL reconstruction is usually recommended in combined ACL/MCL injuries in order to improve healing of the MCL.

Immobilization As discussed earlier, immobilization can lead to detrimental effects on the mechanical properties of ligaments. Joint immobilization in combined ACL/MCL injury reduces knee instability, but has been demonstrated to have negative effects on the structural properties of the FMTC in the rabbit model. Immobilized and nonimmobilized groups were compared at 3, 6, and 14 weeks, postoperatively. The immobilized knees were similar to the normal knee, but the nonimmobilized knees had significant instability. However, the ultimate load for the nonimmobilized MCL was significantly greater than for the immobilized MCL. Although joint immobilization has been proven to be harmful in the isolated MCL, it is still considered as a controversial treatment for the combined MCL/ACL ruptures.

MCL Replacement Allograft replacements for the MCL have been considered for severe injuries. In animal studies, they have been found to have long-term viability; however, the properties of the allograft are diminished from those of normal tissue. Fresh-frozen allograft FMTC was used to replace the MCL in the rabbit model. The highest ultimate load and energy absorbed at failure by the allograft occurred at 3 weeks and gradually decreased over time. Between 12 and 48 weeks after transplantation, the ultimate load was only 50% to 60% of control and the energy absorbed at failure was 30% of that of the control FMTC. The modulus and tensile strength of the allograft were 30% and 30% to 40% of control, respectively, at 12 weeks. The allograft tissue was viable and vascular, but reached an equilibrium that was different from normal. The central portion of fresh-frozen canine patellar tendon allografts has also been studied as an MCL replacement. After a period of immobilization and remobilization, microangiographic and histologic evaluation revealed all reconstructed ligaments to be viable 1 year after implantation. The ultimate load of the FMTC reached 71% of control after 1 year, but the tensile strength of the MCL was only 44% of control.

Clinical and Biomechanical Aspects of Intra-articular Ligament Replacement

The ACL is arguably the most important intra-articular ligament in the body. Specifically, the ACL spans the space between the femur and the tibia within the knee joint without much periligamentous support. Contrary to the success of conservative treatment of isolated MCL injuries, midsub-

stance ACL tears usually do not heal. The long-term sequelae of cruciate-deficient knees include meniscal damage and joint instability with early osteoarthritic changes. Clinically, primary suture repairs of torn ACL ends have been attempted on many occasions, with good short-term (2 to 3 years) but relatively poor longer-term (5 years and beyond) results. Similarly, such lack of success for ACL repair was seen in animal studies.

With poor clinical outcomes for both primary repair and conservative treatment, the focus of how to improve knee function after ACL injury has shifted to surgical reconstruction of the ACL. The most popular surgical replacements for the ACL have been biologic tissue grafts. Both clinical and experimental literature dealing with the clinical, biologic, and biomechanical aspects of these biologic grafts is abundant. Here, the focus will be on a number of factors that have been identified as important and should be considered when performing ligament reconstructions. These factors are the selection of graft material, graft placement, and graft tensioning as well as graft fixation. Interested readers are therefore encouraged to refer to the sources referenced at the end of this chapter.

Graft Material In ligament reconstructions, the replacement graft should have similar tensile properties as well as dimensions of the intact ligament in order to reproduce its in vivo function. Various graft choices have been recommended for ACL reconstructions, but currently the most popular grafts are bone-patellar tendon-bone, and semitendinosus and gracilis. Bone-patellar tendon-bone graft has been popular because of its high ultimate load as well as the possibility for bony fixation. Semitendinosus and gracilis graft provides a multiple-bundle replacement graft that may better reproduce the function of the 2 major bundles of the ACL. Replacement grafts are available either as autografts or allografts (in this latter case, Achilles tendon grafts are also used). During the last few years, autografts have become more popular because of lower risk of adverse inflammatory reaction as well as no risk of disease transmission. However, allografts are often used in failed reconstructions as well as in reconstructions involving multiple ligament injuries.

Autografts After transplantation, the replacement autograft will undergo remodeling in the new environment. For example, the remodeling process of a patellar tendon autograft for ACL reconstruction has been studied in various animal models such as the dog, sheep, goat, rabbit, and monkey. The general trend for the remodeling of patellar tendon autografts is for the ultimate load to reach 20% to 40% of the control FATC after 1 to 2 years, with some degree of increased anterior-posterior joint translation and articular cartilage degeneration. Structural properties of the bone-autograft-bone complex were very low during the first few weeks after transplantation, but increased minimally with time. In a dog model, the grafts were found to have an ultimate load less than 10% of the control FATC at the time of implantation because of fixation site weakness. At 3 months, these load values increased to 20%, and at 20 months to 30% of control. In a long-term study of ACL reconstruction using a goat model, the central third of the patellar tendon was used to replace the ACL. The anterior-posterior translation of the knee, in response to anterior-posterior loads, was highest at 6 and 12 weeks but slowly improved afterward. After 3 years, there was no significant difference in the anterior-posterior knee translation of the grafted knee with that of the intact knee (Fig. 42). The structural properties of the autografts appeared to improve significantly between 12 weeks and 52 weeks, but the improvement was slow afterward. After 3 years, the stiffness and the ultimate load were 44% and 49% respectively, of those of the intact ACL.

In a clinical study on ACL reconstructions using central third patellar tendon autografts and covering more than 800 patients with a follow-up of 2 to 9 years, it was reported that 89% of those reconstructed knees were considered normal or near-normal. Radiographically, 94% of acute knees and 89% of chronic knees had no joint space narrowing. Reports of morphologic and histologic appearance from biopsies of patellar tendon autografts during second-look surgeries describe the process of graft remodeling in 4 phases: synovial envelopment up to 6 months after surgery; fibrous tissue ingrowth at 6 to 12 months; transformation into ligament-like tissue at 12 to 18 months; and maturation of striated ligament-like structure. For the fibrous ingrowth phase, the graft is surrounded by an abundantly vascular synovial tissue with increased cellularity, and the transformation phase is characterized by a decrease in vascularity and longitudinal arrangement of collagen fiber bundles. It should be noted, however, that arthroscopic biopsies are generally obtained from near the surface of the graft, which may not reflect the characteristics of the entire graft. Nevertheless, these reports have enhanced understanding of the graft maturation process.

Allografts The morbidity associated with autograft harvest and the potentially limitless supply of allogenic tissues have increased interest in allografts, especially in ACL surgery for previously failed autografts. Also, allograft usage is still popular for multiple ligament reconstructions, as well as for patients who are not high-performance athletes. The ACL and other tissues, including the Achilles tendon, have been used as allografts. Allografts are usually preserved by deep-freezing or freeze-drying. To date, tissue typically is sterilized using cobalt irradiation, because ethylene oxide gas sterilization has proven to be detrimental to its biomechanical properties. Because these processes can alter the properties of the allograft, a complete understanding of their effects has been pursued.

It has been shown that deep-freezing without drying has little or no effect on the mechanical properties of ligament. No significant differences in the stiffness, ultimate load, or modulus were noted between the treated and control ligaments 26 weeks following treatment. Allograft sterilization by irradiation to reduce the risk of disease transmission, however, can have adverse effects on the tensile properties of ligaments. A decreasing trend in the structural and mechanical properties, which became significant at the 3-Mrad level of dosage, was observed with irradiation. Irradiation also altered tissue morphology, where collagen fascicles were separated and the ligaments were visibly crimped.

Allografts have also been evaluated in animal models. In a goat model, ACL reconstruction using patellar tendon autograft was compared with reconstruction using patellar tendon allograft. The study showed that in 6 months, knees reconstructed with autograft had a smaller increase in anterior-posterior laxity, and higher ultimate load.

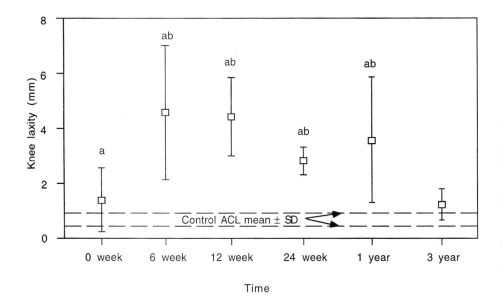

Figure 42

Anterior tibial translation for control and reconstructed knees using an anterior cruciate ligament (ACL) autograft versus different times after surgery. Symbols a and b indicate values that are significantly different from the control and the 3-year groups, respectively. (Reproduced with permission from Ng GY, Oakes BW, Deacon OW, McLean ID, Lampard D: Biomechanics of patellar tendon autograft for reconstruction of the anterior cruciate ligament in the goat: Three-year study. *J Orthop Res* 1995;13:602–608.)

Graft Placement Significant research has been devoted to identifying the ideal position for graft placement with the hope of reproducing the anatomy and, more importantly, the function of the intact ligament. Various methods of graft placement have been evaluated and the 'isometric' placement was favored over other methods in the past. The concept of isometric placement of the graft is to limit the changes in graft length and tension during passive flexion-extension of the knee. In the surgical context, the concept of isometry can be referred only to limit excessive changes in graft length and, thus, graft tension, throughout the range of passive flexion-extension. However, as more basic science knowledge of the ACL and PCL has accumulated, the concept of isometry is now considered. In fact, the cruciate ligaments consist of different fiber bundles that will undergo variable elongation during knee motion. As a result, the anteromedial bundle of the ACL experiences higher stresses and strains during knee flexion while the posterolateral bundle does that during knee extension.

With better understanding of the importance of various bundles of the cruciate ligaments as well as lessons from complications, graft placement in cruciate ligament reconstructions has changed accordingly. For ACL reconstruction, a number of investigators have reported the significance of graft impingement with an anteriorly placed tibial tunnel. This placement could lead to lack of knee extension as well as possible early graft failure. Some authors now recommend the placement of the tibial tunnel at the center or posterior portion of the tibial insertion site of the ACL to avoid this complication. For PCL reconstruction, the anatomic position of the anterolateral bundle is preferred by some surgeons for reconstruction; biomechanical studies revealed that this bundle is significantly bigger and stronger than the posteromedial bundle of the PCL. The ideal position for graft placement for cruciate ligaments is still unknown as more knowledge is gained about their contribution to knee kinematics in order to design an improved clinical approach to cruciate ligament reconstructions.

Initial Graft Tension Tension in the replacement graft at the time of graft fixation will significantly alter joint kinematics as well as forces in the graft in situ during knee motion. A low graft tension will not provide the needed joint stability, and a large tension can cause excessive graft forces that compromise the survivability of the replacement graft as well as restrain joint motion. Clinically, many investigators have empirically suggested an initial tension near 44 N. The subject of initial graft tension is controversial, because the force in the ACL during normal knee function is unknown. Further, it is well known that the initial graft tension decreases shortly after the graft is fixed as a result of viscoelastic stress relaxation.

The effect of an initial tension of 1 N or 39 N on patellar tendon autografts in the dog model was examined. After 3 months, no differences were found in anterior-posterior joint instability or in structural properties (stiffness and ultimate load) of the bone-graft-bone complex. However, the autografts tensioned to 39 N did demonstrate some histologic evidence of degeneration of the articular cartilage. The effect of initial graft tensioning was also examined in a prospective, randomized study on human ACL reconstructions. In this study, patients were randomly divided into 3 groups based on initial graft tension of 20 N, 40 N, and 80 N. At a minimum of 2-year follow-up, anterior laxity over the contralateral control limb was 2.2 ± 2.4 mm, 1.4 ± 1.8 mm, and 0.6 ± 1.7 mm, respectively. However, it should be noted that this is a short-term follow-up report and the long-term effects of graft tensioning on the success of ACL reconstruction remain unknown.

Graft Fixation Graft fixation is also another important factor in cruciate ligament reconstruction. Bone-patellar tendon-bone graft has been a popular ligament graft because of the possibility of fixation of the replacement graft within the bony tunnel. Healing of bone blocks within the bony tunnels are believed to have similarities to those in fracture healing. On the other hand, quadruple semitendinosus and gracilis grafts have also been popular. In the case of bone-patellar tendon-bone grafts, the length of the graft will lead to fixation at different sites along the tibial bone tunnel. As a result, the effective length and stiffness also varied. Thus, various fixation methods have been made available in order to improve initial stiffness and strength of the graft attachment site (Fig. 43).

Significant research has been performed to determine the stiffness and ultimate tensile load because these will have an impact on the function of the graft. In particular, aggressive and early rehabilitation postoperatively is being advocated to date. Recently, much attention has also been directed toward various methods of graft fixation in an effort to increase stiffness of the construction as well as deal with the problem of large graft-tunnel motion. For example, the use of bioabsorbable material as a fixation device within the bone tunnel for soft-tissue grafts has gained popularity. These devices are designed to provide good initial fixation but will be resorbed, thus eliminating difficult hardware removal in the case of revision surgeries. However, what is needed for graft fixation remains an area of great debate. This is an important area in orthopaedics in which new and innovative devices need to be developed based on basic science studies. Only then can definitive improvements on problems related to graft healing fixation and healing in bone tunnels be made.

Summary

In this chapter, many investigations have been presented that were designed to characterize the tensile and viscoelastic properties of tendons and ligaments. Some of the

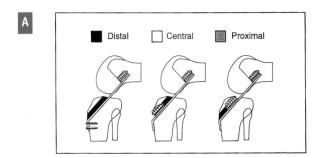

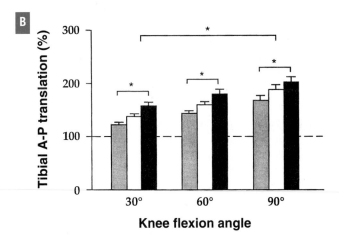

Figure 43

A, Total anteroposterior translation for different fixation locations of the anterior cruciate ligament graft at the tibia. **B,** The proximal site of the graft was secured using an interference screw within the femoral tunnel. The distal site of the graft was fixed sequentially at 3 different locations for each specimen. (Reproduced with permission from Ishibashi Y, Rudy TW, Livesay GA, Stone JD, Fu FH, Woo SL-Y: The effect of anterior cruciate ligament graft fixation site at the tibia on knee stability: Evaluation using a robotic testing system. *Arthroscopy* 1997;13:177–182.)

dons and ligaments during joint motion and activities of daily living remain relatively unknown. Some groups have employed a Hall-effect strain transducer (Microstrain, Burlington, VT) to measure ligament strain during knee motion. This device is attached to the ligament substance parallel to the surface fibers and can be used to determine the in situ strain for both the intact and reconstructed ACL.

Also, with the recent introduction of a robotic/universal force moment sensor (UFS) testing system, it has become possible to study joint kinematics and in situ forces in the tendons and ligaments without contact to the tissue or dissection of the joint. This new technology has led to accurate simulation of multiple DOF of the joint motion and helped obtain realistic data on individual soft-tissue structures in and around the joint in response to an applied load. By using robotic/UFS technology, multiple and combined loading conditions may be applied to the same knee specimen to eliminate interspecimen variation.

It is anticipated that future research will need to focus on the design and improvement of ligament reconstruction and tendon repair in vivo. Thus, efforts on new methodology will be needed. With more precise and accurate methods being developed to characterize functions of ligaments and tendons, it is hoped that in vivo data can be collected. The biomechanics obtained on normal as well as repair tissues in vivo will enable better prediction of the function of surgically repaired tendons and ligaments during daily activities. Concurrently, advances in computer technology will allow simulation of experimental findings based on joint motion. Mathematical models of the human knee joint have been used to predict the biomechanical behavior of individual ligaments. This approach has tremendous potential for understanding mechanism of injury as well as design of appropriate surgical management procedure because realistic yet complex external loading conditions on the joints can be modeled.

More recently, efforts on tissue engineering to enhance healing of ligaments and tendons have also been explored. There is also significant interest in accelerating the healing of soft-tissue tendon grafts within the osseous tunnel after ACL reconstruction. Growth factors such as platelet-derived growth factor, epidermal growth factor, fibroblast growth factors, and transforming growth factor-β1 have been identified to have the potential to upregulate cellular proliferation and elevate protein-sensitive levels by ligament fibroblasts. Gene transfer technology is also being explored as a method of delivering these growth factors repeatedly and at appropriate times after ligament injuries. The collaborative efforts of bioengineers, clinicians, molecular and cell biologists will help yield a better understanding of the healing mechanisms of ligaments and tendons and lead to more successful treatment outcomes.

most important experimental and biologic factors that can affect the measurements of these properties have been identified and elucidated. The data available to date have significantly contributed to the understanding of these living tissues as well as their function in the diarthrodial joints. Furthermore, significant knowledge on the injury and repair of tendons and ligaments has been gained through basic science and clinical research. All of these efforts have helped to advance treatment as well as to prevent soft-tissue injuries.

Although the in vivo properties of tendons and ligaments have also been studied, the forces and strains in situ for ten-

Selected Bibliography

Tendon Biomechanics

Abrahams M: Mechanical behaviour of tendon in vitro: A preliminary report. *Med Biol Eng* 1967;5:433–443.

Berchuck M, Andriacchi TP, Bach BR, Reider B: Gait adaptations by patients who have a deficient anterior cruciate ligament. *J Bone Joint Surg* 1990;72A:871–877.

Betsch DF, Baer E: Structure and mechanical properties of rat tail tendon. *Biorheology* 1980;17:83–94.

Carlstedt CA, Skagervall R: A model for computer-aided analysis of biomechanical properties of the plantaris longus tendon in the rabbit. *J Biomech* 1986;19:251–256.

Cohen RE, Hooley CJ, McCrum NG: Viscoelastic creep of collagenous tissue. *J Biomech* 1976;9:175–184.

Cribb AM, Scott JE: Tendon response to tensile stress: An ultrastructural investigation of collagen: Proteoglycan interactions in stressed tendon. *J Anat* 1995;187:423–428.

Danielsen CC: Mechanical properties of native and reconstituted rat tail tendon collagen upon maturation in vitro. *Mech Ageing Dev* 1987;40:9–16.

Danielson KG, Baribault H, Holmes DF, Graham H, Kadler KE, Iozzo RV. Targeted disruption of decorin leads to abnormal collagen fibril morphology and skin fragility. *J Cell Biol* 1997;136:729–743.

Draganich LF, Vahey JW: An in vitro study of anterior cruciate ligament strain induced by quadriceps and hamstrings forces. *J Orthop Res* 1990;8:57–63.

Fung YC: Stress-strain-history relations of soft tissues in simple elongation, in Fung YC, Perrone N, Anliker M (eds): *Biomechanics: Its Foundations and Objectives.* Englewood Cliffs, NJ, Prentice Hall, 1972, pp 181–208.

Gupta BN, Subramanian KN, Brinker WO, Gupta AN: Tensile strength of canine cranial cruciate ligaments. *Am J Vet Res* 1971;32:183–190.

Hannafin JA, Arnoczky SP, Hoonjan A, Torzilli PA. Effect of stress deprivation and cyclic tensile loading on the material and morphologic properties of canine flexor digitorum profundus tendon: An in vitro study. *J Orthop Res* 1995;13:907–914.

Haut RC, Little RW: A constitutive equation for collagen fibers. *J Biomech* 1972;5:423–430.

Haut RC: The influence of specimen length on the tensile failure properties of tendon collagen. *J Biomech* 1986;19:951–955.

Haut RC: Age-dependent influence of strain rate on the tensile failure of rattail tendon. *J Biomech Eng* 1983;105:296–299.

Hubbard RP, Chun KJ: Mechanical responses of tendons to repeated extensions and wait periods. *J Biomech Eng* 1988;110:11–19.

Itoi E, Berglund LJ, Grabowski JJ, et al: Tensile properties of the supraspinatus tendon. *J Orthop Res* 1995;13:578–584.

Kastelic J, Baer E: Deformation in tendon collagen, in Vincent JFV, Currey JD (eds): *The Mechanical Properties of Biological Materials.* Cambridge, England, Cambridge University Press, 1980, pp 397–435.

Leitschuh PH, Doherty TJ, Taylor DC, Brooks DE, Ryan JB: Effects of postmortem freezing on tensile failure properties of rabbit extensor digitorum longus muscle tendon complex. *J Orthop Res* 1996;14:830–833.

Majima T, Yasuda K, Fujii T, Yamamoto N, Hayashi K, Kaneda K: Biomechanical effects of stress shielding of the rabbit patellar tendon depend on the degree of stress reduction. *J Orthop Res* 1996;14:377–383.

Matthews LS, Ellis D: Viscoelastic properties of cat tendon: Effects of time after death and preservation by freezing. *J Biomech* 1968;1:65–71.

Michna H, Hartmann G: Adaptation of tendon collagen to exercise. *Int Orthop* 1989;13:161–165.

Müller W (ed): *The Knee: Form, Function, and Ligament Reconstruction.* Berlin, Germany, Springer-Verlag, 1983.

Nakagawa Y, Hayashi K, Yamamoto N, Nagashima K. Age-related changes in biomechanical properties of the Achilles tendon in rabbits. *Eur J Appl Physiol* 1996;73:7–10.

Noyes FR, Butler DL, Grood ES, Zernicke RF, Hefzy MS: Biomechanical analysis of human ligament grafts used in knee-ligament repairs and reconstructions. *J Bone Joint Surg* 1984;66A:344–352.

Pins GD, Christiansen DL, Patel R, Silver FH. Self-assembly of collagen fibers: Influence of fibrillar alignment and decorin on mechanical properties. *Biophys J* 1997;73:2164–2172.

Monleon Pradas M, Diaz Calleja R: Nonlinear viscoelastic behaviour of the flexor tendon of the human hand. *J Biomech* 1990;23:773–781.

Pring DJ, Amis AA, Coombs RR: The mechanical properties of human flexor tendons in relation to artificial tendons. *J Hand Surg* 1985;10B:331–336.

Shadwick RE: Elastic energy storage in tendons: Mechanical differences related to function and age. *J Appl Physiol* 1990;68:1033–1040.

Schaefer SL, Ciarelli MJ, Arnoczky SP, Ross HE. Tissue shrinkage with the holmium: Yttrium aluminum garnet laser: A postoperative assessment of tissue length, stiffness, and structure. *Am J Sports Med* 1997;25:841–848.

Smith CW, Young IS, Kearney JN. Mechanical properties of tendons: Changes with sterilization and preservation. *J Biomech Eng* 1996;118: 56–61.

Staubli HU, Schatzmann L, Brunner P, Rincon L, Nolte LP. Quadriceps tendon and patellar ligament: Cryosectional anatomy and structural properties in young adults. *Knee Surg Sports Traumatol Arthros* 1996;4:100–110.

Torp S, Arridge RGC, Armeniades CD, et al: Structure-property relationships in tendon as a function of age, in Atkins EDT, Keller A (eds): *Structure of Fibrous Biopolymers*. London, England, Butterworths, 1975, pp 197–221.

VanBrocklin JD, Ellis DG: A study of the mechanical behavior of toe extensor tendons under applied stress. *Arch Phys Med Rehabil* 1965;46:369–373.

Vangsness CT Jr, Mitchell W III, Nimni M, Erlich M, Saadat V, Schmotzer H: Collagen shortening: An experimental approach with heat. *Clin Orthop* 1997;337:267–271.

Vogel KG, Ordog A, Pogany G, Olah J: Proteoglycans in the compressed region of human tibialis posterior tendon and in ligaments. *J Orthop Res* 1993;11:68–77.

Woo SL: Mechanical properties of tendons and ligaments: I. Quasi-static and nonlinear viscoelastic properties. *Biorheology* 1982;19: 385–396.

Woo SL, Gomez MA, Woo YK, Akeson WH: Mechanical properties of tendons and ligaments: II. The relationships of immobilization and exercise on tissue remodeling. *Biorheology* 1982;19:397–408.

Wood TO, Cooke PH, Goodship AE: The effect of exercise and anabolic steroids on the mechanical properties and crimp morphology of the rat tendon. *Am J Sports Med* 1988;16:153–158.

Yasuda K, Sasaki T: Exercise after anterior cruciate ligament reconstruction: The force exerted on the tibia by the separate isometric contractions of the quadriceps or the hamstrings. *Clin Orthop* 1987;220:275–283.

Yasuda K, Sasaki T: Muscle exercise after anterior cruciate ligament reconstruction: Biomechanics of the simultaneous isometric contraction method of the quadriceps and the hamstrings. *Clin Orthop* 1987;220:266–274.

Tendon Injury, Healing, and Repair

Gelberman RH, Botte MJ, Spiegelman JJ, Akeson WH: The excursion and deformation of repaired flexor tendons treated with protected early motion. *J Hand Surg* 1986;11A:106–110.

Gelberman RH, Woo SL, Lothringer K, Akeson WH, Amiel D: Effects of early intermittent passive mobilization on healing canine flexor tendons. *J Hand Surg* 1982;7A:170–175.

Manske PR, Lesker PA: Biochemical evidence of flexor tendon participation in the repair process: An in vitro study. *J Hand Surg* 1984;9B:117–120.

Noguchi M, Seiler JG III, Gelberman RH, Sofranko RA, Woo SL: In vitro biomechanical analysis of suture methods for flexor tendon repair. *J Orthop Res* 1993;11:603–611.

Nirschl RP: Rotator cuff tendinitis: Basic concepts of pathoetiology, in Barr JS Jr (ed): *Instructional Course Lectures XXXVIII*. Park Ridge, IL, American Academy of Orthopaedic Surgeons, 1989, pp 439–445.

Potenza AD: Concepts of tendon healing and repair, in *American Academy of Orthopaedic Surgeons Symposium on Tendon Surgery in the Hand*. St. Louis, MO, CV Mosby, 1975, pp 18–47.

Seradge H: Elongation of the repair configuration following flexor tendon repair. *J Hand Surg* 1983;8A:182–185.

Wade PJ, Muir IF, Hutcheon LL: Primary flexor tendon repair: The mechanical limitations of the modified Kessler technique. *J Hand Surg* 1986;11B:71–76.

Winters SC, Gelberman RH, Woo SL, Chan SS, Grewal R, Seiler JG III: The effects of multiple-strand suture methods on the strength and excursion of repaired intrasynovial flexor tendons: A biomechanical study in dogs. *J Hand Surg* 1988;23A:97–104.

Ligament Biomechanics

Amiel D, Frank C, Harwood F, Fronek J, Akeson W: Tendons and ligaments: A morphological and biochemical comparison. *J Orthop Res* 1984;1:257–265.

Burks RT: Gross anatomy, in Daniel DM, Akeson WH, O'Connor JJ (eds): *Knee Ligaments: Structure, Function, Injury, and Repair.* New York, NY, Raven Press, 1990, pp 59–76.

Butler DL, Kay MD, Stouffer DC: Comparison of material properties in fascicle-bone units from human patellar tendon and knee ligaments. *J Biomech* 1986;19:425–432.

Danto MI, Woo SL: The mechanical properties of skeletally mature rabbit anterior cruciate ligament and patellar tendon over a range of strain rates. *J Orthop Res* 1993;11:58–67.

Figgie HE III, Bahniuk EH, Heiple KG, Davy DT: The effects of tibial-femoral angle on the failure mechanics of the canine anterior cruciate ligament. *J Biomech* 1986;19:89–91.

Graf BK, Vanderby R Jr., Ulm MJ, Rogalski RP, Thielke RJ. Effect of preconditioning on the viscoelastic response of primate patellar tendon. *Arthroscopy* 1994;10:90–96.

Harner CD, Xerogeanes JW, Livesay GA, et al: The human posterior cruciate ligament complex: An interdisciplinary study: Ligament morphology and biomechanical evaluation. *Am J Sports Med* 1995; 23:736–745.

Hart RA, Woo SL, Newton PO: Ultrastructural morphometry of anterior cruciate and medial collateral ligaments: An experimental study in rabbits. *J Orthop Res* 1992;10:96–103.

Hollis JM, Takai S, Adams DJ, Horibe S, Woo SL: The effects of knee motion and external loading on the length of the anterior cruciate ligament (ACL): A kinematic study. *J Biomech Eng* 1991, 113:208–214.

Kennedy JC, Hawkins RJ, Willis RB, Danylchuck KD: Tension studies of human knee ligaments: Yield point, ultimate failure, and disruption of the cruciate and tibial collateral ligaments. *J Bone Joint Surg* 1976:58A:350–355.

Kennedy JC, Roth JH, Mendenhall HV, Sanford JB: Presidential address: Intraarticular replacement in the anterior cruciate ligament-deficient knee. *Am J Sports Med* 1980:8:1–8.

Kusayama T, Harner CD, Carlin GJ, Xerogeanes JW, Smith BA: Anatomical and biomechanical characteristics of human meniscofemoral ligaments. *Knee Surg Sports Traumatol Arthrosc* 1994:2: 234–237.

Laros GS, Tipton CM, Cooper RR: Influence of physical activity on ligament insertions in the knees of dogs. *J Bone Joint Surg* 1971;53A: 275–286.

Myers BS, McElhaney JH, Doherty BJ: The viscoelastic responses of the human cervical spine in torsion: Experimental limitations of quasi-linear theory, and a method for reducing these effects. *J Biomech* 1991;24:811–817.

Noyes FR: Functional properties of knee ligaments and alterations induced by immobilization: A correlative biomechanical and histological study in primates. *Clin Orthop* 1977;123:210–242.

Noyes FR, DeLucas JL, Torvik PJ: Biomechanics of anterior cruciate ligament failure: An analysis of strain-rate sensitivity and mechanisms of failure in primates. *J Bone Joint Surg* 1974; 56A:236–253.

Tipton CM, Matthes RD, Maynard JA, Carey RA: The influence of physical activity on ligaments and tendons. *Med Sci Sports* 1975; 7:165–175.

Trent PS, Walker PS, Wolf B: Ligament length patterns, strength, and rotational axes of the knee joint. *Clin Orthop* 1976;117:263–270.

Viidik A: Elasticity and tensile strength of the anterior cruciate ligament in rabbits as influenced by training. *Acta Physiol Scand* 1968;74:372–380.

Viidik A, Sandqvist L, Mägi M: Influence of postmortal storage on tensile strength characteristics and histology of rabbit ligaments. *Acta Orthop Scand Suppl* 1965;79:7–38.

Woo SL, Chan SS, Yamaji T: Biomechanics of knee ligament healing, repair and reconstruction. *J Biomech* 1997;30:431–439.

Woo SL, Hollis JM, Adams DJ, Lyon RM, Takai S: Tensile properties of the human femur-anterior cruciate ligament-tibia complex: The effects of specimen age and orientation. *Am J Sports Med* 1991;19: 217–225.

Woo SL, Newton PO, MacKenna DA, Lyon RM: A comparative evaluation of the mechanical properties of the rabbit medial collateral and anterior cruciate ligaments. *J Biomech* 1992;25:377–386.

Woo SL, Ohland KJ, Weiss JA: Aging and sex-related changes in the biomechanical properties of the rabbit medial collateral ligament. *Mech Ageing Dev* 1990;56:129–142.

Woo SL, Orlando CA, Camp JF, Akeson WH: Effects of postmortem storage by freezing on ligament tensile behavior. *J Biomech* 1986;19: 399–404.

Healing and Reconstruction of Ligaments

Anderson DR, Weiss JA, Takai S, Ohland KJ, Woo SL: Healing of the medial collateral ligament following a triad injury: A biomechanical and histological study of the knee in rabbits. *J Orthop Res* 1992;10: 485–495.

Andriacchi TP, Mikosz RP, Hampton SJ, Galante JO: Model studies of the stiffness characteristics of the human knee joint. *J Biomech* 1983; 16:23–29.

Arnoczky SP, Warren RF, Ashlock MA: Replacement of the anterior cruciate ligament using a patellar tendon allograft: An experimental study. *J Bone Joint Surg* 1986;68A:376–385.

Ballock RT, Woo SL, Lyon RM, Hollis JM, Akeson WH: Use of patellar tendon autograft for anterior cruciate ligament reconstruction in the rabbit: A long-term histologic and biomechanical study. *J Orthop Res* 1989;7:474–485.

Batten ML, Hansen JC, Dahners LE: Influence of dosage and timing of application of platelet-derived growth factor on early healing of the rat medial collateral ligament. *J Orthop Res* 1996;14:736–741.

Beynnon BD, Pope MH, Fleming BD, et al: An in-vivo study of the ACL strain biomechanics in the normal knee. *Trans Orthop Res Soc* 1989;14:324.

Beynnon BD, Stankewich CJ, Fleming BC, Pope MH, Johnson RJ: The development and initial testing of a new sensor to simultaneously measure strain and pressure in tendons and ligaments, in *Transactions of the Combined Meeting of the Orthopaedic Research Societies of USA, Japan, and Canada*. Banff, Alberta, Canada, University of Calgary Printing Services, 1991, p 104.

Biden E, O'Connor JJ: Experimental methods used to evaluate knee ligament function, in Daniel DM, Akeson WH, O'Connor JJ (eds): *Knee Ligaments: Structure, Function, Injury, and Repair*. New York, NY, Raven Press, 1990, pp 135–151.

Blankevoort L, Huiskes R: Ligament-bone interaction in a three-dimensional model of the knee. *J Biomech Eng* 1991;113:263–269.

Blankevoort L, Huiskes R: A mechanism for rotation restraints in the knee joint. *J Orthop Res* 1996;14:676–679.

Bray RC, Rangayyan RM, Frank CB: Normal and healing ligament vascularity: A quantitative histological assessment in the adult rabbit medial collateral ligament. *J Anat* 1996;188:87–95.

Bray RC, Shrive NG, Frank CB, Chimich DD: The early effects of joint immobilization on medial collateral ligament healing in an ACL-deficient knee: A gross anatomic and biomechanical investigation in the adult rabbit model. *J Orthop Res* 1992;10:157–166.

Butler DL: Anterior cruciate ligament: Its normal response and replacement. *J Orthop Res* 1989;7:910–921.

Butler DL, Sheh MY, Stouffer DC, Samaranayake VA, Levy MS: Surface strain variation in human patellar tendon and knee cruciate ligaments. *J Biomech Eng* 1990;112:38–45.

Bylski-Austrow DI, Grood ES, Hefzy MS, Holden JP, Butler DL: Anterior cruciate ligament replacements: A mechanical study of femoral attachment location, flexion angle at tensioning, and initial tension. *J Orthop Res* 1990;8:522–531.

Clancy WG Jr, Narechania RG, Rosenberg TD, Gmeiner JG, Wisnefske DD, Lange TA: Anterior and posterior cruciate ligament reconstruction in rhesus monkeys. *J Bone Joint Surg* 1981;63A:1270–1284.

Derscheid GL, Garrick JG: Medial collateral ligament injuries in football: Nonoperative management of grade I and grade II sprains. *Am J Sports Med* 1981;9:365–368.

Feagin JA Jr, Curl WW: Isolated tear of the anterior cruciate ligament: 5-year follow-up study. *Am J Sports Med* 1976;4:95–100.

Fleming BC, Beynonn BD, Nichols CE, Johnson RJ, Pope MH: An in vivo comparison of anterior tibial translation and strain in the anteromedial band of the anterior cruciate ligament. *J Biomech* 1993;26:51–58.

France EP, Paulos LE, Rosenberg TD, et al: The biomechanics of anterior cruciate allografts, in Friedman MJ, Ferkel RD (eds): *Prosthetic Ligament Reconstruction of the Knee*. Philadelphia, PA, WB Saunders, 1988, pp 180–185.

Frank C, Woo SL, Amiel D, Harwood F, Gomez M, Akeson W: Medial collateral ligament healing: A multidisciplinary assessment in rabbits. *Am J Sports Med* 1983;11:379–389.

Frank CB: Ligament healing: Current knowledge and clinical applications. *J Am Acad Orthop Surg* 1996;4:74–83.

Frank CB, Jackson DW: The science of reconstruction of the anterior cruciate ligament. *J Bone Joint Surg* 1997;79A:1556–1576.

Fujie H, Mabuchi K, Woo SL, Livesay GA, Arai S, Tsukamoto Y: The use of robotics technology to study human joint kinematics: A new methodology. *J Biomech Eng* 1993;115:211–217.

Fujie H, Livesay GA, Woo SL, Kashiwaguchi S, Blomstrom G: The use of a universal force-moment sensor to determine in-situ forces in ligaments: A new methodology. *J Biomech Eng* 1995;117:1–7.

Gibbons MJ, Butler DL, Grood ES, Bylski-Austrow DI, Levy MS, Noyes FR: Effects of gamma irradiation on the initial mechanical and material properties of goat bone-patellar tendon-bone allografts. *J Orthop Res* 1991;9:209–218.

Goodfellow J, O'Connor J: The mechanics of the knee and prosthesis design. *J Bone Joint Surg* 1978;60B:358–369.

Grood ES, Hefzy MS, Lindenfield TN: Factors affecting the region of most isometric femoral attachments: Part I: The posterior cruciate ligament. *Am J Sports Med* 1989;17:197–207.

Haut RC, Powlison AC: The effects of test environment and cyclic stretching on the failure properties of human patellar tendons. *J Orthop Res* 1990;8:532–540.

Hefzy MS, Grood ES: Sensitivity of insertion locations on length patterns of anterior cruciate ligament fibers. *J Biomech Eng* 1986;108: 73–82.

Hefzy MS, Grood ES, Noyes FR: Factors affecting the region of most isometric femoral attachments: Part II. The anterior cruciate ligament. *Am J Sports Med* 1989;17:208–216.

Hildebrand KA, Woo SL, Smith DW, et al: The effects of platelet-derived growth factor-BB on healing of the rabbit medial collateral ligament: An in-vivo study. *Am J Sports Med* 1998;26:549–554.

Holden DL, Eggert AW, Butler JE: The nonoperative treatment of grade I and II medial collateral ligament injuries to the knee. *Am J Sports Med* 1983:11:340–344.

Holden JP, Grood ES, Butler DL, et al: Biomechanics of fascia lata ligament replacements: Early postoperative changes in the goat. *J Orthop Res* 1988:6:639–647.

Horibe S, Shino K, Nagano J, Nakamura H, Tanaka M, Ono K: Replacing the medial collateral ligament with an allogenic tendon graft: An experimental canine study. *J Bone Joint Surg* 1990:72B:1044–1049.

Howell SM, Taylor MA: Failure of reconstruction of the anterior cruciate ligament due to impingement by the intercondylar roof. *J Bone Joint Surg* 1993:75A:1044–1055.

Indelicato PA: Non-operative treatment of complete tears of the medial collateral ligament of the knee. *J Bone Joint Surg* 1983;65A: 323–329.

Inoue M, McGurk-Burleson E, Hollis JM, Woo SL: Treatment of the medial collateral ligament injury: I. The importance of anterior cruciate ligament on the varus-valgus knee laxity. *Am J Sports Med* 1987;15:15–21.

Ishibashi Y, Rudy TW, Livesay GA, Stone JD, Fu FH, Woo S L: The effect of anterior cruciate ligament graft fixation site at the tibia on knee stability: Evaluation using a robotic testing system. *Arthroscopy* 1997;13:177–182.

Jackson DW, Arnoczky SP, Woo SLY, Frank CB, Simon TM (eds): The *Anterior Cruciate Ligament: Current and Future Concepts*. New York, NY, Raven Press, 1993.

Jackson DW, Grood ES, Arnoczky SP, Butler DL, Simon TM: Freeze dried anterior cruciate ligament allografts: Preliminary studies in a goat model. *Am J Sports Med* 1987;15:295–303.

Jackson DW, Grood ES, Cohn BT, Arnoczky SP, Simon TM, Cummings JF: The effects of in situ freezing on the anterior cruciate ligament: An experimental study in goats. *J Bone Joint Surg* 1991;73A:201–213.

Johnson DL, Fu FH: Anterior cruciate ligament reconstruction: Why do failures occur?, in Jackson DW (ed): *Instructional Course Lectures 40*. Rosemont, IL, American Academy of Orthopaedic Surgeons, 1995, pp 391–406.

Johnson RJ, Beynnon BD, Nichols CE, Renstrom PA: The treatment of injuries of the anterior cruciate ligament. *J Bone Joint Surg* 1992;74A: 140–151.

Livesay GA, Rudy TW, Woo SL, et al: Evaluation of the effect of joint constraints on the in situ force distribution in the anterior cruciate ligament. *J Orthop Res* 1997;15:278–84.

Lundberg M, Messner K: Long-term prognosis of isolated partial medial collateral ligament ruptures: A ten-year clinical and radiographic evaluation of a prospectively observed group of patients. *Am J Sports Med* 1996;24:160–163.

Mott HW: Semitendinosus anatomic reconstruction for cruciate ligament insufficiency. *Clin Orthop* 1983;172:90–92.

Ng GY, Oakes BW, Deacon OW, McLean ID, Lampard D: Biomechanics of patellar tendon autograft for reconstruction of the anterior cruciate ligament in the goat: Three-year study. *J Orthop Res* 1995;13: 602–608.

Noyes FR, Grood ES: The strength of the anterior cruciate ligament in humans and rhesus monkeys: Age-related and species-related changes. *J Bone Joint Surg* 1976;58A:1074–1082.

O'Brien SJ, Warren RF, Pavlov H, Panariello R, Wickiewicz TL: Reconstruction of the chronically insufficient anterior cruciate ligament with the central third of the patellar ligament. *J Bone Joint Surg* 1991; 73A:278–286.

O'Donoghue DH, Frank GR, Jeter GL, Johnson W, Zeiders JW, Kenyon R: Repair and reconstruction of the anterior cruciate ligament in dogs: Factors influencing long-term results. *J Bone Joint Surg* 1971; 53A:710–718.

Odensten M, Gillquist J: Functional anatomy of the anterior cruciate ligament and a rationale for reconstruction. *J Bone Joint Surg* 1985; 67A:257–262.

Ohno K, Pomaybo AS, Schmidt CC, Levine RE, Ohland KJ, Woo SL: Healing of the medial collateral ligament after a combined medial collateral and anterior cruciate ligament injury and reconstruction of the anterior cruciate ligament: Comparison of repair and nonrepair of medial collateral ligament tears in rabbits. *J Orthop Res* 1995; 13:442–449.

Penner DA, Daniel DM, Wood P, Mishra D: An in vitro study of anterior cruciate ligament graft placement and isometry. *Am J Sports Med* 1988;16:238–243.

Pruitt DL, Aoki M, Maske PR: Effect of suture knot location on tensile strength after flexor tendon repair. *J Hand Surg* 1996;21A:969–973.

Roberts TS, Drez D Jr, McCarthy W, Paine R: Anterior cruciate ligament reconstruction using freeze-dried, ethylene oxide-sterilized, bone-patellar tendon-bone allografts: Two year results in thirty-six patients. *Am J Sports Med* 1991;19:35–41.

Sabiston P, Frank C, Lam T, Shrive N: Transplantation of the rabbit medial collateral ligament: II. Biomechanical evaluation of frozen/thawed allografts. *J Orthop Res* 1990;8:46–56.

Sakane M, Fox RJ, Woo SL, Livesay GA, Li G, Fu FH: In situ forces in the anterior cruciate ligament and its bundles in response to anterior tibial loads. *J Orthop Res* 1997;15:285–293.

Shelbourne KD, Gray T: Anterior cruciate ligament reconstruction with autogenous patellar tendon graft followed by accelerated rehabilitation: A two- to nine-year follow-up. *Am J Sports Med* 1997;25:786–795.

Shino K, Inoue M, Horibe S, Hamada M, Ono K: Reconstruction of the anterior cruciate ligament using allogeneic tendon: Long-term follow-up. *Am J Sports Med* 1990;18:457–465.

Thomas ED, Gresham RB: Comparative tensile strength study of fresh, frozen, and freeze-dried human fascia lata. *Surg Forum* 1963;14:442–443.

Vasseur PB, Rodrigo JJ, Stevenson S, Clark G, Sharkey N: Replacement of the anterior cruciate ligament with a bone-ligament-bone anterior cruciate ligament allograft in dogs. *Clin Orthop* 1987;219:268–277.

Webster DA, Werner FW: Mechanical and functional properties of implanted freeze-dried flexor tendons. *Clin Orthop* 1983;180:301–309.

Weiss JA, Woo SL, Ohland KJ, Horibe S, Newton PO: Evaluation of a new injury model to study medial collateral ligament healing: Primary repair versus nonoperative treatment. *J Orthop Res* 1991;9:516–528.

Woo SL, Inoue M, McGurk-Burleson E, Gomez MA: Treatment of the medial collateral ligament injury: II. Structure and function of canine knees in response to differing treatment regimens. *Am J Sports Med* 1987;15:22–29.

Woo SL, Young EP, Ohland KJ, Marcin JP, Horibe S, Lin HC: The effects of transection of the anterior cruciate ligament on healing of the medial collateral ligament: A biomechanical study of the knee in dogs. *J Bone Joint Surg* 1990;72A:382–392.

Woo SL, Buckwalter JA: Ligament and tendon autografts and allografts, in Friedlaender GE, Goldberg VM (eds): *Bone and Cartilage Allografts: Biology and Clinical Applications.* Park Ridge, IL, American Academy Orthopaedic Surgeons, 1991, pp 103–121.

Woo SL, Smith DW, Hildebrand KA, Zeminski JA, Johnson LA: Engineering the healing of the rabbit medial collateral ligament. *Med Biol Eng Comput* 1998;36:359–364.

Yasuda K, Tomiyama Y, Ohkoshi Y, et al: Arthroscopic observations of autogeneic quadriceps and patellar tendon grafts after anterior cruciate ligament reconstruction of the knee. *Clin Orthop* 1989;246:217–224.

Yasuda K, Tsujino J, Tanabe Y, Kaneda K: Effects of initial graft tension on clinical outcome after anterior cruciate ligament reconstruction: Autogenous doubled hamstring tendons connected in series with polyester tapes. *Am J Sports Med* 1997;25:99–106.

Yoshiya S, Andrish JT, Manley MT, Bauer TW: Graft tension in anterior cruciate ligament reconstruction: An in vivo study in dogs. *Am J Sports Med* 1987;15:464–470.

Chapter Outline

Chapter 25

Peripheral Nerve Physiology, Anatomy, and Pathology

Sue C. Bodine, PhD

Richard L. Lieber, PhD

This chapter at a glance

This chapter discusses the physiology, anatomy, and pathology of peripheral nerves; specifically, neurons and signal generation, sensory and motor systems, and electrodiagnosis.

One or more of the authors or the department with which they are affiliated has received something of value from a commercial or other party related directly or indirectly to the subject of this chapter.

Neurons and Signal Generation

The human brain is a complex biologic structure composed of approximately 10^{11} nerve cells (neurons). Although neurons may be classified into as many as 10,000 different types, they share many common features, including the unique ability to communicate precisely, rapidly, and over long distances with one another and with target tissues, such as muscles.

Nerve Cells—General Description

A typical neuron has 4 morphologically defined regions (Fig. 1, *A*): the cell body, dendrites, axon, and presynaptic terminal. The cell body contains the nucleus and the organelles for making RNA and proteins and is the metabolic center of the neuron although it typically contains less than 10% of the neuron's total volume. The remaining neuron volume consists of the dendrites and the axon. The dendrites are thin processes that branch off the cell body and serve as the main apparatus for receiving synaptic input from other nerve cells.

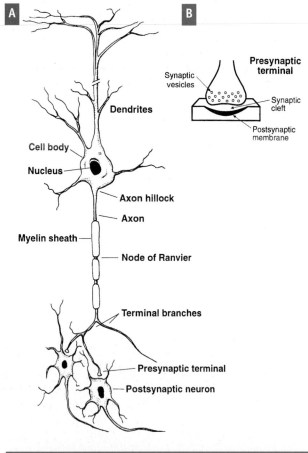

Figure 1

A, Main features of a typical vertebrate neuron. **B,** Presynaptic terminal-postsynaptic receptor.

A cell body gives rise to only 1 axon, which is the main conducting unit of the neuron and is capable of accurately conveying information over long distances by propagating electrical signals known as action potentials. The axon arises from a specialized region of the cell body, the axon hillock, from which the all-or-none action potential is initiated once a critical threshold has been reached. The axon and its terminal branches require proteins to maintain their structural integrity, to support action potential propagation, and to effect the release of neurotransmitters; however, the axon hillock and axon cannot make proteins. To meet the requirements of the neuron, proteins are synthesized in the cell body, assembled into macromolecules, and transported down the axon via axoplasmic transport. The part of the axon nearest its target organ or termination site is divided into fine branches that have specialized endings called presynaptic terminals. These terminals are responsible for transmitting information from the neuron to the dendrites or cell body of another neuron (Fig. 1, *A*) or a postsynaptic receptor such as the neuromuscular junction (Fig. 1, *B*).

Glial Cells and Myelin Formation

Nerve cell bodies and axons are surrounded by glial cells, which are divided into microglia and macroglia. Microglia arise from macrophages and are phagocytes that are mobilized after injury, infection, or disease. The 3 primary types of macroglia are oligodendrocytes, Schwann cells, and astrocytes (Fig. 2).

Oligodendrocytes and Schwann cells insulate the axons by forming a myelin sheath. Myelin is composed of 70% lipid and 30% protein, with a high concentration of cholesterol and phospholipid. Myelinated axons conduct electrical impulses at faster speeds and at higher frequencies with less energy consumption than nonmyelinated axons. Oligodendrocytes and Schwann cells form the sheath by wrapping their membranous processes concentrically around the axon in a tight spiral. Oligodendrocytes occur only in the central nervous system (CNS), and a single cell can myelinate several different axons (on average 15). Schwann cells occur in the peripheral nervous system, and each cell myelinates a region of 1 axon.

A single peripheral axon can be myelinated by as many as 500 Schwann cells. The genes in Schwann cells that code for myelin are turned on by the presence of an axon. Schwann cells line up along the axon at intervals of 0.1 to 1.0 mm. These intervals eventually will become nodes of Ranvier, which are specialized zones for action potential initiation. The external cell membrane of the Schwann cell surrounds the axon and forms a double membrane structure that then elongates and spirals around the axon in concentric layers. Loss of the myelin sheath, called demyelination, can disrupt the conduction of action potentials along axons.

Astrocytes, the most common glial cells, are found only in

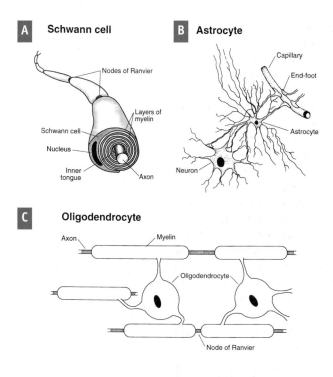

A Schwann cell

Nodes of Ranvier

Layers of myelin

Schwann cell

Nucleus

Inner tongue

Axon

B Astrocyte

Capillary

End-foot

Astrocyte

Neuron

C Oligodendrocyte

Axon

Myelin

Oligodendrocyte

Node of Ranvier

Figure 2

The principal types of glial cells. **A,** Schwann cells line up along the length of peripheral nervous system axons at regular intervals, each forming a segment of myelin sheath about 1 mm long. **B,** Astrocytes are star-shaped and have end feet that contact both capillaries and neurons. **C,** In white matter, oligodendrocytes participate in myelination of axons; a single oligodendrocyte can form myelin around several different axons. In gray matter, they surround the cell bodies of neurons.

the CNS and are thought to serve many functions. They serve as supporting structures, providing firmness and structure to the brain. Some astrocytes have processes that contact blood capillaries and neurons, thus leading to the speculation that they serve a nutritive function (Fig. 2, *B*). Some fulfill a scavenger role, removing neuronal debris after injury. Astrocytes also have been shown to take up excess K^+ in the extracellular space and remove neurotransmitters from the synaptic cleft after synaptic transmission. Astrocytes also turn on the expression of myelin in oligodendrocytes.

Axoplasmic Transport

The neuron is a polarized cell; its cell body and presynaptic terminals often are separated by considerable distances. The proteins required to maintain the structural integrity of the axon, to support action potential propagation, and to enable neurotransmitter release at the presynaptic terminals are produced only in the cell body. Therefore, special intracellular transport systems have been developed to bring molecules synthesized in the cell body to the axon and nerve terminals and to return degradation products from the axon and terminals to the cell body for molecular reprocessing. The importance of these transport systems is

demonstrated by the fact that severance of the axon from the cell body results in degeneration of the distal axon segment. Constituents move within the axon in 3 ways: slow and fast anterograde transport and fast retrograde transport.

Data from isotope labeling experiments reveal that motor and sensory nerves have similar transport rates. The transport rate is sensitive to temperature, slowing down with decreasing temperature and stopping at a temperature of 11°C.

Recent evidence suggests that the mechanisms for slow and fast anterograde transport are the same. Axoplasmic transport has been shown to depend on adenosine triphosphate (ATP) derived primarily from oxidative metabolism. Axon transport is blocked within 10 to 30 minutes after a nerve is made anoxic by switching to a nitrogen atmosphere. The rate of transport recovers when the nerve is reoxygenated after 1.5 hours of anoxia. If, however, a nerve is kept anoxic for 2 to 5 hours, transport recovers very slowly after reoxygenation, although action potential transmission recovers immediately. After 2 hours of tourniquet-induced ischemia, full recovery of axoplasmic transport in the feline sciatic nerve was found to take over 24 hours. Axoplasmic transport also depends on intraneural calcium concentrations. Normally, the level of free Ca^{2+} in the nerve is maintained at 0.1 µM, with the total amount of Ca^{2+} present in the nerve being 0.4 µM. Most of the calcium is sequestered in the mitochondria and smooth endoplasmic reticulum and bound to the calcium-binding protein, calmodulin. In addition to ATP and calcium, axoplasmic transport depends on microtubules. Chemicals that cause the microtubules to disassemble block axon transport.

The model hypothesized for fast and slow transport requires ATP, Ca^{2+}-Mg^{2+} adenosine triphosphatase (ATPase), microtubules, carrier proteins, and a mechanism to control free calcium concentrations in the axoplasm (Fig. 3). An organelle or protein binds to a carrier protein that binds to the microtubule, which has side arms or associated proteins that use ATP via a Ca^{2+}-Mg^{2+} ATPase to cycle and move the carrier along the microtubule. Different carrier proteins are thought to be used in anterograde and retrograde transport. The protein kinesin has been isolated and shown to be important in anterograde transport. The microtubule-associated proteins may also control the direction of transport.

The transport filament model has been used to describe both slow and fast transport. Slow-transported proteins are loosely attached to the carrier and are dropped off early, that is, closer to the cell body, whereas fast-transported proteins remain bound to the carrier all the way to the terminal. Differences in drop-off rates produce what are measured experimentally as slow, intermediate, and fast transport rates.

Fast axon transport also occurs from nerve terminals to the cell body, that is, in the retrograde direction. Retrograde transport is important in the returning of materials, such as empty neurotransmitter vesicles, from the terminals to the cell body either for degradation or for restoration and reuse

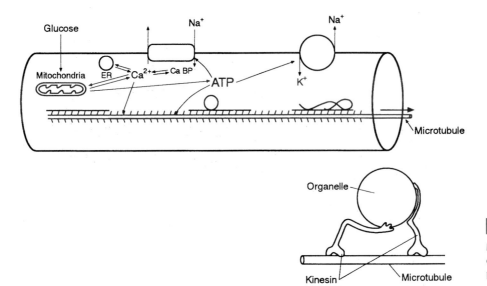

Figure 3

Model for axonal transport. Ca BP = calcium binding protein; ER = endoplasmic reticulum.

(Fig. 4). The materials are packaged in large membrane-bound organelles that are part of the lysosomal system. The rate of retrograde transport is approximately one half to two thirds that of fast anterograde transport.

In addition to its important scavenger function, the movement of molecules from the terminals to the cell body can also be clinically important. For example, nerve growth factors released from the target organ are picked up by the growing axon and transported to the cell body, thereby influencing the direction of growth of regenerating axons after injury and nourishing the neuron. In addition, chromatolysis is initiated in the cell body when the axon is disrupted. This response may be induced by some injury signal that is given off by the target organ, picked up by the damaged axon, and transported to the cell body. Retrograde transport can also have adverse effects. For example, several viruses, including herpes simplex, rabies, polio, and tetanus toxin, are transported from nerve terminals to the cell body via retrograde transport.

Investigators have used the retrograde transport mechanism to trace axonal projections and label cell bodies. Horseradish peroxidase and various fluorescent dyes injected into a target organ or directly into the nerve are transported to the cell body in this manner, allowing the investigator to trace the axonal projection or identify the location of the cell bodies in the spinal cord or spinal ganglion (Fig. 5).

Reductions in axonal transport have been observed in diseases such as diabetes and amyotrophic lateral sclerosis, and recent evidence suggests that abnormal rapid axonal transport may be involved in other peripheral neuropathies. It has not been determined, however, whether the abnormalities in axonal transport caused the associated nerve damage or whether they merely reflected structural damage to the axon from other causes. Secondary failure of axonal transport could determine the course of the neuropathy by inducing axonal atrophy, impaired nerve con-

duction, degeneration of nerve terminals, failure of synaptic transmission, and loss of trophic interactions.

Resting Membrane Potential and the Action Potential

The flow of information within and between neurons is conveyed by electrical and chemical signals. Nerve cells are able to process information because of the special properties of the neuronal cell membrane. Like other cell membranes, the neuronal cell membrane is composed of a lipid bilayer into which various membrane proteins are incorporated. The lipids within the membrane are hydrophobic; that is, they are immiscible with water. In contrast, the ions in the extracellular and intracellular space are hydrophilic; that is, they attract water. Ions are able to pass through the membrane by way of ion channels composed of proteins present in the membrane. These protein channels control the flux of ions across the membrane.

The Resting Membrane Potential

In all neurons there is an electrical potential difference between the 2 sides of the cell membrane, which can be measured by inserting an electrode into the cell and measuring the potential difference between the intracellular electrode and a reference electrode in the extracellular fluid (Fig. 6). By convention the reference electrode is set at 0 volts. In neurons at a resting state there is a negative potential within the cell; the inside of the cell is negative compared to the external environment. The potential difference of a neuron at rest is called the resting potential and usually lies between -50 and -80 mV.

The resting potential results from an unequal distribution of monovalent ions on either side of the cell membrane. The 4 most abundant ions on either side of the membrane are Na^+, K^+, Cl^-, and organic anions (often referred to as A^-).

Early experiments that described the electrical excitability of nerve cells were performed on the giant squid axon, which is a single axon with a very large (1 mm) diameter that enables the placement of macroelectrodes inside it. The distribution of ions inside and outside the membrane of the giant squid axon is given in Table 1. Na$^+$ and Cl$^-$ are concentrated on the outside of the cell, and K$^+$ and A$^-$ are concentrated inside the cell.

A lipid bilayer is negligibly permeable to charged ions; however, in biologic membranes, ion channels or pores in the lipid bilayer increase the permeability of the membrane to ions. Ion channels can have selective permeabilities based on the size, charge, or hydration of the specific ion. In 1902, it was hypothesized that the resting membrane

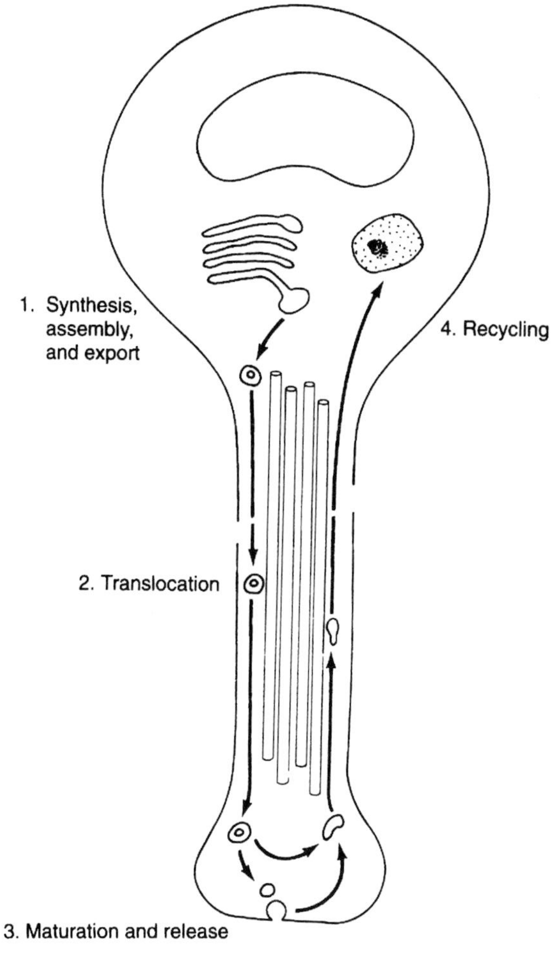

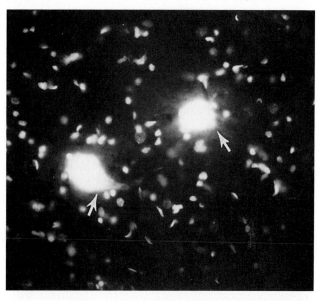

Figure 5

Labeled soleus motoneuron cell bodies in the ventral horn of the rat spinal cord. Motoneurons were labeled by injecting a fluorescent dye (fast blue) in the soleus muscles. The dye is taken up at the neuromuscular junction and transported to the cell body via retrograde axonal transport.

1. Synthesis, assembly, and export

2. Translocation

3. Maturation and release

4. Recycling

Figure 4

Synaptic vesicles and other membranous organelles involved in synaptic transmission at the nerve terminal are returned to the cell body for recycling after they are used at the synapse. 1. Proteins and lipids are synthesized and incorporated into membranes within the endoplasmic reticulum and Golgi apparatus in the neuron's cell body. 2. Organelles are then assembled from these components and exported from the cell body into the axon, where they are rapidly moved toward terminals by fast axonal transport. 3. Synaptic vesicles and their precursors reach the neuron's terminals, where they participate in the release of transmitter substances by exocytosis. At random, a small proportion of the membrane becomes degraded, and this material is returned to the cell body by fast retrograde axonal transport. 4. The degraded membrane is partly recycled, its residue is progressively accumulated in large, end-stage lysosomes that are characteristic of neuronal cell bodies. (Reproduced with permission from Kandel ER, Schwartz JH, Jessel TM: *Principles of Neural Science*, ed 3. Norwalk, CT, Appleton & Lange, 1991, p 57.)

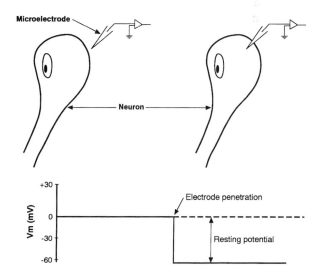

Figure 6

Measurement of the potential across a cell membrane. When a microelectrode connected to an electronic amplifier is placed outside the cell in the extracellular fluid, a potential of zero is measured. When the microelectrode is inserted through the cell membrane into the neuron, a negative potential difference is measured.

Table 1

Distribution of Major Ions in Giant Squid Axon

Ion	Cytoplasm mM	Extracellular mM	Nernst Potential* mV
K+	400	20	−75
Na+	50	440	+55
Cl−	52	560	−60
Organic Anion−	385	—	—

* The membrane potential at which there is no net flux of an ion across the cell membrane

potential was based on the selective permeability of the membrane to potassium. In the 1940s this theory was shown to be acceptable by comparing the actual resting potential measured using intracellular electrodes with that predicted by the Nernst equation, assuming selective permeability to potassium.

The Nernst equation is used to calculate the membrane potential at which the net flux of a specific ion across the membrane is zero. An ion's flux across the membrane depends on its concentration and electrical gradients. If the distribution of ions across a membrane equals those listed in Table 1 and the membrane is permeable only to K+, the K+ ions will diffuse down their concentration gradient from inside to outside the cell. As K+ ions move from inside to outside, an excess of positive ions accumulates on the outside of the membrane, creating a potential difference across the membrane. This potential difference tends to repel the positively charged ions, moving them from outside to inside the cell. The potential difference at which the flow of K+ ions from outside to inside the cell equals the flow from inside to outside is called the equilibrium potential and can be calculated using the Nernst equation:

$$E = \frac{RT}{FZ} \ln \frac{[A]_i}{[A]_o}$$

where E is the membrane potential, R is the universal gas constant (8.303), T is the temperature in absolute degrees Kelvin (0°C = 273°K), F is the Faraday constant, Z is the ion valence, $[A]_o$ represents the concentration of ion A outside the membrane, and $[A]_i$ represents the concentration of ion A inside the membrane.

At 25°C, RT/FZ is 26 mV and the equilibrium potential of K+ equals -75 mV. If a neuron was permeable only to K+, the resting membrane potential would equal the equilibrium potential for K+. The resting membrane potential of the giant squid axon is -68 mV; therefore, the membrane must be permeable to more than a single ion. Measurements of the resting membrane potential with intracellular elec-

trodes and radioactive tracers have shown that nerve cells at rest are permeable to Na+, Cl−, and K+.

Given that the equilibrium potentials of Na+ and K+ are -55 mV and -75 mV, respectively, the inside of the neuron would accumulate Na+ and lose K+ at a resting membrane potential of -68 mV. If this process actually occurred, the concentration gradients and the electrical potential would go to 0 and the neuron would die. The neuron maintains its concentration gradients and resting membrane potential by the use of the sodium-potassium pump.

The sodium-potassium pump is an integral membrane protein that uses energy, in the form of ATP, to pump 3 Na+ out of the neuron for every 2 K+ it brings into the neuron (Fig. 7). When the neuron is at rest, the active fluxes (driven by the pump) and the passive fluxes (driven by diffusion) are balanced so that the net flux of Na+ and K+ is zero. The resting membrane potential is actually a steady-state potential, because energy must be used to maintain ionic gradients across the membrane.

Passive Membrane Properties

Neurons process and transmit information using electrical signals produced by temporary changes in the current flow into and out of the neuron. Electrical signals come in 2 forms: graded potentials and action potentials.

A graded potential is a hyperpolarizing or depolarizing local change in a neuron's membrane potential (Fig. 8). In graded potentials, the amplitude of the voltage change is variable and directly related to the intensity of the external signal. Graded potentials can be one of 3 types: (1) Receptor (or generator) potentials are created in specialized sensory cells called receptors; for example, mechanoreceptors and pain receptors. (2) Pacemaker potentials are not found in mammalian nerve cells, but are found in the heart and smooth muscle. These are spontaneous changes in a cell's own membrane potential caused by intrinsic properties of the cell rather than by external stimuli. (3) Synaptic potentials are changes evoked at a synapse as a result of ionic currents through the membrane of the postsynaptic cell.

The conductance of graded potentials depends on the passive properties of the cell membrane: the membrane resistance R_m, internal resistance R_i, and capacitance C_m of the resting membrane. Because cell membranes act as bar-

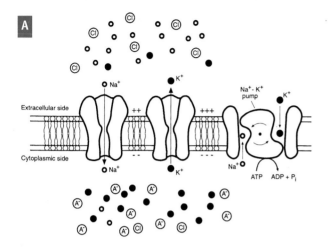

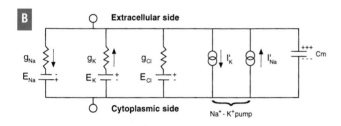

Figure 7

Permeabilities and driving forces of Na^+, K^+, and Cl^-. **A,** When the cell is at rest, the passive fluxes of Na^+ and K^+ into and out of the cell are balanced by the energy-dependent sodium-potassium pump. **B,** The electrical equivalent circuit of a neuron at rest includes the most abundant types of ion channels in parallel. Under steady state conditions, the currents resulting from passive diffusion of Na and K are balanced by active Na and K fluxes (I'_{Na} and I'_K) driven by the sodium-potassium pump.

riers to certain ions, they are able to store charges and can be considered to be capacitors. However, cell membranes are not perfect capacitors because some ions can pass through, and they often are called leaky capacitors because pores make their resistance finite. (Refer to the glossary for definitions of basic electrical terms.)

When current I is injected into a neuron, the voltage V does not rise instantaneously, but rises at an exponential rate. The amplitude of the steady-state voltage is proportional to the intensity of the stimulus because at steady state, V = IR (Ohm's law; R = resistance). The change in voltage is not instantaneous because the membrane has both resistance and capacitance. Although current flows instantaneously through a resistor, it takes time to charge or discharge a capacitor. Once the capacitor has reached a steady state, current can flow through the membrane's resistance. The amount of time it takes to reach 66% of the peak voltage is defined as the time constant t, and is determined by the membrane's resistance and capacitance: t = RC. The time constant increases with the time to reach the steady state voltage (Fig. 9). The time constant can control the rate at which a neuron fires or the speed at which an action potential is propagated down the axon.

As a graded potential travels down the axon it decreases in amplitude (Fig. 10). Within an axon there are 2 types of resistance: the internal resistance R_i, which runs longitudinally down the axon, and the transverse resistance R_m, which is equivalent to the membrane resistance (Fig. 10). When current is injected, the amount of current will be greatest at the point of injection, and the current will go down the path of least resistance. Each time current flows across the membrane, less current flows from the point of injection and the amplitude of the voltage decreases because of the decrease in current. The distance at which voltage has decreased to 37% of its maximum is defined as lambda λ or the length constant. The length constant is dependent on both R_i and R_m: $\lambda = R_m/R_i$. If the membrane

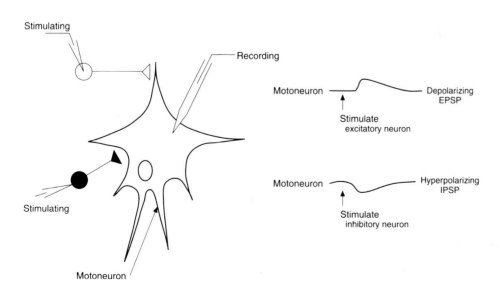

Figure 8

Graded potentials. Stimulation of an excitatory neuron that synapses onto a motoneuron produces a depolarizing synaptic potential in the cell body (excitatory postsynaptic potential, EPSP). Stimulation of an inhibitory neuron that synapses onto a motoneuron produces a hyperpolarizing synaptic potential in the cell (inhibitory postsynaptic potential, IPSP).

resistance is high, the length constant will be high, more current will flow down the axon, and the potential will decay at a slower rate. If the internal resistance is greater than the membrane resistance, the length constant will be low and current will flow out of the cell, causing the graded potential to decay rapidly.

The Action Potential

The action potential transmits coded messages rapidly and over long distances to other neurons or effector organs such as muscle. Graded potentials are good only for communication over short distances within a neuron because they decay over time and distance. An action potential can be described as a brief (~ 1 ms) explosive change in the mem-

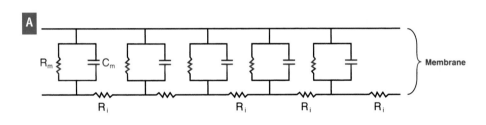

Figure 9

Membrane time constant. **A,** Current-voltage relationship for a cell membrane consisting of resistive as well as capacitive elements. **B,** Time course of the change of membrane potential in response to a step of current. Line c shows the actual response of the membrane potential (ΔVm) to a rectangular current pulse; line a shows the response of a membrane containing only resistive elements; and line b the response of a membrane containing only capacitive elements. The membrane potential approaches a maximum exponentially with a time constant equal to the membrane resistance times capacitance. **C,** The time courses of the total membrane current (I_m), the ionic current (I_i), and the capacitive current (I_c).

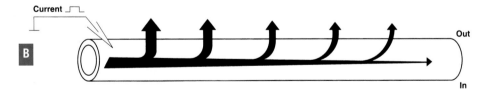

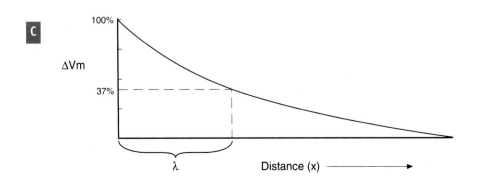

Figure 10

Length constant and passive current flow. **A,** Equivalent circuit of a hypothetical nerve fiber consisting of membrane resistance (R_m) and internal resistance (R_i). **B,** Current injected into a neuronal process by a microelectrode follows the path of least resistance. Current loss results when current flows out of the membrane through R_m instead of down the axon through R_i. **C,** The change in membrane potential (ΔVm) decays exponentially with distance along the length of the axon or dendrite.

brane potential from its normal resting potential to a very positive value. Action potentials are self-regenerating potentials that occur spontaneously when the membrane is depolarized beyond a critical membrane potential called threshold (Fig. 11, *A*). The peak amplitude of the action potential is fixed and independent of the stimulus intensity above threshold. Cells that can produce action potentials are referred to as excitable cells.

Stimuli that are less than threshold create graded potentials. Graded potentials are proportional to the intensity of the stimulus, and different potentials can summate. An action potential is initiated when the graded potentials depolarize the membrane to the threshold potential. At the threshold potential, the neuron membrane resistance begins to change, and the membrane no longer obeys Ohm's law V = IR. The membrane resistance is determined by the number of open channels. At rest the number of open channels remains constant; however, depolarization causes Na^+ membrane ion channels to actively open, allowing Na^+ to flow across the membrane into the cell.

The rising phase of the action potential results from an increase in the permeability (or conductance g) of the membrane to Na^+. The Na^+ conductance increases as a result of structural changes in gated ion channels selective to Na^+. Gated ion channels open or close as a result of structural changes that occur in response to various stimuli. The 3 major signals that can gate ion channels are voltage (voltage-gated channels), chemical transmitters (transmitter-gated channels), and pressure or stretch (mechanically-gated channels) (Fig. 12). Nongated channels are always open and are responsible for the resting membrane poten-

tial. The Na^+ channels responsible for the action potential are voltage-gated. Membrane depolarization causes a conformational change that opens the channels, allowing Na+ to diffuse into the cell according to its electrochemical gradient (Fig. 13).

Action potentials are propagated down the axon by a combination of passive current flow and active membrane changes. For example, once the membrane along any point of the axon has been depolarized beyond threshold, an action potential is generated in that region in response to the opening of voltage-gated Na^+ channels. This local depolarization then spreads passively along the axon, causing the adjacent region of the membrane to reach threshold for generating an action potential (Fig. 14). The depolarization is spread by passive current flow that results from the potential difference between the active and the inactive regions of the axon membrane. Once the depolarization of the inactive region of the membrane approaches threshold, the voltage-gated Na^+ channels in this region open, Na^+ rushes into the axoplasm, and an action potential is initiated. The actively generated depolarization then spreads by passive, local circuit flow to the next region of the membrane, and the cycle is repeated.

The rate at which the action potential is conducted along the axon depends on the passive membrane properties: the capacitance C_m and the internal resistance of the axoplasm R_i. As described, an action potential generated in one segment of the axon supplies the current to depolarize the adjacent segments. According to Ohm's law, the larger the internal resistance, the less the current flow (I = V/R) and, thus, the longer it takes to change the charge on the mem-

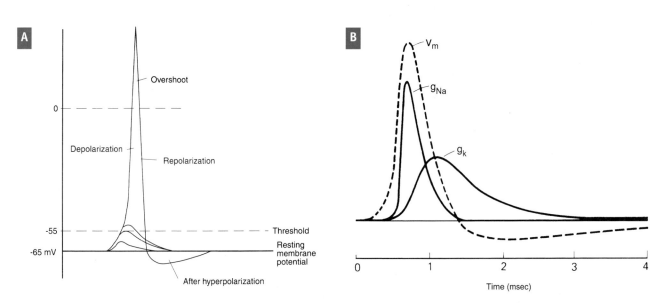

Figure 11

A, Action potentials are generated when the membrane potential reaches a critical threshold voltage. The depolarization phase is due to the active opening of Na channels and repolarization to the active opening of K channels. **B,** The shape of the action potential can be calculated from the changes in g_{Na} and g_K that result from the opening and closing of voltage-gated Na and K channels. (Adapted with permission from Hodgkin AL: *The Conduction of a Nervous Impulse*. Springfield, IL, Charles C. Thomas, 1964.)

brane of the adjacent segment. Additionally, the higher the capacitance, the larger the time constant, and the longer it takes to charge the membrane and to depolarize the membrane. The rate of passive current flow varies inversely with the product R_iC_m. If this product is reduced, the rate of passive current spread and the rate of action potential conduction, that is, conduction velocity, will both increase.

One way to increase the conduction velocity is to increase the diameter of the axon. Because the internal resistance R_i decreases in proportion to the square of the axon diameter, and the capacitance C_m increases in direct proportion to the diameter, the net effect of increasing the diameter is a decrease in R_iC_m. Because of the need for a large number of axons, this adaptation has not taken place in vertebrates. In vertebrates, conduction velocity is increased by increasing the membrane resistance R_m.

Vertebrate axons are wrapped in myelin, which effectively

acts as an insulator, increasing the membrane resistance and decreasing the membrane capacitance. The resulting increase in the length constant and decrease in the time constant increases the rate of passive current flow. Although myelin interferes with action potential initiation, there are specialized regions of the axon that are not wrapped in myelin, the nodes of Ranvier, at which there is a high concentration of voltage-gated Na^+ channels. Action

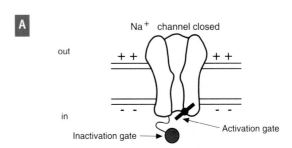

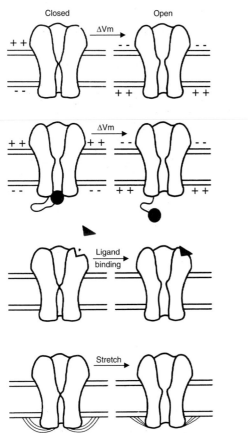

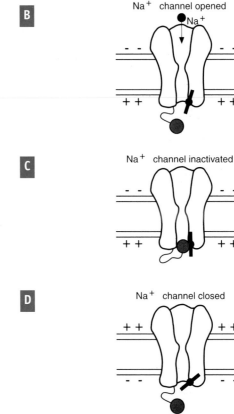

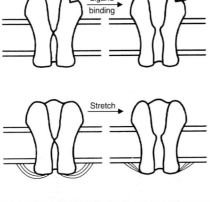

Figure 12

Channel gating is controlled by several types of stimuli. Changes in voltage can regulate a channel by causing a blocking particle to swing into or out of the channel mouth (often referred to as ball and chain model). Binding of a ligand to a receptor located on the channel or stretch or pressure can activate the channel by causing conformational changes in the channel. (Adapted with permission from Kandel ER, Schwartz JH, Jessell TM: *Principles of Neural Science*, ed 3. Norwalk, CT, Appleton & Lange, 1991, pp 75–76.)

Figure 13

Response of gated Na channel during action potential. **A,** When the cell is in the resting state, the Na activation gate is closed and the inactivation gate is open. **B,** Depolarization of the cell causes the Na activation gate to open and Na enters the cell. **C,** As the depolarization is maintained, channels that have opened begin to close because the inactivation gates close. **D,** After the membrane is repolarized, the channel returns to its resting state. (Adapted with permission from Kandel ER, Schwartz JH, Jessell TM: *Principles of Neural Science*, ed 3. Norwalk, CT, Appleton & Lange, 1991, p 14.)

potentials are evoked at the nodes, and local currents flow quickly, largely unattenuated down the myelinated region of the axon (the internode) from one node to the next, where a new action potential is evoked; that is, action potential production jumps via saltatory propagation from node to node. This means of increasing the conduction velocity is very effective.

Several diseases of the nervous system cause demyelination, such as multiple sclerosis and Guillain-Barré syndrome. Demyelinated regions of the axon have a higher capacitance and a lower membrane resistance; therefore, when an action potential is propagated down a myelinated axon and reaches a demyelinated region, its conduction will be slowed or may be stopped completely. A decrease or loss of conduction could have devastating effects on behavior.

External Activation of Axons

To drive an axon to threshold, the current must pass through the membrane. Of the total stimulating current, only a small fraction flows across the membrane of any one axon. The current passes through the membrane, flows along the axoplasmic core, and exits through the membrane in a distant region. Larger diameter axons have a lower current threshold and their axoplasm is less resistant to current flow. Because of this, more current enters the larger axons, where it depolarizes the membrane and brings it to threshold. Once threshold is reached, the action potential is initiated and self-propagated. A gradual increase in stimulus strength will excite the larger axons first and then, at relatively large current strengths, the smaller axons.

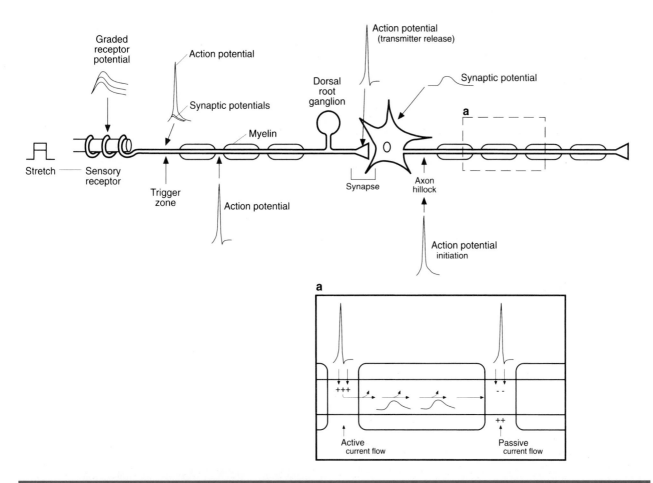

Figure 14

Propagation of action potential and passive current flow. Graded stretching of a muscle produces graded potentials in the terminal fibers of the sensory neuron. This potential spreads passively to the trigger zone and, if the potential is large enough, it will trigger an action potential, which is actively propagated without change along the axon to the terminal region. At the terminal of the afferent fiber, the action potential triggers the release of transmitter that diffuses across the synaptic cleft and interacts with the membrane of the motoneuron to initiate a synaptic potential in the motoneuron. The synaptic potential passively spreads to the axon hillock where an action potential is initiated if the membrane potential is above threshold. Action potential propagation results from the spread of local passive depolarizing currents between the nodes of Ranvier. At the nodes, voltage-gated channels open, producing an action potential.

Sensory and Motor Systems

Classification of Nerve Fibers

The CNS consists of the brain and the spinal cord. All remaining nervous tissue is referred to as the peripheral nervous system (PNS). Peripheral nerves are bundles of axons that are enclosed in sheaths of connective tissue that maintain the continuity of, nourish, and protect the individual axons.

An axon is composed of a core of axoplasm enclosed in an axolemmal membrane. The axoplasm contains subcellular structures including microtubules, neurofibrils, mitochondria, vesicles of the smooth endoplasmic reticulum, and, occasionally, dense bodies and glycogen particles. Every axon in a peripheral nerve is surrounded by a myelin sheath that is formed by Schwann cells. A nerve fiber is defined as the axon and the Schwann cell sheath surrounding it.

The outer sheath of the nerve fiber varies in structure depending on whether or not the axon is myelinated. One myelinated axon is associated with a single Schwann cell at any one level. The Schwann cell wraps spirally around the axon and produces a sheath of alternating layers of lipid and protein that are compressed together, giving the myelin sheath a characteristic laminated structure (Fig. 15, A). In general, an axon becomes myelinated once it reaches a diameter of 1 to 2 μm. The thickness of the myelin sheath increases with the size of the axon. The diameter of peripheral axons, excluding the myelin sheath, varies from 0.5 to 10 μm. In unmyelinated fibers, a single Schwann cell surrounds many axons (Fig. 15, B). Physiologically, the primary difference between myelinated and unmyelinated fibers is the conduction velocity.

Nerve fibers can be classified into different types based on their diameter and conduction velocity or their function. Nerve fibers that transmit information from sensory receptors to the CNS are referred to as afferent. Afferent fibers from the viscera are termed visceral afferents and those from receptors in muscles, skin, and sensory organs of the head are called somatic afferents. Transmission of information from the CNS to the periphery occurs via efferent nerve fibers. Efferent fibers that innervate skeletal muscle fibers are called motor efferents. The remaining efferent nerve fibers are classified as autonomic efferents. Peripheral nerves that innervate the skin, skeletal muscles, and the joints are referred to as somatic nerves, and nerves leading to the viscera are called splanchnic or autonomic nerves. This chapter will focus on somatic nerves.

Two sets of nomenclature have been used to classify axons based on the diameter of the axon and the conduction velocity. The Erlanger/Gasser classification uses an alphabetical scheme to classify afferents in cutaneous nerves. The Lloyd/Hunt classification uses Roman numerals to classify afferents in motor nerves. The axon diameters and conduction velocities for the different types of nerve fibers are given in Table 2. The distribution of afferents in motor and cutaneous nerves is illustrated in Figure 16. Cutaneous nerves have only 3 peaks because the group I (Aα) afferents are absent. Group I afferents are typically primary muscle spindle afferents and afferents from muscle tendon organs. Virtually all mechanoreceptors are Aα and Aβ fibers, whereas thermoreceptors and nociceptors belong to the Aα and C fiber groups.

A compound nerve action potential is produced by electrically stimulating a peripheral nerve at an intensity that activates all motor and sensory fibers; thus, it is the summation of action potentials from all activated nerve fibers. In general, the compound nerve action potential has 2 major deflections corresponding to the Aα (large myelinated) and Aδ (small myelinated) fibers (Fig. 17). Action potentials of unmyelinated fibers (Group C or IV) are conducted slowly and produce a small late peak that typically cannot be recorded in vivo.

Sensory Systems

Sensory systems receive information from the environment and within the body through receptors located at the periphery of the body and transmit this information to the

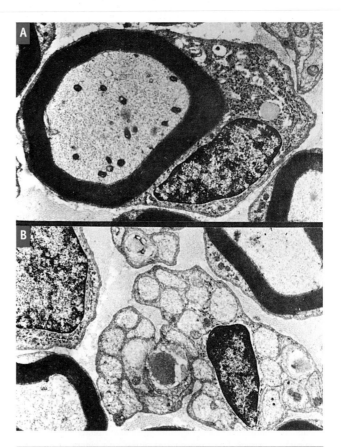

Figure 15

Photomicrograph showing myelinated (**A**) and unmyelinated (**B**) axons.

CNS. This information is used for 3 primary functions: sensation, control of movement, and maintaining arousal. Although sensation is a conscious experience, much of the sensory information used to control movement is not perceived. In addition, much of the sensory information received from within the body and used to regulate such functions as temperature, blood pressure, heart rate, respiratory rate, and reflex movement never reaches consciousness.

Sensory systems extract 4 attributes from a stimulus: modality or quality, intensity, duration, and location. The major modalities are described in Table 3. All sensory systems are organized in a similar manner. External stimuli are recognized by specialized neural structures called sensory receptors. Each receptor is sensitive to a specific form of physical energy: mechanical, thermal, chemical, or electromagnetic (Table 3). The external stimulus or energy is transformed into electrochemical energy through the process of sensory transduction. Sensory information is then transmitted to the CNS by action potentials. The attributes of the stimulus are neurally encoded by the action potentials. In the somatic system, the sensory receptor is a neuron that carries out both sensory transduction and neural encoding of the action potentials.

Sensory information is transmitted to the brain via 2 pathways: the dorsal column-medial lemniscal tract and the anterolateral tract. The receptor neuron, which is referred to as the first-order neuron or the primary afferent, projects to the spinal cord or the brain stem, where it synapses with second-order neurons. The neurons in subcortical regions are referred to as lower-order neurons. The information from lower-order neurons is passed through relay nuclei to higher-order neurons in the cerebral cortex. In the sensory system, the thalamus is an essential relay point. Sensory information is sent from the thalamus to specific sensory regions of the cortex where it is perceived.

The somatic sensory system is distinct because it processes many different types of stimuli and its receptors for somatic sensation are distributed throughout the body rather than confined to a specialized organ such as the eye. The somatic sensory system conveys 3 distinct modalities: mechanical, elicited by mechanical stimulation of the body surface (touch) and mechanical displacements of the muscles and joints (proprioception); pain, elicited by noxious (tissue damaging) stimuli; and thermal sensation, elicited by cool and warm stimuli. Within each modality there are submodalities; for example, superficial and deep touch (pressure).

Each somatosensory modality is mediated by a separate class of receptors (Table 4). However, regardless of the receptor type, all somatosensory information from the body is transmitted to the spinal cord or the brain stem by dorsal root ganglion neurons. The dorsal root ganglion neu-

Table 2

Classification of Nerve Fibers

Group	Function (Examples)	Average Fiber Diameter (μm)	Average CV* (ms)
Erlanger/Gasser Classification			
Aα	Primary muscle-spindle afferents, motor axons to muscle	15	100
Aβ	Cutaneous touch and pressure afferents	8	50
Aγ	Motor axons to muscle spindle	5	20
Aδ	Cutaneous temperature and pain afferents	3	15
B	Sympathetic preganglionic	3	7
C	Cutaneous pain afferents, sympathetic postganglionic	0.5	1
Lloyd/Hunt Classification			
I	Primary muscle-spindle afferents and afferents from tendon organs	13	75
II	Mechanoreceptors	9	55
III	Deep pressure sensors in muscle	3	11
IV	Unmyelinated pain afferents	0.5	1

*   CV = conduction velocity

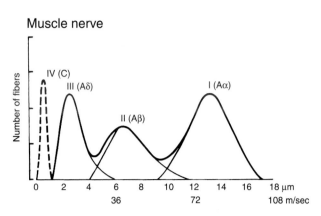

Muscle nerve

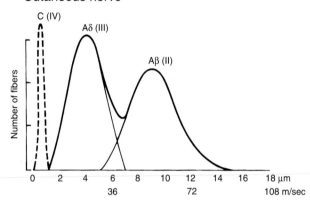

Cutaneous nerve

Figure 16

The distribution of different types of afferent fibers in muscle and cutaneous tissue. Axonal diameters are given in micrometers and conduction velocities are given in meters per second. (Adapted with permission from Boyd IA, Davey MR: *Composition of Peripheral Nerves.* Edinburgh, Scotland, Churchill Livingstone, 1968.)

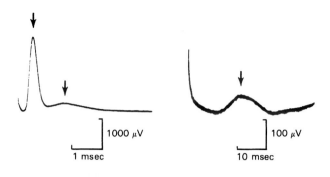

Figure 17

The compound action potential has 3 distinct peaks corresponding to Aα, Aδ, and C fibers. The compound action potential shown here was recorded in vitro because potentials from C fibers cannot be recorded in vivo. The nerve, from an 11-year-old boy whose leg had been amputated above the knee, was placed in a specialized recording chamber. The recording on the left shows peaks produced by Aα (left arrow) and Aδ (right arrow) fibers. The trace on the right is a high-gain, slow time scale recording of a C-fiber peak. (Reproduced with permission from Kimura J: *Electrodiagnosis in Diseases of Nerve and Muscle: Principles and Practice,* ed 2. Philadelphia, PA, FA Davis, 1989.)

ron performs 2 functions: sensory transduction and transmission of encoded stimulus information. The morphology of the dorsal root ganglion neuron is illustrated in Figure 18. Dorsal root ganglion neurons are not all alike and can be distinguished by (1) the morphology of the terminal, (2) sensitivity to a stimulus, (3) the diameter of the axon and cell body, and (4) the presence or absence of a myelin sheath. The terminal of the dorsal root ganglion neuron is the only region that is sensitive to stimulus energy and is either a bare nerve ending or an end organ consisting of a nonneuronal capsule surrounding the axon terminal. Noci-

Table 3			
Sensory Systems			
Modality	**Stimulus**	**Receptor Type**	**Receptors**
Vision	Light	Photoreceptors	Rods, cones
Hearing	Sound	Mechanoreceptors	Hair cells (cochlear)
Balance	Head motion	Mechanoreceptors	Hair cells (semicircular canal)
Somatic	Mechanical Thermal Noxious	Mechanoreceptors Thermoreceptors Nociceptors, chemoreceptors	Dorsal root ganglion cells
Taste	Chemical	Chemoreceptors	Taste buds
Smell	Chemical	Chemoreceptors	Olfactory sensory neurons

(Reproduced with permission from Kandel ER, Schwartz JH, Jessel TM (eds): *Principles of Neural Science,* ed 3. Norwalk, CT, Appleton & Lange, 1991, p 334.)

Table 4
Receptor Types

Receptor type	Fiber type	Quality
Nociceptors		
Mechanical	Aδ	Sharp, pricking pain
Thermal and mechanothermal	Aγ	Sharp, pricking pain
Thermal and mechanothermal	C	Slow, burning pain
Polymodal	C	Slow, burning pain
Cutaneous and subcutaneous mechanoreceptors		
Meissner's corpuscle	Aβ	Touch
Pacinian corpuscle	Aβ	Flutter
Ruffini corpuscle	Aβ	Vibration
Merkel's receptor	Aβ	Steady skin indentation
Hair-guard, hair-tylotrich	Aβ	Steady skin indentation
Hair-down	Aβ	Flutter
Muscle and skeletal mechanoreceptors		
Muscle spindle primary	Aα	Limb proprioception
Muscle spindle secondary	Aβ	Limb proprioception
Golgi tendon organ	Aα	Limb proprioception
Joint capsule mechanoreceptor	Aβ	Limb proprioception

(Reproduced with permission from Kandel ER, Schwartz JH, Jessel TM (eds): *Principles of Neural Science,* ed 3. Norwalk, CT, Appleton & Lange, 1991, p 342.)

ceptors and thermoreceptors are bare nerve endings. Mechanoreceptors are generally specialized end organs. The sensory information is transmitted to the spinal cord or brain stem by the primary afferent fiber. The cell body is located in the dorsal root ganglia in the PNS and gives rise to 2 processes: the peripheral and central branches of the primary afferent. Sensory information regarding touch and limb proprioception is carried by the medial lemniscal tract and information concerned with pain and temperature by the anterolateral tract.

Motor Systems

The motor system is hierarchically organized and consists of 4 major divisions: the spinal cord, the brain stem and reticular formation, the motor cortex, and the premotor cortical areas that include the basal ganglia and cerebellum. Each division contains separate neural circuits that are linked to each of the other divisions. The spinal cord contains the neural circuitry responsible for segmental and proprioceptive reflexes as well as the circuitry responsible for the reciprocal activation of flexor and extensor muscles

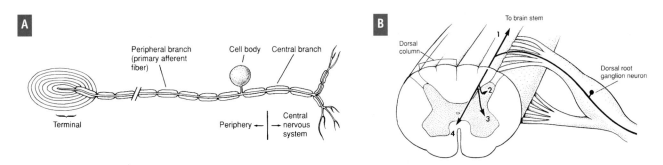

Figure 18

A, Morphology of dorsal root ganglion cells. The cell body lies in a ganglion in the dorsal root of a spinal nerve. The axon has 2 branches, 1 projecting to the periphery and 1 to the central nervous system. **B,** Projections of the central branch. The dorsal root ganglion cells that mediate pressure, touch, and proprioception have several central branches. The principal branch ascends in the dorsal column to the brain stem (1). The other branches terminate locally in the dorsal and ventral horns of the spinal cord (2, 3), or descend a few segments and terminate in the spinal cord (4). Branches 2, 3, and 4 participate in local spinal reflexes. (Adapted with permission from Kandel ER, Schwartz JH, Jessell TM: *Principles of Neural Science,* ed 3. Norwalk, CT, Appleton & Lange, 1991, pp 287–342.)

during locomotion. Spinal cord neurons process information from the peripheral system, from each other, and from descending pathways in the spinal cord to mediate reflexes and control motor output. In addition, they send ascending projections to higher centers. The descending pathways originate from upper motoneurons in the cerebral cortex and brainstem. These pathways often are divided into pyramidal and extrapyramidal tracts. The pyramidal or corticospinal tract originates from neurons in the motor cortex, premotor cortex, and parietal lobe. The extrapyramidal tracts arise from cells in the red nucleus, reticular formation, and vestibular nucleus of the brain stem and give rise to the rubrospinal, reticulospinal, and vestibulospinal tracts, respectively.

Spinal Cord Anatomy

In the adult human, the spinal cord extends from the foramen magnum to the lower border of the first lumbar vertebra. Axons enter and exit the spinal cord via the spinal nerves, each of which consists of a ventral or efferent root and a dorsal or afferent root (Fig. 19, A). The ventral roots carry output to the striated muscles from the myelinated nerve fibers of the α and γ motoneurons in the gray matter of the ventral horn. The dorsal roots carry sensory input from myelinated and unmyelinated nerve fibers that originate from somatic sensory receptors. The cell bodies of the afferent fibers are located in the dorsal root ganglia.

The spinal cord is divided into white and gray matter. The white matter is divided into columns of ascending and descending fiber tracts that contain myelinated and unmyelinated nerve axons. The gray matter, which consists of longitudinally arranged neuronal cell bodies, dendrites, glial cells, and myelinated and unmyelinated axons, is divided into the dorsal horn, intermediate zone, and ventral horn. There are 3 types of neurons present in the spinal gray matter: neurons that send axonal projections out of the CNS via the ventral roots (α and γ motoneurons), those that have axonal projections that remain in the spinal cord (interneurons), and those that send ascending axonal projections to supraspinal centers (tract cells). The spinal gray matter is histologically divided by cell characteristics into 9 different regions or lamina (Fig. 19, C). Each lamina contains a specific type of neuron and receives axonal projections from specific sensory axons and descending pathways.

Lower Motoneurons

Movement is generated by the activation of striated skeletal muscles. Skeletal muscles are innervated by lower motoneurons located in the ventral gray matter of the spinal cord. The motoneurons innervating a specific muscle are arranged in columns that extend through several spinal segments. The α motoneurons are relatively large cells that have body areas ranging from 30 to 70 μm² and motor axons that innervate the extrafusal muscle fibers in striated muscles. Within the ventral horn, the motoneurons

are located in nonoverlapping areas: axial muscles are innervated by medially located motoneurons (lamina VIII), and limb muscles are innervated by more laterally located motoneurons (lamina IX). The most medial of the lateral group of motoneurons tends to innervate the proximal muscles (muscles of the shoulder and hip), while the more lateral motoneurons in lamina IX tend to innervate the distal muscles (the muscles of the extremities and digits). The motoneurons innervating the extensor muscles tend to be located ventral to those innervating flexor muscles. The γ motoneurons are smaller than α motoneurons and innervate intrafusal fibers of the muscle spindles.

The basic functional unit of a muscle is the motor unit, which consists of an α motoneuron, its motor axon, and all the muscle fibers it innervates. The motor unit has been called the final common pathway because all information, both direct and indirect, must be processed by the α motoneuron for muscle contraction to occur. The α motoneuron receives input from 3 major sources: the sensory system, the pyramidal pathways, and the extrapyramidal pathways. Although the motoneuron receives direct inputs from these systems, activity in neural circuits is coordinated primarily by interneurons. The interneurons function as a link between the peripheral nervous system, the descending pathways from the cortex and brain stem, and local spinal neurons and motoneurons.

Motor Unit Types

The function of a muscle is a reflection of the physiologic, morphologic, and biochemical characteristics of its motor units. Characterization of the physiologic properties of the muscle unit (the fibers innervated by 1 motoneuron) has revealed a number of interrelationships that have been the basis of the classification of units into types. Motor units most often are separated into 4 major types based on the physiologic properties of the muscle unit: slow fatigue resistant (type S); fast fatigue resistant (type FR); fast fatigue intermediate (type FI); and fast fatigable (type FF). The physiologic properties most often used to classify units are (1) contraction time, (2) the presence or absence of sag in an unfused tetanus, (3) maximum tension, and (4) the fatigue properties. The relative differences between each type are shown in Table 5. In general, type S units produce the lowest tensions, have the slowest contraction times, and are the most fatigue-resistant. In contrast, units producing the largest force tend to be the fastest contracting and the most fatigable.

The fatigue resistance of a motor unit is related, in part, to the metabolic properties of the muscle fibers within the unit. The presence of 3 muscle fiber types has been established based on qualitative histochemical staining with succinate dehydrogenase, an oxidative marker enzyme; α-glycerophosphate dehydrogenase, a glycolytic marker enzyme; and myosin ATPase, an enzyme that is related to the rate at which ATP can be hydrolyzed. Using these histo-

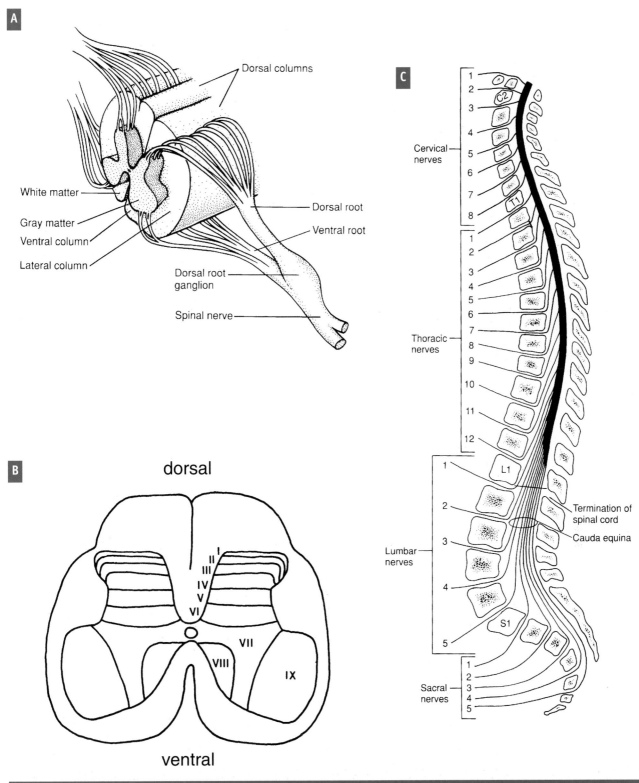

A, Each spinal nerve has a dorsal and ventral root.

Dorsal columns

White matter

Gray matter

Ventral column

Lateral column

Dorsal root

Ventral root

Dorsal root ganglion

Spinal nerve

B

dorsal

ventral

C

Cervical nerves

Thoracic nerves

Lumbar nerves

Sacral nerves

Termination of spinal cord

Cauda equina

Figure 19

Spinal cord anatomy. **A,** Each spinal nerve has a dorsal and ventral root. The dorsal (sensory) root comprises the central branches of the dorsal root ganglion cells; the ventral (motor) root comprises the motor axons emerging from motoneurons in the ventral horn. **B,** Location of Rexed's lamina within the dorsal and ventral horns of the spinal cord. **C,** The individual spinal nerves are related to the 4 levels of the spinal cord. The adult spinal cord terminates at the border of L-1. The dorsal and ventral roots of the lumbar and sacral nerves within the vertebral column are collectively termed the cauda equina. (**A** and **C** reproduced with permission from Kandel ER, Schwartz JH, Jessell TM: *Principles of Neural Science,* ed 3. Norwalk, CT, Appleton & Lange, 1991, pp 285–286.)

chemical stains, fibers have been classified as fast glycolytic, fast oxidative glycolytic, and slow oxidative. Glycogen depletion of physiologically classified motor units shows that type FF units are composed of fast glycolytic fibers, type FR units are composed of fast oxidative glycolytic fibers, and S units are composed of slow oxidative fibers (Table 5). The classification scheme based on the myosin ATPase staining characteristics at different pHs is also shown in Table 5. The relationship between succinate dehydrogenase activity, maximum tension, and fatigue index is shown in Figure 20. In general, there is a direct relationship between succinate dehydrogenase activity and fatigue resistance.

The fibers of the different motor unit types vary in size; fast glycolytic fibers are the largest and slow oxidative fibers are the smallest. However, the fibers of any given type range in size, and the size of the same type of fiber may be quite different in a homogeneous (all the same type) and a het-erogeneous (mixed types) muscle. For example, slow oxidative fibers in a heterogeneous muscle, such as the medial gastrocnemius, are significantly smaller than those in the soleus, a homogeneous muscle. Although fibers within a motor unit had been assumed to be identical in size, recent evidence has shown that there can be a threefold to eight-fold range in cross-sectional area of these fibers.

In a given muscle, the force capabilities of the component motor units differ widely. The observed range in force may be attributed to variations in (1) the number of fibers inner-vated by the motoneurons (the innervation ratio); (2) the size of the muscle fibers belonging to the motor unit; and/or (3) the specific force output per unit area of active muscle (the specific tension). The difference in force poten-tial between slow and fast units had been assumed to be related to differences in the specific tension of slow and fast fibers. However, recent studies have shown that the differ-ence in tension between motor units is primarily a function

Table 5
General Characteristics of Motor Unit Types

Parameter	Motor Unit Types* FF	FR	S
Muscle unit physiology*			
Contraction time	Fastest	Slightly slower	Slowest
Sag	Present	Present	Absent
Maximum tension	Largest	Smaller	Smallest
Fatigue index	< 0.25	< 0.75–1.0	0.7–1.0
Muscle unit anatomy+			
Innervation ratio	2.9	2.1	1.0
Fiber cross-sectional area	1.3	0.98	1.0
Specific tension	1.4	1.2	1.0
Muscle unit metabolism			
Fiber type++	FG	FOG	SO
Myosin heavy chain	IIB	IIA	I
Glycogen	High	High	Low
Hexokinase	Low	Intermediate	High
Glycolytic enzymes	High	High	Low
Oxidative enzymes	Low	High	High
Cytochrome c	Low	High	High
Capillary supply	Sparse	Rich	Very rich
Motoneuron			
Cell body size	Largest	Slightly smaller	Smallest
Conduction velocity	Fastest	Slightly slower	Slowest
After-hyperpolarization duration	Shortest	Slightly shorter	Longest
Input resistance	Lowest	Slightly higher	Highest

*   FF = fast fatigable; FR = fast fatigue resistant; S = fatigue resistant
** Data relative to the FF unit
+   Data relative to the slow unit
++ FG = fast glycolytic; FOG = fast oxidative glycolytic; SO = slow oxidative

of the innervation ratio. Although the specific tension of slow units is lower than that of fast units, the difference accounts for only a small part of the observed differences in maximum tension (-2%) (Table 5). The relationship between innervation ratio and maximum tension is shown in Figure 21, *A*. After the nerve to a muscle has been cut (denervation) and allowed to grow back (Fig. 21, *B*), the motor units often produce larger tensions than normal; however, there is still a direct relationship between tension and innervation ratio. Further, when a portion of the motor

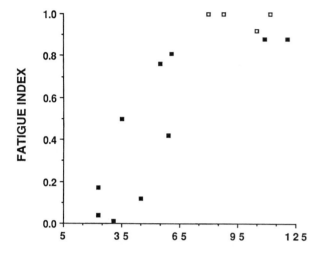

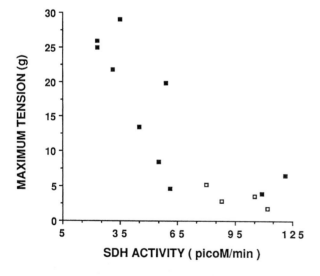

SDH ACTIVITY (picoM/min)

Figure 20

Relationships between succinate dehydrogenase (SDH) activity and fatigue index for 14 motor units isolated from cat tibialis anterior muscle. Fast units are represented as filled squares and slow units as empty squares. (Data taken from Martin TP, Bodine-Fowler S, Roy RR, Eldred E, Edgerton VR: Metabolic and fiber size properties of cat tibialis anterior motor units. *Am J Physiol* 1988;255:C43–50.)

axons innervating a muscle have been lost (as in certain motoneuron diseases, with partial nerve injuries, and in spinal root injuries), the remaining motor axons will sprout and innervate the denervated muscle fibers. Consequently, the tension of the remaining units will increase.

The distribution of muscle fibers belonging to a motor unit has been examined using electromyographic and glycogen depletion techniques. The fibers belonging to a motor unit are not distributed across the entire cross section of a muscle but, in general, are localized to a specific region of the muscle (Fig. 22). The relative size of the motor unit territory, calculated as a percentage of the whole muscle cross section, ranges from 8% to 22% in the cat tibialis anterior muscle and 41% to 76% in the cat soleus muscle. As many as 20 to 30 units may overlap within a given region of the muscle. A motor unit's fibers are distributed such that few fibers belonging to the same unit are adjacent (Fig. 23, *A*). For example, in an average tibialis anterior unit, 71% of the motor unit fibers are not adjacent to another fiber from the same unit, 21% of the motor unit fibers occur in groups of 2, and only 8% occur in groups of 3 or more. After reinnervation, there is often an increase in the number of adjacencies between motor unit fibers (Fig. 23, *B*).

The α motoneurons are among the largest neurons in the mammalian CNS. A single motoneuron can innervate only a few muscle fibers in muscles such as those that control eye movements or fine movements of the hand or it can innervate hundreds to thousands of fibers in muscles of the lower extremity. When a motoneuron is activated, it stimulates all of the muscle fibers that it innervates. Just as muscle unit types differ in their physiologic properties, motoneurons innervating each of the muscle unit types differ in their electrophysiologic and morphologic properties. The total cell membrane area of motoneurons is correlated with the type of muscle unit innervated in the following sequence: type FF > type FR > type S. Moreover, the diameter and conduction velocity of a motor axon are directly correlated with the size of the parent cell body, although the correlation is not precise. Consequently, the motor axons innervating the type S units are generally the slowest conducting and the smallest in diameter.

There is an inverse correlation between the measured sizes of motoneurons and their input resistance. Input resistance is a complex function of membrane area, membrane resistance, and the time and length constants of the neuron. Because slow motoneurons generally have a higher input resistance than fast motoneurons, injecting the same amount of current into each type will cause a greater change in the membrane potential of the slow motoneuron according to Ohm's law, V = IR. The susceptibility of motoneuron types to discharge action potential during intracellular current injection also differs; slow motoneurons generally require less current to be excited than fast motoneurons. Also, slow and fast motoneurons differ in the length of their after-hyperpolarization (AHP) duration, which is important in determining the maximum firing frequency of a motoneuron. Slow motoneurons have a longer AHP than fast motoneurons and fire at a lower maximum frequency. The AHP duration of the motoneuron is directly correlated to the contraction time of the muscle unit (Fig. 24). The relative differences between motoneurons as related to motor unit type are summarized in Table 5. In general, the intrinsic properties of the motoneurons vary such that there is a gradient of increasing excitability: S > FR > FF.

Recruitment Order

The majority of evidence indicates that the motor units within a specific muscle are recruited in an orderly manner. The size principle indicates that the size of the motoneuron dictates its excitability, which determines the degree of use of the motor unit, and its usage, in turn, specifies or influences the type of muscle fiber required. Data from human subjects as well as from experimental animals indicate that recruitment during slow development of force in both vol-

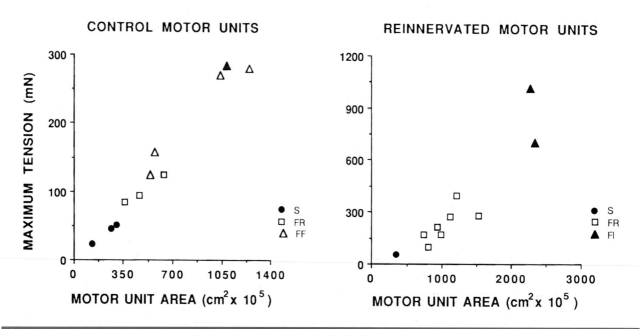

Figure 21

Relationship between motor unit maximum tension and innervation ratio for motor units isolated from control cat tibialis anterior and cat tibialis anterior 6 months after denervation and self-reinnervation. Units were classified into types based on the contractile properties of the muscle unit. (Data taken from Bodine SC, Roy RR, Eldred E, Edgerton VR: Maximal force as a function of anatomical features of motor units in the cat tibialis anterior. *J Neurophysiol* 1987;57:1730-1745, and Unguez GA, Bodine-Fowler S, Roy RR, Pierotti DJ, Edgerton VR: Evidence of incomplete neural control of motor unit properties in adult cat tibialis anterior after self-reinnervation. *J Physiol (Lond)* 1993;472:103–125.)

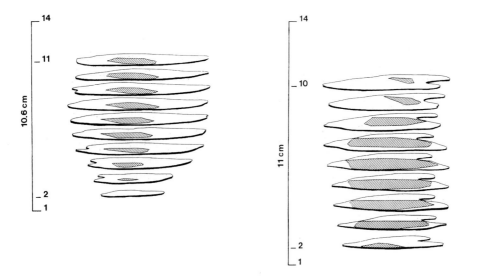

Figure 22

Distribution of motor unit fibers throughout the length of the cat tibialis anterior. The size in centimeters of the block from which each cross-section was taken is indicated. The stippled area represents the location and relative size of the territory over which the motor unit fibers were distributed. Although the motor unit territory may be distributed throughout most of the muscle, the individual muscle fibers often do not extend the length of the muscle. (Reproduced with permission from Bodine-Fowler SC, Unguez GA, Roy RR, Armstrong AN, Edgerton VR: Innervation patterns in the cat tibialis anterior six months after self-reinnervation. *Muscle Nerve* 1993;16:379–391.)

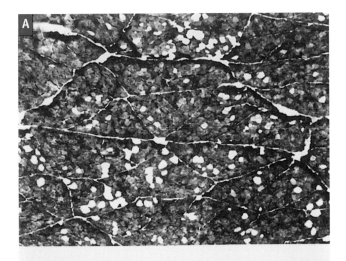

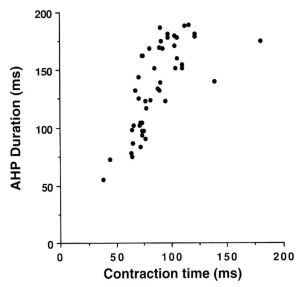

Figure 24

Relationship between motoneuron after hyperpolarization (AHP) duration and muscle unit contraction time from motor units recorded from the cat soleus muscle.

Figure 23

Cross sections from 2 cat tibialis anterior muscles 6 months after denervation (**A**) and self-reinnervation (**B**). In each muscle, a single motor unit was isolated and repetitively stimulated to deplete the muscle fibers of glycogen. Muscle cross sections were stained for glycogen using the periodic acid-Schiff reaction; the unstained fibers were identified as belonging to the stimulated motor unit. Calibration bar = 500 μm. (Reproduced with permission from Bodine-Fowler SC, Unguez GA, Roy RR, Armstrong AN, Edgerton VR: Innervation patterns in the cat tibialis anterior six months after self-reinnervation. *Muscle Nerve* 1993;16:379–391.)

untary and reflex muscle contractions begins with the slowest contracting, lowest force units. As the demand for tension increases, the faster fatigue resistant, intermediate force units are recruited. The last units to be recruited, usually during maximal contractions, are the fastest, most fatigable, largest force units. An example of orderly recruitment in the human first interosseous muscle is shown in Figure 25. Studies using experimental animals have shown that motor units within a muscle are recruited according to increasing maximum tension and increasing conduction velocity (Table 6). In general, the data suggest that units are recruited during normal movements in the following order: S-FR-FF (Fig. 26).

Some investigators have suggested that the recruitment order can be reversed in some situations such that the fast, large-force units are selectively recruited before the slow,

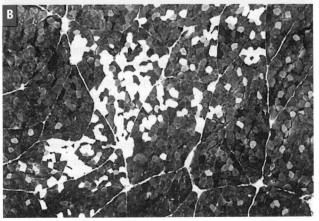

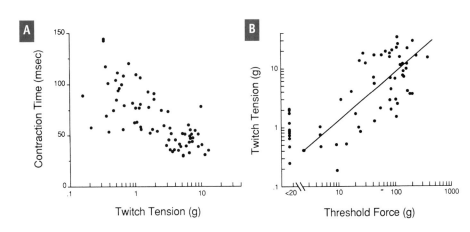

Figure 25

A, Human motor unit twitch contraction time as a function of twitch tension recorded by spike-triggered averaging. Note that as contractile tension increases, contraction time decreases. This suggests that the motor units with larger tension have faster contractile speed, as predicted by the size principle. **B,** Human motor unit twitch tension as a function of threshold voltage. As threshold increases, larger units are recruited, as predicted by the size principle. (Reproduced with permission from Lieber RL: *Skeletal Muscle Structure and Function.* Baltimore, MD, Williams & Wilkins, 1992, p 99.)

Table 6

Relationship of Recruitment Threshold to Axonal Conduction Velocity (CV) and Maximum Tension (P_0) of the Muscle Unit

Type of Units in Pairs	Number of Pairs	Number of Pairs With Lower Threshold Unit Having:			
		Slower CV	Faster CV	Smaller P_0	Larger P_0
Fast, Fast	20	9	10	20	0
Slow, Slow	9	8	1	9	0
Slow, Fast	13	13	0	13	0

(Data from Zajac FE, Faden JS: Relationship among recruitment order, axonal conducted velocity, and muscle-unit properties of type-identified motor units in cat plantaris muscle. *J Neurophysiol* 1985;53:1303–1322.)

low-force units. Preferential activation of normally high threshold units (the FF units) has been reported during very rapid isotonic movements in humans and is implied by observations of rapid alternating isotonic movements in animals. It also has been suggested that a motoneuron may have different thresholds for firing, depending on the specific task being performed; however, this has been found primarily for motor units in multifunctional muscles. During most movements, motor units are recruited in an orderly manner according to the size principle. Thus, it appears that the physiologic and metabolic properties of a unit are matched such that the units recruited most often and required to maintain tension for the longest periods of time have the highest resistance to fatigue.

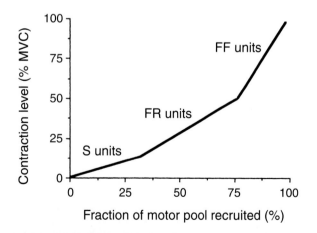

Figure 26

Schematic demonstration of predicted orderly recruitment of motor units during voluntary activity as a function of contractile force. At lower forces S units are recruited, while as force increases FR and FF units are recruited. (Reproduced with permission from Lieber RL: *Skeletal Muscle Structure and Function*. Baltimore, MD, Williams & Wilkins, 1992, p 99. Original adapted from Edgerton VR, Roy RR, Bodine SC, et al: The matching of neuronal and muscular physiology, in Borer KT, Edington DW, White TP (eds): *Frontiers of Exercise Biology*. Champaign, IL, Human Kinetics Publishers, 1983.)

Spinal Cord Reflexes

Spinal cord reflexes involve the final common pathway and are an integral part of the neural circuitry believed to be involved in the maintenance of posture and the production of movement. A reflex is a stereotyped response to a specific sensory stimulus. A reflex pathway consists of the receptor (the sensory organ), the effector (the motoneuron), and the interconnecting neural elements (the interneurons). A reflex that involves only 1 synapse between the receptor and the effector is a monosynaptic reflex; a reflex that involves more than 1 interneuron between the receptor and the effector is a polysynaptic reflex. In general, most reflexes are polysynaptic. Spinal reflex pathways can be modulated by supraspinal pathways either directly, through a mechanism known as presynaptic inhibition, or indirectly, through interneurons.

The following spinal reflexes will be reviewed in this chapter: (1) the stretch reflex, (2) the clasp-knife response, (3) autogenic inhibition, and (4) the flexion withdrawal reflex (Table 7).

The Stretch Reflex

The stretch reflex is a monosynaptic reflex initiated by an afferent discharge from the muscle spindles, which excites the α motoneurons innervating both the muscle from which the afferent discharge originated and synergistic muscles to produce a brisk, transient muscle contraction. The stretch reflex can be produced in both flexor and extensor muscles, but is generally strongest in muscles that function as physiologic extensors, that is, those muscles that oppose gravity. In humans, they are the flexors of the upper extremity and the extensors of the lower extremity.

Muscle spindles are specialized receptors distributed throughout the belly of the muscle and arranged parallel to the extrafusal muscle fibers in striated muscles. Each spindle consists of an encapsulated group of specialized muscle fibers called intrafusal fibers (Fig. 27). The intrafusal fibers are of 2 types, nuclear bag fibers and nuclear chain fibers,

Table 7
Summary of Spinal Reflexes

Segmental Reflex	Receptor Organ	Afferent Fiber
Phasic stretch reflex	Muscle spindle (primary endings)	Type Ia (large myelinated)
Tonic stretch reflex	Muscle spindle (secondary endings)	Type II (intermediate myelinated)
Clasp-knife response	Muscle spindle (secondary endings)	Type II (intermediate myelinated)
Flexion withdrawal reflex	Nociceptors (free nerve endings), touch and pressure receptors	Flexor-reflex afferents: small unmyelinated cutaneous afferents (A-delta, C and muscle afferents, group III)
Autogenic inhibition	Golgi tendon organ	Type Ib (large myelinated)

which differ both morphologically and physiologically. The nuclear bag fibers are larger than the nuclear chain fibers, are fast-contracting, and have clustered nuclei. The nuclear chain fibers are slow-contracting and have nuclei that are arranged in a single row.

Each intrafusal fiber within the spindle is innervated by a γ motoneuron (Fig. 27). Upon activation of the γ motoneurons, the ends or poles of the intrafusal fiber contract, causing the noncontractile equatorial region to stretch. When a muscle is shortened, the intrafusal fibers become slack or unloaded and are unable to monitor length changes. The γ-motoneuron activation provides a means of controlling the length of the intrafusal fibers and the ability of the muscle spindle to detect changes in muscle length. The γ motoneurons are generally coactivated with α motoneurons.

Two types of afferent endings, primary and secondary, are found in muscle spindles. All intrafusal fibers in the spindle have a primary ending located in the center or equatorial

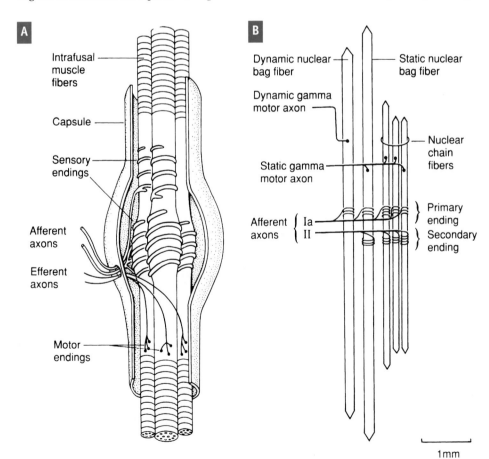

Figure 27

A, The main components of the muscle spindle are intrafusal fibers, sensory endings, and motor axons. The intrafusal fibers are specialized muscle fibers; their central regions are not contractile. The sensory endings spiral around the central regions of the intrafusal fibers and are responsive to stretch. (Original adapted from Hullinger M: The mammalian muscle spindle and its central control. *Rev Physiol Biochem Pharmacol* 1984;101:1–110.) B, The muscle spindle contains 3 types of intrafusal fibers: dynamic nuclear bag, static nuclear bag, and nuclear chain fibers. A single group Ia afferent fiber innervates all 3 types of intrafusal fibers, forming a primary ending. A group II afferent fiber innervates chain and static bag fibers, forming a secondary ending. (Original adapted from Boyd LA: The isolated mammalian muscle spindle. *Trends Neurosci* 1980;3:258–265. Reproduced with permission from Kandel ER, Schwartz JH, Jessell TM: *Principles of Neural Science*, ed 3. Norwalk, CT, Appleton & Lange, 1991, p 566.)

region of the fiber, which gives rise to a large diameter, fast-conducting afferent fiber called a type Ia fiber (Fig. 27, *B*). The primary endings are most sensitive to sudden changes in the length of the muscle and are responsible for the phasic component of the stretch reflex. The secondary endings are located primarily on the nuclear chain fibers and give rise to small diameter, slow-conducting afferent fibers called type II fibers (Fig. 27, *B*). The secondary endings are most sensitive to steady changes in muscle length and are responsible for the tonic component of the stretch reflex.

The phasic stretch reflex is elicited by muscle stretch sufficient to excite the primary afferent (Ia) fibers. Clinically, the stretch reflex is most commonly elicited by tapping on a tendon to produce stretch of the extrafusal muscle fibers, which is detected by the muscle spindle and transmitted to the CNS via the Ia afferent fibers.

The Ia afferent fibers project through the dorsal roots and make the following connections in the spinal cord (Fig. 28): (1) a monosynaptic, excitatory connection with α motoneurons that innervate the muscle from which the fiber originated (homonymous motoneurons); (2) a monosynaptic, excitatory connection with α motoneurons that innervate synergistic muscles (heteronymous motoneurons); and (3) a monosynaptic connection to an inhibitory interneuron referred to as the Ia inhibitory interneuron. The Ia inhibitory interneuron, in turn, connects directly to the α motoneurons that are antagonistic to the muscle from which the Ia afferent fiber originated, providing an inhibitory potential to those motoneurons. Consequently, when a muscle is stretched, the motoneurons innervating the stretched muscle and its synergists are excited, while the motoneurons innervating the antagonist muscles are inhibited. This pattern of simultaneous inhibition of antagonists and excitation of the homonymous and synergistic motoneurons is referred to as reciprocal inhibition.

The type II afferents from the secondary endings have similar connections to the type Ia afferents. In addition, the type II afferent fibers make widespread polysynaptic connections in the spinal cord and are thought to play a role in the flexion reflex. Because they produce a length-dependent inhibition of the stretch reflex, the type II afferent fibers are also thought to participate in the clasp-knife response. This response is characterized by an initial resistance (increase in muscle tone) at the beginning of the stretch, followed by a sudden loss of resistance (decrease in muscle tone) once the muscle has been stretched past a certain point.

Autogenic Inhibition (or Inverse Myotaxic Reflex)

Golgi tendon organs are encapsulated sensory organs located primarily near the myotendinous junction in muscle (Fig. 29). Each Golgi tendon organ is in series with approximately 15 to 20 extrafusal muscle fibers and is innervated by an Ib afferent fiber. When a muscle contracts, the Ib afferent fiber is compressed and activated. The Golgi

tendon organ is most sensitive to active muscle contraction and measures muscle tension.

Activation of Ib afferent fibers results in inhibition of the muscles from which they originated and of synergistic muscles, and in excitation of antagonistic muscles. Because this response is opposite to the stretch reflex, it often is referred to as the inverse myotaxic reflex. This response also is referred to as autogenic inhibition. The Ib afferent fibers make a disynaptic, inhibitory connection to the motoneurons from the homonymous and synergistic muscles, and a disynaptic, excitatory connection to the motoneurons of the antagonistic muscles (Fig. 30). The central connections of the Ib afferent fibers have 3 main features: all connections to motoneurons are through interneurons; connections to flexor muscles are weak, but connections to exten-

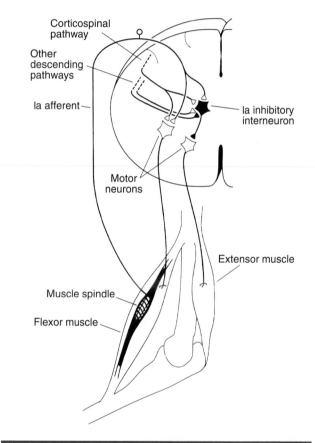

Figure 28

The Ia inhibitory interneuron allows higher centers to coordinate opposing muscles at a joint through a single command. This inhibitory interneuron mediates reciprocal innervation in stretch reflex circuits. In addition, it receives inputs from corticospinal descending axons, so that a descending signal to activate one set of muscles automatically leads to relaxation of the antagonists. Other descending pathways make excitatory and inhibitory connections to this interneuron. When the balance of inputs is shifted to greater inhibition, reciprocal inhibition will be decreased, and cocontraction of opposing muscles will occur. (Only a few of the many inputs to the Ia interneuron and motor neurons are shown in this highly simplified diagram.) (Adapted with permission from Kandel ER, Schwartz JH, Jessell TM: *Principles of Neural Science,* ed 3. Norwalk, CT, Appleton & Lange, 1991, p 584.)

sor muscles are strong; and the central connections are more widespread than those of the Ia afferent fibers.

Renshaw Cell

Another important inhibitory spinal interneuron is the Renshaw cell. α motoneurons give off a collateral that makes a direct, excitatory connection to the Renshaw cell, which projects back to the same motoneuron and to synergistic motoneurons (Fig. 31). The Renshaw cell projection to α motoneurons is inhibitory. This process is called recurrent inhibition, and it regulates the activation of a particular motor pool.

The Renshaw cell also projects to the Ia inhibitory interneuron (Fig. 31). This pathway results in releasing inhibition (or disinhibition) of the antagonist motoneurons by inhibiting of the Ia inhibitory interneuron. The Renshaw cell-Ia inhibitory interneuron pathway may function to limit the duration and magnitude of the Ia afferent mediated reflex response.

Flexion Reflex

The flexion reflex, also referred to as the withdrawal reflex, the cutaneous reflex, or the nociceptive reflex, is a polysynaptic reflex mediated by myelinated group II and unmyeli-

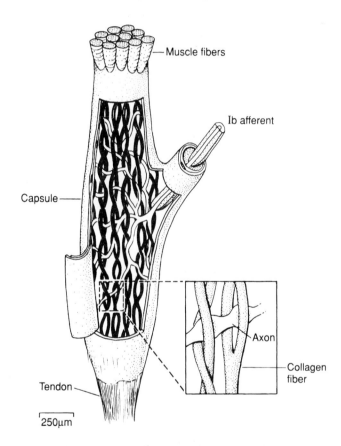

Figure 29

Golgi tendon organs are specialized structures found at the junctions between muscle and tendon. Collagen fibers in the tendon organ attach to the muscle fibers. A single Ib afferent axon enters the capsule and branches into many unmyelinated endings that wrap around and between the collagen fibers. When the tendon organ is stretched (usually because of contraction of the muscle), the afferent axon is compressed by the collagen fibers (see inset at lower right) and increases its rate of firing. (Adapted with permission from Schmidt RF: Motor systems, in Schmidt RF, Thews G (eds): *Human Physiology.* Berlin, Germany, Springer-Verlag, 1983, pp 81–110. Inset adapted with permission from Swett JE, Schoultz TW: Mechanical transduction in the Golgi tendon organ: A hypothesis. *Arch Ital Biol* 1975;113:374–382.)

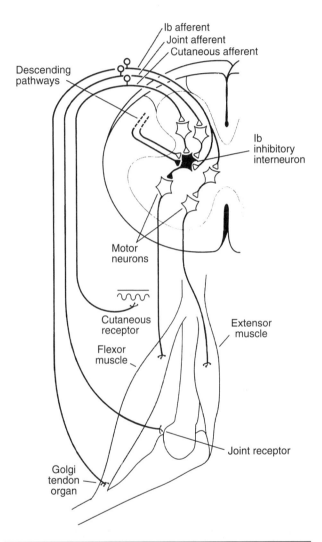

Figure 30

Ib afferent fibers from Golgi tendon organs provide a negative feedback system for regulating muscle tension. Ib afferents inhibit homonymous and synergist motor neurons (not shown) through the Ib inhibitory interneuron. They also excite antagonist motor neurons through an excitatory interneuron. Thus, the reflex effect of stimulating tendon organs is opposite to that of stimulating muscle spindles. The Ib inhibitory interneurons receive convergent input from joint and cutaneous receptors and from descending pathways, and thus mediate control of movements in which integration of different sensory modalities is important, as in touch. (Adapted with permission from Kandel ER, Schwartz JH, Jessell TM: *Principles of Neural Science,* ed 3. Norwalk, CT, Appleton & Lange, 1991, p 586.)

nated group IV afferents. Generally, these afferents carry information from nociceptors, touch and pressure receptors, joint receptors, and muscle receptors. These afferents, which produce flexion responses, are collectively called flexor reflex afferents.

The general response to activation of flexor reflex afferents is excitation of the flexor motoneurons and inhibition of the extensor motoneurons on the ipsilateral side, and inhibition of the flexor motoneurons and excitation of the extensor motoneurons on the contralateral side. Contralateral excitation of the extensor motoneurons (also known as the crossed-extension reflex) stabilizes the body as the ipsilateral limb is flexed. The basic circuitry for the flexion reflex is diagrammed in Figure 32.

Upper Motoneuron Syndrome and Spasticity

Disruption of motor pathways caused by stroke, brain trauma, or spinal cord injury leads to a variety of motor dysfunctions. The term upper motoneuron syndrome is commonly used to describe patients who have abnormal motor functions as the result of lesions to descending pathways at the level of the cortex, internal capsule, brain stem, or spinal cord. Patients who have upper motoneuron syndrome suffer from both negative symptoms or performance deficits and positive symptoms or abnormal behaviors (Tables 8 and 9). Negative symptoms include weakness and/or paresis, loss of dexterity (especially fine motor control of the fingers), and fatigability. Positive symptoms include abnormal posture, exaggeration of proprioceptive reflexes producing spasticity, and exaggeration of cutaneous reflexes produc-

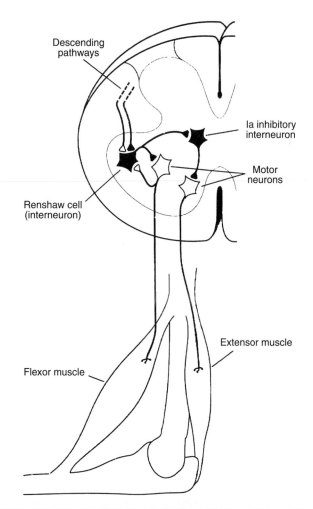

Figure 31

Renshaw cells produce recurrent inhibition of motor neurons. These spinal interneurons are excited by collaterals from motor neurons and then inhibit the same motor neurons. This negative feedback system regulates motor neuron excitability and stabilizes firing rates. Renshaw cells also send collaterals to synergist motor neurons (not shown) and to Ia inhibitory interneurons. Thus, descending inputs that modulate the excitability of the Renshaw cell adjust the excitability of all the motor neurons around a joint. (Adapted with permission from Kandel ER, Schwartz JH, Jessell TM: *Principles of Neural Science,* ed 3. Norwalk, CT, Appleton & Lange, 1991, p 585.)

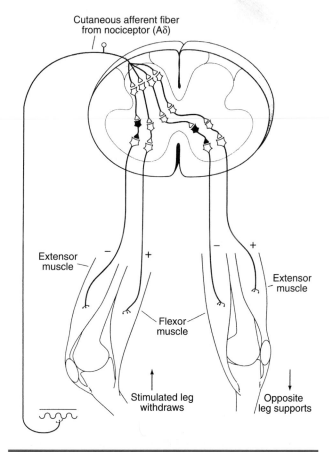

Figure 32

The flexion withdrawal reflex produces flexion of the stimulated limb and extension of the opposite limb. Stimulation of cutaneous afferents, such as an Aδ fiber from a nociceptor, produces excitation of ipsilateral flexor muscles and inhibition of ipsilateral extensor muscles, while producing the opposite response in the contralateral limb (the crossed extensor reflex). The cutaneous input is distributed over many spinal segments, so that the full reflex involves contraction of muscles at all joints of both limbs. The pathways are schematically illustrated here for 1 spinal segment only.

ing flexion withdrawal spasms, extensor spasms, and the Babinski response. These positive symptoms can be caused by the increased excitability of a specific part of the neural circuit or by the release of part of the neural circuit from the inhibitory control of another.

Spasticity, a common component of the upper motoneuron syndrome, is the result of changes in spinal proprioceptive reflexes; its severity and its time course depend largely on the location of the lesion(s) and the CNS pathways involved. For the clinician, the term spasticity often is used to describe such phenomena as (1) increased tendon reflexes; (2) increased resistance to passive movement of the limb; (3) flexor spasms associated with paraplegia; (4) motor dysfunctions, including decreased strength, speed, and range of voluntary movement; and (5) dystonia and rigidity. Spasticity also has been defined as a motor disorder characterized by a velocity-dependent increase in tonic stretch reflexes (muscle tone) with exaggerated tendon jerks, resulting from hyperexcitability of the stretch reflex. Because excitability of the stretch reflex is controlled by many different spinal cord circuits, a change in any one component of those circuits could modify the stretch reflex.

Diagnosis of movement disorders requires an understanding of the organization of the neural networks and pathways that mediate movement as well as an understanding of the integration of the motor system with the sensory system. Because of the intermingling of fibers from the cerebral cortex and brain stem, damage is rarely restricted to a single descending pathway. Selective damage of the corticospinal tract at the level of the medullary pyramids or cerebral peduncles produces only minor movement deficits. In general, the only permanent functional defect is the loss of independent control of the fingers of the affected arm. However, damage to the extrapyramidal fibers

Table 8

Findings in Upper and Lower Motoneuron Lesions

Findings	Upper Motoneuron Lesion	Lower Motoneuron Lesion
Stretch	Decreased	Decreased
Tone	Increased	Decreased
Deep tendon reflexes	Increased	Decreased
Superficial tendon reflexes	Decreased	Decreased
Babinski's sign	Present	Absent
Clonus	Present	Absent
Fasciculations	Absent	Present
Atrophy	Absent	Present

Table 9

Positive and Negative Symptoms Observed in Upper Motoneuron Lesions at Various Levels

Damaged Pathway	Level of Damage		
	Spinal	Brain Stem/Caudal to the Red Nucleus	Brain Stem/Rostral to the Red Nucleus
Pyramidal tract (corticospinal tract)	Weakness, loss of abdominal reflex, Babinski's sign	Weakness, loss of abdominal reflex, Babinski's sign, hyporeflexia, and hypotonia	Weakness, loss of abdominal abdominal reflex, Babinski's sign, seizure, apraxia, hyporeflexia, and hypotonia
Extrapyramidal tract (rubrospinal, reticulospinal, and vestibulospinal tracts)	Hyperreflexia, clonus spasticity, and clasp-knife reflex	Hyperreflexia, clonus spasticity, clasp-knife reflex, and decerebrate posture	Hyperreflexia, clonus spasticity, clasp-knife reflex, apraxia, and decorticate posture

or brain stem pathways is generally associated with the appearance of spasticity.

Spasticity is the result of changes in segmental spinal circuits, in particular, the stretch reflex arc. An enhanced reflex response to muscle stretch (hyperreflexia) could occur as the result of an increase in the excitability of the γ motoneuron and/or an increase in the amount of excitatory input elicited by muscle stretch. A motoneuron is hyperexcitable if it takes less than normal amounts of excitatory input to recruit the motoneuron or alter its discharge frequency, or if the same amount of input generates a greater response. A motoneuron would be at a state of increased excitability if it were constantly depolarized, that is, if the membrane potential were closer to the threshold for action potential generation. A depolarized state could result from a change in the balance of excitatory and inhibitory input to the motoneuron. Lesions to upper motoneurons may result in a reduction in the amount of inhibitory input to the motoneuron from inhibitory interneurons such as the Renshaw cell, the Ia interneuron, or the Ib interneuron. A motoneuron could also exhibit increased excitability if its intrinsic electrical properties were altered such that a given synaptic current generated a larger than normal voltage change in the neuron.

Another possible explanation for the hyperreflexia is that the imposed stretch on the muscle generates greater than normal excitatory input to the motoneuron. An increased synaptic current could result from the same stretch if the Ia afferent fiber showed an enhanced response to stretch, that is, greater rate of firing, because of increased gamma motoneuron bias or if the excitatory interneurons within the neural circuit were more responsive to muscle afferent input. The second alternative could occur as a result of (1) collateral sprouting, leading to an increase in the number of excitatory synapses; (2) denervation supersensitivity; or (3) a reduction in presynaptic inhibition of the muscle afferent, resulting in greater transmission of the excitatory signal.

Of the mechanisms mentioned above, there is no evidence in support of increased fusimotor activity leading to excessive muscle spindle activity, decreased group II inhibition, or decreased recurrent inhibition. There is evidence, however, in support of decreased presynaptic inhibition of Ia afferent fibers, decreased inhibition of antagonists through reciprocal inhibition, and increased motoneuronal excitability. Experimental evidence suggests that motoneuron hyperexcitability is not caused by a significant change in the intrinsic properties of the motoneuron. Therefore, the changes must occur as the result of alterations in the amount of excitatory and/or inhibitory input to the cell.

In summary, patients with upper motoneuron lesions demonstrate varying degrees of spastic hypertonia, in addition to paresis and loss of dexterity, flexor spasm, clasp-knife response, and cocontraction of agonist and antagonist muscles. Changes in reflex responses can, in part, be related to a loss of inhibitory control of segmental reflex circuits by

supraspinal pathways. In addition, local biochemical and/or morphologic changes at the spinal cord level may occur. These local changes could include collateral sprouting of intact dorsal root afferents, shortening of motoneuron dendrites, and/or denervation supersensitivity.

Peripheral Nerve Development, Structure, and Biomechanics

Nerve Trunk Development

The mature nervous system is composed of up to 10,000 different cell types, more than any other tissue in the body. The many classes of neurons in the brain are not randomly mixed, but are highly organized into a 3-dimensional pattern that evolves during development. The functional properties of the nervous system depend on this intricate network of neuronal connections, the development of which begins with the extension of the axon through a complex and mutable environment to reach one of many possible targets. The accuracy with which axons select pathways and synapse with the correct target organ is important not only during development, but also during regeneration after nerve fiber injury in the central and peripheral nervous systems.

Development of the nervous system begins after the formation of the 3 germ layers: the ectoderm, mesoderm, and endoderm. The endoderm gives rise to the gut and many of the major organs associated with the gut; the mesoderm forms muscle, skeleton, connective tissue, and the cardiovascular and urogenital systems; and the ectoderm forms the skin and the nervous system. During the neurulation stage of development in the embryo, the ectoderm further divides to form the neural tube, neural crest, and epidermis. At the same time, mesodermal structures are also formed; the somites form adjacent to the neural tube and provide the first segmentation in the embryo. Each somite is composed of 2 major tissues; the dermamyotome will form the dermis and back muscle, and the sclerotome will form the vertebrae. The neural tube eventually forms the spinal cord and the brain (that is, the CNS), and the PNS originates from a distinct group of neural crest cells. The motoneurons are derived from neuroblasts in the wall of the neural tube, and the afferent neurons are derived from the cells in the neural crest.

Individual axons exit the spinal cord at discrete levels via the spinal nerves; each nerve root consists of a ventral or efferent root and a dorsal or afferent root. In humans there are 31 pairs of spinal nerves: 8 cervical, 12 thoracic, 5 lumbar, 5 sacral, and 1 coccygeal. In a given species, the spinal nerves grow into the limb bud in a highly stereotyped way, collecting first into plexuses from which major branches emerge. From the major branches, axons diverge at highly reproducible anatomic locations to form nerves to individual muscles. In humans, 3 major plexuses—the cervical (C-1 to C-4), brachial (C-5 to T-1), and lumbosacral (T-12 to S-4)—provide innervation to the muscles of the upper and lower extremities. Each muscle is innervated by many motoneurons. These motoneurons are located in a specific and spatially discrete position in the lateral column of the ventral horn of the spinal cord. The motor pool, that is, the motoneurons innervating a specific muscle, forms a longitudinal column extending 2 to 4 spinal segments. Although the axons that innervate a specific muscle exit the cord through different spinal nerves, they converge to form a single nerve.

During development, motoneurons are able to find their appropriate targets with remarkable accuracy. The pathway taken by a nerve to a specific muscle is discrete, with few projection errors occurring. This precise patterning of the neuronal connections emerges, in part, from the interactions between the growing tips of the axons, the growth cones, and their cellular environment.

Spatial Distribution of Axons

The location of the motoneurons innervating individual muscles can be determined through use of retrogradely transported tracers, such as horseradish peroxidase. In general, the position of the individual motor pools within the spinal cord is related to the position of their target in the limb. More proximal muscles in the limb are innervated by more rostral motoneurons in the spinal cord. Analysis of the projection pattern of axons going to a particular muscle shows that, at the spinal nerve level, axons from many motor pools are intermingled. Axons to individual muscles begin to sort out into spatially discrete groups within and beyond the plexus (Fig. 33). The gross anatomic pattern of plexuses and nerve branches in the limb appears to be determined by the surrounding connective tissue matrix. The extracellular matrix material in the limb may provide paths that promote growth and barriers that inhibit growth of the axonal growth cones. Some of the molecules that may promote or inhibit axon growth are discussed in the following section.

Extracellular Matrix Proteins and Axon Guidance

General cell adhesion molecules are expressed on the neural epithelial cells and mesenchymal cells through which the first axons extend, and they appear to provide permissive substrates that promote axon extension. N-cadherin and neural cell adhesion molecule (NCAM), respectively, are integral membrane glycoproteins that are the most abundant Ca^{2+}-dependent and Ca^{2+}-independent adhesion molecules present on vertebrate nerve cells. Both molecules promote cell adhesion via the binding of the same molecular species (homophilic binding) on opposing surfaces of interacting cells. Both N-cadherin and NCAM are expressed on the neural ectoderm and the axons of differentiated neurons.

Laminin, fibronectin, collagen, and tenacin are glycoproteins found in the extracellular matrix. In vitro, laminin has been shown to be the most effective in promoting neurite growth. It is not as widely expressed as N-cadherin or NCAM and, therefore, may play a more specific role in promoting directional outgrowth. Laminin promotes extension by interacting with axonal glycoproteins that are members of the integrin family of receptors. The integrins are transmembrane proteins containing 2 noncovalently linked subunits.

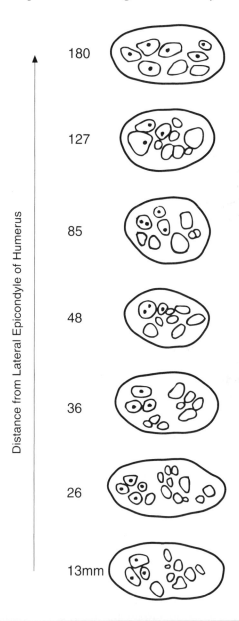

Distance from Lateral Epicondyle of Humerus

180
127
85
48
36
26
13mm

Figure 33

Selected transverse sections from a serially-sectioned radial nerve illustrating the fascicular redistribution of the different branch fiber systems brought about by fascicular plexuses. The levels are in millimeters above the lateral humeral epicondyle. The distribution of the superficial radial nerve fibers is indicated by the filled circles. (Adapted with permission from Sunderland S: *Nerve Injuries and Their Repair: A Critical Appraisal.* New York, NY, Churchill Livingstone, 1991, p 36.)

Several distinct α and β subunits have been discovered, and the types of subunits expressed determine the binding specificities of the integrin receptor. Antibodies against integrins inhibit the extension of central and peripheral axons on laminin or other extracellular matrix substrates.

Molecules that promote adhesion are important for axon extension; however, they may not provide directional cues to the growing axons. Axon guidance probably is derived from contact-mediated inhibitory interactions between the growth cone and surrounding inhibitory molecules that restrict growth across a particular surface and that cause the fasciculation of "like" axons (Fig. 34). Evidence for the existence of cell surface molecules that inhibit axon extension has come from the in vitro analysis of the interaction between neurons and oligodendrocytes. Developing axons will not extend on oligodendrocyte substrates. Mature oligodendrocytes express surface proteins that appear to mediate the inhibitory response because antibodies against these proteins neutralize the inhibitory properties of the oligodendrocytes. The presence of inhibitory proteins on oligodendrocytes is believed to be partially responsible for the inability of CNS axons to regenerate after injury in the adult. Contact-mediated inhibitory mechanisms may contribute to the selection of axonal pathways. For example, the segmentation of spinal nerves appears to be determined by inhibitory/adhesive molecules in the adjacent somites. Before axons reach the plexus region they must travel through the sclerotome of the somites. It has been shown that axons selectively project through the anterior somites and actively grow away from the posterior somites.

The segmental patterning of motor nerves may result from a combination of contract-mediated inhibition and selective adhesion between developing neurons. Glycoproteins, such as L1, G4, neurofascin, and contactin, which tend to be restricted to axonal surfaces, may play a role in the guidance of axons by causing the fasciculation of like axons. As later developing axons grow down the pathways traveled by the first growing axons, they may be attracted to axons with similar surface proteins. This type of mechanism may be important for the fasciculation of axons innervating a particular muscle.

Growth cones also may be oriented by diffusible chemotrophic molecules that are secreted by restricted populations of intermediate or final cellular targets (Fig. 34). Experiments have shown that in the absence of a muscle target, the outgrowth of the axons is random, whereas in the presence of denervated muscle, the outgrowth of the motor axons is directed toward the muscle. Additional experiments suggested that the motor axons were responding to a diffusible substrate being released from the denervated muscle. Extracts of denervated muscle have been shown to increase neuron survival and promote neurite extension of cells in culture. Consequently, diffusible factors that could influence axonal outgrowth may be released from muscle after denervation; however, the distance over

which these factors work is unknown. Additional chemotrophic molecules may be released from the distal stump of the damaged nerve.

Several experiments have shown that substances released from the distal stump of a damaged nerve can promote and direct the outgrowth of regenerating axons. The precise contribution of chemoattractants in vivo, however, remains to be determined. The demonstration of directed growth does not exclude the possibility that other factors, in addition to chemoattractants, are influencing the growth. A complete understanding of directional growth and the role of chemoattractants will require the isolation and biochemical characterization of specific chemoattractants.

Anatomy of the Peripheral Nerve

A peripheral nerve is a complex structure made up of individual nerve fibers, blood vessels, and supporting connective tissue. Individual nerve fibers collect into fascicles, which are surrounded by a connective layer called the perineurium. Within the fascicles, the individual nerve fibers are separated by a connective tissue framework called the endoneurium.

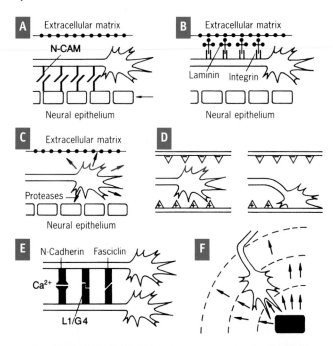

Figure 34

Mechanisms of neuronal navigation. Outgrowing neurites are guided by interactions with their surroundings. **A,** Adhesion between neurons and neural epithelium by homophilic interactions between cell adhesion molecules. **B,** Interactions between glycoproteins of the extracellular matrix and receptor molecules on the axon surface. **C,** Progression of growth cone by release of proteases. **D,** Selective attraction or repulsion between growth cones and cell- or substrate-bound molecules. **E,** Fasciculation of nerve fibers induced by glycoproteins on different growth cones or neurites. **F,** Chemotactic response of a growth cone to diffusible substances (after Dodd and Jessel). (Reproduced with permission from Reichert H: *Introduction to Neurobiology.* Stuttgart, Germany, Georg Thieme Verlag, 1992, p 197.)

Nerve fascicles are embedded in a connective tissue matrix called the epineurium, which provides a supportive and protective framework for the fascicles (Fig. 35).

Fascicular Organization

Individual fascicles are often grouped together into "fascicular bundles" separated by the deep, inner, or interfascicular epineurium. Nerves composed of 1 fascicle are referred to as monofascicular (Fig. 36). Nerves composed of many fascicles are categorized by the number and size of the fascicles: type 1 has few large fascicles; type 2 has many small fascicles that are approximately the same size; and type 3 has large and small fascicles combined together (Fig. 36). The general organization of fascicles in a nerve is summarized as follows: (1) Fascicles repeatedly divide and unite to form fascicular plexuses and, therefore, are not arranged as parallel uninterrupted strands along the entire length of a nerve. (2) No fascicle runs an unaltered course along the length of a nerve; however, at a given level, some fascicles may not participate in plexus formation. (3) The precise form of a plexus varies from nerve to nerve, level to level, side to side, and individual to individual. (4) The size and number of fascicles are inversely related at any given level. (5) The diameters of most fascicles range from 40 μm to 2 mm. (6) Fascicles are smaller and more numerous where a nerve crosses a joint, presumably to allow for nerve deformation without damage. (7) For a given fascicular area, nerve tensile strength increases with the number of fasci-

cles. (8) The fascicular structure of a nerve changes rapidly and frequently along its length; the greatest length of a major nerve with an unchanged fascicular pattern is about 15 to 20 mm (Fig. 37).

Fascicular anatomy is relevant to the consequences of partial injury, the pathology and classification of nerve injuries, and surgical nerve repair. A nerve with many small fascicles, as opposed to a few fascicles of various sizes, may sustain only partial injury after mechanical trauma because of the greater amount of epineurium (Fig. 38). In addition, nerve ends must be properly aligned during repair to maximize the potential for correct reinnervation.

Peripheral Nerve Connective Tissue

Endoneurium The endoneurium is a loose collagenous matrix that surrounds the individual nerve fibers within the fascicle. The matrix has large extracellular spaces and contains fibroblasts, mast cells, and a capillary network. Collagen fibrils predominate within the endoneurium and are closely packed around each nerve fiber to form a supporting framework. The collagen fibrils in the endoneurium of spinal nerves are fewer and finer than those in the endoneurium of peripheral nerves. The endoneurium forms a thin bilaminar sheath around each nerve fiber. This bilaminar sheath forms the wall of the "endoneurial tube," which contains the axon, the Schwann cell layer, and the myelin when it is present.

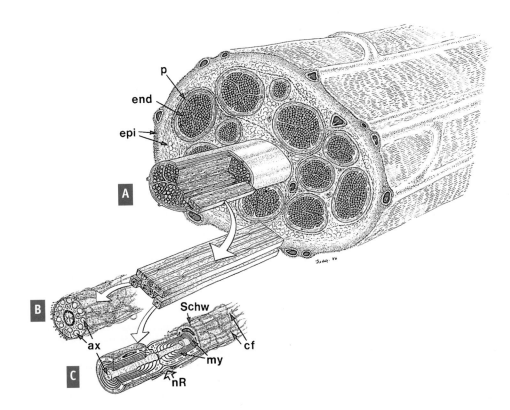

Figure 35

Microanatomy of a peripheral nerve trunk and its components. **A,** Fascicles surrounded by a multilaminated perineurium (p) are embedded in a loose connective tissue, the epineurium (epi). The outer layers of the epineurium are condensed into a sheath. **B** and **C** illustrate the appearance of unmyelinated and myelinated fibers, respectively. Schw = Schwann cell; my = myelin sheath; ax = axon; nR = node of Ranvier; cf = collagen fibrils. (Reproduced with permission from Lundborg G: *Nerve Injury and Repair*. New York, NY, Churchill Livingstone, 1988, p 33.)

Perineurium The perineurium is a thin, dense connective tissue sheath that surrounds each fascicle. The sheath is composed of 3 identifiable layers. The internal layer is composed of a single layer of flattened mesothelial cells that form a smooth inner surface with tight junctions at cell boundaries. The outer layer merges with the epineurium. At this junction, the perineurial cells are replaced by fibroblasts, and the collagen fibers become thicker and their

arrangement is less orderly. The middle layer is composed of flattened perineurial cells arranged in a series of 3 to 15 concentric lamellae. The lamellae are separated by spaces containing longitudinally oriented capillaries, collagen fibrils, and, occasionally, elastin fibers that are aligned longitudinally and obliquely. The perineurial cells in the middle layer have a basement membrane and tight junctions, and they function as a bidirectional diffusion barrier. The perineurium varies in thickness from 1.3 to 100 μm; there is a linear relationship between its thickness and the diameter of the fascicle. The tensile strength of the perineurium is high; the perineurium resists and maintains an interfascicular pressure that can be experimentally raised to 750 mm Hg before it ruptures. The perineurial diffusion barrier protects the fibers in the endoneurial space by preventing the penetration of the epineurial edema caused by ischemia. Spinal nerves do not have perineurial or epineurial tissue, which increases their vulnerability to stretch and compression injuries and to injury resulting from infections and exposure to chemicals.

Epineurium The epineurium is a loose meshwork of collagen and elastin fibers that provides a supportive and protective framework for the fascicles. Collagen fibers in the epineurium are thicker than those in the endoneurium and perineurium. The amount of epineurium varies from nerve to nerve and level to level and is generally thicker where the nerve crosses a joint. The epineurium is thought to protect the nerve from compressive forces. The epineurium contains a well-developed vascular plexus with numerous longitudinal main vascular channels feeding the endoneurial plexus.

The Blood Supply

The nerve fiber requires a continuous energy source to maintain impulse conduction and axonal transport. Consequently, peripheral nerves are supplied by a well-developed intraneural microvascular system consisting of separate but interconnecting microvascular networks within the

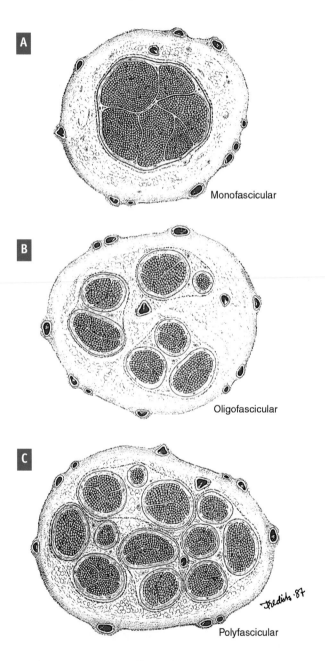

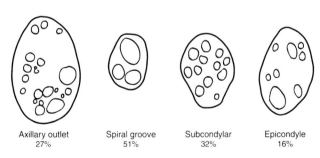

Axillary outlet 27%	Spiral groove 51%	Subcondylar 32%	Epicondyle 16%

Figure 36

Basic patterns of interneural structure. **A,** Monofascicular; **B,** oligofascicular; **C,** polyfascicular. (Reproduced with permission from Lundborg G: *Nerve Injury and Repair.* New York, NY, Churchill Livingstone, 1988, p 198.)

Figure 37

Variations in the size, number, and arrangement of fasciculi in a specimen of the radial nerve between the axilla and the elbow. The figures given are the percentage of cross-sectional area of the nerve devoted to fasciculi. (Adapted with permission from Sunderland S: *Nerve Injuries and Their Repair: A Critical Appraisal.* New York, NY, Churchill Livingstone, 1991, p 33.)

epineurium, perineurium, and endoneurium. The micro-vascular system of human nerves has been studied extensively. The vascular systems, both intrinsic and extrinsic, are characterized by longitudinally oriented vessels that communicate with each other via anastomoses. The intrinsic vascular system consists of the vascular plexuses in the epineurium, perineurium, and endoneurium (Fig. 39). The extrinsic vascular system is made up of segmental regional vessels that approach the nerve trunk at various levels along its course; these vessels run in the loose connective tissue meshwork that surrounds the nerve trunk.

In the epineurium, large arterial and venular vessels,

which run longitudinally along the nerve in close apposition to the fascicles, supply both the superficial and deep layers. The epineurial vessels anastomose with the perineurial vascular plexus, which consists of individual vessels located at various depths between the lamellae of the perineurium. The perineurial vessels travel longitudinally between the perineurial lamellae layers for a long distance before they pierce through the inner layer into the endoneurial space in a characteristic oblique manner. The perineurial vascular plexus and the endoneurial vascular plexus are an anatomically well-defined vascular unit that can be isolated and spared when fascicles are teased apart.

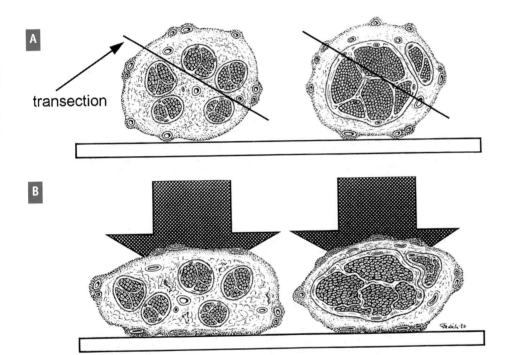

transection

Figure 38

Protective effects of the epineurium when a nerve is subjected to mechanical trauma. Several small fascicles embedded in a large amount of epineurium (**A**) are less vulnerable to transection injuries and compression than large fascicles in a small amount of epineurium (**B**). (Adapted with permission from Lundborg G: *Nerve Injury and Repair.* New York, NY, Churchill Livingstone, 1988, p 65.)

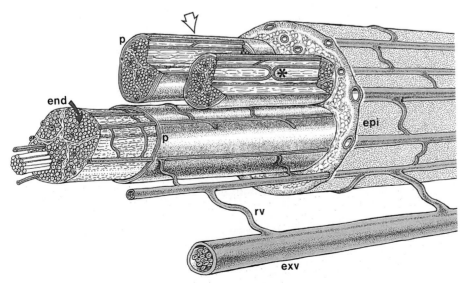

Figure 39

Interneural vascularization. Vessels are abundant in all layers of the nerve, forming a pattern of longitudinally oriented vessels. Extrinsic vessels (exv) are, via regional feeding vessels (rv), supporting vascular plexa in superficial and deep layers of the epineurium (epi), perineurium (p), and endoneurium (end). Note the oblique course of vessels penetrating the perineurium (arrows) and the intrafascicular "double loop formations" (*). (Reproduced with permission from Lundborg G: *Nerve Injury and Repair.* New York, NY, Churchill Livingstone, 1988, p 43.)

The individual fascicles, which often run together as a fascicular group, have a common vascular unit, which also can be defined and spared during surgery.

The endoneurial microvascular network consists of capillaries, arterioles, and venules; their vascular bed appears to form a continuous anastomotic network throughout the length of the fascicles. Their capillaries are unusually large, with the smallest capillaries having diameters of 6 to 10 μm compared to muscle capillaries with diameters of 3 to 6 μm. These capillaries have structural and functional characteristics similar to those of capillaries in the CNS. Consequently, the blood-nerve barrier is similar to the blood-brain barrier, being impermeable to a large range of macromolecules, especially proteins. The blood-nerve barrier and the diffusion barrier of the perineurium are essential for maintaining the appropriate endoneurial environment. The diffusion barrier can be damaged by metabolic and infectious diseases, intoxication, and irradiation, which can bring about changes in the ionic equilibrium, osmotic pressure, and endoneurial fluid pressure.

Response to Trauma

The PNS, like most other highly vascularized systems, responds to trauma with an inflammatory response. The epineurial vessels, which lack a blood-nerve barrier, respond to even slight trauma by increasing their permeability, leading to epineurial edema. The perineurial diffusion barrier prevents the edema from reaching the endoneurial space. However, severe trauma, such as crush or transection lesions, can induce increased vascular permeability of the endoneurial capillaries. This increased vascular permeability probably is caused by direct trauma to the blood vessels, but may also be caused by the liberation of endogenous chemicals that increase permeability. It has been suggested that mast cells, located in both the epineurium and endoneurium, release histamine and serotonin, thereby increasing vascular permeability.

Crush and transection injuries damage the barriers in the endoneurial and perineurial vessels. Compression injuries and ischemia may, under some circumstances, induce vascular changes in the endoneurial vessels without affecting the perineurial vessels. Under these conditions, edema would occur in the endoneurial space and would not be drained because of the functioning perineurial diffusion barrier. Normally, there is a positive pressure inside the fascicles, the endoneurial fluid pressure. However, edema-caused increases in the endoneurial fluid pressure could affect blood flow and the exchange of nutrient and waste products. Changes in the ionic content of the endoneurial fluid or a decrease in oxygen delivery and energy production may affect the nerve fiber conduction of action potentials and axonal transport. Chronic nerve compression or irritation may cause chronic intraneural edema, which could profoundly affect nerve function.

Nerve Biomechanics

Peripheral nerves, like other structures that involve a connective tissue matrix surrounding other structures, have biomechanical properties characteristic of soft tissues. For example, a nerve can be stretched and the load supported by the nerve measured. If such experiments are performed under controlled conditions, it can be demonstrated that nerves have a typical stress-strain relationship (see the chapter on biomechanics), with a compliant toe region observed at low strain and increasing stiffness at higher strains. This type of relationship has been thoroughly defined for other tissues, such as bone, tendon, ligament, and muscle.

A review of the literature reveals a wide variety of values for ultimate strain (that is, the strain at which a nerve fails), ranging from 20% to 60%. Table 10 gives some of the values that have been reported. Unfortunately, many of the ultimate strain values were historically derived by attaching a nerve to a stretching machine and deforming it until it failed. The distance between the clamps at the time of failure was used to calculate strain based on the original length (see the chapter on tendon, ligament, and meniscus). The problem with this approach is that it is difficult to securely fasten nerves to clamps and, as the tissue is deformed, slippage around the clamp occurs. As a result, the distance between the clamps overestimates the actual strain in the nerve material, and many of these ultimate strain values were probably artificially inflated. Several recent biomechanical studies of peripheral nerve, however, have been performed under conditions in which surface strain has been measured directly. In a study of the rabbit tibial nerve in which the nerve was slowly deformed from its "slack" length (defined as zero strain) to failure, ultimate strain was 38% ± 2% and the in situ strain of the material was recorded to be 11% ± 1.5%. In a study of the rat sciatic nerve, zero strain was defined at that point where the load rose above the noise level and continued to rise. In this study, mean ultimate strain was 16% ± 4.3%, and the mean in situ strain was 1.9% ± 0.58% (Fig. 40).

These data indicate that the nerve is under some degree of tension in the resting tissue and suggest that under normal physiologic conditions the nerve functions in the very compliant toe region of the stress-strain curve, where it probably produces low tension. This relationship may be dramatically altered, however, in those cases where nerves are repaired and the retracted stumps of the nerve are brought together under tension. In human nerves, gaps of 3 to 5 cm are often overcome to reappose the proximal and distal nerve stumps. Additionally, although nerves may not rupture until strains approach 20%, the nerve undergoes ischemic damage at strains approaching 15%.

The speed at which the nerve regains its structural strength is important because limbs are often immobilized for periods of 3 to 6 weeks following nerve repair in order to

Table 10

Comparison of Ultimate Elongation and Stress

Reference	Nerve	Ultimate Elongation (%)	Ultimate Stress*
Beel and associates	Mouse sciatic control	43	3.2×10^{-7} dynes/cm^2
	Crush, day 2	63	2.6×10^{-7} dynes/cm^2
	Crush, day 6	55	3.0×10^{-7} dynes/cm^2
	Crush, day 12	51	4.2×10^{-7} dynes/cm^2
	Crush, day 24	40	3.8×10^{-7} dynes/cm^2
Clark and associates	Rat sciatic	17	3.4 N
Denny-Brown and Doherty	Cat peroneal	43–316	NA
Haftek	Rabbit tibial	69.3	NA
Okamoto	Human median	18.4	1.32 kg/mm^2
	Human femoral	18.5	1.30 kg/mm^2
	Human sciatic	18.5	1.28 kg/mm^2
	Pig sciatic	18.8	1.25 kg/mm^2
	Pig median	18.6	1.35 kg/mm^2
	Dog sciatic	18.1	0.83 kg/mm^2
	Dog median	18.3	0.95 kg/mm^2
	Cat sciatic	19.2	0.95 kg/mm^2
	Cat median	19.0	1.12 kg/mm^2
	Rabbit sciatic	22.0	0.67 kg/mm^2
	Rabbit median	22.2	0.94 kg/mm^2
	Mouse sciatic	19.4	0.64 kg/mm^2
Rydevik and associates	Rabbit tibial	38.5	11.7 MPa
Sunderland and Bradley	Human median	19	1.7 kg/mm^2
	Human ulnar	18	1.6 kg/mm^2
	Human tibial	23	1.1 kg/mm^2
	Human peroneal	20	1.3 kg/mm^2
Yoshimura and associates	Rabbit tibial	31.8	NA

* NA, not applicable

protect the repair site. In an experimental study on rat sciatic nerve, end-to-end epineurial repair was performed immediately following a transection injury. The nerve regained 66% of its strength almost immediately after repair (within 7 days) and maintained a relatively constant level of ultimate stress and ultimate strain throughout the testing period, which extended up to 84 days. These data challenge the dogma that extended limb immobilization is required after peripheral nerve repair. However, because the study was performed in rats, which have a higher tissue turnover than primates or humans, it is not clear to what extent these results transfer to the clinical situation. It does appear, however, that nerves repair themselves much faster than ligaments and tendons. More studies are required to define the tensile properties of repaired nerve.

Like many other biologic tissues, nerves demonstrate time-dependent biomechanical properties (viscoelasticity). The familiar tests used to quantify viscoelasticity are the creep test and the stress relaxation test (Fig. 41). In the creep test, a load is rapidly applied to a nerve, and the nerve slowly elongates or "creeps" to a new length. The length of time required for the creep to occur is a measure of the viscoelasticity of the nerve itself. Similarly, a deformation can be applied to a nerve, immediately raising the load on the nerve. When the deformation is held constant, that load slowly decays; this phenomenon is known as stress relaxation, which is another measurement of nerve viscoelasticity. The parameters related to these properties are time constants. These properties have been derived for rabbit tibial nerves and show that nerves are not highly viscoelastic compared to tendon and ligaments. These data indicate that rapid movement of limbs, which results in rapid elongations of nerves, would probably not have a major impact on the stress experienced by the nerve and, therefore, would probably not contribute in a significant way to nerve injury.

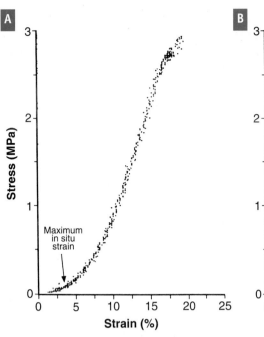

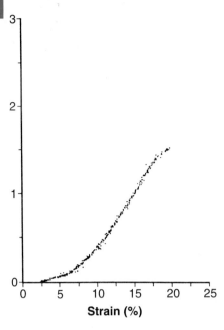

Figure 40

Stress-strain curves showing in situ strain in rat sciatic nerve. Control (A) and 7 days after repair (B).

Electrodiagnosis of Peripheral Nerves

Nerve conduction studies and electromyography can be used to evaluate the function of motor and sensory nerves and skeletal muscle, and have become invaluable tools for the diagnosis of neuropathies and myopathies. The objectives of electrical diagnosis are: (1) differentiation of weakness due to lower motoneuron versus upper motoneuron dysfunction and ventral horn motoneuron lesions versus more peripheral lesions; (2) identification of the involved muscles to determine the level of the injury and degree of dysfunction; and (3) demonstration of (a) muscle denervation to differentiate between a complete lesion and a reversible nerve conduction block, (b) reinnervation as proof of regeneration, (c) aberrant reinnervation following a peripheral nerve lesion, (d) diffuse or localized disturbances of nerve conduction in peripheral nerves, and (e) disturbances of neurotransmission at the motor end plate.

Nerve Conduction Studies

Nerve conduction studies can be used to determine the presence and severity of any peripheral nerve dysfunction, its localization (that is, cell body, spinal roots, plexus, or peripheral nerve), its distribution (focal, multifocal, or diffuse), and its pathophysiology (for example, axonal degeneration versus axonal demyelination). It should be pointed out that nerve conduction studies evaluate only the large myelinated nerve fiber function. Nerve fiber function is routinely evaluated in the following nerves: the ulnar, medial, radial, and tibial nerves (motor and sensory fibers); the sciatic, femoral, and peroneal nerves (motor fibers

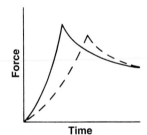

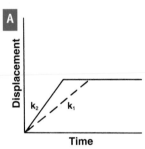

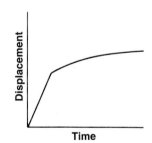

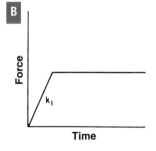

Figure 41

Curves for force relaxation (A) and creep (B) tests. Input loading curves are on the left, and typical output curves are on the right. (Reproduced with permission from Butler DL, Noyes FR, Grood ES: Measurement of the biomechanical properties of ligaments, in Bahnuik G, Burstein A (eds): *Handbook of Engineering and Biology*. West Palm Beach, FL, CRC Press, 1978.)

only); and the musculocutaneous, superficial peroneal, sural, and saphenous nerves (sensory fibers only).

Stimulation and Recording Procedures

Electrical activity can be recorded extracellularly from muscle or nerve using surface electrodes. Surface electrodes come in a variety of shapes and sizes. Commonly used

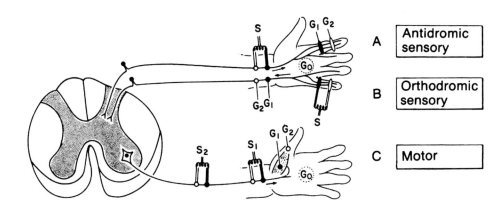

Figure 42

Diagrammatic illustration of electrode placement for nerve conduction studies. Antidromic sensory study (**A**); orthodromic sensory study (**B**); and motor nerve conduction study (**C**). G_1 = active recording electrode; G_2 = reference recording electrode; G_0 = ground electrode; S = stimulating electrode; S_1 = distal stimulation site; S_2 = proximal stimulation site. Cathode is black; anode is white. (Reproduced with permission from Sethi RK, Thompson LL: *The Electromyographer's Handbook*, ed 2. Boston, MA, Little, Brown and Company, 1989, p 4.)

types are small silver disk electrodes that are applied to the skin or ring electrodes that fit around the fingers. Stimulating electrodes come in pairs that usually are placed 2 to 3 cm apart. Several terms used to describe the electrodes are listed in the glossary and are illustrated in Figure 42. The stimulus artifact, which is the deflection from the baseline resulting from direct conduction of the stimulus, is often used for latency measurements as a marker of the onset of a sweep. It often is so large that it masks the onset of the response being measured. This phenomenon is related to excessive cutaneous spread of the stimulating current to the recording electrodes and is particularly noticeable during sensory stimulation in which the higher amplification of the signal is often needed.

The standard stimulus is a 0.1- to 0.2-ms square wave pulse at a slow repetitive stimulation rate of 1 to 2 per second. The intensity is gradually increased to get the maximal response and then increased 20% to 30%. This is referred to as supramaximal stimulation and is used to ensure activation of all the nerve fibers. The action potentials that are recorded have either a biphasic or triphasic configuration (Fig. 43). According to the convention of clinical electrophysiology, an upward deflection reflects a relative negativity of the active electrode (G_1) with respect to the reference electrode (G_2); that is, depolarization, and a downward deflection reflects a relative positivity of the active electrode.

Motor Nerve Conduction

To study motor conduction, the nerve is supramaximally stimulated where it is most superficial at 2 or more points along its course (Fig. 44). The motor response is recorded from a distal muscle that is innervated by the nerve (Fig. 42). In the recording of muscle potentials, the active electrode is placed over or close to the end plate region in the muscle, and the reference electrode is placed over the tendon. The evoked motor response is a sum of the action potentials of the individual muscle fibers and is called a compound muscle action potential (CMAP). It also is referred to as the M-wave. If the recording electrode is directly over the end plate region, the evoked response will be a biphasic potential with an initial large upward (negative) deflection followed by a smaller downward (positive) deflection (Fig. 43). If the initial deflection is downward or positive (Fig. 43), this suggests that (1) the recording electrode is not over the end plate region, (2) the active and reference electrodes have been transposed, (3) stimulation of neighboring nerves has occurred because of incorrect placement of stimulating electrodes or by spread of stimulus as a result of its high intensity, or (4) there is an anomalous innervation. The CMAP is described by its latency,

A Biphasic

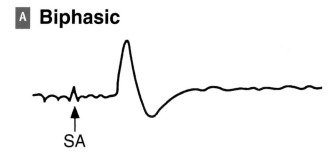

SA

B Triphasic

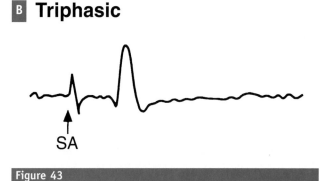

SA

Figure 43

Biphasic (**A**) and triphasic (**B**) wave forms. SA = stimulus artifact.

amplitude, area, and duration, which are measured as shown in Figure 45.

Latency and Conduction Velocity The latency is the time in milliseconds from the application of the stimulation to the initial deflection from the baseline. The onset latency is a measure of the fastest-conducting motor fibers and includes the time required to travel from the site of stimulation to the nerve terminal (nerve conduction time), the time required for the stimulus to activate the postsynaptic terminal on the muscle fibers (neuromuscular transmission time), and the time required for the action potential to propagate along the muscle membrane to the recording electrode. To measure the nerve conduction time, the CMAP is recorded after stimulation from at least 2 sites along the nerve. Because the neuromuscular transmission time and muscle fiber propagation time will be the same, the latency difference between the two represents the time required for the nerve impulse to travel from one stimulation site to the other (Fig. 44). The conduction velocity is calculated using the following equation: CV (m/s) = distance (mm) between proximal and distal stimulating sites/proximal latency (ms) - distal latency (ms).

Normative values for individual nerves in children and adults can be found in several textbooks. Table 11 lists some normative data for a few nerves at different ages.

In myelinated axons, conduction velocity is influenced by myelin thickness, internode distance, age, and temperature. Nerve conduction velocities at birth are about 50% of adult values, increasing to about 75% by 12 months and 100% by 4 to 5 years. The relative increase in speed is caused by myelination and increase in size of axons, which is usually complete by age 5. Temperature has a considerable effect on conduction velocity. As surface temperature decreases below 34°C, there is a progressive increase in latency and a decrease in conduction velocity.

Conduction velocity measurements vary between the upper and lower extremities and between proximal and distal segments of the same nerve. Upper extremity conduction velocities are generally 10% to 15% faster than those of the lower extremity. The lower limit of conduction velocity is approximately 50 m/s in the upper extremity and approximately 45 m/s in the lower extremity. Conduction velocity in the proximal segments is generally 5% to 10% faster than in the distal segments. This variation may be related to lower temperatures and smaller nerve fibers distally. In general, there is an error of about 5% to 10% in the measurement of conduction velocity caused by observer errors in measuring distance and latency.

Amplitude and Duration The amplitude of the CMAP is measured from the baseline to the negative peak or between negative and positive peaks and is expressed in millivolts (Fig. 45). With supramaximal stimulation, the area under the negative peak is directly proportional to the number of muscle fibers depolarized. Both amplitude and area provide an estimate of the amount of functioning axons and muscle, although area is a better measurement than amplitude. The duration of the CMAP is a reflection of the range of conduction velocities and the synchrony of contraction of the muscle fibers. The duration is measured as the time, in milliseconds, from the onset to the end of the initial negative phase. If the axonal conduction velocities vary widely, the muscle fibers will be activated at different times, and the duration of the negative phase will be long. Dispersion of the CMAP, which occurs when some axons conduct slowly (for example, in acute demyelinating diseases), is shown on the recording as an increase in the dura-

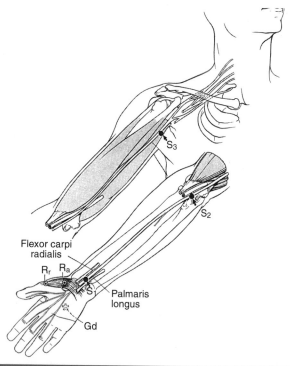

Flexor carpi
radialis

Palmaris
longus

Figure 44

Motor conduction set up for median nerve (motor). (Reproduced with permission from Liveson JA, Ma DM: *Laboratory Reference for Clinical Neurophysiology*. Philadelphia, PA, FA Davis, 1992, p 84.)

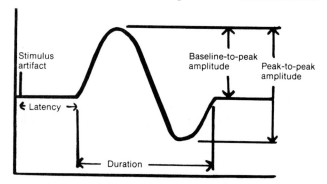

Figure 45

Measured parameters of a compound motor action potential. (Reproduced with permission from Sethi RK, Thompson LL: *The Electromyographer's Handbook*, ed 2. Boston, MA, Little, Brown and Company, 1989, p 10.)

tion and number of turns (spikes without baseline crossings) or phases (spikes with baseline crossings).

Sensory Nerve Conduction

Sensory potentials are unaffected by lesions proximal to the dorsal root ganglion even though there is sensory loss. Consequently, sensory potentials are useful in localizing a lesion either proximal (root or spinal cord) or distal (plexus or nerve) to the dorsal root ganglia. Sensory nerve action potentials (or compound nerve action potentials) are much smaller in amplitude than CMAP and are often obscured by other electrical activity and artifacts. Consequently, techniques that use digital averaging of multiple potentials and high amplification are often required.

Sensory axons are evaluated by (1) stimulating and recording from a cutaneous nerve, (2) recording from a cutaneous nerve while stimulating a mixed nerve, (3) recording from a mixed nerve while stimulating a cutaneous nerve, or (4) recording from the spinal column while simulating a cutaneous or mixed nerve. The recording electrodes are placed 3 to 4 cm apart, with the active recording electrode (G1) placed 10 to 15 cm from the cathode of the stimulating electrode (Fig. 46). Larger distances tend to increase dispersion and decrease the amplitude. Potentials recorded by an electrode that is placed closer to the spinal cord than the stimulating electrode are said to be orthodromic potentials (in the direction of the physiologic conduction), whereas those recorded by an electrode that is distal to the stimulating electrode are antidromic (in the direction opposite the physiologic conduction). The speed of conduction is the same in both directions; however, the amplitude is generally larger with antidromic recording because the recording electrode is closer to the nerve (Fig. 46).

An orthodromically recorded compound nerve action potential typically is a triphasic wave with an initial small downward (positive) deflection (Fig. 47). Antidromic recordings typically have a biphasic wave with an initial large upward (negative) deflection. The sensory latency is measured from the stimulus onset to the onset of the negative peak or to the top of the initial positive peak (Fig. 47). This latency measurement represents the conduction in the fastest sensory fibers. Latencies to the peak of the negative phase (peak latency) are often used because they are more easily defined, especially in noisy recordings. The conduction velocity (m/s) is calculated by dividing the conduction distance (in mm) by the sensory latency (in ms).

The amplitude of the response is measured from the positive to negative peak and is an estimate of the total number of fibers activated, although it is heavily influenced by the distance between the recording electrode and the nerve. The area under the peak is often difficult to measure because of the difficulty in defining the measurement points.

The F-Wave

The F-wave is a long-latency motor response to antidromic activation of α motoneurons in the spinal cord. The F-wave is evoked by supramaximal stimulation of peripheral nerves and can be recorded in almost all skeletal muscles. Supramaximal stimulation of a nerve results in an impulse that travels orthodromically toward the muscle and antidromically toward the spinal cord (Fig. 48). The short latency orthodromic response is called the M-wave and the late response occurring after the M-wave is called the F-wave. The latency of the F-wave includes the time required for the evoked potential to travel antidromically to the ventral horn of the spinal cord, the delay time to activate the α motoneurons (~ 1 ms), and the time required for the signal to travel orthodromically from the spinal cord to the muscle. With more proximal stimulation, the latency of the M-wave increases and the latency of the F-wave decreases (Fig. 48). The F-wave is small in comparison to the M-wave because not all of the motor axons activated in the M-wave are activated in the F-wave. The F-waves usually vary considerably in amplitude, latency, and shape with repeated stimulation because different groups of motoneurons are activated with each stimulus (Fig. 49). In general, the motor unit potentials activated in the F-waves represent the highest threshold, largest amplitude motor units. The shortest latency in a series of recorded F-waves is a measure of the fastest conducting fibers. The percentage of stimuli that

Table 11				
Mean Motor Nerve Conduction Velocities at Different Ages				
Average Age	**Ulnar Nerve** **m/sec**	**Median Nerve** **m/sec**	**Peroneal Nerve** **m/sec**	**Tibial Nerve** **m/sec**
5 weeks	34.5	33.1	37.2	34.2
1 year	46.1	41.8	44.1	38.3
4 years	52.4	49.4	44.2	43.1
6 years	56.1	54.9	52.2	48.4

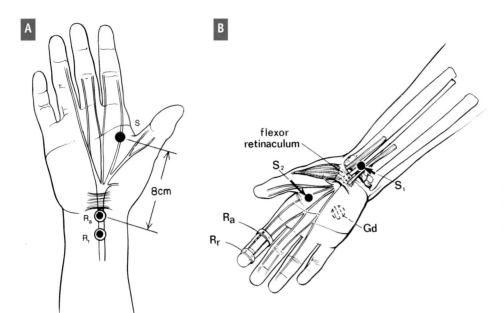

Figure 46

Carpal tunnel studies. **A,** Orthodromic palmar stimulation. **B,** Antidromic palmar stimulation. S = stimulating electrode; R_a = active recording electrode; R_r = reference recording electrode; Gd = ground. (Reproduced with permission from Liveson JA, Ma DM: *Laboratory Reference for Clinical Neurophysiology*. Philadelphia, PA, FA Davis, 1992, pp 116, 120.)

elicits an F-wave is termed F-persistence and is normally 90% to 100%. Inconsistency of F-waves may be an early sign of a neuropathy.

To record the F-wave, 2 sets of recording electrodes are placed over the end plate region of the muscle and over the tendon. The M- and F-waves must be recorded from different electrodes because a higher gain and different time base are required to record the F-wave. Usually 10 or more F-waves are recorded, and the shortest latency is measured. Other parameters of the F-wave that are measured are minimum-maximum latency differences, F-wave amplitude, F-wave persistence, and duration of the F-wave complex.

The F-wave is often measured to supplement routine nerve conduction studies because the F-wave permits evaluation of the proximal segments of peripheral nerves. F-waves are valuable in evaluating disorders involving the nerve roots, plexuses, and the proximal segments of peripheral nerves. Determination of F-wave latencies is particularly valuable in evaluating patients with demyelinating polyradiculoneuropathies.

The H-reflex

The H-reflex is an electrically evoked spinal monosynaptic reflex involving the Ia afferent fibers from the muscle spindles and motor axons. A submaximal stimulus activates the Ia afferents (large myelinated fibers with the lowest threshold for activation) in a mixed nerve, which in turn evokes a monosynaptic reflex contraction in the corresponding muscle. The motoneurons activated in the H-reflex are the lowest threshold, slow-conducting motoneurons. In contrast, the axons activated by the peripheral stimulation and recorded in the M-wave are the large, fast-conducting motor axons. The amplitude of the H-reflex is indirectly related to the amplitude of the M-wave (Fig. 50) and is maximal near the threshold for the M-wave. With increasing

stimulation intensity, motor fibers in the nerve are activated, with the resulting antidromic motor impulse colliding with the reflex impulse and obliterating it.

The H-reflex has several characteristics that differ significantly from the M-wave: (1) the stimulus threshold is lower than that required to elicit an M-wave; (2) the latency and waveform tend to be constant at a fixed stimulus intensity because the same motoneurons are activated each time; (3) the amplitude often exceeds that of the M-wave at low stimulus intensity, and the mean amplitude can be 50% to 100% of the M-wave; and (4) after the first year of life, the H-reflex is consistently found only in the calf muscles and flexor carpi radialis.

The H-reflex from the soleus is primarily mediated by the S1 spinal root and is the analog of the ankle reflex. A unilateral abnormality is useful in differentiating an S1 from an

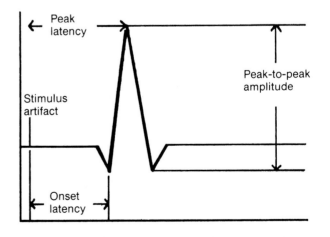

Figure 47

Measured parameters of a sensory nerve action potential. (Reproduced with permission from Sethi RK, Thompson LL: *The Electromyographer's Handbook*, ed 2. Boston, MA, Little, Brown and Company, 1989, p 16.)

L5 radiculopathy. The H-reflex in the quadriceps is used to study the L3 and L4 spinal roots. Bilateral H-reflex abnormalities are a sensitive indicator of a peripheral polyneuropathy, but must be differentiated from bilateral S1 radiculopathies. H-reflex abnormalities occur early in the course of demyelinating neuropathies.

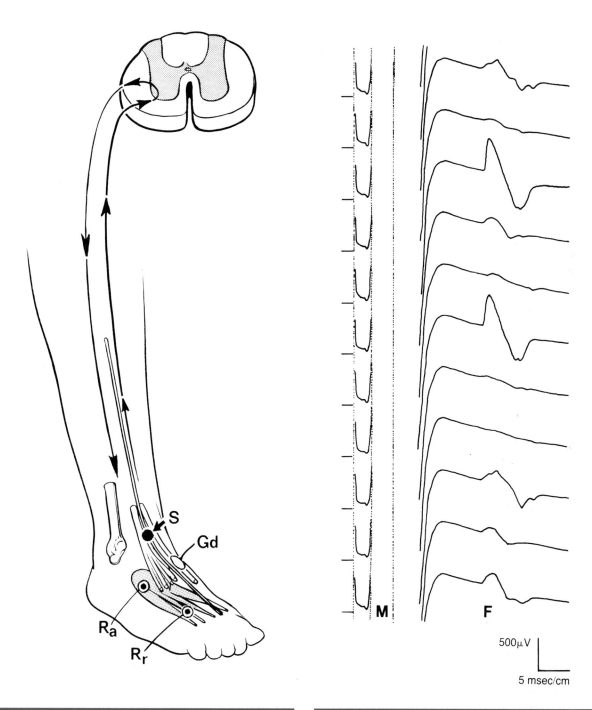

Figure 48

F-wave test. S = stimulating electrode; Gd = ground; R_a = active recording electrode; R_r = reference recording electrode. (Reproduced with permission from Liveson JA, Ma DM: *Laboratory Reference for Clinical Neurophysiology.* Philadelphia, PA, FA Davis, 1992, p 250.)

Figure 49

F waves. Median nerve stimulation at wrist with surface recording from abductor pollicis brevis. Calibration: 500 μV, 5 ms/cm. M = direct response, F = F waves. Note intermittent and varying configuration of F waves. (Reproduced with permission from Liveson JA, Ma DM: *Laboratory Reference for Clinical Neurophysiology.* Philadelphia, PA, FA Davis, 1992, p 253.)

Electromyography

Electromyography refers to the methods used to study the electrical activity of individual muscle fibers and motor units. Electromyographic (EMG) examination often is used in conjunction with nerve conduction studies and permits determination of the origin of the lesion as neural, muscular, or junctional. If the lesion is of neural origin, EMG studies can help localize the level of the lesion to the motoneuron, spinal root, nerve plexus, or peripheral nerve. EMG studies also can assist in determining the prognosis of a peripheral nerve lesion.

The electrical activity of a muscle is studied by inserting a recording electrode directly into the muscle. In screening patients for EMG studies attention should be paid to bleeding tendencies and unusual susceptibility to recurrent systemic infections. In addition, repeated EMG studies should not be done before muscle biopsies because the repeated insertion and movement of the electrodes will induce local muscle damage and inflammation that could interfere with the interpretation of subsequent muscle biopsies and histologic evaluation.

EMG Electrodes

Two types of electrodes are commonly used for EMG studies: the concentric needle electrode and the monopolar needle electrode (Fig. 51). The concentric needle consists of an outer stainless steel cannula through which runs a single wire that is insulated except at the tip. The inner wire serves as the recording electrode, the outer cannula serves as the reference electrode, and the patient is grounded by a separate surface electrode. The potential difference between the outer cannula and inner wire is recorded. Monopolar electrodes consist of a needle of solid steel, usually stainless, that is insulated except at the tip. The potential difference is measured between the tip of the needle and a reference electrode that is either a conductive plate attached to the skin or a needle inserted subcutaneously. The concentric needle records from a smaller area in the muscle than the monopolar needle and has an asymmetric pickup area as opposed to the circular pickup area of the monopolar needle. The electrode records motor unit action potentials with biphasic or triphasic waveforms.

A typical EMG recording session generally proceeds as follows. A needle is inserted into a muscle while the muscle is relaxed so that the presence and extent of any insertion activity can be noted. Then, the muscle is explored systematically with the electrode for the presence of spontaneous activity. The patient is then asked to contract the muscle voluntarily to submaximal force levels, and the parameters of individual motor units are studied at several different sites within the muscle. The parameters that are measured are the shape and dimensions of the potentials, the initial firing frequency, the rate at which a unit must fire before additional units are recruited, and, finally, the number of units recruited.

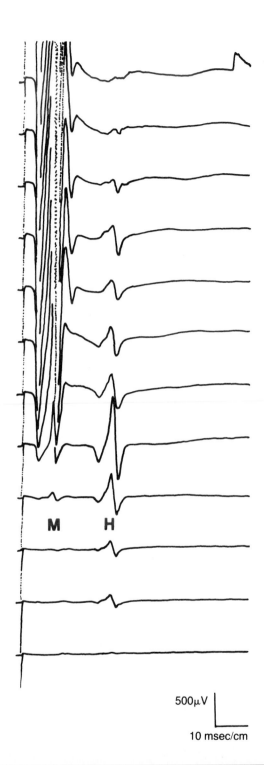

500μV

10 msec/cm

Figure 50

H-reflex. Popliteal stimulation of tibial nerve; surface recording from soleus. Calibration: 500 μV, 10 ms/cm. M = direct response, H = H-reflex. Increasing stimulus strength progressing from lowest to highest sweep. Note appearance of H reflex at low stimulus intensity, and its subsequent inverse relationship to the M wave with increasing stimulus intensity. (Reproduced with permission from Liveson JA, Ma DM: *Laboratory Reference for Clinical Neurophysiology*. Philadelphia, PA, FA Davis, 1992, p 240.)

Insertional Activity

When a needle is inserted into or moved within a muscle, there is a single burst of activity that usually lasts 300 to 500 ms. The activity is related to movement of the electrode and is thought to result from mechanical stimulation or injury of the muscle fibers. Insertional activity that lasts longer than 300 to 500 ms may be an early sign of denervation and is found in polymyositis, the myotonic disorders, and some of the other myopathies. In contrast, a reduction of insertion activity is found after prolonged denervation when muscle fibers have been replaced by connective tissue and with fibrosis.

EMG Activity in Resting Muscle

In healthy muscles, EMG activity usually cannot be measured at rest, except at the end plate region where 2 types of end plate activity can be identified. Table 12 lists the characteristics of end plate activity that can be recorded in normal muscle. End plate noise represents nonpropagated end plate depolarization (miniature end plate potentials) caused by random release of transmitter from the motor nerve terminals. End plate spikes are nonpropagated single muscle fiber discharges caused by excitation in the intramuscular nerves.

Spontaneous activity recorded from relaxed muscles that is not from the end plate and continues after the insertional activity has ceased is abnormal. The basic types of spontaneous activity that can be recorded include fibrillation potentials, positive sharp waves, fasciculation potentials, myokymic discharges, and complex repetitive discharges.

Fibrillations are action potentials that arise spontaneously from single muscle fibers. These potentials usually occur rhythmically and are thought to be caused by oscillations of the resting membrane potential in denervated fibers. They are typically biphasic or triphasic waveforms that are distinguished from end plate potentials by their initial positive phase and the high-pitched repetitive click that can be heard when the recordings are listened to over the loudspeaker. Other waveform characteristics are listed in Table 13. Positive sharp waves often are found in association with fibrillation potentials, but tend to precede them in appearance after a nerve lesion. Positive sharp waves arise from single fibers that have been injured. Their waveform consists of an initial positive phase followed by a slow negative phase that is much lower in amplitude and much longer (~ 10 ms) in duration.

Fibrillation potentials and positive sharp waves are found in denervated muscle, but may not appear for 3 to 5 weeks after the nerve lesion. They are most often seen in neurogenic lesions affecting the motoneurons, spinal roots, plexus, or peripheral nerves. They remain until the muscle fibers become reinnervated or the fibers become fibrotic. Fibrillation potentials alone are not diagnostic of denervation, because they occur in primary muscle diseases such as polymyositis and muscular dystrophy. Because these potentials can be found in healthy muscles, pathologic significance should not be attributed to their appearance

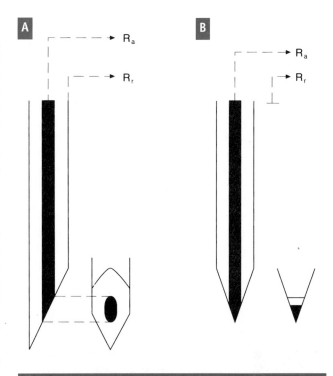

Figure 51

Concentric (**A**) and monopolar (**B**) needles. R_a = active electrode; R_r = reference electrode.

unless they are detected in at least 3 different sites within the muscle.

Fasciculation potentials are caused by the spontaneous discharges of a group of muscle fibers representing a whole or part of a motor unit, and usually produce a visible twitching in the muscle. Fasciculation potentials most commonly occur in diseases of the anterior horn cells. Grouped fasciculation potentials result from the discharge of multiple units and commonly occur in amyotrophic lateral sclerosis, progressive spinal muscular atrophy, or other degenerative diseases of the anterior horn cells such as poliomyelitis and syringomyelia. These discharges are referred to as myokymic discharges. During these discharges, multiple units fire repetitively, usually 2 to 10 spikes at a frequency of 30 to 40 Hz, recurring at regular intervals of 0.1 to 10 seconds. Myokymic bursts are thought to be generated ectopically in demyelinating motor nerve fibers.

EMG Activity During Voluntary Movements

Individual motor unit potentials can be measured during submaximal voluntary contractions using EMG electrodes. The motor unit action potential (MUAP) represents the summated electrical activity of the muscle fibers innervated by a single motoneuron that are within the recording range of the electrode. MUAPs are generally triphasic waveforms (Fig. 52) that are characterized by their shape, amplitude, and duration. With careful electrode placement and a patient who is able to produce a consistent submaximal voluntary contraction a single MUAP can be recorded.

For quantitative measurements, 2 to 3 motor units that can be clearly identified are recorded from each site. Several sites can be examined from a single needle insertion by advancing or withdrawing the needle in small steps and changing the direction of the needle. Typically, amplitude, duration, and shape of the waveform are measured for 20 or more MUAPs in a single patient during mild voluntary contractions. These values are compared with data from the same muscle in age-matched normal subjects examined in the same laboratory under similar recording conditions. The general characteristics of MUAPs in normal subjects are listed in Outline 1.

The rise time is measured from the initial positive to the subsequent negative peak (Fig. 52) and is a measure of the distance between the EMG electrode and the muscle fibers generating the major spike potentials. It should be less than 500 ms for the MUAP to be acceptable for measurements.

The amplitude of the major spike is determined primarily by those muscle fibers that are within a 1-mm radius of the recording electrode. In general, the higher the amplitude, the closer together are the muscle fibers belonging to the unit. Hence, the amplitude assists in determining the muscle fiber density within a motor unit. The duration measured from the initial deflection from the baseline to final return to the baseline reflects the activity of most of the muscle fibers in the motor unit and is a good indicator of motor unit territory. The shape of the waveform is also used for diagnostic purposes. An increase in the percentage of polyphasic potentials suggests desynchronized discharge or dropoff of individual fibers within a motor unit. The changes in the motor unit potential in myopathic and neuropathic disorders will be discussed at the end of this section.

Another way to measure changes in the structural and functional properties of motor units is to assess recruit-

Table 12
Normal Spontaneous Activity

Parameter	End Plate Noise	End Plate Spikes
Amplitude	10–15 µV	100–200 µV
Duration	1–2 ms	3–5 ms
Frequency	20–40 Hz	5–50 Hz
Firing interval	Irregular	Irregular
Sound	Hissing	Crackling
Waveform	Monophasic (negative)	Biphasic (initial negative)

(Reproduced with permission from Sethi RK, Thompson LL: *The Electromyographer's Handbook*, ed 2. Boston, MA, Little, Brown and Company, 1989, p 128.)

Table 13
Spontaneous Activity with Denervation

Parameter	Fibrillations	Positive Sharp Waves
Amplitude	20–300 µV (< 1 mV)	20–300 µV (< 1 mV)
Duration	1–5 ms	10–30 ms (< 100 ms)
Frequency	1–50 Hz	1–50 Hz
Firing interval	Usually regular	Usually regular
Sound	Crisp clicks	Dull popping
Waveform	Biphasic and triphasic (initial positive, then sharp negative)	Biphasic and triphasic (initial positive, then long negative wave)

(Reproduced with permission from Sethi RK, Thompson LL: *The Electromyographer's Handbook*, ed 2. Boston, MA, Little, Brown and Company, 1989, p 129.)

ment patterns during submaximal and maximal voluntary contractions. According to the size principle, small tension units are recruited before large tension units. As the demand for tension increases, the units that already are recruited increase their rate of firing, and additional units are recruited. The recruitment frequency is defined as the firing frequency of a unit at the time an additional unit is recruited. In normal subjects, the recruitment ratio (the average firing frequency divided by the number of active units) should not exceed 5. An increase in the ratio suggests a loss of motor units.

The interference pattern is the electrical activity recorded from a muscle during full effort. With maximal contractions, a complete or full interference pattern is recorded, implying that individual units cannot be recognized. The average amplitude of the cumulative response is an estimate of the number of firing units. In disorders that reduce the number of excitable motor units, the recruitment of additional units as force demand increases is limited; therefore, the surviving units must fire at an inappropriately high rate to compensate for the loss in number of units. In paralysis resulting from upper motoneuron lesions, the firing frequency during maximal contractions is generally lower than expected. In myopathies, the motor units are smaller in size than normal; consequently, a greater number of units are recruited to produce a given submaximal force. In advanced myogenic disorders, recruitment patterns are similar to those observed in neurogenic disorders because of the loss of entire motor units.

Single-Fiber EMG

In conventional EMG, a concentric or monopolar electrode is used to study the temporal and spatial relationship of action potentials from a restricted number of muscle fibers within a motor unit. Several other techniques recently have been developed to examine the activity of individual muscle fibers and motor end plates, the territory of a motor unit, and the cumulative activity of the whole motor unit. These techniques include single-fiber, scanning, and macro EMG.

Single-fiber EMG can be used to assess both the density of motor unit fibers and neuromuscular transmission. The electrode consists of a 0.5-mm steel cannula with 1 to 14 platinum wires, each 25 μm in diameter, exposed in a side port a few millimeters behind the tip (Fig. 53). The small size of the electrode surface allows selective recording of a single muscle fiber. Under certain conditions, the activity from 2 fibers belonging to the same unit can be recorded and neuromuscular transmission can be studied (Fig. 53). The time interval between the 2 action potentials varies between consecutive discharges. This variability, called jitter, results primarily from the variability in transmission time in the 2 motor end plates being recorded. Jitter is expressed as the mean consecutive difference (MCD). The MCD is the mean value of the differences between interpotential intervals of consecutive discharges and is calculated as

$$MCD = [D1 - D2] + [D2 - D3] + ... + [D(n-1) - Dn]/n - 1$$

where D = individual interpotential intervals and n = the number of discharges.

At least 50 discharges for each fiber pair and a minimum of 20 pairs should be analyzed when the abnormalities are minimal. Normal values for jitter range from 20 to 50 μs, but occasionally can be as low as 5 μs. Increased jitter is observed in myasthenia gravis and following reinnervation.

Single-fiber EMG can also provide information regarding

Outline 1

Characteristics of Motor Unit Action Potentials in Normal Subjects

Amplitude	Variable (up to 3 mV)
Duration	Variable (< 15 ms)
Frequency	Depends on degree of effort (up to 50 per second)
Shape	Biphasic or triphasic, 5% to 12% polyphasic (more than 4 phases)
Firing pattern	Semirhythmic
Sound	Sharp and crisp

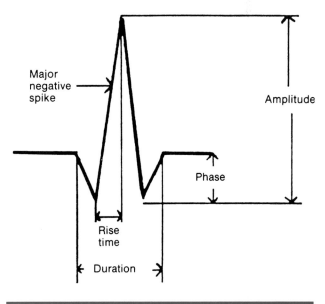

Figure 52

Measured parameters of a motor unit action potential. (Reproduced with permission from Sethi RK, Thompson LL: *The Electromyographer's Handbook*, ed 2. Boston, MA, Little Brown and Company, 1989, p 136.)

the local distribution or density of motor unit fibers that are within a 300-μm uptake radius of the recording electrode. The electrode is placed close to 1 active fiber, and the number of synchronously firing fibers is counted. To be counted, an action potential must have an amplitude exceeding 200 μV and a rise time less than 300 μs. The fiber density of a unit is calculated by taking measurements at 20 different sites within the motor-unit territory. In the extensor digitorum communis in young adults, the density is normally less than 1.5. After reinnervation, the density of motor unit fibers usually increases (Fig. 54).

Evaluation of Neuromuscular Disorders

Nerve lesions can affect either the axon or the myelin and can predominate in motor or sensory axons. Localized peripheral nerve lesions are characterized by 3 basic types of abnormalities: (1) reduced amplitude with normal or slightly increased latency; (2) increased latency with relatively normal amplitude; and (3) absent responses. Table 14 summarizes some of the patterns observed.

Axonal Neuropathies

Axonal neuropathies involve axonal degeneration and are characterized by reduced sensory and motor amplitudes with only mild slowing of the conduction velocities and latencies. The reduction in conduction velocity is generally less than 40% of the normal mean. Diabetes and alcohol abuse are the most common causes of axonal neuropathies. Most neuropathies affect motor and sensory fibers, but selective involvement of sensory fibers can occur with lesions affecting only the dorsal root ganglia.

Demyelinating Neuropathies

Demyelinating neuropathies are characterized by slowing of conduction velocities and latencies, including those of late responses such as F-waves. The slowing of conduction velocity is often greater than 40% of the normal mean. Values < 40 m/s in the upper extremity and < 30 m/s in the lower extremity are suggestive of demyelinating neuropathy. Slow conduction and dispersion can also be observed in immature regenerating axons.

Myopathies

Myopathies are polyphasic and are characterized by motor unit potentials that have small amplitudes and short duration (Table 15). These changes are related to a loss of muscle fibers within the motor units. There is rapid recruitment of motor units with a complete interference pattern of reduced amplitude on weak effort. Fibrillations and positive sharp waves can be seen in inflammatory myopathies, muscular dystrophies, and some toxic myopathies.

The electrophysiologic approach to the diagnosis of specific clinical disorders will be outlined next. These descriptions are taken from *The Electromyographer's Handbook*.

Motoneuron Diseases

EMG examination is the most useful test for evaluating motoneuron diseases. To diagnose diffuse degenerative diseases of α motoneurons, widespread and progressive neurogenic changes must be demonstrated, which could not

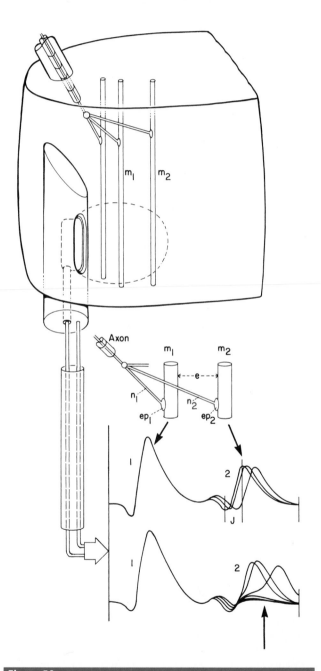

Figure 53

Single-fiber electromyography. Paired single-fiber action potentials are studied by using one to trigger a sweep. This permits the variation between the pair (J = "jitter") to be measured (upper record), and "blocking" to be demonstrated (arrow, bottom record). (Reproduced with permission from Liveson JA, Ma DM: *Laboratory Reference for Clinical Neurophysiology*. Philadelphia, PA, FA Davis, 1992, p 373.)

result from a focal structural spinal cord lesion. The following criteria can be used as guidelines.

The EMG shows abnormal spontaneous activity with fibrillations, positive sharp waves, and fasciculations. The motor unit potentials are reduced in number and increased in amplitude and duration, and there is an increased incidence of polyphasic potentials. These changes should be demonstrated in at least 3 extremities based on study of 2 or 3 muscles in each limb innervated by different nerves and roots.

In addition, motor conduction, including F-wave and H-reflex latencies, is either normal or shows mild slowing, and reduction of conduction velocity is less than 40% of the normal mean. Finally, sensory nerve conduction studies are normal.

Radiculopathy

The relative inaccessibility of roots and plexuses make radiculopathies difficult to diagnose. EMG examination is generally used rather than nerve conduction studies. Objective abnormalities on EMG may be absent if only the sensory roots are involved or if the lesion is purely demyelinating. Positive EMG examinations have a 70% to 95% correlation with myelograms. Clinical and EMG abnormalities caused by single-root lesions are generally partial because of multisegmental innervation. The following criteria can be used as guidelines.

The EMG diagnosis must demonstrate that denervation activity or chronic motor unit recruitment changes are restricted to a single root. The abnormalities should be documented in at least 2 or more limb muscles innervated by the same root but different peripheral nerves and absent in muscles not innervated by that root. Fibrillation potentials take 2 to 5 weeks to develop, whereas reinnervation changes take at least 6 to 8 weeks after the onset of symp-

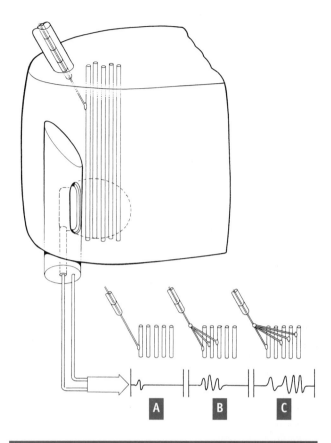

Figure 54

Fiber density studies. With the use of a single-fiber electromyography needle, multiple readings are taken of the number of single-fiber action potentials subtended by the field of the needle. These reflect the number of muscle fibers triggered by a single axon. Increasing reinnervation is represented in the figure from left (**A**) to right (**C**). (Reproduced with permission from Liveson JA, Ma DM: *Laboratory Reference for Clinical Neurophysiology*. Philadelphia, PA, FA Davis, 1992, p 378.)

Table 14

Patterns of Abnormality in Nerve Conduction Studies of Peripheral Neuromuscular Disorders

Disorder	Motor Nerve Studies Action Potential*				Sensory Nerve Studies Action Potential		
	Amplitude	Duration	Conduction Velocity	F-Wave Latency	Ampitude	Duration	Conduction Velocity
Axonal neuropathy	↓	Normal	> 70%	Mild ↑	↓↓	Normal	> 70%
Demyelinating neuropathy	↓ proximal	↑ proximal	< 50%	↑	↓	↑ proximal	< 50%
Mononeuropathy	↓	↑	↓	↑	↓↓	↑	↓
Regenerated nerve	↓	↑	↓	↑	↓	↓	↓
Motor neuron disease	↓↓	Normal	> 70%	Mild ↑	Normal	Normal	Normal
Neuromuscular transmission defect	(↓)	Normal	Normal	Normal	Normal	Normal	Normal
Myopathy	(↓)	Normal	Normal	Normal	Normal	Normal	Normal

* ↑, increase; ↓, decrease; ↓↓, greater decrease; (↓), occasional decrease

toms. Neurogenic changes start in the more proximal muscles and progress to the distal muscles. Reduced recruitment with increased firing frequency may be seen even before other EMG findings have developed.

Paraspinal muscle involvement is corroborative evidence of a proximal lesion, but its absence does not exclude a radiculopathy. Segmental sensory stimulation of appropriate cutaneous nerves is normal in spite of any sensory loss, because the peripheral sensory axons remain intact with preganglionic lesions. F-wave latencies are usually normal because the short involved segment is diluted by a long, normally conducting distal segment, but the H-reflex is often abnormal in S1 root lesions.

Entrapment Neuropathies

Mononeuropathies resulting from mechanical compression are referred to as entrapment neuropathies. The pathophysiology is focal demyelination, with secondary axonal degeneration as severity of compression increases. The 3 most common entrapment neuropathies are median nerve at the wrist, ulnar nerve at the elbow, and common peroneal nerve at the fibular head. A combination of a nerve entrapment and a radiculopathy (for example, carpal tunnel and a C6 or C7 radiculopathy) is not uncommon and is sometimes referred to as the double crush syndrome. Entrapments are characterized by the following electrophysiologic findings.

Focal slowing of conduction and/or conduction block is seen across the suspected site of the entrapment (Fig. 55). Sensory conduction studies across the entrapment are generally more sensitive than motor studies. Reduced motor and sensory amplitudes to stimulation distal to the entrapment indicate the severity of compression because they are a reflection of the amount of axonal degeneration. Moreover, with axonal degeneration, EMG evidence is seen of denervation and/or reinnervation restricted to the muscles innervated by the entrapped nerve distal to the site of entrapment.

Traumatic Neuropathies

Nerve conduction studies can assist in distinguishing between the 3 major types of nerve injuries: neurapraxia, axonotmesis, and neurotmesis. Table 16 lists the sequence of posttraumatic findings on electrophysiologic testing.

With neurapraxia there is immediate conduction block across the site of injury with normal conduction distally. With severe trauma, there is focal demyelination without disruption of the axons, and slowing of the conduction velocity can be demonstrated across the lesion.

With axonotmesis, there is interruption of the axons, resulting in immediate conduction failure across the site of injury. Axonal degeneration occurs distally; however, conduction velocity is preserved distal to the injury site for up to 7 days. There is a decline in amplitude of evoked responses on distal stimulation during the first week, progressing to complete failure of neuromuscular transmission. Denervation activity with fibrillation and positive sharp waves appears in the affected muscle in 2 to 5 weeks, depending on the distance from the injury site.

With neurotmesis, there is interruption of the entire nerve trunk. The electrophysiologic findings are identical to those seen with axonotmesis, but regeneration does not occur as expected and, therefore, surgical repair of the nerve is required.

Traumatic Nerve Injury

Localized nerve injuries fall into 2 main categories: those causing a temporary block of nerve conduction at the site of injury without loss of axon continuity, and those in which axons are severed or damaged to a degree that causes axonal degeneration below the site of injury and for a variable distance above the injury. The reaction to the second category of injury proceeds in 2 phases. In the first phase, the axon and the myelin sheath disintegrate along the entire distance distal to the site of injury and for some distance proximal to the site of injury. These changes, referred to as wallerian degeneration, result in the separation of the neuron cell body from the target organ; that is, denervation. Depending on both the injury's location along the axon and its severity, the cell body may respond by regeneration of the injured axon or by its own degeneration; that is, cell death. In most instances, the cell body's reaction is one of

Table 15

Typical Motor Unit Action Potential Characteristics

	Myopathy	Normal	Neuropathy
Duration	< 5 ms	5–16 ms	> 16 ms
Amplitude (mean)	< 200 μV	200–400 μV	> 400 μV
Waveform	Polyphasic	Triphasic	Polyphasic

(Reproduced with permission from Sethi RK, Thompson LL: *The Electromyographer's Handbook*, ed 2. Boston, MA, Little, Brown and Company, 1989, p 142.)

axonal elongation and restoration of axon continuity with the peripheral target organ. The details of axonal degeneration and regeneration will be discussed in a later section. The degree to which functional recovery occurs depends on several variables, including whether or not the endoneurial tubes have been transected or damaged.

Classification of Nerve Injuries

Prior to World War II, nerve injuries were categorized according to general terms such as contusion, concussion, stretch, compression, laceration, and division. In 1943, 3 classifications—neurapraxia, axonotmesis, and neurotmesis—were introduced based on the pathology of the nerve fiber and nerve trunk. In 1951, a classification scheme was introduced that included the 3 types listed above, but with 2 additional categories. This classification scheme describes 5 degrees of nerve injury increasing in severity from loss of conduction through loss of continuity of the entire nerve trunk (Fig. 56). This classification scheme is based on the histopathology of the nerve rather than the cause of the injury. Each of these injuries can be caused by a variety of agents: mechanical, thermal, chemical, and ischemic. The site of injury may be localized to a short segment of the nerve or it may extend over a considerable length. A description of the degrees in this scheme follows.

First-Degree Injury

The first-degree injury corresponds to neurapraxia and is characterized by an interruption of conduction at the site of injury. The severity of the injury, as measured by the duration of the conduction loss, is influenced by the magnitude of the deforming force, the rate of application of the force, the time over which it acts, and the manner in which it is applied. Conduction blocks are classified as either brief, mild, or severe, and have the following characteristics in common: the lesion is localized; the continuity of the axon is preserved; there is no wallerian degeneration; and all changes are reversible providing the offending agent is removed. As a general rule, motor fibers are more susceptible to injury than sensory fibers, and large myelinated fibers are more susceptible than fine or nonmyelinated fibers. Motor and sensory nerve fibers generally fail sequentially in the following order: motor, proprioceptor, touch, temperature, and pain. Recovery occurs sequentially in the reverse order.

The principal causes of conduction block are mild compression and ischemia. The mechanisms responsible for the cessation of conduction across a localized segment of nerve are not fully understood. This cessation is probably related to pathologic changes resulting from mechanical trauma and/or impaired blood supply, which could produce segmental demyelination and alter the ionic composition, nutrient supply, energy metabolism, and/or axonal transport.

In first-degree injury, there is conduction above and below the lesion, but not across the lesion. There is complete or partial loss of motor function depending on the number of motor nerves affected. However, there are no fibrillation or denervation changes in the affected muscles. In a severe first-degree injury, in addition to loss of motor function, there may be loss of all forms of sensation in those areas innervated by the injured nerves. Frequently, however, the

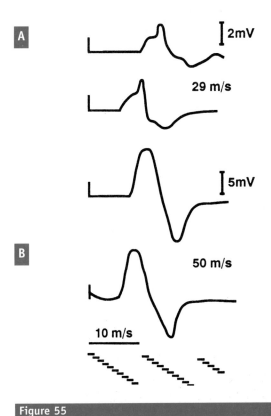

A 2mV

29 m/s

5mV

B 50 m/s

10 m/s

Figure 55

A, Ulnar entrapment neuropathy with stimulation 6 cm above and 4 cm below the ulnar sulcus. **B,** Normal ulnar nerve conduction with same stimulation site is shown below for comparison. (Adapted with permission from Sethi RK, Thompson LL: *The Electromyographer's Handbook,* ed 2. Boston, MA, Little, Brown and Company, 1989, p 165.)

Table 16	
Sequence of Events After Traumatic Nerve Injury	
Electrophysiologic Abnormality	**Timing of Onset**
Conduction block across injury site	Immediate
Reduced amplitudes on distal stimulation	> 7 days
Denervation changes on EMG	2–5 weeks
Reinnervation on EMG (partial lesion)	> 6–8 weeks

EMG, Electromyography. (Reproduced with permission from Sethi RK, Thompson LL: The Electromyographer's Handbook, ed 2. Boston, MA, Little, Brown & Company, 1989, p 166.)

only sensory defect that can be detected is loss of proprioception. There is complete functional recovery after first-degree injuries because axonal continuity is preserved and the changes responsible for the conduction loss are fully reversible. Full restoration of function may take as long as 3 to 4 months after the injury. A residual motor deficit indicates a loss of axons and suggests a more severe injury.

Second-Degree Injury

The second-degree injury corresponds to axonotmesis. These injuries involve severe damage or severance of the axon, leading to wallerian degeneration. The continuity of the endoneurial sheath and the basal lamina of the Schwann cell layer is maintained. Consequently, the axon regenerates within its original endoneurial tube and is guided back to its original target, thereby ensuring complete and functional restoration of motor and sensory functions.

A second degree injury results in complete loss of motor and sensory functions. The distal segment can be electrically activated immediately after the lesion; however, conduction distal to the lesion is lost within 24 to 72 hours after the injury. Fibrillation and other EMG signs of denervation are evident in the muscles, and the denervated muscles begin to atrophy. The interval between injury and the onset of recovery is influenced by the severity and the level of the injury because regenerating axons must elongate over a greater distance after proximal as opposed to distal lesions.

The next 3 classifications correspond to divisions of the neurotmesis classification of nerve injury. The injuries progress from damage to the axon and endoneurial tube, to damage to the perineurium and fascicular organization, to complete severance of the epineurium.

Third-Degree Injury

The third-degree injury involves degeneration of the axons and loss of endoneurial tube continuity. The internal struc-

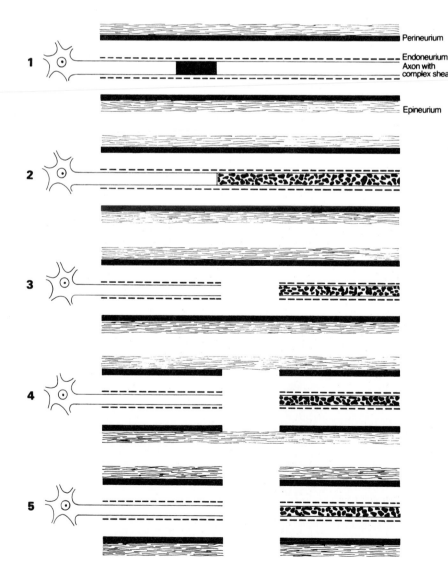

Figure 56

Diagram illustrating the 5 degrees of nerve injury. (**1**) Conduction block. (**2**) The lesion confined to the axon within an intact endoneurial sheath and resulting in wallerian degeneration. (**3**) Loss of nerve fiber continuity (axon and endoneurial sheath) inside an intact perineurium. (**4**) Loss of fascicular continuity with nerve trunk continuity depending solely on epineurial tissue. (**5**) Loss of continuity of the entire nerve trunk. (Adapted with permission from Sunderland S: *Nerve Injuries and Their Repair: A Critical Appraisal.* New York, NY, Churchill Livingstone, 1991, p 222.)

ture of the fascicle is disorganized, but the arrangement of the individual fascicles is preserved; that is, the perineurium remains intact. Intrafascicular damage may include hemorrhage, edema, and ischemia. Intrafascicular fibrosis may occur, which can seriously impede axon regeneration and elongation across the injury site. If the axons are injured at proximal levels (close to the spinal roots), loss of axons may be caused by degeneration of the cell bodies within the spinal cord.

A third-degree injury results in complete loss of motor and sensory functions in the region served by the nerve. The onset of recovery is delayed for longer periods than in second-degree injuries because of the more severe retrograde disturbances to the cell body and the additional time taken by the regenerating axons to traverse the disorganized and possibly fibrotic internal structures of the fascicles. In addition, the muscles remain in a denervated state for a longer period of time and, consequently, additional time may be required for functional recovery when the muscles are reinnervated.

The outcome of third-degree injuries varies depending on the loss of axons, the extent and severity of intrafascicular fibrosis, and the extent of incomplete and incorrect reinnervation of the denervated muscles. Because of the loss of continuity of the endoneurial tube, axons may be misdirected and reinnervate inappropriate targets. The degree to which inappropriate reinnervation occurs depends on the nerve fiber composition of the affected fascicles. If the nerve fibers within the fascicles innervate the same or functionally similar targets, then the functional outcome will be minimally affected. However, if the fascicles are composed of nerve fibers from functionally unrelated targets and, in particular, if motor and sensory fibers are intermingled, the reinnervation is often misdirected and incorrect, leading to poor functional recovery. In general, the more proximal the injury, the worse the prognosis for functional recovery because the nerve fibers from distal targets are intermingled and more widely distributed over the fascicles.

Fourth-Degree Injury

In the fourth-degree injury, the continuity of the nerve trunk is preserved; however, the fascicles are ruptured or so disorganized that they can no longer be demarcated from the epineurium. Wallerian degeneration follows the usual pattern. The retrograde neuronal effects are more severe than in third-degree injuries and, consequently, there is a higher incidence of neuronal cell-body degeneration and axon loss. In addition, axon regeneration and elongation are complicated by extensive intraneural scarring and complete disruption of the fascicular structure. Thus, the number of axons that make it back to their original targets is greatly reduced.

A fourth-degree injury results in complete loss of motor and sensory functions in the region served by the nerve.

There may be spontaneous regeneration; however, it rarely proceeds in a useful manner. Generally, this type of injury requires excision of the damaged segment and surgical repair of the nerve.

Fifth-Degree Injury

A fifth-degree injury is one in which there is loss of continuity of the nerve trunk. Generally, the nerve ends remain separated, and varying amounts of scar tissue may form between the cut ends. Often, a neuroma forms on the proximal stump. Wallerian degeneration occurs in the distal stump. Although some axons may regenerate and elongate along the distal stump, the chances for restoring function are minimal because the number of axons that regenerate across the lesion are few in number and the reinnervation is usually incorrect. These types of injuries require surgical nerve repair.

Causes of Nerve Injuries

Nerve injuries can be caused by a variety of agents. A nerve can be damaged by physical trauma in the form of compression, stretch, or friction. Compression is defined as a force applied to the nerve that results in an alteration in the cross-sectional dimensions of the nerve. Stretch or traction is a deforming force applied along the long axis of the nerve, resulting in increases in its length. Friction is applied to a nerve when it rubs across a rough surface or structure. Compression and stretch injuries can be open or closed and can be first- through fifth-degree injuries. Friction-based injuries are closed injuries; the most common are entrapment nerve lesions.

Nerve injuries can also be caused by ischemia, a reduction in blood supply to the nerve resulting from constriction or obstruction of a blood vessel. Ischemia is often a component of nerve injuries that result from physical trauma. A nerve can be damaged by therapeutic agents (such as phenol and lidocaine) that are inadvertently injected into the nerve or purposely injected into the nerve with the intention of decreasing abnormal activity in the nerve fibers. Other miscellaneous causes of nerve injury include dislocations, closed and open fractures, high velocity and other missile wounding, childbearing, and compression injuries caused during anesthesia, coma, drug narcosis, and the undisturbed sleep of the fatigued and wasted individual.

Compression Nerve Injury

Nerve compression injuries fall into 2 major categories: acute injuries of immediate onset and chronic injuries of delayed and gradual onset. The deforming force can be from either an external or internal source. The primary underlying cause of the impaired nerve function in acute and chronic compression lesions is related to a combination of mechanical and ischemic factors.

Categories of Compression Injuries

The extent and severity of the compression lesions are determined by the magnitude and rate of application of the force, the duration over which the force is applied, and the manner in which it is applied. The magnitude of the force can be mild, intermediate, or severe. Mild compression produces first- and second-degree injuries, intermediate forces produce third-degree injuries, and severe forces can cause damage resulting in fourth- and even fifth-degree injuries. Nerves can tolerate greater magnitudes of force when the deforming force is applied gradually and slowly increases over long periods of time (months and years versus milliseconds and seconds). The manner in which the force is applied (Fig. 57) will also influence the severity of the lesion. The force may be localized to a point on the surface of the nerve, leading to a penetrating or puncture injury; it may slice obliquely or transversely across the nerve; or it may be applied to a length of the nerve and crush or lacerate that segment.

Features That Increase the Vulnerability to Compression Injury

Not all nerve fibers respond the same way to compression. Nerve fibers that are collected into a single or a few large closely packed fascicles with little epineurium are more susceptible to compression injuries than nerve fibers collected into several small fascicles embedded in a large amount of epineurium. This phenomenon is thought to be related to the manner in which the compressive forces are dispersed through the epineurium (Fig. 38). Spinal nerve roots are more vulnerable to compression injury than peripheral nerves because they lack epineurial and perineurial tissues. Within a fascicle, the damage to a nerve fiber may be related to its position, with fibers situated near the surface of the fascicle suffering more than fibers situated more centrally, and its size, with large fibers more susceptible than small fibers.

A nerve is at particular risk in areas where (1) it is in direct contact with an unyielding surface against which it can be compressed, for example, the ulnar nerve behind the medial humeral epicondyle, the radial nerve in the musculospiral groove of the humerus, and the common peroneal nerve near the head of the fibula; (2) it passes through, or is contained within, a compartment with unyielding walls, for example, the median nerve in the carpal tunnel and the lumbar plexus in the psoas compartment; or (3) it is intimately related to a structure that would stretch or compress the nerve if enlarged; for example, aneurysmal swelling of a vessel in contact with the nerve.

Biologic Effects of Pressure

The effects of compression on intraneural tissues are illustrated in Figure 58. In severe acute injuries, the mechanical deformation of the nerve fibers is primarily responsible for the pathologic changes in the nerve. In chronic compression, ischemia becomes a significant factor in the genesis of the injury. Delayed secondary effects include edema, hemorrhage, neural fibrosis, and the formation of adhesions that impair the gliding of the nerve.

The mildest compression injury is the prolonged conduction block or first-degree injury. In these injuries, the block is rapidly reversible when the deforming force is released, suggesting that it is associated with impaired oxygenation caused by partial or total occlusion of intraneural vessels. Extended periods of vascular occlusion may result in edema, which will extend the period required for recovery. Under higher compressive forces, there is not only vascular obstruction, but also mechanical deformation of nerve fibers and blood vessels. Examples of this type of injury include unrelieved pressure on the radial nerve and tourniquet compression. In these instances, long-lasting conduction block may result from local intraneural edema and segmental demyelination. Severe compressive forces may lead to further damage to the various connective tissues, resulting in third- and fourth-degree injuries.

Recent studies have addressed the question of critical pressure levels for peripheral nerve viability in humans. Patients who have carpal tunnel syndrome have intracarpal canal tissue pressures of 32 mm Hg as compared to an average pressure of 2.5 mm Hg in control subjects. Based on these data, a human model was developed to study the effects of induced intracarpal pressures of various levels on sensory and motor function of the median nerve. At a tissue pressure of 30 mm Hg in the carpal tunnel, mild neurophysiologic changes and symptoms were found, including paresthesia and a slight increase in latencies. Complete blockage of motor and sensory conduction was found at tissue fluid pressures of 50 to 60 mm Hg. The sensory action potential decreased rapidly and disappeared after 25 to 50 minutes, and the motor potential disappeared 10 to 30 minutes after the disappearance of the sensory potential.

There is experimental and clinical evidence that tourniquet ischemia can cause compression lesions and nerve dysfunction. Cuff pressures sufficient to occlude blood flow in the upper arm will also block nerve conduction within 15 to 45 minutes. At a cuff pressure of 150 mm Hg, sensory loss and paralysis develop at the same rate as when a pressure of 300 mm Hg is used, suggesting that ischemia rather than

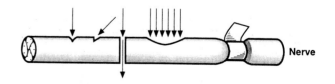

Figure 57

Manner in which compressive force can be applied to nerve. (Adapted with permission from Sunderland S: *Nerve Injuries and Their Repair: A Critical Appraisal.* New York, NY, Churchill Livingstone, 1991, p 131.)

mechanical pressure is the underlying cause of the conduction block. Reported complications vary from slight disturbances in sensibility to total paralysis involving the median, ulnar, and radial nerves in the forearm and hand. In most cases, complete recovery occurred within 3 to 6 months. The majority of cases involved faulty pressure gauges, with the actual applied pressures varying from 350 to 1,200 mm Hg.

There are also reports of nerve injuries following the use of a tourniquet to the lower extremity. In a study of 48 arthrotomy patients where the cuff pressure was between 350 and 450 mm Hg, more than 50% had EMG changes postsurgery. In those surgeries that exceeded 1 hour, 85% of the patients had abnormal EMGs postsurgery. To minimize the effects of tourniquet ischemia on muscle and nerve, it is recommended that the pressure in the cuff used for upper extremity surgery be no more than 50 to 100 mm Hg above the systolic pressure. For lower extremity surgery, twice the systolic pressure is recommended. Tourniquets should not be applied for more than 2 hours to minimize neural and muscular injury.

External compression of a nerve causes obstruction of intraneural blood vessels, jeopardizing the microcirculation in the nerve. Ischemia induced by compression may cause anoxic and mechanical damage to endothelial cells of the intraneural microvessels, resulting in increased permeability to water, various ions, and proteins. Consequently, ischemia may lead to intraneural edema when the blood flow is restored. The extent of the edema is influenced by the magnitude and duration of the compression. In the rab-

bit tibial nerve, compression at 50 mm Hg for 2 hours induced edema that was restricted to the epineurium. Increasing the pressure to 200 mm Hg caused endoneurial edema at the edge of the nerve segment, but not in the center. When the duration was increased to 4 and 6 hours at a pressure of 200 mm Hg, endoneurial edema was observed in the center as well as the edges of the compressed segment.

Endoneurial fluid pressure can be measured following ischemia/compression. A threefold increase of pressure was observed in rabbits after compression at 30 or 80 mm Hg for 8 hours. The endoneurial fluid pressure was still elevated to the same level 24 hours after the compression was removed. The increase in pressure was associated with a marked endoneurial edema, with separation of nerve fibers and nerve fiber injury of varying degrees beneath the perineurium. Demyelination of superficial fibers within the fascicles could be seen at pressures of only 30 mm Hg. At higher pressures (80 mm Hg), axonal damage was observed.

The results show that compression causes increases in endoneurial fluid pressures, which parallel the occurrence of endoneurial edema. If sustained, such pressure increases have been shown to cause nerve fiber damage, changes in the electrolyte composition of the endoneurial fluid, and impairment of endoneurial capillary blood flow. Compression may also influence nerve function by impairing axonal transport directly through production of a mechanical block or secondarily through induction of anoxia, because both slow and fast transport depend on ATP derived from oxidative metabolism. Several studies have shown that both slow and fast transport are impaired in a graded manner with compression. These results indicate that pressures comparable to those found in patients with carpal tunnel syndrome may interfere with both the slow and fast axonal transport systems. Impairment of axonal transport systems is thought to be partially responsible for the double crush syndrome.

Compression could also induce nerve injury via direct mechanical trauma to the nerve. Extreme tourniquet pressures (1,000 mm Hg) have been shown to cause nerve injury to single fibers by displacement of the nodes of Ranvier. The damage was found to be restricted to large, myelinated fibers under the edge of the cuff. In summary, the majority of the data suggest that in chronic compression nerve lesions, the primary pathology is based on vascular complications. However, the contribution of direct physical deformation cannot be disregarded.

Double Crush Syndrome

Patients who have symptoms of a nerve entrapment at one level commonly also have symptoms that indicate compression of the same nerve at another level of the same extremity. Of 115 patients with either carpal tunnel syndrome or ulnar neuropathy, 70% also showed evidence of cervicothoracic root lesions. The term double crush syndrome was introduced to describe this phenomenon. From

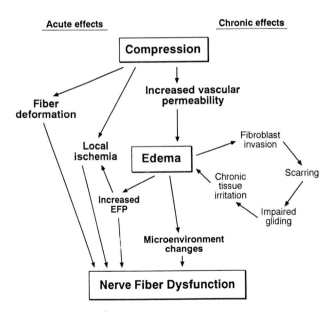

Figure 58

Effects of compression on intraneural tissues. (Adapted with permission from Lundborg G: *Nerve Injury and Repair.* New York, NY, Churchill Livingstone, 1988, p 64.)

the clinical observations, it was postulated that a partial lesion at one level of nerve makes the nerve more susceptible to compression at another site. These ideas are not universally accepted, but have raised interesting questions that are being studied.

One of the postulated mechanisms is that proximal compression of a nerve fiber leads to impairments in slow and fast transport. The disruption of axonal transport systems decreases the delivery of cytoskeletal components, such as tubulin, actin, and other membrane proteins, to the distal axons. This decrease impairs the quality of the axoplasm as well as the axonal membrane in the distal segment, making the distal nerve more vulnerable to physical trauma, such as compression. The reverse situation may also occur; that is, a distal impingement of a peripheral nerve may contribute to the development of an entrapment neuropathy at more proximal levels. A typical example is ulnar nerve entrapment at the wrist level caused by a local blow to the wrist, which later changes in nature, resulting in symptoms that indicate ulnar nerve compression at the elbow level. Additional explanations for the occurrence of multiple compressive injuries in a nerve include: (1) endoneurial edema proximally affecting neural circulation distally; (2) intrinsic susceptibility of the nerve to compression as a result of diabetes or other peripheral neuropathies; (3) mechanical effects of loss of nerve elasticity; and (4) connective tissue abnormalities.

Nerve Stretch Injuries

Categories and Causes of Stretch Injuries

Nerve injuries caused by traction or stretch fall into 2 major categories: the acute injury caused by an abrupt application of force of considerable magnitude, and the chronic injury caused by slowly stretching the nerve over an extended period of time. Stretch-induced nerve injuries can range from first- to fifth-degree, and the extent and severity of the damage are determined by the magnitude of the force and the rate of deformation. The deforming forces can be arbitrarily assigned a magnitude of mild, intermediate, or violent. In general, mild stretch produces first- and second-degree injuries, intermediate stretch produces structural damage leading to third-degree injuries, and violent stretch causes widespread trauma and tearing, resulting in fourth-degree injuries, or complete loss of continuity (fifth-degree injuries). When a nerve is slowly stretched over months or years, it can be stretched well beyond its normal limits and deformed to a remarkable degree without showing symptoms of loss of function. However, if this same nerve is rapidly stretched over milliseconds or seconds, conduction and structural failure can be instantaneous. For example, human nerves stretched at an elongation rate of 7.5 cm/min have an elastic limit of approximately 20% elongation. With rapid tstretch the elastic limit may be as low as 2% to 4% elongation.

Stretch injuries have a variety of causes. A stretch injury can be caused by the severe displacement of 2 parts of the body that have a nerve passing between them. For example, stretch injuries of the brachial plexus occur when the arm and shoulder girdle are forcibly displaced in relation to the trunk. Stretch injuries can also occur with joint dislocation or fractures. The passage of a high velocity missile through the limb can create a range of forces within the limb that can stretch the nerves, creating injuries ranging from first-degree conduction blocks to gross lacerations and loss of continuity. Stretch on the nerve ends brought together during end-to-end nerve repair may produce stretch lesions at other levels along the nerve. Premature and forcible postoperative extension of a joint immobilized in flexion to permit tension-free nerve repair may induce stretch lesions along the nerve or cause rupture at the repair site. Nerve fibers may also experience stretch and compression forces leading to injuries at a point where the nerve is in direct contact with a slowly enlarging aneurysm, cyst, ganglion, or tumor.

Features That Increase the Vulnerability to Stretch Injury

Certain anatomic features increase the susceptibility of a nerve to stretch injuries. Nerve fibers in a nerve with a single or a few large fascicles with minimal epineurial tissues are more susceptible to stretch injuries than nerve fibers in a nerve with many small fascicles embedded in a lot of epineurial tissue. A nerve that crosses the extensor aspect of a joint is under tension during full flexion and vulnerable to injury. Examples of this include the ulnar nerve at the elbow and the sciatic nerve at the hip joint. A nerve in close proximity to a joint is predisposed to stretch injury when the joint is dislocated. Nerves at risk include the axillary nerve with dislocation of the shoulder, the median and ulnar nerves at the elbow, and the common peroneal nerve at the knee joint.

Nerve Elasticity

Information regarding the sequence of events that occurs with nerve stretch is important in understanding the nature and prognosis of the lesion (Fig. 59). When first stretched, a nerve elongates rapidly and easily as the slack in the nerve trunk and its fascicles is taken up and the undulations are eliminated. Although the epineurium assists in maintaining the undulations in the nerve trunk, the component primarily responsible for the tensile strength and elasticity of the nerve is the perineurium. As stretching continues, the nerve fibers become taut and are stretched with the perineurium. As the fascicles are stretched, their cross-sectional area is reduced, raising the intrafascicular pressure and leading to compression deformation and ischemia (first-degree injury). As elongation approaches the elastic limit, nerve fibers begin to rupture inside the fascicles (second-degree injury). With increasing stretch, the endoneurial tubes rupture within the fascicles (third-degree injury), and then the perineurium tears (fourth-degree injury). Further stretching results in tearing of the epineurium and loss of continuity (fifth-degree injury). The rupture of nerve fibers and fascicles can occur over a considerable length of the nerve. These injuries are associated with extensive intrafascicular damage and fibrosis, which can impede regeneration.

A contrasting sequence of events in which the epineurium is the first tissue to rupture has been presented based on experimental data. According to this theory, damage to the nerve caused by stretching up to the elastic limit corresponds to neurapraxia or axonotmesis. At the limit of elasticity, the epineurium ruptures but the fascicles remain intact and continue to elongate. Further elongation ruptures the perineurium. Ultimately, the nerve fibers rupture, resulting in a loss of continuity.

Neural Degeneration

Trauma to peripheral nerve trunks results in various degrees of nerve fiber injury as described in the previous section. The most serious injury is the complete severance of the nerve trunk. Healing of nerve injuries is unique in that it consists of a process of cellular repair as opposed to tissue repair. In order to reestablish function, the neuron cell body must send out new axonal processes, which find the appropriate target organ and establish synaptic connection. Although the number of neurons does not increase, the repair occurs in an environment of intense cellular prolifer-

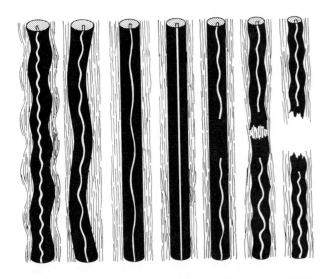

Figure 59

Diagram illustrating the changes occurring in a nerve as it is gradually stretched to mechanical failure. For simplification only 1 fasciculus and 1 nerve fiber are shown. (Reproduced with permission from Sunderland S: *Nerve Injuries and Their Repair: A Critical Appraisal.* New York, NY, Churchill Livingstone, 1991, p 148.)

ation (fibroblasts, endothelial cells, Schwann cells, etc). The initial response to nerve injury is axonal degeneration followed by regeneration (Fig. 60). This section will review changes that occur immediately after the injury, particularly those changes that occur after the complete severance of a nerve trunk.

Zone of Injury

When a nerve trunk is severed, the 2 ends retract, and a gap is left between the proximal and distal nerve stumps. Within the first 24 hours after the injury, capillary permeability increases and reaches a peak between days 7 and 14. The increase in capillary permeability is thought to be mediated by serotonin and histamine, which are released from the mast cells during degranulation of the axoplasm. A swelling composed of a disorganized edematous matrix of Schwann cells, fibroblasts, capillaries, macrophages, and collagen fibers soon develops at the end of each nerve stump. Eventually, the growing tips of the proximal axons will enter this swelling and must navigate through this matrix to the distal stump. Many of the axons will be arrested, forming whorls, spirals, and other abnormal endings; others will be deflected back to the proximal stump; and some will find the way to the distal stump. With the passage of time, the zone between the 2 stumps is converted into scar tissue. During secondary surgical repair of an injury that has severed the 2 ends, this traumatized zone of injury is resected and the stumps are reapposed with sutures or a nerve graft.

Wallerian Degeneration

When a nerve fiber is disconnected from its cell body, a series of metabolic and structural events occur in the segment distal to the lesion. The process of wallerian degeneration involves changes in the axon, myelin sheaths, Schwann cells, and endoneurial collagen.

Axonal Degeneration

The first stage of wallerian degeneration involves granular disintegration of axoplasmic microtubules and neurofilaments as a result of proteolysis. This process is initiated within hours of the injury. Neural conductance within the distal segment is completely lost within 48 to 96 hours after the injury. All traces of the axon debris are usually lost within 2 weeks of the injury. The disintegration of the axoplasm appears to be triggered by a large increase in axoplasmic calcium and mediated by calcium-sensitive proteases. In normal nerves, intra-axonal calcium concentration is very low (~ 0.3 μM). Transection of the nerve fiber results in a rise in the intra-axonal calcium throughout the distal stump. Chelation of calcium in the extracellular fluid delays the time of granular disintegration, suggesting that the entry of extracellular calcium is involved in initiating the axoplasmic degradation.

The breakdown of myelin follows the disintegration of the axoplasm by only hours. Within 36 to 48 hours of the injury, myelin breakdown is well advanced, and within 3 days myelin fragments are collecting into ovoids. The myelin debris is removed by the phagocytic action of macrophages and Schwann cells, occurring over a 1-week to 3-month period. In the final stages of wallerian degeneration, the interior of the nerve fiber is occupied by an amorphous mass of axon and myelin debris. Axon degeneration begins at the site of injury and progresses distally to the peripheral target organ.

Schwann Cell Response

The Schwann cells of normal intact myelinated fibers do not divide. Within 24 hours of nerve transection, Schwann cells throughout the distal segment undergo a series of mitoses. Schwann cell proliferation peaks around day 3 after the injury, and slowly declines during the following weeks. A second wave of Schwann cell proliferation occurs during the regenerative phase. The stimulus for Schwann cell proliferation is unknown; however, the onset of Schwann cell mitogenesis is synchronous with that of other endoneurial cells, including fibroblasts, endothelial cells, and mast cells. The newly divided Schwann cells maintain cytoplasmic processes that interdigitate and line up in rows beneath the original basal lamina of the nerve fiber. These tubes are referred to as the bands of Büngner. The Schwann cell basal lamina produces fibronectin and laminin, which have been shown to promote the growth of neurites in culture. The proliferating Schwann cells also synthesize nerve growth factor and nerve growth factor receptors. In the absence of axonal growth down the endoneurial tubes or bands of Büngner, the tubes atrophy.

Macrophage Response

After nerve injury (day 1 to 3), there is an accumulation of macrophages around the degenerating fibers. The early macrophages express Ia, the major histocompatibility class II antigen, and are not phagocytic. Once the cells pass through the basal lamina of the degenerating fiber, they lose their Ia expression and become phagocytic. Throughout their cycle, macrophages in wallerian degeneration express interleukin-1, a cytokine that influences the behavior of the Schwann cells. In particular, macrophage-derived interleukin-1 is required to stimulate Schwann cells to produce nerve growth factor.

Nerve Cell Body Response

When an axon is severed, the nerve cell body goes through structural and functional changes reflecting an alteration in metabolic priority from the production of neurotransmitters needed for synaptic transmission to the production of proteins needed for axonal repair and growth. The degree of the response varies with age, species, the severity of the injury, the level of the injury, the type and size of the neuron

and whether functional connections are restored. The closer the injury is to the cell body (or the greater the loss of axoplasm), the more severe the reaction. In general, the reaction occurs more rapidly and to a greater degree in sensory than in motor neurons. Within the sensory neuron population, the cell body reaction is more severe in nonmyelinated than in myelinated axons.

The response of the cell body can be divided into several phases: a reactive or chromatolytic phase, a recovery phase, and a degenerative phase. The reactive phase includes an increase in cell body volume, displacement of the nucleus to the periphery, and the disappearance of basophilic material from the cytoplasm. This phase is followed by the complete or incomplete recovery of the cell or its degrada-

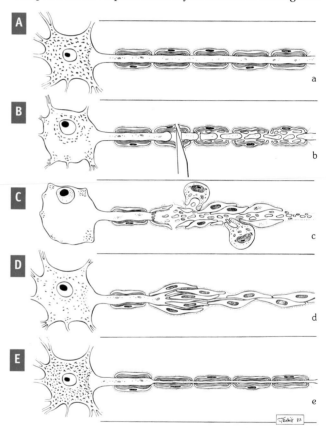

Figure 60

Degeneration and regeneration of myelinated fiber. **A,** Normal appearance. **B,** Transection of the fiber results in distal fragmentation of axon and myelin. In the proximal segment degeneration occurs at least to the nearest node of Ranvier. **C,** In the distal segment Schwann cells proliferate. Macrophages and Schwann cells phagocytose debris material. **D,** The Schwann cells in the distal segment have lined up in bands of Büngner. Sprouting occurs from the cut axonal stump. Advancing sprouts are embedded in Schwann cell cytoplasm. **E,** "Axonal" connection with periphery, maturation of nerve fiber. Sprouts that do not link up with the periphery may atrophy and disappear. The cell body response during these phases includes swelling, migration of the nucleus to the periphery, and condensation of basophilic material (chromatolysis). (Reproduced with permission from Lundborg G: *Nerve Injury and Repair.* New York, NY, Churchill Livingstone, 1988, p 151.)

tion. The synthesis of neurotransmitters and neurofilament proteins is decreased, and the synthesis of cytoskeletal proteins such as tubulin and actin is increased. In addition, there is an increase in the synthesis of several growth-associated proteins (GAPs) that promote axonal growth and extension. One specific growth-associated protein that is enhanced is GAP-43.

Proximal Segment Response

With transection of the nerve, axonal degeneration occurs over one or several internodal segments in the proximal stump, leaving the endoneurial tubes of the last centimeter or so of the proximal stump occupied only by Schwann cells. The fate of the axons above the injury depends on whether the cell body survives and regenerates a new axon or degenerates. If the cell body degenerates, the entire proximal length of the axon undergoes wallerian degeneration. If the cell body survives, the proximal nerve fibers undergo a reduction in axon diameter and myelin thickness that proceeds distally from the cell body. As regeneration proceeds and the axons make functional contact, axon diameter increases but remains smaller than normal. This permanent reduction in axon diameter and myelin thickness is accompanied with a slowing of the conduction velocity.

Within the first few days after transection, proximal myelinated axons produce a great number of collateral and terminal sprouts that advance distally and are confined to the endoneurial tubes until they reach the injury site. The behavior of the axons at this point depends on the degree of the injury. Collateral sprouts arise from the nodes of Ranvier at the level where the axons are still intact, whereas terminal sprouts arise from the tips of the remaining axons (Fig. 61). The growing sprouts from a single axon form an anatomic unit called the regenerating unit. The regenerating units consist of clusters of nonmyelinated axons originating from the same myelinated axon and surrounded by a single Schwann cell and its basal lamina. Occasionally, regenerating units are found that contain several Schwann cells surrounded by a single basal lamina. With time, the average number of sprouts per group diminishes. The reduction in the number of sprouts occurs because some axons fail to make functional contact with a peripheral target.

Axonal Regeneration

Axon Elongation Across the Zone of Injury

Regenerating axons from the proximal stump must cross a critical zone to reach the distal stump. The final success of regeneration depends largely on what happens at this level. When a nerve trunk has been severed, the nerve ends are left separated by a gap or are reunited surgically. In either case, the tissue that develops between the ends is essentially the same, except that the tissue between separated nerve ends is more extensive, denser, and more disorganized than is the tissue between surgically reunited nerve ends.

The zone between the stumps is similar to other wound-healing environments. It is characterized by exudation, cell proliferation, and collagen synthesis. Initially, the gap is filled with an exudate containing blood corpuscles and macrophages, and then a fibrin clot is formed. Subsequently, there is an ingrowth of capillaries and fibroblasts from the nerve stumps as well as from surrounding tissues. Schwann cells migrate into the gap from the proximal and distal stumps, forming columns and groups. The tissue that forms between the stumps is generally not as suitable for growth as that in the endoneurial tubes of the distal segment. In general, the tissue is obstructive to axonal growth and results in delays and misdirection of axonal growth. The direction taken by each growing axon tip is influenced by the structural organization of the medium through which it regenerates. Resistance is minimal where collagen fibrils are organized in parallel. The direction of axonal growth may also be influenced by chemotropic molecules released into the microenvironment of the growing axons. This topic will be discussed in greater detail in the next section.

The overall effect of scar tissue in the zone between the nerve stumps is to: (1) obstruct the advance of some regenerating axons, thereby reducing the number of axons that reinnervate denervated end organs; (2) delay the advance of regenerating axons; (3) retard the development of those axons that have regenerated by delaying and limiting their maturation; and (4) misdirect axons into functionally unrelated endoneurial tubes.

Axon Elongation in the Distal Segment

Regenerating axons that make it across the zone of injury enter endoneurial tubes in the distal segment. Generally, an excess number of sprouts invade the distal segment, resulting in endoneurial tubes occupied by multiple axons (usually from the same parent neuron). The original basal lamina eventually disintegrates, releasing new fibers into the fascicle. With time, however, the number of axons in the distal segment decreases as axons that do not make functional connections with the periphery atrophy and disappear. The excess sprouts in the distal segment suggest that axon counting is not a reliable method for assessing regeneration. In fact, an excess number of axons in the distal segment may be a response to obstacles in the zone of injury and, therefore, is an indication of poor regeneration.

The signal for myelination comes from the regenerating axon. The regenerating axon of an originally myelinated neuron instructs the enveloping Schwann cells of the distal segment to form myelin, while unmyelinated fibers remain unmyelinated even when regenerating into a distal segment originally containing myelinated fibers. The maturation of an axon depends on its innervating the appropriate peripheral target.

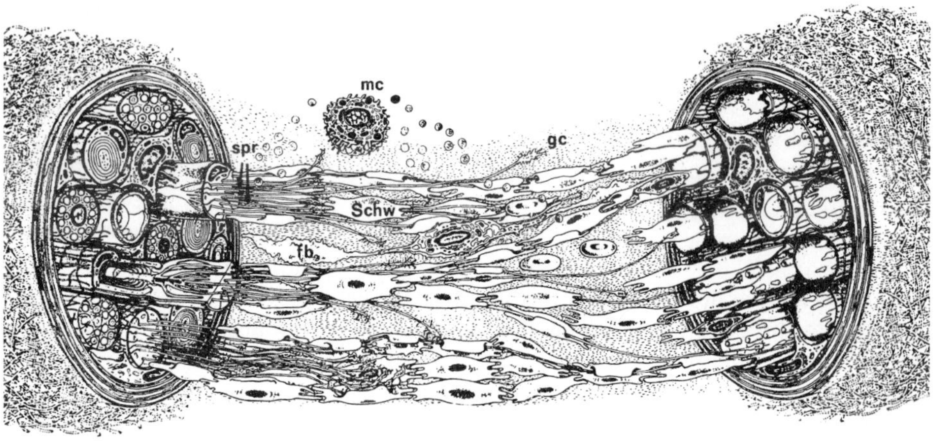

Figure 61

Local cellular response to nerve transection. Schw = Schwann cells; spr = sprouts; fb = fibroblasts; gc = growth cone. (Reproduced with permission from Lundborg G: *Nerve Injury and Repair*. New York, NY, Churchill Livingstone, 1988, pp 152-153.)

The rate of regeneration varies depending on the type and location of the injury. In general, axonal elongation is slower after a complete nerve lesion than after a crush injury. Regeneration rates in nerves from experimental animals range from 2.0 to 3.5 mm/day after transection and repair, and from 3.0 to 4.4 mm/day after crush. Regeneration of human peripheral nerves has been reported to be nonlinear, with a gradually decreasing regeneration rate in more distal regions of the limb (Table 17). For example, regeneration rates are faster in the axilla than in the wrist. In humans, an average outgrowth of 1 to 2 mm/day is generally quoted.

Functional Recovery After Nerve Injury

The outcome of peripheral nerve injuries varies greatly. Variables hypothesized to have an important role in determining the outcome of nerve repair include: (1) age of the patient; (2) type of nerve injured; (3) distance the regenerating axons must grow to reach the target organ; (4) length of the injury zone; (5) timing of the nerve repair; (6) status of the target organ at the time it is reinnervated; and (7) technical expertise of the surgeon.

Functional recovery is generally complete after a crush injury because the basement membrane and endoneurium are left intact, and the damaged axons can regenerate within their original endoneurial tubes and reinnervate their original target organ. After a complete lesion to the nerve, however, functional recovery of movement is often quite poor. The loss of functional recovery is probably related to the failure of axons to regenerate and the misdirection of regenerating axons, which leads to inappropriate innervation of denervated muscles. Inappropriate innervation is thought to result in a loss in the ability to accurately recruit individual muscles and motor units within a muscle, resulting in the loss of motor control.

Specificity of Reinnervation

Although regeneration of axons across a lesion is a prerequisite for recovery, it is generally believed that axon misdirection is primarily responsible for the lack of functional recovery. Specificity of reinnervation can occur at many levels. Specificity at the tissue level is characterized by growth of an axon toward the severed nerve segment as opposed to tendon, muscle, or visceral organs. Once inside the nerve, the axon must move in the appropriate direction at those intersections where the nerve branches, that is, toward a sensory or motor branch or toward 1 of 2 major motor branches, such as the peroneal or tibial branch of the sciatic nerve. The axon must then be attracted toward the target organ it is to innervate. Motor nerves may innervate different muscles and sensory nerves may attach to various types of sensory receptors. The final attachment(s) must be made within the target organ. For example, once a motor axon has innervated a muscle, the number and type (that is, fast versus slow) of fibers to be innervated must be determined.

During development, motoneurons find their appropriate

Table 17	
Axonal Regeneration Rate	
Location of Injury	**Rate (mm/day)**
Rates of uncomplicated axon regeneration	
Root of limb	6
Elbow	4–5
Wrist	1–2
Hand	1–1.5
Lower limb	1–2
Ankle	1
Rates of axon regeneration after nerve suture	
Lower forearm	2
Wrist and hand	1
Upper leg	2
Lower leg	1.5
Ankle	1

targets with remarkable accuracy. This precise patterning of neuronal connections emerges, in part, from the interactions between the growth cones and their cellular environment. The question is, can damaged axons in the adult reach the correct target with the same specificity as developing axons? If not, what can be done to increase the probability of correct reinnervation after injury? Some of the mechanisms thought to be responsible for the generation of specific connections are shown in Figure 62.

Traditionally, the surgeon has attempted to improve specificity by operative alignment of the proximal and distal nerve stumps. The mechanical approach forces axons to take a certain path. If the axon is allowed to explore its environment, humeral mechanisms may also be available to guide it to the appropriate target. Contact recognition permits an axon to select the appropriate path based on the molecular composition of the environment. Axons would selectively propagate down distal tubes that had the appropriate molecular signature. Neurotropism refers to an active process in which axons select or are guided to the appropriate target based on diffusible factors that are released from the distal targets. Neurotrophy refers to a mechanism in which axons randomly grow to a target, and only those entering a correct pathway or innervating the correct target receive a trophic or nutritive factor that allows the axon to continue to develop and become myelinated. Axons that receive no trophic support would degenerate.

Selectivity of reinnervation has been reported to occur after the transection of motor axons in the neonatal rat, whereas reinnervation in adult rats appeared to be random. It has been suggested that during development there are target-derived cues that serve to guide the motor axons to their correct targets. Target-specific regeneration, however, has been considered impossible in the mammalian adult peripheral nervous system. A high degree of nonselectivity has been shown to occur in rats after section and resuture of the sciatic nerve, as well as in humans after severance and surgical repair of the ulnar nerve branch at the wrist.

Recent evidence suggests that injured axons in mature animals may be capable of detecting and following specific neurotropic cues. A neurotropic factor is a substance that provides directional cues. Studies have shown that a regenerating sprout will preferentially grow towards a tube that contains nerve as opposed to tendon or muscle. Additional evidence of target-specificity has been provided by experiments that demonstrated that motor axons in the proximal portion of a Y-shaped silicone tube preferentially reinnervated the distal branch that contained the motor stump rather than the sensory stump. Moreover, the distance between the proximal and distal stumps was found to be important. Motor axons in the proximal stump of a cut nerve would selectively grow into a distal tube containing a motor stump as opposed to a sensory stump if the cut ends were separated by 5 mm; however, selective innervation was not apparent if the distance between the stumps was only 2 mm.

Several investigators also have shown that selectivity of axon growth occurs at the level of the nerve trunk. Using a Y-shaped Silastic tube, they demonstrated that the proximal stump of the tibial and peroneal branches of the sciatic nerve of the rat and cat preferentially innervated that portion of the tube containing the appropriate distal stump, that is, proximal tibial to distal tibial and proximal peroneal to distal peroneal. These studies raise the possibility that target-specific reinnervation can occur in the adult, given the appropriate conditions.

Other Factors

Neuronotropic factors are macromolecular proteins derived from various sources that promote the survival and growth of specific neuronal populations. These factors are present in the target of innervation (muscle or sensory receptor) or in the distal structure to be innervated (distal nerve segment). These factors may function to enhance regeneration by increasing the survival of neurons or the rate of regeneration, and they may also provide directional cues to regenerating axons. Additional research is needed to determine the exact function of these factors in regeneration.

Several other agents have been shown to promote nerve regeneration. Exogenous application of gangliosides, which are a major structural component of the neuronal plasma membrane, has been reported to stimulate axonal sprouting in vivo, to stimulate sprouting at the neuromuscular junction in vivo, and to promote axon extension in vitro. Hormones also have been reported to enhance the rate of regeneration. Testosterone has been shown to stimulate regeneration of transected hypoglossal and facial nerves and crushed sciatic nerves. Administration of thyroid hormone (T3) has been reported to increase protein synthesis in the nerve cell body, increase the rate of axonal outgrowth, and improve maturation of regenerating axons. However, it also has been reported that experimentally induced hyperthyroidism does not enhance peripheral nerve regeneration. It has been hypothesized that the protease inhibitor, leupeptin, may enhance regeneration because of its ability to inhibit wallerian degeneration in the distal segment and reduce the amount of atrophy in denervated skeletal muscles. Administration of leupeptin after transection of the rat sciatic nerve or primate median nerve has been reported to lead to an increase in the number of regenerating axons. Table 18 lists some of the factors thought to play a role in axon elongation and survival. Clearly, axonal growth is influenced by numerous factors. The discovery of factors that can increase the rate of regeneration, the number of surviving axons, and the specificity of reinnervation should lead to better functional recovery after nerve injury.

Muscle Recovery After Denervation

Partial recovery of muscles is thought to be a major factor that limits the recovery of motor function after long-term denervation. An inability of the muscle to recover its tension-producing capabilities after reinnervation may be related to (1) a loss of muscle fibers, (2) a loss of motor units, or (3) a loss in the ability to increase muscle fiber size and reverse the atrophy that occurs after denervation. Long-term denervation has been shown to result in both a loss of muscle fibers and increased connective tissue proliferation within the muscle. The ability of a muscle to recover from denervation is thought to be related, in part, to the number of motor axons that reinnervate the muscle. A decrease in the number of axons that reinnervate a muscle may result in fibers remaining denervated and, subsequently, a loss of muscle fibers. However, a reduction in motor axons may not necessarily lead to denervated muscle fibers. The motor axons that reinnervate the muscle may have the capacity to sprout and maintain synaptic connections with more fibers than they would in a normal muscle. This should lead to an increase in the number of large motor units. An increase in motor unit size, that is, mean motor unit tension, has been observed after injury to the sciatic nerve and in muscles that have been partially denervated. A change in the distribution of motor unit tensions may influence the manner in which units are recruited, which, in turn, may cause a deficit in motor control.

The reason for a lack of muscle recovery may also reside in the muscle itself. If the muscle tissue cannot reverse the atrophy that occurs after denervation, the fibers will remain smaller than normal, and tension will not be fully recovered. The inability to recover muscle mass may reside in the satellite cells and their ability to proliferate and increase fiber size. Growth factors such as fibroblast growth factor (FGF), insulin-like growth factor (IGF), and transforming growth factor-β have been suggested to have a role in myogenesis and satellite cell proliferation and differentiation. FGF and IGF have both been shown to stimulate satellite cell proliferation. Moreover, the expression of IGF has recently been shown to be increased in muscles during regeneration after ischemic injury. Further studies are needed to determine the exact role of growth factors during muscle degeneration and regeneration.

Surgical Nerve Repair

Prior to World War II, nerves were still regarded as cord-like structures and were treated the same as other tissues during surgery. The period following World War II marked the beginning of many breakthroughs in trauma surgery and peripheral nerve repair. The effective control of wound infection by antibiotics was a major advance. In addition, a better understanding of the internal structure of nerves and the physiology of the nervous system, along with improved surgical techniques and surgical instruments, made nerve repair potentially more successful.

This period of technical achievement can be attributed to several factors including: (1) clinicians' recognition of the significance of basic science data; (2) the realization that nerve repair involved far more than the simple restoration of nerve trunk continuity; (3) the recognition that nerve repair had become a highly specialized undertaking, demanding a detailed knowledge of the internal anatomy of nerves and regenerative processes and calling for great technical skill and experience, meticulous observance of atraumatic techniques, and the use of surgical methods, instruments, and suture materials specially designed for this type of work; (4) the application of microsurgical techniques to the repair of nerves; and (5) the emergence of hand surgery as a recognized specialty.

The objectives of surgical repair of a damaged nerve are to maximize (1) the number of axons that regenerate across the lesion site and (2) the accuracy with which these axons reinnervate denervated peripheral targets. The surgeon can influence the result by the way the damaged tissue is

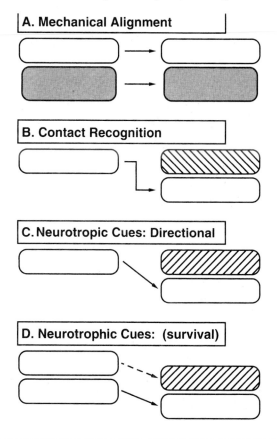

Figure 62

Guidance mechanisms. (Adapted with permission from Brushart T: The mechanical and humoral control of specificity in nerve repair, in Gelberman RH (ed): *Operative Nerve Repair and Reconstruction.* Philadelphia, PA, JB Lippincott, 1991, p 217.)

handled and by the method used to reapproximate the severed ends.

The 4 basic steps of nerve repair are: preparation of the stumps, often involving resection or interfascicular dissection with separation of individual fascicles or groups of fascicles; approximation, with special reference to the length of the gap between the stumps as well as the amount of tension present; coaptation of the nerve stumps; and maintenance of coaptation, involving the use of, for example, stitches, glue, or a natural fibrin clot. Coaptation describes the apposition of corresponding nerve ends with special attention to bringing the cross-section of the fascicles into optimal contact. A direct coaptation (neurorrhaphy) can oppose stump to stump, fascicle to fascicle, or fascicle group to fascicle group in the corresponding ends. An indirect coaptation can be performed by interposing a nerve graft. Other factors that may influence the results are the timing of the surgery and the postoperative rehabilitation. These topics have been addressed extensively in several textbooks.

Table 18
Factors Reported to Enhance Nerve Regeneration

Factor	Proposed Mechanism*
Nerve growth factor (NGF)	NTF
Ciliary neuronotropic factor (CNTF)	NTF
Motor nerve growth factor (MNGF)	NTF
Fibronectin	NPF
Laminin	NPF
Neural cell adhesion molecule (NCAM)	NPF
N-cadherin	
Hormones Estrogen Testosterone Thyroid hormone Insulin	IPS
Acidic fibroblast growth factor (aFGF)	NTF
Basic fibroblast growth factor (bFGF)	NTF
Insulin-like growth factor (IGF)	NTF
Forskolin	IPS
Leupeptin	ITD
Gangliosides	?

* NTF: promotes neuro survival; NPF: promotes axonal extension; IPS: increased protein synthesis; ITD: inhibits traumatic degeneration

Selected Bibliography

Neurons and Signal Generation

Goldman DE: Potential, impedance, and rectification in membranes. *J Gen Physiol* 1943;27:37–60.

Hirokawa N, Pfister KK, Yorifuji H, Wagner MC, Brady ST, Bloom GS: Submolecular domains of bovine brain kinesin identified by electron microscopy and monoclonal antibody decoration. *Cell* 1989;56:867–878.

Hodgkin AL: Chance and design in electrophysiology: An informal account of certain experiments on nerve carried out between 1934 and 1952. *J Physiol (Lond)* 1976;263:1–21.

Hodgkin AL, Huxley AF: A quantitative description of membrane current and its application to conduction and excitation in nerve. *J Physiol (Lond)* 1952:117;500–544.

Hodgkin AL, Katz B: The effect of sodium ions on the electrical activity of the giant axon of the squid. *J Physiol (Lond)* 1949:108:37–77.

Kandel ER, Schwartz JH, Jessell TM (eds): *Principles of Neural Science*, ed 3. New York, NY, Elsevier Science Publishing, 1991.

Nicholls JG, Martin AR, Wallace BG (eds): *From Neuron To Brain: A Cellular and Molecular Approach to the Function of the Nervous System*, ed 3. Sunderland, MA, Sinauer Associates, 1992.

Ochs S: Fast transport of materials in mammalian nerve fibers. *Science* 1972;176:252–260.

Ochs S, Brimijoin WS: Axonal transport, in Dyck PJ, Thomas PK, Griffin JW, Low PA, Poduslo JF (eds): *Peripheral Neuropathy*, ed 3. Philadelphia, PA, WB Saunders, 1993, vol 1, pp 331–360.

Rall W: Core conductor theory and cable properties of neurons, in Kandel ER (ed): *Handbook of Physiology, Section 1: The Nervous System: Volume I: Cellular Biology of Neurons, Part 1*. Bethesda, MD, American Physiological Society, 1977, pp 39–97.

Reichert H (ed): *Introduction to Neurobiology*. New York, NY, Oxford University Press, 1992.

Sensory and Motor Systems

Bodine SC, Garfinkel A, Roy RR, Edgerton VR: Spatial distribution of motor unit fibers in the cat soleus and tibialis anterior muscles: Local interactions. *J Neurosci* 1988;8:2142–2152.

Bodine SC, Roy RR, Eldred E, Edgerton VR: Maximal force as a function of anatomical features of motor units in the cat tibialis anterior. *J Neurophysiol* 1987;57:1730–1745.

Brandstater ME, Lambert EH: Motor unit anatomy: Type and spatial arrangement of muscle fibers, in Desmedt JE (ed): *New Developments in Electromyography and Clinical Neurophysiology.* Basel, Switzerland, S Karger, 1973, vol 1, pp 14–22.

Brown AG (ed): *Organization in the Spinal Cord: The Anatomy and Physiology of Identified Neurones.* Berlin, Germany, Springer-Verlag, 1981.

Burke D: Spasticity as an adaptation to pyramidal tract injury. *Adv Neurol* 1988;47:401–423.

Burke RE: Motor units: Anatomy, physiology, and functional organization, in Brooks VB (ed): *Handbook of Physiology, Section I, The Nervous System: Volume 2: Motor Control, Part 1.* Bethesda, MD, American Physiological Society, 1981, pp 345–422.

Daube JR, Reagan TJ, Sandok BA, Westmoreland BF (eds): *Medical Neurosciences: An Approach to Anatomy, Pathology, and Physiology by Systems and Levels,* ed 2. Boston, MA, Little, Brown and Company, 1986.

Delwaide PJ, Young RR (eds): *Clinical Neurophysiology in Spasticity: Contribution to Assessment and Pathophysiology.* Amsterdam, The Netherlands, Elsevier, 1985.

Edstrom L, Kugelberg E: Histochemical composition, distribution of fibres and fatiguability of single motor units: Anterior tibial muscle of the rat. *J Neurol Neurosurg Psychiatry* 1968;31:424–433.

Guyton AC (ed): *Basic Neuroscience: Anatomy and Physiology,* ed 2. Philadelphia, PA, WB Saunders, 1991.

Henneman E, Mendell LM: Functional organization of motoneuron pool and its inputs, in Brooks VB (ed): *Handbook of Physiology: Section 1, The Nervous System: Volume 2: Motor Control, Part 1.* Bethesda, MD, American Physiological Society, 1981, pp 423–507.

Jansen JK, Fladby T: The perinatal reorganization of the innervation of skeletal muscle in mammals. *Prog Neurobiol* 1990;34:39–90.

Katz RT, Rymer WZ: Spastic hypertonia: Mechanisms and measurement. *Arch Phys Med Rehabil* 1989;70:144–155.

Kugelberg E: Properties of the rat hind-limb motor units, in Desmedt JE (ed): *New Developments in Electromyography and Clinical Neurophysiology.* Basel, Switzerland, S Karger, 1973, vol 1, pp 2–13.

Lance JW: The control of muscle tone, reflexes, and movement: Robert Wartenberg Lecture. *Neurology* 1980;30:1303–1313.

Matthews PBC: Muscle spindles: Their messages and their fusimotor supply, in Brooks VB (ed): *Handbook of Physiology, Section 1, The Nervous System: Volume II: Motor Control, Part 1.* Bethesda, MD, American Physiological Society, 1981, pp 189–228.

Nickel VL, Botte MJ (eds): *Orthopaedic Rehabilitation,* ed 2. New York, NY, Churchill Livingstone, 1992.

Park TS, Phillips LH II, Peacock WJ (eds): *Neurosurgery: State of the Art Reviews: Management of Spasticity in Cerebral Palsy and Spinal Cord Injury.* Philadelphia, PA, Hanley and Belfus, 1989, vol 4.

Purves D, Lichtman JW (eds): *Principles of Neural Development.* Sunderland, MA, Sinauer Associates, 1985.

Romanes GJ: The motor cell columns of the lumbo-sacral spinal cord of the cat. *J Comp Neurol* 1951;94:313–363.

Schmidt RF (ed): *Fundamentals of Neurophysiology,* ed 2. New York, NY, Springer-Verlag, 1978. Translated by Biederman-Thorson, MA.

Van Essen DC: Neuromuscular synapse elimination: Structural, functional, and mechanistic aspects, in Spitzer NC (ed): *Neuronal Development.* New York, NY, Plenum Press, 1982, pp 333–376.

Wernig A (ed): *Plasticity of Motoneuronal Connections.* Amsterdam, The Netherlands, Elsevier, 1991.

Peripheral Nerve Development, Structure, and Biomechanics

Beel JA, Groswald DE, Luttges MW: Alterations in the mechanical properties of peripheral nerve following crush injury. *J Biomech* 1984;17:185–193.

Clark WL, Trumble TE, Swiontkowski MF, Tencer AF: Nerve tension and blood flow in a rat model of immediate and delayed repairs. *J Hand Surg* 1992;17A:677–687.

Denny-Brown D, Doherty MM: Effects of transient stretching of peripheral nerve. *Arch Neurol Psychiatry* 1945;54:116–129.

Dodd J, Jessell TM: Axon guidance and the patterning of neuronal projections in vertebrates. *Science* 1988;242:692–699.

Haftek J: Stretch injury of peripheral nerve: Acute effects of stretching on rabbit nerve. *J Bone Joint Surg* 1970;52B:354–365.

Hall ZW (ed): *An Introduction to Molecular Neurobiology.* Sunderland, MA, Sinauer Associates, 1992.

Lance-Jones C: Motoneuron axon guidance: Development of specific projections to two muscles in the embryonic chick limb. *Brain Behav Evol* 1988;31:209–217.

Landmesser LT: The generation of neuromuscular specificity. *Annu Rev Neurosci* 1980;3:279–302.

Landmesser L: The development of specific motor pathways in the chick embryo. *Trends Neurosci* 1984;7:336–339.

Lundborg G: The intrinsic vascularization of human peripheral nerves: Structural and functional aspects. *J Hand Surg* 1979;4A: 34–41.

Lundborg G (ed): *Nerve Injury and Repair.* Edinburgh, Scotland, Churchill Livingstone, 1988.

Okamoto T: Study on strength of peripheral nerve tissue of human beings and various animals. *J Kyoto Pref Med Univ* 1955;58: 1007–1029.

Rydevik BL, Kwan MK, Myers RR, et al: An in vitro mechanical and histological study of acute stretching on rabbit tibial nerve. *J Orthop Res* 1990;8:694–701.

Sanes JR: Extracellular matrix molecules that influence neural development. *Annu Rev Neurosci* 1989;12:491–516.

Sanes JR, Schachner M, Covault J: Expression of several adhesive macromolecules (N-CAM, L1, J1, NILE, uvomorulin, laminin, fibronectin, and a heparan sulfate proteoglycan) in embryonic, adult, and denervated adult skeletal muscle. *J Cell Biol* 1986; 102:420–431.

Sunderland S (ed): *Nerve Injuries and Their Repair: A Critical Appraisal.* Edinburgh, Scotland, Churchill Livingstone, 1991.

Sunderland S, Bradley KC: Stress-strain phenomena in human peripheral nerve trunks. *Brain* 1961;84:102–119.

Yoshimura M, Amaya S, Tyujo M, Nomura S: Experimental studies on the traction injury of peripheral nerves. *Neuro-Orthop* 1989;7:1–7.

Electrodiagnosis of the Peripheral Nerve

Aminoff MJ (ed): *Electrodiagnosis in Clinical Neurology,* ed 3. New York, NY, Churchill Livingstone, 1992.

Kimura J (ed): *Electrodiagnosis in Diseases of Nerve and Muscle: Principles and Practice.* Philadelphia, PA, FA Davis, 1983.

Kugelberg E, Edstrom L, Abbruzzese M: Mapping of motor units in experimentally reinnervated rat muscle: Interpretation of histochemical and atrophic fibre patterns in neurogenic lesions. *J Neurol Neurosurg Psychiatry* 1970;33:319–329.

Liveson JA (ed): *Peripheral Neurology: Case Studies in Electrodiagnosis,* ed 2. Philadelphia, PA, FA Davis, 1991.

Liveson JA, Ma DM (eds): *Laboratory Reference for Clinical Neurophysiology.* Philadelphia, PA, FA Davis, 1992.

Luff AR, Hatcher DD, Torkko K: Enlarged motor units resulting from partial denervation of cat hindlimb muscles. *J Neurophysiol* 1988;59: 1377–1394.

Mumenthaler M, Schliack H (eds): *Peripheral Nerve Lesions: Diagnosis and Therapy.* New York, NY, Thieme Medical Publishers, 1991.

Peyronnard J-M, Charron L: Muscle reorganization after partial denervation and reinnervation. *Muscle Nerve* 1980;3:509–518.

Sethi RK, Thompson LL (eds): *The Electromyographer's Handbook,* ed 2. Boston, MA, Little, Brown and Company, 1989.

Stalberg E: Single-fiber electromyography and some other electrophysiologic techniques for the study of the motor unit, in Dyck PJ, Thomas PK, Griffin JW, Low PA, Poduslo JF (eds): *Peripheral Neuropathy,* ed 3. Philadelphia, PA, WB Saunders, 1993, vol 1, pp 645–657.

Traumatic Nerve Injury

Dahlin LB, McLean WG: Effects of graded experimental compression on slow and fast axonal transport in rabbit vagus nerve. *J Neurol Sci* 1986;72:19–30.

Flatt AE: Tourniquet time in hand surgery. *Arch Surg* 1972;104: 190–192.

Gasser HS, Erlanger J: The role of fiber size in the establishment of a nerve block by pressure or cocaine. *Am J Physiol* 1929;88:581–591.

Gelberman RH, Hergenroeder PT, Hargens AR, Lundborg GN, Akeson WH: The carpal tunnel syndrome: A study of carpal canal pressures. *J Bone Joint Surg* 1981;63A:380–383.

Gelberman RH, Szabo RM, Williamson RV, Hargens AR, Yaru NC, Minteer-Convery MA: Tissue pressure threshold for peripheral nerve viability. *Clin Orthop* 1983;178:285–291.

Klenerman L: The tourniquet in operations on the knee: A review. *J R Soc Med* 1982;75:31–32.

Lundborg G, Gelberman RH, Minteer-Convery M, Lee YF, Hargens AR: Median nerve compression in the carpal tunnel: Functional response to experimentally induced controlled pressure. *J Hand Surg* 1982;7A:252–259.

Lundborg G, Myers R, Powell H: Nerve compression injury and increased endoneurial fluid pressure: A "miniature compartment syndrome." *J Neurol Neurosurg Psychiatry* 1983;46:1119–1124.

Myers RR, Powell HC: Endoneurial fluid pressure in peripheral neuropathies, in Hargens AR (ed): *Tissue Fluid Pressure and Composition*. Baltimore, MD, Williams & Wilkins, 1981, pp 193–207.

Ochoa J, Fowler TJ, Gilliatt RW: Anatomical changes in peripheral nerves compressed by a pneumatic tourniquet. *J Anat* 1972;113:433–455.

Rorabeck CH: Tourniquet-induced nerve ischemia: An experimental investigation. *J Trauma* 1980;20:280–286.

Rydevik B, Lundborg G, Bagge U: Effects of graded compression on intraneural blood flow: An in vivo study on rabbit tibial nerve. *J Hand Surg* 1981;6A:3–12.

Seddon HJ: Three types of nerve injury. *Brain* 1943;66:237–288.

Seddon H (ed): *Surgical Disorders of the Peripheral Nerves*, ed 2. Edinburgh, Scotland, Churchill Livingstone, 1975.

Sunderland S: A classification of peripheral nerve injuries producing loss of function. *Brain* 1951;74:491–516.

Sunderland S (ed): *Nerves and Nerve Injuries*, ed 2. Edinburgh, Scotland, Churchill Livingstone, 1978.

Neural Degeneration, Axonal Regeneration, and Functional Recovery After Nerve Injury

Anzil AP, Wernig A: Muscle fibre loss and reinnervation after long-term denervation. *J Neurocytol* 1989;18:833–845.

Archibald SJ, Krarup C, Shefner J, Li ST, Madison RD: A collagen-based nerve guide conduit for peripheral nerve repair: An electrophysiological study of nerve regeneration in rodents and nonhuman primates. *J Comp Neurol* 1991;306:685–696.

Bain JR, Mackinnon SE, Hunter DA: Functional evaluation of complete sciatic, peroneal, and posterior tibial nerve lesions in the rat. *Plast Reconstr Surg* 1989;83:129–138.

Brushart TM: Preferential reinnervation of motor nerves by regenerating motor axons. *J Neurosci* 1988;8:1026–1031.

Brushart TM, Mesulam MM: Alteration in connections between muscle and anterior horn motoneurons after peripheral nerve repair. *Science* 1980;208:603–605.

Brushart TM, Seiler WA IV: Selective reinnervation of distal motor stumps by peripheral motor axons. *Exp Neurol* 1987;97:289–300.

Brushart TM, Tarlov EC, Mesulam MM: Specificity of muscle reinnervation after epineurial and individual fascicular suture of the rat sciatic nerve. *J Hand Surg* 1983;8A:248–253.

Cabaud HE, Rodkey WG, McCarroll HR Jr: Peripheral nerve injuries: Studies in higher nonhuman primates. *J Hand Surg* 1980;5A:201–206.

Cabaud HE, Rodkey WG, McCarroll HR Jr, Mutz SB, Niebauer JJ: Epineurial and perineurial fascicular nerve repairs: A critical comparison. *J Hand Surg* 1976;1A:131–137.

Danielsen N, Pettmann B, Vahlsing HL, Manthrope M, Varon S: Fibroblast growth factor effects on peripheral nerve regeneration in a silicone chamber model. *J Neurosci Res* 1988;20:320–330.

Daniloff JK, Levi G, Grumet M, Rieger F, Edelman GM: Altered expression of neuronal cell adhesion molecules induced by nerve injury and repair. *J Cell Biol* 1986;103:929–945.

Dellon AL, Mackinnon SE: Selection of the appropriate parameter to measure neural regeneration. *Ann Plast Surg* 1989;23:197–202.

Evans PJ, Bain JR, Mackinnon SE, Makino AP, Hunter DA: Selective reinnervation: A comparison of recovery following microsuture and conduit nerve repair. *Brain Res* 1991;559:315–321.

Fawcett JW, Keynes RJ: Peripheral nerve regeneration. *Annu Rev Neurosci* 1990;13:43–60.

Fields RD, Ellisman MH: Axons regenerated through silicone tube splices: I. Conduction properties. *Exp Neurol* 1986;92:48–60.

Fields RD, Ellisman MH: Axons regenerated through silicone tube splices: II. Functional morphology. *Exp Neurol* 1986;92:61–74.

Fields RD, Le Beau JM, Longo FM, Ellisman MH: Nerve regeneration through artificial tubular implants. *Prog Neurobiol* 1989;33:87–134.

Hardman VJ, Brown MC: Accuracy of reinnervation of rat internal intercostal muscles by their own segmental nerves. *J Neurosci* 1987;7:1031–1036.

Harsh C, Archibald SJ, Madison RD: Double-labeling of saphenous nerve neuron pools: A model for determining the accuracy of axon regeneration at the single neuron level. *J Neurosci Methods* 1991;39:123–130.

Hollowell JP, Villadiego A, Rich KM: Sciatic nerve regeneration across gaps within silicone chambers: Long-term effects of NGF and consideration of axonal branching. *Exp Neurol* 1990;110:45–51.

Irintchev A, Draguhn A, Wernig A: Reinnervation and recovery of mouse soleus muscle after long-term denervation. *Neuroscience* 1990;39:231–243.

Keynes RJ: Schwann cells during neural development and regeneration: Leaders or followers? *Trends Neurosci* 1987;10:137–139.

Knoops B, Hurtado H, van den Bosch de Aguilar P: Rat sciatic nerve regeneration within an acrylic semipermeable tube and comparison with a silicone impermeable material. *J Neuropathol Exp Neurol* 1990;49:438–448.

Kuffler DP: Regeneration of muscle axons in the frog is directed by diffusible factors from denervated muscle and nerve tubes. *J Comp Neurol* 1989;281:416–425.

Kuno M: Target dependence of motoneuronal survival: The current status. *Neurosci Res (NY)* 1990;9:155–172.

Laskowski MB, Sanes JR: Topographic mapping of motor pools onto skeletal muscles. *J Neurosci* 1987;7:252–260.

Laskowski MB, Sanes JR: Topographically selective reinnervation of adult mammalian skeletal muscles. *J Neurosci* 1988;8:3094–3099.

Le Beau JM, Ellisman MH, Powell HC: Ultrastructural and morphometric analysis of long-term peripheral nerve regeneration through silicone tubes. *J Neurocytol* 1988;17:161–172.

Lieberman AR: The axon reaction: A review of the principle features of perikaryal responses to axon injury. *Int Rev Neurobiol* 1971; 14:49–124.

Longo FM, Hayman EG, Davis GE, et al: Neurite-promoting factors and extracellular matrix components accumulating in vivo within nerve regeneration chambers. *Brain Res* 1984;309:105–117.

Lundborg G, Dahlin LB, Danielsen N, Nachemson AK: Tissue specificity in nerve regeneration. *Scand J Plast Reconstr Surg* 1986;20: 279–283.

Mackinnon SE, Dellon AL, Lundborg G, Hudson AR, Hunter DA: A study of neurotrophism in a primate model. *J Hand Surg* 1986;11A: 888–894.

Madison RD, Da Silva CF, Dikkes P: Entubulation repair with protein additives increases the maximum nerve gap distance successfully bridged with tubular prostheses. *Brain Res* 1988;447:325–334.

Manthorpe M, Engvall E, Ruoslahti E, Longo FM, Davis GE, Varon S: Laminin promotes neuritic regeneration from cultured peripheral and central neurons. *J Cell Biol* 1983;97:1882–1890.

Nurcombe V, Hill MA, Eagleson KL, Bennett MR: Motor neuron survival and neuritic extension from spinal cord explants induced by factors released from denervated muscle. *Brain Res* 1984;291:19–28.

Politis MJ: Specificity in mammalian peripheral nerve regeneration at the level of the nerve trunk. *Brain Res* 1985;328:271–276.

Politis MJ, Ederle K, Spencer PS: Tropism in nerve regeneration in vivo: Attraction of regenerating axons by diffusible factors derived from cells in distal nerve stumps of transected peripheral nerves. *Brain Res* 1982;253:1–12.

Rosario CM, Fry KR, Madison R: Rabbit retinal ganglion cells survive optic transection and entubulation repair with type I collagen nerve guide tubes. *Restor Neurol Neurosci* 1989;1:31.

Seckel BR: Enhancement of peripheral nerve regeneration. *Muscle Nerve* 1990;13:785–800.

Seckel BR, Chiu TH, Nyilas E, Sidman RL: Nerve regeneration through synthetic biodegradable nerve guides: Regulation by the target organ. *Plast Reconstr Surg* 1984;74:173–181.

Seckel BR, Ryan SE, Gagne RG, Chiu TH, Watkins E Jr: Target-specific nerve regeneration through a nerve guide in the rat. *Plast Reconstr Surg* 1986;78:793–800.

Sumner AJ: Aberrant reinnervation. *Muscle Nerve* 1990;13:801–803.

Tessier-Lavigne M, Placzek M: Target attraction: Are developing axons guided by chemotropism? *Trends Neurosci* 1991;14:303–310.

Thomas CK, Stein RB, Gordon T, Lee RG, Elleker MG: Patterns of reinnervation and motor unit recruitment in human hand muscles after complete ulnar and median nerve section and resuture. *J Neurol Neurosurg Psychiatry* 1987;50:259–268.

Wasserschaff M: Coordination of reinnervated muscle and reorganization of spinal cord motoneurons after nerve transection in mice. *Brain Res* 1990;515:241–246.

Williams LR: Exogenous fibrin matrix precursors stimulate the temporal progress of nerve regeneration within a silicone chamber. *Neurochem Res* 1987;12:851–860.

Williams LR, Danielsen N, Muller H, Varon S: Exogenous matrix precursors promote functional nerve regeneration across a 15-mm gap within a silicone chamber in the rat. *J Comp Neurol* 1987;264: 284–290.

Woolley AL, Hollowell JP, Rich KM: Fibronectin-laminin combination enhances peripheral nerve regeneration across long gaps. *Otolaryngol Head Neck Surg* 1990;103:509–518.

Yamada S, Buffinger N, DiMario J, Strohman RC: Fibroblast growth factor is stored in fiber extracellular matrix and plays a role in regulating muscle hypertrophy. *Med Sci Sports Exerc* 1989;21(suppl 5): S173–S180.

Surgical Nerve Repair

Brunelli G, Monini L, Brunelli F: Problems in nerve lesions surgery. *Microsurgery* 1985;6:187–198.

Gelberman RH (ed): *Operative Nerve Repair and Reconstruction*. Philadelphia, PA, JB Lippincott, 1991.

Mackinnon SE, Dellon AL (eds): *Surgery of the Peripheral Nerve*. New York, NY, Thieme Medical Publishers, 1988.

Millesi H: Nerve grafting. *Clin Plast Surg* 1984;11:105–113.

Millesi H: The nerve gap: Theory and clinical practice. *Hand Clin* 1986;2:651–663.

Millesi H: Brachial plexus injuries: Nerve grafting. *Clin Orthop* 1988; 237:36–42.

Millesi H: Progress in peripheral nerve reconstruction. *World J Surg* 1990;14:733–747.

Moberg E: Nerve repair in hand surgery: An analysis. *Surg Clin North Am* 1968;48:985–991.

Nicholson OR, Seddon HJ: Nerve repair in civil practice: Results of treatment of median and ulnar nerve lesions. *Br Med J* 1957;2: 1065–1071.

Orgel MG, Terzis JK: Epineurial vs. perineurial repair: An ultrastructural and electrophysiological study of nerve regeneration. *Plast Reconstr Surg* 1977;60:80–91.

Omer GE Jr: The evaluation of clinical results following peripheral nerve suture, in Omer GE Jr, Spinner M (eds): *Management of Peripheral Nerve Problems*. Philadelphia, PA, WB Saunders, 1980, pp 431–442.

Suematsu N: Tubulation for peripheral nerve gap: Its history and possibility. *Microsurgery* 1989;10:71–74.

Sunderland S: The intraneural topography of the radial, median and ulnar nerves. *Brain* 1945;68:243–299.

Sunderland S: Funicular suture and funicular exclusion in the repair of severed nerves. *Br J Surg* 1953;40:580–587.

Terzis JK, Smith KL (eds): *The Peripheral Nerve: Structure, Function and Reconstruction*. New York, NY, Raven Press, 1990.

Yahr MD, Beebe GW: Recovery of motor function, in Woodhall B, Beebe GW (eds): *Peripheral Nerve Regeneration: A Follow-Up Study of 3,656 World War II Injuries*. Washington, DC, US Government Printing Office, 1956.

Chapter Outline

Chapter 26

Anatomy, Physiology, and Mechanics of Skeletal Muscle

William E. Garrett, Jr, MD, PhD

Thomas M. Best, MD, PhD

This chapter at a glance

This chapter discusses the anatomy, physiology, and mechanics of skeletal muscle; specifically, muscle structure and function, growth and development, injury and repair, energetics, fiber types, and training effects.

One or more of the authors or the department with which they are affiliated has received something of value from a commercial or other party related directly or indirectly to the subject of this chapter.

Introduction

Skeletal muscle constitutes the single largest tissue mass in the body, making up 40% to 45% of the total body weight. It is a composite structure that consists of muscle cells, organized networks of nerves and blood vessels, and an extracellular connective tissue matrix (Fig. 1). This framework is necessary to support and protect the structure against injury and to organize the individual units into tissues and organs that can contract efficiently to produce joint movement and locomotion. With its enormous adaptive potential, variability, and dependability, skeletal muscle has been the subject of many theories and complex philosophic schemes to explain the fascinating aspects of animal movement. In the last few centuries, and particularly in recent years, knowledge of skeletal muscle has expanded rapidly.

Muscle Structure and Function

Histologic Organization

The basic structural element of skeletal muscle is the muscle fiber. It is a syncytium of many cells fused together with multiple nuclei. The fiber runs from tendon or bone across 1 or more joints into a tendon of insertion, which connects to bone. The fiber is a single very long "cell," but usually is much shorter than the length of the muscle because of its oblique orientation to the muscle axis. Fiber arrangement can be parallel or oblique to the long axis of the muscle (Fig. 2). The latter arrangement includes pennate, bipennate, multipennate, or even more complex fiber arrangements.

Muscle fibers are organized histologically by the surrounding connective tissue. This framework binds the contractile units together to provide for integrated motion among the fibers. The endomysium is the delicate connective tissue surrounding individual fibers. In turn, fibers are arranged together as fascicles, which are large enough to be visible to the naked eye. The connective tissue surrounding fascicles is called the perimysium and that surrounding the whole muscle is called the epimysium. This membrane covers the muscle loosely to allow for the length changes that occur in muscle. Blood vessels supplying the fibers also are arranged in the connective tissue with enough redundancy to allow for changes in length during the contraction-extension cycle of a muscle.

In addition to a highly organized pattern at the microscopic level, muscle fibers have a highly organized architectural arrangement. Fiber arrangement within the muscle is an important determinant of its functional and contractile properties (Fig. 3). As muscle fibers shorten, the muscle's volume usually is assumed to be constant. Consequently, the tendon moves only along the axis of pull, and fibers become more pennated (α increases, Fig. 3, *D*). Therefore, the fiber and tendon shortening are not colinear, and the force along the axis of the tendon is reduced by cos α. Although this pennated arrangement results in a reduction

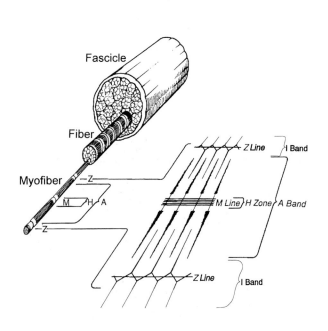

Figure 1

Schematic drawing of the structural design of human skeletal muscle.

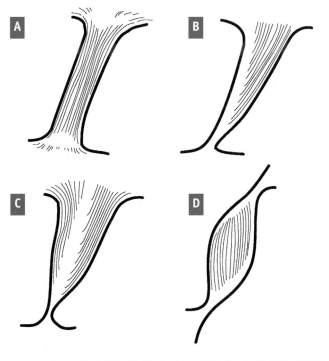

Figure 2

Muscle fiber architecture. **A,** Parallel. **B,** Unipennate. **C,** Bipennate. **D,** Fusiform.

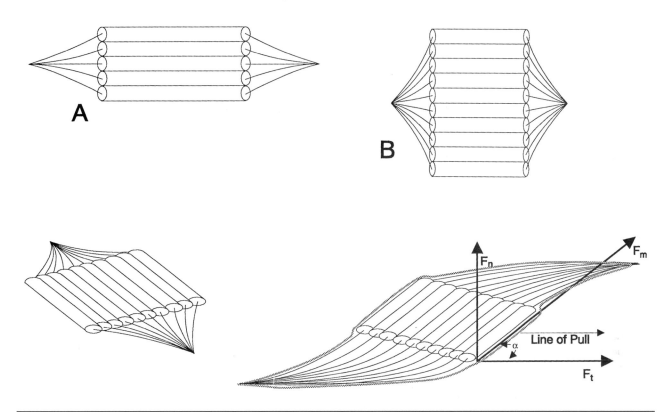

Figure 3

The effects of muscle architecture on force development and length change. **Top,** The length of A is twice that of B; the cross-sectional area of A equals that of B; the maximum force of A is one-half that of B and the maximum length change of A is twice that of B. **Bottom left,** The force is diminished only by a small factor when fibers are arranged in a pennate fashion. **Bottom right,** The effect of fiber angle pennation on whole-muscle force. α = angle of pennation; F_m = muscle force; F_n = normal component; F_t = tangential component.

of the muscle fiber force transmitted to the tendon, it permits a larger number of fibers to be packed in a smaller cross-sectional area.

In general, maximal force production of a muscle is proportional to its physiologic cross-sectional area (PCSA), but the total amount and speed of shortening are proportional to individual muscle fiber length. A muscle needed more for force production might have many short fibers arranged in a pennate fashion. However, the same amount of muscle tissue could be arranged in fewer but longer fibers when more shortening and less force are required of the muscle. In general, the architectural arrangement of its muscle fibers is quite specific to the task of a muscle in the body and is one of the primary mechanisms used for specificity of function.

In clinical practice a muscle made ineffective by direct trauma or denervation may be substituted by the transfer of another muscle-tendon unit. It is necessary to have a tendon with suitable size and length to allow transfer. Because the ability of the muscle to shorten and to generate force is largely determined by the number, size, and architectural arrangement of the muscle fibers within the muscle belly, it is important to match the characteristics desired of the deficient muscle with those of the transferred muscle.

Cytology of the Muscle Fiber

Individual muscle fibers are surrounded by a plasma membrane known as the sarcolemma. External to this membrane is a separate basement membrane that is a connective tissue structure 100 to 200 nm thick. Electron microscopy shows that this membrane consists of an inner layer, the lamina rara or lucida, and an outer, more dense layer, the lamina densa. The basement membrane then merges with a reticular layer and the extracellular matrix. This basement membrane contains a number of protein and carbohydrate components contributed by both the muscle fiber and fibroblasts. Among its components are collagen, laminin, fibronectin, and other specific glycoproteins. The basement membrane, the reticular layer, and the close layer of matrix and collagen fibers together constitute the endomysium, which is well supplied with capillaries.

Each striated muscle fiber contains numerous nuclei, which typically are located at the periphery of the fiber immediately beneath the sarcolemma. In addition, separate cells called satellite cells lie along the surface of the muscle at the periphery of each fiber. These cells are thought to be stem cells capable of proliferation and regeneration in the event of damage to the muscle fibers.

A muscle fiber contains a sarcoplasm that includes the

contents of the sarcolemma exclusive of the nuclei. The sarcoplasm is similar to the cytoplasm of other cell types and, therefore, contains a cellular matrix and organelles. These organelles include the Golgi apparatus found near many of the nuclei and the mitochondria, which are abundant near the nuclei. The other important organelle is the sarcoplasmic reticulum, a continuous system of membrane that corresponds to the endoplasmic reticulum of other cell types. Other components of the sarcoplasm include lipid droplets, glycogen, and myoglobin.

Nerve-Muscle Interaction

Skeletal muscle is under the control of a nerve that enters the muscle at its motor point. Each nerve cell axon then branches many times, and every muscle fiber is contacted by a single nerve terminal. This point of contact is called the motor end plate (Fig. 4) and is the site of cellular communication between the nervous system and skeletal muscles. Together a single nerve axon and all muscle fibers it contacts constitute a motor unit. Muscle fibers belonging to a single motor unit are not necessarily adjacent; adjacent muscle fibers can belong to different motor units. Both the number of muscle fibers within a motor unit and the number of motor units within a given muscle are quite variable. Where fine motor control and coordinated movements are necessary, as in the extraocular muscles, there may be as few as 10 muscle fibers per motor unit. Yet in large muscles

such as the gastrocnemius there may be more than 1,000 muscle fibers in a single motor unit. The size of the motor unit is also related to the size of the motor axon and to the size of the cell body in the anterior gray horn of the spinal cord. In addition, motor unit size is related to the fiber type and physiology of muscle, as will be discussed below.

A motor unit is stimulated to contract by an electrical impulse, or action potential, which originates from the cell body of the nerve. This potential is propagated down the entire length of the axon from the spinal cord to the peripheral skeletal muscle. The nerve forms a synapse with the muscle at a specialized region known as the motor end plate. An electrical impulse passing along the cell membrane of the axon is transformed to a similar electrical signal in the membrane of the muscle fiber. This transmission is not achieved by direct electrical transmission; the process involves chemical transmission across a gap of extracellular space separating the 2 membrane systems. As the axon approaches the muscle at the synapse, it loses its myelin sheath and the entire terminal axon is covered by a Schwann cell, a connective tissue cell surrounding nerve fibers (Fig. 4). The nerve terminal spreads out over an area of the muscle membrane called the sole plate. An axon terminal and muscle membrane interdigitate across a series of membrane foldings called primary synaptic folds, which greatly amplify the area of membrane juxtaposed between nerve and muscle. At all times the muscle membrane is separated from the nerve membrane by a space of approximately

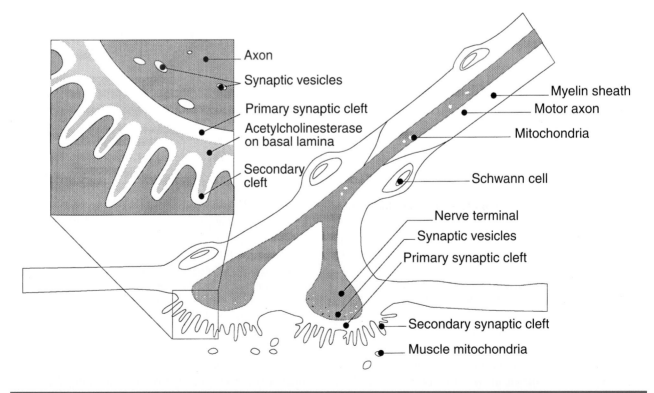

Figure 4

Schematic representations of the motor end plate.

50 nm, called the synaptic cleft.

The nerve and muscle membranes are not in direct contact, and signals are passed from nerve to muscle by chemical transmitters. The chemical acetylcholine is stored in the presynaptic axon in small membrane-bound sacs called vesicles. When the electrical impulse arrives in the terminal axon, the membrane allows the flow of calcium ions into the cell. An increase in the intracellular calcium concentration causes the vesicles to fuse with the terminal axon membrane and to release acetylcholine into the synaptic cleft. The acetylcholine must then diffuse across the synaptic cleft and bind to a specific receptor on the surface of the muscle membrane. The binding of the acetylcholine to its receptor allows currents to flow into the muscle membrane and depolarize the cell. Depolarization triggers an action potential that passes the length of the muscle membrane. The action potential in the muscle membrane is similar to the action potential in a nerve. The acetylcholine is deactivated by the enzyme acetylcholinesterase or other less specific cholinesterases located in the extracellular space and associated with the basement membrane. The breakdown products may be reabsorbed by the terminal axon to be used in the resynthesis of additional transmitter.

Various pharmacologic and physiologic processes influence the neuromuscular junction. Alpha-tubocurarine binds to the acetylcholine receptors and makes impulse transmission impossible. This agent was discovered initially as a poison used on the arrows of South American Indian tribes to paralyze an animal, and today it is commonly used as a paralyzing anesthetic agent. Succinylcholine and many other compounds can exert a similar effect on muscle by various interactions with the receptor. Succinylcholine actually binds to the receptor and causes temporary depolarization of the muscle membrane, followed by failure of impulse transmission.

Other pharmacologic agents can inhibit acetylcholinesterase and lead to continued high concentrations of acetylcholine at the synapse. These agents can be used to help reverse the effects of paralyzing agents or to treat diseases characterized by deficient interactions between acetylcholine and its receptor. Myasthenia gravis is a disease characterized by severe muscle weakness that is particularly evident following muscle fatigue. The basic pathophysiology is a shortage of acetylcholine receptors, which probably is caused by an autoimmune reaction against the receptors. Cholinesterase inhibitors, such as neostigmine and edrophonium, allow a longer life for acetylcholine and, therefore, more chance for it to interact with receptors before hydrolysis of the molecule. The effects of these medically useful agents are, of course, reversible. There are also compounds that alter the cholinesterase irreversibly. These anticholinesterase compounds include the highly toxic nerve gases used in chemical warfare and in certain insecticides. The toxicity of these irreversible agents limits their clinical usefulness.

Muscle Membrane System

Muscle fibers are long cells, and electrical activity at the surface is far away from the central portions of these fibers. Following depolarization of the end plate, the electrical impulse passes down the muscle membrane to reach the interior of the muscle by an intricate membrane system (Fig. 5). This extensive system facilitates communication of the surface signals into the depths of the muscle fiber, permitting rapid signal impulse throughout the cell. Transverse tubules, generally directed perpendicularly to the axis of the cells, penetrate from the surface into the fibers near the level of the A-band and I-band junction in mammalian muscle. The transverse tubules interact with another large system of membrane-bound sacs called the sarcoplasmic reticulum, which stores calcium inside its membrane system and, therefore, out of the muscle cytoplasm. The membranes of the sarcoplasmic reticulum actively accumulate calcium from the muscle cytoplasm.

An electrical impulse originating within the muscle membrane and tubular systems causes the momentary release of calcium from the sarcoplasmic reticulum into the muscle cytoplasm. Calcium release is the trigger that causes the contractile proteins to interact and to generate force. The membrane system, including the surface membrane, transverse tubules, and sarcoplasmic reticulum, provides a mechanism for rapid conduction of an electric signal from the cell surface throughout the entire fiber. This system allows for more concurrent release of calcium, synchronized interactions of muscle proteins, and subsequent production of force.

The sarcoplasmic reticulum is specialized for somewhat different functions. The portion that abuts the transverse

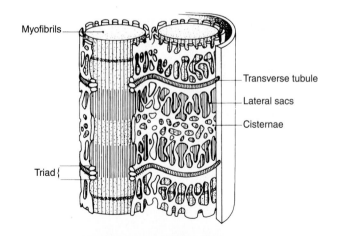

Figure 5

Details of the sarcoplasmic reticulum (SR), the system of membranes responsible for transmission of the electrical signal from one muscle cell to the next. An action potential moving over the surface of the fiber passes down the transverse tubules and causes Ca^{2+} release from the outer vesicles of the SR.

tubules is called the junctional sarcoplasmic reticulum. Usually the transverse tubule is linked to 2 sacs of the junctional reticulum in a structure called a triad. Bridging structures connect the 3 separate membrane systems. Electrical impulses in the tubules will cause calcium release from this sarcoplasmic reticulum. Other specializations of the sarcoplasmic reticulum include fenestrated and tubular membranous structures placed throughout the cell.

The sarcoplasmic reticulum contains specific enzymes for sequestration of calcium into the membrane system and out of the sarcoplasm. Control of the intracellular calcium concentration is the mechanism for regulating the on-off contractile function of the contractile proteins. The calcium adenosine triphosphatase (ATPase) protein is a distinct membrane protein. Calsequestrin and another glycoprotein with a high affinity for calcium are other protein components of the sarcoplasmic reticulum.

Structural Proteins of Muscle

The proteins responsible for force production in the presence of calcium form highly ordered structures in the muscle cytoplasm. Observation of histologic sections of muscle shows that a high degree of order exists, and that there is a repeating structural array of longitudinal fibers with a discrete cross-striated appearance. If the plasma membrane and basement membranes of a muscle fiber are disrupted, the internal structures of the cell are seen to consist of many long, slender, parallel elements called myofibrils. The long myofibrils are about 1 μm in diameter and have a distinct banding pattern. The patterns in the individual myofibrils are usually in register in the muscle fiber. This gives the entire fiber a striated appearance by light microscopy, giving rise to striated muscle as the descriptive term for skeletal muscle. Within the fiber and within the

individual myofibrils, there is a regular arrangement of alternating light and dark bands with a repeating period of 2 to 3 μm. The ordered structure is explained by the molecular structure of the contractile proteins.

The fibril is composed of repeating units called sarcomeres (Fig. 6). The fine structure of the sarcomere can be seen with the electron microscope. There are repeating light and dark bands; each of the bands is bisected by a more darkly staining line. The dark band or A-band is composed primarily of parallel thick filaments in register with a central set of interconnecting filaments called the M-line. The thick filaments are composed primarily of the protein myosin. Myosin is a hexameric molecule, molecular weight of about 500,000 daltons, composed of 2 large isomers known as heavy chains and 4 smaller polypeptides called light chains (Fig. 7). The molecule has a long relatively insoluble helical portion that polymerizes to form the backbone portion of the thick filament. There are also 2 associated globular portions of the molecule called cross-bridges, which project from the backbone of the thick filament. These globular proteins can be enzymatically cleaved from the helical portion of the myosin molecule and are soluble in physiologic solutions. The myosin projections are the enzymatic portion of the molecule; they are capable of binding to the thin filaments and are capable of hydrolyzing adenosine triphosphate (ATP).

In addition to myosin, there are other proteins that make up the thick filaments. Among these are C-protein, M-protein, and titin. Titin is a large (10^6) protein that is involved in the tiny filamentous connections between the ends of the thick filaments to the Z-line. Additionally, M-protein, myosin, and creatine kinase are associated with thick filaments at the M-line. Creatine kinase catalyzes the phosphorylation of adenosine diphosphate (ADP) to form ATP and may be important in maintaining the supply of energy

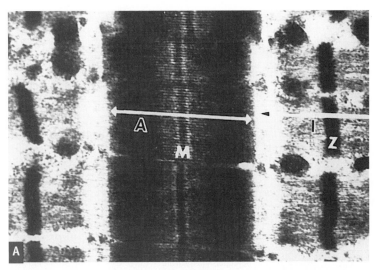
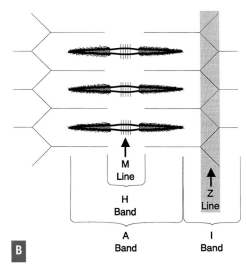

Figure 6

A, Electron micrograph of skeletal muscle illustrating the striated, banded appearance. A = A-band; M = M-line; I = I-band; 2 = 2-line. **B,** The basic functional unit of skeletal muscle, the sarcomere.

molecules to the cross-bridges. The functions of the minor proteins of the A-band are not well characterized.

The I-band is composed of thin filaments in register and joined at their axial center by the interconnecting Z-line (Fig. 8). The thin filaments are made up primarily of molecules of the protein actin. The thin filaments are approximately 1.0 μm long; the protein and the filament size are highly conserved. Actin monomers are arranged in a helical fashion on the thin filaments with an axial separation of 5.5 nm between subunits and a helical repeat of approximately 77 nm. Two other proteins associated with the thin filaments are troponin and tropomyosin, which will be discussed below. Other proteins associated with the Z-line include α-actinin, desmin, zeugmatin, and filamin. The Z-line is a highly organized structure that interconnects the thin filaments in a very precise array. The thick filaments of the A-band are arranged in a hexagonal lattice. A-bands and I-bands interdigitate so that the thin filaments are located at the trigonal points of the hexagonal lattice of thick filaments. The cross-bridges project from the thick filaments toward the thin filaments at regular intervals of approximately 14.3 nm.

The guiding hypothesis for muscle shortening calls for the cross-bridges from the thick filaments to reach out and attach to the thin filaments. Cross-bridges use the energy made available from the hydrolysis of ATP to undergo a conformational change and, by some mechanism, cause the thick filaments to slide past the thin filaments. The cross-bridges cycle many times as they release from the actin on the thin filament, spring back to their initial conformation, and are ready to repeat the process in rapid succession. Both actin and myosin molecules have a recognizable polarity, which is essential to muscular contraction. To allow shortening of the sarcomere, the polarity must be different in the thick filaments on either side of the M-line so

that the thick filament arrays of the I-bands on either side of the A-band are pulled toward each other and toward the center of the A-band. Similarly, the thin filaments must have opposite polarity on either side of the Z-line so that they are pulled in between the thick filaments by the cross-bridges to allow shortening and force production (Fig. 8). These features form the basis of the well-known sliding filament-swinging cross-bridge theory of muscle contraction.

How does calcium regulate this process? Troponin and tropomyosin are regulatory proteins linked to the actin molecules (Fig. 9). Tropomyosin is an approximately 41-nm long helical molecule that is situated on the thin filament in such a manner that it prevents the cross-bridges from binding to the actin. The 2 main subunits of the molecule are the α and β polypeptide chains, which differ mainly in their cysteine content and electrophoretic mobility. The ratio of these 2 subunits varies among fiber types. Troponin is the calcium-sensitive regulatory protein that can induce a conformational change in tropomyosin and, thereby, allow cross-bridge association with actin. Troponin has 3 subunits: troponin-I is inhibitory and can block actin-myosin interaction; troponin-T binds to tropomyosin; and troponin-C can bind calcium. A high enough concentration of

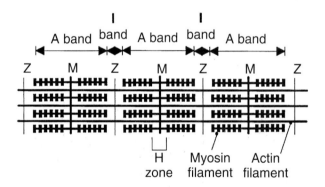

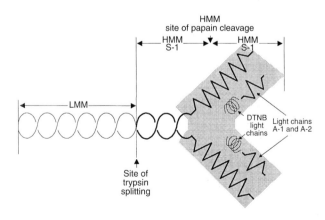

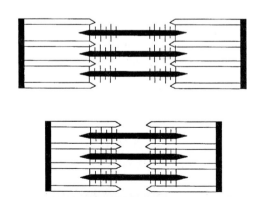

Figure 7

Schematic drawing of myosin molecule showing subunit structure. The heavy-chain component possesses the ATPase activity and the light chain confers solubility properties of the molecule. HMM = heavy meromyosin; LMM = light meromyosin.

Figure 8

Schematic drawing indicating the sliding of thick and thin filaments that occurs when a muscle is stretched. Note the constancy of the lengths of both thick and thin filaments. (Adapted with permission from Carlson FD, Wilkie DR: *Muscle Physiology.* New Jersey, Prentice Hall, 1974.)

calcium in the sarcoplasm will allow binding of calcium to troponin-C. A conformational change then removes the troponin-I from its inhibitory position and allows for actin and myosin interaction, with subsequent ATP hydrolysis and initiation of muscle contraction. When calcium is no longer available to the troponin, its conformation reverts and the tropomyosin shifts back to create a stearic block to the cross-bridges.

The physiology of muscle cell activation can be summarized as follows. A single electrical impulse passes down an axon to its motor end plates, chemical transmission occurs at the synapses, and electrical potentials are generated in the muscle membranes. These electrical potentials pass along the muscle surface and into the fibers via the transverse tubules, resulting in calcium release from the sarcoplasmic reticulum. Calcium binds to the thin filaments and causes conformational changes that allow interactions between thick and thin filaments. Using the energy from the hydrolysis of ATP, the cross-bridges cycle and cause the sarcomeres to attempt to shorten or to resist stretch by pulling the thin filament arrays into the thick filament arrays. The contractile proteins interact, resulting in muscle contraction and force production. Following completion of the electrical event, muscle relaxation occurs by active transport of the calcium into the longitudinal tubules of the sarcoplasmic reticulum. This results in calcium dissociation from troponin and a conformational change in tropomyosin to prevent further cross-bridge attachment.

Muscle Contraction or Action

The cellular events in the process of muscle activation can now be considered at the level of the whole neuromuscular organ system along with the physiologic basis for muscle contraction. Traditionally, it has been important to define the conditions under which muscle is activated, because many parameters are believed to influence its contraction.

For the most part, muscle has been studied under conditions of controlled length or tension. In isometric (same length) testing, muscle length is held constant, and the resultant force is measured. Alternatively, in isotonic (same load) testing, a muscle is activated to shorten against a constant load, while length changes with time are assessed. More recently, muscle has been evaluated under isokinetic (same speed) activation, which the load accommodates to maintain a constant velocity of shortening or lengthening.

Muscle activation results in force generation within the muscle. If the resisting load is less than the force generated by the muscle, then the muscle will shorten; this condition is termed concentric action (or contraction). If the resisting force is greater than that generated by the muscle, the muscle will lengthen; this is termed eccentric action (or contraction). Some confusion has been generated by the traditional use of the term muscle contraction. Muscle can be activated and lengthened simultaneously. Rather than call this condition an eccentric (or lengthening) contraction, it is, perhaps, less confusing to call it eccentric action. However, contraction usually refers to the action of activated muscle whether its length is decreasing, constant, or increasing.

Conditions of nerve activation can be controlled to produce a single stimulus, repetitive stimuli at constant frequencies, or stimuli in other desired modes. For a single activation, the muscle tension can be seen to rise quickly and then fall back to baseline in a variable amount of time, usually less than 200 ms. This physiologic event is called a muscle twitch, the tension response by a muscle to a single nerve stimulus (Fig. 10). There is no increment in tension as a result of repetitive stimuli if a second nerve action potential arrives after the tension in response to the first action potential has returned to the baseline and the membrane has stabilized. All that happens is that another twitch occurs. However, if the nerve stimulation frequency increases such that successive action potentials arrive before the contractile tension resulting from the previous stimulus has returned to the baseline, the tension can rise above the tension of a single twitch. As the stimulation frequency increases, the tension in the muscle displays a summation effect that, with higher frequencies of stimulation, approaches a maximum level called a tetanus. The tension generated during tetanus can be several times that of a twitch, making the alteration of stimulation frequency a powerful mechanism under control of the central nervous system (CNS) for altering tension. Stimulation frequencies needed to achieve tetanic stimulation vary from 40 to 300 Hz for different muscles and species.

The force of muscle contraction can be increased either by altering the frequency of stimulation to make the same motor units work harder or by involving more motor units (recruitment). It is now believed that these phenomena occur together, resulting in a very ordered and sequential recruitment of motor units and regulation of activation frequency to optimize muscle contraction and limb motion. The relative contribution of these 2 mechanisms to increasing force production varies among different muscles. For example, in muscles such as the abductor pollicis, motor

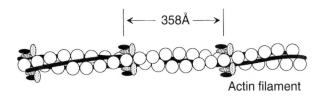

<!-- 358Å --> 358Å

Actin filament

Figure 9

Features of regulation of muscle contraction. Structure of actin is represented by two chains of beads in a double helix. The troponin complex consists of calcium-binding protein (TN-C, black); inhibitory protein (TN-I, cross-hatched); and protein binding to tropomyosin (TN-T, stippled). The tropomyosin (dark line) lies in each groove of the actin filament.

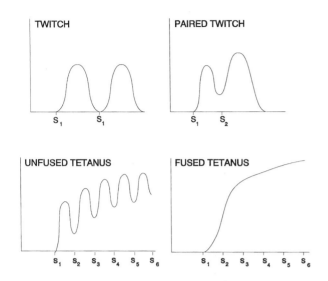

Twitch and tetanus. As the frequency of stimulation is increased, muscle force rises to an eventual plateau level known as fused tetanus.

unit recruitment is probably maximum when the force reaches about 30% of maximum; whereas, in muscles such as the biceps brachii, motor unit recruitment is believed to occur up to 85% of the maximum force.

Myotendinous Junction

The force generated within muscle fibers must be transmitted to the tendon to produce limb movement and human locomotion. The area responsible for this force transmission is the myotendinous junction, a region of highly folded membranes at the muscle-tendon interface (Fig. 11). This folding increases junctional surface area by 10 to 20 times. Because stress is proportional to force and inversely related to contact area, the large increase in membrane area within this region results in a corresponding decrease in the stresses. In addition, the stresses are changed from tensile to shear because the membranes are aligned nearly parallel with the axis of the muscle and the tendon.

The structural and molecular organization of the myotendinous junction is being studied in more detail. The thin filaments appear to terminate beneath the muscle plasma membrane within subsarcolemmal densities that seem to be involved with the binding of the contractile proteins to the cell membranes. At least 2 cytoskeletal proteins, vinculin and talin, are thought to be involved in the molecular chain linking the thin filaments to the extracellular structural proteins. A separate structural link must actually traverse the cell membrane of the muscle. The likely molecular link is a large transmembrane glycoprotein called integrin, which has an affinity for both the intracellular and extracellular structural proteins and exists within the cell

membrane at the myotendinous junction. On the extracellular side of the junction is a well-developed basement membrane seen easily by electron microscopy. At this region, the forces generated by the myofibrils and passed across the cell membrane are thought to be linked to the extracellular collagen fibers of the tendon. Among the proteins present in the basement membrane are fibronectin, laminin, and type IV collagen. Some of these proteins have a molecular affinity for the collagen of the tendon.

Fiber Types and Adaptability of Muscle

The Motor Unit

A motor unit includes a single alpha motoneuron axon and the muscle fibers it innervates. All muscle fibers in a single motor unit have the same contractile and metabolic properties, implying that the muscle fiber type is related to its interaction with its motor nerve. Different fiber or motor unit types are widely recognized, and they have distinctly different physiologic, structural, and histochemical proper-

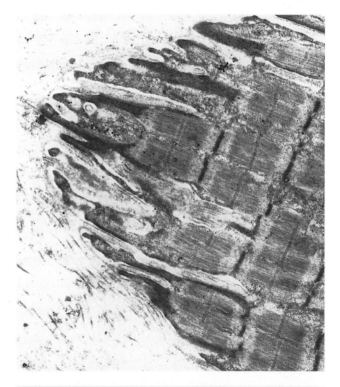

The myotendinous junction. Electron micrograph of a myotendinous junction section longitudinally. Myofilaments distal to the terminal Z disk end in a series of filaments bounded by a folded plasmalemma. (Reproduced with permission from Tidball JG: Myotendinous junction: Morphological changes and mechanical failure associated with muscle cell atrophy. *Exp Mol Pathol* 1984;40:1–12.)

ties (Table 1). For example, chicken muscle exists in distinctly different fiber types as noted by color (dark or white) and taste. More recent observations of different muscle fiber types have been aided greatly by the use of histochemical stains. Histochemical staining allows differentiation of muscle fibers based on the reactivity of muscle structural proteins and metabolic pathways in response to incubation in appropriate chemical reactants. Serial sections can then be used to compare the properties of the same fiber after exposure to other histochemical stains and to routine histologic techniques.

The most useful histochemical techniques for distinguishing fiber types are those based on the ability of myosin to hydrolyze ATP and those based on the enzymes and substrates of the different metabolic pathways in muscle fibers. The enzyme that hydrolizes ATP is referred to as actomyosin ATPase, or more commonly the myosin ATPase. Differences in the specific ATPase activities of myosin are a result of the existence of several forms of this protein. Myosin from muscles that develop tension slowly (slow twitch muscles) is acid stable and alkaline labile, whereas the opposite is true for myosin from muscles that develop tension quickly (fast twitch muscles). According to the sliding filament hypothesis, myosin is the most important contractile protein because it hydrolyzes the ATP to yield the energy for formation of the actomyosin complex. Furthermore, the activity of the myosin ATPase correlates closely with the intrinsic speed of muscle shortening. Much of the regulation and alteration of skeletal muscle phenotypes involves the myosin molecule, and the relative size of a muscle fiber appears to be related to the type of myosin expressed. Relatively large fibers express primarily fast myosin, whereas relatively small fibers express slow myosin.

Histochemical stains have allowed profiling of several sets of fibers according to the structural, biochemical, and physiologic characteristics of the fiber types. There are also subtle differences in the myofibrillar structure. At least 3 separate motor unit profiles are widely accepted, although available evidence and classification schemes make it clear that there is significant overlap and that other fiber types might also be considered.

The type I or slow-oxidative fiber is characterized histochemically by a light reaction to myosin ATPase stains at alkaline conditions and a heavy reaction to the enzymes and substrates of oxidative metabolic pathways. Physiologically this fiber type has slower contraction and relaxation times than other fiber types. The contraction time of a muscle relates to the rate at which force is developed after electrical stimulation (for example, fast or slow), and relaxation time relates to the rate of decline of force in the muscle following cessation of stimulation. Type I motor units, those with type I fibers, are extremely resistant to fatigue. Structurally, there are more mitochondria in these fibers as well as more capillaries per fiber.

Type II motor units can be subdivided into several subgroups; however, 2 main subgroups usually are considered, types IIA and IIB. The type IIB or fast glycolytic motor unit has the fastest contraction time and is the least resistant to fatigue. As expected from its physiologic characteristics, this type has a well-developed glycolytic metabolic capacity and a less well-developed oxidative system. The type IIB motor unit has the largest number of muscle fibers per motor unit, the largest axon, and the largest cell body.

Intermediate between type I and type IIB motor units are the type IIA or fast oxidative glycolytic motor units. Their contraction times are faster than type I but slower than type IIB. Similarly, their fatigue resistance lies between that of types I and IIB motor units. In IIA motor units, both the

Table 1
Characteristics of Human Skeletal Muscle Fiber Types

	Type I	Type IIA	Type IIB
Other Names	Red, slow twitch (ST) Slow oxidative (SO)	White, fast twitch (FT) Fast oxidative glycolytic (FOG)	Fast glycolytic (FG)
Speed of contraction	Slow	Fast	Fast
Strength of contraction	Low	High	High
Fatigability	Fatigue-resistant	Fatigable	Most fatigable
Aerobic capacity	High	Medium	Low
Anaerobic capacity	Low	Medium	High
Motor unit size	Small	Larger	Largest
Capillary density	High	High	Low

oxidative and glycolytic pathways are well developed. Axon size and the number of muscle fibers per motor unit in type IIA motor units also rank between types I and IIB motor units. Distinctions in physiologic, histochemical, and biochemical properties are less distinct between IIA and IIB fibers than between either of them and type I fibers. Biochemically, the structural proteins in the sarcomere are also distinct. Myosin, tropomyosin, and troposin have distinct structural isomers with different fiber types. Recent investigations have shown more heterogeneity in the structural proteins than had been expected.

Most mammalian carnivores, including humans, also have a type IIC fiber, which is most prominent in the jaw muscle. It has a unique myosin with physiologic and histochemical properties intermediate in the spectrum, between type IIA and type IIB fibers. At birth, up to 10% of muscle fibers may be type IIC; this declines to approximately 2% after the first year of life. As a result, it is often thought that the type IIC fiber is an undifferentiated fiber. During physical training there may be as many as 10% of these fibers present in some muscles of endurance athletes. Their presence has yet to be explained, although it is thought by some that this fiber type represents a transitional form between types I and II fibers.

Motor units and fiber types are recruited into activity by the CNS in an orderly fashion according to size. The smaller motor units, composed predominantly of type I fibers, are recruited first, whereas the largest motor units, composed of type IIB fibers, are recruited primarily with exercise of higher intensity, and the type IIA fibers or motor units are intermediate in size and order of recruitment. Biochemistry studies of muscle glycogen depletion patterns in man have supported this concept. It has been shown that low intensity exercise results in significant glycogen depletion in the type I fibers with little change in type II fibers. Conversely, high intensity exercise produces glycogen depletion in both fiber types, but it is more severe in the type II fibers.

Correlation of Fiber Type With Performance

Most human muscles are composed of a mixture of the muscle fiber types discussed above, whereas some animal muscles are composed of a single muscle fiber type. The tonic or postural muscles such as the soleus are usually situated closer to the bony skeleton and have a greater proportion of type I fibers. In contrast, the phasic or faster contracting muscles lie in a more superficial position and have a higher proportion of type II fibers. However, individual variations in fiber type composition are often quite large, and biopsies of the vastus lateralis muscle may vary to the extent that more than 90% of the muscle fibers are either type I or type II fibers. In addition, significant variations in fiber type percentages occur at different locations within the same muscle for a given individual. Thus, significant skepticism should be displayed when interpreting the results of studies showing changes in fiber type proportions in response to different exercise regimens.

The physiologic properties of a muscle largely reflect the specific types and concentrations of proteins within the muscle. Inherent fiber type differences appear to be related to performance capacity, especially where speed of contraction and endurance or fatigability are concerned. Muscle biopsies from successful sprinters are much more likely to show a preponderance of type II fibers. Similarly, distance runners are highly inclined toward having predominantly type I fibers. Athletes in those sports requiring the extremes of speed and endurance often display a fiber type profile that is consistent with current knowledge of fiber type differences. However, it remains unknown at this time if these fiber distributions are genetically based or are a response to sustained extremes of training.

In addition, isokinetic dynamometers can be used to evaluate the ability of individuals to perform motor tasks requiring speed or endurance for which they have not trained, and muscle biopsy indicates a correlation between performance and fiber type. Those with a higher percentage of type I fibers will generally exhibit more endurance, whereas those with more type II fibers will demonstrate more torque at higher speeds. There is overlap, however, and fiber type is only one of many factors relevant to performance capacity. Most sports are neither purely speed nor endurance oriented, and fiber type percentage provides little correlation with performance. In addition, athletes without a fiber type composition that might be considered ideal are still able to excel at speed and endurance sports. Therefore, the use of biopsy results in selecting athletes for sport is not generally accepted.

Mutability of Fiber Types

Various forms of overload can bring about adaptation of all components of the motor unit including the muscle fiber itself, the neuromuscular junction, and the corresponding α-motoneuron. This biologic plasticity of muscle typically results in a logical alteration of both the morphology and the function of the muscle fiber, which is consistent with the hypothesis that muscle adapts to the function it performs. This polymorphism of the skeletal muscle fiber also exists in smooth muscle and cardiac muscle. A variety of stimuli including cross-reinnervation, electrical stimulation, hypergravity stress, thyrotoxicosis, compensatory hypertrophy, and exercise have been studied to elucidate mechanisms for this adaptive response.

Extreme conditions, beyond those usually encountered in rigorous training, can lead to fiber type interconversions. Studies have shown that a nerve to predominantly type I muscle can be cut and reconnected to the distal cut end of a predominantly type II muscle. Similarly, the proximal end of a nerve to a type II muscle can be connected to a type I muscle. Both result in a logical alteration in the expression of fiber types. With time, there is an extensive, but not complete, conversion of the fiber type characteristics of the muscle to reflect the fiber types usually supplied by the new motor nerve. Even without interchanging the nerves, the fiber type characteristics of a muscle can be altered to a new profile by changing the frequency at which the muscle is stimulated. Type II muscles driven by external stimulation of the nerve at the low frequencies characteristic of type I muscles can undergo fiber type interconversions. Clearly, there is a complex interaction between the nerve, the muscle, and their pattern of use by the CNS that can lead to interconversions between type I and II fibers.

Caution must be taken in drawing conclusions about the potential adaptive response of human muscle to exercise. The experimental protocols used in the above studies bear little resemblance to physical activity of humans. It is generally accepted that in humans the relative percentages of type I or type II fibers are established genetically without a great deal of capacity for change. However, within the type II fiber population there is ample evidence for interconversion of types IIA and IIB fibers. For example, endurance training appears to be able to increase the percentage of type IIA fibers at the expense of type IIB fibers. Strength training without an emphasis on endurance conditioning may correspondingly increase the percentage of type IIB fibers. Certainly, the differences and boundaries between types IIA and IIB fibers are less than those between types I and II fibers.

Energetics of Muscle

Phosphagens

The immediate chemical energy source for muscle contraction is the ATP molecule (Fig. 12). This molecule consists of an adenosine moiety attached to 3 serial inorganic phosphate moieties; the terminal 2 phosphate bonds are high-energy bonds that, on hydrolysis, make a significant amount of chemical energy available to support biologic reactions. When the terminal phosphate of ATP is hydrolyzed, ADP and inorganic phosphate are formed, and energy is released. The second high-energy phosphate bond may be hydrolyzed, resulting in the formation of adenosine monophosphate (AMP) and inorganic phosphate and, again, the release of the energy of the phosphate bond.

Although ATP is used as the energy source for muscle contraction, most studies show little change in the level of ATP in activated muscle even after enough time to hydrolyze all available ATP. The muscle cell has mechanisms for maintaining the concentration of ATP. Another source of high-energy phosphate bonds, the molecule creatine phosphate

(CP), has a bond energy even higher than that in ATP. However, CP cannot be used directly by the cells as a source of energy; instead, it is used to synthesize ATP from ADP. The enzyme creatine kinase found in muscle catalyzes transfer of the high-energy phosphate bond of CP to ADP by the reaction

$$ADP + CP \rightarrow ATP + Creatine$$

In addition, a second enzyme, myokinase, maintains ATP concentration by the reaction

$$ADP + ADP \rightarrow ATP + AMP$$

The total energy available from ATP hydrolysis is approximately enough to allow a person to sprint for less than 50 yards. If the energy available from all the stored forms of high-energy phosphate compounds (phosphagens) is considered, there is enough energy to run approximately 200 yards.

Normal activity levels and, especially, the extremely high activity levels of athletic participation rely on metabolic processes that can replenish the supply of phosphagens to support muscle contraction. For many aspects of athletic performance, the ability of these metabolic systems to replenish ATP is the limiting factor in the level of performance. Two metabolic pathways are available to maintain the energy supply. The aerobic system relies on the availability of oxygen, and the anaerobic system can proceed in the absence of oxygen at the cellular level.

Aerobic Metabolism

When oxygen is available, aerobic metabolism is the primary source for replenishment of ATP. The aerobic system may use glucose or fatty acids to produce large quantities of ATP (Fig. 13). In aerobic metabolism, glucose is broken into 2 molecules of pyruvate, which then enter the Krebs cycle. Basically, in the Krebs cycle hydrogen atoms are removed from the pyruvate and combined with oxygen to produce water and liberate energy, which is made available to processes that transform low-energy phosphates into high-energy phosphates. In turn, these high-energy phosphates are coupled with ADP to produce ATP. In this manner, a

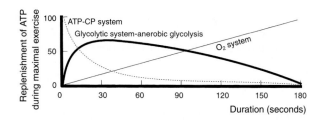

Figure 12

Energy sources for anaerobic activity.

molecule of glucose can be oxidized to result in 38 molecules of ATP by the overall reaction:

$$C_6H_{12}O_6 + 6O_2 + 38P + 38\ ADP \rightarrow 6CO_2 + 6H_2O + 38\ ATP$$

Glucose, considered the initial energy source, exists in the cell as a limited quantity of its phosphorylated form, glucose-6-phosphate. After the digestion of carbohydrates and sugars, glucose enters the bloodstream, from which it can enter the cell. Glucose not converted to glucose-6-phosphate can be stored in the form of glycogen. The quantity of stored glycogen is a product of the use and storage of glucose. Diets rich in carbohydrate may lead to a higher store of glycogen, which can prolong the cellular ability to continue energy production at a given rate. In addition, the use of glycogen could be diminished if there were other potential sources of energy for oxidative metabolism of muscle. Muscle glycogen levels, unlike those in liver, remain quite stable and usually do not decline during fasting. In cardiac muscle, glycogen levels may actually increase during fasting.

Anaerobic Metabolism

Anaerobic metabolism involves the hydrolysis of glucose molecules by a succession of steps to lactic acid; therefore, this system is sometimes referred to as lactic acid metabolism (Fig. 14). By anaerobic metabolism, glucose can be rapidly transformed into 2 molecules of lactic acid plus sufficient energy to convert 2 molecules of ADP to ATP. However, the lactic acid produced is a relatively toxic substance,

which causes acidosis and fatigue. Additionally, anaerobic metabolism uses the potential energy in a molecule of glucose very inefficiently. However, it is the energy system relied on by the muscle when a lot of energy is needed for a relatively short period of time.

Fat and Protein

Fat stores are abundant in the body and provide by far the largest potential source of energy. Fats usually are stored in the body as triglycerides, which consist of 3 separate fatty acids bound to the molecule glyceraldehyde. Triglycerides can be cleaved into free fatty acids, which can be cleaved by a process called beta-oxidation into successive 2-carbon fragments called acetyl coenzyme A (acetyl CoA). Acetyl CoA can then enter the Krebs cycle, in which it is hydrolyzed, as are the products of glucose metabolism. The breakdown of a single free fatty acid molecule can yield sufficient energy to convert a variable amount of ADP to ATP, depending on the length of the carbon chain. For example, a fatty acid molecule with 16 carbon atoms can yield sufficient energy to convert as many as 129 molecules of ADP to ATP after complete oxidation.

Fatty acids can be stored within the muscle or supplied via the bloodstream. They can enter the bloodstream immediately after digestion or following mobilization from tissue sources such as adipose tissue. Their availability is quite unlikely to be a limiting factor in metabolism, except in unusual circumstances of malnutrition.

Under normal conditions, proteins never provide the primary fuel for metabolism, but they serve as an accessory source. Protein is hydrolyzed in the alimentary system into its constituent amino acids. Deamination of amino acids produces ketoacids, which can enter into the Krebs cycle for energy production. Ketoacids can also go through a process, called gluconeogenesis, by which they can be converted to glucose; this process occurs in conditions of severe glucose depletion when body proteins are hydrolyzed to provide energy substrate.

Use of Energy Sources

Aerobic and anaerobic metabolism take place simultaneously, and there is a well-ordered interaction between the 2 systems. It is not true that exercise of different intensity levels results in the use of 1 system exclusively; aerobic and anaerobic pathways are both used, and both carbohydrate and fat are used as energy sources for exercise of virtually any intensity. However, the 2 systems are quite distinct and can respond quite differently to stresses applied to muscle. Exercises designed to work the body at an intensity level that will not result in rapid fatigue because the energy demand can be met by the oxidative energy system are called aerobic exercises. Conversely, anaerobic exercise refers to exercise of high enough intensity and duration to

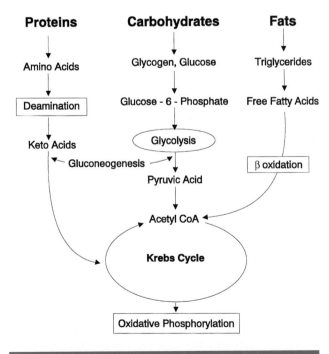

Figure 13

Foodstuffs (fats, carbohydrates, proteins) containing carbon and hydrogen for glycolysis, fatty acid oxidation, and the Krebs cycle in a muscle cell.

cause the anaerobic system to produce enough by-products to cause fatigue and lead to cessation or reduction of exercise.

The different motor unit types have different levels of enzymes needed for the aerobic and anaerobic energy systems. Histochemical stains show that type I fibers have a higher concentration of the aerobic system enzymes and that type IIB fibers have a higher concentration of enzymes involved with anaerobic energy supply. Type IIA fibers generally have intermediate levels of both types of enzymes.

The intensity and duration of muscular activity greatly influence the use of the separate energy sources and metabolic systems. Brief exercises of high intensity, such as a short sprint, rely on stored phosphagens. As the intensity falls and the length of activity increases, the anaerobic system is more involved because it replenishes the supply of ATP. The production of acidosis induces fatigue and limits the duration of activity. As the exercise intensity falls further, such as in walking or jogging slowly, the metabolic demands can be met by aerobic metabolism. The level at which the body can meet its metabolic demands without developing acidosis is influenced by the rate at which the cardiovascular system can supply oxygen and by the metabolic capacity of the fibers. The metabolic pathways and energy sources are very much influenced by the state of training.

Aerobic metabolism uses either glucose derived from stored glycogen or fatty acids derived from stored triglycerides. An acute response during prolonged aerobic exercise is the shift to oxidation of fatty acids, which in turn conserves the limited carbohydrate stores in the body. That carbohydrates are the limiting factor is easily appreciated on realization that 1 lb of stored fat can produce more than enough energy to run a marathon.

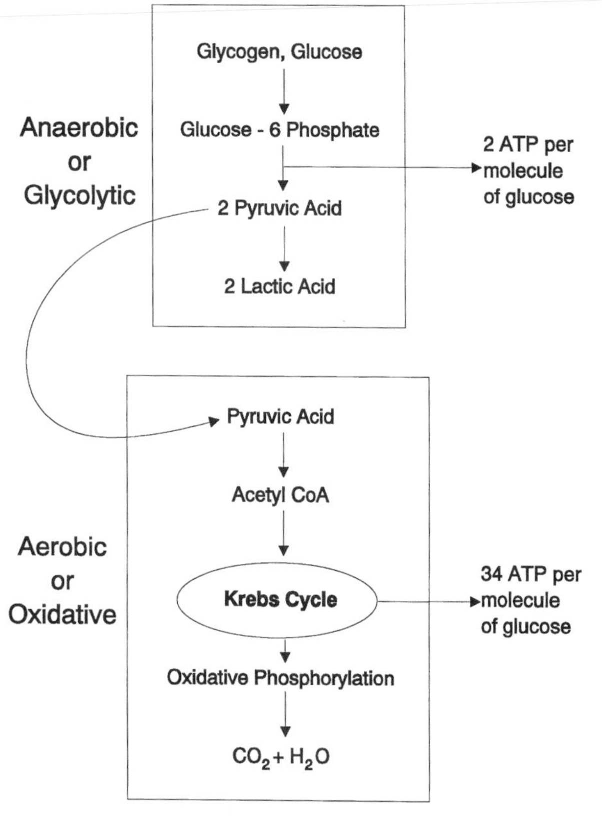

Muscle Mechanics

The mechanical properties of muscle have in the past been subject to extensive investigation. Most of the research in the field has concerned the study of isolated muscle or muscle fibers. Although some intricacies of muscle are not yet fully understood, the major properties of this tissue, both active and passive, are now clearly defined.

The forces produced by muscles will be considered, including their relationship to muscle length, shortening speed, time, and state of activation. Muscle can actively shorten, and it can resist lengthening by active or passive means. In classic mechanics, muscle has been considered to consist of contractile elements that respond to stimulation of the muscle and passive or elastic elements that can passively resist stretching, similarly to a spring. It was useful in previous models characterizing the load-deformation relationship of muscle to consider that there are elastic elements both in parallel and in series with the contractile element. Much of the pioneering work in this area was initiated by A.V. Hill, who proposed the famous 3-element model of skeletal muscle (Fig. 15). This model consists of an active contractile element, which represents the muscle's response to stimulation, in series with an elastic element, the series elastic component. The series elastic component and the contractile element are in parallel with another elastic element, the parallel elastic component. The tension exerted by the parallel elastic component is independent of the contractile element and is believed to represent the tension in the connective tissue of the muscle. The series elastic component is located in the tendon as well as in the cross-bridges between the actin and myosin filaments. The dynamic performance of a muscle is dominated primarily by the properties of the muscle fibers and the aponeurosis; the tendon (another series elastic component) is probably too stiff.

It has been known for some time that muscle demonstrates nonlinear, time-dependent viscoelastic responses similar to those of other biologic tissues. Although Hill's model is useful in providing a general picture of muscle behavior, it must be treated as somewhat idealized. An accurate model of muscle would include a much more

Figure 14

A summary of the adenosine triphosphate yield in the anaerobic and aerobic breakdown of carbohydrates. Glycolysis and anaerobic metabolism occur in the cytoplasm while oxidative phosphorylation occurs in the mitochondria.

complex design describing its nonlinear and time-dependent functions. Because muscle consists of 75% water by weight and much of what remains is amorphous, long-chain polymer-like material, it is not surprising that this tissue demonstrates quite a bit of viscous behavior. Various mechanical models have been developed to account for these phenomena.

Length-Tension Relationship

Muscle can be stretched and its tension can be recorded mechanically. When this is done with unstimulated muscle, there is a period of length change before any tension is recorded. From that point there is a nonlinear increase in tension, which is similar to the (toe region) response of ligament and tendon. If the muscle is activated by tetanically stimulating the motor neuron, the tension produced is higher, especially at relatively small stretches in the muscle. At larger stretches, the tension in activated muscle approaches that in passively stretched muscle (Fig. 16).

Subtracting the tension in passively stretched muscle from the tension in actively stretched muscle at each length gives the portion of the tension that results from contractile muscle forces alone. Often, the onset of the rise in passive tension occurs near the peak of active tension production. There is considerable variability between muscles, but the active force is often high at muscle lengths that are not associated with significant passive tensions.

The tension in a passively stretched muscle can be quite significant at higher strains. In fact, the passive tension developed in muscle before mechanical failure occurs can be several times higher than that of the maximal active force of the muscle. The viscoelastic properties of muscle are largely responsible for the tension in passively stretched muscle. This tension is due primarily to the connective tissue around muscle fibers and to the fascial components of the muscle belly. Recent studies indicate that some passive tension may come from the myofibrillar proteins themselves.

The passive stretch of a muscle can limit motions about joints, especially with muscles that span 2 joints and can be stretched by either. In most people, the hamstrings can easily limit knee extension with the hip flexed more than 90°. Similarly, the gastrocnemius can limit ankle dorsiflexion when the knee is extended. In both examples, the passive tension developed is sufficient to limit further muscle stretch without pain and high forces.

Myofibrillar ultrastructure provides an explanation for the length-tension relationship for active muscle. Force can be produced only when the cross-bridges of the thick filaments can interact with the thin filaments. Therefore, in the lengthened position the thick filaments are not overlapped by the thin filaments. As sarcomere length decreases, there is initially more overlap of thick and thin filaments. At more shortened positions the thick filaments of adjacent sarcomeres begin to abut the 2 lines and the tension begins to fall

again. More shortening causes further collision of the filaments and successive loss of contractile force.

Blix Curve and Joint Torque

For a given degree of neurologic stimulus, the active force possible as a function of muscle length displays an ascending, then a descending, curve as noted above. Although the force that a muscle exerts may change with muscle length, human movement results primarily from the torques pro-

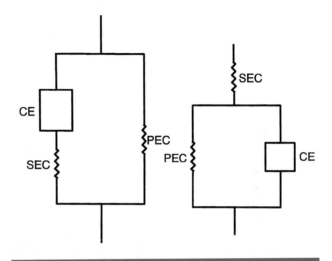

Figure 15

Hill's 3-element model. Classical representations for the Hill model of muscle are CE = contractile element; SEC = series elements; PEC = parallel element.

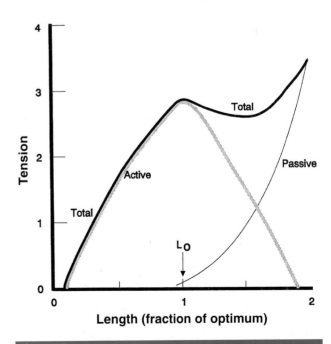

Figure 16

Representative isometric tension-length curve of skeletal muscle.

duced by this force. Thus, torque is defined as: $T = r \times F$, where T is torque, r is the moment arm or the perpendicular distance from the line of action of the muscle-force vector to the axis of rotation, and F is the applied force. Therefore, torque is a vector quantity having both a magnitude and a direction; it is measured in Newton•meters (N•m). The direction of a torque is along the axis of rotation and, thus, is perpendicular to the plane in which the twisting force is applied; it is given by the right-hand rule.

Variations in muscle torque represent the interaction of moment-arm and muscle-length effects. The torque produced by muscles around a joint is related both to the relationship of muscle tension versus length and to the moment arm determined by the perpendicular distance from the line of action of the muscle to the joint center of rotation. In many cases, torque can be predicted relatively well if joint mechanics are considered alone, and the neurologic stimulus to muscle force is considered to be a constant.

There are at least 3 strategies for altering torque production under this condition: change the force produced by the muscle, change the moment arm over which the muscle acts, and vary the angle between the line of force of the muscle and the joint access. In effect, the third strategy actually changes the length of the moment arm. At a constant neurologic stimulation, production of muscle force can be changed by altering the position on the length-tension curve at which the muscle is acting. Concentric action describes that situation in which the muscle, regardless of its length, is shortening and, hence, the muscle moment is in the same direction as the change in joint angle. In eccentric action, the muscle is lengthened, and the net muscle moment is in the opposite direction to the change in joint angle.

The effect of changing the moment arm must be known to determine whether the torque produced will be greater in an eccentric contraction as compared with a concentric contraction. For example, in early swing, flexion is produced by a concentric action of the iliopsoas about the hip joint. This action produces an increasing torque with increasing flexion despite progressive shortening of the muscle because the moment arm is increasing. In contrast, at the end of swing as flexion of the hip and extension of the knee produces an eccentric action of the hamstrings, the moment arm of the iliopsoas about the knee joint is decreasing. The torque thus produced could be approximately the same throughout the muscle's action.

For some muscles, such as the elbow flexors and extensors, the greatest torque seems to occur when the joint is in a midrange position, and the torque falls when the joint is in full flexion or extension. At either extreme, the force of 1 of these 2 muscles may actually be maximal but the moment arm may be minimal. Such is the case of biceps action in resisting elbow moment from flexion to extension (eccentric) or in attempting to lift a weight with the elbow going from maximum extension to flexion (concentric). In both of these actions, the muscle changes its length and the moment arm continually changes. For muscles with pulley systems for their tendons or retinacular sheaths maintaining the tendon close to or at a relatively constant distance from the joint access, the part that the moment arm plays in the changing torque as the muscle exerts its force may be less important.

Force-Velocity Relationship

Muscles are the primary tools for providing human motion; therefore, a consideration of muscle function and its relation to velocity can be valuable. When muscle is stimulated by its motor nerve, it generates force and attempts to shorten. Classic muscle physiology experiments have shown that the velocity at which a muscle can shorten is related to the load on the muscle. With low loads, muscle shortens at a higher velocity than with heavy loads. The relationship between force and velocity is hyperbolic and was described by Hill. Unlike the length-tension relationship, the force-velocity relationship does not have an anatomic basis. As the velocity of shortening approaches zero, muscle generates increasing force. Similarly, as the load approaches the maximal isometric force of the muscle, the velocity of shortening approaches zero. Based on this relationship, which applies only to tetanically-stimulated amphibian muscle, Hill developed the force-velocity relationship for the contractile elements as shown below.

$$(F + a)(v + b) = (F_{max} + a)b$$

where F is the muscle tensile force, v is the velocity of contraction, F_{max} is the maximum (tetanic) isometric force, and a and b are constants (usually about 0.25).

According to this equation, there is an inverse relationship between muscle force F and velocity of contraction (Fig. 17). This equation describes the force-velocity relationship of tetanically-stimulated skeletal muscle upon its immediate release from an isometric condition. It cannot describe the force-velocity relationship when a tetanically-stimulated muscle is slowly released. Furthermore, the theory described in this equation applies to the individual muscle fiber, thus limiting the direct extrapolation to clinical practice and the study of whole muscle systems.

Isokinetic dynamometers are popular in training and rehabilitation programs. These machines contain a servomechanism that permits motion with a constant angular velocity. The servomechanism regulates the joint torque to whatever torque is needed to maintain the joint velocity at the level selected. Because the resistance offered by the machine matches that of the individual, this type of exercise is also known as accommodating resistance exercise. Of course, constant angular velocity of the joint does not mean that the muscle itself is shortening at a constant velocity. However, it is apparent from the clinical application that there is an inverse relationship between velocity of

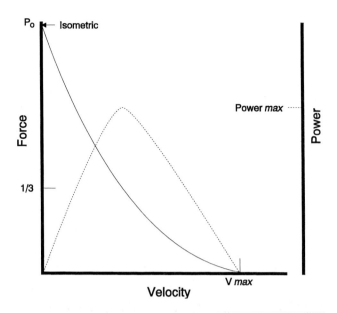

Figure 17

The classic force-velocity curve (dashed line) in an isolated muscle, showing the velocity of muscle contraction is maximal with zero load. The solid line gives the muscle power (muscle force x velocity of contraction).

movement and force production (as in Hill's equation). The muscles about the knee, for example, generate approximately 120% more joint torque at 60° than at an angular velocity of 360°.

Muscle that is activated eccentrically can produce more force and do more work (actually negative work) for the same velocity of movement than muscle that is activated concentrically. Kinesiology studies show that a very large portion of muscle activity occurs in an eccentric fashion. For example, gait studies show that many of the lower extremity muscle activities are eccentric and function to decelerate or control joint motion. The major portion of quadriceps activity occurs at heel strike while the knee is flexing rather than later during the gait cycle when the knee is extending. The potentially advantageous mechanisms of increased force production and diminished energy consumption are often at work as muscles function eccentrically.

The eccentric action of muscle can be contrasted to concentric action (Fig. 18). The shape of the force-velocity relationship is different; the velocity of lengthening is less than the velocity of shortening for a given increment of force. The muscle, therefore, acts as a stiffer material when it is resisting shortening. This changes abruptly near a force 50% greater than the maximal isometric force. The hyperbolic relationship between force and velocity is important clinically, because the force drops off rapidly as velocity increases.

Isokinetic dynamometers that can function in an eccentric fashion are now being used for training and rehabilitation routines. Of course, this requires a robotic capacity for the exercise device, because it must have power to gen-erate motion of the lever arm in excess of what the muscle can resist.

The possibilities of eccentric training and rehabilitation, as long as they are performed properly and safely, are promising and are being investigated. Mechanical efficiency is higher and oxygen consumption lower with eccentric than with concentric action. This difference results in a lower energy cost during eccentric exercise and may make this training mode attractive in patients with low capacity to deliver energy to the muscles. Other favorable features of eccentric muscle action include submaximal neural activities during maximal voluntary activity and higher maximal torque values at the same corresponding velocity compared with concentric action. It also appears that repeated exposure to eccentric muscle action can result in adaptations leading to increased resistance to muscle soreness following exercise.

Training Effects on Muscle

Muscle is a tissue capable of significant adaptation as can be seen in the extremes of muscle capacity observed in the severely ill and the world-class athlete. The type and magnitude of the tissue response vary tremendously, based on the nature of the training. Muscle training can involve exercises aimed at increasing strength, endurance, and anaero-

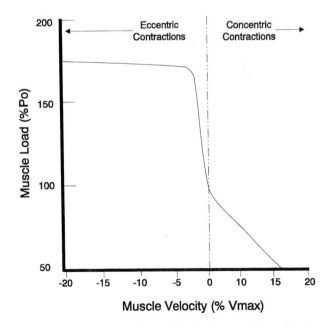

Figure 18

The highest force can be developed in a fast eccentric contraction and then declines to a minimum when the muscle is activated in a concentric contraction at high speeds. Note that force increases significantly in forced muscle lengthening (eccentric) contractions. P_0 = isometric muscle force; V_{max} = maximum muscle velocity.

bic fitness. Although most training regimens involve a mixture of these possibilities, it is instructive to consider them separately at first. Changes in muscle structure, function, and metabolism can thus be evaluated.

Strength Training

Observation of the muscles of competing power lifters and bodybuilders might lead to the idea that strength training results in relatively striking changes in muscle. High-force, low-repetition training results in an increase in muscle strength, which is proportional to the cross-sectional area of the fibers in the muscles. Whether this increase in muscle size is a result of muscle hypertrophy, that is, an increase in the size of muscle fibers, or of hyperplasia, that is, an increase in the number of fibers, is still under debate. Experimental data exist in support of both arguments. Although the applicability to humans of data obtained using animals is somewhat limited, it appears likely that the majority of change that occurs with strength training is a result of hypertrophy. With an increase in fiber size, there is an increase in the amount of contractile proteins.

There also is a strong neurologic component to strength training. An accumulating body of evidence suggests that motor-unit recruitment provides an important contribution to the strength gains commonly seen following weight training. In an untrained person, it has been estimated that approximately 80% of the motor units can be stimulated voluntarily. Training is believed to result in an alteration of CNS firing of motor neurons to achieve better synchronization of muscle activation.

Metabolic changes in response to strength training are less remarkable than the changes in muscle size. There are increased amounts of phosphagens, the immediate source of muscle energy; however, there is little or no change in oxidative enzyme levels. In fact, the volume density of mitochondria may decrease with pure strength training. As the fiber size increases without a significant stimulus for an increase in mitochondrial density or size, the volume fraction of mitochondria decreases.

An increase in the force or tension on a muscle is needed to increase its strength over time. A technique called synergist ablation is often used in animal studies. It involves the surgical excision of a muscle with a function very similar to that of the muscle being tested. For example, if the gastrocnemius is removed, the remaining soleus has more work to do and it must resist more force.

In humans, strength training involves increasing the resistance against which the muscle shortens. A resistance generally is chosen such that the muscle can move through a prescribed range of motion for only a few times (1 to 15 repetitions) before being unable to repeat the movement. It is considered important to continue repeating until fatigue prevents continuing the exercise. A relatively high resistance and a low number of possible repetitions lead to

increases in the strength and size of the muscle rather than an improved capacity for endurance, which would be the result of training against a resistance that could be repeated, for example, 20 times or more before fatigue. In general, strength training will involve several sets of repetitions to fatigue. Exercises are often arranged to work on separate muscle groups sequentially to allow the exercised muscle groups some recovery time before their next set. There are many different programs altering the number of sets and repetitions (or reps) to achieve the desired effect.

Strength training involves adaptations in all fiber types. These adaptations promote greater capacity of fibers to resist external loads, primarily through an increase in contractile protein content. Because the intensity of exercise is near maximal, all fiber types are recruited in the exercise. However, studies have shown that the type II fibers show a more pronounced hypertrophy than do the type I fibers. Type I fibers apparently can generate as much specific tension, or force per cross-sectional area, as type II fibers when tested under isometric conditions. Under high velocity conditions, individuals with a higher percentage of type II fibers may have an advantage. The overall result is the distribution of load across a greater muscle mass, which leads to a reduction of stress on these fibers. Again, there is a strong neurologic component to strength training; it is believed that in a poorly conditioned muscle as few as 60% of the fibers are firing simultaneously, whereas a well-conditioned muscle may have over 90% active fibers.

Endurance Training (Aerobic Training)

Training to increase muscle endurance and aerobic fitness involves a very different challenge to the muscle and an entirely different set of adaptations by the muscle and the cardiovascular system. Strength training involves presenting the muscles with a task they are not strong enough to perform; the adaptation is to get stronger, which involves getting larger. However, endurance training typically does not involve high forces or resistance-type exercises. For example, distance running involves forces no higher than those required to take steps at a fast rate. The challenge presented to muscles during aerobic training is to take more and faster steps before fatigue. The adaptations, then, are those involved with the supply of energy rather than the size of the muscle. Therefore, the improvements in endurance as a result of aerobic training appear to result from changes in both central and peripheral circulation and muscle metabolism. Specifically, the contractile machinery of muscle adapts to use energy more efficiently.

Specific changes in the cardiovascular system occur with aerobic training; the body cannot rely exclusively on anaerobic processes for prolonged exercise. Aerobic training results in a greater reliance on oxidative metabolism to provide energy to skeletal muscle; therefore, the cardiovascular system must adapt to supply oxygen to the muscles at an increased rate. The heart develops a larger stroke volume and a larger ventricular size to accommodate this increase in stroke volume. More importantly, increases in pressure, work, and heart rate are minimized in favor of this increase in stroke volume. The heart rate at rest falls because the increased stroke volume means that fewer beats are required to deliver the same amount of blood. The circulatory system also adapts to improve blood flow to the muscles through control of the arterioles in the muscle. In addition, there is an increased number of capillaries within the muscle after endurance training. This is especially true for the type I fibers.

Changes in the muscle fiber itself are also noteworthy. Because oxidative metabolism involves the mitochondria, it is perhaps not surprising that mitochondrial size, number, and density are increased. The physiologic significance of these changes has been debated. Some believe that the capillarization of skeletal muscle is not the limiting factor to whole body maximal aerobic power in humans. The enzyme systems of the Krebs cycle and the respiratory chain also show marked increases as do the enzyme systems involved with the supply and processing of fatty acids for use by the mitochondria. The increase in mitochondrial enzymes leads to a marked increase in the ability to oxidize pyruvic acid from glycogen and acetyl CoA from fats. There is also a decrease in glycolytic enzymes following aerobic training, which appears to be limited to fast-twitch muscles. For the most part, however, these adaptations in enzyme activity have only been shown in animal models of intense endurance training.

With training, the metabolic pathways adapt to use a higher portion of fatty acids for fuel instead of glycogen. In long-duration exercise, the supply of glycogen can limit endurance; this is particularly true for exercise lasting more than 2 hours. The relative use of different fuel sources can be estimated using indirect calorimetry. This technique monitors expired oxygen and carbon dioxide, thereby allowing determination of the ratio of oxygen consumed and carbon dioxide produced. The general formula for carbohydrate (glucose) use is $C_6H_{12}O_6 + 6O_2 \rightarrow 6CO_2 + 6H_2O$. The ratio of $CO_2/O_2 = 6/6 = 1.0$. For fats the general formula calls for the use of successive 2-carbon fragments. An estimate of this formula is $3(CH_2–CH_2) + 9O_2 \rightarrow 6CO_2 + 6H_2O$. The ratio of $CO_2/O_2 = 6/9 = 0.7$. Respiratory gas measurements can be used to determine CO_2 production, O_2 consumption, and the CO_2/O_2 ratio during exercise. From this ratio it has been possible to demonstrate that aerobic training involves increased use of fat for energy.

Different muscle fiber types respond differently to endurance training. The oxidative capacity of all 3 fiber types increases. Very intense exercise in animals can lead to a conversion of type II to type I fibers; however, it has been more difficult to prove this conversion in man. Study results have generally indicated a change within type II fibers such that the percentage of more highly oxidative IIA fibers increases.

Specific responses are also possible in muscle as a result of dietary manipulations. The endurance capacity of muscle is related to the available stores of glycogen in the muscle fibers and in the liver. Glycogen, as the storage vehicle for glucose, is used extensively, especially in exercises of moderate to high intensity. Muscle and liver glycogen stores can be increased by the consumption of high carbohydrate, low-fat diet for several days prior to competition or testing. In addition, exercise that effects a relative depletion of muscle glycogen prior to the high carbohydrate diet may increase the storage of glycogen in muscles. This routine of a high carbohydrate diet prior to an event involving endurance stresses is called carbohydrate loading.

Anaerobic (Sprint or Power) Training

Exercises of a high intensity that last for a few seconds to approximately 2 minutes require metabolic support primarily from anaerobic pathways. Such exercises rely primarily on the availability of ATP in the form of phosphagens and on the ability to supply energy through anaerobic glycolysis. The requirements for ATP use are higher than the ability of the aerobic system to supply ATP.

Although there have been far fewer investigations on the effects of anaerobic training, several adaptations have been documented. One of the primary adaptations is an increase in the level of stored phosphagens. In addition, there are elevations in some of the enzymes controlling glycolysis, such as phosphofructokinase and succinate dehydrogenase; however, these changes in enzyme levels are far less pronounced than with aerobic training. These changes appear to be confined primarily to fast-twitch muscle fibers.

Growth and Development of Muscle

Skeletal muscle cells develop from a mesodermal cell population arising from the somite. Muscle progenitor cells derive from mesoderm and are termed myoblasts early in the developmental period. These fusiform cells respond to molecular messengers in development to undergo mitosis. When sufficient numbers of cells exist, they undergo fusion to form long multinucleate cells called myotubes. These cells are the precursors of the eventual muscle fibers. The myotubes continue to differentiate into muscle fibers, which are large multinucleate cells. The fusion of myoblasts into myotubes is also a time of nearly synchronous differentiation of the muscle cells. Many of the contractile proteins appear synchronously; however, it appears that many of the specific genes coding for muscle proteins are regulated, coordinated, and influenced by a large number of factors. By the seventh week of gestation, distinct muscle and tendinous structures can be identified.

In addition, it is apparent that even embryonic muscle cells exhibit a number of isoforms of the myofibrillar proteins. Different isoforms may exist during different stages of development as well as in mature muscle. The further differentiation of the myotubes involves the production of structural proteins, the proteins and enzymes of the metabolic pathways, the association of the myotubes with the extracellular connective tissue matrix of muscle, and innervation.

Growth and Changes in Muscle Length

The development of muscle and hypertrophy associated with training or adaptation to stress have been discussed. There remains the question of how muscle grows in length. Bone, of course, has growth plates that increase its length. Muscles have no such specific structural adaptation, yet they are able to increase in length to accommodate for skeletal growth. The possibilities include increased tendon length, increased muscle length, or both. In immature animals it appears that both muscle fibers and tendons increase in length. Elongation of the muscle fiber while the sarcomere length remains relatively stable can be explained by the addition of more sarcomeres to the muscle fibers during longitudinal growth. The region of the muscle-tendon junction shows a great deal of activity and adaptability during growth; fibers grow in length at this region rather than near the middle of the muscle fiber.

In mature animals, elongation of the muscle belly is the primary mechanism for changing the length of the muscle-tendon unit. Because skeletal length is not increasing in mature animals, studies have dealt with the response of muscle to immobilization in various positions that put the muscle-tendon unit under different degrees of stretch. Data from such studies are important because muscle growth may often be the limiting factor in surgical skeletal lengthening.

When muscle fibers are immobilized under stretch, the immediate effect is that the fibers are longer and the constituent myofibrils lengthen. The sarcomeres are longer initially as a result of the stretch that separates the A-bands and I-bands more than at normal rest length. After several weeks, the sarcomeres return to their normal rest lengths, although the whole muscle and fibers maintain their stretched length. This return to normal sarcomere length is effected by an increase in the number of sarcomeres in series in the myofibrils and, therefore, in the fiber. The additional sarcomeres are added at the region of the muscle-tendon junction.

Mechanically, the active portion of the length-tension diagram shifts so that the peak of force production occurs at a longer length. The addition of more sarcomeres in series implies an increase in the amount of skeletal muscle protein and an increase in muscle weight, even in the presence of immobilization. The increased weight comes from longer fibers rather than from an increase in cross-sectional area.

Adaptations also occur in the passive properties of mus-

cle. If a muscle is held in a stretched position for as little as 2 weeks, the length-tension relation shifts to the right such that less passive force is generated in response to the same stretch. The opposite occurs for muscles immobilized in or restricted to a shortened position. After several weeks of being held shortened, muscles will generate more resistance for a given stretch or a given change in joint angle when the muscle length is increasing.

These concepts of changing muscle length in response to immobilization are not appreciated by many physicians who treat musculoskeletal conditions. The problem has not been widely studied in humans; however, data from animal studies make it clear that the muscle-tendon unit length is dynamic and can respond to length changes imposed by a growing skeleton or by external fixation of muscle length. In skeletally mature individuals, most of the length change occurs within the muscle tissue rather than in the tendon. A better understanding of the response of muscle to long-term length changes will improve results obtained from tendon and muscle transfers, limb length alterations, and even immobilization in muscle. Clinically, patients demonstrate reduced flexibility, decreased range of motion, and reduced tolerance to muscle work following immobilization. Although these findings appear to be consistent from patient to patient, it is only recently that the detrimental effects of total immobilization have been appreciated. Clearly, proper muscle function depends on a number of factors, including intact proprioceptive activity, motor innervation, mechanical load, and mobility of the joints. Interruption of any of the above can lead to reduced motion, and if severe enough, total immobilization.

Muscle Injury and Repair

Muscle injury can occur by a variety of mechanisms ranging from ischemia to direct injury by crush or laceration. The injury and repair processes appear to be regulated by a number of cytokines and growth factors that are just beginning to be appreciated and understood in animal models and human studies. Potential sources of cytokines in injured skeletal muscle include infiltrating neutrophils and monocytes/macrophages, activated fibroblasts, and stimulated endothelial cells. In addition, muscle precursor cells and myotubes can synthesize certain cytokines. It also appears that oxygen-derived free radicals are produced early following injury although their significance is yet to be determined. Injured muscle undergoes processes of degeneration and regeneration; when muscle fibers undergo necrosis for any reason, the damaged fibers are removed by macrophages and other cells from the circulatory system. New muscle cells appear within the connective tissue framework of damaged muscle. These cells are thought to arise from a population of relatively undifferentiated satellite cells that exist in a quiescent state beside the original muscle syncytium. Many progenitor cells begin to form myoblasts, which fuse to form myotubes. Myotubes coalesce and become muscle fibers. At the same time, a connective tissue basal lamina surrounding the muscle fiber and an extracellular matrix are formed. The muscle tissue regenerates simultaneously with the proliferation of fibrous connective tissue. The connective tissue proliferation may interfere with the ability of muscle to regenerate into normally functioning tissue. In rodents and other animals, regeneration of entire muscles may occur following revascularization. However, the regeneration process is generally less effective for muscles that weigh more than 1.5 g and, therefore, is unlikely to occur in a significant fashion in most human muscles. The response of human muscle varies with the nature and severity of the injury.

Recovery of muscle depends on revascularization from surrounding viable tissue. The regenerating myotubes and the neovascularization may influence one another's development. The process of reinnervation is also interesting from a cellular point of view. Part of the structural specialization of the synapse is the organization of the connective tissue basal lamina surrounding the muscle fibers. The specialized region of the basal lamina at the motor end plate may persist after death of the muscle fiber. Even without regeneration of the nerve, the site of the preexisting motor endplate region of basal lamina influences the development of muscle fibers regenerating within the basal lamina. Clearly, the regeneration of nerve fibers, muscle cells, and the connective tissue basal lamina have special and complex interrelationships in reinnervating muscle.

An important factor in regeneration of human muscle is the simultaneous and often more exuberant and predominant formation of connective tissue in the form of fibrosis or scar. The connective tissue regeneration can be extensive enough to interfere with muscle regeneration. A number of specific examples of muscle injury and the recovery processes are discussed below.

Muscle Laceration

Direct laceration of muscle is not uncommon in trauma. Several studies demonstrate the potential for recovery of lacerated muscle and the problems that often prevent recovery of normal tissue. Complete transection of a muscle can lead to a normal-appearing tissue only in very small muscles of animal models.

Lacerations in skeletal muscle usually result from direct trauma by a sharp object. Surgical exposures may require division of muscles. For normal function following lacerations, muscle must regenerate across the repair site, and tissue denervated by laceration of the muscle belly and separated from the intramuscular nerve supply must be reinnervated. Clinical experience has shown that functional recovery following muscle laceration is rarely complete,

although partial recovery is usually possible.

Following complete laceration and suture repair of rabbit skeletal muscle, the muscle fragments healed primarily by dense connective tissue scar (Fig. 19). A small number of myotubes penetrated the scar tissue, but good regeneration of muscle tissue across the laceration was not seen. The muscle fragment isolated from the motor point had histologic findings of denervation. Recovery of muscle function was evaluated by measuring the isometric muscle tension following motor-nerve stimulation. Muscles lacerated near the midbelly recovered approximately 50% of their ability to produce tension and could shorten about 80% of their normal amount. Recovery of muscle function after partial lacerations was proportional to the degree of laceration.

A recent clinical study showed good correlation with these experiments. Muscle lacerations were repaired by connecting the proximal portion of the lacerated muscle to the distal portion by tendon grafts. At a mean follow-up period of 14 months, approximately 40% of the mean grip strength was recovered. Over half of the muscles achieved grade 4 or grade 5 strength by manual muscle testing.

Muscle Contusion

Muscle contusions usually result from nonpenetrating blunt injury. They occur frequently in accidents and sports and can cause significant disability and pain. The best method of treatment has not been clearly defined, but animal experiments provide some insight into the natural history of the injury. An inflammatory reaction and hematoma occurred soon after production of consistent lesions in rat gastrocnemius muscles. Later, scar formation consisting of dense connective tissue with variable amounts of muscle regeneration was seen. Mobilized muscle was compared to immobilized muscle in the recovery process. The inflammatory reaction in mobilized muscle was greater, but it disappeared more rapidly with more scar formation than in the immobilized muscle. The speed of tissue repair was related directly to vascular ingrowth during the repair

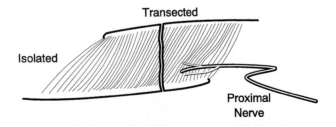

Figure 19

Schematic drawing of lacerated muscle. The laceration leaves fibers intact proximally and distally while dividing the central fibers. Scar tissue isolates the distal segment from its nerve supply. (Reproduced with permission from Garrett WE, Seaber AV, Boswick J, et al: Recovery of skeletal muscle following laceration and repair. *J Hand Surg* 1984;9A:683–692.)

process. Biomechanical testing showed faster recovery of tensile strength in mobilized muscles. The quality of repair following blunt trauma varied with age; young rats demonstrated a more intense inflammatory reaction and hematoma formation than older rats. Incorporation of radioactively labeled proline demonstrated synthesis of extracellular connective tissue by 2 days after trauma, with most intensive synthesis occurring between days 5 and 21. The appearance and distribution of collagen types I, III, IV, and V and of fibronectin have also been studied using histologic and immunofluorescent techniques.

Severe blunt injury to muscle may result in bone formation within the muscle, referred to as myositis ossificans (Fig. 20). A prospective study of patients with quadriceps hematoma showed subsequent myositis ossificans in approximately 20% of cases. The new bone formed after blunt trauma can be contiguous with normal bone or periosteum or can be completely free of any connection with existing bone. Some animals, including rabbits, appear to develop primarily periosteal new bone; however, other animals, such as sheep, develop both periosteal new bone and heterotopic bone. Periosteal reactive new bone developed in all sheep receiving blunt trauma to the anterior thigh muscles, whereas heterotopic bone occurred in 17% of the sheep. Multiple episodes of injury and hematoma formation increased the likelihood of formation of heterotopic bone.

Following direct injury, there is early swelling associated with bleeding and inflammation. The mass may enlarge or be symptomatic for several months before stabilizing. The mass may be associated with the possible appearance of heterotopic bone, if there is a history of a previous muscle contusion. This condition may also mimic osteogenic sarcoma with its mass effect and the appearance of irregular new bone. The histologic features may also be similar if a

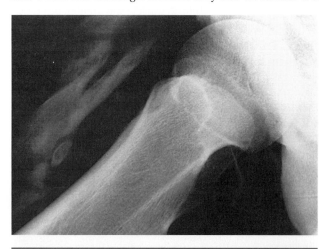

Figure 20

Radiograph of myositis ossificans of the rectus femoris. This 22-year-old patient suffered a quadriceps contusion which resulted in the above roentgenographic findings. The heterotopic bone gradually resorbed over time without consequence.

biopsy is performed early in the course of myositis ossificans. The heterotopic bone may absorb with time. Recovery of normal function is possible with the presence of myositis ossificans, but the recovery period is longer than that following an uncomplicated contusion. No specific treatment is recommended in addition to the treatment for contusions. Early surgery is to be avoided because it may exacerbate the heterotopic bone formation and prolong disability. Surgery should be considered only after the heterotopic bone is mature and no changes are occurring in both the clinical and radiologic evaluation of the patient.

Indirect Muscle Strain Injury

Indirect muscle injuries are caused by excessive force or stress on a muscle rather than by any direct trauma. This injury has been called a strain, muscle pull, muscle tear, and various other names. Indirect muscle injuries occur frequently, and are a major reason for time lost from athletic or occupational pursuits. Interest in the basic pathophysiologic characteristics of this injury has been relatively slow to develop despite its clinical significance.

Complete Muscle Tears

In one of the earliest studies of failure of the muscle-tendon unit in response to stretch, the gastrocnemius muscle-tendon unit of rabbits was stretched to failure. The healthy tendon did not fail even after partial transection of the tendon. Failure occurred at the bone-tendon junction, the myotendinous junction, or within the muscle.

Rabbit muscle-tendon units stretched to failure consistently fail near the myotendinous junction. The tendons of origin and insertion of most muscles extend well into the length of the muscle, and the muscle fibers have an oblique angle of insertion into the tendons. The fiber architecture is quite variable in different muscles. Rabbit hindlimb muscles were strained to failure without any direct nerve or muscle activation. For all muscles and for a wide range of strain rates, failure consistently occurred near the myotendinous junction.

The exact site of failure has not been clearly determined. The muscle fiber can avulse from the tendon at the precise muscle-tendon junction; however, failure usually occurs within the muscle fiber within several millimeters of the junction. The terminal sarcomeres near the myotendinous junction are stiffer than the middle sarcomeres of a muscle fiber. The injury to muscle occurs within this region of relatively limited extensibility. There are structural differences in the region, but detailed studies of the region of injury are lacking.

The response of activated muscle to stretch has been investigated using rabbit muscles stretched to failure during activation by motor-nerve stimulation. Activated muscle tore at the same increase in length as submaximally stimulated or unstimulated muscle, but slightly greater forces were recorded at failure for the stimulated muscles. The ability of stimulated muscle to maintain a higher force during stretching allowed a stimulated muscle to absorb much more energy than an unstimulated muscle, suggesting that the active component of a muscle protects against injury through energy absorption (Fig. 21). Muscle often contracts eccentrically to absorb energy, as in the case of the quadriceps muscle in landing from a jump. Joint control and protection from injury may be better when muscles are able to absorb more kinetic energy.

Trainers and athletes have traditionally believed that weak or fatigued muscles were more likely to be injured. It might seem paradoxical that the lower force-generating capacity of weakened or fatigued muscle results in more injury; however, muscles often are activated as energy absorbers or motion controllers, actions requiring higher muscle forces. Clinically, muscle strains usually occur in the setting of powerful eccentric muscle activity. Weakened or fatigued muscles might absorb less energy or be less able to resist stretching.

Incomplete Muscle Tears

Although complete muscle tears are seen clinically, incomplete injuries are much more common. Only a few studies have addressed the pathophysiologic features of incomplete muscle injury. Nondisruptive muscle injuries, produced by stretching rabbit anterior tibial muscles well into the elastic region of the load-deformation relation, resulted in a characteristic lesion near the myotendinous junction.

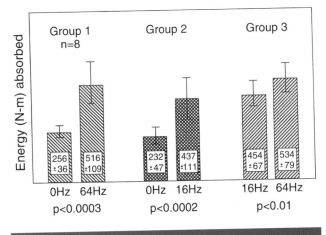

Figure 21

Energy absorbed by muscles strained to failure under varying conditions. In group 1, 1 rabbit extensor digitorum longus is strained to failure without muscle activation while the contralateral muscle is activated by nerve stimulation at 64 Hz. In group 2, 1 muscle is not activated and the other is activated by nerve stimulation at 16 Hz. In group 3, muscles are stimulated by the tetanic frequency (64 Hz) and by the submaximal frequency (16 Hz). (Adapted with permission from Garrett WE, Safran MR, Seaber AV, et al: Biomechanical comparison of stimulated and nonstimulated skeletal muscle pulled to failure. *Am J Sports Med* 1988;15:448–454.)

Fiber disruption and a small amount of hemorrhage were initially present (Fig. 22). During the next 1 to 4 days, a cellular inflammatory response occurred with the appearance of edema and granulation tissue containing fibroblasts and inflammatory cells. After a week, a significant amount of scar tissue and repair were present. Physiologically, there was a consistent decrease in the ability of the injured muscles to produce active tension for the first few days. After 7 days, the muscle approached normal tension production (Fig. 23).

Clinical studies of acute muscle strains reflect the changes seen in basic laboratory studies. Computed tomography and magnetic resonance imaging demonstrate muscle abnormalities in the region of the muscle-tendon junction. Acute changes include evidence of inflammatory changes and edema at the site of injury. Among the frequently injured muscles are the hamstrings, the rectus femoris, and the gastrocnemius; they all cross at least 2 joints and may be subject to more stretch. Studies of the muscle architecture demonstrate the extensive length of the muscle-tendon junction in these muscles. The region of the proximal or distal muscle-tendon junction extends the entire length of the muscle belly in the hamstring muscles.

Delayed Muscle Soreness

Delayed muscle soreness (DMS) is defined as muscular pain that generally occurs 24 to 72 hours after intense exercise. The damage is associated primarily with eccentric exercise and varies with both the intensity and duration of the exercise. DMS should be distinguished from discomfort during exercise that often is associated with muscle fatigue and from painful involuntary cramps caused by strong contractions of susceptible muscles, such as the gastrocnemius. DMS is characterized by a variable sense of discomfort in the muscle beginning several hours after exercise and reaching a maximum after 1 to 3 days. Clinically, patients usually demonstrate reduced activity and often display firm and swollen muscles. Peak swelling typically occurs 1 day or more following exercise. These findings strongly suggest that an increase in intramuscular pressure is present. Strength loss in the affected muscles is also common. In some cases, there can be up to a 50% loss in isometric strength immediately postexercise. This loss in strength usually lasts only a short time; however, measurable deficits can persist for up to 10 days.

Many of the concepts of DMS were introduced by Hough at the beginning of this century. He showed that forceful jerky movements produced muscle discomfort 24 to 48 hours after exercise, particularly in someone unaccustomed to such exercise. Measurable muscle weakness accompanied the muscle soreness. Even after a brief conditioning period allowing for resolution of the soreness, the weakness persisted for several days. The soreness was considered the result of intramuscular damage to the structural elements of the muscle. This injury was readily reversible.

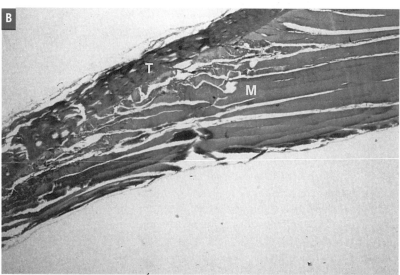
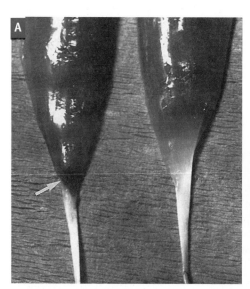

Figure 22

A, Gross appearance of tibialis anterior (TA) muscle following controlled passive strain injury. A small hemorrhage (arrow) is visible at the distal tip of injured muscle at 24 hours. The muscle on the right is the control. **B,** Histologic appearance of TA muscle immediately after passive strain injury. Note the rupture of fibers at the distal muscle-tendon junction, along with hemorrhage. T = tendon; M = intact muscle fibers (Masson's stain, ×100).

Current studies using muscle biopsies and animal models show that the original hypothesis of structural damage is indeed correct.

A number of theories have been proposed to explain the damage and subsequent repair that occur with DMS. Perhaps the most widely accepted is the hypothetical model that argues that mechanical factors are largely responsible for the initial events of the injury. This hypothesis is based on the assumption that high tensile stresses within the

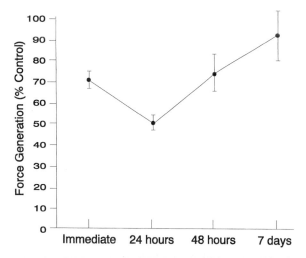

Figure 23

Percent of control force generation over range of frequencies versus time after controlled passive injury; immediately after injury (n = 30), 24 hours (n = 7), 48 hours (n = 8), 7 days (n = 8). All values I SEM. (Reproduced with permission from Nikolaou PK, Macdonald BL, Glisson RR, Seaber AV, Garrett WE Jr: Biomechanical and histological evaluation of muscle after controlled strain injury. *Am J Sports Med* 1987;15:9–14.)

muscle result in structural injury. Sarcolemmal damage is accompanied by an influx of Ca^{2+}. The mitochondria accumulate this Ca^{2+}, leading to a reduction in cellular respiration. Further injury to the sarcolemma is accompanied by diffusion of intracellular components into the interstitium and plasma. Shortly thereafter, the phagocytic phase predominates as monocytes are converted to macrophages. Further accumulation of histamine and kinins as well as elevated pressure from tissue edema leads to an activation of receptors resulting in the painful sensation of DMS.

The structural abnormalities that accompany DMS are well documented and typically include Z-band streaming, A-band disruption, and myofibril misalignment. Soreness does not appear immediately after exercise despite muscle biopsies showing structural damage within an hour after exercise. These structural abnormalities are most severe 2 to 3 days after exercise and seem to occur primarily in the fast-twitch glycolytic (type IIB) fibers. Magnetic resonance images have demonstrated increased T_2 relaxation times lasting 2 to 3 months after the bout of exercise. Early changes in T_2 relaxation probably reflect changes in cell water resulting from edema and swelling. Recently, it has been suspected that muscle fiber disruption leads to a leakage of protein-bound ions, which in turn creates edema. Muscle soreness has been shown to be directly associated with swollen muscle fibers and elevated resting muscle pressures 2 days after a single bout of eccentric exercise.

Serology studies have shown that exhausting exercise may be associated with increased levels of intramuscular enzymes in the serum. The increased levels of common indicators of muscle damage, such as creatine kinase, myoglobin, and lactate dehydrogenase (LDH), may correlate with the presence of muscle soreness. In addition, there are indications that connective tissue breakdown is also a part of the syndrome of delayed muscle soreness. Increased levels of urinary hydroxyproline excretion, which are indicative of collagen or connective tissue breakdown, have been associated with delayed muscle soreness.

Recent studies have shown that the structural damage that occurs with eccentric exercise is repairable. Furthermore, it appears that change takes place, which allows the involved muscles to become more resistant to damage from a subsequent bout of eccentric exercise. The exact time course of these adaptations is not clear at this point. One theory regarding the protection effect of excessive training is the "fragile fiber" hypothesis, which argues that fibers which are most susceptible to injury are damaged during an initial burst of eccentric contractions and replaced with stronger fibers that are resistant to subsequent damage.

Muscle Cramps

In spite of its frequency and impact on active exercise and work, the common muscle cramp is not well understood. Some muscles in certain individuals are susceptible to a very painful active contraction in a spasmodic fashion. The cramp begins when the susceptible muscle is in a shortened position and can usually be interrupted by stretch of the muscle by its antagonists or by external forces. For example, a cramp in the gastrocnemius can be stopped by active contraction of the ankle dorsiflexors and knee extensors or by standing on the toes and allowing the body weight and gravity to stretch the triceps surae. For many minutes after resolution of the cramp, the muscle shows evidence of altered excitability and fasciculations. Muscle cramps can occur after fatigue, prolonged muscle activity, dehydration, or even at night during sleep when the muscle remains in a shortened position. Cramping also occurs in clinical conditions such as renal failure, especially in the face of fluid and electrolyte disturbances. Susceptible muscles include the gastrocnemius, the hamstrings, the abdominal muscles, and a number of other muscle groups.

The electrical activity in the affected muscles is characteristic of that of motor units rather than that of individual muscle fibers, suggesting that the electrical activity responsible for cramps is coming from the nerve rather than from the mass action of individual muscle fibers. Specifically, it has been suggested that the active contractions of muscles are initiated from motor nerves once they have entered the belly of the muscles.

The etiology of abnormal action potentials is not well understood. Data from studies of athletes are ambiguous. Dehydration or loss of water and sodium are likely when cramps occur. Hydration and sodium replacement are frequently recommended for athletes. In studies of patients with renal failure it seems that the cramping condition can be ameliorated by correcting an abnormally low serum potassium. Lowered levels of serum Ca^{2+} and Mg^{2+} have also been implicated. However, data from these studies cannot be applied to cramps during athletic participation.

Immobilization and Disuse

When muscle is held immobilized for any significant length of time, there are a number of changes in its size and structure, physiologic properties, and metabolic properties. Disuse also can have many effects similar to those of immobilization. Disuse can occur without immobilization as a voluntary response to painful conditions or it can occur as a result of force deprivation by suspension, bed rest, or hypogravity states. In models of disuse or immobilization, muscle does not undergo its usual force production and its length changes because of lack of CNS drive, presence of motion restrictions, or deprivation of forces. For instance, disuse resulting from a painful condition may lead to motion limitation caused by voluntary CNS disuse. However, immobilization prohibits movement even though there may be near-normal activation of the muscle by the CNS. The muscle does not develop the normal stresses and strains but it may experience similar activation patterns, especially when a normal limb is temporarily immobilized.

Among the first changes occurring with immobilization is muscle atrophy; the weight of the entire muscle declines. The rate of loss of weight is not linear; it is more nearly exponential with more weight loss in the initial days than in subsequent days. The weight loss can be seen on a microscopic level as atrophy of individual muscle fibers. In general, all fibers demonstrate some atrophy. Depending on the experimental model, some muscles atrophy more than others; for example, the anti-gravity muscles from animals suspended and not allowed to bear weight atrophy more than other muscles.

Concomitant with loss of muscle mass is a loss of strength. Because strength or force production by muscle is a function of its cross-sectional area, it seems evident that loss of mass and cross-sectional area would result in strength decrements. When force production is normalized as strength per cross-sectional area, disuse and atrophy produce no change or a decrease in strength. Not only are mass and strength diminished by immobilization and disuse; the capacity of muscle to do prolonged work also decreases, or the fatigability of muscle increases. Fatigability can be assessed by physiologic techniques, showing a decline in force with continued use. There are also biochemical correlates of fatigability, including lower energy supplies and increased amounts of lactic acid. The increased fatigability is associated with a diminished ability to use fats in aerobic metabolic pathways.

The changes that accompany immobilization of muscle are related to the lengths at which muscles are immobilized. Atrophy and strength loss are much more prominent in muscle immobilized under no tension than in muscles immobilized under some stretch. This factor may explain the clinical observation of quadriceps atrophy greater than hamstring atrophy in thigh musculature. Immobilization or even disuse occurring with the knee being held in extension results in shortened quadriceps with some degree of hamstring stretch. Immobilization in a stretched position leads to a decrease in strength and cross-sectional area, but a less pronounced change in mass because muscle fibers held under stretch synthesize new contractile proteins, and sarcomeres are added to the ends of the existing fibrils. Therefore, changes in cross-sectional area are somewhat offset by increasing numbers of sarcomeres in the length of the muscle. In addition to the fibrillar changes, muscle immobilized with some stretch of the fibers maintained its strength better without a decrement in force production per cross-sectional area.

There also are significant changes in the passive properties of immobilized muscle. Changes relating to muscle growth have been discussed above. The passive length-tension relationship of muscle varies with the position of immobilization. Muscle immobilized in a shortened position develops more tension in response to passive stretch to a given length than muscle held in a lengthened position. Muscle extensibility may be a significant cause of the limitation of joint motion after injury or immobilization.

Some research has been directed toward the cellular and molecular mechanisms of the changes seen with disuse or atrophy. The rate of protein synthesis in muscle decreases within hours of the initiation of immobilization. Hormonal effects also occur very early. The insulin sensitivity of immobilized muscle decreases relatively quickly, and it is, therefore, more difficult for glucose to enter the muscle. In addition, immobilization increases levels of corticosteroids, which should decrease muscle protein synthesis. A better understanding of these mechanisms may provide significant improvements in the clinical ability to prevent or reverse loss of muscular function accompanying disease or injury.

Hormonal Effects on Skeletal Muscle

The effects of insulin, growth hormone, and testosterone on skeletal muscle will be considered. In addition, the use of these agents as potential anabolic-androgenic agents by athletes will also be discussed.

Insulin

Insulin, a polypeptide hormone secreted by the islet cells of the pancreas, plays an important role in the regulation of the intermediary metabolism of carbohydrates, proteins, and fats. Its primary role in metabolism is anabolic, increasing the storage of glucose, fatty acids, and amino acids. Glucagon, which is also secreted by the islet cells, has an action reciprocal to that of insulin, causing glucose, fatty acids, and amino acids to be mobilized into the bloodstream.

The principal actions of insulin in muscle include increased glucose entry into the cell, increased glycogen synthesis, increased amino acid uptake, increased ribosomal protein synthesis, decreased protein catabolism, and decreased release of gluconeogenic amino acids. Therefore, insulin has a net anabolic effect on muscle as it promotes the storage of both carbohydrate and protein and leads to the use of glucose. Growth hormone and insulin have synergistic effects to increase protein stores within the body. These effects are counteracted by the glucocorticoids, which accelerate protein degradation and amino acid release and inhibit amino acid transport and conversion to protein.

In humans, insulin deficiency is a common and often pathologic state leading to diabetes mellitus, which can lead to polyuria, polydipsia, weight loss, hyperglycemia, glycosuria, ketosis, acidosis, and coma. It appears that regular physical exercise can have positive effects on individuals with diabetes mellitus. Exercise is typically recommended for persons who have type I diabetes, particularly if they do not suffer from complications such as proliferative retinopathy, nephropathy, or autonomic neuropathy. Adaptive effects occur in muscle because physical training in persons with diabetes can lead to increased hexokinase levels and decreased LDH activity. In persons with type II diabetes who engage in regular physical exercise, the activity of the oxidative enzymes can be increased similarly to that of healthy persons.

Growth Hormone (Somatotropin)

Growth hormone is a single-chain peptide hormone synthesized in the anterior segment of the pituitary gland. Its production is under both stimulatory and inhibitory hypothalamic control. Growth hormone exerts its anabolic effects on muscle by increasing amino acid transport into the cell and by incorporating these amino acids into proteins, resulting in an increase in skeletal muscle synthesis. The exact mechanism by which this increased protein synthesis occurs in muscle remains unknown. There is evidence that growth hormone may bind to receptors on the plasma membrane of muscle tissue and have a direct anabolic action. Other data suggest that these effects are indirect and result from the action of somatomedins or insulin-like growth factors (IGF). A number of these growth factors have been identified, and they differ in their growth-promoting activity. IGF-I, a peptide produced by the liver and other tissues, including skeletal muscle, is responsible for increased protein and mRNA synthesis, amino acid uptake, and growth of cartilage and muscle. It appears that the secretion of both IGF-I and IGF-II is influenced by growth hormone, because concentrations of both factors seem to fall with its deficiency.

The presence of growth hormone is crucial to the growth and development of various tissues including bone, connective, visceral, adipose, and skeletal muscle. Excessive production of growth hormone before closure of the epiphyses produces gigantism, whereas deficiency of the hormone leads to dwarfism. After epiphyseal closure, the main effect of growth hormone hypersecretion is cortical thickening and periosteal overgrowth leading to the well-known condition of acromegaly. Complications include increased mortality, diabetes mellitus, atherosclerosis, neuropathy, and proximal myopathy of the hypertrophied muscles. These patients demonstrate selective type I fiber hypertrophy with atrophy of the type II fibers. Individuals often have skeletal muscle hypertrophy, but this is accompanied by weakness and fatigue, which probably is related to the atrophy of the type II fibers.

In addition to its growth-stimulating effects, growth hormone plays an important role in the regulation of metabolism. The general metabolic (lipolytic) effects are to reduce glucose and protein metabolism by shifting oxidative metabolism toward the use of fatty acids while sparing glucose and amino acids.

Testosterone

Androgens are synthesized primarily in the testicular interstitial cells of Leydig. Small amounts are produced by the ovaries and by the adrenal cortices of both sexes. Testosterone is the principal steroid hormone produced by the testes and has a considerable anabolic effect on muscle tissue. It is a 19-carbon steroid, which is synthesized from cholesterol in the Leydig cells and is also formed via progesterone and 17-hydroxyprogesterone. Small amounts are also formed in the adrenal cortex. The vast majority of this hormone is bound either to sex hormone-binding globulin or to albumin. Its plasma concentration is increased by estrogens and decreased by androgens. A small percentage (2%) exists in the unbound free form and exerts its anabolic effects by increasing protein synthesis and decreasing the rate of protein catabolism within the muscle fiber. The free, active hormone is used rapidly or is converted, primarily by the liver, into relatively inactive androgens that are excreted in the urine as neutral 17-ketosteroids, with small quantities also exiting through the bile (feces) and the skin.

Testosterone and other androgens exert a feedback inhibitory effect on pituitary gland secretion, develop and maintain the male secondary sex characteristics, and exert an important anabolic, growth-promoting action on both skeletal muscle and bone. This anabolic action of androgens has led to their use in counteracting effects of prolonged bed rest, disease, and surgical trauma. Androgen therapy can convert a mild negative nitrogen balance to a net retention of nitrogen. These effects are brought about by an increase in the synthesis and a decrease in the breakdown of protein. Androgens also promote physeal closure of the long bones.

Anabolic Steroids

It has been known for some time that the administration of testosterone to animals and humans can produce an increase in both muscle weight and strength. Testosterone has the effect of increasing body and muscle size (the "anabolic" effect) and the effect of virilization (the "androgenic" effect) or the expression of male sexual characteristics such as a lowered voice, increase in facial and body hair, and genital enlargement. A group of compounds have been developed in attempts to maintain the anabolic effects and avoid the virilizing effects. These compounds have been called anabolic steroids. None have ever really avoided the virilizing effects. These compounds have received a great deal of attention recently because of their use in sports. Although their use is considered both illegal and unethical, they are frequently used by athletes in particular sports and their effectiveness and risks are highly controversial.

Anabolic steroid use has become popular among athletes attempting to improve performance in events involving a large anaerobic energy requirement (for example, weightlifting and sprinting) as well as to increase strength and body weight. It has been reported that such athletes use 400% to 1,000% of the recommended medical dose of these agents. Whether or not these compounds are, in fact, effective remains controversial. The 1987 American College of Sports Medicine position statement on anabolic steroids concluded that "the gains in muscular strength achieved through high-intensity exercise and proper diet can be increased by the use of anabolic-androgenic steroids in some individuals." The 1991 American Academy of Orthopaedic Surgeons® position statement emphasizes that the use of anabolic steroids "can cause serious harmful physiological, pathological, and psychological effects."

A number of investigations have been conducted to characterize the potential biochemical, physiologic, and performance-enhancing effects of anabolic steroids in animal models under both acute and chronic conditions. Perhaps because of the different forms of exercise and treatment protocols used, these studies have yielded conflicting evidence as to the potential performance-enhancing capability of these agents. Further studies are needed to critically evaluate the effects of anabolic steroids on muscle mass and strength. While the positive effects of anabolic steroids on muscle protein synthesis have been well documented, evidence relating exercise and steroid treatment to muscle fiber hypertrophy and enhanced performance needs to be more critically studied.

Although the long-term effects of high doses of anabolic-androgenic agents are not entirely clear, several facts have been well established. There are CNS effects that may include a sensation of well-being or euphoria and increased levels of aggression, which may lead to intense antisocial or psychotic behavior, in individuals taking large doses of these agents. Cardiovascular effects include decreased high-density-lipoprotein levels, stroke, and cardiomyopathy; myocardial infarctions have been documented in individuals administered large doses of anabolic steroids. Hepatic and endocrine dysfunction, negative reproductive effects (oligospermia; azospermia; testicular atrophy; reductions in testosterone and gonadotropic hormones; and decreased levels of luteinizing hormone, follicle-stimulating hormone, estrogens, and progesterone), and other adverse effects (renal dysfunction) have also been implicated as possible side effects of these agents. Premature epiphyseal closure has been reported in youths. Because of this irreversible halt in growth, these compounds are especially contraindicated prior to skeletal maturity.

The effects of these agents on skeletal muscle and tendon are less well documented. Changes in the morphology of the muscle-tendon unit have also been studied in animals. Anabolic agents used concurrently with swimming produced slow-twitch fiber hypertrophy in the rat. Exercise and steroid protocols by themselves increased the fast oxidative glycolytic fiber population and decreased the fast glycolytic subtype. Clinically, several cases of spontaneous tendon rupture have been reported in athletes taking large doses of anabolic steroids. Laboratory studies have shown that administration of large doses of anabolic steroids to rats produced inhibitory effects on collagen biosynthesis. None of these studies, however, conclusively confirm the use of these agents as the causative problem.

Another ergogenic aid is human growth hormone. The development of synthetic agents has led to a dramatic increase in the use of these potentially anabolic agents. Similar to the use of other anabolic agents, the use of growth hormone is potentially widespread with serious side effects, including diabetogenic effects, cardiomegaly, and acromegaly.

The physiologic mechanism responsible for exercise-induced muscle growth is unknown. Muscle hypertrophy can be induced by overload in castrated, hypophysectomized, and diabetic animals. Therefore, at least in some experimental animal models, the presence of testosterone, growth hormone, or insulin does not seem to be required to produce muscle hypertrophy. Maintenance of, as well as increases in, muscle size and strength can be achieved in actively exercising elderly humans, although advanced age and malnutrition can decrease levels of certain growth factors, a concept true in animals as well. There has been tremendous recent interest in exercise enhancement and specific benefits of creatine and prostaglandin supplementation to athletes. The creatine/pcr system plays an essential role in the normal injury metabolism of muscle because it acts as a buffer for the ATP within muscle. Although the potential for long-term side effects has not been studied, it does appear that under certain circumstances, creatine supplementation may yield certain benefits to enhance athletic performance.

Muscle Stretching and Viscoelasticity

Muscle stretching exercises or routines are frequently used by athletes before and during sports. They are also a part of many rehabilitation and fitness programs. Few scientific data address the efficacy of stretching in injury prevention and rehabilitation or in the enhancement of performance. Various reflexes involving the CNS and motor control of skeletal muscle are frequently mentioned as the scientific rationale for stretching. These reflexes are very important in the motor control of dynamic movement, but their effects on static stretching are unknown.

The effects of chronic stretching may be related to the previous discussions of longitudinal growth of muscle or to the effects of immobilization in extension. In these situations, the stretch is maintained long enough to allow time for biologic growth or rearrangement of muscle tissue. The acute effects of stretching have only recently been evaluated. Skeletal muscle exhibits the same viscoelastic effects seen in dense connective tissue and bone. These viscoelastic effects explain many of the effects of stretching.

Viscoelasticity, discussed in more detail in Chapter 5, Biomechanics, describes the stress and strain relationship and its time-dependent nature. When muscle is stretched to a given length, it develops a certain tension. The tension does not remain constant with time. Instead the stress diminishes with time; this phenomenon is called stress relaxation. Muscle can lose more than 20% of the initial force in as little as 30 s. Muscle also exhibits creep behavior, meaning that when a given load is applied to a muscle it reaches an initial length and then will slowly stretch out with time. Viscoelastic phenomena can account for the diminished stiffness of muscle after stretching and for the increased range of motion allowed by stretching.

Another property of viscoelasticity that relates to muscle stretching is the dependence of stress developed in muscle to the rate of strain. Muscle stretched quickly is stiffer than muscle stretched slowly. Temperature effects also are important. Cold muscle is stiffer than warm muscle; therefore, warm muscle will develop less force than cold muscle when stretched to a given length. Viscoelasticity in muscle can certainly help to explain the common benefits attributed to stretching.

Common stretching routines usually advocate slow static stretching of the muscle-tendon unit. Under these conditions it appears that the electrical activity within muscle is minimal. This means that the resistance of muscle to stretch comes primarily from the mechanical properties of the muscle-tendon unit rather than from active contraction of the muscle. Therefore, the viscoelastic properties of muscle are probably more important to static muscle stretching than reflex-mediated relaxation controlled by the CNS.

Electromyography

Muscles and tendons can be thought of as the interface between the CNS and the skeleton. Communication between these effectors occurs through electrical activity. The electrical currents passing across the membranes of the muscle cells can be detected and measured by methods similar to those by which electrical currents in the heart are recorded as an electrocardiogram. The electromyographic (EMG) signal is the electrical representation of the neuromuscular activation associated with a contracting muscle. A number of uses for this technique have been developed to study normal muscle function and to assist in the diagnoses of muscle abnormalities.

Basically, the electrical signals within the muscle are detected by electrodes, amplified, and subsequently recorded or processed (Fig. 24). Surface electrodes are placed on the skin surface and can detect underlying muscle currents. These electrodes are simple and convenient for the study of large surface muscles. Needle electrodes, in contrast, are inserted through the skin into the muscle. Insulated wire inside a needle-like cannula allows for the detection of a myoelectric signal from a smaller volume of muscle and may be used to study individual muscles and muscles not on the surface. Fine wire electrodes are very small and can be inserted into muscles and left for kinesiological studies. They are small enough and painless enough to cause little perturbation of the normal use of the muscle. The signals detected by the electrodes are amplified and recorded with appropriate electrical considerations to ensure that the recorded signal most closely resembles the myoelectric signal generated within the muscle.

Central Nervous System Control

The study of electrical signals in the muscle has led to a tremendous insight into the nature of CNS control of muscle activity. Appropriate electrodes can actually evaluate the distribution and activity of single motor units. Sophisticated techniques of signal acquisition and decomposition have allowed researchers to analyze how the many motor units interact under conditions such as varying force and time of excitation. The CNS control depends on the type of muscle; small muscles and muscles needing fine control are somewhat different from the larger muscle groups. Small muscles are capable of higher frequencies of muscle activation with plateaus near 60 Hz compared to approximately 25 Hz for larger muscles. The smaller muscles, thus, have a larger range of control.

Data from EMG studies have provided information necessary to understand the control of force in muscle. Basically, force is increased in a muscle both by increasing the recruitment of motor units and by increasing the frequency of stimulation of recruited motor units. The changes in both recruitment and frequency are under the influence of a common drive from the CNS. The common drive allows the CNS to control motor units as a pool rather than as single units. The addition and subtraction of motor units is an orderly process based in large part on the size of the motor unit. The smallest motor units are recruited initially, followed by larger and larger motor units.

The recruitment pattern differs among muscles. In small muscles, the motor units are often fully recruited at force levels below 50% of a maximum contraction. Alterations in frequency provide additional control above this level. Larger muscles may not recruit all motor units until forces near maximum are achieved. The varying relationship between maximum force in a muscle and the mechanism of force control, that is, alterations in recruitment and stimulation frequency, might imply that there is not a strict relationship between muscle force output and the EMG signal. Although it is true that an increasing EMG signal is usually accompanied by increasing force, this relationship is not necessarily linear. In addition, the relationship varies among subjects and among different muscles. In general, the smaller muscles have a more linear relationship between force and the integrated EMG signal; larger muscles often demonstrate less linearity, with the signal increasing more than the force.

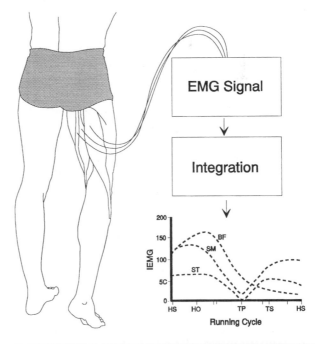

Figure 24

An averaged integrated electromyogram from biceps femoris (BF), semimembranosus (SM), and semitendinosus (ST). HS = Heel strike; HO = immediately prior to the heel lofting off treadmill; TP = thigh perpendicular to treadmill; TS = toe strike; IEMG = integrated electromyogram.

Electromyography has also been important in arriving at the present understanding of local muscle fatigue. An isometrically activated muscle might be expected to maintain a constant EMG signal; however, the EMG signal depends on time of activation, intensity of activation, and fatigue. In general, the integrated EMG signal increases with time when a constant force is achieved by a muscle. Although the amplitude of the signal increases, the mean and median frequencies of motor unit firing rates decrease. This shift in frequency begins very quickly after initiation of a sustained isometric contraction and continues with time. This measurable change provides an excellent parameter for studying the state of local muscle fatigue.

Clinical applications of the EMG signal to provide information regarding the state of muscle and its CNS control are increasing. EMG can provide an excellent measure of the degree of muscle activation; however, the EMG signal may not be a direct measure of the force output of the muscle. In addition, EMG may be able to provide information about the state of fatigue in muscle. Application of EMG techniques is increasing in the fields of athletic training and rehabilitation; these techniques are being applied to muscles of the limbs and of the axial skeleton.

EMG in Kinesiology

Kinesiology, or the study of movement, has benefited greatly from EMG techniques. Movement studies can be correlated with EMG studies to show when and to what extent the muscle is active in a particular movement. The use of EMG techniques to study gait has been invaluable. The combined effects of kinetic and potential energy, the interdependence of joint movements, and the influences of ground contact make it impossible to know about the state of muscle activity without a direct means of detection. Studies of gait in normal and pathologic states have benefited greatly from combining kinesiology and EMG.

EMG has been used in gait studies with increasing sophistication over the last 55 years. At present more applications are becoming apparent; complex motor activities such as throwing, swimming, and even a golf or tennis swing are being understood as never before. The data obtained are useful in understanding the movement and its disorders, and with time EMG techniques hold the promise of improving performance and of guiding and assessing rehabilitation. Implantable fine-wire electrodes and methods of telemetry have allowed increasing applications of these techniques.

EMG in Diagnosis of Neuromuscular Disease

Diagnostic EMG has made significant strides recently and is now a sophisticated tool in the diagnosis of neuromuscular pathology. Although primarily used by neurologists to study neurologic disease, EMG has significance for orthopaedics and the study of musculoskeletal problems. These applications specifically concern the presence and chronicity of injury to nerves and nerve roots.

Following injury to its motor nerve, the muscle is deprived of its normal control mechanism. In the case of a neurapraxia, the nerve distal to the site of injury does not undergo necrosis. However, the muscle is electrically silent even in response to efforts to activate the muscle. If the injury is an axonotmesis or a neurotmesis, the axon distal to the injury undergoes necrosis. The motor end plate eventually degenerates after several weeks, depending on the length of nerve between the injury and the synapse. After the synapse undergoes degeneration, changes occur within the membrane system of the muscle. The individual muscle fibers spontaneously depolarize and give rise to axonal action potentials. The spontaneous discharges are in single muscle fibers rather than in an entire motor unit; therefore, the potentials are smaller and occur intermittently. Needle electrodes detect these changes as fibrillations, which are indicative of denervation. If the nerve injury is due to an incomplete lesion to the nerve or to a single ventral root, as in a radiculopathy from the level of the spinal cord, apparently normal action potentials or action potentials of reduced magnitude exist, with fibrillations also evident when the muscle and nerve are at rest.

After denervation and distal axonal necrosis, reinnervation may occur. This may be the result of regrowth of axons across the site of injury, or sprouting of collateral branches from axons reaching the muscles. The regrown axons and the sprouts give rise to large and atypical motor units. The action potentials of these motor units are large and complex in contrast to the normal motor unit action potential. These abnormal action potentials are called giant polyphasic action potentials and are a sign of reinnervation.

Selected Bibliography

Muscle Structure and Function

Burke RE: Motor unit properties and selective involvement in movement. *Exerc Sport Sci Rev* 1975;3:31–81.

Carlson FD, Wilkie DR (eds): *Muscle Physiology*. Englewood Cliffs, NJ, Prentice Hall Inc, 1974.

Huxley AF, Simmons RM: Proposed mechanism of force generation in striated muscle. *Nature* 1971;233:533–538.

Huxley AF: Muscle structure and theories of contraction. *Prog Biophys Biophys Chem* 1957;7:255–318.

Huxley HE: Electron microscope studies on the structure of natural and synthetic protein filaments from striated muscle. *J Mol Biol* 1963;7:281–308.

Huxley HE: The mechanism of muscular contraction. *Science* 1969;164:1356–1365.

Schaub MC, Watterson JG: Control of the contractile process in muscle. *Trends Pharmacol Sci* 1981;2:279–282.

Wickiewicz TL, Roy RR, Powell PL, et al: Muscle architecture of the human lower limb. *Clin Orthop* 1983;179:275–283.

Fiber Types and Adaptability of Muscle

Baldwin KM, Winder WW, Holloszy JO: Adaptation of actomyosin ATPase in different types of muscle to endurance exercise. *Am J Physiol* 1975;229:422–426.

Barany M, Close RI: The transformation of myosin in cross-innervated rat muscles. *J Physiol* (Lond) 1971;213:455–474.

Buchthal F, Schmalbruch H: Motor unit of mammalian muscle. *Physiol Rev* 1980;60:90–142.

Buller AJ, Eccles JC, Eccles RM: Interactions between motoneurones and muscles in respect of the characteristic speeds of their responses. *J Physiol* (Lond) 1960;150:417–439.

Close RI: Dynamic properties of mammalian skeletal muscles. *Physiol Rev* 1972;52:129–197.

Dubowitz V, Brooke MH (eds): *Muscle Biopsy: A Modern Approach.* London, England, WB Saunders, 1973, vol 2.

Gauthier GF: Skeletal muscle fiber types, in Engle AG, Banker BQ (eds): *Myology: Basic and Clinical.* New York, NY, McGraw-Hill, pp 255–283.

Henneman E: Relation between size of neurons and their susceptibility to discharge. *Science* 1957;126:1345–1347.

Johnson MA, Polgar J, Weightman D, et al: Data on the distribution of fibre types in thirty-six human muscles: An autopsy study. *J Neurol Sci* 1973;18:111–129.

Kugelberg E: Histochemical composition, contraction speed, and fatiguability of rat soleus motor units. *J Neurol Sci* 1973;20:177–198.

Lowey S, Risby D: Light chains from fast and slow muscle myosins. *Nature* 1971;234:81–85.

Martin WD, Romond EH: Effects of chronic rotation and hypergravity on muscle fibers of soleus and plantaris muscles of the rat. *Exp Neurol* 1975;49:758–771.

Pette D (ed): *Plasticity of Muscle.* Berlin, Germany, Walter de Gruyter, 1980.

Roy RR, Meadows ID, Baldwin KM, et al: Functional significance of compensatory overloaded rat fast muscle. *J Appl Physiol* 1982;52:473–478.

Salmons S, Sreter FA: Significance of impulse activity in the transformation of skeletal muscle type. *Nature* 1976; 263:30–34.

Samaha FJ, Guth L, Albers RW: Differences between slow and fast muscle myosin: Adenosine triphosphatase activity and release of associated proteins by p-chloromercuriphenylsulfonate. *J Biol Chem* 1970;245:219–224.

Sreter FA, Seidel JC, Gergely J: Studies on myosin from red and white skeletal muscles of the rabbit: I. Adenosine triphosphatase activity. *J Biol Chem* 1966;241:5772–5776.

Muscle Mechanics

Hill AV: The heat of shortening and the dynamic constants of muscle (1938): *Proc R Soc Lond* (Biol) 1938;126:136–195.

Huxley AF: Muscular contraction. *J Physiol* (Lond) 1974;243:1–43.

Kulig K, Andrews JG, Hay JG: Human strength curves. *Exerc Sport Sci Rev* 1984;12:417–466.

Woittiez RD, Huijing PA, Boom HB, et al: A three-dimensional muscle model: Quantified relation between form and function of skeletal muscles. *J Morphol* 1984;182:95–113.

Training Effects on Muscle

Gollnick PD, Armstrong RB, Saltin B, et al: Effect of training on enzyme activity and fiber composition of human skeletal muscle. *J Appl Physiol* 1973;34:107–111.

Gollnick PD, Matoba H: The muscle fiber composition of skeletal muscle as a predictor of athletic success: An overview. *Am J Sports Med* 1984;12:212–217.

Green HJ, Reichmann H, Pette D: Fibre type specific transformations in the enzyme activity pattern of rat vastus lateralis muscle by prolonged endurance training. *Pflugers Arch* 1983;399:216–222.

Holloszy JO: Biochemical adaptations in muscle: Effects of exercise on mitochondrial oxygen uptake and respiratory enzyme activity in skeletal muscle. *J Biol Chem* 1967;242:2278–2282.

Howald H, Hoppeler H, Claassen H, et al: Influences of endurance training on the ultrastructural composition of the different muscle fiber types in humans. *Pflugers Arch* 1985;403:369–376.

Komi PV, Rusko H, Vos J, et al: Anaerobic performance capacity in athletes. *Acta Physiol Scand* 1977;100:107–114.

Milner-Brown HS, Stein RB, Yemm R: Changes in firing rate of human motor units during linearly changing voluntary contractions. *J Physiol* (Lond) 1973;230:371–390.

Saltin B, Henriksson J, Nygaard E, et al: Fiber types and metabolic potentials of skeletal muscles in sedentary man and endurance runners. *Ann N Y Acad Sci* 1977;301:3–29.

Taylor NA, Wilkinson JG: Exercise-induced skeletal muscle growth: Hypertrophy or hyerplasia? *Sports Med* 1986;3:190–200.

Tesch P, Karlsson J: Isometric strength performance and muscle fibre type distribution in man. *Acta Physiol Scand* 1978;103:47–51.

Thorstensson A, Hulten B, von Dobeln W, et al: Effect of strength training on enzyme activities and fibre characteristics in human skeletal muscle. *Acta Physiol Scand* 1976;96:392–398.

Tipton CM, Schild RJ, Tomanek RJ: Influence of physical activity on the strength of knee ligaments in rats. *Am J Physiol* 1967;212:783–787.

Growth and Development of Muscle

Dix DJ, Eisenberg BR: Myosin mRNA accumulation and myofibrillogenesis at the myotendinous junction of stretched muscle fibers. *J Cell Biol* 1990;1:1885–1894.

Griffin GE, Williams PE, Goldspink G: Region of longitudinal growth in striated muscle fibres. *Nature* (New Biol) 1971;232:28–29.

Williams PE, Goldspink G: Changes in sarcomere length and physiological properties in immobilized muscle. *J Anat* 1978;127:459–468.

Williams PE, Goldspink G: Connective tissue changes in immobilised muscle. *J Anat* 1984;138:343–350.

Williams PE, Goldspink G: The effect of immobilization on the longitudinal growth of striated muscle fibres. *J Anat* 1973;116:45–55.

Muscle Injury and Repair

Armstrong RB: Mechanisms of exercise-induced delayed onset muscular soreness: A brief review. *Med Sci Sports Exerc* 1984;16:529–538.

Asmussen E: Observations on experimental muscular soreness. *Acta Rheum Scand* 1956;2:109–116.

Best TM, Fiebig R, Curr DT, et al: Free radical activity, antioxidant enzyme, and glutathione changes with muscle stretch injury in rabbits. *J Appl Physiol,* in press.

Besson C, Rochcongar P, Beauverger Y, et al: Study of the valuations of serum muscular enzymes and myoglobin after maximal exercise test and during the next 24 hours. (author's translation) *Eur J Appl Physiol* 1981;47:47–56.

Byrnes WC, Clarkson PM, White JS, et al: Delayed onset muscle soreness following repeated bouts of downhill running. *J Appl Phys* 1985;59:710–715.

Cannon JG, St. Pierre BA: Cytokines in exercise-induced skeletal muscle injury. *Mol Cell Biochem* 1998;179:159–167.

Denny-Brown D: Clinical problems in neuromuscular physiology. *Am J Med* 1953;15:368–390.

Friden J, Sjostrom M, Ekblom B: Myofibrillar damage following intense eccentric exercise in man. *Int J Sports Med* 1983;4:170–176.

Garrett WE Jr, Safran MR, Seaber AV, et al: Biomechanical comparison of stimulated and nonstimulated skeletal muscle pulled to failure. *Am J Sports Med* 1987;15:448–454.

Garrett WE Jr, Seaber AV, Boswick J, et al: Recovery of skeletal muscle after laceration and repair. *J Hand Surg* 1984;9A:683–692.

Hough T: Ergographic studies in muscular soreness. *Am J Physiol* 1902;7:76–92.

Hughston JC, Whatley GS, Stone MM: Myositis ossificans traumatica (myo-osteosis). *South Med J* 1962;55:1167–1170.

Jackson DW, Feagin JA: Quadriceps contusions in young athletes: Relation of severity of injury to treatment and prognosis. *J Bone Joint Surg* 1973;55A:95–105.

King JB: Post-traumatic ectopic calcification in the muscles of athletes: A review. *Br J Sports Med* 1998;32:287–290.

Lieber RL, Friden J: Selective damage of fast glycolytic muscle fibres with eccentric contraction of the rabbit tibialis anterior. *Acta Physiol Scand* 1988;133:587–588.

Lieber RL, Woodburn TM, Friden J: Muscle damage induced by eccentric contractions of 25% strain. *J Appl Physiol* 1991;70:2498–2507.

Maughan RJ: Exercise-induced muscle cramp: A prospective biochemical study in marathon runners. *J Sport Sci* 1986;4:31–34.

Moss HK, Herrmann LG: Night cramps in human extremities: Clinical study of physiologic action of quinine and prostigmine upon spontaneous contractions of resting muscles. *Am Heart J* 1948;35:403–408.

Nikolaou PK, Macdonald BL, Glisson RR, et al: Biomechanical and histological evaluation of muscle after controlled strain injury. *Am J Sports Med* 1987;15:9–14.

Parrow A, Samuelsson SM: Use of chloroquine phosphate—a new treatment for spontaneous leg cramps. *Acta Medica Scand* 1967;181:237–244.

Sacco P, Jones DA: The protective effect of damaging eccentric exercise against repeated bouts of exercise in the mouse tibialis anterior muscle. *Exp Physiol* 1992;77:757–760.

Schwane JA, Johnson SR, Vandenakker CB, et al: Delayed-onset muscular soreness and plasma CPK and LDH activities after downhill running. *Med Sci Sports Exerc* 1983;15:51–56.

Shellock FG, Fukunaga T, Mink JH, et al: Exertional muscle injury: Evaluation of concentric versus eccentric actions with serial MR imaging. *Radiology* 1991;179:659–664.

Speer KP, Lohlnes J, Garrett WE Jr: Radiographic imaging of muscle strain injury. *Am J Sports Med* 1993;21:89–95.

Stauber WT: Eccentric action of muscles: Physiology, injury, and adaptation. *Exerc Sport Sci Rev* 1989;17:157–185.

Stewart WK, Fleming LW, Manuel MA: Muscle cramps during maintenance haemodialysis. *Lancet* 1972;1:1049–1051.

Tidball JG: Myotendinous junction: Morphological changes and mechanical failure associated with muscle cell atrophy. *Exp Mol Pathol* 1984;40:1–12.

Tidball JG: Inflammatory cell response to acute muscle injury. *Med Sci Sports Exerc* 1995;27:1022–1032.

Immobilization

Alford EK, Roy RR, Hodgson JA, et al: Electromyography of rat soleus, medial gastrocnemius, and tibialis anterior during hind limb suspension. *Exp Neurol* 1987;96:635–649.

Appell HJ: Morphology of immobilized skeletal muscle and the effects of a pre- and post-immobilization training program. *Int J Sports Med* 1986;7:6–12.

Booth FW: Physiologic and biochemical effects of immobilization on muscle. *Clin Orthop* 1987;219:15–20.

Booth FW, Seider MJ: Recovery of skeletal muscle after 3 months of hind limb immobilization in rats. *J Appl Physiol* 1979;47:435–439.

Jansson E, Sylven C, Arvidsson I, et al: Increase in myoglobin content and decrease in oxidative enzyme activities by leg muscle immobilization in man. *Acta Physiol Scand* 1988;132:515–517.

Lieber RL, Friden JO, Hargens AR, et al: Differential response of the dog quadriceps muscle to external skeletal fixation of the knee. *Muscle Nerve* 1988;11:193–201.

Lipschütz A, Audova A: The comparative atrophy of the skeletal muscle after cutting the nerve and after cutting the tendon. *J Physiol* (Lond) 1921;55:300–304.

MacDougall JD, Elder GC, Sale DG, et al: Effects of strength training and immobilization on human muscle fibres. *Eur J Appl Physiol* 1980; 43:25–34.

Max SR: Disuse atrophy of skeletal muscle: Loss of functional activity of mitochondria. *Biochem Biophys Res Commun* 1972;46: 1394–1398.

Roy RR, Bello MA, Bouissou P, et al: Size and metabolic properties of fibers in rat fast-twitch muscles after hind-limb suspension. *J Appl Physiol* 1987;62:2348–2357.

Sargeant AJ, Davies CT, Edwards RH, et al: Functional and structural changes after disuse of human muscle. *Clin Sci Mol Med* 1977;52: 337–342.

Solandt DY, Partridge RC, Hunter J: The effect of skeletal fixation on skeletal muscle. *J Neurophysiol* 1943;6:17–22.

Thomason DB, Herrick RE, Surdyka D, et al: Time course of soleus muscle myosin expression during hindlimb suspension and recovery. *J Appl Physiol* 1987;63:130–137.

Tomanek RJ, Lund DD: Degeneration of different types of skeletal muscle fibres. II Immobilization. *J Anat* 1974;118:531–541.

Hormonal Effects

Alen M, Hakkinen K, Komi PV: Changes in neuromuscular performance and muscle fiber characteristics of elite power athletes self-administering androgenic and anabolic steroids. *Acta Physiol Scand* 1984;122:535–544.

AMA Council on Scientific Affairs: Drug abuse in athletes: Anabolic steroids and human growth hormone. *JAMA* 1988;259:1703–1705.

American College of Sports Medicine position stand on the use of anabolic-androgenic steroids in sports. *Med Sci Sports Exerc* 1987; 19:534–539.

American Academy of Orthopaedic Surgeons Position Statement: Anabolic Steroids to Enhance Athletic Performance. Park Ridge, IL, American Academy of Orthopaedic Surgeons, 1991.

Apostolakis M, Deligiannis A, Madena-Pyrgaki A: The effects of human growth hormone administration on the functional status of rat atrophied muscle following immobilization. *Physiologist* 1980:23 (suppl):S111–112.

Bach BR Jr, Warren RF, Wickiewicz TL: Triceps rupture: A case report and literature review. *Am J Sports Med* 1987;15:285–289.

Breuer CB, Florini JR: Amino acid incorporation into protein by cell-free systems from rat skeletal muscle: IV. Effects of animal age, androgens, and anabolic agents on activity of muscle ribosomes. *Biochemistry* 1965;4:1544–1550.

Clark JF: Creatine and phosphocreatine: A review of their use in exercise and sport. *J Athl Train* 1997;32:45–51.

Dimauro J, Balnave RJ, Shorey CD: Effects of anabolic steroids and high intensity exercise on rat skeletal muscle fibres and capillarization: A morphometric study. *Eur J Appl Physiol* 1992;64:204–212.

Egginton S: Effects of an anabolic hormone on striated muscle growth and performance. *Pflugers Arch* 1987;410:349–355.

Exner GU, Staudte HW, Pette D: Isometric training of rats: Effects upon fast and slow muscle and modification by an anabolic hormone (nandrolone decanoate). I. Female rats. *Pflugers Arch* 1973;345:1–14.

Exner GU, Staudte HW, Pette D: Isometric training of rats: Effects upon fast and slow muscle and modification by an anabolic hormone (nandrolone decanoate). II. Male rats. *Pflugers Arch* 1973; 345:15–22.

Florini J: Hormonal control of muscle growth. *J Anim Sci* 1985;61:21–37.

Goldberg AL, Goodman HM: Relationship between growth hormone and muscular work in determining muscle size. *J Physiol* (Lond) 1969;200:655–666.

Greenhaff PL, Casey A, Short AH, Harris R, Soderlund K, Hultman E: Influence of oral creatine supplementation of muscle torque during repeated bouts of maximal voluntary exercise in man. *Clin Sci* (Colch) 1993;84:565–571.

Haupt HA, Rovere GD: Anabolic steroids: A review of the literature. *Am J Sports Med* 1984;12:469–484.

Herrick RT, Herrick S: Ruptured triceps in a powerlifter presenting as cubital tunnel syndrome: A case report. *Am J Sports Med* 1987;15:514–516.

Hill JA, Suker JR, Sachs K, et al: The athletic polydrug abuse phenomenon: A case report. *Am J Sports Med* 1983;11:269–271.

Kibble MW, Ross MB: Adverse effects of anabolic steroids in athletes. *Clin Pharm* 1987;6:686–692.

Kreider RB, Ferreira M, Wilson M, et al: Effects of creatine supplementation on body composition, strength, and sprint performance. *Med Sci Sports Exerc* 1998;30:73–82.

Michna H, Stang-Voss C: The predisposition to tendon rupture after doping with anabolic steroids. *Int J Sports Med* 1986;4:59.

Perlmutter G, Lowenthal DT: Use of anabolic steroids by athletes. *Am Fam Physician* 1985;32:208–210.

Muscle Stretching and Viscoelasticity

Best TM, McElhaney J, Garrett WE Jr, Myers BS: Characterization of the passive responses of live skeletal muscle using the quasi-linear theory of viscoelasticity . *J Biomech* 1994;27:413–419.

Dalton JD Jr, Seaber AV, Garrett WE Jr: Biomechanics of passively stretched muscle: Viscoelasticity vs. reflex effects. *Surg Forum* 1989;40:516–518.

Inman VT, Ralston HJ, de Saunder JB, et al: Relation of human electromyogram to muscular tension. *EEG Clin Neurophysiol* 1952;4:187–194.

Lippold OCJ: The relation between integrated action potentials in a human muscle and its isometric tension. *J Physiol* (Lond) 1952;117:492–499.

Taylor DC, Dalton JD Jr, Seaber AV, Garrett WE Jr: Viscoelastic properties of muscle-tendon units: The biomechanical effects of stretching. *Am J Sports Med* 1990;18:300–309.

Chapter Outline

Chapter 27

Spinal Mechanisms for Control of Movement

William Z. Rymer, MD, PhD

Jacquelin Perry, MD

This chapter at a glance

This chapter discusses the mechanical properties of muscle that provide a basis for understanding the neural factors that regulate movement.

Introduction

When performing a task related to motion or posture, all motor commands from the central nervous system are expressed through changes in the magnitude of neural excitation of skeletal muscle. The response of the activated muscle is force generation for the purpose of creating or restraining motion. The magnitude and mode of the resulting muscle force depends on the properties of muscle, the mechanical load experienced by the muscle, the nature of the neural excitation, and feedback from the muscle receptors. Although the physiology of muscle is a separate topic, there are mechanical properties of muscle that provide a basis for understanding the neural factors that regulate movement and, thus, this chapter will begin with a short description of muscle mechanics.

Mechanical Properties of Whole Muscle

Length-Tension Relationships: The Spring-Like Behavior of Muscle

Stimulation of a resting muscle activates its contraction mechanics to create a force. For a given level of neural excitation, the muscle force increases with increasing muscle extension until a length is reached where further stretch does not generate additional contractile force (Fig. 1) and a temporary peak occurs. This end point, designated L_0, marks the muscle's "maximum physiologic length." With further stretch of the muscle, the contraction force progressively declines while stiffness of the noncontractile structures within the muscle (parallel-elastic elements) introduces passive tension. Hence, additional stretch continues to increase total muscle tension but it now represents the sum of increasing passive tension and waning contractile muscle force. The pattern of passive stretch is actually determined by stretch testing relaxed muscle. Tissue flexibility within the muscle's physiologic length provides little resistance to stretch, but beyond L_0 passive resistance rapidly rises. Stretch beyond the optimum length (L_0) is not normally seen in the intact limb where both ends of the muscle are attached to the limb's bones. Also, in an intact limb the increase in muscle force with lengthening is obscured by the overlay of skeletal leverage from changes in joint position.

As the muscle is stretched within its physiologic length, the force rises smoothly and approximately in proportion to the degree of muscle extension. Conversely, when the muscle is allowed to shorten the reduction in force is essentially proportional to the decrease in muscle length. These features are characteristic of a spring. Furthermore, when the muscle stretch is maintained, the increase in force also

is maintained. This is additional verification of the muscle's spring-like property, because a metal spring continues to resist when extended.

The form of the length-tension relationship varies with the rate of neural excitation. The differences are in the length at which the muscle force begins its steep increase and the muscle length when peak tension occurs.

Experiments to demonstrate the length-tension phenomenon are performed with the muscle's insertion detached from bone to allow unlimited stretch. (Muscle tension, or force, is measured with a transducer fastened to the free tendon end). This phenomenon also is seen in humans with cineplasties. In this clinical situation the muscle's insertion has been released from bone so the muscle can serve as an independent motor to control a prosthesis, rather than act on the joint. The customary experiment uses a series of isometric states. However, a more precise spring-like quality of muscle mechanics is seen when a continuous slow stretch is induced.

These length-dependent changes in muscle force primarily relate to the change in the number of bonds between myosin cross-bridges and the receptor sites on actin filaments (described in Chapter 26). Calcium ion release also is a critical element in cross-bridge cycling related to length-tension increases. A clinical benefit of these spring-like properties is that the muscle forms a compliant interface with the external world and acts somewhat as a shock absorber.

Force-Velocity Relationship

The magnitude of the force generated during active muscle shortening is determined primarily by the speed with which the shortening occurs. For example, when a muscle is activated by stimulation of its motor nerve and allowed to

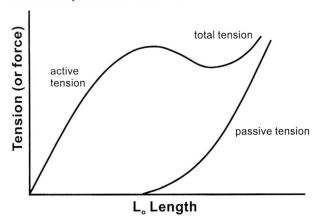

Figure 1

Force-length relationship of an active whole muscle. The left ascending curve represents the increase in contraction force as the muscle is stretched to greater length. L_0 indicates the peak of the active force increase that occurs at the natural rest length of the muscle. It also denotes the onset of passive tension created by stretch of the noncontractile, in parallel elements in muscle. Total tension is the sum of the 2 forces.

shorten against a load, the speed of that action will increase with declining loads. A typical force-velocity relationship for a mammalian skeletal muscle shows that the decline in force (relative to the isometric state of zero velocity) is very steep, even at modest shortening velocities (Fig. 2, *A*). Hence, the effect of movement on muscle force is quite profound.

In a typical shortening experiment (Fig. 2, *B*), there is an initial isometric phase before the muscle force becomes sufficiently intense to overcome the opposing load. During this period the force is increasing without an accompanying reduction in muscle length, and there is no motion. Once the generated force exceeds the magnitude of the opposing load, the muscle begins to shorten progressively at a constant velocity. The shortening velocity is rapid when loads are small and decline when the applied load is increased.

Although the classic force-velocity relationship experiments used muscle shortening against controlled loads, the converse also applies. That is, there is a well-defined relationship between the speed with which a muscle can shorten and the load it can carry. Maximum muscle force generation falls steeply when muscle velocity is increased by the experimenter. These force-velocity relationships are very important in regulating the speed of human movement and they ultimately limit motor performance.

Muscle Fiber Contraction Mechanics

The skeletal muscles that control body motion are composed of thousands of muscle fibers. In the human medial gastrocnemius, for example, 1 million have been identified. Each muscle fiber is a force-generating structure with specific timing, intensity, and endurance qualities.

Fiber Types

The basic action of a muscle fiber is a twitch of force in response to a single neural stimulus. Anatomic and physiologic differences divide the fibers into 2 fundamental types, fast and slow. Fast fibers are further classified as fast fatigable (FF) and fast fatigue resistant (FR). Their functional differences are rate of contraction, force magnitude, and fatigue susceptibility (Fig. 3).

Twitch Contraction Speed and Force

Muscle fibers vary greatly in the rate at which they contract. In the cat medial gastrocnemius, the time boundary between fast and slow is 55 ms. Twitch contraction time is measured from the onset of the twitch transient to its peak. Twitch contraction times longer than 55 ms are called slow twitch (S). These motor units are able to generate only small twitches and modest levels of force. The fast twitch (F) motor units have a contraction time less than 55 ms and usually are able to generate larger twitch forces. This speed of contraction turns out to be an important marker of muscle fiber specialization.

The force generation capacity is greater for F fibers than S fibers. Calculations of specific tension (force/unit area) shows about a twofold to threefold difference between fiber types.

Muscle Fiber Fatigability

The ability to sustain a tetanic force in response to repetitive activation is the measure of the muscle fiber's fatigability. When a motor unit (group of like muscle fibers with a common neuron) is subjected to repetitive activation at high frequency (such as 30 pulses/s for 10s) the unit generates a sustained tetanus. The resulting force may be several times greater than that of a twitch.

When a slow type motor unit is activated repetitively, the

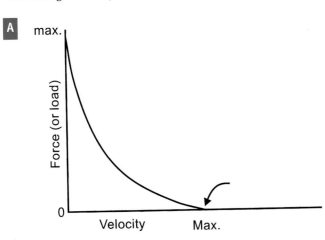

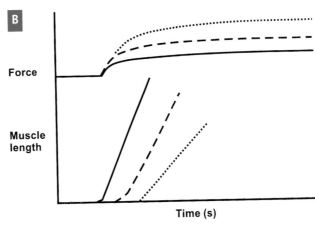

Figure 2

Force-velocity relationship of active whole muscle. **A,** Total curve. At zero velocity (isometric) muscle force is maximum. Even with small increases in velocity, muscle force production rapidly declines. At maximum velocity, muscle force is minimal. **B,** Muscle shortening against 3 different loads: small (solid line), intermediate (dashed line), and large (bulleted line). Note that the largest load is associated with the slowest shortening relocity.

force response reaches a sustained tetanus, and remains at the same level, sometimes up to several hours. After 2 minutes (the time chosen arbitrarily for evaluation) the force will have dropped by less than 25%.

In contrast, F fibers fail to sustain the tetanic force for even 2 minutes, falling to less than 25% of the initial level by that time. They are classified as FF. Other F fibers are better able to sustain their tetanic force, with their 2-minute level being 25% to 75% of the initial tetanic force. These are called FR. The durability of the force response to prolonged repetitive activation has proved to be a helpful classification tool.

Muscle Fiber Energy Production

Adenosine triphosphate (ATP) is the basic source of energy used in each muscle contraction and the metabolic processes muscles use have been identified as significant characteristics for muscle fiber classification. The enzyme ATPase is located in the myosin head, and appears to be a significant component in regulating the speed of cross-bridge recycling during muscle fiber excitation. Myosin ATPase levels have been found to be directly proportional to the rate of contraction (V_{max}).

Through selective histochemical staining techniques, the chemistry muscle fibers use to provide the energy for contraction has been identified. There are 2 basic processes, oxidative phosphorylation (energy with oxygen) and glycolysis (energy without oxygen).

S fibers use oxidative phosphorylation and by the metabolic classification scheme they are named slow oxidative (SO). Anatomically, SO fibers are prepared for sustained activation. They contain many mitochondria and supporting enzymes. The SO fibers also contain substantial concentrations of myoglobin and are surrounded by a dense capillary network. Because this is an efficient means to generate ATP, muscle contraction can continue without decre-

ment for prolonged periods of time, provided that blood flow is sufficient to deliver the needed substrates.

FF muscle fibers rely on glycolysis to generate the necessary ATP for sustaining contraction and therefore are called fast glycolytic (FG) in the current metabolic classification scheme. Histochemical analysis of the FF (FG) fibers show high concentrations of myosin ATPase, few mitochondria, a meager capillary network and substantial glycogen stores.

FR fibers, showing an intermediate degree of fatigability, reveal residual oxidative machinery on histochemical analysis, including mitochondria and associated enzymes, in addition to a glycolytic ability. Because their histochemical profile is mixed, these fibers are classified as fast, oxidative, glycolytic (FOG).

The degree of fatigue, defined as the loss of force generation capacity, appears to be related to the muscle fiber's capacity to sustain high levels of ATP production. In the FF (FG) fibers ATP synthesis declines when glycogen stores are depleted, causing muscle contraction to decline. In the fibers classified as FR (FOG), the residual oxidative contributions delay fatigue onset.

S or SO fibers have little glycogen stored. Instead they depend on transported blood glucose or free fatty acids from which to generate the necessary ATP. With adequate circulation, their fatigability is low.

Neural Excitation of Muscle

Motoneurons and the Motoneuron Pool

A spinal motoneuron is the neuron responsible for directly innervating skeletal muscle. Each neuron includes a cell body (soma) in the ventral horn of the gray matter in the spinal cord, and its axon exits via the ventral root of the peripheral nerve to travel to the muscle. The soma of spinal

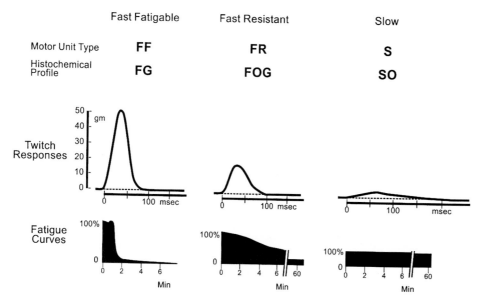

	Fast Fatigable	Fast Resistant	Slow
Motor Unit Type	FF	FR	S
Histochemical Profile	FG	FOG	SO

Figure 3

Muscle fiber contraction types. FF = Fast fatigable, FR = fast (fatigue) resistant, S = slow, FG = fast glycolytic, FOG = fast oxidative and glycolytic, SO = slow oxidative. Twitch response is the reaction to a single stimulus. Fatigue curves identify magnitude and duration of muscle force to a sustained tetanic stimulus.

motoneurons may be large (100 microns). Its dendritic arbor is even larger and may extend several millimeters radially from the cell body, reaching out into the white matter and far up into the dorsal gray matter.

Most extremity muscles are composed of thousands of muscle fibers. These muscle fibers are clustered into groups that are served by a common motor axon. The motoneuron, together with the muscle fibers it innervates, is called the motor unit. For the previously mentioned medial gastrocnemius, the 1 million muscle fibers are divided into approximately 580 motor units. All of the motoneurons innervating a given muscle are termed the motoneuron pool.

Motor Units: The Functional Units of Motor Control

All of the muscle fibers innervated by the same motoneuron are of the same type (SO, FG, or FOG). Hence, individual motor units are homogenous in function, though they vary in size. Most muscles contain a mixture of fiber types, but there may be a dominant type. Balanced function throughout a muscle is gained by broad dispersion of motor unit fibers. In the cat soleus, the area of a single motor unit spans 60% of the muscle; in the anterior tibialis the average motor unit area is 16%.

When the twitch responses of different units in a given muscle are compared, the force amplitude varies from several grams to only a few milligrams. The reason for these differences are complex but there are a number of contributing factors. First, large motor units have more muscle fibers innervated by their axons, that is, their innervation ratio is different. In the case of the medial gastrocnemius of the cat, the innervation ratio of the larger twitch units is greater than for smaller units, but the difference is not enough to explain the difference in twitch force. For example, the innervation ratio may vary threefold but the difference in force may be 50- or even 100-fold.

A second factor is the cross-sectional diameter of the muscle fiber, which reflects the number of myofibrils that can contribute to force generation. The myofibrils are arranged in parallel and can add to net fiber force individually. The average cross-sectional area of individual fibers in large twitch motor units is substantially greater than that of small twitch units. The difference in area, however, is not quite enough to explain the differences in twitch and tetanic force.

The third and final factor is the specific force-generating capacity of each fiber type. In other words, the force/unit area (which is the measure of specific tension) is potentially greater in F than S fibers. Attempts to calculate the specific tension of different muscle fiber have shown, at most, a threefold difference, with twofold being considered more likely.

Stimulation Frequency and Muscle Force

When the motor axon is activated by a single electrical pulse, a single action potential is transmitted from nerve to muscle, and a transient increase in muscle force is produced. This is described as a muscle twitch (Fig. 4, *A*). There is a substantial delay between the arrival of the excitatory potential in the muscle and the beginning of the muscle force generation. This delay, called an excitation-contraction delay, may reach 3 to 5 ms or more, depending on the type of muscle being studied. In all mammalian muscle the twitch has a characteristic form with a relatively rapid rise from onset to peak followed by a more gradual decay. The times to peak force and half peak decay force vary greatly in different types of muscles but the twitch is routinely asymmetric.

When muscle is activated repeatedly by a train of action potentials, the mean force level that is generated varies with the rate of neural activation (Fig. 4, *A*). If the excitation rate is so slow that it allows the twitch force to return to baseline between each twitch, there is no net force increase and the maximum force reached is simply that generated at the

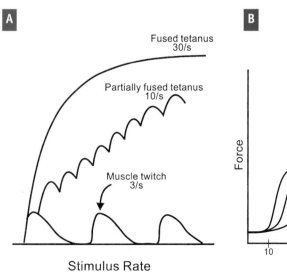

A

Fused tetanus
30/s

Partially fused tetanus
10/s

Muscle twitch
3/s

Stimulus Rate

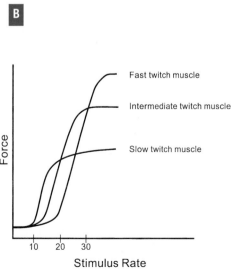

B

Force

Fast twitch muscle

Intermediate twitch muscle

Slow twitch muscle

10 20 30

Stimulus Rate

Figure 4

Stimulation rate effect. **A,** The typical magnitude and pattern of force responses to 3 representative stimulation rates, that is, number of stimuli per second: 3/s, 10/s, 30/s. **B,** The characteristic sigmoid force patterns of the 3 basic types of muscle fibers in response to activation. Note the slow fiber initiates its force sooner but it attains the lowest tetanic force. This is consistent with the lower stimulation rate required for activation. Fast fibers show the reverse characteristics, that is, the higher rate of stimulation needed introduces a delay.

peak of each twitch. When the rate of stimulation has increased sufficiently for the new nerve impulse to arrive before the force generated by the previous twitch has completely dissipated, there is force summation. Now the successive twitches generate a progressively increasing force level. After the initial force level is increased by the first few stimulating pulses a plateau is reached. This is called partially fused tetanus when the individual twitches are still discernible. A further increase in stimulation rate produces a smooth force trace without evidence of individual twitch transients. This response is described as fused tetanus.

There is a nonlinear relationship between stimulus rate and the resulting mean muscle force, which has a sigmoid curve when plotted on a graph (Fig. 4, *B*). The faster the rate of stimulation, the more rapid is the rise in force. At very low stimulation rates (usually between 3 to 6 pulses per second) relative increases in rate produce only small gains in force. After rates of 8 to 10 impulses per second are reached, a substantial increase in mean forces is realized. Stimulation rates of 30 to 40 pulses per second provide the highest force. In most instances, the nervous system generates motoneuron discharge rates that lie within the steep rising portion of these sigmoid relationships for each motor unit (Fig 4, *B*). Slowly contracting muscle fibers reach the steep portion of their sigmoid curve at relatively low discharge rates, whereas rapidly contracting fibers need more frequent neural activation to achieve full tetanus. As a consequence, in rapidly contracting muscles, the sigmoid curve is moved (relatively) to the right on the stimulus rate graph.

The means by which motoneuron discharge rate is tuned to match the contractile properties of the associated muscle fibers are not entirely clear. Yet this matching must be achieved acutely to accommodate the changing contractile properties of muscle fibers during repetitive activation. For example, with fatigue, chemical changes within the muscle fiber substantially slow contraction and relaxation times, necessitating lower motoneuron discharge rates to achieve maximum muscle force. Conversely, repeated activation of other fibers may increase twitch force (a state called potentiation) and contraction times may change.

The practical implication of this relationship between stimulation frequency and force generation is the ease of modulating the rate of force generation by activating different muscle fiber types. Conversely, this nonlinear relationship between stimulation frequency and muscle force generation requires that the motor units be activated at particular rates in order for the muscle to be an optimally effective force generator.

Regulation of Muscle Force

There are 2 broadly different ways in which activation of the motoneuron pool can increase muscle force (Fig. 5). The first mode is by recruitment of motoneurons, which is, simply, the transition of an increasing number of motoneurons from a quiescent to an excited state. The second mode of force regulation is achieved by increasing the rate of discharge of individual motoneurons (rate modulation).

In effect, recruitment progressively activates additional motoneurons (and muscle fibers) until the pool is completely activated. Rate modulation alters the individual force output of single motor units by inducing a partially fused tetanus. The mean force output becomes progressively greater with increasing rates of motoneuronal discharge (Fig. 4, *B*). These 2 regulatory mechanisms are closely interwoven. Recruitment is the dominant source of force increase in low levels of motoneuron pool excitation, while rate modulation is used for the higher forces. Rate modulation also generates a relatively greater impact on muscle force output as more motoneurons are activated.

The Size Principle of Motoneuron Recruitment

In response to increasing excitatory synaptic input, the resulting recruitment of different motoneurons is very orderly and virtually stereotypic. The governing rule is called the size principle. Motoneurons are recruited in a defined order with small sized motoneurons being activated first. These are followed by progressively larger motoneurons (Fig. 5). Conversely, if motoneurons in a pool are already active, increasing inhibitory input (from Ia inhibitory interneurons, for example) will cause a derecruitment by size, with the largest motoneurons being the first to drop out, continuing progressively to the smallest being the last to be silenced.

The size principle of recruitment also applies to rapid, even ballistic movement. It is thought that this sequence of motoneuron activation protects the muscle from injury. By graduating the force, the probability of an abrupt stretch is lessened. Experience with sports injuries, however, identifies a limit to this protection.

The physiologic mechanism governing the size principle of recruitment has not been determined despite intensive investigation. Two mechanisms regulating the firing rate of motoneurons have been identified. The major factor is the afterhyperpolarization (AHP): the hyperpolarizing voltage swing that follows the occurrence of the action potential. This AHP limits the firing rate by controlling motoneuron excitability. Another factor is the varying electrical resistance of different motoneurons; smaller neurons display higher resistance to injected current, and produce larger synaptic potentials.

Muscle Receptors

Skeletal muscles contain specialized receptors designed to continually sense the status of muscle action and help regulate its stiffness by monitoring the qualities of muscle stretch. At the same time, the tendon and other series elastic elements are elongated. The 3 main classes of muscle receptors are muscle spindle receptors, Golgi tendon organs, and free nerve endings (Fig. 6).

Muscle Spindle Receptors

Muscle spindles consist of a cluster of slender muscle fibers (called intrafusal fibers) that are contained within a fluid-filled capsule (Fig. 6). The muscle spindle lies adjacent to the regular (extrafusal) muscle fibers and traverses the length of the muscle from the tendon of origin to the tendon of insertion. By this arrangement the muscle spindle is "in parallel" with regular skeletal muscle fibers. This allows the spindle afferent system to sense the stretch being experienced by the skeletal muscles. Conversely, spindle tension is reduced by active contraction of the skeletal muscle. This state is most apparent under isometric conditions, and the spindle receptors are unloaded. A basic function of the efferent system of intrafusal fibers is to reset the spindle to a sensitive length so afferent feedback is preserved.

The intrafusal fibers of the muscle spindle are classified according to the anatomic arrangement of their nuclei. The majority of the intrafusal fibers (4 to 6 per spindle) have their nuclei arranged along the length of the fiber and are called nuclear chain fibers. A small fraction of intrafusal fibers (1 or 2 per spindle) have their nuclei clustered in a bulbous center or equatorial region. These are called nuclear bag fibers. (Recent investigations have identified further subdivisions that are not pertinent to this chapter).

Afferent Muscle Spindle Function

The afferent component of the muscle spindles consists of 2 types of specialized sensory terminals (Fig. 7, A). The primary ending is a large, typically annulospiral-shaped ending wrapped around the central portion of all intrafusal fibers in the spindle (nuclear bags and nuclear chains). The afferent nerve from the primary sensor is called Ia. A smaller, often branching sensory terminal, called the secondary ending, is located toward the polar region of the spindle, and its nerve is named II.

Sensitivity of the muscle spindle's receptor terminals to stretch appears to be determined by the biophysical properties of intrafusal fiber structure. For example, the nuclear bags have little contractile material in the equatorial area; instead, the contractile regions are confined to the intrafusal fiber poles, making them stiffer. Consequently, the more rapid stretches would extend the equatorial regions disproportionately compared to the more viscous poles. This anatomic difference appears to make the primary ending site more sensitive to stretch than the secondary ending. Although more prominent in the nuclear bags, this difference also exists in the nuclear chains.

In response to a relatively slow, constant velocity stretch of the parent muscle, the primary endings (Ia) show a prompt and substantial rate increase during the dynamic phase of the stretch that then drops in rate once a constant length is achieved. In contrast, the signal from the secondary ending rises slowly and with lesser magnitude. These responses suggest that the primary spindle afferent is a velocity sensor

while the secondary spindle afferent more closely follows the length change (Fig. 7, B). Recording at much higher velocities failed to show this difference. Also, a proportional sensitivity to velocity has been not identified. A 100-fold increase in stretch velocity induced only a twofold increase in signal rate in either kind of receptor. Amplitude of the stretch showed a strong influence on muscle spindle receptor discharge, with a 1- to 2-mm stretch initiating an immediate, afferent signal that is larger than could be sustained with increasing amplitudes.

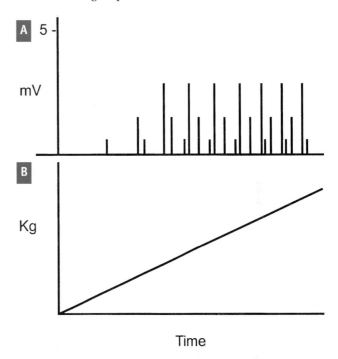

Figure 5

Motor unit recruitment. **A**, Vertical lines indicate electromyographic signal of fiber activation. Three motor units of different sizes are shown. Note recruitment order from smallest to largest and the progressive increase in rate of activation. **B**, Force diagram denoting increase in force from both number and rate of motor unit recruitment.

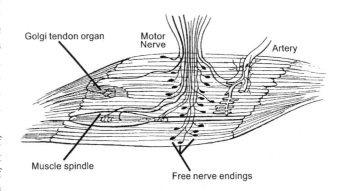

Figure 6

Muscle receptors. Diagram of a longitudinal section of muscle showing the muscle spindles and Golgi tendon organs.

Other studies have shown that the primary muscle spindle afferents (Ia) are also highly active during voluntary skeletal muscle (extrafusal) contraction (Fig. 8). The activation is very strong at the lowest force levels and it may increase slightly with increased force. In intact subjects, muscle afferent recordings have shown a consistent pattern of increased rate of spindle afferent excitation in concert with motoneuron activation. This action allows the spindle to compensate for muscle fiber shortening to a large degree, except when the muscle shortening is rapid.

Efferent Innervation of the Muscle Spindle

All muscle spindles receive efferent (motor) innervation by small diameter, slow conducting myelinated fibers that arise in the ventral horn of the spinal cord. These are called gamma (γ) fibers (Fig. 6). Some efferent innervation also may arise as branches from the large diameter, faster conducting skeletomotor fibers, called alpha or α. These are classed as β fibers. The actions of the γ and β fibers appear comparable. Together they comprise the fusimotor innervation.

During an isometric contraction, the increase in muscle force will reduce tension on the spindle and spindle receptors as the 2 ends of the tendon are pulled toward each other. The effect is a potential reduction in the afferent discharge rate, which is called unloading. This is compensated by increases in fusimotor activity accompanying the increased skeletomotor activity to reset the spindles' monitoring capability. Thus, fusimotor input is quite powerful in its effects on spindle afferent discharge.

The γ fibers are activated before the α skeletomotor activity begins giving rise to α-γ coactivation. Other times γ neurons may be activated without concurrent α motoneuron activation. At present the rules governing fusiomotor activation are not entirely clear. Whether or not there is the capacity for independent fusimotor control remains to be verified. Studies in human limb function (upper and lower) show substantial variation in the level of fusimotor input during most naturally-occurring movement.

The effect of the fusimotor innervation on spindle afferent discharge depends essentially on the particular type of intrafusal fiber it innervates. Those acting on the nuclear bag fibers enhance the dynamic response of their primary endings (gamma dynamic, γd). Fusimotor fibers that innervate the nuclear chain fibers enhance both length sensitivity and static background by their effect on both primary and secondary endings (gamma static, γs).

Studies of both human and animal models suggest that γ dynamic and γ static fusimotor activation take place together. Fusimotor input to the spindles serves 3 functions: (1) Activation takes up the slack in muscle spindles as the muscle shortens during contraction; that is, the spindles reset their length, which allows both the primary and secondary ending to respond with critical sensitivity. It is thought that the fusimotor input allows the spindle receptors to maintain a broad dynamic range and still be sensitive to small length perturbations. (2) Fusimotor innervation may serve to match muscle spindles to the changing mechanical properties of muscle; that is, adaptation to increased mus-

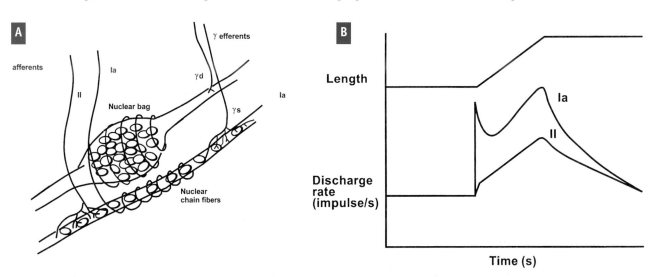

Figure 7

Muscle spindles. **A,** Anatomy and nerves. Note the nuclei (small ovals) clustered in the dilated center of the nuclear bag. Note the nuclei spread lengthwise in the intrafusal nuclear chain fibers. Gamma (γ) efferents are subclassified as gamma dynamic (γd) to nuclear bag and gamma static (γs) to nuclear chain. Primary afferents (Ia) arise from coiled ending around the midsection of both the nuclear bag and nuclear chain. Secondary afferents (II) arise from the nuclear chain only. **B,** Muscle spindle afferent response to muscle stretch. Length diagram indicates accompanying length increase by height of line; relaxed state (low line), increasing stretch (rising line), sustained stretch force (high line), electronic discharge record of afferent nerve response (bottom line). Initial low line indicates quiescence before stretch occurs. Ia line shows an immediate intense response that is not sustained. The group II discharge pattern shows a slow, gradual rise that parallels the change in muscle length, which implies the secondary afferent endings are sensitive to a change in length, not the rate of change.

cle stiffness with higher levels of activity. (3) γd input induces a substantial increase in dynamic spindle response during muscle stretch but has much less effect during shortening. Fusimotor activation may be important for maintaining asymmetry of reflex stretch and release.

Golgi Tendon Organs as Force Transducers

The tendon organ is an encapsulated receptor that consists of a branching nerve terminal interwoven with collagen and elastic fibers. The organ lies between a group of muscle fibers and the tendon (Fig. 9, *A*). Thus, it is "in-series" with the muscle-tendon boundary and is subjected to mechanical strain when the muscle fibers are active. The number of muscle fibers sampled by a tendon organ is quite small, typically 12 to 16 in the large limb muscle of a cat. Tendon

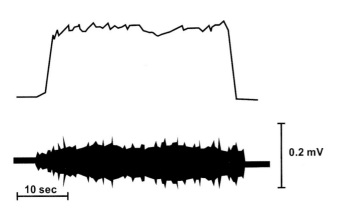

0.2 mV

10 sec

Figure 8

Rapid and substantial increase in muscle spindle afferent discharge (*top*) accompanying the onset of voluntary isometric contraction (electromyogram, lower trace). Data from an intact human subject, showing α-γ coactivation during voluntary muscle contraction.

organs also may be scattered through many muscle regions quite distant from the tendon, though these locations are usually near collagenous tissue planes.

Tendon Organ Response to Muscle Force Change

The means by which muscle force is transduced by the tendon organ is not yet known, but it is likely mediated by regional strain on nerve terminals as they are compressed among the tendinous fascicles. Tendon organs are excited most readily by active muscle force, such as is produced by neural excitation, rather than passive force increases by muscle stretch. Typically, under conditions of physiologic activation, tendon organ discharge increases more or less proportionally with increased muscle force (Fig. 9, *B*). At low muscle forces, their rate increases irregularly and is dependent on recruitment of the related subset of muscle fibers. Once many muscle fibers are active, the tendon organ follows the changing force quite accurately. Despite their limited muscle fiber sample, the response patterns of individual tendon organs are surprisingly close to the force variations of the whole muscle, except with very low forces when only 1 or 2 fibers attached to the tendon organ have been activated.

Free Nerve Endings and Other Muscle Mechanoreceptors

The major muscle spindle and tendon organ afferents usually constitute less than 50% of the total sensory innervation from a typical muscle. The rest of the afferent fibers contained in the muscle's nerve lack specialized terminal structures yet they exhibit a range of functional specializations; hence, the name free nerve ending (Fig. 6, *A*). Some respond to nociceptive input. Others react to mechanical stimulation but with less sensitivity to pressure and tension than the spindles and tendon organs. Additional functions

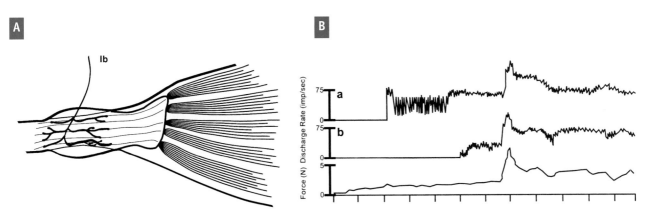

Figure 9

Golgi tendon organ response to muscle force increase. Diagram of Golgi tendon organ (**A**). Note this encapsulated structure is located between a group of muscle fibers and the beginning of the tendon, that is, at a musculotendinous junction. Traces of 2 tendon organ signal discharges (**B**), upper 2 lines are patterns of the initiating tendon force. Initial variability of tendon organ response is attributed to each being attached to only a few muscle fibers.

are thermal and metabolic changes (perhaps related to exercise or fatigue). These nerves vary in size, myelinization, and conduction velocity.

Comparison of Reflex and Areflex Behavior of Active Muscle

As identified in the initial discussion on the length-tension relationship of muscle, increasing stretch of an active muscle with an intact reflex system is accompanied by an increase in muscle force. When a muscle is stretched at a constant velocity, however, there is a force overshoot at the end of the stretch that suggests some degree of dynamic or velocity sensitivity (Fig. 10, *middle*).

Repetition of the stretch experiment with a muscle devoid of reflex feedback presents a much more irregular force response (Fig. 10, *bottom*). This is interpreted as displaying the mechanical properties of muscle without the advantage of reflex modulation.

Three major changes in the areflexic muscle response to a rapid stretch from its initial isometric state have been identified. The first is a disruption in the spring-like behavior. The spring-like response is replaced with a sharp change in muscle stiffness. Once the stretch exceeds a fraction of a millimeter (300 to 400 µm) the initial steep rise in force is interrupted by a yield point, causing an irregular force response to emerge (Fig. 10, *bottom*). The initial high stiffness region is called the short range stiffness and the early sharp decline in force is the muscle yield. The sustained stretch also fails to hold its tension, sometimes even falling below the initial preset level. Although the short range stiffness and yield responses are most distinct in slow-twitch muscles (such as the soleus) there also is a routine change in stiffness in fast twitch muscle. The initial high stiffness is attributable to the stiffness of the population of actin-myosin cross-bridge bonds, whereas the subsequent steep decline in force is considered a result of stretch-induced cross-bridge rupture.

The second difference in the force response to stretch of a muscle lacking reflex control is profound asymmetry. A mechanical spring, when released from its stretch force, retraces its stretch pattern in reverse. This also is characteristic of normally innervated muscle. The force patterns of stretch and release in a normally innervated muscle are highly symmetrical.

A third discrepancy is the irregular response of the release of the stretch. If the response of a deafferented muscle to stretch and release is matched to the normal reflex response with the same initial force, the early force response to stretch in both cases is virtually identical, indicating that the response was initially governed by the intrinsic mechanical properties of active muscle. However, the deafferented muscle follows a much more irregular course after its yield point (Fig. 10, *bottom*). In contrast, the reflex intact muscle continues smoothly without disconti-

nuity, indicating that the response is initially governed by the intrinsic mechanical properties of active muscle but at the point that yielding should have occurred, the reflex response continues smoothly without discontinuity, indicating that effective compensatory mechanisms must have been operating (Fig. 10, *middle*).

The shortening response of an areflexive muscle, by contrast, is much more similar to a reflex response. This indicates that the requirement for neurally mediated compensation is less for the shortening phase of motion.

The findings that the more complex mechanical properties of muscle, such as the yield, are obscured in the presence of reflex action indicate that the reflexes serve to linearize and to smooth the mechanical behavior of muscle. It also is clear that in the absence of reflex action, the onset of muscle yield occurs very early in relation to stretch onset, approximately within 20 to 50 ms of stretch onset. This rapid change is likely to impose severe time constraints on compensatory responses, which may take an

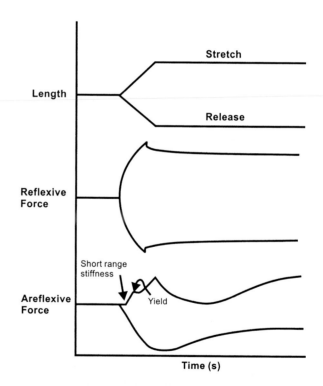

Figure 10

A comparison of force response to stretch and release in a reflexive muscle (reflex feedback is intact) and an areflexive muscle (reflex control is lacking). **Top,** Pattern of muscle length change. Initial line indicates starting state. Rise in level indicates progressive stretch. Final high line indicates sustained stretch. For the release, the initial line segment indicates the preexisting stretched state, the drop in level implies a reduction in muscle length. The final level line identifies relaxation. **Middle,** Reflex controlled muscle. Both the stretch and release response display a brief force level overshoot during the length change, which is followed by a sustained force plateau. **Bottom,** An areflexive muscle response to stretch. The initial stiffness is interrupted by a yield in force production and the force response to sustained stretch is irregular.

additional 25 to 50 ms to elicit an appropriate mechanical response. A second issue is the substantial reflex input required to compensate for the mechanical muscle response to stretch compared to relatively modest differences in the responses to shortening. These mechanical characteristics of muscle devoid of reflex control pose substantial difficulty for any neural control mechanisms. The major problem is in slow twitch muscles, where the force changes are profound and develop quickly.

The debate about the nature and consequences of reflex action is still ongoing; however, it is believed that much of the compensatory response for muscle yield is built into the response characteristics of the muscle spindle receptors. This is an unexpected solution to the problem of controlling muscle force because muscle spindle receptors are usually designated as primary length sensors. The latter interpretation may be a result of the experimental practice of controlling muscle length. Muscle spindle receptors are the only candidate with a short onset time for activation and it also has the requisite pattern of asymmetric response to stretch release. Thus, it appears that the neural mechanisms mediating stretch reflex action act predictably, at least initially, in that the muscle spindle receptor issues a response appropriate for correcting impending changes in muscle properties such as yielding and asymmetrical stiffness.

Although tendon organ responses could contribute to and promote the improvement in muscle properties, the speed of tendon organ-mediated feedback is too slow to prevent the manifestation of rapid onset mechanical changes, such as yielding. Furthermore, appropriate compensatory muscle mechanical responses occur even when Golgi tendon organ afferent (Ib) interneuron responses are very modest or even absent.

Afferent Pathways to the Spinal Cord

Muscle afferent neurons with a range of diameters have been classified by their size and their organ of origin. The largest (group I) are also the fastest, and typically conduct at velocities up to 100 m/s or more. Primary afferent (Ia) conduction velocities may reach 120 m/s in the cat, whose fibers have been the most extensively studied. The Ib afferents also are large. Secondary spindle afferents (group II) are of intermediate size and conduct at velocities ranging from 24 to 72 m/s, although these boundaries may differ in man. Small myelinated and unmyelinated fibers (groups III and IV) from muscle and skin have conduction velocities from less than 1 m/s to 24 m/s. Conduction boundaries for the different fiber populations are not as well defined in man. In particular, there is not a clearly defined conduction velocity boundary between primary and secondary spindle afferents, although spindle morphologic studies indicate both receptor populations are present in man.

Central Connections and Central Projections of Afferent Pathways

Sensory fibers enter the spinal cord primarily via the dorsal roots of the peripheral nerves, where their cell bodies lie. A small number of unmyelinated nerve fibers and even a few myelinated fibers turn from the dorsal root to enter the cord through the ventral roots (Fig. 11).

Large myelinated muscle afferents (groups Ia and II), after entering through the dorsal root, tend to segregate medially and then travel ventrally in the gray matter. Some fibers terminate by making synaptic connections with regional interneurons while a few continue on to synapse directly with motoneurons in the ventral horn. Large myelinated afferents from muscle, joint, or skin also may branch to send fibers into dorsal columns (gracilis, cuneatus) and dorsolateral column white matter where they may travel rostrally for many centimeters; others may reenter dorsal gray matter in proximal segments and synapse with regional neurons. Muscle afferents in particular may make a separate relay in the brain stem. Fibers from the gracilis, cuneate nuclei, or brain stem then pass the signals to higher centers, including thalamus, cerebellum, and eventually the cortex.

Muscle Ia afferents make extensive monosynaptic connections with virtually all motoneurons innervating the muscle from which the spindle afferents originate (the homonymous motoneuron pool) as well as with many motoneurons from nearby synergists. The result is extensive divergence of afferents to many motoneurons and

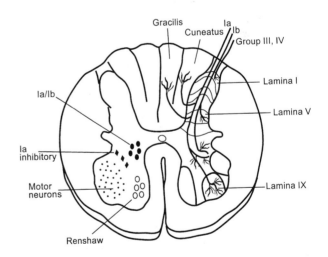

Figure 11

Spinal cord cross-sectional anatomy showing structures pertinent to reflex muscle control. Ia, Ib afferent nerves enter spinal cord via the posterior root and extend to interneuron and motoneuron cell body areas. Branches also enter dorsal columns. Group III, IV fibers go to Lamina I. Location of interneuron cells identified (Ia/Ib, Ia Inhibitory, Renshaw). Motoneurons indicate area of anterior horn cell bodies of primary (alpha, α) muscle efferent neurons.

extensive convergence of Ia afferents onto individual motoneurons.

Small myelinated (Aσ) and unmyelinated (C) fibers make synaptic connections with neurons in dorsal gray matter such as the superficial lamina I, which is largely concerned with pain-related or nociceptive information. Other mechanoreceptor afferents (group III and IV) project to deeper regions of the dorsal gray (lamina IV, V) (Fig. 11).

Spinal Interneuronal System

Spinal interneurons are defined as neurons that arise and end within the spinal cord. Their axons extend a relatively short distance within the cord, usually no more than a few spinal segments. The cell bodies of these neurons are usually small, less than 50 μm. Almost all afferents, including those from the primary and secondary endings, make their first synapse with neurons in the dorsal or intermediate spinal gray matter.

Interneurons perform several important computational operations, the most common being a signal change. For example, an afferent originating from muscle or skin produces synaptic excitation at the first synaptic relay but the activated interneuron is an inhibitory type, so the product is inhibition at subsequent postsynaptic sites (Fig. 12). Excitatory interneurons may act to amplify information received from the periphery, may change the spatial distribution of that information by the pattern of divergence of their nerve terminals, or change the time course and frequency content of incoming signals. In summary, the primary role of interneurons appear to be summing or integrating elements in which convergent input from various sources (including different sensory modalities) is integrated and passed on to the next step of information processing.

Actions of Identified Interneurons

Most of the interneuronal systems of the mammalian spinal cord are not fully identified. Interneuron naming generally is dependent on some distinctive electrophysiologic feature that may have little relation to its functional role.

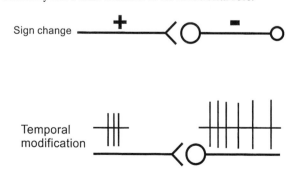

Figure 12

Examples of Ia afferent input modifications by synapses with interneurons. Temporal modification: Ia input (+++) altered by interneuron (+++++). Sign change: Excitatory stimulus (+) changed to inhibitory (-) input.

Renshaw neurons are small interneurons located in the ventral horn, medial to the spinal motor nuclei (Fig. 11). The Renshaw interneurons receive excitatory input from motor collaterals and make inhibitory synapses on regional spinal motoneurons, other interneurons, and regional Ia inhibitory interneurons (Fig. 13).

Ia inhibitory interneurons receive input from Ia afferents in 1 muscle and then make inhibitory synaptic connections to motoneurons of opposing, antagonistic muscles (Fig. 12). Through these connections the Ia interneuron is believed to promote reciprocal innervation in which agonists and antagonists acting about 1 joint are prevented from being active simultaneously. In other words, an interneuron activated by Ia afferents of a particular muscle is silenced by ventral root stimulation.

Ib afferents make synaptic relays in the intermediate gray matter of the spinal cord, producing autogenic inhibition of homonymous and synergist motoneurons. They also project to Clark's column neurons. These interneurons also receive afferent input from Ia spindle receptor afferents. This raises the possibility of a force regulatory role. These Ia/Ib interneurons lie in the proximal lumbar segment and give rise to axons traveling as the dorsal spinocerebellar tract.

Several human studies have provided indirect evidence of a force regulator. Fatigue has been used as the test probe to evaluate force feedback compensation based on the fact that fatigue induces a substantial short-term loss of muscle contractile force. Although such a loss of force-generating capacity would be registered by the Golgi tendon organs, substantial changes in afferent inflow from several types of muscle receptors (such as changes in muscle temperature, pH and metabolic rate) are likely. All of these factors may change the spontaneous discharge patterns and the responsiveness of group III and IV muscle afferents that may converge on the same Ib interneuron and alter its responsiveness pathway.

Group II excitatory interneurons receive selective input from secondary spindle afferents and synapse with lumbosacral spinal interneurons. The functional role of these interneurons is not well understood but they may be important contributors to increased motoneuron excitability in spastic muscles.

Presynaptic inhibitory interneurons depolarize the presynaptic terminal, reducing the amount of transmitter released. Part of the action is a reduction in the amount of calcium that enters the terminal with the arrival of each action potential.

Reflex Regulation of Movement

The spinal cord is engaged in 3 aspects of movement regulation. In information transmission the spinal cord relays afferent information to higher centers in the spinal cord, brain stem, and beyond. In the opposite direction efferent commands are transmitted from higher centers to the motor nuclei within the spinal cord. During reflex action, spinal cord neurons and their connections form the substrates for a variety of sensory-motor reflexes.

Reflexes

A reflex is a stereotypic motor response to a particular sensory input. Reflexes vary broadly in the complexity of their motor response and in the number and diversity of neural elements used. A simple reflex may be Ia afferents from a single muscle inducing activation of motoneurons innervating the same muscle. Such reflexes, which include the tendon jerk and tonic stretch reflex, are often called autogenic or homonymous. Reflexes elicited by afferents of 1 muscle acting on motoneurons of a neighboring muscle are often described as heteronymous. When such reflexes result in coordinated responses between 2 or more muscles with similar mechanical action, the muscles are said to be acting as synergists.

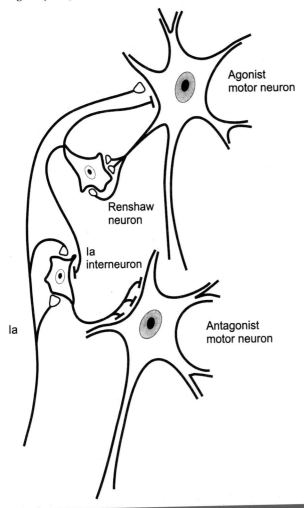

Figure 13

Example of interneuron ties between agonist and antagonist motoneurons. Afferent Ia synapses with Ia inhibitory interneuron and agonist motor neuron. Ia inhibitory interneuron synapses with antagonist motor neuron. Renshaw neuron receives input from agonist motor collateral and also Ia interneuron.

At a somewhat higher level of the reflex organization hierarchy, there is a reciprocal pattern of activation. Inhibition is exerted by Ia afferents of a single muscle on motoneurons of the antagonist muscle via the inhibitory interneurons.

The next level involves a more complex array of reflexes in which the response to a sensory input activates motoneurons at several levels. One example is the flexor withdrawal reflex, where a noxious or high-intensity stimulus to the skin or other deep tissue elicits a broad-scale, coordinated withdrawal of a limb. There is systematic activation of flexor muscles at several joints, coupled with inhibition of the opposing extensors. Although the range of afferent input is diverse, the ultimate effect is relatively stereotypic and primarily via the Ia inhibitory interneuronal system.

Beyond the flexor withdrawal reflex, there is an array of complex goal-directed reflexes such as scratching, in which local excitation of skin surface gives rise to a coordinated and often repetitive motion to remove the irritant. The fact that the action attempting to eradicate the irritant is repetitive and rhythmical in character suggests that the response may also involve an oscillator or pattern generator, which gives rise to rhythmical excitation of spinal circuits.

Role of Force Feedback: An Assessment of the Hypothesis of "Stiffness Regulation"

The dual and competing actions of muscle length feedback (which would promote increased stiffness of muscle) and force feedback (which would induce reduced muscle stiffness) are simultaneously present under many conditions. This suggests that regulation of stiffness to some predetermined level could be a possible function of stretch reflex mechanisms. However, the evidence in support of the stretch reflex having a primary role as a stiffness regulator is limited because muscle stiffness does not remain constant, or even approximately constant under most operating conditions. Nevertheless, it is clear that force and length sensors together with their reflex connections give rise to a much more spring-like behavior of muscle, and this characteristic of muscle is likely to be important in the control of movement. For example, the presence of reflex compensation means modulation of the potentially sharp extension of the ankle by the soleus during the stance phase of locomotion into a smooth force increase and enhanced dampening of the contact point.

Pattern Generators

The term pattern generation refers to the spinal cord and brain stem interneurons forming the basis for oscillatory neuronal discharge, which underlies rhythmical behavior such as locomotion, respiration, and mastication.

Virtually all nervous systems contain groups of neurons with the capacity to generate rhythmical bursting behavior, even when isolated from other neuronal systems. The action may be spontaneous or may need a gating signal such as provided by a monoaminergic agent such as norepinephrine, but the pattern of discharge is not dependent on any incoming afferent or descending signals, hence the term pattern generator.

On the basis of extensive studies from acute and chronic spinally transected models (including the cat and turtle), it is evident that such neuronal clusters can induce repetitive discharge sufficient to drive locomotion. Furthermore, the finding that locomotion-like patterns of motoneuronal discharge are not dependent on either descending, ascending, or peripheral afferent inputs supports the view that locomotion emerges from activities of a discrete oscillator located primarily within the interneurons of the spinal cord.

In the presence of appropriate tonic pharmacologic drive provided by norepinephrine or other adrenergic agonists (such as clonidine) these interneuronal systems will continue to discharge, showing the essential features responsible for rhythmical bursting.

The pattern generators appear to be activated by descending input from locomotion control regions in the mesencephalon and other areas of the brain stem. Some of these brain stem regions release norepinephrine in the spinal cord, and others may trigger norepinephrine release directly.

The discharge of the spinal pattern generators is subject to peripheral modulation in that it can be modified by appropriate segmental afferent inflow. Specifically, cutaneous stimulation of a foot in a quadruped during swing phase of locomotion gives rise to avoidance behavior in which the leg is caused to circumvent the obstruction. When the leg is still weightbearing, similar cutaneous stimulation is ineffectual, indicating that there is a substantial phase-dependent modulation of the effects of sensory input.

Summary

Spinal neural mechanisms control movement first by activating motor units. Then muscle receptors, after sensing the effects of muscle stretch and tension, impose stimulating or inhibitory modulations to assure optimum motor effectiveness. Reflex mechanisms within the spinal cord, in response to afferent input, initiate movement patterns that may involve a single muscle, agonist and antagonist, multiple muscle synergies, multiple joint synergy within the limb, or reciprocal limb action as a basic pattern for locomotion.

Selected Bibliography

Bodine-Fowler S, Garfinkel A, Roy RR, Edgerton VR: Spatial distribution of muscle fibers within the territory of a motor unit. *Muscle Nerve* 1990;13:1133–1145.

Bottinelli R, Pellegrino MA, Canepari M, Rossi R, Reggiani C: Specific contributions of various muscle fibre types to human muscle performance: An in vitro study. *J Electromyogr Kinesiol* 1999;9:87–95.

Burke D: Muscle spindle function during movement. *Trends Neurosci* 1980;3:251-253.

Burke RE, Levine DN, Tsairis P, Zajac FE III: Physiological types and histochemical profiles in motor units of the cat gastrocnemius. *J Physiol (Lond)* 1973;234:723–748.

Burke RE, Tsairis P: Histochemical and physiological profile of a skeletofusimotor (beta) unit in cat soleus muscle. *Brain Res* 1977;129: 341–345.

Burke RE: Physiology of motor units, in Engle AG (ed): *Myology; Basic Clinical*. New York, NY, McGraw-Hill, 1986; vol. 1, pp 419–443.

Crago PE, Houk JC, Rymer WZ: Sampling of total muscle force by tendon organs. *J Neurophysiol* 1982;47:1069–1083.

Gordon AM, Huxley AF, Julian FJ: The length-tension diagram of single vertebrate striated muscle fibres. *J Physiol* 1964;171:28P–30P.

Hunt CC: Mammalian muscle spindle: Peripheral mechanisms. *Physiol Rev* 1990;70:643–663.

Huxley A: Muscular contraction. *Annu Rev Physiol* 1988;50:1–16.

Huxley A, Niedergerke R: Structural changes in muscle during contraction: Interference microscopy of living fibres. *Nature* 1954;173: 971–973.

Huxley H, Hanson J: Changes in the cross-striations of muscle during contraction and stretch and their structural interpretation. *Nature* 1954;173:973–976.

Jami L: Golgi tendon organs in mammalian skeletal muscle: Functional properties and central actions. *Physiol Rev* 1992;72:623–666.

Lieber RL (ed): *Skeletal Muscle Structure and Function: Implications for Rehabilitation and Sports Medicine*. Baltimore, MD, Williams & Wilkins, 1992.

Nichols TR, Houk JC: Improvement in linearity and regulation of stiffness that results from actions of stretch reflex. *J Neurophysiol* 1976;39:119–142.

Vallbo AB: Discharge patterns in human muscle spindle afferents during isometric voluntary contractions. *Acta Physiol Scand* 1970;80: 552–566.

Chapter Outline

Chapter 28

Kinesiology

Sheldon R. Simon, MD

Hannu Alaranta, MD, PhD

Kai-Nan An, PhD

Andrew Cosgarea, MD

Richard Fischer, MD

Joel Frazier, MD

Christopher Keading, MD

Michael Muha, MD

Jacquelin Perry, MD

Malcolm Pope, PhD, DMSc

Peter Quesada, PhD

This chapter at a glance

This chapter describes the role and function of the components of the musculoskeletal system in the creation of human motion.

Introduction

Kinesiology is the study of motion of the human body and encompasses such acts as walking or throwing a baseball. Although such motions are quite complex, they are governed by the movements of each separate component of the musculoskeletal system. The biologic and biomechanical/structural properties of these components have been described in previous chapters. This chapter describes the role and function of each of these components in the creation of human motion. It will show how biologic form and structure result from function and how the sum of the individual parts of this system create human functional abilities that far exceed those of any one part.

Kinematics

Kinematics is the study of the movements of rigid structures, independent of the forces that might be involved. Two types of movement, translation (linear displacement) and rotation (angular displacement), occur within 3 orthogonal planes; that is, movement has 6 degrees of freedom.

Humans belong to the vertebrate portion of the phylum Chordata, and as such possess a bony endoskeleton that includes a vertebral spine and paired extremities. Each extremity is composed of articulated skeletal segments linked together by connective tissue elements and surrounded by skeletal muscle. Motion between skeletal segments occurs at joints. Most joint motion is minimally translational and primarily rotational. The deviation from absolute rotatory motion may be noted by the changes in the path of a joint's "instantaneous center of rotation." These paths have been measured for most of the joints in the body and vary only slightly from true arcs of rotation. For human motion to be effective, a comparatively rigid limb segment must not only rotate its position relative to an adjacent segment, but many adjacent limb movements must interact. Whether the hand reaches for a cup or the foot must be lifted high enough to clear an obstacle on the ground, the activity is achieved via coordinated movements of multiple limb segments.

Kinesiology, thus, is first a study of kinematics between each of many limb segments. To provide for the greatest possible function of an extremity, the proximal joint must have the widest range of motion to position the limb in space. This joint must allow for rotatory motions of large degrees in all 3 planes about all 3 axes. A means is also provided to alter the length of the limb, so that an extremity can function at all locations within its global range. Rotational motion of the elbow and knee joints allows such overall changes as adjacent limb segments move. Finally, to fine-tune the use of this mechanism with respect to the extremities, for their functional purposes, the hand and foot are required to have a vast amount of movement about all 3 axes, although the rigid segments are relatively small.

Such movement requires the presence of relatively universal joints at the terminal aspect of each extremity.

Kinetics

The study of the forces that bring about these movements is part of the mechanical discipline called kinetics. Because kinetics provides insights into the cause of the observed motion, it is essential to the proper interpretation of human movement processes. Forces and loads are not visually observable; they must be either measured with instrumentation or calculated from kinematics data. Kinetic quantities studied include such parameters as the forces produced by muscles; reaction loads between body parts as well as their interactions with external surfaces; the load transmitted through the joints; the power transferred between body segments; and the mechanical energy of body segments. Inherent to such studies are the functional demands imposed on the body.

The structure and stability of each extremity and its joints reflect different systems and functional demands. The functional demands on the upper extremity are quite different from those on either the upper and lower axial skeleton or those on the lower extremity. Depending on which joint and/or structure is addressed, different types and degrees of rotational motion are allowed and are functional. How much structural strength is needed versus how much movement is allowed in each area dictates the nature of the material, size, shape, and infrastructure of the joint system established to perform a given movement. Kinesiology depends upon anatomy in that anatomy is a study that covers the appearance, structure, and location of the various parts of the body, and kinesiology is a study of the function of the musculoskeletal elements.

Joint Stability

Human motion is governed by Newton's 3 laws of motion: (1) an object will change velocity only if a force is applied; (2) the change in velocity is proportional to the force; and (3) forces always exist in pairs that are equal and opposite in direction, such that if one body pushes against another, the second body will push back against the first with a force of equal magnitude if the state of motion is constant. Newton's third law is especially significant because purposeful functional movements could not exist without it. Many movements of limb segments and the motion of the body as a whole could not take place without interaction with external surfaces based on Newton's third law. Applied to human internal movement, this law suggests muscles cannot impart movement to a limb segment without the segment's interaction with another bone and without a joint structure that will allow the desired rotational direction and force. If stability or directional constraints are provided through such a mechanism, translational movements, which serve to "dislocate" one rigid bony limb segment from another, are avoided.

Joint stability is created by bony configurations, ligaments, and muscles; combinations of these constructs differ between joints. Bone primarily constrains translational motions. Where rotation is needed, there is no bony blockage. Because bone is the most rigid anatomic structure, the greater the circumference of the joint enclosed by bone, the greater the amount of inherent translational stability that exists in the joint. This point is illustrated by the contrast between the spherical head of the femur (which is enclosed by a hemispheric arc of bony acetabulum) and the flatter radius of curvature of the glenoid (which encloses little of the humeral head) and the relative ease of dislocation or subluxation of the latter as compared to the former.

Ligaments can restrict or constrain rotational or translational motions. By the tension developed in it when it is stretched, a ligament resists motion along the axes in which it lies. Unlike bone, however, ligaments allow some motion to occur, and thus, cannot be considered rigid constraints. The position of the ligament is the key to the type of motions it limits. For example, at the knee, the cruciate ligaments limit the anteroposterior (AP) translation of the tibia on the femur, while at the ankle, the interosseous ligament prevents translational motion between the tibia and fibula, as compared to the deltoid or talocalcaneofibular ligaments, which prevent rotational motions as well as translational motions between these two bones and the calcaneus.

Muscle-tendon complexes are also semirigid restraints and complement the action of ligaments to stabilize joints. However, because ligaments are only passive stabilizers, muscles, which are active in controlling joint motion, have an obvious advantage. Muscle action, in fact, can protect ligaments from tearing in most instances. Muscle contraction produces compressive force across the joint tending to squeeze the joint together. This compressive force maintains stability against forces that might pivot a joint open. Where the compressive forces of a muscle are parallel to those exerted by the tensile forces occurring in the ligament, they provide load sharing. Where their direction of force is opposite, muscles can work in concert with the ligaments and serve to protect the joint when disruption of the ligament occurs. An example of this interaction is the protection the hamstrings provide when the anterior cruciate ligament (ACL) is torn. Thus, not only are muscles the force actuators at joints that initiate or prevent a desired movement, but they also can limit motions caused by external body weight or antagonist muscles harmful to joint stability.

Without joint stability, true functional motion cannot exist because much displacement will occur between the 2 rigid members at the joint surface. The extent to which each of the 3 structures—bone, ligaments, and muscles—contributes to joint stability differs at each joint. These differences are illustrated throughout this chapter with the discussions of the various joints. The spine, perhaps, illustrates the most intricate balance of contributions between the 3 structural stabilizers.

Control of Movement

Kinesiology also concerns understanding how the musculoskeletal system provides the means to initiate a movement, control the movement's magnitude and direction, and, when the desired goal is achieved, end the movement. This implies interactions not only of adjacent limb segments, but also between multiple segments. Human motions require the use of force actuators and a control mechanism to determine the placement, timing, and magnitude of force generation. These determinations are made via a dynamic system related not only to the muscle, but also to all aspects of the neurologic system. The energy causing joint rotation is not merely the contracting force produced by the muscle, but is a product of the perpendicular distance between the joint center of rotation and the tendon (the moment). The magnitude of the muscle force depends on the mode of muscle action (eccentric or concentric), the speed at which it occurs, and which body segment is to be moved. For example, during locomotion activities, quadriceps activation is needed to prevent the knee joint from collapsing during initiation of weightbearing. The amount of force required differs markedly during walking, running, initiating the next step during stair climbing, or getting up from a chair. With walking and running, the quadriceps restrains falling body weight by an eccentric response at very different speeds. During stair climbing or when rising from a chair the quadriceps operates in a concentric mode to lift body weight with the knee at different angles of flexion. During kicking, concentric quadriceps action moves the lower leg at high speed. The magnitude of force required will vary depending on whether the kicking is part of a game of soccer or that required to score a field goal in a football game.

The nature of how much effort a single muscle or several muscles acting about 1 or more joints produces is dictated by neurocontrol. For many types of functions, the exact mechanism of neurocontrol remains a puzzle; it is the subject of intensive basic research in the field of neurophysiology. The amount of effort needed at each joint can also be viewed as a mechanical problem that has an almost infinite number of solutions. Yet, the body does not use an infinite number of solutions; it operates in a finite way, thereby suggesting that human biologic systems have developed an optimal way of performing these tasks. This area has aroused intense interest in fields of engineering and modeling, not only because of interest in biologic systems, but also because of efforts in robotics. For example, in a 2-legged robot similar to humans, with hip, knee, and ankle joints, appropriate activations of springs or brakes at each of these joints would be required to maintain the robot in an upright position. If fully understood, this neurocontrol system would benefit not only the treatment of a variety of human disorders, but also the creation of mechanical robotic systems. These aspects of human movement are discussed more fully below when the mechanisms of throwing, standing, and walking are described.

Kinesiology is thus a study of how the musculoskeletal system has adapted to kinetics and kinematics on a microscopic and macroscopic scale between adjacent and across multiple limb segments. It is a study and understanding of how motions are produced by forces at individual joints as well as what characterizes their integration when a specific function is desired. Like any movement involving multiple parts, it requires different types of contributions from different components and a means for controlling and integrating the various activities of the individual parts. This chapter will present current knowledge of various representative parts of the process. This is not a comprehensive representation of the entire subject of kinesiology as it relates to human movement. For that, the reader is advised to refer to the many existing texts that discuss various aspects of the system.

Structure and Function of the Shoulder Joint

The shoulder joint allows the arm to move with respect to the thorax. This motion normally occurs through a complex interaction of the individual motions of the acromioclavicular, sternoclavicular, and glenohumeral joints as well as the scapulothoracic articulation. The biomechanics of the shoulder joint really is a study of these 4 different articulations that make up the shoulder complex.

The shoulder complex allows the greatest range of motion of any "joint" in the body. Traditional descriptions of humeral thoracic motion involve measuring the angle formed by the humerus and the thorax in the sagittal plane (flexion and extension) and the coronal plane (abduction). Axial rotation of the humerus is conventionally described by the measurement in degrees of internal or external rotation when the humeral axis is parallel to the thorax (Fig. 1), or perpendicular to the thorax (abducted 90°). Horizontal abduction and adduction, also known as horizontal extension and flexion, respectively, are commonly used to describe arm position when the axis of the humerus is perpendicular to the thorax.

Theoretically, 180° of elevation of the arm is possible, but very few individuals ever attain this degree of motion. Normal arm elevation in men has been reported as 167° or 168° and in women from 171° to 175°. Average extension or posterior elevation has been shown to be approximately 60° (Fig. 2). With the arm adducted by the side of the body, approximately 180° of rotation is possible. With abduction of the arm to 90°, however, the total arc of rotation is reduced to 120° with relatively more internal rotation

possible at that arm position. The range of motion of the shoulder decreases with normal aging. A comparison of two groups of males whose mean collective ages differed by only 12.5 years indicated that the younger group averaged 3.4° greater flexion, 3.4° greater internal rotation, 8.4° greater external rotation, and 10.2° greater extension.

Although measurements of the range of motion of the shoulder have commonly been made in specific planes such as flexion and extension, very few activities of daily living or recreation involving humeral thoracic motion are limited to these single planes. The most common plane for

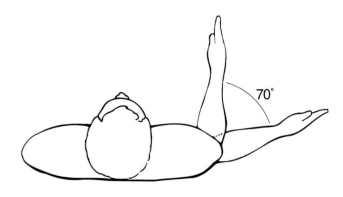

Figure 1

External rotation of the shoulder from 0° to 70° with the arm adducted.

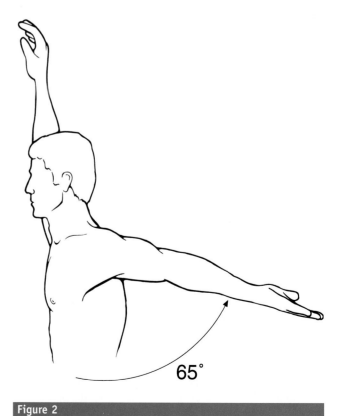

Figure 2

Extension of the shoulder to 65°.

humeral elevation in daily living is 50° to 60° anterior to the coronal plane. This approximates the line of the scapula or the scapular plane (also called scaption), which is described as being any where from 30° to 50° anterior to the coronal axis (Fig. 3). The act of combing one's hair requires an average of 148° of elevation in this plane, whereas the act of eating requires only an average of 52° of elevation in the same plane.

Clinical terms such as flexion, adduction, horizontal adduction, and extension are descriptive, but insufficient in their ability to portray the position of the arm with respect to the thorax, because more than one modifying word applies to virtually every arm position in space. In order to describe the position of a military salute, for example, conventional terminology would include 80° of abduction, 30° of horizontal adduction or horizontal flexion, and 40° of internal rotation of the humerus. Conversely, it could be described as forward flexion to 80°, 30° anterior to the coronal plane, with 40° of internal rotation of the humerus. Such language can be cumbersome and inconsistent. A cornerstone to the understanding of the kinematics of a joint is the ability to measure and describe its motion in an accurate and reproducible fashion. One method to achieve this accuracy in description is to designate various vertical planes available for elevation of the humerus similar to the segments of an orange or the longitudinal demarcations of a globe. The plane of pure abduction in the coronal plane is defined as the 0° plane and pure flexion in the anterior sagittal plane is +90° (Fig. 4). Maximum horizontal adduc-

tion of the shoulder occurs at +124° with maximum extension and horizontal abduction occurring at -88° (Fig. 5). Therefore, 212 different planes of humeral elevation are possible. Humeral elevation within a given plane is then quantified by measuring the angle formed between the unelevated humerus and the elevated humerus. Pure

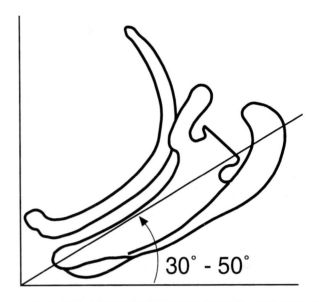

Figure 3

The plane of the scapula is approximately 30° to 50° anterior to the coronal plane of the body.

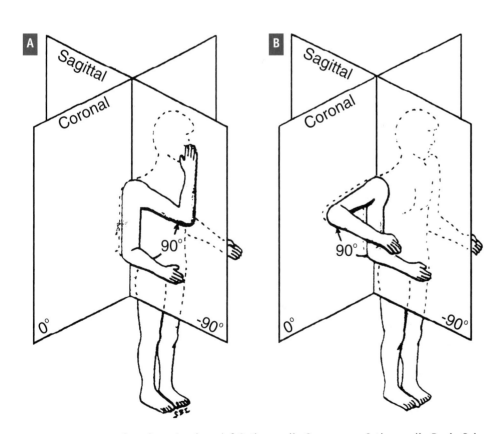

Figure 4

A, Elevation of the arm in the sagittal plane (flexion) may be defined as occurring in the +90° plane. Flexion to an angle of 90° within that plane is then described as (+90, 90). **B**, Elevation of the arm in the coronal plane (abduction) may be defined as occurring in the 0° plane. Abduction to an angle of 90° within that plane is described as (0, 90). (Reproduced with permission from Pearl ML, Harris SL, Lippitt SB, et al: A system for describing positions of the humerus relative to the thorax and its use in the presentation of several functionally important arm positions. *J Shoulder Elbow Surg* 1992;1: 113–115.)

abduction to 90° is described as (0, 90) whereas pure flexion to 90° is described as (+90, 90). For example, the act of washing the contralateral axilla requires the 104° plane as well as 52° of elevation of the humerus within that plane (+104, 52).

The final determinant of shoulder position is the axial rotation of the humerus described by the angle formed between the forearm (elbow flexed to 90°) and a line perpendicular to the plane of elevation (Fig. 6). If the forearm is perpendicular to the plane of elevation, rotation is defined as 0°. External rotation from that position is designated as positive (+), and internal rotation from that position is designated as negative (-). In this system, the military salute position previously discussed can be described as (+30, 80, +40). The act of combing the hair requires 57° of external rotation and could be described in this system as (+50, 110, +57).

Biomechanics of the Glenohumeral Joint

The glenohumeral joint demonstrates a normal range of laxity in virtually every direction. Average passive glenohumeral translation of 11.5 mm, both anteriorly and posteriorly, has been demonstrated in cadaver shoulders. A study of normal unanesthetized volunteers has demonstrated that passive humeral translation on the glenoid averaged 8 mm anteriorly, 9 mm posteriorly, and 11 mm inferiorly. Up to 2 cm of glenohumeral translation has been documented in some unanesthetized volunteers with no history

of shoulder instability. These evaluations of glenohumeral laxity were performed in the absence of any significant compressive force across the glenohumeral joint. They represent possible passive translation when an externally applied passive force acts on the humerus and, therefore, do not represent normal physiologic glenohumeral kinematics. These studies do demonstrate the great potential laxity in the glenohumeral joint.

Glenohumeral translation occurs to a significantly smaller degree during arm elevation and rotation than during drawer or laxity testing. In cadaver shoulders with a rigidly fixed scapula, passive forward elevation of the humerus up to 55° in the sagittal plane has demonstrated no translation between the center of rotation of the humeral head and the center of rotation of the glenoid. Up to 35° of passive extension was also possible without any translation. Throughout this total arc of 90°, essentially pure rotation between the humerus and glenoid occurred. Translation began to occur beyond 55° of flexion or 35° of extension. However, the rigidly fixed scapula prevented normal scapular motion. Simulated active forward elevation of the cadaver shoulder using cables attached to the deltoid and rotator cuff insertions has demonstrated an initial superior translation of 1 mm, from 0° to 30° of forward elevation. However, between 30° and 180° of elevation, the center of rotation of the humer-

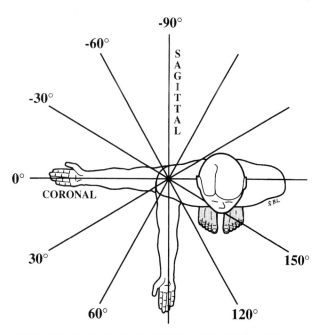

Figure 5

Planes of elevation of the arm. In normal individuals, the available planes of elevation are from -88° to +124°; therefore, there are 212 different planes of humeral elevation. (Reproduced with permission from Pearl ML, Harris SL, Lippitt SB, et al: A system for describing positions of the humerus relative to the thorax and its use in the presentation of several functionally important arm positions. *J Shoulder Elbow Surg* 1992;1:113–115.)

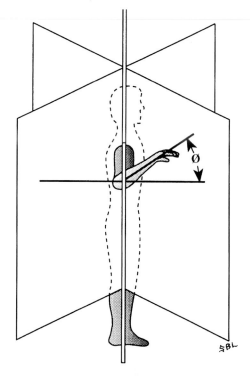

Figure 6

Rotation of the humerus is described by the angle formed by the forearm and a line perpendicular to the plane of elevation. (Reproduced with permission from Pearl ML, Harris SL, Lippitt SB, et al: A system for describing positions of the humerus relative to the thorax and its use in the presentation of several functionally important arm positions. *J Shoulder Elbow Surg* 1992;1:113–115.)

al head has been shown to translate only 0.94 mm in the AP direction and 1.29 mm in the superoinferior direction.

Radiographic analysis of normal volunteer subjects has shown that precise centering of the humeral head in the glenoid is maintained in all positions in the horizontal plane except when the arm is in maximum horizontal extension and simultaneous external rotation. At that point, 4 mm of posterior translation with respect to the center of the glenoid occurred. Radiographic analysis of active elevation in the plane of the scapula has shown that superior humeral head translation of 1 mm occurs for each 30° increment of forward elevation of the arm. These studies demonstrate in various ways that the center of rotation of the humeral head stays within a few millimeters of the center of rotation of the glenoid during normal glenohumeral range of motion despite the great potential for passive laxity in the glenohumeral joint. Rotational motion predominates in the glenohumeral joint despite the great potential for translation. The structure and methods for stabilizing the glenohumeral joint provide the basis for explaining how this potentially large translation is held to a minimum in this joint.

Anatomy of the Glenohumeral Joint

The glenoid is an oval or bean-shaped shallow socket that is retroverted approximately 7° with respect to the plane perpendicular to the plane of the scapula (Fig. 7). However, because the plane of the scapula is anterior to the coronal plane, the glenoid is anteverted 30° to 40° with respect to the coronal plane of the body (Fig. 3). The glenoid also faces superiorly approximately 5° when the scapula is in the normal resting position (Fig. 8). This superior inclination has been shown to contribute significantly to inferior stability of the glenohumeral joint, probably because of a cam effect that potentiates tightening of the superior capsule during inferiorly directed stress on the humerus. The surface area

of the glenoid socket is approximately one third that of the surface area of the humeral head. The depth of the glenoid socket has been measured to be 9 mm in a superoinferior direction and 5 mm in the AP direction. Of the total depth of the glenoid socket, 50% is provided by the surrounding glenoid labrum and 50% is provided by the configuration of the bone and articular cartilage. The articular cartilage of the glenoid is thicker peripherally than centrally, and this further deepens the glenoid socket (Fig. 9). Thus, the actual joint surface of the glenoid is more concave than the concavity of the subchondral bone seen on radiographic analysis of the glenoid.

The articular surface of the proximal humerus is approximately one third of a sphere and it is retroverted 30° to 40° with respect to the intercondylar plane of the distal humerus (Fig. 10). Stereophotogrammetric studies of the curvature of fresh frozen human cadaver shoulders have demonstrated that the deviation from sphericity of the convex humeral articular surface and concave glenoid articular surface was less than 1%. Therefore, these 2 articular surfaces are highly congruent. Traditionally, the glenohumeral joint has been likened to a large ball articulating with a small flat platform; for example, a golf ball on a tee. The glenohumeral joint, however, is actually composed of 2 closely fitting spherical surfaces. The lack of stability of the humeral surface against the glenoid surface is not caused by a discrepancy in radii, but rather is a reflection of the smaller surface area of the glenoid, which cannot capture the humeral head. Because of the decreased articular

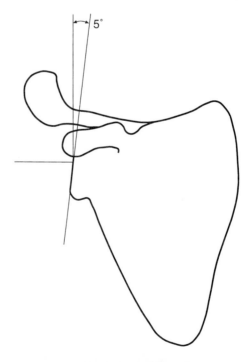

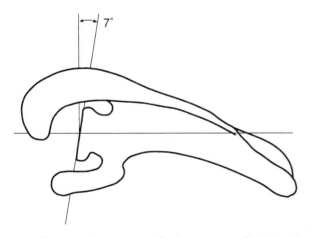

Figure 7

The glenoid is retroverted 7° with respect to the plane perpendicular to the scapular plane.

Figure 8

The glenoid faces superiorly approximately 5°, with reference to the vertical plane.

surface area of the glenoid, the glenohumeral joint depends primarily on soft tissues for maintenance of a stable articulation. A combination of muscles, capsule, and ligamentous forces is necessary for normal glenohumeral motion to occur, but a variety of passive mechanisms enhance the stability of the glenohumeral articulation as well.

Glenohumeral Stability

Passive Constraints

Because of the conformity of the radii of curvature of the glenoid and the humeral articular surfaces, and because of the synovial fluid present, adhesion and cohesion act together to stabilize the glenohumeral articulation. Synovial fluid adheres to the articular cartilage via the principle of adhesion, and this thin film of fluid between the 2 joint surfaces allows sliding motion to occur between these surfaces. Concomitantly, because of the principle of cohesion, the 2 joint surfaces cannot easily be pulled apart. This works in the same way that a drinking glass can slide in a film of water on a glass tabletop, but momentarily sticks during attempts to lift the glass off the tabletop. In the glenohumeral joint, the compliant glenoid labrum that surrounds the rim of the glenoid further potentiates this passive stabilizing effect.

The intra-articular pressure in the glenohumeral joint is slightly negative under normal conditions. This negative intra-articular pressure probably arises as a result of high osmotic pressure in the surrounding tissues, which acts to draw water from the joint. The glenohumeral joint normally contains less than 1 cc of fluid, although it can accommodate more than 30 cc of fluid. The watertight capsule of the glenohumeral joint is pulled inwardly by this negative intra-articular pressure, thereby keeping the capsule and ligaments under continuous stretch and helping to maintain the stability of the joint. Joint effusions or venting of the capsule interferes with this mechanism. If an inferiorly directed translation force of 16 N is applied to the humerus in a cadaver shoulder, an inferior translation of 2 mm has been demonstrated. If the capsule of that cadaver shoulder is then punctured, the resultant inferior translation increases to 28 mm during application of the same 16-N force. The integrity of the capsule around the shoulder is important for the maintenance of this negative intra-articular pressure.

Considering that the arm is one twelfth of body weight, it would seem that in the normal resting position, with the arm hanging by the side, some degree of muscular activity would be necessary to maintain the glenohumeral joint in a reduced position. Electromyographic (EMG) analysis of the deltoid, supraspinatus, infraspinatus, triceps, and biceps muscles in young male volunteers has demonstrated that no activity occurs in these muscles when the arm is quietly maintained by the side. Inferior translation of the humerus is not present on normal AP radiographs of the shoulder. Spontaneous translations of the humerus on the glenoid do not occur when patients in the operating room are administered general anesthesia. Therefore, either passive stabilizing mechanisms or the ligamentous and capsule static constraints are responsible for maintaining the reduction of the glenohumeral articulation. An examination of the static capsular ligamentous constraints of the glenohumeral joint will augment understanding of how the glenohumeral joint maintains a stable reduction during resting posture.

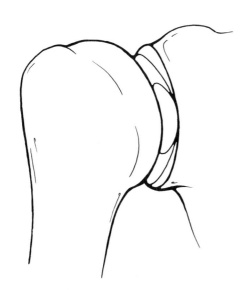

Figure 9

The glenoid labrum provides 50% of the depth of the glenoid socket. The articular cartilage is thicker peripherally than centrally, which increases the concavity of the articular surface of the glenoid.

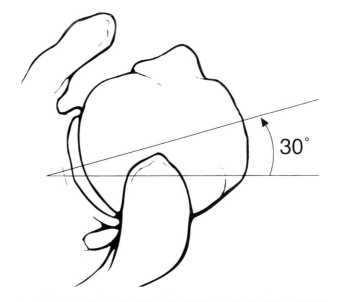

Figure 10

The humeral head is retroverted 30° to 40° with respect to the intercondylar plane of the humerus.

Static Constraints

The capsule and ligaments are the most important stabilizers in preventing dislocation of the glenohumeral joint. The capsuloligamentous structures form a truncated cone of collagenous tissue with the smaller of the 2 circular attachments surrounding the glenoid and the larger of the 2 circular attachments surrounding the humeral head. The glenohumeral ligaments are thickenings or condensations of the glenohumeral capsule and are located primarily anteriorly and inferiorly in the capsule itself. The coracohumeral ligament represents a folded thickening of the glenohumeral capsule in the area of the rotator interval between the subscapularis and supraspinatus muscles. Although the capsule extends circumferentially around the glenoid, the posterosuperior quadrant of the capsule is devoid of ligamentous condensations.

Superior Glenohumeral Ligament The superior glenohumeral ligament (SGHL) originates just anteriorly to the long head of the biceps origin on the superior glenoid, and it inserts on the proximal aspect of the lesser tuberosity of the humerus. The SGHL is present in approximately 90% of shoulders, and is well developed in approximately 50% of shoulders. However, there is variability in its development. It is the main capsular structure resisting inferior translation of the humerus in the adducted shoulder. It is less important in stabilizing the glenohumeral joint against AP translation.

Middle Glenohumeral Ligament The middle glenohumeral ligament (MGHL) demonstrates the greatest variability of the glenohumeral ligaments and, in fact, is absent in up to 30% of shoulders. The MGHL originates from the glenoid or the labrum just inferior to the SGHL and inserts just medial to the lesser tuberosity of the proximal humerus (Fig. 11). It acts as a secondary restraint to inferior glenohumeral translation in the adducted and externally rotated shoulder as well as to anterior glenohumeral translation in the shoulder abducted to 90°. The MGHL limits anterior translation of the humerus on the glenoid to a more significant degree when the arm is abducted 45° than when the arm is either at 90° or 0° of abduction.

Inferior Glenohumeral Ligament The inferior glenohumeral ligament (IGHL) is the most important static restraint in the glenohumeral joint. The IGHL is a complex structure consisting of anterior and posterior thickenings or bands with a sling-like pouch in between (Fig. 11). This pouch is referred to as the axillary pouch. The anterior band of the IGHL originates on the anterior aspect of the glenoid or glenoid neck at approximately the 3 o'clock position. The posterior band of the IGHL originates from the glenoid at approximately the 9 o'clock position. The IGHL is the primary stabilizer of the abducted shoulder against AP translation. The stabilizing role of this complex ligament increases with increasing arm abduction. During external rotation of the humerus, the anterior band of the IGHL fans out and tightens, whereas the posterior band fans out and tightens during internal rotation of the arm (Fig. 12). This reciprocal tightening and loosening of the anterior and posterior bands of the IGHL, with respect to various arm positions, has been likened to the function of a hammock during asymmetric loading. The IGHL is also an important structure in providing superoinferior stability to the glenohumeral joint, especially with increasing amounts of abduction. In fact, the IGHL is the primary restraint to inferior translation of the humerus on the glenoid in a position of 90° of abduction of the arm.

Mechanical testing performed on the anterior glenohumeral capsule and IGHL has indicated that the tensile strength of the anterior capsular attachment in cadavers is approximately 70 N. When tested in tension, the IGHL complex undergoes significant plastic deformation prior to failure. The strain-to-failure of the IGHL in cadaver shoulders averages 27.9%, with a range of 15% to 61.2%.

Coracohumeral Ligament The coracohumeral ligament (CHL) originates from the base of the coracoid process and attaches to the lateral aspect of the bicipital groove on the greater tuberosity of the humerus. The importance of the CHL in limiting inferior translation of the adducted humerus is unclear. Some have demonstrated that the CHL has little significance in stabilizing the adducted shoulder, although others have found that it significantly limits inferior humeral translation.

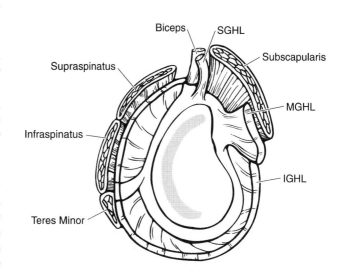

Figure 11

The relationship of the glenohumeral ligaments as they attach to the glenoid. Although the posterosuperior capsule is devoid of ligamentous condensations, this portion of the glenohumeral joint is bolstered by the presence of the rotator cuff tendons. SGHL = superior glenohumeral ligament; MGHL = middle glenohumeral ligament; IGHL = inferior glenohumeral ligament.

The Relationship of Static and Passive Constraints

Ligaments function in tension and are of little stabilizing effect when lax. To limit anterior translation of the humerus on the glenoid, capsuloligamentous structures would have to be under tension. If the ligamentous structures around the glenohumeral joint were responsible for eliminating translation of the humerus on the glenoid during normal motion, these structures would have to be taut. Yet, large amounts of translation are possible in the glenohumeral joint in virtually all directions. Moreover, the center of rotation of the humeral head varies only a few millimeters from the center of rotation of the glenoid during glenohumeral motion. Therefore, some mechanism exists to maintain the pure rotation of the glenohumeral joint through a great

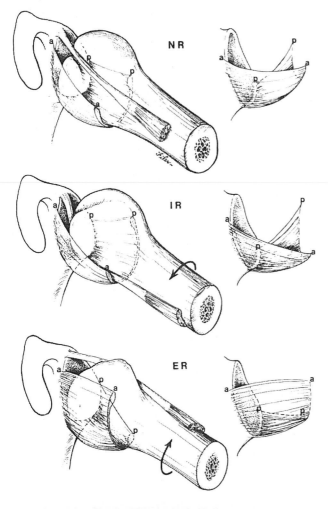

Figure 12

The anterior and posterior portions of the inferior glenohumeral ligament (IGHL) complex reciprocally tighten and loosen depending on the rotation of the humerus. With external rotation (ER), the anterior band (a) of the IGHL tightens and moves superiorly on the humeral head. During internal rotation (IR) of the humerus, the posterior band (p) of the IGHL tightens and moves superiorly. NR = no rotation. (Reproduced with permission from Warner JP, Caborn DM, Berger R, et al: Dynamic capsuloligamentous anatomy of the glenohumeral joint. *J Shoulder Elbow Surg* 1993;2:115–133.)

range of motion while the ligaments remain relatively lax. This pure rotation is maintained by the passive stabilizing mechanisms, such as adhesion, cohesion, and negative intra-articular pressure, as well as by the dynamic stabilizing forces (muscles) that cross the glenohumeral joint when those forces are combined with the ability of the glenoid to move in space in synchrony with the humerus.

The complex bony architecture and muscular arrangement of the shoulder girdle allow the minimally constrained glenohumeral joint to maintain concentric reduction throughout the huge range of motion necessary for activities of daily living. However, pathologic translation of the humerus on the glenoid certainly occurs, especially in clinical instability of the shoulder. Most joints in the human body dislocate only when ligamentous structures are torn or periarticular fractures occur. The glenohumeral joint can dislocate without actual tearing of ligamentous tissue if capsuloligamentous structures are significantly stretched. It can be safely stated, however, that glenohumeral dislocations do not occur in the presence of efficiently functioning glenohumeral ligament structures. Selective cutting experiments have helped to clarify the role of the various capsuloligamentous structures around the glenohumeral joint.

The Role of Selective Cutting Experiments The primary stabilizer of the glenohumeral joint in the superoinferior direction of the adducted arm appears to be the superior capsular structures, especially the SGHL. With increasing abduction of the arm, however, the inferior capsular structures, especially the IGHL, become the most significant stabilizers against inferior translation. The primary stabilizer of the glenohumeral joint against anterior translation is the IGHL; at lower degrees of abduction, the MGHL and subscapularis also contribute. The primary stabilizer of the glenohumeral joint against posterior translation also appears to be the IGHL. If the entire posterior capsule of the glenohumeral joint is incised, posterior translation increases, but posterior dislocation does not occur. With an additional incision anteriorly, from 12 o'clock to 3 o'clock, through the anterosuperior capsule (SGHL, MGHL), posterior dislocation of the flexed and internally rotated humerus can occur. Posterior humeral translation increases when the anterior band of the IGHL is incised, if the arm is maintained in 30° of extension. Posterior translation increases when the anterior portion of the IGHL is detached from the glenoid (Bankart lesion).

Bankart's concept of a single essential lesion producing shoulder instability is attractive, but too simplistic. The creation of a Bankart lesion in the cadaver shoulder leads to increased glenohumeral translation of several millimeters, although anterior glenohumeral dislocation does not occur. Translation of the glenohumeral joint increases with injury to the capsule on one side of this joint, but in order for dislocation to occur, the capsule must be injured or stretched on both sides of the glenohumeral joint. This fact is important during surgical reconstruction of the ligaments around the unstable shoulder. Individuals demonstrating increased clinical laxity in the musculoskeletal system become more at risk for glenohumeral dislocation with minor trauma to their glenohumeral ligaments. In an individual with generalized joint laxity, inherent laxity of the posterior capsule combined with a small amount of injury to the IGHL anteriorly may allow a dislocation of the glenohumeral joint anteriorly. In another individual with normal ligamentous laxity, a relatively greater degree of trauma to the IGHL anteriorly would be required to effect an anterior glenohumeral dislocation.

When interpreting selective cutting experiments, it is important to remember that the interaction of muscle forces, intra-articular pressure, and the degree of plastic deformation of the capsuloligamentous structures are clinically important and are difficult to replicate during experiments in cadaver shoulders. Dynamic stabilizers of the glenohumeral joint, that is, muscular forces, significantly affect glenohumeral stability as well. Selective cutting experiments in the shoulder, as opposed to some of the other joints in the human body, help to clarify ligamentous function, but must be interpreted cautiously regarding the etiology of clinical instability.

Unlike the acetabulum of the hip joint, the glenoid socket is quite mobile. This allows the relatively shallow glenoid to be placed advantageously so that it can most effectively resist the joint reaction forces generated by the muscle contractions crossing the glenohumeral joint. In this way, the glenoid can be likened to a mobile backstop. The motion required for this effect is possible because of the complex architecture of the clavicle and scapula, the coordinated activities of the musculature controlling the scapula, and the relatively unconstrained acromioclavicular and sternoclavicular joints.

The Clavicle The clavicle acts as a strut that effectively maintains the scapula and glenoid lateral to the thorax despite a variety of arm and body positions. This strut allows muscles, such as the pectoralis major and latissimus dorsi, to powerfully move the humerus without effectively changing the position of the glenoid in relation to the midline of the body. The prime movers of the humerus compress the humeral head against the glenoid and, in so doing, cause a chain reaction across the acromioclavicular joint, the scapular thoracic articulation, and, finally, the sternoclavicular joint.

The Acromioclavicular Joint The acromioclavicular (AC) joint is a true diarthrodial joint that allows the articulation of the medial aspect of the acromion with the lateral aspect of the clavicle. The joint surfaces are not perfectly congruent, and a fibrocartilaginous meniscus is interposed between the clavicle and the acromion. The AC capsule is thickened superiorly, forming the AC ligament. The AC lig-

ament and AC capsule are the initial stabilizers of the AC joint in the AP direction and for axial rotation of the clavicle. The AC capsule and ligaments are the primary stabilizers of the AC joint when this joint is subjected to relatively light loads of daily activity and recreation; however, when greater forces are applied to the AC joint, the most important stabilizing structures become the coracoclavicular ligaments composed of the trapezoid and conoid ligaments.

The scapula is essentially suspended from the clavicle by way of these two strong ligaments that span from the undersurface of the clavicle to the coracoid process of the scapula. Although the trapezoid is larger and stronger, it has been shown that during large displacements of the AC joint, the conoid resists almost four times as much force (70%) as does the trapezoid (18%). The trapezoid ligament, because of its oblique fibers, more effectively resists AC joint compression during loading of the glenohumeral joint, such as in weight lifting. This tough sling of ligamentous tissue effectively decreases the compression of the acromion against the lateral end of the clavicle.

The Sternoclavicular Joint The sternoclavicular joint forms the only true skeletal articulation or bridge between the upper extremity and the thorax. This diarthrodial joint is composed of reciprocally saddle-shaped, but incongruous, articular surfaces with an interposed fibrocartilaginous disk or meniscus. Ligamentous restraints surround the sternoclavicular joint anteriorly, posteriorly, superiorly, and inferiorly.

Motion of the Clavicle The clavicle moves in the AP and superoinferior directions and also rotates about its long axis both anteriorly and posteriorly during normal motion of the arm. Greater motion occurs at the sternoclavicular joint than at the AC joint. Approximately 35° of superior rotation, anterior rotation, and posterior rotation occurs in the sternoclavicular joint, and this unconstrained, saddle-shaped articulation allows 45° to 50° of axial rotation to occur. The clavicle has been shown to rotate 40° to 50° during active forward elevation of the arm. Although the clavicle rotates this amount with respect to the fixed sternum, it rotates only 5° to 8° with respect to the acromion at the AC joint because of the concomitant synchronous rotation of the scapula during forward elevation of the arm.

Biomechanics of the Shoulder

Muscular Activity of the Shoulder Joint Complex
Twenty different muscles act on the shoulder girdle. Some of these muscles can be further subdivided according to differing functional heads into the 3 heads of the deltoid, 2 heads of the biceps brachii, 2 portions of the pectoralis major, and 3 portions of the trapezius. The muscles affecting the shoulder girdle can be classified as glenohumeral, scapulothoracic, or thoracohumeral based on their origins and insertions (Outline 1).

The effectiveness of any muscle depends on its physiologic cross-sectional area, angle of pull, and intensity of contraction. EMG can demonstrate and quantify the amount of activity in a particular muscle group during dynamic conditions. The percentage of recorded EMG activity indicates the level of activity of a given muscle, but does not indicate the force generated by that muscle. For complete understanding of the force generated by a particular muscle about the shoulder, the moment arm (distance between the insertion of that muscle into the bone and the instantaneous center of joint rotation) and the physiologic cross-sectional area (the volume of the muscle divided by the muscle length) must be known. In the shoulder, the bones and both the origins and insertions of the muscles all move simultaneously. Therefore, changes in the muscle volume, length, and moment arms occur constantly throughout the entire range of motion. The great arcs of motion in multiple planes with multiple arm rotations produce constant changes in the relationship of a given muscle to the joint's instantaneous center of rotation. The quantification of muscle forces about the shoulder is, therefore, an arduous task.

The relatively unconstrained glenohumeral joint and "floating" scapula critically depend on finely balanced muscle forces to maintain rhythm and synchrony of arm motion relative to the thorax as the arm moves through space to lift and throw. This is particularly true at the glenohumeral joint as the alignment of the prime mover, the deltoid, causes the muscle to challenge joint stability as it elevates the humerus.

Specific muscular activity about the shoulder complex has been studied anatomically and through stereophotogrammetry and dynamic EMG. The change in lever arms and orientation of musculature for the different positions of the arm with respect to the thorax have been demonstrated. The cross-sectional area of some of the musculature around the shoulder girdle has been studied (Table 1). By combining knowledge of the cross-sectional area and the orientation of particular muscles, muscle forces can be approximated.

Elevation of the arm with respect to the thorax has been studied more than any other specific shoulder motion. Forward elevation of the humerus has been studied using a combination of stereophotogrammetry to analyze motion during forward elevation and EMG to record muscular activity.

The interrelationship between the supraspinatus and the deltoid muscles during elevation of the arm has been studied by a variety of investigators. In 1944, it was demonstrated that the supraspinatus muscle acts synergistically with the deltoid during elevation of the arm, while the infraspinatus, teres minor, and subscapularis muscles provide the humeral depressor effect necessary to prevent cephalic migration of the humeral head during forward elevation. The deltoid muscle possesses a dominant pull that is oriented vertically and amounts to 89% of the muscle's total

Outline 1
Muscles Affecting the Shoulder Girdle

Glenohumeral muscles
Deltoid
Supraspinatus
Infraspinatus
Teres minor
Subscapularis
Teres major
Coracobrachialis
Biceps brachii (short head)
Triceps brachii (long head)

Scapulothoracic muscles
Trapezius
Serratus anterior
Rhomboid major
Rhomboid minor
Levator scapulae
Pectoralis minor

Thoracohumeral muscles
Pectoralis major (sternal head)
Latissimus dorsi

Other
Biceps brachii (long head)
Pectoralis major (clavicular head)
Subclavius
Omohyoid
Sternocleidomastoid

Table 1
Cross-Sectional Area of Shoulder Girdle Musculature

Muscle	Area (cm^2)
Deltoid	18.17
Deltoid posterior	5.00
Supraspinatus	5.72
Subscapularis	16.30
Infraspinatus and teres minor	13.74
Pectoralis major	13.34
Latissimus dorsi	12.00
Teres major	8.77
Triceps (long head)	2.96
Biceps (long head)	2.01
Biceps (short head)	1.11
Coracobrachialis	1.60

force. This results in a vertical sheer force imparted by the deltoid. The infraspinatus, teres minor, and subscapularis have a net inferior sheer force that amounts to 71% to 82% of the total force of these muscles.

The specific contributions of the supraspinatus and the deltoid muscles, respectively, have been reported variably. The supraspinatus muscle has been thought to initiate abduction of the arm, allowing the deltoid to continue this abduction once it gained an advantageous moment arm. Dynamic EMG investigations have demonstrated that the deltoid and all 4 rotator cuff muscles are active throughout the full range of forward elevation in the scapular plane: flexion, as well as abduction. Investigators, using selective local anesthetic nerve blocks of either the axillary or suprascapular nerves to study torque production in the arm during flexion and abduction, demonstrated that the deltoid and the supraspinatus muscles were equally responsible for torque production. Others demonstrated that full arm abduction was possible under the influence of an axillary nerve block; however, the strength of such abduction was approximately 50% of normal. Suprascapular nerve block, by eliminating the supraspinatus and infraspinatus, still allowed full abduction of the arm, although it was significantly weaker. Under suprascapular nerve block, the remaining teres minor and subscapularis muscles provide glenohumeral compression and humeral depression.

Simultaneous axillary and suprascapular nerve blocks render active abduction of the arm impossible; this observation supports the concept of the essential muscles for elevation of the arm. Under suprascapular nerve block, isometric strength in abduction decreases approximately 50% at 30° of forward elevation in the scapular plane, and 35% at 90° of forward elevation in the scapular plane. At 120° of forward elevation, suprascapular nerve block produces a decrease in isometric abduction strength of approximately 25%.

Both the supraspinatus and deltoid are necessary for normal elevation of the arm, and although both muscles are active through the entire range of motion, the deltoid becomes progressively more effective with increasing elevation as the moment arm of the deltoid progressively improves. The required lifting force of the deltoid muscle drops from 50% of maximum at 30° elevation to 43% of maximum at 90° of elevation and becomes only 18% of maximum at 150° of elevation. At 0° of abduction, the percentage of deltoid force that is directed vertically is 90%. However, as the arm is elevated to the horizontal, the percentage of vertical force of the deltoid decreases to 55% owing to the improvement of pull of the deltoid muscle (Fig. 13). The supraspinatus, however, maintains a consistent 75° angle between its line of pull and the glenoid surface. Of the muscle force of the supraspinatus, 97% is directed toward compression of the glenohumeral joint (Fig. 14). The subscapularis and infraspinatus have an angle of pull of approximately 45° directed inferiorly, and the teres minor has an angle of pull directed inferiorly approximately 55° (Fig. 14). These vectors of pull result in muscle forces that are nearly equally divided between glenohumeral joint compression and humeral head depression.

Pure arm abduction and pure arm flexion demonstrate the same basic synergy between the rotator cuff and the deltoid. In flexion, the prime movers are the anterior and middle deltoid, with 73% and 62% activity, respectively. The prime stabilizers are the infraspinatus, supraspinatus, and the latissimus dorsi. The latissimus dorsi demonstrates up to 25% activity as flexion continues above the horizontal plane. In pure abduction, a very similar relationship is demonstrated; however, the subscapularis assumes a more important stabilizing role and the posterior deltoid is moderately active.

External Rotation The infraspinatus muscle is the primary external rotator of the humerus. It is assisted by the teres minor and the posterior deltoid. EMG studies have indicated that the infraspinatus is the most active of all shoulder muscles during external rotation in all positions of arm abduction. The activity of the infraspinatus is approximately 50% throughout external rotation; that of the subscapularis is just below 50%, indicating its importance as the primary stabilizer during external rotation.

After suprascapular nerve block, isometric external rotation strength, performed at 30° of abduction, decreased by 74%. In these same shoulders, however, the decrease in external rotation strength after suprascapular nerve block became less noticeable as the amount of abduction increased. The posterior deltoid becomes a more efficient external rotator of the humerus with increasing abduction

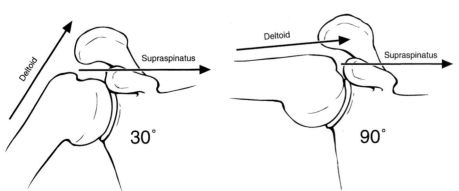

Deltoid
Supraspinatus
30°

Deltoid
Supraspinatus
90°

Figure 13

As the arm is abducted to 90°, the direction of pull of the deltoid approximates that of the supraspinatus. Therefore, patients with a large tear of the rotator cuff can often actively maintain the arm abducted to 90°, but may not be capable of actively abducting to 90°.

of the arm, especially when combined with some degree of extension of the arm. The deltoid accounts for 60% of the strength in horizontal abduction of the arm.

Internal Rotation The prime movers for internal rotation of the arm with respect to the thorax are the pectoralis major (especially the sternal head), the latissimus dorsi, and the subscapularis muscle groups. In addition, the teres major assists in this internal rotation. The subscapularis demonstrates activity in all positions during internal rotation, but its activity tends to decrease with increasing abduction. At

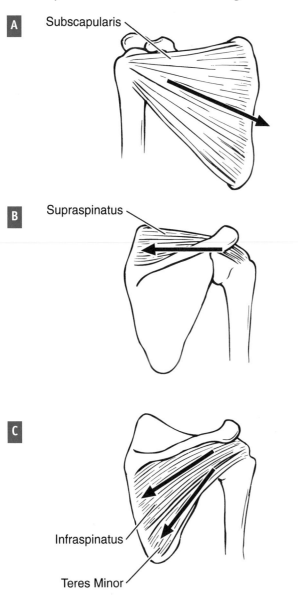

A Subscapularis

B Supraspinatus

C

Infraspinatus

Teres Minor

Figure 14

The angle of pull of the subscapularis (**A**) is approximately 45°. The angle of pull of the infraspinatus (**C**) is also approximately 45°, and the teres minor (**C**) is approximately 55°. These vectors result in nearly equal glenohumeral joint compression and humeral head depression. The supraspinatus (**B**) is essentially horizontal in its orientation, resulting in compression of the glenohumeral joint.

0° of abduction, the subscapularis activity has been shown to be 34%; whereas at 90° of abduction, it decreases to 21%. Activity in the pectoralis major during internal rotation also decreases with increasing abduction from 30% at 0° of abduction to 2% at 90° of abduction. The latissimus dorsi demonstrates a similar activity during internal rotation with a decrease from 20% at 0° of abduction to 7% at 90° of abduction. During internal rotation, EMG activity in the middle and posterior deltoid tends to increase when tested at positions of increased abduction of the arm.

Extension During extension of the arm, the prime movers are the posterior and the middle deltoid. The posterior head of the deltoid has demonstrated 70% to 74% activity on EMG during extension, with the middle head demonstrating 57% activity. The subscapularis is active throughout extension with 53% activity. The supraspinatus demonstrates increasing activity (35%) as the degree of extension increases. The subscapularis and supraspinatus are considered the prime stabilizers during extension of the arm.

Scapulothoracic Motion The glenoid and, therefore, the scapula, rotate in an upward fashion as elevation of the arm occurs (Fig. 15). This rotation is important for maintenance of a relatively constant fiber length of the deltoid muscle, thereby allowing the deltoid to remain powerful despite a variety of arm positions. Upward rotation of the scapula increases the stability of the glenohumeral joint in overhead activities and also decreases the tendency for impingement of the rotator cuff tendons beneath the coracoacromial arch. The upper trapezius, levator scapulae, and upper portion of the serratus anterior muscles contract concomitantly with the lower trapezius and lower digitations of the serratus anterior to produce a scapular rotating force couple (Fig. 16). The synergistic action of the serratus anterior and trapezius must be present for a full forward elevation of the arm to occur.

The relative contributions of scapular, thoracic, and glenohumeral motion during forward elevation have been studied extensively. The ratio of glenohumeral motion and scapulothoracic motion has been determined to be from 1.1:1 to 4.3:1. Most of the variability in this ratio occurs during the initial 30° of arm elevation. Scapulothoracic motion during this phase of elevation is highly variable and sometimes is even absent. Once the scapulothoracic motion is underway, the rhythm becomes more linear, and the relationship between glenohumeral and scapulothoracic becomes more constant. The setting phase of scapulothoracic motion during the first 30° of abduction is more pronounced and longer than during forward flexion. The variability observed in scapulothoracic motion during elevation of the arm can occur in an individual. This motion has been shown to be 3-dimensional (3-D), complex, and task-dependent. Optimal scapular position for heavy lifting or pushing may require a different glenoid orientation to minimize glenohumeral sheer, as well as to optimize muscle length/tension relationships. Therefore, the ratio of glenohumeral scapulothoracic motion seems to be variable, but roughly 2° of glenohumeral motion occurs for each 1° of scapulothoracic motion during elevation of the arm.

Structure and Function of the Elbow Joint

Introduction

The elbow is a complex joint that acts as a component link of the lever arm system in placing the hand. As a fulcrum for the forearm lever, its muscles provide the power to perform lifting activities. With crutch walking, the elbow is a weightbearing joint. In power and fine work activities, the elbow stabilizes the upper extremity linkage. Thus, the biomechanics of the elbow relate to the kinematics, forces across the joint, and stability.

Kinematics and Joint Stability

The elbow has 2 degrees of freedom: flexion-extension and axial rotation, or pronation-supination. The normal range of motion is between 0° and 140° to 160° of flexion-extension and forearm rotation with about 70° to 80° of pronation and 80° to 85° of supination. The functional arc of motion for most activities of daily living is 100° from 30° to 130° of flexion-extension with 50° of pronation and 50° of supination (Figs. 17 and 18).

The rotational axis of flexion-extension occurs about a tight locus of points (instantaneous axes of rotation), measuring only 2 to 3 mm in the broadest dimension, and is

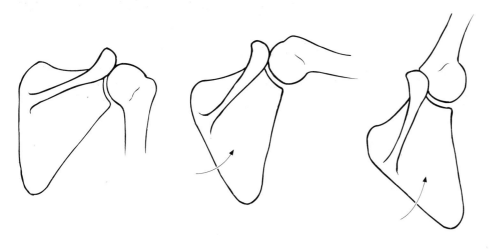

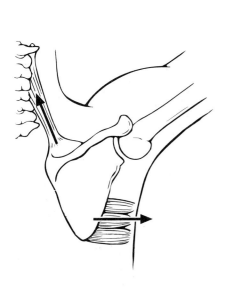

Figure 15

Forward elevation or abduction of the arm requires synchronous rotation of the scapula.

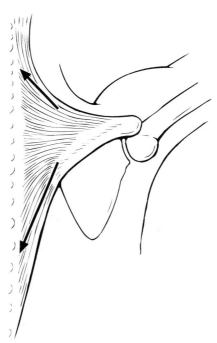

Figure 16

Rotation of the scapula is produced by the synergistic contractions of the lower portion of the serratus anterior and the lower trapezius, with the upper trapezius, levator scapulae, and upper serratus anterior.

located at the center of the lateral projected curvature of the trochlea and capitellum (Fig. 19). The axis of forearm rotation passes through the capitellum and head of the radius, extending to the distal ulna, and defines a cone (Fig. 20). The carrying angle, the angle between the long axis of the humerus and the long axis of the ulna, is measured in the frontal plane with the elbow extended, and averages 7°

in men and 13° in women. This angle decreases with elbow flexion and there is a slight axial rotation of about 5°, first internal and then external rotation of the ulna with reference to the humerus (Fig. 21).

Varus/valgus rotational motions at the elbow are restricted. Motion produced in this plane constitutes joint instability. The greatest resistance to rotational forces exists at the elbow on the medial side, where the medial collateral ligament is the most important stabilizer, especially the anterior oblique fibers. The anterior oblique ligament is taut throughout the flexion-extension range, whereas the posterior oblique ligament is taut only during flexion. At 90° of flexion, the medial collateral ligament contributes 54% of the resistance to valgus stress. The remainder is supplied by the shape of the articular surface and the anterior capsule. The articular congruity provides partial stability. The radial head provides about 30% of valgus stability and is more important in 0° to 30° of flexion and pronation. In extension, the olecranon becomes locked in its fossa. Equal contributions from the medial collateral ligament, shape of joint surfaces, and anterior capsule are important to resisting valgus stress in extension.

Stability to varus stress is provided by the lateral collateral ligament, anconeus, and joint capsule. The lateral ligament

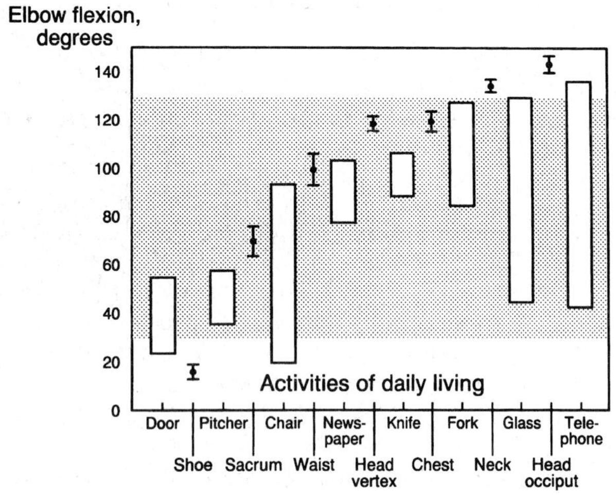

Figure 17

Functional arc of elbow motion for activities of daily living is approximately 100°, between 30° and 103°. (Adapted with permission from Morrey BF, Askew LJ, An KN, et al: A biomechanical study of functional elbow motion. *J Bone Joint Surg* 1981;63A:872.)

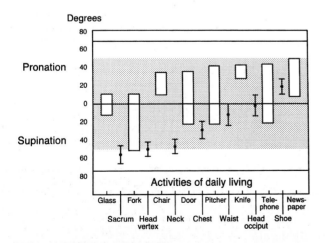

Figure 18

Functional arc of forearm rotation is approximately 50° of pronation and 50° of supination for most activities of daily living. (Adapted with permission from Morrey BF, Askew LJ, An KN, et al: A biomechanical study of functional elbow motion. *J Bone Joint Surg* 1981;63A:872.)

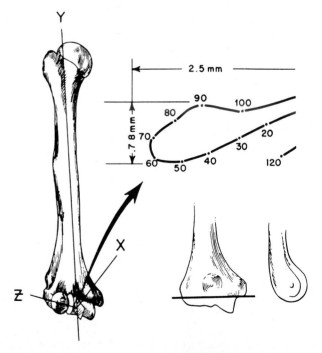

Figure 19

The very small locus of instant center of rotation for the elbow joint demonstrates that the axis may be replicated by a single line drawn from the inferior aspect of the medial epicondyle through the center of the lateral epicondyle, which is in the center of the lateral projected curvature of the trochlea and capitellum. (Adapted with permission from Morrey BF, Chao EY: Passive motion of the elbow joint. *J Bone Joint Surg* 1976;58A:501.)

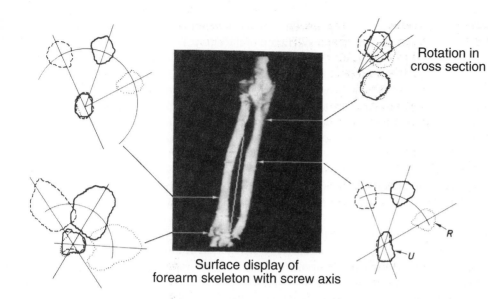

Rotation in cross section

Surface display of forearm skeleton with screw axis

Figure 20

Three-dimensional shaded surface display of the forearm showing the rotation of the radius, R; about the ulna, U; in supination (dashed line), neutral (solid line), and pronation (dotted line). (Reproduced with permission from Robbin, ML, An KN, Linscheid RL, et al: Anatomic and kinematic anaylsis of the human forearm using high-speed computed tomography. *Med Biol Eng Comput* 1986;24: 164–168.)

contributes only 9% of restraint to varus stress at 90° of flexion. Approximately 78% is provided by joint articulation and 13% by the joint capsule. In extension, the lateral ligament contributes 14% of restraint to varus stress, with 54% provided by the joint surface shape and 32% by the capsule.

Because the elbow functions as a link to position the hand in space, no single position is considered optimal for function. To understand this it is important to recognize that the shoulder functions as a ball joint, allowing the hand to describe a portion of a surface of a sphere in space. With each successive change in the degree of rotational flexion/extension position of the elbow, a sphere of a different radius is described. The elbow thus allows the upper extremity to operate at different distances away from the body. Loss of motion at the elbow can then be described as a loss of reach length. This reach length can be described as the cosine of the angle of elbow flexion multiplied by the length of the forearm and hand. If the elbow is in full extension, then the cosine function is 1 and the reach length is at its maximum. With an elbow flexion contracture smaller than 30° the cosine function remains near 1, but as the angle progresses past 30° the cosine function rapidly decreases, as does the ability to reach in space. In actuality, the ability to reach not only is related to the diameter of the sphere but also affects the amount of the circumference of the sphere in which the hand can operate; that is, the volume of the sphere (Fig. 22). Thus, reach capacity is not linear, but is calculated as a function of the third power of the radius. Patients can tolerate flexion contractures of about 30° with about a 20% functional loss; when loss is more than 30° of extension, patients readily complain of functional impairment. Extension contractures at the elbow also limit function, particularly if the dominant arm is involved. Inability to flex the elbow more than 100° restricts such self-care activities as dressing, feeding, and hygiene for the face and head.

Elbow Kinetics

Muscle forces that act about the elbow have short lever arms; thus, they are relatively inefficient kinetically but very

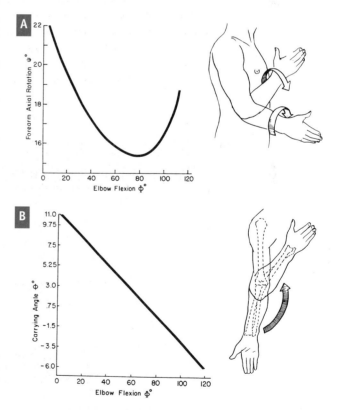

Figure 21

A, During elbow flexion, the ulna demonstrates a slight axial rotation referable to the humerus with an amplitude of less than 10°. **B,** During elbow flexion and extension, a linear change in the carrying angle is demonstrated, typically going from valgus in extension to varus in flexion. (Reproduced with permission from Morrey BF, Chao EY: Passive motion of the elbow joint. *J Bone Joint Surg* 1976;58A:501.)

efficient kinematically—that is, a small muscle excursion can produce a large arc of motion at the hand. Rapid distal motion of the limb is possible by short excursions of proximal muscles lying close to the axis of joint rotation to permit actions such as throwing. Conversely, large muscle forces are needed to produce large flexion or extension torques for lifting and pushing. Because the flexor moment arm is shortest at full extension, a large muscle force is necessary to initiate a flexion movement, and the joint compressive load at this position is relatively large.

For elbow flexion, the maximum isometric torque created at the elbow joint is, on average, 7 kg•m for men and 3.5 kg•m for women. Overall, men are about 50% stronger than women and the dominant extremity is 5% to 10% stronger than the nondominant side (Table 2). Muscle force is greatest during flexion at joint positions between 90° and 110°. At elbow angles of 45° to 135°, only approximately 75% of the maximum elbow flexion strength is generated. Maximum flexion strength is generated in forearm supination. The mean pronation strength is 86% of supination. Most of the flexor torque occurs from the biceps, brachialis, and brachioradialis function.

The isometric force of the flexors is about 40% greater than the isometric force of the extensors. The maximum flexor muscle force per unit cross-sectional area is in the range of 10 to 14 kg/cm². About one third or one half of the maximum lifting force can be generated with the elbow in the extended or 30° flexed position. At these positions, a compressive force 3 times the body weight can be encountered in the elbow joint during strenuous lifting. Thus, the magnitude of the force crossing the elbow joint justifies consideration of the elbow as a weightbearing joint.

The distribution of force transmission on ulna and radius with the elbow extended and axially loaded is approximately 40% across the ulnohumeral joint and 60% across the radiohumeral joint. The greatest force transmission occurs between 0° and 30° of flexion, and it consistently decreases with increased flexion. Force transmission is also greater with the forearm in pronation (Fig. 23). The varus-valgus pivot point with the elbow extended is also noted to closely approximate the line of action of the brachial muscle, which crosses near the center of the lateral portion of the trochlea.

The orientation of the resultant joint force is quite sensitive to changes of the muscle force line of the upper arm muscles. The orientation of the resultant joint force moves from the central portion of the trochlea toward the rim as the direction of muscle pull relative to the forearm changes from perpendicular to parallel. The direction of force produced by the forearm muscles with respect to the trochlear notch, on the other hand, is relatively constant, so the direction of the resultant joint forces is reasonably constant. For example, when the forearm muscles (eg, brachioradialis) carry the dominant forces, the resultant joint force on the proximal ulna is consistently toward the rim of the coronoid process throughout the elbow flexion angle.

The average maximum torque strength for elbow extension is 4 kg•m for men and 2 kg•m for women. Although peak extension strength occurs between 60° and 140°, the 90° position generates the greatest isometric extension force. Elbow extension strength obtained from the pronated position is

Table 2

Isometric Elbow Strength of 104 Normal Subjects

		Men	Women	M − WM M	Dom − NonDom Dom
Flexion	Dom	725 ± 154	336 ± 80	0.54	
(Kg-cm)	Non	708 ± 156	323 ± 78	0.54	0.03
Extension	Dom	421 ± 109	210 ± 61	0.50	
(Kg-cm)	Non	406 ± 106	194 ± 50	0.52	0.04
Pronation	Dom	73 ± 18	36 ± 8	0.51	
(Kg-cm)	Non	68 ± 17	33 ± 10	0.51	0.07
Supination	Dom	91 ± 23	44 ± 12	0.52	
(Kg-cm)	Non	80 ± 21	41 ± 10	0.49	0.089
Grip	Dom	53 ± 12	30 ± 10	0.43	
(kg)	Non	51 ± 11	27 ± 9	0.47	0.06

Dom = Dominant; Non = Nondominant

(Reproduced with permission from Askew LJ, An KN, Morrey BF, Chao EYS: Isometric elbow strength in normal individuals. *Clin Orthop* 1987;222:261–266.)

significantly greater than that in the supinated position.

Measurements during forearm supination and pronation demonstrate a linear relationship between strength and forearm rotation. The greatest supination strength is generated from the pronated position; the converse is also true. The average torque of supination exceeds that of pronation by about 15% to 20% for men and women throughout the majority of shoulder-elbow positions. The average pronation and supination strengths for men are 80 and 90 kg·cm, respectively, and for women, 35 and 55 kg·cm, respectively. The difference between dominant and nondominant strength averages about 10%.

Structure and Function of the Hand and Wrist

The Hand

The 2 primary functions of the hand as an organ are touch and prehension. Prehension has been defined as the grasping or taking hold of an object between any 2 surfaces of the hand, or when an object is seized within the cup of the hand. Prehension may or may not include the thumb. The fundamental requirement of prehension is a firm grip. It is performed in different fashions according to the purpose of the grip, and it is described as either power grip or precision grip.

Power grip is defined as forceful finger flexion used to maintain an object against the palm. The ulnar 2 digits, which are innervated by the ulnar nerve, are more related to power grip; they provide support instead of control during power grip.

Precision grip requires fine kinesthetic control and usually is associated with fine tactile sensibility at the finger tips. It is formed by the clamp of the fingers and thumb, with the object held at the tips of the digits such that the palm is not involved. In this position, maximum sensation and speedy movement are available. The thumb, index, and middle fingers, which have medial nerve innervation, are more related to precision grip. This radial side of the hand has been referred to as the "dynamic tridactyl" and is concerned with balance, such as in holding a coffee cup.

Power and precision grips can be further differentiated according to the way that each grip is performed or by describing the individual phases composing the grip. Power grip involves the formation of a finger-palm vise and, therefore, has been described as proceeding through a sequence of 4 stages. The first 3 are dynamic; that is, during these stages muscles act to change the wrist and finger positions. Stage 1 consists of opening the hand; this is primarily a function of the long extensors and lumbricals. Stage 2 involves positioning of the fingers for closure about the object, and stage 3 is the actual finger closure to grasp the object. Stages 2 and 3 will be described in the finger kinetics section. Stage 4 involves the use of muscles to maintain the grip on the object; because there is no motion, this activity can be considered static. In this final static phase, the digits surround the object and maintain a flexed posture. In power grip, the palm is cupped and the fingers are flexed against the thenar eminence, producing an oblique grip at approximately 45° to the transverse axes of the hand. The obliquity is produced in part by the ulnar deviation and rotation of the digits at the metacarpophalangeal (MP) joints of the fingers together with flexion at the carpometacarpal (CMC) joints of the ring and little fingers. The thumb base provides the fixed buttress, with the thumb itself usually controlling the leverage of the object being gripped.

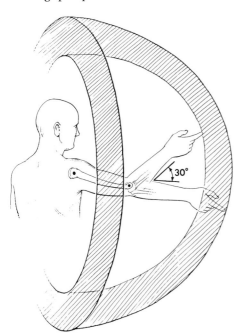

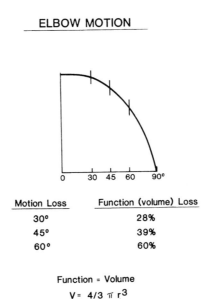

ELBOW MOTION

Motion Loss	Function (volume) Loss
30°	28%
45°	39%
60°	60%

Function = Volume

$$V = 4/3 \ \pi \ r^3$$

Figure 22

Restricted elbow motion limits the sphere of influence of the hand in space. Flexion contractures over 30° are associated with a rapid loss of effective reach area. (Reproduced with permission from An K-N, Morrey BF: Biomechanics, in Morrey BF, Chao EYS (eds): *Joint Replacement Arthroplasty*. New York, NY, Churchill Livingstone, 1991, p 261.)

The steps of precision grip are similar to the first 3 steps of power grip; however, it does not include a final static gripping phase that is either similar in appearance or prolonged in time. Rather, there is a constant alteration at the fingertips between static activity to grip the object and a dynamic component to manipulate the object. Hence, precision grip is often termed precision handling.

Power grip has been divided into 3 subtypes: cylindrical grip, spherical grip, and hooked grip (Fig. 24). Lateral prehension is also included under power grip because it involves a static holding phase.

In cylindrical grip, the hand makes a fist around a handle such as a baseball bat. The fingers are flexed with the thumb flexed over the index and middle fingers. This involves primarily function of the flexor digitorum profundus. The flexor digitorum sublimis and interosseous muscles assist when greater force is required. The interossei are important in providing MP flexion as well as abduction and rotation of the phalanges to accommodate the objects. The hypothenars are active and lock the little finger into positions. The flexor pollicis longus and thenars are active.

Spherical grip is used when gripping a baseball. It is similar to cylindrical grip except that there is greater spread at the fingers. MP joints are more abducted, resulting in more interosseous activity.

Hooked grip usually involves flexion of the proximal interphalangeal (PIP) joints of all the fingers, with an abducted thumb. This is the grip normally used to carry a suitcase and is specialized in that it can be maintained for long periods of time. It is the function, primarily, of the flexor digitorum profundus and superficialis muscles of the fingers. Thumb use is excluded.

In lateral prehension, between the fingers, the MP and interphalangeal (IP) joints of adjacent fingers are extended. Simultaneous abduction or adduction of the adjacent MP joints brings the digits together to produce a static holding phase such as that commonly used in holding a cigarette. This form of prehension is relatively weak. It is unique in that it is the only form of prehension in which the extensors play a role in sustaining posture.

Precision grip or handling requires finer control and sensibility using the radial digits; static holding is kept to a minimum. Precision grip is divided into 3 subtypes: pad-to-pad, tip-to-tip, and pad-to-side prehension (Fig. 25).

Pad-to-pad prehension involves true opposition of the pulp of the thumb to that of the fingers. It is commonly referred to as 2- or 3-point pinch or chuck pinch through opposition of the thumb to the index or index and middle fingers, respectively, and is responsible for nearly 80% of precision handling. The pulps of the fingers supinate when the MPs are flexed or the index finger is abducted for optimum opposition and function. Pad-to-pad prehension normally involves dynamic manipulation in which the volar and dorsal interossei work reciprocally to move the objects among the fingertips. This is in contrast to power grip in which the interossei work synergistically (at the same time).

Tip-to-tip prehension is the most precise of all the prehensions. It differs from pad-to-pad prehension in that there is full IP joint flexion of the fingers and thumb. The flexor digitorum profundus, the pollicis longus, and interosseous muscles are all active.

Pad-to-side prehension, also known as key pinch, involves an adducted and extended thumb opposed to the radial side of the index. It differs from other precision handling in that the thumb is more adducted and less rotated. There is increased activity of the flexor pollicis brevis and adductor pollicis with decreased activity in the opponens pollicis. Pad-to-side prehension has more power available than in the pulp-to-pulp pinch, but it is the least precise prehension.

Power grip force is applied primarily by the extrinsic mus-

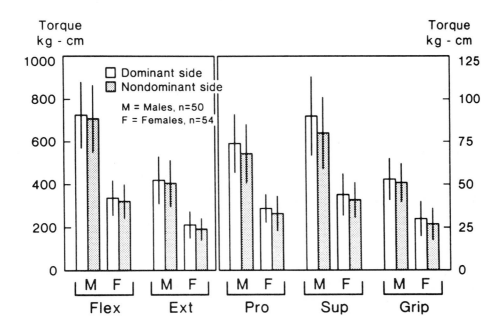

Figure 23

Isometric elbow strength in normal individuals. (Reproduced with permission from Morrey BF: Functional evaluation of the elbow, in Morrey BF (ed): *The Elbow and Its Disorders*, ed 2. Philadelphia, PA, WB Saunders, 1993.)

culature, with the flexors playing the major role. The interossei serve to act as MP joint flexors and rotators of the proximal phalanges. The lumbricals are not normally involved in power grip.

Precision handling also uses the extrinsic muscles to transmit force to the objects being grasped. However, the interossei act reciprocally to adduct and abduct the digits to rotate the objects at the fingertips. The lumbricals are active as are the extensors of the IP joints. Also, the thumb is motored primarily by the superficial 3 thenar muscles, which receive predominantly median nerve innervation as opposed to power grip, which usually involves the adductor pollicis and receives ulnar nerve innervation.

It is an important general principle to realize that, like many other places in the body during a coordinated functional movement, the flexors and extensors to the hand are in balanced opposition so that all hand movements are synergistic; that is, many muscles having opposing actions are active at the same time.

The extrinsic wrist and finger muscles, in a somewhat oversimplification, can be divided into 3 systems of agonist-

antagonist forces. The extensor carpi ulnaris muscle acting at the same time as the abductor pollicis longus and extensor pollicis brevis muscles prevents radial deviation of the wrist and allows the action of these muscles to be directed entirely to the thumb. The action of the extensor digitorum communis, the extensor indicis proprius, and extensor digiti minimi opposed by simultaneous activity of the flexor carpi radialis and flexor pollicis longus muscles allows finger extension without causing these muscles to dissipate energy in producing wrist extension. The third group of forces involve the extensor carpi radialis brevis and longus. These are antagonized by cocontractile activity of the flexor carpi ulnaris, preventing radial deviation with the occurrence of wrist extension.

Additionally, the extensor carpi radialis brevis and longus, functioning synergistically, cocontract with the flexor digitorum profundus and superficialis muscles. Because the wrist's position optimizes the power of finger flexors through its tenodesis effect, maintaining extension of the wrist through this cocontraction enhances the excursion of the long flexor tendons required for efficient flexion of the fingers.

Optimal hand function is, therefore, the result of mobile balance of the wrist and fingers with their respective muscles. Motions occur around variable axes to facilitate precise positioning of the digits for prehension. Optimal hand function thus requires a complex interaction between the wrist, thumb, and fingers. Each of these 3 components will

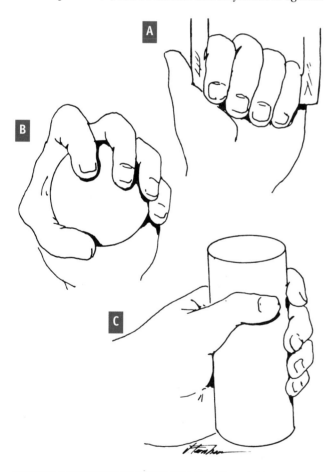

Figure 24

Power grip: hook grip (**A**), spherical grip (**B**), and cylindrical grip (**C**). (Reproduced with permission from Norkin C, Le Vangie P: *Joint Structure and Function: A Comprehensive Analysis*. Philadelphia, PA, FA Davis, 1990, p 243.)

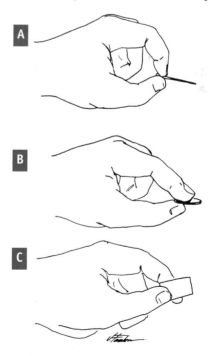

Figure 25

Precision grip or handling: tip-to-tip prehension (**A**), pad-to-pad prehension (**B**), and pad-to-side prehension (**C**). (Reproduced with permission from Norkin C, Le Vangie P: *Joint Structure and Function: A Comprehensive Analysis*. Philadelphia, PA, FA Davis, 1990, p 243.)

be addressed separately below for the ease of discussion. However, it must be emphasized that their functions are quite integrated and are difficult to separate clinically. Included within each section is a description of wrist and hand anatomy so essential to the comprehension of wrist and hand kinematics and kinetics. Because the scope of this section is limited, only the relevant anatomy is reviewed.

The Wrist

The wrist or carpus provides a stable support for the hand, allowing for the transmission of grip forces as well as positioning of the hand and digits for fine movements. The main function of the wrist is to fine-tune grasp by controlling the length-tension relationship in the extrinsic muscles to the hand. For example, the self-selected wrist position for maximal power grip has been shown to be 35° of extension with 7° of ulnar deviation. Furthermore, full wrist flexion reduces the efficiency of the finger flexors and the grip strength to 25% of that available when the wrist is in extension. Martial arts experts have used this finding for a long time to disarm assailants. When the wrist is positioned in flexion, the combination of a passive extensor tenodesis effect, increasing resistance to flexion, and decreasing excursion of the flexors results in a weakened grip. The assailant, therefore, is unable to maintain a grip on the weapon.

Wrist Stability

Traditionally, the carpal bones are described as being arranged in 2 anatomic rows. The proximal carpal row consists of the scaphoid, lunate, and triquetrum, and the distal row is formed by the trapezium, trapezoid, capitate, and hamate. The pisiform lies within the flexor carpi ulnaris tendon and, through its articulation with the trapezium, functions as a sesamoid; therefore, it is not included as a functional member of the proximal carpal row. The scaphoid links the proximal and distal rows. Both rows move with respect to each other in the midcarpal joint, and the proximal row moves on the radius in the radiocarpal joint.

The carpus may also be considered in terms of 3 functional columns (Fig. 26). The central or flexion-extension column is formed by the distal carpal row and the lunate. This column functions as a longitudinal link between the radius and metacarpals and its integrity depends on the carpal ligaments because the muscles that produce wrist motion attach distal to the central column. The lateral or mobile column is the scaphoid. The medial or rotational column is the triquetrum.

The arrangement of the carpal bones and their ligaments is crucial to wrist stability. The 2 carpal rows articulate to form the midcarpal joint, which consists of 3 different types of articular surfaces. On the radial side, the trapezium and trapezoid (of the distal row) are concave with their articulations to the distal scaphoid and lateral capitate. The head of the capitate in the center of the midcarpal joint is convex.

The ulnar-sided hamate-triquetral articulation is helicoid in nature.

The proximal carpal row has a single biconvex joint surface that articulates with a shallower, concave distal radius with 2 facets and a triangular fibrocartilage complex. The radiocarpal joint, therefore, appears relatively incongruent. The distal radius has an average of 14° of palmar tilt, and 22° of radial inclination. This structure probably contributes to the limitation of motion such that flexion is greater than extension and ulnar deviation greater than radial deviation. The radial articular surface of the wrist affords no real bony stability; stability is provided primarily by the soft-tissue envelope of the wrist.

Ligaments are the primary stabilizers of the wrist. They usually are classified into palmar and dorsal ligaments as well as extrinsic and intrinsic ligaments (Fig. 27). The palmar ligaments, which are more numerous and substantial than the dorsal ligaments and are considered the principle stabilizers of the wrist, function principally to resist hyperextension forces. The majority of the extrinsic ligaments, which arise from the radius and ulna and attach to the carpus, insert on the proximal carpal row. The important extrinsic ligaments are the radioscaphocapitate, radiolunotriquetral, and ulnolunate. The radioscapholunate ligament is relatively thin and offers little stability, but contains blood vessels. The palmar and dorsal radiocarpal ligaments are obliquely oriented to resist the tendency of the proximal carpal row to slide down the palmar and ulnar inclined surface of the distal radius.

The intrinsic ligaments originate and insert on the carpus. The scapholunate ligament and the lunotriquetral ligament

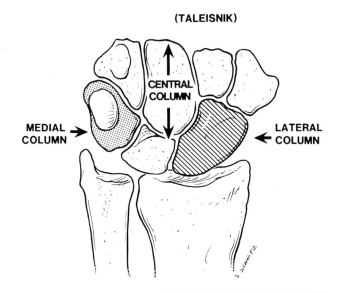

Figure 26

Three columns of the wrist with the bones in each are as follows: central, lunate and entire distal carpal row; lateral, scaphoid; and medial, triquetrum. (Reproduced with permission from *Regional Review Courses in Hand Surgery,* ed 4. Aurora, CO, American Society for Surgery of the Hand, 1991.)

are important links in the proximal carpal row and provide additional stability to the wrist.

The stability provided by the volar intrinsic and extrinsic ligaments may be best described by the double V configuration that they form (Fig. 28). The arcuate ligaments, consisting of the radioscaphocapitate and ulnocapitate ligaments, converge on the capitate to form the distal V. The proximal V is formed by the radiolunotriquetral, radioscaphoid, ulnolunate, and ulnotriquetral ligaments. With ulnar deviation, the proximal V changes to an L configuration. The ulnolunate ligament assumes a more transverse orientation to essentially limit lunate displacement, and the radiolunate ligament assumes a more longitudinal configuration to limit lunate extension. The distal V ligamentous configuration similarly assumes an L configuration, but in the opposite direction. The scaphocapitate ligament becomes transverse to limit ulnar translation of the capitate, and the triquetral capitate ligament assumes a longitudinal configuration to prevent capitate flexion. The opposite is believed to occur in radial deviation.

In addition to creating movement, the extrinsic muscles of the wrist offer a dynamic component to wrist stability. There are 6 dedicated wrist muscles: the extensor carpi radialis brevis and longus, extensor carpi ulnaris, flexor carpi radialis, flexor carpi ulnaris, and palmaris longus muscles. The extensor carpi radialis brevis and longus are usually considered in combination, and there is agreement that together they generate the largest fraction of wrist extension torque. The extensor carpi radialis brevis is the key extensor of the wrist. It inserts onto the base of the third metacarpal and is essentially a pure wrist extensor that has a minimal radial deviation moment. Although the tendon of the extensor carpi radialis brevis has a larger extension moment than that of the extensor carpi radialis longus, there is some controversy about which generates greater overall torque. This controversy exists because the extensor carpi radialis longus inserts onto the second metacarpal, and some of the torque it produces generates a radial deviation moment along with an extension moment. When the radial deviation force of the extensor carpi radialis longus is balanced by the extensor carpi ulnaris, some consider this combination of muscles to be the most effective manner of producing wrist extension.

The extensor carpi ulnaris tendon is unique in that its fulcrum and moment arm relative to the ulna are fixed by the extensor compartment; it thus maintains a relatively con-

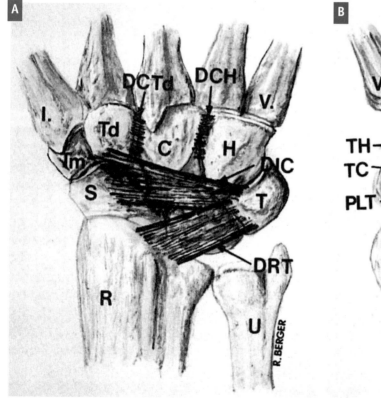
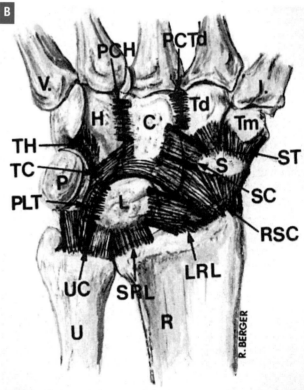

Figure 27

A, Extrinsic ligaments of the wrist (dorsal): dorsal intercarpal ligament (DIC) and dorsal radiotriquetral ligament (DRT). **B,** Extrinsic ligaments of the wrist (volar): scaphotrapezial (ST), radioscaphocapitate (RSC), scaphocapitate (SC), long radiolunate (LRL), short radiolunate (SRL), ulnocarpal (UC), palmar lunotriquetral (PLT), triquetral-capitate (TC), triquetral-hamate (TH), lunate (L), scaphoid (S), pisiform (P). Trapezium (Tm), trapezoid (Td), capitate (C), hamate (H), scaphoid (S), triquetrum (T). (Reproduced with permission from Cooney WP III, Linscheid RL, Dobyns JH: Fractures and dislocations of the wrist, in Rockwood CA Jr, Green DP, Bucholz RW (eds): *Rockwood and Green's Fractures in Adults*, ed 3. Philadelphia, PA, JB Lippincott, 1991, p 564.)

stant relationship and is also an important stabilizer of the ulnar head. It is felt to be an effective wrist extensor only when the wrist is supinated, because, in pronation, the extensor carpi ulnaris tendon lies lateral to the carpus and provides an ulnar deviation moment.

The flexor carpi ulnaris is a flexor and ulnar deviator of the wrist. It inserts into the pisiform with an extension into the hook of the hamate. The intratendinous pisiform functions as a sesamoid to increase the flexion and extension moments, thus allowing the flexor carpi ulnaris to achieve the highest tension of any muscle crossing the wrist, with the least excursion. This is the muscle that powers karate chops and hammer strokes, as well as resisting the radial deviation forces produced by firing a handgun. Its ulnar deviation forces are second only to those of the extensor carpi ulnaris in a pronated wrist.

The flexor carpi radialis, through its insertion onto the base of the second metacarpal, flexes the wrist and is also active during radial deviation. It is approximately 60% as strong as the flexor carpi ulnaris.

The palmaris longus is a pure, but relatively weak, wrist flexor. It is absent in approximately 15% of the population. Its insertion into the palmar fascia often spreads over the thenars and may assist in thumb abduction. The wrist flexors, as a group, have approximately greater than twice the work capacity of the extensors (Table 3).

The long flexors and extensors of the fingers and thumb are secondary wrist muscles. To effect motion at the wrist, these muscles depend on the antagonistic forces to prevent their action on distal joints.

Wrist Kinematics

Although the wrist is usually described as having 3 degrees of freedom with flexion-extension rotational movement, radioulnar deviation, and pronosupination, these isolated movements do not occur around three fixed mutually perpendicular axes. The primary axis of motion is an oblique screw axis within the head of the capitate (Fig. 29).

The average amount of flexion-extension motion of the wrist is variable (Table 4) with a range of 84° to 169° and an average of 140°. The average range of flexion is 65° to 80° and of extension, 55° to 75°. Flexion usually exceeds extension by approximately 10°. The average combined radioulnar deviation is 65°, with a range of 15° to 25° of radial deviation and 30° to 45° of ulnar deviation. At rest, there is physiologic ulnar deviation of the wrist. The average arc of pronation-supination is 150° with a pronation range of 60° to 80° and a supination range of 60° to 85°. For most activities of daily living, the functional range of motion for the wrist is 5° to 40° of flexion, 30° to 40° of extension, and 10° of radial deviation to 15° to 30° of ulnar deviation.

Studies have shown that there appears to be less than 12° of intercarpal motion among the distal carpal row, supporting the theory that this row can be viewed as a single functional unit. Intercarpal motion between the scaphoid and lunate has been shown to range between 24° and 34°. Similarly, motion between the lunate and triquetrum has been shown to range between 12° and 18°. This mobile proximal carpal row, with its lack of tendon or muscle attachments, is

Table 3
Relative Muscle Power

Muscle	Relative Power
Flexor digitorum pollicis	4.5
Flexor carpi ulnaris, brachioradialis, extensor digitorum communis	2.0
Palmaris, flexor pollicis longus, extensor carpi ulnaris, extensor carpi radialis longus	1.1
Extensor carpi radialis brevis, flexor carpi ulnaris, flexor carpi radialis	0.9
Palmaris longus, abductor pollicis longus	0.1

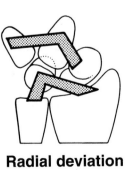

Radial deviation

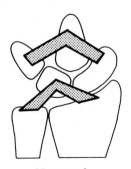
Neutral

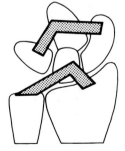
Ulnar deviation

Figure 28

Diagrammatic representation of changes in orientation of palmar radiocarpal ligaments. (Illustration by Elizabeth Roselius, © 1985. Reproduced with permission from Taleisnik J: *The Wrist*. New York, NY, Churchill Livingstone, 1985, p 26.)

an intercalated segment, which readily responds to transmitted angular forces from the more rigid distal row and CMC joints where the wrist muscles attach at the metacarpal bases. The row's stability depends on the complex ligament structure and articular surface contours described above. With flexion-extension motion (Fig. 30), there is synchronous angulation of each carpal row in the same direction. The radiocarpal joint contributes 66% of wrist extension with 34% from the intercarpal joint. With flexion, the radiocarpal joint contributes 40%, with 60% at the intercarpal joint.

As a result of the relative strength of the wrist extensors and flexors, the wrist does not normally move on a single axis of flexion and extension in respect to the forearm; instead, it rotates about an axis creating dorsal-radial extension to the ulnar-palmar flexion axis. This motion is described as a dart-thrower's motion. Flexion and extension are closely integrated with radial and ulnar deviation in the wrist, and their separation in describing the kine-

matics of the wrist is somewhat of an oversimplification.

All the primary muscles of the wrist except the flexor carpi ulnaris are attached to the metacarpals. It is hypothesized that the mechanism of flexion-extension of the wrist is initiated at the distal carpal row. In proceeding from flexion to extension, the distal carpal row rotates on the proximal row. At neutral, the radioscaphocapitate ligament is thought to functionally link the scaphoid with the distal carpal row so that they move as a unit. With further extension, the intercarpal ligament brings the scapholunate joint into a closed packed position so that the entire distal and proximal rows now essentially move as one. Further extension then proceeds at the radiocarpal joint. The reverse occurs in proceeding from extension to flexion. The scaphoid travels through an arc of about 40° during flexion and extension. This motion exemplifies how the scaphoid is a link between the proximal and distal rows.

A similar complex interaction between the proximal and carpal distal rows occurs with radioulnar deviation. During

Table 4
Range of Motion (Axis Middle Finger)

Motion*	Wrist	Finger	Thumb
Extension**	55°–75°		
MP		30°–45°	0°
PIP		0°	
DIP		10°–20°	
CMC			0°
IP			0°–20°
Flexion	65°–80°		
MP		85°–100°	0°–90°
PIP		100°–115°	
DIP		80°–90°	
CMC			44°–70°
IP			85°–90°
Ulnar deviation	30°–45°		
Radial deviation	15°–25°		
Supination	60°–85°		
Pronation	60°–80°		
Abduction/adduction		20°–60°/0°	
Palmar abduction			
CMC			40°–70°
MP			0°–20°
Dorsal adduction			
CMC			0°–30°
MP			0°
Axial rotation			
CMC			17°–20°

MP = metacarpophalangeal; PIP = proximal interphalangeal; DIP = distal interphalangeal; CMC = carpometacarpal; IP = interphalangeal

** Thumb extension is radial abduction

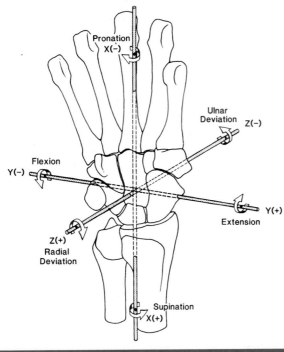

Figure 29

A coordinate system to describe the screw axis of the wrist, which passes through the head of the capitate for flexion Y(-) and extension Y(+); radial deviation Z(+) and ulnar deviation Z(-); and pronation X(-) and supination X(+). (Reproduced with permission from Cooney WP III, Linscheid RL, Dobyns JH: Fractures and dislocations of the wrist, in Rockwood CA Jr, Green DP, Bucholz RW (eds): *Rockwood and Green's Fractures in Adults*, ed 3. Philadelphia, PA, JB Lippincott, 1991, p 564.)

radioulnar deviation, each carpal row demonstrates not only synchronous motion in the AP/coronal plane, but also conjoint rotation in the sagittal plane (Fig. 30). In radial deviation (Fig. 31, *B*), the obliquely oriented scaphoid flexes as the trapezium approaches the radius. During the return towards full ulnar deviation, the proximal row extends, including the scaphoid. More importantly, the hamate migrates proximally forcing the triquetrum to displace volarly and extend the lunate. This variable geometry of the proximal carpal row, which includes varying length and contour, allows for the excursion of the wrist with longitudinal stability. During radial deviation, there is primarily intercarpal motion with the distal row moving radially and negligible proximal row motion ulnarly. During ulnar deviation (Fig. 31, *A*), there is both intercarpal and radiocarpal motion, with the distal row moving ulnarly and the proximal row radially. In proceeding from ulnar deviation to radial deviation, the distal carpal row rotates in a radial direction and translates from a dorsal to a palmar direction. Simultaneously, the proximal carpal row flexes and, in a reciprocal motion, slides ulnarly on the distal radioulnar joint.

One theory holds that with radial deviation, the scaphoid initiates movement of the proximal carpal row. It flexes to avoid impingement against the radial styloid and, thus, allows greater motion. The remaining carpals of the proximal row follow in flexion by virtue of their intercarpal ligamentous attachments. The second theory holds that motion proceeds from the ulnar side of the wrist at the triquetral-hamate joint with radioulnar deviation. With radial deviation, the tri-

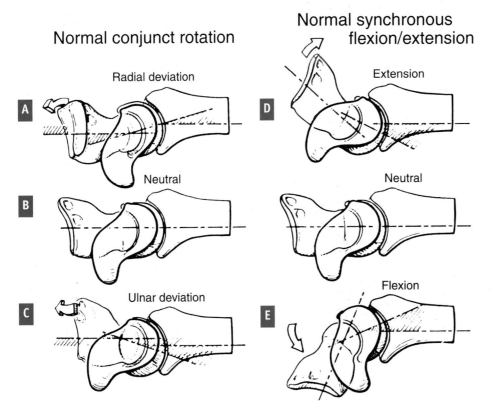

Figure 30

Conjunct rotation of the proximal carpal row occurs in flexion during radial deviation (**A**). The axes of the radius and carpal rows are colinear in neutral (**B**), and the proximal row extends with ulnar deviation (**C**). Angulatory excursions of the proximal and distal rows are essentially equal in amplitude and direction during extension (**D**) and flexion (**E**). This may be described as synchronous angulation. (Reproduced with permission from Cooney WP III, Linscheid RL, Dobyns JH: Fractures and dislocations of the wrist, in Rockwood CA Jr, Green DP, Bucholz RW (eds): *Rockwood and Green's Fractures in Adults,* ed 3. Philadelphia, PA, JB Lippincott, 1991, p 578.)

quetrum is felt to slide radially, dorsally, and proximally through its articulation with the hamate. Through its intercarpal attachment, the lunate flexes followed by the scaphoid. The reverse occurs with ulnar deviation. The triquetrum slides palmarly only distal on the hamate accompanied by lunate and scaphoid extension. The proximal carpal row as a whole slides on the radial carpal joint in a direction opposite that of the hand movement.

While 90% of the pronation-supination motion occurs in the forearm, the remaining 10% (15°) is divided between the radiocarpal and intercarpal motion.

Wrist Kinetics

To further understand the kinematics of the wrist, a tendon-shift mechanism has been described in which the wrist continuously rebalances its flexion and extension forces by controlling their moment arms. As previously noted, the axis of motion of the wrist is normally from extension with radial deviation to flexion with ulnar deviation. With radial deviation, the scaphoid flexes to increase the diameter on the radial side of the wrist. As the scaphoid flexes, the distal pole acts as a pulley to increase the moment arm of the flexor carpi radialis tendon. This action optimizes the force for return from extension and radial deviation to flexion. With ulnar deviation, the scaphoid extends and the wrist AP diameter decreases on the radial side. The flexed proximal carpal row and radius form a convex pulley over which the extensors pass (Fig. 32). The extensors are thus moved away from the wrist, increasing their moment arm for return to extension. The tendon-shift mechanism ensures large moment arms by maintaining a given distance between the flexors and extensors, thereby ensuring optimal wrist stability and function.

To further this concept, with radial deviation-extension the flexed scaphoid distal pole forms a pulley for the finger flexors to create a moment for return to ulnar deviation (Fig. 33). The hook of the hamate similarly forms a pulley for the finger flexors when the wrist is ulnarly deviated. This tendon-shift mechanism would be disturbed by limited carpal fusions, proximal row carpectomies, or other surgeries that alter normal carpal movement.

The distal radius in the ulnar neutral wrist normally bears about 80% to 85% of the load across the distal radioulnar carpal complex and the distal ulna, 15% to 20%. Of the force transmitted across the radiocarpal joint, 46% to 50% of total radioulnar carpal complex force has been shown to be transmitted by the radioscaphoid fossa and the remaining 30% to 35% by the radiolunate fossa. The amount of force transmitted across the lunate fossa can be increased, and a slight increase can be produced in ulnocarpal force through ulnar deviation of the wrist. The ulnocarpal force also increases with the increase in the ulnar variance associated with forearm pronation.

The triangular fibrocartilage complex (TFCC) essentially serves as a spacer between the distal ulna and carpus. An inverse linear relationship between ulnar variance and the thickness of the TFCC has been demonstrated. Forced transmission through the distal ulna changes significantly only when two thirds or more of the horizontal portion of the TFCC is excised. Therefore, partial TFCC debridement or excision is recommended in central perforations.

The total surface area of the radiocarpal joint from the carpal aspect ranges from 320 to 480 mm². The lunate fossa accounts for 46%, the scaphoid fossa for 43%, and the TFCC for 11% of the area. The contact area of the radiocarpal joint covers only approximately 20.6% of the total joint surface, with a range from 14% in radial deviation, pronation, and either neutral or 20° of flexion to 32% in radial deviation, supination, and 20° of extension. The separate and distinct scaphoid contact area is 1.47 times that of the lunate. The scaphoid contact area generally is greatest in ulnar deviation, when the scaphoid is vertical. The scaphoid-lunate contact area ratio usually increases as the wrist moves from radial to ulnar deviation and/or flexion to extension. The contact area is palmar when the wrist is in flexion and dorsal when the

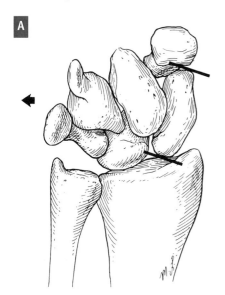
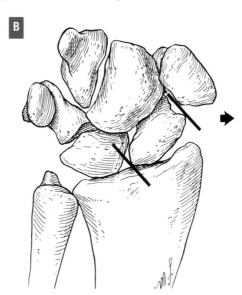

Figure 31

Scaphoid displacement. **A,** Extension with ulnar deviation. **B,** Flexion with radial deviation. (Reproduced with permission from *Regional Review Courses in Hand Surgery,* ed 4. Aurora, CO, American Society for Surgery of the Hand, 1991.)

wrist is in extension at 40°, but initially from 20° of flexion to 20° of extension, the contact area shifts palmarly. The area will increase to a maximum of 40% of the available articular surface with increasing pressure. In a similar fashion, the midcarpal joint pressure contact area covers an average of 8%, up to a maximum of 15%, of the available contact area. Of this area, approximately 50% proceeds on a path from the capitate to its articulations with the scaphoid and the lunate.

Carpal instabilities can significantly alter the joint contact areas and pressures. A scapholunate dissociation with an associated dorsal intercalated segmental instability deformity and palmar flexed scaphoid will result in decreased joint contact area and increased scaphoid fossa pressure. However, the lunotriquetral dissociations that have an associated palmar intercalated segmental instability are not significantly altered for the pressure distribution in the radiocarpal joint. This fact is consistent with the clinical course of this instability.

Similarly, limited intercarpal fusions for these disorders change force transmission. Scaphotrapezial-trapezoid and scaphocapitate fusions transfer loads to the scaphoid fossa. The scaphoid essentially acts as a component at the distal carpal row and is unable to flex or extend with radial and ulnar deviation. This results in increased compressive stresses at the radiocarpal joint with radial deviation that leads to assumed degenerative changes. In ulnar deviation, these limited intercarpal fusions produce a tensile stress on the scapholunate ligament, resulting in increased gapping between the scaphoid and lunate. This gapping is caused by the inability of the scaphoid to extend. Scapholunate, scapholunocapitate, and capitolunate intercarpal fusions all have less effect on load distributions at the radial carpal

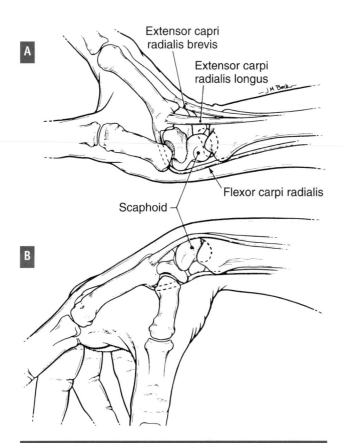

Figure 32

A, The wrist extensors bowstring for maximal extensor moment arms while the vertical scaphoid carries the flexor carpi radialis (FCR) tendon palmarward with the radial side of the carpus. **B,** Wrist flexion creates a "convex pulley" from the combined shape of the distal radius and the repositioning of the scaphoid. This convex pulley lifts the radial wrist extensor tendons to preserve their moment arms for the return cycle into wrist extension. Simultaneously, the repositioned scaphoid moves the FCR tendon dorsally, shortening its moment arm to complement hand opening, precision digital functions, and so forth. (Reproduced with permission from Brand PW, Hollister A: *Clinical Mechanisms of the Hand*, ed 2. St. Louis, MO, CV Mosby, 1993.)

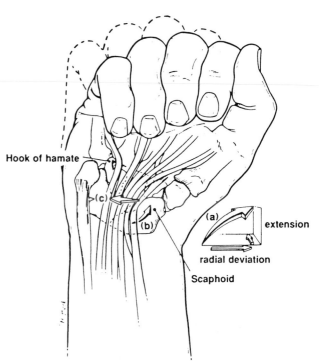

Figure 33

Radial deviation in extension (a) positions the scaphoid as a vertical "finger" of bone to define the dorsal radial wall of the carpal tunnel as a fulcrum for the digital flexor tendons. By actively sweeping into a vertical position (b), it displaces all 9 digital flexor tendons toward the palmar ulnar border of the wrist (c), thereby widely separating the wrist flexion effect of the digital flexors from the radial wrist extensor tendons. Wide separation of the high tension forces transmitted by these tendons is an essential element in creating the stable wrist necessary for forceful grasp by the digits. (Reproduced with permission from Brand PW, Hollister A: *Clinical Mechanisms of the Hand*, ed 2. St. Louis, MO, CV Mosby, 1993.)

joint, but still are not entirely normal. Load distribution is further affected by the relative position at which the carpals are fused. On the other hand, alteration of load transmission across the radiocarpal joint may be desirable. Joint leveling by radial shortening or ulnar lengthening is a viable treatment option in the Kienböck's disease associated with a negative ulnar variant. Two and one half millimeters of ulnar lengthening have been shown to increase the ulnar load to 42%. The remaining 58% of the load transmission across the radiocarpal joint is redistributed to increase pressure across the radioscaphoid joint and decrease the pressure across the radiolunate facet.

Experimentally, the total transmitted force though the radiolunate joint can be significantly decreased by an average of 45% by a joint leveling procedure. Although this procedure results in an increased force through the TFCC, the radioscaphoid joint slightly increases and the lunocapitate force decreases to about 13% of the normally transmitted force. Reciprocally, when distal ulnar decompression is needed, ulnar shortening of 2.5 mm results in a decrease from an average of 20% to 4% of the total radioulnar force.

The Thumb

The thumb is undeniably the most important digit on the hand because of its ability to oppose the fingers as a result of its movable metacarpal.

Kinematics and Joint Stability

The thumb ray is thought to start with the trapezium and its articulation with the first metacarpal because there is no significant motion among the carpals with thumb motion. The flexion-extension plane of motion for the thumb is described as being approximately parallel to the palm. Flexion is motion toward the hypothenar eminence, whereas palmar abduction-adduction occurs in a plane perpendicular to the flexion-extension plane. The trapeziometacarpal joint allows approximately 45° to 70° of flexion, accompanied by some pronation. Overall thumb motion also includes approximately 0° to 30° of adduction to 40° to 70° of palmar abduction. The palmar abduction is divided between the CMC joint with an average of 42° and the MP joint with a range of 0° to 20°.

Thumb opposition consists of the composite motions of abduction, which lifts the thumb away from the hand, and rotation of the thumb into pronation. Thumb pronation is rotation of the thumb so that the pulp surfaces of the thumb and fingers face one another. Opposition occurs as a unit involving the IP, MP, and trapeziometacarpal joints, and sequentially proceeds through abduction, flexion, and adduction accompanied by simultaneous pronation. The motion of the thumb forms a cone. The rotation is not around the axis of the first metacarpal, but is the result of an arc around a central point in the palm. It is this swinging movement in abduction that is used to draw the thumb in front of the palm and then hold an object between the thumb and finger. Full opposition proceeds approximately through 110° from full extension to complete abduction-flexion and rotation. Opposition occurs primarily at the trapeziometacarpal joint, making it the most important joint in the hand.

The trapezium is angled volarly; placing the rest of the thumb in a position palmar to the plane of the hand. In a resting position, the first metacarpal then forms an angle of approximately 45° to 60° with the second metacarpal.

The trapeziometacarpal joint is a double-saddle configuration with a ridge on the surface of the trapezium; it is concave in one plane and convex in another. This geometry permits primarily 2 degrees of freedom, flexion-extension and abduction-adduction; however, with distraction an average of 17° of axial rotation occurs. The prime stabilizer of the trapeziometacarpal joint is the anterior-oblique ligament, which is taut in abduction, extension, and pronation. The first intermetacarpal, ulnar-collateral, and posterior-oblique ligaments make up the secondary stabilizers. The dorsal-radial facet provides the main resistance to dorsal subluxation and becomes eroded early in degenerative arthritis.

The MP joint of the thumb has a condylar configuration with 2 degrees of freedom. It has variable flexion-extension ranging from 0° to 90° and an average flexion of 55°. Although these motions at the MP joint aid in opposition, if MP joint motion is lost or the joint is fused, the adjacent joints in the thumb will compensate. Similarly, if the CMC joint is lost or fixed in an opposed position, the MP joint, having good intrinsic control, can take over as the prime mobile joint. The MP joint is statically stabilized by the collateral ligaments and volar plate. In addition, the thenar intrinsics, by inserting onto the 2 sesamoids and the extensor mechanism, provide dynamic restraints to hyperextension and excessive abduction and adduction.

The IP joint is a true hinge joint with 1 degree of freedom. It is similarly stabilized by a volar plate and 2 collateral ligaments. It allows an average of 85° to 90° of flexion, which is accompanied by slight pronation. The joint also allows an average of 0° to 20° of hyperextension to increase the surface area of the thumb pad available to pinch.

Kinetics

The thumb is powered by 4 extrinsic and 4 intrinsic muscles. The extrinsic muscles consist of the abductor pollicis longus, extensor pollicis brevis, extensor pollicis longus, and flexor pollicis longus. Excluding the flexor pollicis longus, the main function of these extrinsic muscles is to retrieve the position of the thumb from the opposed position in the palm. The abductor pollicis longus tendon inserts by a variable number of tendinous slips into the base of the first metacarpal. There is approximately an 80% occurrence of multiple slips. This tendon acts as a dynamic stabilizer of the CMC joint when the thumb metacarpal is adducted. With reference to the plane of thumb motion, the abductor pollicis longus primarily extends the first metacarpal, but its direction of pull also allows it to flex the wrist.

The extensor pollicis brevis inserts into the dorsal base of the proximal phalanx. Its action is to extend the proximal phalanx and secondarily abduct the thumb. The extensor pollicis brevis is always narrower than the abductor pollicis longus and is absent in 5% to 7% of people. Both the extensor pollicis brevis and abductor pollicis longus will assist in radial deviation of the wrist. The extensor carpi ulnaris normally functions synergistically with these two muscles to prevent radial deviation of the wrist and allow strong function of the thumb.

The extensor pollicis longus inserts into the base of the distal phalanx to extend the IP joint. On continued action, the extensor pollicis longus will extend the proximal phalanx, metacarpal, and wrist. The extensor pollicis longus is the most powerful of the 3 extrinsic muscles inserting on the dorsum of the thumb; its unique position around Lister's tubercle allows it to secondarily adduct the thumb. The extensor pollicis longus primarily positions the thumb in extension to produce a flat, open hand such as is used in clapping, slapping, or pushing. This muscle's secondary actions of adduction and supination make it the direct antagonist to opposition. It is important to note that all 3 dorsal extrinsics (abductor pollicis longus, extensor pollicis brevis, and extensor pollicis longus) also supinate or rotate the pulp surface of the thumb away from the finger pulp surfaces, so that the thumb pulp faces flat and parallel with the palm surface.

The flexor pollicis longus is the only extrinsic muscle on the flexor surface of the thumb. It inserts into the base of the distal phalanx, and it not only flexes the IP joint, but also flexes and adducts the first metacarpal. It is the strongest of the extrinsic muscles and provides power to thumb flexion once the thenar muscles have set the direction.

The 4 intrinsic muscles, collectively referred to as the thenar muscles, include the abductor pollicis brevis, opponens pollicis, flexor pollicis brevis, and the adductor pollicis. They may best be viewed as a fan of muscles originating from the carpals, metacarpals, and the transverse carpal ligament and inserting on the thumb to produce a continuum of motion from flexion-abduction to the stronger flexion-adduction. The thenar muscles are primarily responsible for producing opposition of the thumb.

There is extensive interaction between the muscles of the thumb to facilitate opposition. The abductor pollicis longus, extensor pollicis brevis, abductor pollicis brevis, and opponens pollicis work in conjunction to open the first web space. The addition of the extensor pollicis longus further opens the thumb. The extrinsics (abductor pollicis brevis, extensor pollicis brevis, and extensor pollicis longus) are responsible primarily for repositioning the thumb by extension and supination away from the palm. The intrinsics (abductor pollicis brevis and opponens pol-

licis) serve to position the thumb in abduction and pronation with the maximally functional force of the flexor pollicis brevis.

The activity of each of the thumb muscles varies with the force of opposition. With simple opposition in which the thumb gently contacts the finger, the activity of the opponens pollicis predominates followed by that of the abductor pollicis brevis, and then the flexor pollicis brevis. In forced opposition against the index and middle fingers, the activity of the flexor pollicis brevis exceeds that of the opponens pollicis. However, activity of the opponens pollicis increases to approximately equal that of the flexor pollicis brevis, as opposition proceeds ulnarly toward the little finger, because of the increased requirement for thumb metacarpal abduction and pronation.

Similarly, adductor pollicis activity increases as resistance increases and as opposition progresses toward the ulnar digits. With further resisted opposition, the extrinsics (flexor pollicis longus, abductor pollicis brevis, extensor pollicis brevis, and extensor pollicis longus) assist the maximal joint control of the thenars. Thumb involvement in power grip can be distinguished from that during precision handling by high activity of the adductor pollicis. The limiting factor in grip strength may be related to the ability of the thumb to oppose loads. Thumb position is most variable during cylindrical grip. In hooked grip, thumb use is excluded.

During simple pinch, it has been shown that compressive forces averaging 3, 5.4, and 12 kg develop in the IP, MP, and CMC joints of the thumb, respectively. During power grip, however, the compressive force in the thumb's CMC joint can increase up to tenfold. Average grip strength is 50 to 53 kg and 25 to 30 kg in men and women, respectively; 3 point pinch strengths are 8 kg for men and 5 kg for women. Grip and pinch strengths required for activities of daily living are 4 kg and 1 kg, respectively. This may be significant in the predilection of this joint to osteoarthritis.

The abductor pollicis brevis is the most important muscle of opposition and weakest of the thenars. Through its insertion into the radial side of the proximal phalanx, lateral MP joint capsule, and extensor apparatus, the abductor pollicis brevis functions to abduct and flex the first metacarpal, slightly flex the proximal phalanx, and extend the IP joint. It acts to position the thumb for function.

The opponens pollicis inserts into the radial side of the metacarpal and is the only thenar to insert on the metacarpal. It positions the metacarpal by means of abduction, flexion, and slight pronation.

The flexor pollicis brevis consists of 2 parts: (1) a superficial head innervated by the median nerve and inserting via the radial sesamoid into the radial base of the proximal phalanx and extensor apparatus; and (2) a deep-ulnar head innervated by the ulnar nerve and inserting into the ulnar base of the proximal phalanx. The action of the flexor pollicis brevis is to flex the metacarpal and proximal phalanx and, through the insertion on the extensor apparatus, to extend the IP joint. Secondarily, it assists in adduction and, with the thumb in a flexed position, provides slight pronation. The flexor pollicis brevis adds power to both forced opposition and abduction.

The adductor pollicis muscle usually assists in reinforcing grip. It has 2 heads (transverse and oblique) that converge and insert via the ulnar sesamoid into the ulnar aspect of the volar plate and proximal phalanx. It acts to adduct the metacarpal and slightly flex the MP joint. By its aponeurosis inserting into the dorsal extensor mechanism, the adductor pollicis muscle also contributes to IP joint extension.

The Fingers

Kinematics and Joint Stability

Each of the 4 finger rays is composed of a metacarpal, its 3 phalanges, and their interposed articulations.

The metacarpals themselves provide a space, in length and width, to allow objects of size to be grasped. Palmar cupping allows the hand to conform to objects to increase the surface area of contact and improve application of gripping forces. This cupping is made possible by 3 arches of the hand. A longitudinal arch is formed by the metacarpals and flexed fingers. This arch is supplemented by 2 transverse arches. The first is a relatively immobile structural arch, formed by the carpals and supported by the transverse carpal ligament. The second transverse arch is distal, is formed by the metacarpal heads, and allows the hand to have greater adaptability. The progressive motion of the ulnar digits, along with the hypothenar muscles, flex and adduct the fifth metacarpal and finger to assist in cradling objects. The palm cups with metacarpal flexion and, reciprocally, the palm flattens with metacarpal extension.

Proximally, the metacarpals of each digit articulate with the wrist via the CMC joints. The primary function of the these joints is to stabilize the metacarpals and, on the ulnar side, control hollowing of the palm. Those of the index through the ring fingers are considered to be plain synovial joints with 1 degree of freedom, flexion and extension. The fifth CMC joint is described as a shallow saddle joint with 2 degrees of freedom. The CMC joints are stabilized by tough transverse intermetacarpal and longitudinal CMC ligaments. The dorsal CMC ligaments are stronger than the volar ligaments. The second CMC joint is relatively immobile, but progressively more mobility is seen in the fourth and fifth metacarpals. The fourth CMC joint exhibits 8° to 10° of motion, whereas the fifth exhibits 15° to 20° of flexion with supination.

The MP joints are considered the key element in the kinematic chain of the fingers as they position the IP joints in space. Their surfaces are described as being condyloid, with predominantly 2 degrees of rotational freedom. Motion is primarily in the flexion-extension axis followed by abduction-adduction and accompanied by slight rotation. The metacarpal head has an eccentric articular surface that is broader on the palmar surface. This structure combined with the eccentric insertion of its collateral ligaments permits more abduction and adduction with the joint in extension than flexion. Collateral ligaments tighten with flexion, making this the most stable position. This eccentricity of the metacarpal head is the major reason the MP joints are more likely to become stiff in extension than in flexion.

In addition to the collateral ligaments, the MP joints are stabilized by the volar plate, sagittal bands of the extensor apparatus, and the deep transverse metacarpal ligament. The deep transverse metacarpal ligament or intervolar plate ligament is continuous with the volar plate and holds them together. These joints show a slight increase in the range of motion into flexion proceeding from the radial side to the ulnar side with the index showing approximately 90° of flexion and the fifth MP showing approximately 110° of flexion. The MP joints have an average passive hyperextension range of 30° to 45°. Although this is relatively constant between digits, it varies greatly between individuals and is commonly used as a measure of general flexibility.

In full extension, the tips of the fingers lie on the circumference of a circle formed in the plane of the hand, the center of which is the head of the third metacarpal. In closing the hand, the fingers flex and adduct to converge towards the base of the thenar eminence. This movement is facilitated by increased motion in the ulnar digits.

There are 2 separate functional positions that exist as the fingers flex to grasp an object. The first is the formation of the placement arc, which occurs at a position where there is full MP flexion and is responsible for 77% of total finger flexion. The position when the fingers grasp an object, known as the final encompassment, arises from motion of the PIP and distal IP (DIP) joints and makes up the remaining 23% of finger flexion. The PIP joint contributes 85% and the DIP joint 15% of this motion. Thus, it can be deduced that the PIP joint is the critical joint in final encompassment, emphasizing the importance of its motion.

The IP joints, both PIP and DIP, are true hinge joints with 1 degree of freedom in flexion-extension. These joints are stabilized by collateral ligaments as well as by a strong volar plate that prevents hyperextension. The collateral ligaments of the IP joints are relatively taut in all positions of flexion, such that the joint is relatively stable throughout its range of motion. Consistent with the other joints of the finger rays, the IP joints show a similar pattern of increased range of motion from radial to ulnar. PIP joint flexion averages 100° to 115° at the index finger and progressively increases to approximately 135° at the little finger. Similarly, the DIP joint of the index finger has a flexion mean of 80°, which increases to 90° at the small finger. The adjacent condyles of the heads of the proximal phalanges vary such that with flexion, the middle through small fingers deviate radially at the PIP joints while the index finger's IP joint deviates ulnarly. This deviation, along with the progressive range of motion in the ulnar digits, helps to angulate these digits when flexed toward the scaphoid tubercle, thereby assisting in the opposition to the thumb as well as providing a tighter ulnar grip.

The joint orientation angles for index finger functions are presented to reinforce the overall range that is required in different joints for various functions (Table 5).

Kinetics

The muscles of the fingers can be divided into flexors and extensors, both extrinsic and intrinsic. The flexor digitorum profundus and flexor digitorum superficialis make up the long extrinsic flexors of the fingers.

The flexor digitorum profundus inserts on the distal phalanx of each finger and is the only flexor at the DIP joint. Although the long flexors provide synchronous flexion of the proximal and distal phalanges, they contribute little to MP joint flexion. The profundus tendon also assists in adducting the finger during flexion. The tendon to the index finger is relatively independent, allowing this to be the only digit that can generate maximum profundus force even while the others are extended. The ulnar 3 digits have limited independent motion because of the common origin of the flexor digitorum profundus tendons as well as common origins of the third and fourth lumbricals. This conjoined nature of the profundi and lumbricals is responsible for the limited independent extension of the ring finger that is commonly annoying to piano players.

The flexor digitorum superficialis inserts on the base of the middle phalanx and flexes the PIP joints. Each superficialis can act in isolation from each other and the profundus. By preventing hyperextension, the action of the sublimis contributes to PIP joint stability. Hook or baggage grip is essentially IP flexion, is a load bearing grip, and can be sustained for long periods. Most of the sustained power comes from the flexor digitorum superficialis, which keep the PIP joints at about 90° with DIP control as necessary from the profundi.

Extrinsic finger extension is provided through the 4 tendons of the extensor digitorum communis, assisted by the extensor indicis proprius and the extensor digiti quinti (Fig. 34). The extensor digitorum communis tendon is centered by sagittal bands that insert into the deep transverse

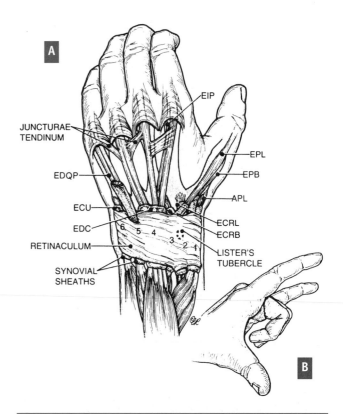

Figure 34

A, The extensor tendons gain entrance to the hand from the forearm through a series of 6 canals, 5 fibro-osseous and 1 fibrous (the latter is the fifth dorsal compartment, which contains the extensor digiti quinti proprius [EDQP]). The first compartment contains the abductor pollicis longus (APL) and extensor pollicis brevis (EPB); the second, the radial wrist extensors; the third, the extensor pollicis longus (EPL), which angles around Lister's tubercle; the fourth, the extensor digitorum communis (EDC) to the fingers, as well as the extensor indicis proprius (EIP); the fifth, the EDQP; and the sixth, the extensor carpi ulnaris (ECU). The communis tendons are jointed distally near the MP joints by fibrous interconnections called juncturae tendinum. These juncturae are usually found only between the communis tendons and may aid in surgical recognition of the proprius tendon of the index. The proprius tendons are always positioned to the ulnar side of the adjacent communis tendons. Beneath the retinaculum, the extensor tendons are covered with a synovial sheath. **B,** The proprius tendons to the index and little fingers are capable of independent extension, and their function may be evaluated as depicted. With the middle and ring fingers flexed into the palm, the proprius tendons can extend the ring and little fingers. Independent extension of the index, however, is not lost following transfer of the indicis proprius. ECRB, extensor carpi radialis brevis; ECRL, extensor carpi radialis longus. (Illustration by Elizabeth Roselius, © 1993. Reproduced with permission from Doyle JR: Extensor tendons: Acute injuries, in Green DP (ed): *Operative Hand Surgery*, ed 3. New York, NY, Churchill Livingstone, 1993, vol 2, pp 1925–1954.)

Table 5

Joint Orientation Angles for Index Finger Functions

Function	Joint Flexion Angle (°)*		
	DIP	PIP	MP
Tip pinch	25	50	48
Key pinch	20	35	20
Pulp pinch	0	50	48
Grasp	23	48	62
Baggage/hook grip	44	72	23
Holding glass	20	48	5
Opening big jar	35	55	50

DIP = distal interphalangeal; PIP = proximal interphalangeal;
MP = metacarpophalangeal

(Reproduced with permission from An KN, Chao EY, Cooney WP, et al: Forces in the normal and abnormal hand. *J Orthop Res* 1985;3:202–211.)

metacarpal ligament and volar plate complex. This circumferential sling extends the MP joint, because the extensor digitorum communis has no direct insertion into the proximal phalanx. It has an indirect insertion via connections to the dorsal capsule of the MP joint and via the volar sling formed by the sagittal bands to the volar plate. The extensor tendon proceeds through the extensor expansion to insert on the middle phalanx base as the central slip. The central slip's lateral fibers and intrinsic tendons form the lateral bands that insert at the base of the distal phalanx as the terminal tendon (Fig. 35).

The extensor indicis proprius inserts in a similar fashion on the index finger ulnar to the dorsally central extensor digitorum communis. The extensor digiti quinti also inserts ulnar to the midline on the fifth digit. It is considered the main extensor because the extensor digitorum communis tendon is absent more than 50% of the time and is replaced by a junctura tendinum from the ring finger extensor digitorum communis.

The primary function of the long extensors is to extend the MP joints. There is some controversy as to their contribution in extending the PIP joint. When the long extensors are isolated anatomically, full hyperextension of the MP joints is required before the PIP joints will start to extend. The extrinsic extensors stabilize the proximal phalanx so that the intrinsics can function and can abduct with extension of the fingers as the hand opens. The extensor indicis proprius and extensor digiti quinti allow independent extension of the index and small fingers, respectively.

The intrinsic muscles of the fingers are made up of the palmar and dorsal interossei, lumbricals, and hypothenars. The interossei arising from the metacarpals pass palmar to the MP joint axis to insert into the proximal phalanx and extensor hood. As a group, the interossei most consistently produce MP joint flexion with simultaneous extension of the IP joints. In addition, adduction of the digits is provided by the 4 dorsal interossei, whereas the 3 palmar interossei are responsible for adducting the digits. The middle finger is the accepted axis of reference for these motions.

The dorsal interossei as a group are stronger, having twice the muscle mass of the palmar interossei. The first dorsal interosseous, being the strongest, provides the main resistance to ulnar directed forces applied by the thumb. The first dorsal interosseous is unique among the interossei in that its insertion is entirely into the base of the proximal phalanx. In addition to abducting, it also supinates the finger to facilitate opposition to the thumb.

The 4 lumbricals are unique in that they all arise and insert via tendons. The lumbricals take origin from the flexor digitorum profundus tendons, pass palmarly to the MP joint axis, and insert into the radial aspect of the extensor apparatus at a point distal to that of the interossei. Their unique origin provides them with a greater contractile range. In fact, their origin actually moves more than their insertion during motion. In referring to the intrinsics as a group, it can

be said that the interossei are more effective as MP flexors, while the lumbricals are more effective as IP extensors.

The hypothenar muscles are made up of the abductor digiti minimi, the flexor digiti minimi brevis, and the opponens digiti minimi. The abductor digiti minimi has a dual insertion into the ulnar base of the proximal phalanx and into the extensor apparatus of the fifth digit. It is a strong abductor and slight flexor of the proximal phalanx and secondarily extends the 2 phalanges of the fifth digit. The flexor digiti minimi brevis inserts into the ulnar base of the proximal phalanx and is a strong flexor of the MP joint. It also slightly adducts and flexes the metacarpal. The opponens digiti minimi, simi-

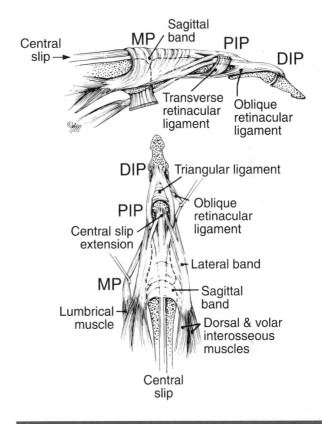

Figure 35

The extensor tendon at the metacarpophalangeal (MP) joint level is held in place by the transverse lamina or sagittal band, which tethers and centers the extensor tendons over the joint. This sagittal band arises from the volar plate and the intermetacarpal ligaments at the neck of the metacarpals. Any injury to this extensor hood or expansion may result in subluxation or dislocation of the extensor tendon. The intrinsic tendons from the lumbrical and interosseous muscles join the extensor mechanism at about the level of the proximal and midportion of the proximal phalanx and continue distally to the distal interphalangeal joint of the finger. The extensor mechanism at the proximal interphalangeal (PIP) joint is best described as a trifurcation of the extensor tendon into the central slip, which attaches to the dorsal base of the middle phalanx, and the 2 lateral bands. These lateral bands continue distal to insert at the dorsal base of the distal phalanx. The extensor mechanism is maintained in place over the PIP joint by the transverse retinacular ligaments. (Illustration by Elizabeth Roselius, © 1993. Reproduced with permission from Doyle JR: Extensor tendons: Acute injuries, in Green DP (ed): *Operative Hand Surgery*, ed 3. New York, NY, Churchill Livingstone, 1993, vol 2, pp 1925–1954.)

lar to the opponens pollicis, inserts entirely onto the fifth metacarpal to flex and adduct it. It is the most active muscle during opposition of the thumb to the fifth finger. The activity of the opponens digiti minimi exceeds that of the flexor pollicis brevis with resisted opposition. The hypothenar muscles combine to flex and adduct the metacarpal, flex the proximal phalanx, and extend the middle and distal phalanges to cup the palm and enhance opposition.

It is important to mention that 3 primary retinacula in the hand (the extensor, flexor, and digital sheath) act as pulleys and are responsible for all direction changes of the tendons. They serve to maintain functional axes of motion and contribute to stability of the wrist and digits by preventing bow stringing, thereby ensuring functional moment arms in the hand.

Finger flexion is a combination of active muscle forces opposing the passive viscoelastic forces of the extensor apparatus. The flexor digitorum profundus is the primary flexor during synchronous flexion of the fingers. EMG studies have shown that when such flexion is produced without external resistance, the flexor digitorum profundus is the only active flexor at the IP joints. The flexor digitorum sublimis is activated when flexion against resistance is required. In a similar fashion, the interossei are responsible for MP flexion against resistance. Passive forces are primarily provided by the oblique retinacular ligament (Fig. 35). This ligament arises from the palmar aspect of the proximal phalanx and the adjacent flexor sheath, passing volar to the axis of PIP flexion and then dorsal along the sides of the middle phalanx, and dorsal to the axis of the DIP joint to insert into the distal lateral bands. The ligament's function is to coordinate motion of the middle and distal phalanges.

Finger flexion occurs first at the PIP joint by the action of the flexor digitorum profundus. This is followed by flexion at the MP and then the DIP joints. These motions are quite integrated and are difficult to separate clinically. Action of the flexor digitorum profundus produces tension in the oblique retinacula ligament, which in turn prevents DIP flexion as long as the PIP is extended. The pull of the profundus, thus, does not first cause DIP flexion; instead, its action is transferred proximally causing flexion of the PIP joint. This motion pulls the extensor apparatus distally, placing the intrinsic tendons on stretch and subsequently leading to MP joint flexion via passive viscoelastic forces. With continued flexion of the PIP joint, the oblique retinacula ligament relaxes to allow flexion at the DIP joint. Flexion of the PIP joint then proceeds along with that of the DIP joint, but does so at a faster rate. DIP joint flexion is complete only at the end, producing a locking grip.

Flexion of the fingers also is regulated by a synergistic activity of the long extensors as well as the passive forces of the lumbricals. The extensor digitorum communis acts to restrain MP and PIP flexion, effectively causing motion at these 2 joints to occur in a synchronous fashion. The lumbricals do not actively participate in producing flexion, but play a significant coordinating role. When finger flexion occurs unopposed by an external resistance, the passive viscoelastic forces of the lumbricals, via their insertion into the extensor apparatus, prevent full IP joint flexion prior to MP joint flexion. This allows the hand to surround an object. The importance of lumbrical function is evident in ulnar nerve palsy with intrinsic paralysis. In this situation, the finger flexes at the IP joints before flexing the MP joints, preventing the hand from grasping any object of a reasonable size.

Extension of the fingers is less well understood and more involved than flexion. Digital extension is similar to flexion in that it is a combination of active and passive forces. EMG studies confirm that the lumbricals and extensor digitorum communis provide the active component of extension. As with flexion, a passive component of extension is provided by the viscoelastic forces of the oblique retinacula ligament that coordinate extension of the middle and distal phalanges. In a fully flexed finger, the proximal phalanx serves as a kinetic link to extension.

With full finger flexion, the sagittal band connecting the extensor digitorum communis to the proximal phalanx is distal to the MP joint (up to 16 mm) and lax (Fig. 36). The extensor digitorum communis is thus unable to directly extend the MP joint at the beginning of extension. Extension begins at the MP joint by an indirect mechanism, which occurs through the combined forces of the central slip of the extensor digitorum communis and the flexor digitorum sublimis acting on the base of the middle phalanx. With the PIP flexed, action of these muscles transmits a force from the base of the middle phalanx through the PIP joint to the head of the proximal phalanx, which will tend to rotate this bone into extension about the MP joint. Simultaneous action of the flexor digitorum superficialis is essential to prevent extension of the PIP joint and allow the generation of the compressive force at the head of the proximal phalanx.

As the MP joint extends, the extensor aponeurosis shifts proximally. The extensor digitorum communis insertion becomes tense and allows it to act directly through the sagittal band on the proximal phalanx to further extend the MP joint. At the same time, the lumbricals actively extend the IP joints. As the PIP joint extends, the oblique retinacula ligament coordinates the extension of the distal phalanx. Lumbrical muscle contraction pulls the flexor digitorum profundus tendons distally, decreasing their passive resistance to extension. The lumbricals are often considered the workhorses of finger extension, because of their dual role. As in digital flexion, the interossei are inactive during unopposed extension.

Because hand function depends intimately on the balance of its muscles, it is more appropriate to be concerned with the relative power of these muscles with respect to each other than with their individual absolute strengths (Tables 6 and 7). In general, the flexors, with regard to physiologic cross-sectional area of muscles and their ability to generate work, have a work capacity 3 times that of the extensors (Table 8). The flexor digitorum profundus muscles are on an average 50% stronger than the flexor digitorum superficialis. Tension in the flexor digitorum profundus tendons varies little from the second to the fifth digit, whereas the superficialis strength varies widely. The strength of the flexor profundus is approximately equal to that of the sublimis in the middle finger, whereas, in the small finger, the profundus is approximately 3 times as strong as the sublimis. It follows that the middle finger is the strongest of all the fingers to flex and resist extension. In fact, for the middle finger, the strength of the flexor digitorum profundus and superficialis together is equal to the strength of all the extensors.

When examining finger muscle forces (Table 8) the flexor digitorum profundus and flexor digitorum superficialis consistently demonstrate high force potential (cross-section) (Table 9) in comparison to other muscles in most functions. In lateral key pinch, the flexor digitorum superficialis has minimal load, but the extensor digitorum communis and 2 radial intrinsic muscles contribute large forces. In key pinch the radial interosseous balances the MP joint by preventing ulnar deviation. This high force-generating ability of the flexor digitorum profundus, flexor digitorum superficialis, and radial interosseous is reflected in their higher physiologic cross-sectional area. The ulnar deviation force of the radial interosseous creates a large

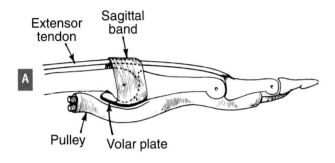

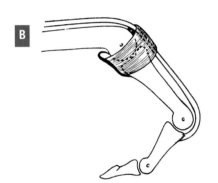

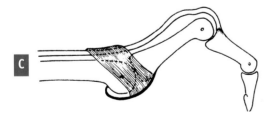

Figure 36

Diagrammatic representation of the sagittal bands. The sagittal bands are attached dorsally to the extensor tendon and volarly to the volar plate. **A,** In extension, the bands overlie the metacarpophalangeal (MP) joint. **B,** With flexion, the bands migrate distally. In this position the extensor tendon can extend the proximal interphalangeal (PIP) joint. **C,** In hyperextension, the extensor tendon distal to the MP joint is lax and the PIP joint falls into flexion. (Reproduced with permission from Smith RJ: Balance and kinetics of the fingers under normal and pathological conditions. *Clin Orthop* 1974;104:92–111.)

Table 6	
Muscle Excursion	
Muscle	**Excursion (cm)**
Finger flexors	7
Finger and thumb extensors	5
Wrist muscles	3
Extensor pollicis brevis, abductor pollicis longus	3
Tendonesis effect of wrist*	2.3

* Increases tendon excursion

Table 7		
Ratios and Aggregate Muscle-Tendon Forces Generated by the Flexor Digitorum Profundus and Superficialis in 40 Normal Hands		
Finger	**Mean (kg)**	**SD***
Profundus: superficialis		
Index	0.97	0.45
Middle	0.79	0.32
Ring	0.95	0.58
Little	1.50	0.73
Profundus + superficialis		
Index	13.22	3.87
Middle	13.40	4.26
Ring	11.75	5.95
Little	9.01	3.15

* Standard deviation

flexion moment at the MP joint that is counteracted by the extensor digitorum communis for balance. The intrinsic muscles appear to produce more force during pinch function than grasp function to stabilize the MP joint. The muscle forces in simulated activities of daily living are similar to those of basic pinch functions.

The joint constraint forces (Table 10) are comparable in both the PIP and MP joints. In lateral (key) pinch, such forces become significantly larger in the MP joint than in the PIP joint because of muscle forces that prevent ulnar deviation of the MP joint (radial interosseous in association with the balancing force of the extensor digitorum communis). The constraint forces are large for both tip and pulp pinch, and should not be overlooked. Volar-dorsal shear forces are directed dorsally, implying that under most activities of daily living the proximal phalanx tends to sublux volarly on the metacarpal head. The radial-ulnar shear forces at the MP joint are directed radially to counteract the slight tendency to shift ulnarly. The proximal phalanx also tends to shift ulnarly, loading the radial support structures.

The actual average forces in the index finger (Table 11), particularly with pinching, are considerable. Especially important are the relatively higher forces at the distal phalanx, which contribute to the etiology of osteoarthritis at the DIP joint, sparing the PIP and MP joints.

Loss of the flexor digitorum superficialis force (Table 12) has more than an additive effect on flexor digitorum profundus force required for tip pinch. With flexor digitorum superficialis loss, the flexor digitorum profundus force requirement more than doubles and the previously inactive extensor digitorum communis contributes very high forces with the increased force from the IP extensors (lumbrical and ulnar interosseous) to balance the finger.

Structure and Function of the Spine

The spine is a flexible column with a multicurved shape that is important in absorbing energy. It is a dynamic system composed of motion segments and having 4 major functions: support, mobility, housing, and control. The spine supports the mass of the body and withstands external forces. At the same time it allows for mobility and enough flexibility to absorb energy and to protect against impact. The spine architecture protects the spinal cord and nerves and the vertebral artery in the cervical area. Trunk muscles and ligaments, acting on individual vertebrae, provide postural control and spinal stability. Trauma, dysfunction, pain, or surgical intervention can affect any of these functions. Healthy spine function depends on the interplay among spinal structure, stability, and flexibility, as well as on muscular strength, endurance, and coordination.

Kinematics of the Spine

General Kinematics

The normal curves of the spine include cervical lordosis, thoracic kyphosis, and lumbar lordosis. This curvature arises naturally from the shape of the vertebrae and disks, the rib cage, and the inclination of the sacral end plate. However, variation in the inclination of the sacral end plate produces considerable individual variation in the shape of vertebrae and disks and, thus, in the curvatures of the spine.

In the spine, 2 types of motion, translation and rotation, are possible about each of the 3 orthogonal planes. These motions are usually coupled. For example, in a flexion move-

Table 8						
Muscle Forces of Index Finger Under Isometric Hand Function						
	Muscle Forces*					
Function	**FDP**	**FDS**	**RI**	**LU**	**UI**	**EDC**
Tip pinch	1.93 – 2.08	1.75 – 2.16	0.0 – 0.99	0.0 – 0.72	10.21 – 0.65	—
Pulp pinch	1.53 – 3.14	0.32 – 1.32	0.0 – 1.61	0.0 – 1.17	0.62 – 1.19	—
Lateral key pinch	1.37 – 5.95	—	1.01 – 7.04	0.0 – 6.10	—	7.45 – 15.95
Grasp	3.17 – 3.47	1.51 – 2.14	0.0 – 1.19	0.0 – 0.91	0.0 – 0.49	—
Baggage/hook grip	0.0 – 0.02	1.70 – 1.78	0.0 – 0.45	0.0 – 0.33	0.11 – 0.27	—
Holding glass	2.77 – 2.99	1.29 – 1.57	—	0.48 – 0.53	-.28 – 0.38	—
Opening big jar	3.50 – 5.49	—	4.2 – 4.53	0.0 – 1.15	0.0 – 1.00	9.48 – 16.23

* Forces in units of applied force; that is, magnitude or multiple times the applied force and not the exact applied force. FDP = flexor digitorum profundus; FDS = flexor digitorum sublimis; EDC = extensor digitorum communis; EIP = extensor indicis; RI = radial interosseous; LU = lumbrical; UI = ulnar interosseous

ment, the vertebra rotates in the sagittal plane and simultaneously undergoes AP translations. In general, in vitro measurements can be made more accurately and under more controlled loading conditions than in vivo measurements, but they may not duplicate in vivo conditions (that is, muscle excitations, fluid environment, temperature, etc).

Figure 37 shows the relative motion in vivo within and between the different parts of the spine, as summarized from the literature. The main determinant for range of motion is the orientation of the facet or zygapophyseal joints and intervertebral disks. Flexion-extension predominates in the cervical region, but considerable axial rotation and lateral bending are possible. Flexion-extension and lateral bending mainly occur in the midcervical region, and axial rotation occurs primarily in the upper part of the cervical spine.

The thoracic region is stabilized by the rib cage and there is generally little motion. The lumbar spine permits considerable lateral bending in the middle portion, while flexion-extension is greatest in the lumbosacral motion segment. Rotation is minimal in the lumbar region because of the orientation of the facet joints. Compared with the thoracic spine, the greater mobility in the cervical and lumbar regions corresponds with greater stresses and more clinical complaints.

Clinical measurement of spine mobility is difficult because the hips and lumbar spine move together. Simple goniometric techniques are most commonly used, but reliability can be improved with the dual inclinometer and flexicurve techniques. The latter method involves reproducing a curve and

Table 9
Physiologic Cross-Sectional Areas (PCSA) of Muscles Across Index Finger Joint

Muscle	PCSA (cm²)
Flexor digitorum profundus	4.10
Flexor digitorum sublimis	3.6
Extensor digitorum communis	1.39
Extensor indicis	1.12
Radial interosseous	4.16
Lumbrical	0.36
Ulnar interosseous	1.60

Table 10
Joint Constraint Forces of Index Finger Under Isometric Hand Function

Function	Compressive Force *X	Dorsal Shear Force* Y	Radial Shear Force* Z
Distal interphalangeal joint			
Tip pinch	2.4–2.7	0.2–0.3	-0.1– -0.1
Key pinch	2.9–12.5	0.7–3.2	0.7–0.9
Pulp pinch	3.0–4.6	0.0–0.2	-0.1– -0.2
Grasp	2.8–3.4	0.5–0.7	-0.2– -0.2
Baggage/hook grip	0.0–0.0	0.0–0.0	0.0–0.0
Holding glass	2.5–2.9	0.2–0.3	-0.2– -0.2
Opening big jar	5.2–9.5	1.7–3.3	0.3–0.5
Proximal interphalangeal joint			
Tip pinch	4.4–4.9	0.9–1.1	0.0–0.1
Key pinch	4.9–19.4	1.1–4.5	0.3–1.1
Pulp pinch	4.8–5.8	1.1–1.4	0.0–0.0
Grasp	4.5–5.3	1.0–1.3	0.0– -0.1
Baggage/hook grip	1.7–1.9	0.0–002	0.0–0.0
Holding glass	4.3–4.4	1.1–1.1	0.0– -0.1
Opening big jar	7.2–14.2	2.4–4.9	0.2–0.8
Metacarpophalangeal			
Tip pinch	3.5–3.9	2.1–2.3	0.1–0.2
Key pinch	14.7–27.1	3.9–5.7	0.0–0.1
Pulp pinch	4.0–4.6	2.2–2.4	0.1–0.1
Grasp	3.2–3.7	2.9–3.1	0.3–0.4
Baggage/hook grip	1.0–1.3	0.6–0.7	0.0–0.0
Holding glass	4.0–4.1	0.9–0.9	02.–0.2
Opening big jar	14.8–24.3	6.5–9.9	0.2–0.3

* In units of applied force; negative sign represents force in the opposite direction

taking tangents to it. Segmental axial rotation is the most difficult motion to study in vivo; however, reasonably accurate results are obtained with pins inserted into the vertebrae, or with biplane or stereo radiography.

Most researchers report less mobility of the spine among older subjects. For example, using a dual inclinometer technique, measurements of spinal mobility have been made among white- and blue-collar workers, ranging in age from 35 to 54 years. Range of motion was found to be lower among the older subjects. Women had a slightly greater range of motion in the cervical area and men showed greater mobility in the lumbar area, but not all measurements followed this pattern. A large industrial study in the United States found no evidence of a relationship between mobility and subsequent back disability. Reduced spinal mobility in combination with pain or tenderness, however, is useful in predicting subsequent disability. Increased sagittal plane translation and coupled translatory and axial motion may be an early sign of disk degeneration and low back problems.

Understanding the movements of the spine, like those of other joints of the body, requires an appreciation of instantaneous axes of rotation (IARs). IARs based on in vitro

studies in the cervical, thoracic, and lumbar regions are presented in Figure 38.

The Motion Segment

The motion segment is the basic anatomic unit of the spine. It comprises 2 adjacent vertebrae and their intervening soft tissues. This structure, sometimes called a functional spinal unit (FSU), is viscoelastic and absorbs energy. It moves with 6 degrees of freedom (3 translations and 3 rotations) (Fig. 39, A). However, because each motion segment depends on its 2 bony elements with 6 articulate faces and multiple ligamentous components for its stability, its motions are complex. Loads and torques applied to an FSU along or about the AP, lateral, or axial axes not only produce pure simple motions but also coupled translations and rotations about several axes. This coupling behavior is present in most functional movements and varies greatly among individuals, depending on such factors as age and (where pathology exists) the level of degeneration.

It is convenient to divide the motion segment into anterior and posterior elements or columns (Fig. 39, B). The dividing line is just behind the vertebral body. The anterior elements include the vertebral body, the disk, and the anterior and posterior longitudinal ligaments. These provide the major support for the spinal column and absorb impact. In so doing they restrict vertical translational motion. The neural arch and its processes and the zygapophyseal joints lie to the posterior and, with the disk, control patterns of motion about the other axes.

Table 11
Average Strengths of Index Finger in Isometric Hand Functions

Function	Average Strength (N)
Tip pinch	224-95
Key pinch	37-106
Pulp pinch	30-83
Grasp: distal phalanx	38-109
Middle phalanx	7-38
Proximal phalanx	23-73

Table 12
Muscle Forces (in Units of Applied Force) in Index Finger During Tip Pinch With and Without Laceration of Flexor Sublimis

	Normal	FDS Laceration
Flexor digitorum profundus	2.20	5.46
Flexor digitorum sublimis	1.77	—
Radial interosseous	1.26	1.43
Lumbrical	0.15	1.85
Ulnar interosseous	0.74	2.37
Extensor digitorum commands	—	7.38

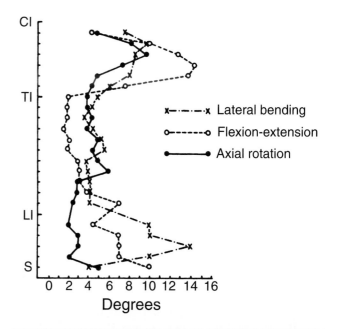

Figure 37

Range of motion within and between the different motion segments of the spine. (Reproduced with permission from Pope MH, Frymoyer JW, Lehmann TR: Structure and function of the lumbar spine, in *Occupational Low Back Pain: Assessment, Treatment, and Prevention*. St. Louis, MO, CV Mosby, 1991.)

Intervertebral Disk The disk forms the primary articulation between the vertebral bodies and is the major constraint to motion of the FSU. The disk is composed of 2 morphologically separate parts. The outer part, the annulus fibrosus, is made up of about 90 collagen sheets bonded to each other. Each sheet is made of collagen fibers oriented vertically at the peripheral layer, but becoming progressively more oblique with each underlying layer (Fig. 40). The fibers in adjacent sheets run at approximately 30° angles to each other. The lamination of these layers strengthens the annulus. The inner or central part of the disk is the nucleus pulposus. In young individuals, it is nearly 90% water, with the remaining structure comprising collagen and proteoglycans, which bind water. Normally, the adult disk is avascular, but end-plate microfractures can result in vascular ingrowth, the formation of granulation tissue, and alterations in the chemistry and mechanical behavior of the disk.

In young, healthy disks, positive pressure within the nucleus pulposus increases as loads are applied to the spine. This pressure is approximately 1.5 times the mean applied pressure over the area of the end plate. The disk is actually quite flexible at low compression loads, but provides increasing resistance at high loads. Its major role in weightbearing is reflected by the fact that disk area increases as a direct function of body mass in all mammals.

Many relationships have been reported between disk height, disk bulge, pressure, and mobility. When the disk is loaded, the nucleus deforms and transfers the force to the anulus. In axial compression, the increased intradiskal pressure is counteracted by annular fiber tension and disk bulge, rather analogous to the bulging in the sides of a tire. Some disk space narrowing also occurs. To describe the internal displacements of the intervertebral disk, with only minimal disruption of normal function, the displacement of injected radiopaque beads can be determined from sagittal plane radiographs taken before and during load application. For the intact disk in compression, the intradiskal bead displacements are predominantly anterior. In flexion, the beads in the center of the disk move posteriorly, whereas the beads closer to the periphery of the disk move anteriorly. In extension, the central beads move anteriorly and the beads closer to the periphery of the disk move posteriorly. After denucleation, the bead displacements for compression and flexion suggest an inward bulging of the inner wall of the anulus, despite outward bulging of the disk surface.

Flexion, extension, and lateral bending all produce a small displacement of the nucleus. Asymmetric and cyclic loading in combined lateral bend, compression, and flexion are risk factors for disk herniation. The lumbar motion segment can resist a combination of bending moment and shear

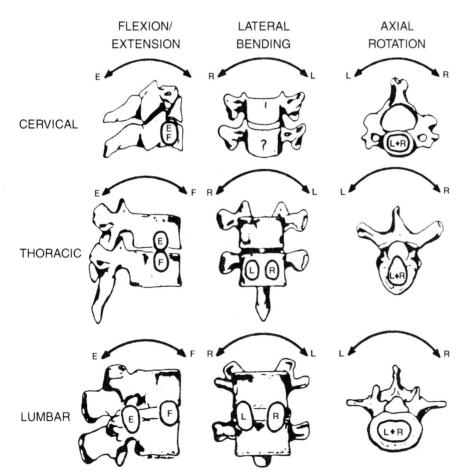

Figure 38

Approximate locations of instantaneous axes of rotation (IAR) in the 3 regions of the spine undergoing rotation in the 3 traditional planes. E = approximate location of IARs in extending from neutral position. F = IARs in flexion from neutral position. L = IARs in left lateral bending or left axial rotation. R = IARs in right lateral bending or right axial rotation. (Reproduced with permission from White AA III, Panjabi MM (eds): *Clinical Biomechanics of the Spine.* Philadelphia, PA, JB Lippincott, 1978.)

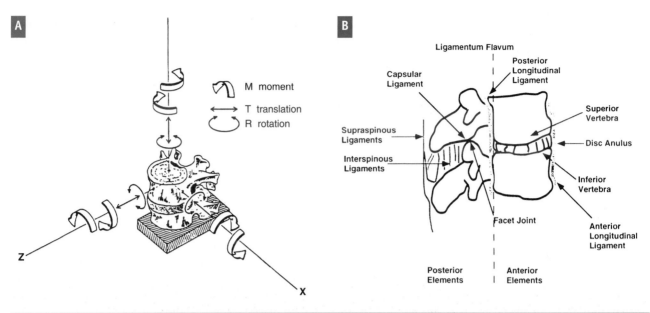

Figure 39

A, The basic structure unit of the spine—the motion segment. (Reproduced with permission from White AA III, Panjabi MM (eds): *Clinical Biomechanics of the Spine*. Philadelphia, PA, JB Lippincott, 1978.) **B,** The division of a motion segment into its two functional elements.

force of 156 N·m and 620 N, respectively, before complete disruption occurs. This is much less than the failure load in compression. The tension force acting on the posterior structures is 2.8 kN. The bone mineral content in the vertebrae appears to be a good predictor of ultimate strength of the lumbar motion segment. About 35% of its torque resistance is provided by the disk and the remaining resistance by the posterior elements and ligaments. Therefore, any defect in the posterior structures increases the risk of disk failure. Several reports have emphasized that little or no nucleus should be removed in surgery so as to maintain stability.

An increase in fluid content increases the stiffness of the

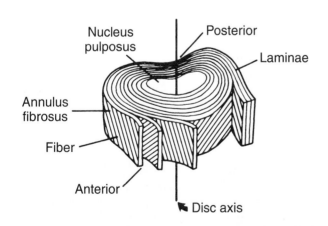

Figure 40

The intervertebral disk. (Reproduced with permission from Pope MH, Frymoyer JW, Lehmann TR: Structure and function of the lumbar spine, in *Occupational Low Back Pain: Assessment, Treatment, and Prevention*. St. Louis, MO, CV Mosby, 1991.)

disk. The disk is separated on both sides from the vertebral bodies by hyaline cartilage end plates. The condition of the end plates influences the nutrition of the disk. Nutrients and fluid enter the disk by diffusion through the end plates or the anulus, which is essential because the disk lacks vascular tissue. Glucose diffuses mainly through the end plates, whereas sulfate ions diffuse mainly through the anulus. The diffusion is influenced by mechanical factors. When the load on the disk increases, there is an outflow of fluid and there is a fluid influx when load decreases. Disk nutrition can also be affected by changes in end-plate permeability. Smoking and vibration decrease nutrition and dynamic exercise enhances it.

Range of motion usually is measured on the basis of a brief force application. However, if a force is applied to a collagenous viscoelastic structure for a prolonged period, further movement can be detected. This movement is small in amplitude, occurs slowly, and is known as creep. Creep is not just a laboratory phenomenon; it occurs in static postures, such as prolonged sitting or standing. Many workers must assume positions that subject the lumbar spine to prolonged load bearing or vibration in a fixed bent or stooped posture.

Time-dependent (viscoelastic) intervertebral disk changes have been demonstrated both in vitro and in vivo. It is postulated that an increase in height occurs if there is a reduction in the overall disk compressive pressure; the reduced intradiskal osmotic pressure allows water to flow into the intervertebral disk. The reverse is true if intradiskal pressure is increased. Reported diurnal changes in the overall height of individuals range from 6.3 mm to 19.3 mm, with an average of 15.7 mm. The average person is 1% shorter in the evening than in the morning; children are 2% shorter in the evening; and the elderly are 0.5% shorter in the evening.

Fifty percent of total length change occurs during the first 2 hours in the upright posture. Thus, for most people, the first 2 hours out of bed in the morning are critical for disk metabolism. Additionally, some have recommended that those who do heavy manual work have short rest periods during which they can recline. Higher loads produce greater creep, which might be associated with long-lasting, higher intradiskal pressure (Fig. 41). Healthy disks creep slowly as compared to degenerated disks, which have less ability to absorb shock; thus, degeneration can increase risk of back disorders.

Physical changes, including disk herniations, have also been caused in lumbar motion segments by exposure to cyclic loading at high loads. In vivo whole-body vibration studies have established the motion characteristics and natural frequency of the lumbar region. The tissues of the motion segment may be at risk for injury at the whole-body natural frequency of 5 Hz. Many vehicles produce vibration at the body's natural frequency, possibly placing drivers at risk for low back pain or injury. The behavior is that of a classic fatigue curve: at loads above 70%, specimens sustain only a few cycles; at loads below 30%, almost all specimens sustain 5,000 load cycles without fracture. Under axial compression, fracture invariably occurs in the end plates, but the anulus is not damaged. Repetitive loading of a flexed lumbar column and cyclic torsional loads may exaggerate failure in the end plates, facets, laminae, and capsular ligaments.

Compression failures promote disk degeneration. A degenerated disk has increased mobility and increased bulge, and appears to behave like a thick-walled cylinder rather than a pressure vessel. In such cases, the stresses in the anulus become large compressive stresses instead of relatively small tensile stresses, and the anulus becomes distorted. Similar types of changes can occur in the denucleated disk and those that have undergone chemonucleolysis.

The Vertebral Bodies

When a pure compressive load is applied to a healthy motion segment, translational motions within an FSU will cause the 2 vertebral bodies to come closer together. Failure of the unit occurs first in the end plate, then in the vertebral bodies, and then in the disk. During compressive loading, pressure is higher in the center of the end plate than in the periphery. This higher concentration of pressure in the center often results in failure from the nucleus rupturing the end plate. However, as noted above, considerably higher loads are needed to disrupt the FSU by compressive loading than by any other type of loading. This is because the vertebral body is well designed for weightbearing, as reflected in its superior and inferior surfaces and internal structure.

If a vertebra had only an outer layer of cortical bone, it would not be strong enough to sustain longitudinal compression, and would tend to collapse like a cardboard box. To complete the metaphor of the box, the outer structure can be reinforced by vertical struts, similar to the vertical trabeculae between the superior and inferior surfaces. A strut can sustain high longitudinal loads, provided it does not buckle. By introducing a series of crossbeams, such as the horizontal trabeculae, the strength of a box can be further increased. When a load is applied, the crossbeams hold the struts in place, preventing them from deforming and preventing the box from collapsing.

The type of failure resulting from an injury depends on whether the spine is loaded in flexion or extension, with flexion tending to cause anterior collapse where the trabeculae are weaker. This phenomenon occurs because the basic structure just described is modified by Wolff's law (Fig. 42) in that oblique trabeculae sweep up or down to aid in load bearing. These trabeculae come together at the pedicles to resist the tensile forces. The trabeculae sweep toward the superior and inferior facets to support the compressive and shear forces in the facets, and outward to the spinous process to withstand the tensile and bending forces applied to the spinous process. Additionally, in vivo, the vertebrae are filled with blood and, thus, they behave like hydraulic shock absorbers, providing greater strength.

Compression tests reveal decreases in vertebral body load and stress with age in both men and women. However, because of their greater cross-sectional area, load failure values are higher in men than in women up to the age of 75. The load-to-failure actually increases with age, with men showing a significantly greater cross-sectional area and a significant increase in vertebral body size, as a result of con-

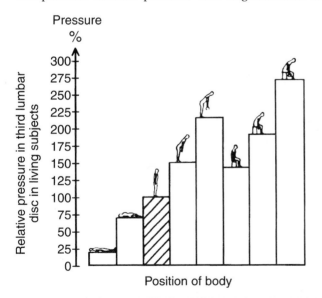

Figure 41

Relative increase and decrease in intradiskal pressure in different supine, standing, and sitting postures compared to the pressure in upright standing (100%). (Reproduced with permission from Nachemson A: Lumbar mechanics as revealed by lumbar intradiscal pressure measurements, in Jayson MIV, Dixon AS (eds): *The Lumbar Spine and Back Pain*, ed 4. Edinburgh, Scotland, Churchill Livingstone, 1992, pp 157–171.)

tinuous periosteal growth. This phenomenon is particularly significant for older people who have diminished bone strength, usually as a result of osteoporosis. Osteoporosis involves a reduction of bone volume, which is inversely related to the load to fracture. Measured bone mass thus should not be the sole index of the biomechanical competence (that is, stiffness and stress) of trabecular bone. Measurements of bone density must be considered in combination with a detailed description of the architecture.

Posterior Elements and Facet Joints (Zygapophyseal Joints)

The posterior elements are the components of the vertebral arch: pedicles, lamina, facet joints, and spinous and transverse processes. The spinous, transverse, accessory, and mammillary processes are levers with muscle attachments. The longer levers are the transverse and spinous processes. Every muscle acting on the lumbar vertebral column is attached somewhere on the posterior elements. The forces acting on the spinous and articular processes are ultimately transmitted to the lamina. Thus, the stability of the

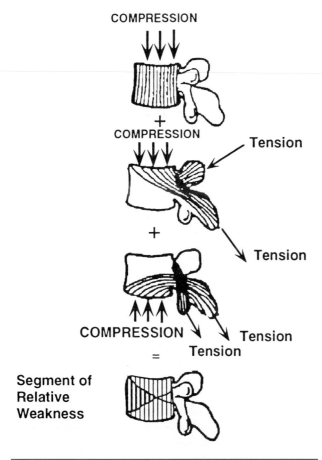

COMPRESSION

COMPRESSION

Tension

Tension

COMPRESSION   Tension

=   Tension

Segment of Relative Weakness

Figure 42

Trabecular directions in the vertebrae. (Reproduced with permission from Pope MH, Frymoyer JW, Lehmann TR: Structure and function of the lumbar spine, in *Occupational Low Back Pain: Assessment, Treatment, and Prevention*. St. Louis, MO, CV Mosby, 1991.)

lumbar spine can be compromised if a lamina is weakened by disease, injury, or surgery.

The pedicles transmit all forces sustained by the posterior elements, such as tension and bending, to the vertebral bodies. If a vertebra slides forward, the inferior articular processes of that vertebra are resisted by the superior articular processes of the inferior vertebra. This resistance is transmitted to the vertebral body through the pedicles. In addition, all muscles that act on a lumbar vertebra pull downward. This action is transmitted to the vertebral body through the pedicles, which are subjected to bending. The lower parts of the pedicle are compressed, but the upper parts are under tension. The pedicles are designed to withstand these moments because they are thick-walled cylinders.

The lamina between the superior and inferior articular process on each side is the pars interarticularis, meaning "interarticular part." Because it must withstand considerable bending forces, the pars is generally thicker than the rest of the lamina. The pars is a common site of fatigue (stress) fracture, or spondylolysis, perhaps because the cortical bone is thin. Such fractures may heal by fibrous union, which weakens the motion segment and sets the stage for spondylolisthesis. Whether failure occurs primarily because of flexion or extension is widely debated. Excessive loading of the spine in extension, however, is more likely to cause loads transmitted through the facet joints to produce high strain in the pars interarticularis, eventually leading to spondylolysis.

The zygapophyseal joints, found between the articular processes, are usually called facet joints, or facets. These articulations of the superior and inferior articular processes are lined with hyaline cartilage. The facets have a major role in controlling motion. They are important in resisting torsion and shear, and they have a role in compression. Normally, the lumbar facets and disks together contribute about 80% of the torsional load resistance, with the facets contributing one half of that amount. The remaining 20% of resistance is from the passive ligamentous structures.

Load sharing between facet and disk also occurs under shear loads and axial compressive loads. This load bearing is markedly reduced by excision of a single facet. The amount of load bearing by the facet joints is related to whether the motion segment is loaded in flexion or extension. In a seated position, lumbar lordosis is often unsupported and reduced, and intradiskal pressure is higher than in a standing position. The increase in lumbar flexion reduces the load-bearing ability of the facets.

Ligaments

The 7 ligaments of the spine can be divided into 3 systems. The nonsegmental longitudinal system includes the anterior and posterior longitudinal ligaments and the supraspinous ligaments. The segmental longitudinal system includes the interspinous, intertransverse ligaments, and the ligamenta flava (yellow ligaments). The articular, or capsular, system comprises the capsular ligaments. At the cephalad and caudal ends of the spine, there are specialized ligaments that attach the skull and the iliac bones, respectively.

Ligaments aid in the control of motion and are vital for the structural stability of the motion segment. The ligaments are also the primary tensile load-bearing structures, acting as passive elements to prevent excessive motion. Ligaments are viscoelastic, which means that their deformation and type of failure depend on the rate at which loads are applied. Their strength also depends on the number of deformations applied. Repetitive loading cycles may cause fatigue failure.

The posterior and anterior longitudinal ligaments traverse the length of the spine, further supporting the vertebral body and disk (Fig. 39). They are interlinked at each level by the disk. These ligaments are richly supplied by pain-sensitive nerve endings. The tensile strength of the anterior longitudinal ligament is about twice that of the posterior longitudinal ligament.

The remaining ligaments support and link the posterior elements. Of great functional importance is the ligamentum flavum, which joins the lamina of adjacent vertebrae. The ligamentum flavum is highly elastic and strong compared to other ligaments, and has a large number of elastic fibers. Its elastic properties allow it to lengthen with spine flexion and shorten with extension. Considerable flexion is required before permanent failure occurs. The ligamentum flavum is normally pretensed to about 6% to 15% of its tensile strain. In patients with severe spinal degeneration the ligamentum flavum becomes thickened and less elastic. These changes produce narrowing of the spinal canal in extension, because the ligament buckles into the spinal canal.

The tip and edges of the spinous process are joined by the interspinous and supraspinous ligaments. Because they are far from the disk, and therefore act on long moment arms, these ligaments play an important role in resisting spine flexion. The ligamenta flava and lumbodorsal fascia are more important in resisting flexion. The iliolumbar ligament, at the lumbosacral junction, also resists flexion-extension and axial rotation. Intertransverse ligaments join the transverse processes of the vertebra. Capsular ligaments limit the excursion of the facet joints. Like all other joints, they are richly supplied with pain-sensitive nerve endings.

Specialization of the Functional Spinal Unit

Cervical Spine

There is an almost infinite number of possible head postures, each produced through the action of different combinations of cervical muscles. The spinous processes increase in length between C-3 and T-1 or T-2. This is consistent with morphologic adaptation to an increase in torque along the spine that is needed to resist a given load on the head. The longer the spinous process, the greater the leverage of the attached muscle.

The orientation of the articular surfaces is almost transverse at C-1 to C-2. At C-2 to C-4, the articular surfaces are aligned 45° to the longitudinal axis, and this remains approximately constant to C-7 to T-1. Below C-3 to C-4, the facet joint plates are perpendicular to the sagittal plane. At C-2 to C-3, however, the joint planes also slope downward laterally by 10° to 20°. The occipitoatlantoaxial complex is a specialized articulation that allows a relatively large range of motion between the head and torso without any intervertebral disks. Flexion-extension predominates at C-3 to C-7. Lateral bend also is greatest in this segment. Axial rotation predominates at C-1 to C-2.

Approximately 60% of the axial rotation of the entire cervical spine and occiput is found in the upper region (occiput to C-1 to C-2), and 40% is found in the lower region (C-3 to C-7). Axial rotation for the occiput to C-1 region requires that 1 occipital condyle slide anteriorly on C-1 and that the contralateral condyle slide posteriorly. This is difficult because of the relatively deep fit of the condyles. In contrast, axial rotation is a major function for C-1 to C-2. The IAR is close to the spinal cord, permitting rotation without bony impingement on the spinal cord. Motion after alar ligament transection increases at both the occiput to C-1 and C-1 to C-2 joints.

In flexion and extension of the neck, there is a sliding movement between vertebrae. The flexion-extension for occipital to C-1 occurs about an axis approximately at the center of curvature of the occipital condyles. It also includes translation of the anterior arch of C-1 cephalad and slightly posteriorly, because of the curved anterior surface of the odontoid. It is possible to gain additional motion by exerting external forces on the fully flexed or extended neck (Fig. 43). Most of the motion in flexion-extension is in the central region. The largest range and the highest incidence of cervical spondylosis is found in C-5 to C-6. For flexion-extension, the location of the IAR for each pair of vertebrae is generally within the body of the lower vertebra, but gradually shifts from a position in the lower dorsal quadrant of C-3 to the middle of the upper end plate of C-7. The IAR is at the center of a circle passing through the articular surface of the facet joint. In extension, the posteroinferior margin of the upper vertebral body approximates the arch of the subjacent vertebra and protrudes into the cervical canal, narrowing the sagittal diameter by 1 to 2 mm. The posterior longitudinal ligament and the ligamenta flava are lax in extension, becoming stretched and thinner in flexion. The value for the intradural sagittal diameter is 2 to 3 mm lower in extension than in flexion. This, coupled with the fact that the cord is thicker in extension than in flexion, is important clinically because the cord has less play in extension than in flexion. Fortunately, the canal is widest at the atlanto-axial level and narrows at C-5. A generally accepted average figure for the sagittal diameter of C-4 to C-7 is 17 mm, whereas that for the transverse diameter is 30 mm (measured on AP radiographs as the interpedicular distance).

Full extension can cause enough foraminal closure to produce increased arm symptoms in a patient with disk herniation or osteophytic encroachment into the foramen.

Lateral bending occurs only to a small extent between occiput to C-1 because the alar ligaments force rotation about the odontoid. This, in turn, requires some stretching out of the transverse ligament.

For lateral bending and axial rotation in C-3 to C-7 vertebrae, there is a smaller range of motion in the more caudal segments. The maximum sagittal plane translation occurring in the lower cervical spine under simulated flexion-extension is in the middle and lower cervical spine. The middle cervical spine region has a distinct characteristic coupling pattern, in which lateral bending and axial rotation are coupled. The coupling occurs in such a way that the spinous processes point in the direction opposite to the lateral bend, as a result of either soft-tissue tensions or the orientation of the facet joints. For lateral bending, the IAR is located in the upper vertebral body. For axial rotation, both the uncinate processes and the facet joints constrain motion. Because the facet joint plates are perpendicular to the sagittal plane, these joints must either open up slightly (for example, the right joint opens with right axial rotation) or must undergo some coupled lateral bending.

Thoracic Spine

The thoracic spine is a transition between the more mobile cervical and lumbar regions. It is relatively rigid and facili-

tates the mechanical activities of the lungs and rib cage. The vertebral bodies and disks are larger in the lower thoracic spine. The spatial orientation of the facets in the thoracic spine changes from the upper to the lower region. In a given individual, the orientation of the facet joints may change abruptly to that of the lumbar region anywhere between T-9 and T-12. In flexion-extension, there are 4° of motion in the upper portion of the thoracic spine and 6° in the middle segments. In the lower portion, there are 12° of motion at each segment. In lateral bending, there are 6° of motion in the upper thoracic spine, with 8° or 9° in the two lower segments. In axial rotation, there are 8° of motion in the upper half of the thoracic spine and 2° for each interspace of the three lower segments.

Abnormalities in coupling of the thoracic spine between lateral bending and axial rotation may be relevant in scoliotic deformities. In the upper and lower thoracic spine, the 2 motions are strongly coupled, but in the middle portion of the thoracic spine, the coupling is inconsistent. In vitro studies have shown that all 6 degrees of freedom demonstrate coupling patterns of varying degrees.

Lumbar Spine

The lumbar spine, in conjunction with the hips, is responsible for much of the mobility of the trunk. The flexion-extension range of motion may be attributed to the sizable intervertebral disk coupled with a lack of facet constraint. Sagittal plane translation is frequently used to determine whether or not there is instability. In symptom-free subjects, 2 to 3 mm or even larger translation in the anterior sagittal plane is normal for the lumbar spine. Some reports mention that even 5-mm translational motion in the L-3 to L-4 and L-4 to L-5 segments and 4 mm in the L-5 to S-1 segment may be normal.

There are several coupling patterns in the lumbar spine such as coupling of axial rotation with +y-axis translation, coupling of 3 degrees of freedom translation with axial rotation (Fig. 44) and coupling of axial rotation and lateral bending with flexion-extension. Because the spinal column is symmetrical about the sagittal plane, coupled rotations in association with sagittal plane motions might not be expected. The observed coupled motions may be due to facet asymmetry, disk degeneration, or suboptimal muscle control.

One of the strongest coupling patterns is that of lateral bending with axial rotation. The pattern is such that the spinous processes point in the same direction as the lateral bending, the opposite of that in the cervical spine and the upper thoracic spine. There is also a coupling pattern of lateral bending with axial rotation at the lumbosacral joint, which is the opposite of that found in the lumbar spine and the same as that observed in the cervical and upper thoracic spine (below C-2). In vitro experiments have shown that coupling patterns are affected by the preload in the spine and by posture.

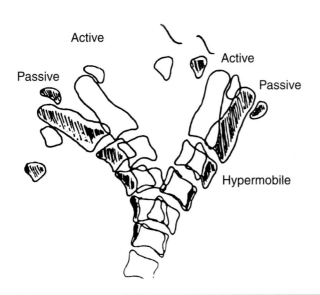

Figure 43

This diagram depicts the active and passive motions of the cervical spine. (Reproduced with permission from Dvorak J, Fraeklich D, Penning L, et al: Functional radiographic diagnosis of the cervical spine. *Spine* 1988;13:748.)

Recent analyses of in vivo flexion-extension radiographs have determined that the center of rotation lies somewhere in the posterior half of the disk near the inferior end plate (Fig. 45). However, there is considerable disagreement regarding its precise location, possibly because the center of rotation moves during flexion-extension. The path described by the moving center of rotation is called the centrode. The axes are in the right side of the disk during left lateral bending and in the left side of the disk during right lateral bending. An in vivo study of lateral bending shows much scatter in the computed instantaneous axes of rotation.

For axial rotation, the IARs are located in the region of the posterior nucleus. In the presence of disk degeneration, there is a tendency for the axes to be spread out. It might be possible to use abnormalities in the IARs to diagnose disk degeneration or other disorders.

Experiments on whole, cadaveric lumbar spines and on male volunteers have been conducted to determine whether axial rotation changes when subjects bend forward and whether rotation is affected by articular tropism. Axial rotation of implanted wires was measured while the spine was rotated in a torsion apparatus. Pins were inserted into the spinous processes of L-3, L-4, and L-5 of the volunteers, and the axial rotation of the pins was measured while the subjects rotated in a torsion apparatus. Axial rotation was found to be less when combined with forward flexion, and articular tropism did not influence the amplitude of rotation.

The Sacroiliac Region

The kinematics of the sacroiliac (SI) joint is poorly understood despite the importance of this joint. The SI joint is partly synovial and partly syndesmotic. It is completely ankylosed in as many as 76% of subjects older than 50 years of age. However, even among normal subjects, these are rather stiff joints, the overall motion and stability of which are affected by the coarse interdigitating articular surfaces.

A pelvic shift that occurs when an individual supports his weight on 1 leg suggests that there may be SI joint motion in the stance phase of gait. Vertical translations of 2 to 3 mm and rotations of up to 3° are reported at the pubic symph-

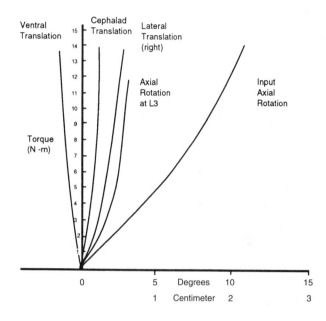

Figure 44

This illustration further demonstrates coupling of motion. Input axial rotation referred to L-3 produces axial rotation at L-3, lateral translation to the right, cephalad translation, and ventral translation. (Reproduced with permission from Pope MH, Wilder DG, Matteri RE, et al: Experimental measurements of vertebral motion under load. *Orthop Clin North Am* 1977;8: 155–167.)

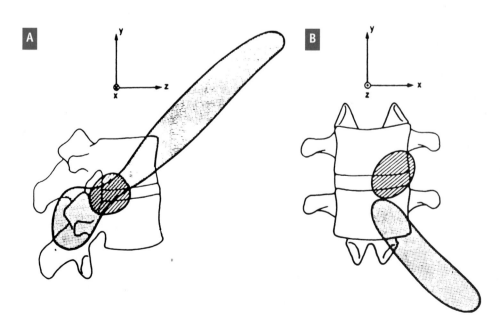

Figure 45

The changes in the location of the instantaneous axes of rotation in the lumbar spine motion segment, with and without degenerative disk disease in flexion (**A**) and right lateral bending (**B**). The axes for the normal disks are shown in the dark areas with longitudinal lines, and those for the degenerated disks are shown in the lighter gray areas. (Reproduced with permission from Rolander SD: Motion of the lumbar spine with special reference to the stabilizing effect of posterior fusion. *Acta Orthop Scand* 1966;90:1–144.)

ysis with standing. The symphysis motion is slightly greater in multiparous females. Patients with sacroiliac joint disorders have been studied with roentgen stereophotogrammetry. The rotations have been small, averaging 2.5°, with translations averaging 0.7 mm. Because of these very small motions, it has been suggested that external fixation of the pelvis is useful in assessing painful sacroiliac joint instability and should precede surgical intervention.

There is scatter of the IARs of the SI joint in both the sagittal and frontal plane motions. Because of the irregular contour of a portion of the joint surface, it is believed that separation must occur with enough force to overcome ligamentous resistance.

Table 13
Vertebral Muscles and Their Motor Functions

Function	Muscles
Anterior	
Muscles in front flex the spine.	Longus collis*

If the muscle runs a little obliquely and contracts independently of the corresponding muscle on the opposite side, it rotates and bends the spine laterally, as well as flexes it.	Longus capitis
	Rectus capitis anterior
	Rectus capitis lateralis+
	Obliquus externus abdominis*
	Obliquus internus abdominis*
	Psoas major+
	Psoas minor+
	    Iliacus
	        Quadratus lumborum

Posterior	
Muscles in back extend the spine.	Superficial stratum

If the muscle runs a little obliquely and contracts independently of the corresponding muscle on the opposite side, it rotates and bends the spine laterally, as well as extends it.	Splenius capitis*+
	Splenius cervicis+
	Erector spinae (sacrospinalis)
	Iliocostalis*+
	Longissimus*
	Spinalis*+
	Deep stratum
	    Semispinali
	        Thoracis*
	        Cervicis*
	        Capitis*
	    Multifidi*
	        Rotatores*
	        Interspinales
	        Intertransversaril*

Lateral	

Muscles on the side bend the spine laterally	Trapezius
	Sternocleidomastoid*
	Quadratus lumborum
	Scalenus*
	    Anterior
	    Medial
	    Posterior

*   Muscles with axial rotation function

+   Muscles with lateral bending function

Spine Kinetics

Kinetics of the spine is best understood in terms of the spine's response to external load moments. The spine is unstable without the support of the muscles. An osteoligamentous spine without the muscles buckles under very small compressive forces. Although clinical and radiographic criteria are increasingly accurate for predicting instability, there is no consensus regarding a definition of segmental instability. Instability is defined biomechanically as a decreased stiffness of the motion segment, increased mobility, or abnormal motions. Segmental instability also has been defined in terms of a loss of stiffness such that the application of force produces pain and greater displacements than would otherwise be seen. However, there are considerable individual differences in spinal structures and motions. In order to understand low back problems, the spine must be understood as more than the sum of its parts.

Muscles allow the trunk to move and retain the position of the spinal segments. Vertebral muscles can be classified as anterior, posterior, or lateral (Table 13). The muscles of the back also can be distinguished as deep or superficial. In addition to the dorsal muscles, the anterior and lateral abdominal muscles and the gluteal muscles help to control trunk motion and support the ligamentous spine.

Cervical Muscles

The role of muscles in the neck is to control head position. The passive elements (bone, disk, ligament, joints) exert important control over translations, as well as the location of the centers of rotation. However, angle rotation is controlled by the muscles, except at the end of the range of motion.

The general structure of the neck is similar to that of the rest of the axial skeleton: some gross-function muscles span several motion segments and fine-function muscles cross only 1 or 2 segments. The anterior gross-function muscles are the longus colli, longus capitis, and scalenes, which attach either to the vertebral bodies or to transverse processes. The anterior fine-function muscles are the intertransversarii, which span just 1 segment. The posterior gross-function muscles attached to the spinous processes are the splenius capitis and semispinalis cervices. Muscles oriented parallel to the longitudinal axis can efficiently extend or bend laterally, but other muscles are needed to produce other motions. Determination of muscle site attachments and measurements of muscle forces in vivo and in vitro have provided a basis for developing biomechanical models of the neck.

The longissimus is made up of the longissimus cervices, which inserts into transverse processes, and the longissimus capitis, which inserts into the mastoid process. The spinalis muscle, absent in the lumbar region, is also divided into 2 parts: spinalis cervices, which connects the transverse processes, and spinalis capitis, which inserts into the occipital. The erector spinae controls movements of both the neck and head. It lies superficial to the semispinalis, multifidus, and rotator muscles, covering them completely. The interspinales connect the adjacent spinous process, and the intertransversarii connect adjacent transverse processes. They provide intrinsic stability to individual spinal levels.

The sternomastoid muscle is the most prominent of the anterior neck muscles arising from the sternum and the clavicle and inserting into the mastoid process. This muscle is a strong rotator and lateral flexor of the head; in addition, when acting together, the sternomastoid muscles flex the neck.

Thoracolumbar Muscles

The small intersegmental muscles found at every lumbar intervertebral joint are the interspinalis and intertransversarii. The polysegmental muscles of the lumbar spine are the multifidus and the longissimus thoracis, the iliocostalis lumborum, and the spinalis thoracis (or spinalis dorsi). The lumbar multifidus is the most medial of the lumbar back muscles and consists of 5 segmental bands. Each segmen-

tal band stems from a spinous process and consists of several individual fascicles with various caudal insertions (Figs. 46 and 47). The spinalis thoracis is relatively small and is principally a muscle of the thoracic region. Only its lowest fibers enter the lumbar region to insert onto the L-1 to L-3 spinous processes. It has little functional role in the lumbar region.

The longissimus thoracis and iliocostalis lumborum are massive muscles and major extensors of the lumbar spine (Fig. 48). Only the thoracic fibers of the longissimus thoracis and iliocostalis lumborum contribute to the erector spinae aponeurosis. The lumbar fibers that form the lumbar erector spinae arise from individual lumbar vertebrae and insert into the iliac crest independent of the erector spinae aponeurosis.

The 4 abdominal muscles are the rectus abdominis, the external and internal obliques, and the transverse abdominal muscle. The rectus abdominis runs as a wide strong band from the xiphoid process to the pubic arch. The external oblique is the largest of the 3 lateral muscles and runs from the ribs to the inguinal ligament, rectus sheath, and

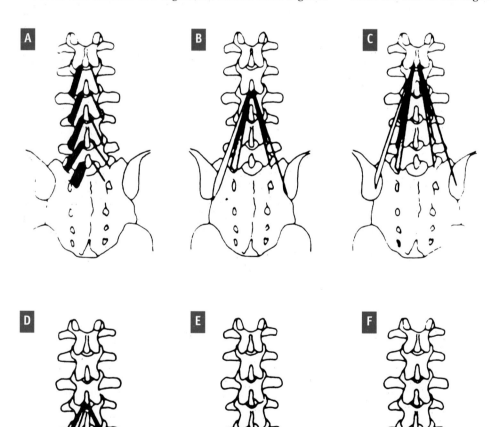

Figure 46

Schematic illustrations of the fascicles of the lumbar multifidus as seen in a posteroanterior view. **A** illustrates the laminar fibers at every level. **B-F** illustrate the longer fascicles from the caudal edge and tubercles of the spinous processes at levels L-1 to L-5. (Reproduced with permission from McIntosh JE, Bogduk N: The biomechanics of lumbar multifidus. *Clin Biomech* 1986;1:205–213.)

ilium. The internal oblique is fan-shaped, running caudolaterally in the superior aspect and mediolaterally in the inferior aspect. The transversus abdominis muscle is deep to the obliques and runs transversely from the rectus sheath to the 6 lower ribs, the thoracolumbar fascia, and the ilium.

Several other muscles that are functionally important to the spine are the quadratus lumborum, psoas, trapezius, and latissimus dorsi. The quadratus lumborum and the psoas muscle attach to the dorsal part of the vertebral bodies of T-12 to L-5 as well as to the disks. The psoas then combine with the iliacus muscle to form the iliopsoas, which attaches to the lesser trochanter. The latissimus dorsi arises from the iliac crest and lower vertebral spinous processes and ribs to insert into the humerus.

Muscle Strength Strength is the ability of a muscle or a group of muscles to exert force. The type of contraction determines the force output and, therefore, calls for different measurement techniques. Strength is measured concentrically, isometrically (static strength), eccentrically, isotonically (concentric strength), isokinetically, and isoinertially. Maximum strength is the most frequently used clinical measure. Because strength varies as a function of joint angle, it can be defined as a curve displaying the force output as a function of the angle (Fig. 49). Strength curves are affected by such factors as age, gender, motivation, pain, and muscle and joint physiology and geometry.

Isometric techniques include manual muscle testing and

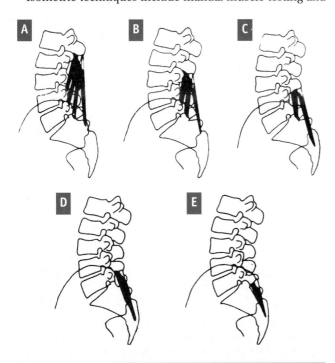

Figure 47

Schematic illustrations of the fascicles of the lumbar multifidus as seen in lateral views. **A-E** show the fascicles present at levels L-1 to L-5, respectively. (Reproduced with permission from McIntosh JE, Bogduk N: The biomechanics of lumbar multifidus. *Clin Biomech* 1986;1:205–213.)

involve the use of spring and strain gauges as well as dynamometers. Typically, the pelvis is strapped in and the subject is fitted with a harness; the subject is then asked to exert force against resistance. Isotonic strength measurement techniques, most of which are concentric, include using free weights in a controlled movement system or using a constrained system that allows unequal effort. Both the lever arm and speed of movement are important to an isotonic strength measurement. Because isotonic means the same force, a pure isotonic exercise requires changing the resistance throughout the range of motion in proportion to changes in moment arm, referred to as a variable resistance exercise. Assessment occurs throughout the range of motion, but reliability is a problem, and isotonic resistance tasks often are unfamiliar to those being tested. Isokinetic assessment requires a subject to move the trunk or limbs at a controlled speed. The systems are controlled with a dynamometer, which is either passive, allowing only concentric movement, or active, allowing both concentric and eccentric movement.

Approximately half of all compensable low back injuries are associated with manual lifting tasks. Some studies suggest a relationship between lifting strength and back injury rates. In jobs that require heavy lifting, workers with inadequate strength are probably at a higher risk of injury.

Muscle Endurance Another important attribute of muscle is endurance. Endurance is defined as the point at which muscle fatigue is observable; for example, when a contraction can no longer be sustained at a certain level (isometric fatigue), or when repetitive work can no longer be maintained at a certain output (dynamic fatigue). The mechanical events are preceded by biochemical and physiologic changes within the muscle, but these changes do not necessarily immediately influence the mechanical performance of the muscle.

Mechanical tests of trunk muscle fatigue generally include maintaining a posture or performing an activity repeatedly. Endurance studies sometimes use a dynamic test in which, for example, subjects move a padded bar connected to an isokinetic dynamometer at a paced rate. In these studies, trunk flexor muscles fatigue more rapidly than trunk extensor muscles, and women have a higher endurance level than men. The trunk muscles fatigue more easily when isometric contractions are performed and the abdominal muscles fatigue more readily than the back muscles.

In postural endurance tests, in which subjects maintain an unsupported trunk in a horizontal position for a defined period of time, patients with ongoing low back pain have significantly less endurance than healthy controls. Patients with injured backs also fatigue faster than do volunteers with unaffected backs when asked to maintain 60% of a maximum isometric voluntary contraction of the trunk muscles. Some studies have used an isoinertial device to study force output and movement patterns in three dimen-

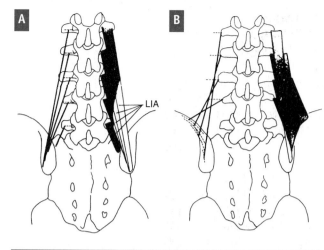

Figure 48

A, A schematic illustration of the fascicles of the longissimus thoracis pars lumborum. Fascicles L-1 to L-4 have long caudal tendons that form the lumbar intermuscular aponeurosis (LIA). The dotted lines marked the extent of the rostral attachments. **B,** A schematic illustration of the lumbar fascicles of iliocostalis lumborum. The dotted lines mark the extent of each attachment. (Reproduced with permission from MacIntosh JE, Bogduk N: The morphology of the lumbar erector spinae. *Spine* 1987;12:658–668.)

sions when subjects performed a flexion-extension movement. Out-of-plane movements increased with fatigue and torque, angular excursion, and angular velocity decreased. The neuromuscular adaptation to fatigue appears to include reduced accuracy, control, and speed of contraction.

EMG data analysis holds much promise as an objective method of measuring muscle fatigue. Early EMG studies relied on the amplitude of the signal as an index of muscle fatigue. However, recent developments indicate that the power density spectrum is a better index of fatigue. Lower frequencies are produced by sustained isometric contractions. Also, back pain patients can be distinguished from pain-free controls by both the initial value of the median frequency and by the rate of change in median frequency over time.

Coordination Musculoskeletal performance capacity implies not only joint stability, but also flexibility, strength, and endurance. Impairment of neuromuscular coordination may also lead to musculoskeletal disability and some suspect that poor coordination plays a role in back pain. Because no single test measures coordination, it is assessed through several independent motor ability components.

Muscular response includes both preparatory muscle activity and anticipatory postural adjustments. The body's center of gravity is shifted so as to offset the resultant forces and moments generated in an upcoming movement. Muscles have been found to be activated in anticipation of a loading event. Under sudden loading conditions, muscle activity begins earlier when adequate warning time is available. Muscle activation might be considered a

pretensioning response analogous to preloading springs. Thus, slack is removed from the system, allowing for a quicker and stiffer response.

The standing human can be modeled in the sagittal plane as a 3-segment linkage. The model predicts that a specific proportional relationship is necessary between the hip, knee, and ankle torques in order to maintain balance. Moreover, a fixed relationship between joint torques may be required to restore balance.

Electromyographic Activity

An understanding of the internal loading of the spine requires the estimation of the tensions in the trunk muscles in addition to considering the external forces and moments acting on the body. Both in vivo experimental and mathematical modeling studies have been performed to characterize the trunk muscle recruitment patterns during various work- or leisure-related activities. For the latter studies, time domain analysis of EMG signals, consisting of quantifying the temporal and amplitude patterns of muscle activities, has been used. The underlying premise is that the tension developed in the muscle has a monotonic relationship with the EMG. Hence, with appropriate signal processing, the biologic EMG signals measured by noninvasive surface electrodes can be used to indicate muscle tension. This topic will be considered in the next section.

The majority of the EMG studies reported in the spine literature address the identification of motor control strategies for execution of trunk movement and/or biomechanical considerations, such as estimation of the compression and shear forces during physical activities. Ergonomists have used EMG studies as a tool to reduce the stresses in

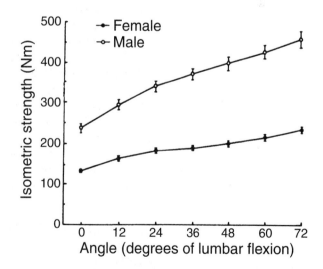

Figure 49

Isometric trunk strength as a function of joint angle. (Reproduced with permission from Graves JE, Pollock ML, Carpenter DM, et al: Quantitative assessment of full range-of-motion isometric lumbar extension strength. *Spine* 1990;15:289–294.)

the spine by modifying the workplace or redesigning the task. The studies of optimal inclination angles between seat and backrest, or the beneficial role of the lumbar support are examples of how seat design has evolved. Rehabilitation experts have also used EMG of trunk muscles in addition to intra-abdominal pressure (IAP) measurements to optimize physical exercises in the treatment of low back pain. These studies have led to modification of exercises to tax the intended muscles maximally while reducing the load in the spine; for example, sit-up with flexed hip and knee joints. The following is a brief overview of recent literatures on EMG studies of the trunk musculature during relaxed standing, slow trunk flexion and extension, lifting, axial rotation, and fast movements against the resistance.

During upright standing, slight myoelectric activity in the paraspinal muscles has been reported. Because postural sway is present, small activities are recorded in either paraspinal or abdominal muscles, but not simultaneously in both. The internal and external oblique muscles show very low activities during relaxed standing. The activities of muscles during unsupported sitting are very similar to those during standing. The inclination of the seat has been shown to influence trunk muscle activities. A marked reduction in activities of trunk muscles is reported as the back inclination is increased to 110°.

EMG activity in back muscle increases as a function of the trunk flexion angle, because the moment generated by the weight of the head, arm, and trunk is progressively increased at more flexed postures (Fig. 49). At the same flexion angle, the higher the external load the greater the back muscle activity. These observations lead to one of the few universally accepted lifting recommendations: keep the load close to your body to lower the stresses in the spine. The large mass of the upper body poses postural perturbations that are anticipated and compensated by the central nervous system (CNS). During slow spinal flexion or extension movements, after a brief agonist activity initiates the movement, body weight is used to maintain the movement while antagonist muscles control the movement by their eccentric action.

The pelvis and spine rhythm has been considered an important clinical sign and should be considered during routine spine mobility measurement. This coordination pattern is controlled by the trunk, pelvic, and thigh muscles. An orderly recruitment of the lower extremity muscles has been found, ensuring stability of the pelvis and lower spine during flexion or extension of the spine. At full flexion, healthy subjects will have reduced activities in the back muscles, and in some cases complete silence is observed. Patients with low back problems may not present this flexion-relaxation phenomenon. Possible explanations include loss of reflex inhibition, abnormal muscle reaction to lengthening, and inability to fully flex because of pain. In one study, a positive relation was found between the disability and the loss of flexion-relaxation among patients.

Such relaxation has been documented during lateral bending for the trunk muscles.

Lateral bending and axial rotation movements are produced by a higher level of coactivation than sagittal plane movements. This is partly caused by the higher trunk stabilization required and the complex line of actions of trunk muscles. During lateral bending, the EMG activities of ipsilateral trunk muscles in the lumbar region increase, but the contralateral muscles have a larger increase. However, in the thoracic region, the ipsalateral muscles show the main increase in activity. The highest activities during axial rotations are found in the external oblique and erector spinae muscles.

Because of the association between manual material handling tasks and low back injuries, the interest shown in examining and quantifying trunk muscle activities during lifting has been considerable. Recent investigations using computerized dynamometers have shown that trunk muscle activities are affected by the trunk posture (including its postural asymmetry), velocity, and level of resisted force. The muscles of the back, buttocks, and hamstring are all active during the lift. The lifting mode is less important than where the load is placed and the speed of lifting. However, whether lifting should be done with the back in a position of lordosis, kyphosis, or in the straight position continues to be debated. During the fast movement of the spine, with or without external resistance, a more impulsive loading takes place with a set of agonist and antagonist recruitment patterns showing a predominantly reciprocal pattern. A very task-specific recruitment pattern is evident in these studies. The level of coactivation, in particular among the latissimus dorsi and oblique muscles, is a function of the speed, amplitude of movement, and resistance levels.

Determination of Muscle, Ligament, and Joint Forces

Figure 50 provides the computations necessary to evaluate the forces in the lumbar spine in simple sagittal plane lifting. The muscles are the primary internal source of force resulting in motion of the vertebrae. Any shift in the center of gravity of the trunk must be balanced by muscle force to maintain equilibrium. Muscle forces also are required to balance the moment caused by an arm, an external weight, or any other force applied to the trunk, head, and upper extremities. If the combined effect of all the body weight and external forces on the spine are assumed to produce a moment that must be balanced by a single spinal muscle group to maintain equilibrium, the force in that muscle group can be calculated. Such representations provide valuable information. For example, such a model illustrates that to maintain low muscle forces, and consequently low stresses, on the spine structures when standing, an upright symmetric posture is preferred and all loads should be as close to the body as possible.

However, there are a number of 3-D models in the literature—most of which determine equilibrium through a cutting plane, usually at the L-3 level—in which the weights of the body segments, the moments of those weights, and any forces and moments externally applied superior to that plane are equilibrated (resisted) by moments provided by the passive tissues; that is, disks, ligaments, and several active muscle forces. These models are a more accurate representation of the problem and are used to acquire information regarding the stresses arising in each of the components sharing the load. When the load moment is applied in asymmetric postures, a much more complex situation occurs. However, in such cases, without further information, the distribution of load among the active muscles is statically indeterminate because the number of unknown muscle forces is larger than the 6 available equations describing the static equilibrium condition. Therefore, additional means must be provided to solve the problem.

Optimization techniques are used to select the optimal solution among the infinite number of solutions resulting from the statically indeterminate condition. An objective function (that is, the energy expenditure of muscular effort is to be minimized, the force produced by each muscle is proportional to its cross-sectional area) is chosen and a set of internal loads is calculated to minimize that function. The most common means of validating muscle activity in these

models is by EMG signals. The second validation technique is to measure intradiskal pressures. The latter technique has been shown to relate directly to spine compression; however, such measurements are both invasive and difficult.

Recently, dynamic models have been considered to calculate a resultant moment at the L-4 to L-5 or L-5 to S-1 levels as a means of predicting disk compression and shear forces at the same time as considering the inertial effects caused by body acceleration.

Representation of more realistic anatomic lines of action of muscles in these models has improved the fidelity of the results. For example, L-4 to L-5 compression estimates were reduced by up to 35% with a more realistic anatomic model of the erector spinae muscle group. The shear force estimates could be altered from more than 500 N, with L-4 tending to shear anteriorly on L-5, to less than 300 N, with L-4 tending to shear posteriorly on L-5. A single "equivalent" extensor soft-tissue moment arm of 7.5 cm, rather than 5 cm, would be needed to equate the compression.

More recently, the temporal and amplitude patterns of measured muscle activity have been quantified by integrating the rectified EMG signal (IEMG) to infer muscle tensions. The resulting measurements have been used in

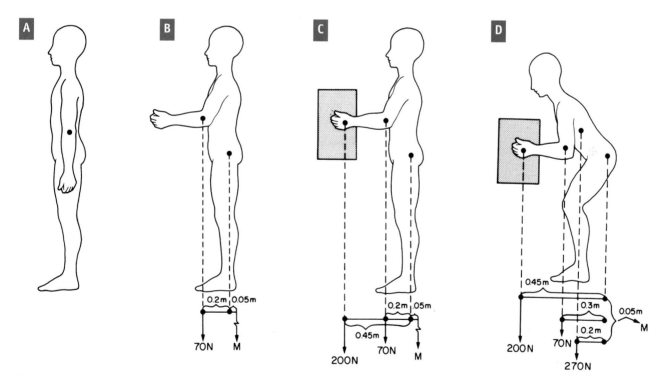

Figure 50

A, In upright standing the body segments are well aligned with respect to the center of gravity and little muscular effort is required to maintain equilibrium. **B,** An elevated arm causes a load moment of about 70 N x 0.2 m (14 N•m), which must be equilibrated by the back muscles acting with an average moment arm of 0.05 m (muscle tension = 280 N). **C,** An additional object with a weight of 200 N held at 0.45 m causes an additional moment of 90 N•m (total muscle tension = 2,080 N). When leaning forward holding no weight (**D**), the trunk moment (270 x 0.21 = 54 N•m), arm moment (70 x 0.3 = 21 N•m), and with hand weight of 37 N•m, the hand moment (37 x 0.45 = 17 N•m) act together, causing a total load moment of 92 N•m (muscle tension = 1,840 N). (Reproduced with permission from Pope MH, Andersson GBJ, Frymoyer JW, et al: Occupational biomechanics of the lumbar spine, in *Occupational Low Back Pain: Assessment, Treatment, and Prevention*. St. Louis, MO, CV Mosby, 1991.)

mathematical models to estimate the internal loading of the spine given the anatomic line of actions of the muscles and their cross-sectional areas. This class of models is called EMG-driven models. Some controversy exists with regard to the nature of the relationship between the IEMG and the muscle force because both linear and nonlinear relationships have been reported and actual measurements of muscle force have not been verified.

Nevertheless, these EMG-driven models have been used to quantify the loads (compression and shear forces) during dynamic activities. The main advantage of these models is their ability to account for coactivation of muscles, which is not predicted by optimization-based models. Thus, EMG-driven models will not underestimate the loads because they incorporate any coactivation that may be present. In addition, they capture interindividual and intraindividual variations present in the recruitment patterns during performance of the repetitive tasks. Finally, there is no need to assume that a mathematical criterion or an objective function is being maximized (or minimized). The advantage of the optimization models is that they are suitable for simulation and design because the changes in the loading conditions can be handled by varying the input to the mathematical model. EMG-driven models, on the other hand, require an elaborate experimental setup to collect the necessary muscle activities. The future may well belong to the hybrid systems.

Intra-Abdominal Pressure

For many years IAP has been widely believed to have a beneficial role in spine biomechanics. During lifting, the amount of weight lifted is linearly related to IAP as measured in the stomach or rectum. This correlation between IAP and trunk effort forms the basis for supposing that IAP reduces loads in the trunk. IAP may help reduce compression in 2 ways: by directly decreasing the contribution of the muscular extensor and/or by creating a spinal tensile force on the diaphragm. The belief that abdominal pressure is a source of spinal support provides the rationale for flexion exercises and for the wearing of corsets and support belts during weightlifting. Some have proposed that spinal support and alleviation of compression are achieved through action on the lumbodorsal fascia, but other researchers maintain that the theory reflects inaccurate assumptions about anatomy.

Because it is not possible to increase abdominal pressure without abdominal wall activity and a closed glottis, the associated costs of contracting the muscles cannot be neglected. The extensor forces and moments created by IAP do not offset the compression and flexor moment generated by abdominal activation. The frontal muscles must contract, producing a flexion moment in order to produce an increase in IAP. A Valsalva maneuver contracts the internal and external obliques, but the rectus abdominis contracts to a much lesser degree. There is still no direct evidence to support the hypothesis that intra-abdominal pressure

reduces tension in the back muscle and compressive loads on the disk during trunk effort. Currently most of the evidence appears to be growing against the suggested role of IAP to relieve activity of the back muscles by providing an extension moment. However, the literature does point to the significance of IAP to provide stability for the trunk during peak external loading.

Structure and Function of the Hip Joint

Introduction

The hip joint is a ball-and-socket joint in which the head of the femur resides in the acetabulum of the pelvis. The surface area and the radius of curvature of the articular surface of the acetabulum closely match those of the articular surface of the femoral head. The hip joint is a highly constrained joint. Because of the inherent stability conferred by its bony architecture, this joint is well suited for performing the weightbearing supportive tasks that are required of it. The femoral ball is captured by the acetabular socket, allowing rotation to occur with virtually no translation. The constraint imparted by the bony architecture minimizes the need for ligamentous and soft-tissue constraints to maintain the stability of the hip articulation. Although this increased constraint confers stability on the hip, it does so at the expense of limiting the global range of motion of this joint at the fulcrum of the lower extremity. Fortunately, the lower extremities do not need to be placed in a variety of positions in space during activities of daily living. During most ambulatory activities, the lower extremity is positioned anteriorly in the sagittal plane with only small rotations necessary in the other 2 planes. Activities such as sitting, rising from a chair, and dressing require greater degrees of flexion and rotation at the hip joint.

Anatomic Structure

The acetabulum has a hemispheric shape and is composed of portions from all 3 sections of the pelvis (the ilium, ischium, and pubis). It faces in an inferior and anterolateral direction (Fig. 51). The articular cartilage is situated about the anterior, lateral, and posterolateral acetabular periphery, encompassing approximately two thirds of the surface of the hemisphere. With its underlying bone it is more prominent than the recessed medial acetabular fossa and defines a diameter that is approximately equal to that of the femoral head. The acetabular labrum is a fibrocartilaginous lip around the rim of the acetabulum; it contributes to the shape and depth of the acetabulum and provides additional femoral head coverage. The matching size and spherical shape of the femoral head and acetabulum provide for a highly stable articulation. This stability and the large size of this joint are consistent with the substantial loads that must be borne by the hip. The femoral head forms approximately a 125° angle of inclination with the femoral shaft. This angle is greater in the child, often 140° at 5 years of age. The angle of femoral torsion is the angle between the transverse axes of the head and neck and that of the condylar axes at the lower end of the femur. In the adult this measures 12° to 15° whereas it measures approximately 40° at birth. Together these two angles cause the femoral neck and head to face cephalad medially and anteriorly. Thus, this direction is not in line with that of the acetabulum as both face anteriorly.

The articulation of the femoral head in the acetabulum permits 3 degrees of rotational freedom of the femur about the pelvis, while essentially eliminating relative translation between the femoral head and acetabulum. A smooth articulation is provided by articular cartilage. The cartilage on the femoral head is thickest at the center, while the acetabular cartilage is thickest at the superior portion of the acetabular wall. This cartilage orientation is consistent with the load-bearing and translational requirements anticipated at the hip joint. The smooth relative rotation between the acetabulum and femoral head is aided by synovial fluid lubrication as well as by the articular cartilage.

Although the bony constituents of the hip joint provide conformity and much of the joint's stability, other passive anatomic structures are required to completely restrain relative translation between femoral head and acetabulum. The capsule, reinforced by ligaments, is one of the strongest

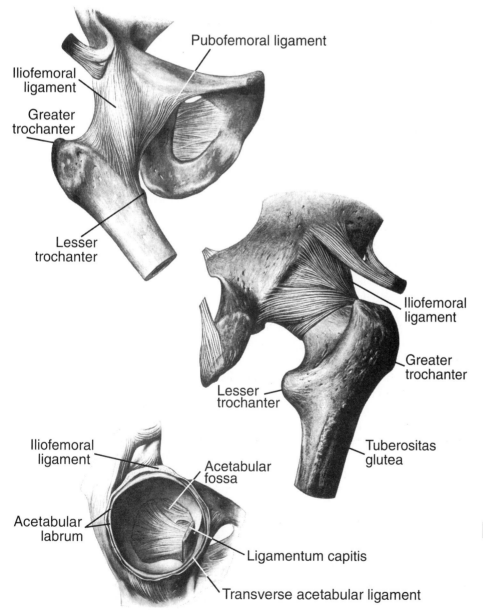

Figure 51

Anatomy of the hip. (Reproduced with permission from Sobotta J, Figge FHJ: *Atlas der Anatomie des Menschen*, ed 20, Vol. I. Munich, Germany, Urban & Schwarzenberg, 1993.)

joint capsules in the entire body. External to its synovial membrane it is composed of fibers oriented in a deep circular and a superficial longitudinal layer extending from the rim of the acetabulum to the femoral neck (Fig. 51). The deep obicular band derives some of its fibers from the deep tendons of the gluteal region as well as the reflected head of the rectus. The longitudinal fibers cover the circular zone anteriorly forming a mass that varies in thickness and direction. Additional passive restraint is provided by several ligaments connecting the pelvis and femur. The ligamentum capitis (ligamentum teres) is a weak synovial attachment extending from the acetabular fossa and transverse acetabular ligament to the fovea capitis on the femoral head. The exceedingly thick band termed the iliofemoral band (or Y ligament of Bigelow) extends from the anterior superior iliac spine to the femoral intertrochanteric line. The bands extending from the upper pubic ramus to the lower intertrochanteric line are thinner and termed the pubofemoral band. The iliofemoral, pubocapsular, and ischiocapsular ligaments lie external to the articular capsule and connect the iliac, pubic, and ischial portions of the acetabular rim to the femur. Together these tissues form an exceedingly strong group of soft tissues, preventing relative acetabular/femoral head translation. These passive restraints do not prevent rotation, but they do limit it to some extent.

Musculature

Requiring movement and strength in all rotational planes about the joint, the hip is enclosed circumferentially by a large mass of 20 muscles. Their origin is from a broad spherical volume of the pelvis located anterior, medial, superior, and posterior to the hip joint. The range of excursion and power of these muscles is increased by the length of the neck, the prominence of the trochanters, and the relatively long moment arms produced by their origin and insertional positions relative to the center of the hip joint.

Anatomically these muscles may be classified by their source of innervation, the quadrant (anterior, posterior, medial, or lateral) in which they cross about the hip joint, or their primary rotational function. As in the case of the ligaments, the actions of these muscles depend significantly on the rotational position of the hip joint. This relates not only to the location of the origin of these muscles but also to their insertion.

Although muscles encapsulate the hip joint, their insertions onto the femur are at small sites about the femur and their line of action is not directly oriented parallel to the longitudinal axes of the femur when the hip joint is in a neutral position. For example, when the hip is in a neutral position, the iliopsoas, which inserts into the lesser trochanter of the femur (posteromedially), has a line of section that is directed anteromedially as it crosses the joint.

Just distal to the posterior aspect of the femoral neck and slightly laterally is the gluteal ridge, where the gluteus maximus tendon inserts. This tendon insertion continues distally as the intermuscular septum. This septum with its bony ridge attachment (linea aspera) extends almost to the lateral supracondylar ridge and biceps septum. Along the linea aspera on the posterior aspect of the femur is the insertion site for the hip adductors. The iliacus and pectineus insert just medial to the linea aspera at the level of insertion of the gluteus maximus. The adductor longus, brevis, and magnus all insert below this along its ridge, extending almost halfway down the femur. Thus, these muscles not only adduct the thigh, but produce external rotation. The adductor longus creates hip flexion if the limb is flexed. The greater trochanter, which has a wide circumference anterolaterally to posterolaterally, provides the insertion area for the gluteus medius. The gluteus minimus inserts closer to the joint, but in line with the gluteus medius and combines with the ligamentous portion of the capsule. Depending on the relative position of the hip, these muscles can be internal or external rotators or assist in hip flexion, extension, or abduction. These muscles are listed in Table 14.

Kinematics

Kinematic measurements at the hip joint typically focus on describing only joint rotations, because relative translations between the articulating components are generally small and difficult to measure dynamically. These joint motions are described, commonly, in terms of flexion-extension rotation, internal-external rotation, and abduction-adduction rotation.

To quantify the 3-D motion of a body segment relative to a global reference, or the relative motion between 2 body segments as a joint, the local coordinate system (LCS) for the segments must be defined. Specification of an LCS for a given segment requires that the positions of at least 3 points on the segments be known (Fig. 52). The first axis of an LCS can be obtained along a line connecting 2 known points. The second axis then can be defined along a line that is mutually perpendicular to the first axis and connecting the third point and 1 of the first 2 points. The third axis then could be defined as mutually perpendicular to the first 2 axes.

The most common means of expressing lower limb joint motions is through Cardan angles. Cardan angles essentially quantify the relative positions of 2 segments (for example, thigh and lower leg), or perhaps more specifically, the relative positions of the LCSs of 2 segments (Fig. 53). The vectors in Figure 52 are the unit vectors that describe the segments' LCSs. Each LCS unit vector has a magnitude of 1 and a direction that is mutually perpendicular to the other 2 LCS unit vectors for the given segment. The directions of the LCS unit vectors can be obtained as described above. The 3 Cardan angles represent the deviations of the LCS for the segments' 3 axes (Fig. 53). These axes include 1 axis from each of the 2 segments' LCS axes. The third axis is determined as being mutually perpendicular to the first two axes. The selection of the first two axes is arbitrary; however, a common convention in motion biomechanics is to select the mediolateral axis of the more proximal segment as the flexion-extension axis, and the longitudinal axis of the more distal segment as the internal-external rotation axis. Consequently, the axis that is mutually perpendicular represents an abduction-adduction axis (Fig. 53).

Clinically, flexion rotation of the femur with respect to the trunk averages approximately 135° (knee to chest), and extension averages approximately 30°. Although this is commonly described as the range of hip flexion-extension, some of this motion relates to pelvic-vertebral motion. Clinically, with the pelvis stabilized at neutral, hip flexion averages 120° and extension 10°. Estimates as to the true range of hip joint flexion-extension vary; this variance is related partly to the definition of the reference axes of the pelvis with respect to its anatomic landmarks. The anatomic axes of the pelvis commonly used clinically are the line connecting the 2 anterior superior iliac crests and a line

Table 14
Hip Muscles

Action	Muscle	Origin	Insertion
Flexor	Iliopsoas	Entire medial aspect of the ilium to the anterolateral vertebral column L-3 to L-5	Lesser trochanter
	Sartorius	Anterior iliac spine	Medial margin of tibial tuberosity
Extensor	Gluteus maximus	Anterior inferior iliac spineposterior lateral ilium to post aspect of sacrum, coccyx, and sacrotuberous ligament	Gluteal tuberosity of the posterior femur and iliotibial tract of fascia lata
	Biceps femoris long head	Ischial tuberosity	Head and lateral condyle of the tibia
	Semitendinosus	Ischial tuberosity	Tibial tuberosity
	Semimembranosus	Ischial tuberosity	Oblique popliteal ligament posterior knee capsule to medial condyle of the tibia
Adductor	Obturator externus	Lateral side of obturator membrane and medial and caudal margins of obturator foramen	Floor of trochanteric fossa
	Pectineus	Pectin of pubis	Pectineal line
	Adductor brevis	Inferior public ramus near symphyses	Pectineal line and proximal third of medial lip of linea aspera
	Adductor longus	Between superior and inferior pubic rami near symphyses	Middle third of medial lip of linea aspera
	Adductor magnus	Lower part of inferior pubic ramus; ramus of ischium; ischial tuberosity pubic rami near symphyses	Medial side of gluteal tuberosity along entire length of linea aspera to the medial supracondylar ridge and strong tendon to the adductor tubercle
	Gracilis	Inferior pubic ramus near symphyses	Anterior medial surface of tibia near tibial tuberosity
Abductor	Gluteus medius	Broad origin spanning external aspect of linea asperaof entire ilium between the anterior of linea asperaand posterior gluteal lines	Cephalocaudal oblique ridge on greater trochanter
	Gluteus minimus	Broad and deep origin across lateral of linea asperaexternal surface of ilium caudal to of linea asperagluteus medius	Greater trochanter and hip joint capsule
	Tensor fascia latae	Iliac crest to anterior superior	Iliotibial tract
External rotator	Piriformis	Sacrum at S-2, S-3, S-4	Greater trochanter
	Quadratus femoris	Ischial tuberosity	Greater trochanter and quadrate line of femur
	Obturator internus	Posterior aspect of obturator foramen and membrane	Medial surface of greater trochanter
	Superior and inferior gemelli	Ischial spine and ischial tuberosity	Conjoint tendon with obturator internus to greater trochanter

perpendicular to it connecting the midpoint of the pubis symphyses and the midline of the sacrum at the level of the posterior-superior iliac spines. The third axis is difficult to define anatomically; Nelaton's line, the line between the anterior superior iliac spine and the ischial tuberosity, is commonly used. Viewed from a lateral perspective, the proximal tip of the greater trochanter usually passes through this line. When the hip is in maximum extension and considered 0°, the long axis of the femur forms a 50° angle with Nelaton's line. The maximum possible position of hip flexion when the pelvifemoral angle is measured using these same axes is 125°. Thus, the true range of hip flexion-extension is considered to be about 75° to 80°. This is truly less than the range of motion that can be achieved by rotating the femur in the acetabulum in the absence of the joint capsule and ligaments and illustrates the passive restraining action of these tissues during normal motions. In actuality, because of the orientation and strength of these tissues (architecture), the range of motion about any axis can vary with the position of the thigh.

Internal-external rotation of the femur at the hip joint occurs around a longitudinal axis passing through the head of the femur and intercondylar region at the lower end. With the the axis of the femur parallel to the trunk, the femur can rotate through a possible total arc of approximately 50°. In most circumstances, this is composed of about 35° of external rotation and 15° of internal rotation. This rotation varies depending on whether the axis of the femur is parallel or perpendicular to the trunk. When the

joint is in more "flexion" the range of these movements may be increased to 40° and 60°, respectively. Finally, rotation of the femur with respect to the midline of the trunk in the coronal plane, termed abduction and adduction, also occurs. Abduction averages approximately 45° and adduction approximately 25°. With the joint in flexion, a greater range of abduction-adduction rotation is permitted.

The kinematics of the hip joint during functional activities requires a knowledge of joint positions at multiple intervals of time. As the time interval between joint position measurments decreases, the kinematic profiles of the joint become more complete. For cyclic activities, such as walking, kinematics typically are reported for a single cycle. Although the determination of the beginning and end of a periodic activity is generally somewhat arbitrary, for walking and other locomotor functions initial foot-floor ontact at the onset of stance is the cycle end point.

For a number of common activities, nonpathologic hip joint motion is confined primarily to a single rotation. Daily tasks involving the hip joint, such as walking, running, cycling, sitting, and bending primarily involve motion in the sagittal plane in the form of flexion and extension. "Jumping jack" exercises generally involve abduction-adduction rotation. At times, however, flexion-extension, internal-external, and abduction-adduction rotations can be present in a single activity, such as soccer style kicking. Tasks that involve a single primary rotation under non-pathologic conditions can include 2 or all 3 rotations in substantial quantities under certain pathologic, or even

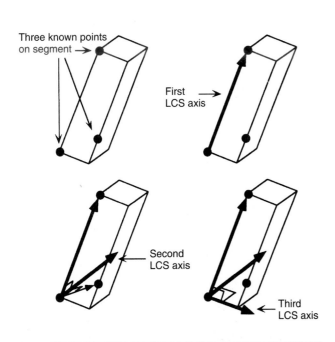

Figure 52

Local coordinate system (LCS) axes.

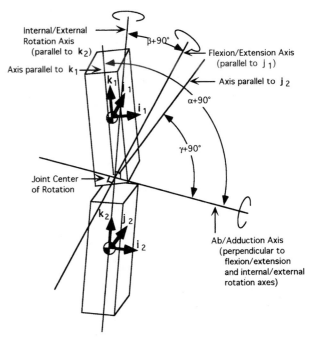

Figure 53

Cardan angles. α represents the flexion-extension angle, β represents the internal-external rotation angle, and γ represents the abduction-adduction angle.

suboptimal states. Walking for an individual with arthritis at the hip might include a raising of the contralateral hip during stance, which would be measured as a hip abduction. Increasing hip abduction during swing phase of walking could be used to compensate for reduced knee flexion in order to obtain foot clearance.

The motion at the nonpathologic hip and knee joints associated with typical daily activity (for example, walking, stair climbing) illustrates the substantial consistency between anatomic structure and essential function (Table 15). Similarly, the right-left symmetry of joint anatomy and common daily motions is not a matter of pure coincidence. Conversely, the motions of hip and knee joints with pathologic conditions (for example, arthritis, muscle spasticity or contracture, hip dislocation) often can be related directly to the specific pathology, as well as involve dramatic asymmetries. The process of relating abnormal joint motions to pathologies, however, is not always a straightforward matter, because such primary abnormal joint motions are associated, typically, with secondary compensatory motions at otherwise nonpathologic joints.

Kinetics

The kinetics at the hip joint relate to the loads associated with this joint. These loads include the forces between the articulating components of the joint, as well as the torques acting about the joints to generate or oppose rotational motion.

In addition to quantifying the relative motion between two segments at a joint, it is also beneficial to quantify, independently, the motions of body segments. Such information is particularly useful for subsequent calculations of joint reaction loads and moments. Euler angles and screw operators are techniques that have been applied frequently to motion biomechanics for representing the positions of body segments.

The Euler angles refer to a set of 3 specific rotations of a body in space (Fig. 54, A). These rotations follow after a translation of the body segment that places the LCS origin coincident with the global coordinate system (GCS) origin. As a common convention, the first rotation is by an angle ϕ about the initial local coordinate system z-axis; the second rotation is by an angle θ, about the local coordinate system x´-axis (the orientation of the LCS x-axis after the first rotation); and the third rotation is by an angle ψ, about the local coordinate system z´´-axis (the orientation of the LCS z-axis after the second rotation). In biomechanics, applications of the Euler angle rotations are intended to align the segment LCS with the GCS. Consequently, the values of the Euler angles quantify the position of the segment in the GCS. To align the LCS and the GCS with the 3 Euler rotations, the first rotation, ϕ about the GCS z-axis, must bring the GCS x´-axis coincident with a "line of nodes" that is defined as a line mutually perpendicular to the GCS z-axis and the initial orientation of the LCS z-axis.

The screw operator involves the displacement of a body from an initial position to a final position via a rotation, ϕ, about a single axis with unit vector u and a translation δ parallel to the same axis (Fig. 54, B). This axis is referred to as the screw axis or the helical axis. Subsequently, by determining the proper direction for the screw axis, angle for the rotation, and distance for the translation, a segment can be moved in a way that aligns its LCS with the GCS. Thus, the screw operator also can be used to define the position of a segment with respect to a GCS. The screw operator is used less commonly than Cardan and Euler angles. This descriptive approach is often used at the knee joint.

Determination of joint kinetics requires considerably greater information than does the calculation of joint kinematics. In addition to body segment positions, the calculation of joint kinetics requires knowledge of body segment parameters, external loading, and segment velocities and accelerations. Body segment parameters that are typically used include mass, volume, length, diameter, and moment of inertia. External loading generally includes ground-reaction forces and gravity during weightbearing portions of activities (for example, stance phase of walking), although only gravity is involved in most nonweightbearing activities. Segment velocities and accelerations are obtained commonly by numerically differentiating positional data; however, these data can be measured directly at times.

Joint torques can be in the direction of motion, in the direction opposite to motion, or in directions for which motion is negligible. Muscles at the hip joint can contribute to joint torques in any of these generally described directions. Muscular torque contributions about the hip joint can be concentric (muscle shortening during contraction), eccentric (muscle lengthening during contraction), or isometric (muscle length constant). Hip joint torques also may have contributions from passive structures (for example, ligamentous and capsular restraints); however, such contributions are generally in directions from which motion is restrained.

At the hip joint, active muscular contraction is primarily responsible for joint torque generation. During many less strenuous activities (for example, walking), lengthening or stretching of the passive elements on a nonactivated muscle, or ligamentous stretch, is all that is required for much of the hip joint torque generated. In other more demanding tasks (for example, stair climbing), active hip torque generation must be used throughout most of the activity. As with the joint kinematics, however, much of the commonly observed hip joint kinetics can be substantially altered in the presence of pathology.

Hip Joint Forces

Joint torques at the hip are calculated more reliably than joint forces. The difficulty of calculating the joint forces arises from the indeterminancy of the individual muscle forces resulting from the large number of muscles acting at the hip joint. Although a number of techniques have been devised for apportioning the loads among the various muscles, none of these techniques have been incorporated into widespread clinical use. While hip joint forces are difficult to calculate directly, it is evident that muscular contractions can contribute substantially to the generation of compressive hip joint forces, if the forces of gravity are to be neutralized by the counterforces of muscles. This is discussed in the chapter on biomechanics. For example, in the presence of arthritis at the hip, compensations such as Trendelenburg lurch or hip hike reduce the muscular exertion about the hip, and, thereby, reduce the compressive force.

Forces that act across the hip joint during dynamic activities have been investigated by several authors. Two approaches have been used. Some have made external measurements of kinetic and kinematic quantities and inferred the internal forces via the use of mathematical computation and models. Others have used internal measurement, affixing the proper instruments to a total joint prosthesis, nail plate, or femoral endoprosthesis. Although neither approach ideally depicts the exact forces present in the average person, their similarities suggest the magnitude of the forces incurred during different activities.

During quiet single-leg stance, the forces transmitted across the hip joint are estimated to be between 2 and 2.8 times body weight. Some have predicted this force to be as high as 6 times body weight. During 2-legged stance, the forces in each hip joint are about half that in single-leg stance. During gait, these forces can be as high as 3 times body weight, although estimates as high as 6 times body weight again have been suggested. The difference in results relates in part to the speed at which the subject walks. In addition, internal instrumented measurements are often lower than mathematically predicted values because the former are based on early postoperative measurements of subjects who had pathologic conditions (for example, arthritis), whereas the latter use data from healthy subjects.

Two peaks usually are noted in these studies; the first just after foot strike at the inception of single-limb stance and the other just preceding opposite foot strike. Forces also exist in swing phase and, generally, have been determined to be about half of the average force seen in stance phase. Getting in and out of bed, raising onto a bedpan, and transferring to a wheelchair all involve high forces of at least 2 times body weight. A summary of the range of motions and estimates of joint forces for the hip and the knee gleaned from the literature for different activities is presented in Tables 15 and 16.

In quiet standing and in gait, the joint-contact force varies over a limited range of the anterosuperior aspect of the femoral head, bounded by a cone. In quiet standing, the direction of this cone closely parallels that of the femoral neck. For activities that require greater hip flexion, the polar angle undergoes a greater anterior excursion consistent with altered out-of-phase increased muscular forces. The joint-contact force, however, does not seem uniform in its pressure distribution and area of contact on the acetabular or femoral cartilage. Although these surfaces represent parts of spheres of identical radius, it has been demonstrated in vivo that, at low loads, the contacting area of the acetabulum is about its periphery. As the load is increased, the contacting area spreads to more central areas with a "flaring out" of the acetabular wall. This flaring, in association with the configuration of the hip joint, explains the constant changes, with changing hip position and activity level, in size and location of femoral surface contacting area.

These changes are significant to "hip containment" and actual surface pressures. Hip containment generally implies either a relative increase in acetabular coverage of the lateral femoral head or an absolute increase in contact of the femoral head with the acetabulum. The maximum potential area of the femoral head that can be in contact with the acetabulum has been estimated to be approximately 65% to 75%. This percentage changes little with changes in hip position, ie, abduction. However, the area of the femoral surface in contact does change.

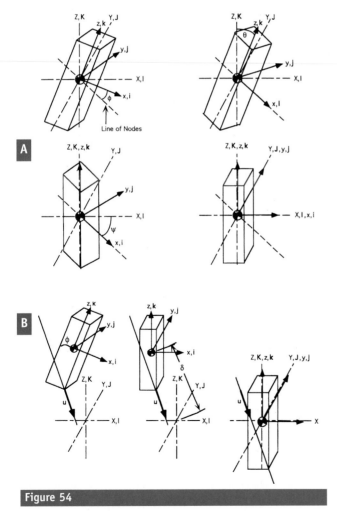

Figure 54

A, Euler angles. B, The screw operator.

Structure and Function of the Knee

The knee actually consists of 2 joints: the femorotibial joint and the patellofemoral joint. The femorotibial joint is the largest joint in the body and is considered to be a modified hinged joint containing the articulating ends of the femur and tibia. The patellofemoral joint consists of the patella, the largest sesamoid bone, and the trochlea of the femur. Taken together, the knee joints function to control the distance between the pelvis and the foot. Because of the role of the knee in weightbearing and its location between the 2 longest bones in the body, tremendous forces are generated across it. During activities such as running, landing, and pivoting, the knee functions to maintain a given leg length and acts as a shock absorber. During stair climbing, crouching, and jumping, large propulsive forces at the knee are generated to control the degree and speed of shortening and lengthening of the leg. In these situations, knee stability is a dynamic process maintained through fixed bony and ligamentous constraints and modified by the action of the muscles crossing the joint.

The bony architecture of the femur, tibia, and patella contributes to joint stability, but to a lesser extent than that of other more constrained joints such as the hip. But in contrast to the shoulder, where stability is maintained through the dynamic action of the surrounding muscles, static constraints play a very significant role in knee stability. The cruciate and collateral ligaments are the major structures limiting motion at the knee. The posteromedial and posterolateral capsular complexes augment the 4 primary ligaments, with the menisci playing a lesser role. The muscles crossing the knee contribute to dynamic stability and are particularly important in the presence of pathologic laxity.

Femorotibial Joint

Architecture

Bone The femoral condyles can be thought of as having separate patellar and tibial articular surfaces. Although the femoral condyles have a variable radius of curvature, if the tibial and patellar articular surfaces are considered separately, each radius of curvature is more uniform. The condyles of the femur can be thought of as having 2 distinct, nearly circular cams. The central portion between these cams is flatter (has a greater radius of curvature) than either the anterior or posterior portions.

The lateral condyle is smaller than the medial in both the AP and proximodistal directions and contributes to the valgus and AP alignment of the knee joint. This configuration, in conjunction with only a slight lateral inclination of the tibial plateau in relation to the joint line (3° valgus and 9° posterior slope), creates an overall valgus and slightly posterior inferior alignment of between 10° and 12° in most knees. The shape of the condyles also plays a critical role in maintaining tension in the ligamentous structures about the knee in all positions of flexion and extension. Disruption of normal architecture can lead to abnormal ligament function with significant alteration in joint stability and biomechanics.

In cross section, the medial and lateral tibial plateaus are roughly ovoid in shape. In the coronal plane they are nearly flat; even when considered in conjunction with the menisci, they are only slightly concave.

Menisci The fibrocartilaginous medial and lateral menisci are thick peripherally and taper to thin edges centrally.

Table 15								
Hip and Knee Kinematics During Various Activities								
Activity Joint	Maximum Flexion	Maximum Extension	Maximum Range	Maximum Adduction	Maximum Abduction	Ab/Adduct Range	Maximum Internal Rotation	Maximum External Rotation
Walking								
Hip	20°–40°	0°–20°	40°–52°	2°–10°	0°–8°	8°–14°	2°–12°	4°–10°
Knee	57°–65°	(–3)°–0°	54°–65°	2°–18°	0°–7°	5°–18°	(–5)°–10°	5°–20°
Cycling								
Knee	110°	(–45)°	65°					
Stair Ascending								
Hip	40°	(–5)°	35°					
Knee	80°	(–5)°	75°					
Stair Descending								
Hip	30°	5°	35°					
Knee	90°	(–5)°	85°					

Table 16

Hip and Knee Kinetics During Various Activities

Acitivity Joint	Max. Joint Force (BW)	Max. Flexion Moment (N·m)	Max. Exten. Moment (N·m)	Max. Adduct. Moment (N·m)	Max. Abduct. Moment (N·m)	Max. Internal Rot. Moment (N·m)	Max. External Rot. Moment (N·m)	Max. Conc. Power (W)	Max. Ecc. Power (W)	Max. Ener. Generation (J)	Max. Ener. Absorption (J)
Walking											
Hip	3–8.5	40–80	30–130	10–100	10–105	3–20	0–13				
Knee	1.2–7.7	20–40	15–47	0–30	0–45	2–10	10–20	42	92	3.7	9.6
Cycling											
Hip		35	10					70–150		20	5
Knee	1.2	10–30	25–40	3	25			110–190		30	3
Stair Ascent											
Hip		10	125	5	60	5	15				
Knee		60	125	15	30–40	10	5				
Stair Descent											
Hip		20	115	15	85	5	20				
Knee		20–30	125–150	15	30–60	5–15	5–15				

Although they deepen the tibial plateaus only slightly, this deepening provides for a somewhat more congruent and constrained surface with the femoral condyles.

Cruciate Ligaments Although the cruciate ligaments are intracapsular, they are covered by a synovial fold; therefore, strictly speaking, they are extra-articular. Many authors have studied the bony attachments of the ACL and posterior cruciate ligament (PCL). The origin of the ACL is posterior in the femoral notch and oriented primarily in the longitudinal axis of the femur. Its insertion is wide and oriented in the AP axis of the tibia; it occupies about a third of the width of the tibia between the anterior and middle thirds. As the ACL passes from its origin to insertion, its fibers rotate approximately 90° on their longitudinal axis. This rotation leads to the development of differential tension in the ACL fibers and causes the ligament to twist as the knee flexes (Fig. 55). The ACL can be differentiated functionally into 2 bundles: anteromedial and posterolateral. With flexion, the anteromedial fibers develop more tension; in extension, the posterolateral bundle is tighter. Likewise, the PCL's femoral origin lies in an AP orientation in the anterior portion of the femoral notch. The PCL inserts, in a broad mediolateral span, into the posterior sulcus of the tibia between the medial and lateral joint surfaces. It can be differentiated into anterolateral and posteromedial bands. Anterolateral fibers become taut in flexion and posteromedial fibers become taut in extension.

Identification of the ACL and PCL origin and insertion is necessary to optimize kinematics when reconstructing torn cruciate ligaments. because of the complex anatomy and presence of multiple functional ligament bundles, it is not possible to position grafts in a perfect "isometric" position. The best the surgeon can do is place tunnels in the position that minimizes changes in graft tension during knee motion. Recent modifications in surgical technique, including changes in tunnel placement and the use of multiple bundle grafts, are being developed to address these issues.

Capsuloligamentous Restraints The capsule, ligaments, and fascia surrounding the joint play a primary role in controlling normal joint motion. These structures include the medial collateral ligament (MCL), lateral collateral ligament (LCL), the joint capsule, and the posteromedial and posterolateral complexes. These supporting structures surrounding the knee can be divided into 3 discrete layers. On the medial side, the most superficial layer (layer 1) is the deep fascia. Posteriorly this layer overlies the 2 heads of the gastrocnemius and serves as a support for the neurovascular structures in the popliteal fossa. Anteriorly it blends with layer 2 and the medial patellar retinaculum.

Layer 2 contains the superficial MCL. Of the 2 components that make up the MCL (superficial and deep), the superficial MCL is clinically more important, and it is the primary medial stabilizer of the knee. It originates on the medial epicondyle and runs approximately 10 cm to its insertion on the tibia, deep to the gracilis and semitendinosus tendons. The posterior oblique fibers of the MCL blend posteriorly into the capsule (layer 3) and, along with contributions from the semimembranosus tendon, form the oblique popliteal ligament.

Layer 3 is the knee joint capsule. It is composed of fibrous tissues of varying thickness, many of which have been identified as specific ligaments. The capsule is quite thin anteriorly. Medially there is a distinct capsular thickening, the deep MCL, which lies under the superficial MCL. This short band of vertical fibers extends from the femur to the periphery of the medial meniscus and tibia. Along the posterior margin of the deep MCL, layer 3 merges with layer 2, forming the reinforced posteromedial capsule.

The lateral structures of the knee are also divided into 3 layers. The most superficial layer, the lateral retinaculum, is made up of superficial oblique and deep transverse components and provides strong lateral support for the patella. The middle layer is made up of the LCL, the fabellofibular ligament, and the arcuate ligament. The LCL originates on the lateral epicondyle of the femur and inserts on the lateral surface of the fibular head. The arcuate ligament is a complex mass of fibers running in various directions. The most consistent fibers form a triangular sheet diverging proximal from the fibular head. The strong lateral limb attaches proximally to the femur, whereas the weaker medial limb arcs over the popliteus muscle. Both blend into the posterior capsule. The popliteofibular ligament has been shown to be important in resisting posterior translation, varus rotation, and external rotation. The deepest lateral layer is again the capsule. It is a thin, weak layer anteriorly that is reinforced posteriorly by the arcuate ligament complex.

Kinematics

The femorotibial articulation has 6 degrees of freedom in 3 geometric axes. In each of these axes (longitudinal, AP, and mediolateral), the tibia can either translate or rotate with respect to the femur, which results in the following 6 paired motions: flexion-extension, varus-valgus, and internal-external rotation; compression-distraction, AP translation, and mediolateral translation. Although this very complex joint is far from being a pure hinged joint, its rotation in the sagittal plane (flexion-extension) greatly dominates both clinical and kinematic study of the knee joint.

Sagittal Range of Motion In the sagittal plane, the arc of flexion-extension is greatly affected by the individual's generalized ligamentous laxity status as well as body habitus. In a normal population, knee extension varies from a few degrees short of 0° to as much as 20° of recurvatum. Knee flexion varies from 125° to 165°. A consensus normal functional range of knee motion would be from approximately 3° to 4° of hyperextension to 140° of flexion.

Like that of other joints in the body, functional range of knee motion varies with specific activities. For example,

during normal walking the knee is flexed approximately 15° at heel strike and has a maximum of 65° of flexion in swing. In contrast, with sprinting the knee is flexed about 35° at foot strike and requires about 130° of maximal flexion in swing. At intervening speeds, knee flexion increases both at heel strike and at maximum flexion during swing phase, and there is a smooth correlation of increasing flexion requirements for the knee with increasing speed of gait. Actually, 130° of flexion are required for most competitive athletic activities. Studies also have shown that for other routine activities of daily living, such as getting in and out of chairs and stair climbing, 115° of knee flexion is required.

Total anterior and posterior translation of the tibia on the femur in an uninjured knee is also variable based on anatomy and the general ligamentous laxity of the individual. Measurement of translation of the tibia with respect to the femur is affected by the position of the knee at the time of the measurement. The degree of flexion of the knee, the amount of its internal or external rotation, and the concomitant amount of joint compression all influence the result. The measurement also depends on the amount of force used to create the translational motion. The AP translation of the tibia on the femur is minimal at full extension, increasing with flexion as the screw home mechanism (see below) unlocks. Anterior translation of the tibia from its neutral position is maximal at approximately 30° of flexion when the anterior restraints are most lax. Posterior translation is greatest at 90° of flexion. These observations support ACL laxity testing at 30° flexion (Lachman test) and PCL testing at 90° knee flexion (posterior drawer test).

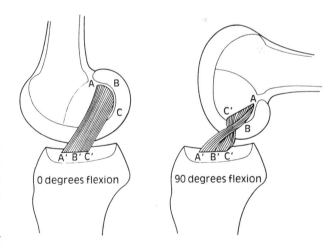

Figure 55

Schematic drawing representing changes in shape and tension of anterior cruciate ligament components in flexion and extension. In flexion, there is lengthening of the anteromedial band (A-A') and shortening of the posterolateral aspect of the ligament (C-C'). Also present, however, is an intermediate component (B-B'), which represents transition between the anteromedial band and posterolateral bulk, with fascicles in varying degrees of tension. (Adapted with permission from Girgis FG, Marshall JL, Monajem ARS: The cruciate ligaments of the knee joint: Anatomical, functional and experimental analysis. *Clin Orthop* 1975;106:216–231.)

Tibiofemoral translation is measured in the AP plane using instrumented laxity measurement devices such as the KT-1000 arthrometer (Medmetric, San Diego, CA). Translation is measured with the knee flexed 20° to 30° and in neutral internal-external and varus-valgus rotation. Standardized anterior forces are applied through the arthrometer. The normal knee is always compared to the injured knee. The manual maximum side-to-side difference has become the standard for evaluating and reporting laxity. Greater than 90% of normal subjects have a side-to-side difference of no more than 2 mm.

Intra-articular Movement A common convention used to describe the relative motion between the femur and tibia is that of the tibia remaining stationary while the femoral surface rolls and slides on the surface of the tibia. Rolling is defined as the translation of the joint axis equaling that of the contact point on the articular surface. With sliding, the joint axis remains stationary while the articular contact point translates. As the knee moves from full extension to flexion, the surface contact point moves posteriorly on both the tibia and the femur but to different extents as the ratio of rolling and sliding does not remain constant through all degrees of flexion. The femoral condyles by sliding anteriorly diminish the posterior progression of the rolling effect, otherwise the condyles would roll off the back of the tibia. Rolling is most prominent in the initial 15 degrees of flexion with the rolling-sliding ratio approximating 1:2. Then sliding becomes more prominent, increasing the rolling-sliding ratio until it reaches 1:4 by the end of flexion (Fig. 56). Clinically this indicates the knee flexion that accompanies weight acceptance is primarily rolling; whereas a deep knee bend would involve considerable joint sliding. The exact ratio of rolling to gliding differs between individuals.

With knee flexion the menisci also move posteriorly. Posterior translation of the medial meniscus is aided by its attachments to the MCL and semimembranosus. Anterior meniscal translation with extension is caused in part by the larger surface area of the anterior femoral condyles pushing the anterior horns forward. The extent of translation is limited by the size of the condyle as well as by increased tension in the capsule posteriorly. Translation of the meniscus allows for maximum contact area and distributes compressive loads evenly across the joint during most positions of femoral rotation.

The direction of movement of the femoral surface contact with the tibia is perpendicular to a line connecting the instant center of rotation with the point of surface contact (Fig. 57). In the normal knee, as the femur rolls and glides on the tibial surface, the instantaneous directional lines generated always remain parallel to the tibial surface. If, for any reason, the relationship between the instant center and surface contact point is altered, femoral movement will be directed either tinto the plateau, crushing the surfaces together, or away from the plateau, producing a lift-off (Fig.

58). Displacement of either the instant center or the normal contact point can occur with an internal derangement, nonphysiologic ligament reconstruction, or abnormal external constraints such as a knee brace. This displacement results in disruption of the normal roll-glide mechanism. The result is analogous to an improperly hung door in which the 2 hinges are not parallel to each other. A knee in which the path of the instant center has been altered will experience changes in joint compressive forces, limitation of motion, or stretching of its surrounding soft-tissue constraints, with consequent loss of normal function.

Frontal Plane Rotation of the tibia on the femur in the frontal plane, more commonly known as varus and valgus angulation, varies in a normal knee depending on the degree of flexion as well as the general ligamentous status of the patient. In the normal knee during passive testing, minimal varus-valgus movement of the tibia exists at terminal extension. Maximal varus and valgus rotation of the tibia occur at approximately 30°. As a general rule, varus motion is greater than valgus rotation because the LCL is lax in flexion, whereas parts of the MCL remain tight. Medial joint distraction with a valgus stress ranges from 1 mm to 10 mm, with an average of 4 mm. Lateral joint opening to a varus stress has been found to be 2 mm to 14 mm, with an average of 6 mm. During the dynamic activity of walking at a freely selected speed, maximum valgus rotation occurs at

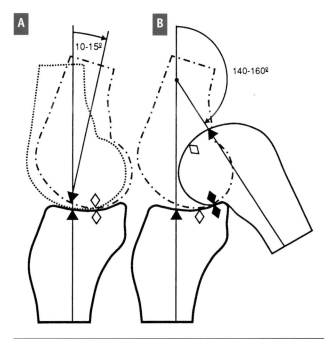

Figure 56

Anteroposterior intra-articular motion (rolling versus sliding). **A,** First 15° arc with rolling dominant. Triangles indicate initial contact points on surface of tibia and femur. White diamonds indicate surface contacts at 15° of flexion. **B,** Remainder of arc, sliding is dominant. Displacement of black femoral triangle indicates the magnitude of femoral sliding. Black diamonds identify contact points at end of range.

heel strike and maximum varus movement occurs during swing phase with an average total varus-valgus rotation during gait of 11°. No significant mediolateral translation of the tibia on the femoral condyles occurs in the normal knee, passively or actively.

Transverse Plane Internal-external rotation of the tibia on the femur is minimal at full extension. The amount of internal tibial rotation on the femur increases progressively, reaching a maximum between 90° and 120° of flexion on passive testing. No significant rotation becomes apparent until after the first 10° to 20° of flexion. The range of maximum external rotation can vary from 0° to 45°, whereas maximum internal rotation ranges from 0° to 25°. During normal gait, the tibia undergoes internal rotation during the swing phase and external rotation during the stance phase. When skeletal pins were used to measure total tibial rotation in normal gait, total rotation was found to be between 4° and 13°, with an average of 8°.

Obligatory external rotation of the tibia on the femur occurs during the terminal degrees of knee extension and is caused, in part, by the differential in radius between the medial femoral condyle and the smaller lateral femoral condyle. This phenomenon has been referred to as the screw home mechanism. Because the medial femoral condyle is larger than the lateral, the distance from the extreme flexion contact point to the extreme extension contact point of the medial femoral condyle has been found to be approximately 17 mm greater than that of the lateral femoral condyle. As the tibia travels from flexion into extension, the medial tibial plateau must cover a greater distance, and thus the tibia externally rotates. This screw home mechanism in terminal extension results in a tightening of both cruciate ligaments and locks the knee such that any movement of the tibia on the femur is minimized and the knee is in the position of maximal stability.

Kinetics

Theoretically, the tibia has 6 degrees of freedom in relation to the femur. In practice, the dynamic and static constraints limit motion to sagittal rotation (flexion-extension) and minimize sagittal translation (AP translation), coronal rotation (varus-valgus), and rotation in the transverse plane (internal-external rotation). The range of motion normally allowed at the knee is limited by the forces developed by bony and joint surface congruity to prevent axial compressive displacement and, primarily, by the tensile strength of the ligaments augmented by muscle contraction to limit all other types of motion.

Ambulatory use of the lower extremity results in ground-reaction forces being transmitted through the tibia. The direction and magnitude of the moment created by these forces depends on the magnitude of the force and the distance of the force line from the instant center of rotation. In order to limit adverse motions of the knee, this externally

generated moment is to some extent counteracted by the moments generated by muscle contraction (Fig. 59). Muscle forces so generated in combination with the ground-reaction force create the joint-reaction force. If this joint-reaction force is perpendicular to the joint surfaces, a joint compressive load results. If the joint-reaction force is not perpendicular to the joint surfaces, translation of the tibia on the femur will also occur, creating a shear force unless restrained by other passive soft-tissue structures. It is a combination of ligament-joint-reaction loads and muscle forces that resist the applied loads and limit the motions about the knee.

For example, the most stable position for the knee is full extension. Extension brings the flatter distal femoral articular surface into contact with the tibial plateaus. This contact makes the joint surfaces more congruent, allowing body weight to be distributed over a greater surface area of the joint and menisci and providing greater resistance to shear. The bony shapes of the femoral condyles and tibial plateau create forces to resist translational motion, when the joint reactive forces are compressive. The menisci, in association with their soft-tissue attachments to the tibia, are believed to also help limit femoral translation by acting as a buttress. This stabilizing buttress effect is even greater with increas-

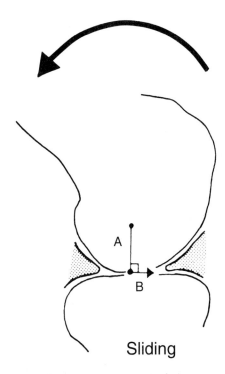

Sliding

Figure 57

In the normal knee, a line drawn from the instant center of the tibiofemoral joint to a tibiofemoral contact point (line A) forms a right angle with a line tangential to the tibial surface (line B). The arrow indicates the direction of displacement of the contact points. Line B is tangential to the tibial surface, indicating that the femur slides on tibial condyles during a measured interval of motion. (Reproduced with permission from Frankel VH, Nordin M: *Basic Biomechanics of the Skeletal System.* Philadelphia, PA, Lea & Febiger, 1980.)

ing axial loads. An anteriorly directed force on the tibia produces greater displacement of the lateral tibial plateau than of the medial tibial plateau. This difference may be a reflection of the firmer fixation of the medial meniscus via the coronary and posterior oblique ligaments versus the greater mobility of the lateral meniscus and the less congruent surface of the lateral tibial plateau. In an ACL-deficient knee, the posterior horns of the menisci act as a buttress to prevent further anterior translation (Fig. 60). Stability in extension is augmented by increased tension in the collateral and cruciate ligaments as well as the posterior capsule. During standing, the knee is further stabilized by the body vector. With the weight line (vector) lying anterior to the knee joint, the posterior capsule offers resistance to hyperextension.

Specific Restraints Conceptually, the same interplay between the various soft tissues about the knee exists regardless of the nature of rotational forces present and the position of the knee. The concept of primary and secondary ligamentous restraints has been developed to explain how the soft tissues about the knee provide shared forces to restrict motion and maintain joint stability. By sectioning knee ligaments and measuring the resultant motion, and varying the order of sectioning, the relative importance of specific ligaments in preventing abnormal motion can be identified. The ligament with the greatest role in preventing motion is designated as the primary restraint, whereas those with a less important role are considered secondary restraints.

AP Translation, 4-Bar Cruciate Linkage, and the Roll-Glide Mechanism The ACL is the primary restraint to anterior translation. The deep MCL (middle medial capsule) is a major secondary restraint. The primary restraint to posterior translation is the PCL. The LCL, posterolateral complex, and superficial MCL are minor secondary restraints.

The rotation of the tibia about the femur in the sagittal plane can be described by a 4-bar mechanical linkage system. In this model, the 2 ligamentous links are the ACL and PCL. The 2 bony links are the horizontal lines connecting the ACL and PCL attachments on the femur and their attachments on the tibia (Fig. 61). The femoral link roughly describes the roof of the intercondylar notch. Computer simulation studies of this 4-bar linkage system have shown how the femur can roll and slide on the tibia and still allow full flexion and extension while not creating undue compressive force across the articular surfaces. Each of the cruciate ligaments as a unit is isometric during the arc of motion, although no single fiber of the cruciate ligament may be truly isometric. Thus, none of the 4 bars in the linkage change in length during flexion and extension of the knee, although the angles between the bars vary. It can be shown that in full extension, the ACL is nearly parallel with the roof of the intercondylar notch or femoral link, whereas in full flexion, the PCL link is nearly parallel with the femoral link. During 140° of flexion, the ACL moves through an angle of approximately 100° with respect to its femoral link and approximately 40° with respect to the tibial link.

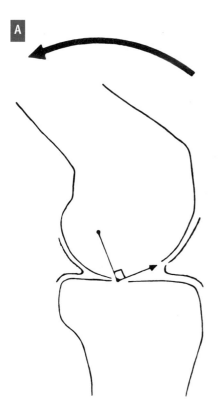

A

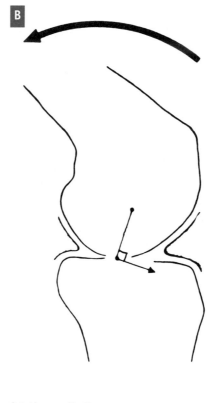

B

Figure 58

Surface motion in two tibiofemoral joints with displaced instant centers. In both joints, the line that is at a right angle drawn between the instant center and the tibiofemoral contact point describes the direction of displacement of the contact points. **A,** The arrow in the joint indicates that the tibiofemoral joint will become distracted with further flexion. **B,** The arrow in the joint indicates that the tibiofemoral joint will become compressed with further flexion. (Reproduced with permission from Frankel VH, Nordin M: *Basic Biomechanics of the Skeletal System.* Philadelphia, PA. Lea & Febiger, 1980.)

During 140° of knee flexion, the PCL moves through an arc of approximately 100° with respect to the femoral link and 40° with respect to the tibial link.

The center of rotation (or instant center) in the 4-bar linkage model is where the 2 cruciate ligament links cross. Because both cruciates pass through the instantaneous axis of rotation and not anterior or posterior to it, they do not generate a flexion or extension moment in the knee during normal range of motion (Fig. 62). Although the cruciates are unable to produce a rotational force in the sagittal plane, they do play a major role in restraining translation in this plane. Because neither the ACL nor the PCL is parallel to the tibial surface, they resist AP translation in 2 ways. The component of the resultant tension force in these ligaments provides a force that directly resists translation. In addition, the component of the ACL resultant force vector perpendicular to the tibia produces a compressive force that increases joint congruency (Fig. 62).

Varus-Valgus The LCL is the primary restraint to varus angulation. Because it is located posterior to the axis of flexion-extension rotation, it is tightest in extension and relaxes with flexion beyond 30°. In extension, the fibers of the iliotibial band are probably the most important lateral stabilizers. The posterolateral capsule is the major secondary restraint. The superficial and deep components of the MCL are the primary restraints to valgus angulation. Increasing tension in the MCL is a manifestation of the geometry of the femoral condyles and origin of the collateral ligaments. The tension in the MCL increases beyond a certain flexion angle as the distance between the origin and insertion increases. With knee flexion, the femur and proximal end of the superficial MCL translate posteriorly relative to the proximal tibia. As flexion progresses, the anterior fibers of the superficial MCL develop increased tension,

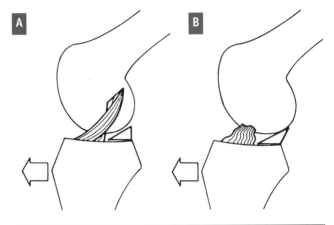

Figure 60

A, With an intact anterior cruciate ligament (ACL), forward translation of the tibia stops before contact with the medial meniscus. **B,** However, with disruption of the ACL, the posterior horn contacts the femoral condyle and acts as a wedge that resists further anterior tibial translation. (Reproduced with permission from Levy IM, Torzilli PA, Warren RF: The effect of medial meniscectomy on anterior-posterior motion of the knee. *J Bone Joint Surg* 1982;64A:883–888.)

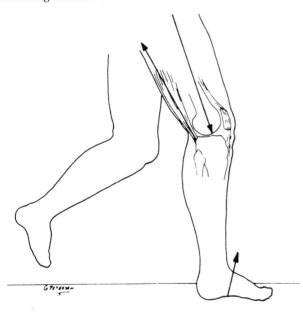

Figure 59

When the foot is in midstance, the foot-floor reaction lies anterior to the bone joint. This force tends to extend the knee and is resisted by muscle forces that tend to flex the knee. These forces in combination require a joint reaction force on the tibial plateau, which is located in the anterior region of the plateau. (Reproduced with permission from Daniel DM, Akeson WH, O'Connor JJ (eds): *Knee Ligaments: Structure, Function, Injury, and Repair.* New York, NY, Raven Press, 1990, p 44.)

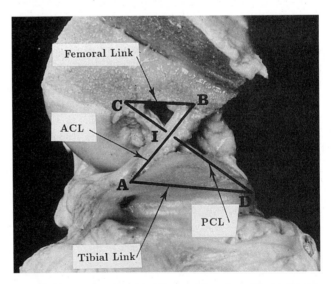

Figure 61

A human knee with the lateral femoral condyle removed, exposing the cruciate ligaments. Superimposed is a diagram of a 4-bar linkage comprising the anterior cruciate ligament (ACL) AB, the posterior cruciate ligament (PCL) CD, the femoral link CB joining the ligament attachment points on the femur, and the tibial link AD joining their attachment points on the tibia. (Reproduced with permission from O'Connor J, Shercliffe T, Fitzpatrick D, et al: Geometry of the knee, in Daniel DM, Akeson WH, O'Connor JJ (eds): *Knee Ligaments: Structure, Function, Injury, and Repair.* New York, NY, Raven Press, 1990, pp 163–169.)

whereas the obliquely oriented posterior fibers show decreased strain. With loss of either of the collateral ligaments, secondary restraints to varus-valgus stresses come from the cruciate ligaments.

Internal-External Rotation The superficial and deep MCL are the primary restraints to internal rotation of the tibia on the femur. The ACL is a secondary restraint. The LCL, posterolateral capsule, and popliteofibular ligament are the primary restraints to external rotation. The PCL is a major secondary restraint.

Dynamic Restraints As the knee moves through a given arc of motion, forces acting across the knee constantly change. In addition, the magnitude of forces acting on the knee for a given knee motion varies greatly with the specific activity involved. For example, forces acting on the knee during supine knee extension are different from the forces generated during a squat or a running jump. Such requirements mandate constant changes in muscle activity for the 14 muscles that cross the knee joint.

The dynamic action of the muscles always occurs in conjunction with static ligamentous restraints. An obvious example of this muscle-ligament interaction is the effect of the knee flexor-extensor muscle groups on anterior and posterior tibial translation. Anterior knee translation is strongly influenced by the quadriceps muscles. When the quadriceps contract to extend the knee, they create a line of force along their tendinous insertion into the tibia. There is an angle at which the tendon's force is perpendicular to the tibial plateau and no translational force is created. This angle has been termed the critical angle. For the quadriceps, this is approximately 70° to 80° of flexion. Quadriceps

contraction in a knee fixed at an angle smaller than the critical angle results in a force with an anterior vector tending to cause anterior tibial translation. This force will be counteracted by the component of the tensile forces developed in the ACL parallel to the tibial plateau as well as by a joint contact force. Similarly, when the knee is actively flexed, the hamstrings and gastrocnemius exert a posteriorly directed force with translation counteracted by the PCL.

When active knee extension is initiated by quadriceps contraction, concomitant anterior translation of the tibia occurs. This translation shifts the starting point of the surface contact point on the tibia and instant center posteriorly, resulting in an initial increased quadriceps lever arm. Hamstring contraction during active knee flexion pulls the tibia posteriorly, moving the initial surface contact point and instant center anteriorly, increasing the lever arm and mechanical advantage. This ability of the human knee to shift its instant center anteriorly and posteriorly to increase or decrease the moment arm of the extensors or flexors decreases the magnitude of muscle force required to overcome the externally applied load, and results in a reduction in joint compressive and shear loads when it is most needed. It would seem that this phenomenon is important in both energy and muscle efficiency as well as in protecting the joint from excessive loads.

If an externally applied load to the lower extremity produces a flexion moment at the knee, this rotational force will be counterbalanced by quadriceps contraction. This phenomenon occurs, for example, during the initiation of stance phase in walking or running, where the ground-reaction force is located posterior to the knee joint. If the knee is flexed less than its critical angle, the patellar tendon force will also produce an anteriorly directed vector on the tibia, resulting in adverse shear stress at the joint. Cocontraction of the knee flexor and extensor muscles is the primary mode of dynamic knee stabilization to external flexion-extension, as well as to the concomitant varus-valgus and internal-external rotational forces. This cocontraction maintains stability of the joint during times of marked changes in stresses. However, as stated earlier, the passive ligamentous contribution to stability in these directions is clinically more important. At foot strike and early stance phase, the knee progresses to about 20° of flexion, with the body's weight tending to be directed posterior to the knee joint. Both the hamstrings and quadriceps muscle groups are active at this time. Such activity has the overall effect of increasing the joint's reactive force and, hence, the importance of static components, such as the bony congruence and the buttress effect of the menisci, in providing joint stability. It is important to realize that this complex interplay of joint reaction and muscle and tendon forces occurs in all 3 planes simultaneously and that this interplay is different at each position of the tibia on the femur.

The ability of muscle contraction to stabilize the knee is readily apparent to anyone who has tried to evaluate an

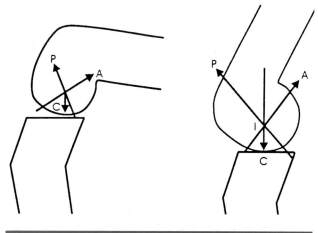

Figure 62

The cruciate ligament forces A and P and the tibiofemoral contact force C intersect at the flexion axis I. They have no moment about that axis. (Reproduced with permission from Daniel DM, Akeson WH, O'Connor JJ (eds): *Knee Ligaments: Structure, Function, Injury, and Repair.* New York, NY, Raven Press, 1990, p 202.)

acute knee injury. Involuntary muscle contraction or spasm may minimize abnormal anterior translation when stress is applied to an ACL-deficient knee, making it difficult to appreciate pathologic laxity. Likewise, the subject's inability to relax the muscles during knee arthrometer testing is the major cause of spurious ligament laxity measurements.

Patellofemoral Joint

The patellofemoral joint is important to knee stability primarily through its role in the extensor mechanism. The patella increases the mechanical advantage of the extensor muscles by transmitting the force across the knee at a greater distance (moment) from the axis of rotation. Stability of the patella in the trochlear groove is a function of bony, ligamentous, and muscular components.

The patella is a sesamoid bone in the quadriceps tendon, which increases the functional lever arm of the quadriceps as well as changes the direction of the pull of the quadriceps mechanism. The quadriceps force needed to achieve full knee extension against gravity increases 15% to 30% after patellectomy. The patella articulates with the trochlear groove of the femoral condyle as it slides a distance of approximately 7 cm from full extension to full flexion. Geometric congruence between the patella and femoral trochlea varies during the flexion arc. In addition, there is considerable anatomic variation at the patellofemoral joint. Significant patellofemoral contact does not occur until approximately 20° of flexion, and "capture" of the patella between the trochlear ridges may require even more flexion. Individuals with abnormalities of the bony architecture, such as patella alta, a flat trochlear groove, or hypoplastic lateral condyles, are predisposed to patellar instability.

The role of the patella in increasing the quadriceps muscle lever arm varies depending on the degree of knee flexion. In full flexion, when the patella is entirely in the intercondylar notch, it increases the lever arm of the quadriceps by only 10%. As the knee starts to come into extension, the patella's contribution to the extensor lever arm increases until approximately 45° of flexion, at which the patella lengthens the lever arm by approximately 30%. From 45° of flexion to full extension, the patella's contribution to the lever arm slowly decreases. Study results have indicated that greater quadriceps muscle force was required for the last 15° of knee extension.

The patellofemoral joint reaction force is determined not only by the magnitude of the quadriceps contraction, but also by the amount of knee flexion at the time of the contracture. If the leg is positioned to eliminate the effect of gravity and a constant resistance is applied to the distal tibia, as the knee is extended from 90° of flexion to 0°, quadriceps muscle force increases and the joint reaction force decreases. The location of greatest contact force differs on both the patellar and trochlear articular surfaces at various knee flexion angles. As the knee goes from 90° of flexion to 0°, maximum patellofemoral forces move proximal on the trochlea and distal on the patella (Fig. 63).

Normal walking has been estimated to create joint compressive forces of approximately half of body weight. Walking upstairs increases joint compression loads to between 2.5 to 3.3 times body weight, and doing deep knee bends produces loads up to 7 to 8 times body weight across this joint. The articular cartilage of the patella has evolved to become very thick in order to accommodate these great compressive loads.

Structure and Function of the Foot and Ankle

The ankle and foot have long been thought of as an unsophisticated appendage that joins the leg to the ground. While the foot may have fewer functions than the hand, in many respects its intricate construction and complex dynamic organization, which provide shock absorption, stability, and propulsion for the body during upright posture and ambulation, are more elaborate than those of the hand.

Ground-reaction forces are a response to the muscular actions and the weight of the body transmitted through the feet. As the foot hits the ground during bipedal locomotion, forces transmitted to the foot begin at the heel, rapidly shift to the entire foot, dwell there during midsupport, and then rapidly move to the forefoot and end at the medial aspect of the forefoot as the leg ends stance and prepares for swing. The direction of the ground-reaction force varies as stance phase progresses. Up and down oscillations of the vertical-reaction force occur during stance as the body decelerates and then accelerates. Changes in the horizontal shear reaction forces correlate with progressional and lateral accelerations of the eccentrically placed body and provide additional force to initiate and bring to an end periods of locomotion and to change the speed or direction of walking. At the initiation of stance, the supporting foot is ahead of the body's center of mass, requiring a backward shear as well as vertical force to brake the movement of the foot and absorb shock. As the body passes medially over the supporting foot, lateral shear forces persist; fore-aft shear forces drop to zero, then are directed forward as the body's center of mass moves ahead of the foot. As the horizontal distance between the supporting foot and the body's center of mass increases, an increase in walking speed, which normally increases both the step length and width (distance between the right and left feet), results in an increase in the peaks of all components of the ground-reaction forces. Changes in functional activities (running, jumping, and stair climbing) or terrain will also alter the magnitude, direction, and primary location of these forces on the foot.

Thus, for proper function, the foot and ankle must with-

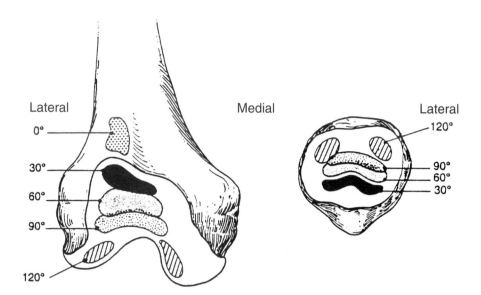

Figure 63

The patellofemoral contact areas at various knee flexion angles. (Reproduced with permission from Aglietti P, Insall JN, Walker PS, Trent P: A new patella prosthesis: Design and application. *Clin Orthop* 1975;107:175–187.)

stand high loads at different times and locations during various body speeds, changes of direction, and conditions of terrain. It successfully performs this task by forming a kinematic chain with the lower leg. This chain transmits forces and motions in the sagittal direction via translations and rotations, the axes of which are not in the body's orthogonal axes. Furthermore no true hinge joints exist in the foot; rather, through the constrained and unconstrained interaction of 26 bones, 21 functional joints, 30 muscles, and over 100 ligaments, the foot and ankle illustrate how form is dictated by function.

The Ankle Joint

General Description

The ankle joint consists of the saddle-shaped lower end of the tibia and fibula, and its inferior transverse ligament encloses the superior aspect of the body of the talus (the trochlea) (Fig. 64). The tibial surface forming the superior dome of the ankle is concave sagittally, is slightly convex from side to side, and is oriented about 93° from the long axis of the tibia (is higher on the lateral than the medial side). The shape of the cavity formed by the tibiofibular mortise appears to match closely that of the upper articulating surfaces of the talus. The superior part of the body of the talus (trochlea) is wedge-shaped; it is about one-fourth wider in front than behind, with an average difference of 2.4 mm; anteriorly a minimal difference of 1.3 mm and a maximal difference of 6 mm. From front to back, the articular surface spans an arc of about 105°. This surface contour has been likened to a section or rostrum of a cone, having a smaller diameter medially than laterally.

The primary motion of the ankle joint is dorsiflexion-plantarflexion. Its axis of rotation is obliquely oriented with respect to all 3 anatomic planes (Table 17). Passing through the inferior tips of the malleoli, the axis extends from ante-

rior, superior, and medial to inferior, posterior, and lateral. It is at angles of 93° with respect to the long axes of the tibia and about 11.5° to the joint surface. However, rather than a true single IAR, the ankle has been noted to have multiple instant centers, all of which fall very close to a single point within the body of the talus. Through a complete arc of ankle rotation, the center may shift anywhere from 4 to 7 mm. Because the axis of rotation is obliquely oriented to the sagittal, coronal, and transverse planes, translation of the talus in the mortise can occur in all 3 directions.

The talus has been observed in vitro to rotate easily in the ankle mortise implying relative movement between the malleoli. Because the trochlea is wider anteriorly than posteriorly, some believe that lateral play of the talus within its mortise occurs only when the ankle is in plantarflexion. Others believe that instability exists in dorsiflexion, while still others believe that with intact ligaments translation occurs only in the sagittal direction. These differences can be explained by behavior of the ligaments and by the roles played by the subtalar joint, the kinematic chain of the hindfoot, and the muscles that traverse this area in transmitting forces across this area during plantarflexion and dorsiflexion.

The talus is unique because this bone, which lies between the foot and the leg, contains no muscular attachments and has seven articulations that connect it to four other bones. The stability of the talus and its articulations, therefore, relies heavily on the ligamentous attachments and musculotendinous complexes that traverse the talus and attach distally. Passive stability of the ankle joint, thus, results from a variety of factors. First is the bony stability provided by contact of the trochlea with the tibial plafond. Second are the medial and lateral cartilaginous slightly concave surfaces that articulate with the 2 malleoli. Third are the ligamentous connections between the tibia, fibula, talus, and calcaneus.

Ligaments of the Ankle Joint

The ankle joint has a fibrous capsule that encircles the joint completely and is thickened laterally. The posterior and anterior tibiofibular ligament (Fig. 65) attaches the fibula to the tibia to strengthen the tibiofibular syndesmosis. The origin of the posterior tibiofibular ligament is broad, covering most of the horizontal distal surface of the tibia. As the ligament fibers sweep laterally and distally to insert on the fibula they fit over the trochlea. The deltoid (medial collateral) ligament is a strong triangular ligament made up of superficial and deep components that arise from the anterior, distal, and posterior borders of the medial malleolus (Fig. 66). The superficial portion consists of three parts; the tibionavicular, tibiocalcaneal (inserting onto the sustentaculum tali of the calcaneus), and posterior tibiotalar ligaments. The deep portion consists only of the anterior tibiotalar ligament.

From the lateral malleolus, 3 ligaments fan out to provide stability. The relatively weak anterior talofibular ligament passes from the anterior surface of the fibula malleolus to the talus. The calcaneofibular ligament, which is attached proximally to the lateral malleolus and distally to the tubercle of the lateral surface of the calcaneus, is long and strong, resembling a collateral ligament of other hinged joints. The posterior talofibular ligament runs horizontally from the posterior process of the talus to the posterior process of the fibula malleolus. Thus, of 7 ligaments arising from the 2 malleoli, only 4 connect to the talus, and none of these 4 are the strongest ligaments surrounding the ankle joint. The

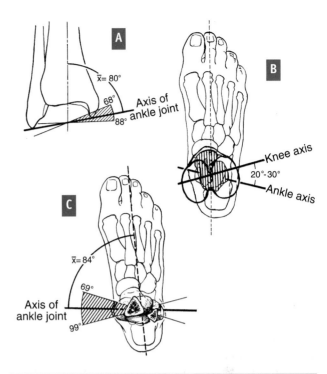

Figure 64

A, Variations in the frontal axis of the ankle joint. **B,** Relationship of the knee and ankle axes. **C,** Relationship of the ankle axis to the long axis of the foot. (Reproduced with permission from Mann RA: Biomechanics of the foot, in *American Academy of Orthopaedic Surgeons: Atlas of Orthotics*, ed 2. St. Louis, MO, CV Mosby, 1985.)

Table 17

Type and Position of the Axis of Rotation for the Ankle

Investigators	Frontal	Position With Respect to the Anatomic Planes		
		Sagittal	**Transverse**	
Elftsman (1945)		67.6° ± 7.4°		
Isman and Inman (1969)	8 mm anterior, 3 mm inferior to the distal tip of the lateral malleolus to 1 mm osterior, 5 mm inferior to the distal tip of the medial malleous	84° ± 7°	10° ± 4°	
Inman and Mann (1979)		78° ± 12°		
Allard and associates (1987)	95.4° ± 6.6°	77.7° ± 12.3°	17.9° ± 4.5°	
Parlasca and associates (1979)	96% within 12 mm of a point 20 mm below the articular surface of the tibia along the long axis			
Hicks (1953)	Dorsiflexion 5 mm inferior to tip of lateral malleolus to 15 mm anterior to tip of medial malleolus Plantarflexion: 5 mm superior to tip of lateral malleolus to 15 mm anterior, 10 mm interior to tip of medial malleolus			

(Adapted with permission from Allard P, Stokes IA, Salathe EP, et al: Modeling of the foot and ankle, in Jahss MH (ed): *Disorders of the Foot and Ankle: Medical and Surgical Management*, ed 2. Philadelphia, PA, WB Saunders, 1991, pp 432–468.)

other 3 ligaments connect more distally to the calcaneus, and are the strongest. This structure has led to the concept that the subtalar joint must be considered a constrained joint and its inversion-eversion movements are integrally involved in the stability of the ankle. This concept will be discussed further after the stability of the foot is described.

Stabilizing Mechanisms of the Foot

Arches of the Foot

The longitudinal vault structure of the foot is considered to be built up by medial and lateral longitudinal arch systems (Fig. 67). The lateral arch system, the lower and shorter one, is composed of the calcaneus, the cuboid, and 2 lateral rays. This system is the more stable, weightbearing portion of the arch; it carries the longer and higher medial arch system. The medial arch consists of the calcaneus, talus, navicular, cuneiforms, and 3 medial rays. Both arches are prolonged into the 5 shorter kinematic chains of the toes. A transverse arch configured by the shape of the midtarsal bones (cuneiforms and cuboid) and the bases of the metatarsals also described. A second transverse arch is suggested to exist at the metatarsal heads when no weight is being borne; it does not exist during weightbearing.

The longitudinal arch is not intrinsically stable owing to the shape of the bones and their intervening joints; it is, in fact, stabilized by heavy ligamentous structures surrounding the joints. This arch is reduced somewhat during weightbearing. However, for short periods, the tension developed in the large mass of ligamentous structure on the plantar surface of the foot can protect it from completely collapsing. EMG studies performed during quiet standing reveal minimal to no activity of intrinsic muscles.

Plantar Aponeurosis

The longitudinal arch is passively stabilized further by the plantar aponeurosis. The plantar aponeurosis arises from the tubercle of the calcaneus, passes distally, and inserts into the base of the proximal phalanges of all the toes. Classically, its mechanism of action has been described as a windlass type. This aponeurosis is most functional on the medial side of the foot; excision of the proximal phalanx or the metatarsal heads causes loss of its function. The breaking load of the aponeurosis varies between 1.7 and 3.4 times body weight, depending on which toe insertion is broken.

If stance is simulated by applying a downward force to the tibia and an upward force in the Achilles tendon, it has been suggested that the applied load is carried partially by a bending moment in the tarsometatarsal arch and partially by tension in the plantar aponeurosis. The plantar aponeurosis may account for about one quarter of the applied load. If the plantar aponeurosis is divided, at least 3 times body weight can be supported by the bony ligamentous arch without damage to the metatarsal bones or attachments.

Dynamic Support

The intrinsic muscles of the foot, like the plantar aponeurosis, help stabilize the longitudinal arch. The flexor digitorum brevis helps to stabilize both the medial and lateral arches; the abductor hallucis and abductor digiti minimi help stabilize the medial arch and the lateral arch, respectively. Thus, when the toes are forced into dorsiflexion, this enhances the function of the plantar aponeurosis and the intrinsic muscles.

The flexor hallucis longus and flexor digitorum longus (extrinsic muscles) do not directly stabilize the arch. These

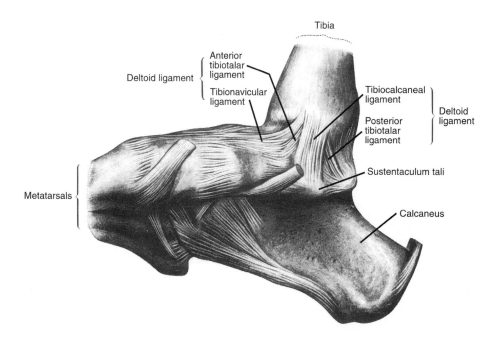

Figure 65

Ligaments of the ankle and foot. (Reproduced with permission from Sobotta J, Figge FHJ: *Atlas der Anatomie des Menschen*, ed 20, Vol. I. Munich, Germany, Urban & Schwarzenberg, 1993.)

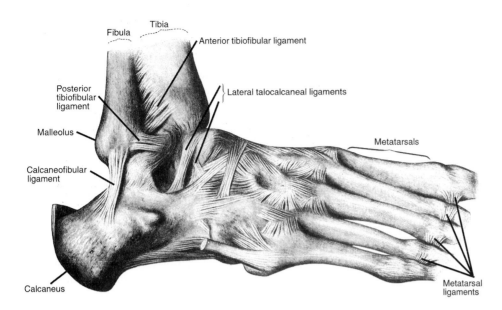

Figure 66

Ligaments of the foot. (Reproduced with permission from Sobotta J, Figge FHJ: *Atlas der Anatomie des Menschen*, ed 20, Vol. I. Munich, Germany, Urban & Schwarzenberg, 1993.)

muscles help to produce inversion of the heel and to maintain the ankle in plantarflexion. However, contributions from the posterior and anterior tibialis and the peroneus longus may serve a more direct function in maintaining the arch. Tendons from these muscles run parallel to the ligaments and insert in an area of the first cuneiform and base of the first metatarsal. By enveloping its medial, plantar, and lateral aspects, they strongly assist in constraining movement of the proximal half of the foot. The peroneus longus, and the slip of the posterior tibialis inserting onto the cuboid, in association with the oblique and transverse heads of the adductor hallucis brevis, maintain the transverse arch and stabilize the link between the medial and longitudinal arches. Added support of the arch can be obtained by small rotations of the individual joints via external rotation of the tibia, inversion of the calcaneus, and adduction of the forefoot.

Kinematics and Kinetics of the Foot

The axis of rotation of the subtalar joint is obliquely oriented (Fig. 68). The joint forms angles of about 41° to the horizontal in the sagittal plane and 23° to the midline axis of the foot in the transverse plane. Forces transmitted across this joint, thus, tend to create inversion with slight plantarflexion and adduction or eversion with slight dorsiflexion and abduction with respect to orthogonal axes about the tibia. However, translational motions occur with rotational motions about this joint. As high as a 10-mm lateral shift in the axis has been noted between maximum eversion and inversion, resulting in variations of up to 13° with respect to the position of the rotational axis. Although this shift suggests a variable axis rather than a fixed one, there is still

controversy about whether its movement is about a hinge or a screw-like mechanism.

The transverse tarsal joints lying distal to the subtalar joint are 2 joints that form a continuous line across the foot. Medially and superiorly, the talonavicular joint can be characterized as a ball-and-socket joint that has considerable rotational mobility (Fig. 69). Inversion induces the greatest rotation in this joint. Laterally and inferiorly, the calca-

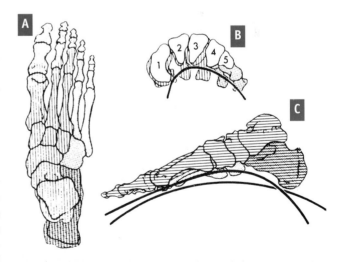

Figure 67

The arches of the foot. **A,** The medial longitudinal arch (lines) is the active portion of the arch. The lateral longitudinal arch (stippled) is the static portion of the arch. The calcaneus is common to both arches. **B,** Curvature of the transverse arch. **C,** Curves of the medial and lateral longitudinal arches. (Reproduced with permission from Mann R, Inman VT: Structure and function, in DuVries HL (ed): *Surgery of the Foot*, ed 2. St. Louis, MO, CV Mosby, 1965.)

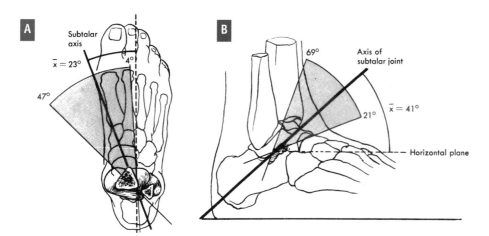

Figure 68

Variations in the axes of the subtalar joint. **A,** Transverse plane. **B,** Horizontal plane. (Reproduced with permission from Mann RA: Biomechanics of the foot, in American Academy of Orthopaedic Surgeons: *Atlas of Orthotics*, ed 2. St. Louis, MO, CV Mosby, 1985.)

neocuboid joint can be classified as a saddle joint that allows mostly translation.

Proximally, the plantar calcaneonavicular (spring) ligament is the most important ligament supporting the medial arch (Fig. 70). The short and long plantar ligaments, the strongest ligaments of the foot, connect the calcaneus, cuboid, and lateral metatarsals. Predominantly vertically oriented fibers that belong not only to the talocalcaneal ligaments, but also to the tarsal crural ligaments, keep the medial and lateral arches together where the medial arch is mounted on the lateral arch. Oblique and some transverse fibers, especially in the region of the navicular, cuboid, and cuneiform bones and at the bases of the metatarsals, keep the parallel rows of the arch systems together.

In the proximal part of the foot composed of the tarsal bones, the static longitudinal arch system is integrated

Talonavicular joint

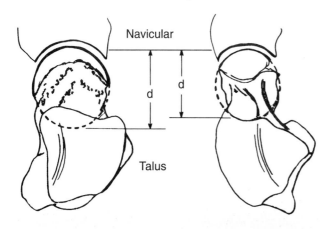

Figure 69

Superior view (**left**) and lateral view (**right**) of the relationship of the head of the talus to the navicular bone showing differing diameters of the head of the talus. (Reproduced with permission from Mann RA: Biomechanics of running, in Nicholas JA, Hershman EB (eds): *The Lower Extremity and Spine in Sports Medicine*. St. Louis, MO, Mosby-Year Book, 1986.)

kinematically into what can be called a closed kinematic chain with interdependent movements at the different joints. The mechanical coupling of the talus, calcaneus, cuboid, and navicular as a result of their arrangement in a closed kinematic chain is known as the tarsal mechanism. The ligaments surrounding these joints, especially horizontal fibers of the talofibular ligament, are crucial structural elements in this mechanism.

During activities of daily living, motions at these joints are induced primarily by varus-valgus ground-reaction force and forces tending to rotate the lower leg in internal-external rotation. The transverse rotation of the leg alone or in combination with sideward swaying motions is converted by the tarsal mechanism into inversion-eversion motions of the foot.

These rotational as well as dorsiflexion-plantarflexion motions are transmitted from the leg to the rest of the foot through a number of different but closely cooperating osteoligamentous mechanisms in addition to the tarsal mechanism. These mechanisms include: (1) the midtarsal mechanism; (2) the tarsometatarsal mechanism; and (3) the metatarsophalangeal mechanism.

Tarsal Mechanism

The subtalar, talonavicular, and calcaneocuboid joints are most involved with the mechanics of inversion and eversion. The navicular and cuboid bones move as a single unit, whereas the calcaneus articulates with both the talus and the cuboid navicular piece by means of separate hinges. Although this mechanism is structurally complex, it is routinely conceptualized mechanically as a simple hinge of the midtalar joint. In actuality, the axis of rotation of motions of these tarsal joints are best described as a fan-shaped or cone-shaped bundle of discrete axes representing the successive positions of a moving axis in reference to the subtalar joint. All of the axes have an oblique direction with respect to the foot.

In vivo the foot inverts in response to external rotation of the leg. Starting from a neutral position, this response has been found to be far more extensive than the limited eversion response to internal rotation. In addition, a delayed response of relative external rotation of the talus during external rotation of the leg occurs, resulting from a "lock" of the tarsal mechanism that prohibits further eversion.

Because no muscles can move the talus directly, forces transmitted through the contact surfaces and the ligaments of the talocrural joint must impose the input motion on the talus. The horizontally running fibers of the anterior talofibular ligament play a crucial role in bringing the talus into an external rotation, which is converted into inversion by the tarsal mechanism. Thus, in stance, via this mechanism the tibialis posterior is an effective invertor together with the flexor digitorum longus, whereas the peronei and the extensor digitorum longus have the opposite effect. Under these conditions, the tibialis anterior seems to be a less effective invertor. The abductor hallucis muscle is an example of an intrinsic foot muscle acting directly on the tarsal mechanism. Through its attachments toward distal elements and proximally to the calcaneus, it has a notable inversion effect.

These features support the clinical experience that patients with permanent ligament defect after injury may regain stable joint function through specific and careful muscle training. It has also been noted during the initial phase of external rotation of the tibia that the talus does not follow the tibia immediately, and this has been described as the tibial talar delay. This delay may be ascribed to a variable laxity in the horizontal talocrural ligament fibers and it is supposed that these fibers have to build up an initial tension before they can transmit the pulling forces from the leg to the talus. After this initial delay, talar rotation increases generally. In most cases, after having reached a plateau, talar rotation decreases again during the last phase of tibial rotation.

The anterior talofibular ligament thus plays an important role in talocrural transmission; this ligament permits different people to have different degrees of rotational motion. Joints with rather lax talocrural ligaments seem to be characterized by a delay that is greatest from 0° to 10° of external rotation of the tibia and increases with the increase of plantarflexion. Joints with rather stiff talocrural ligaments feature a delay that occurs mainly at the end of external rotation and especially in 25° to 30° of plantarflexion. Tibial talar delay can increase markedly after severing the anterior talofibular ligament with its adjacent capsular structures.

Ankle joint stability can now be viewed in light of this tarsal mechanism. One commonly accepted theory is that, because of the talar mechanism, ligaments play the following role during plantarflexion. The stability of the ankle is achieved mainly by the tibionavicular fibers of the deltoid and the lateral ligaments. The lateral ligaments maintain the intrinsic stability of the talus and its mortise by developing a fairly uniform ligamentous force about it. As plantarflexion occurs, all the lateral ligaments remain taut, and because of this passive talar mechanism, movement of inversion and adduction occurs. This movement is assisted dynamically in the early phases of gait by the intrinsic plantarflexors on the medial side of the ankle, which are active throughout stance as are all the extrinsic ankle and foot plantarflexors (Fig. 71).

Because of this talar mechanism, in the absence of muscular contracture the talus still cannot move freely in its

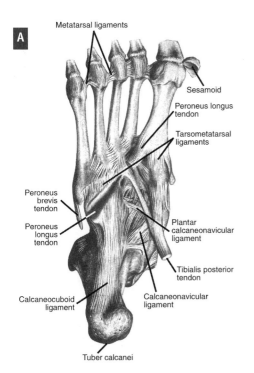

A

Metatarsal ligaments

Sesamoid

Peroneus longus tendon

Tarsometatarsal ligaments

Peroneus brevis tendon

Peroneus longus tendon

Plantar calcaneonavicular ligament

Tibialis posterior tendon

Calcaneocuboid ligament

Calcaneonavicular ligament

Tuber calcanei

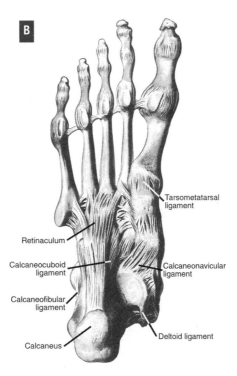

B

Tarsometatarsal ligament

Retinaculum

Calcaneocuboid ligament

Calcaneonavicular ligament

Calcaneofibular ligament

Deltoid ligament

Calcaneus

Figure 70

A, Ligaments of the foot and ankle. B, Ligaments of the plantar surface of the foot. (Reproduced with permission from Sobotta J, Figge FHJ: *Atlas der Anatomie des Menschen*, ed 20, Vol. I. Munich, Germany, Urban & Schwarzenberg, 1993.)

mortise during passive plantarflexion. The anterior talo-fibular ligament and the similarly oriented fibers of the del-toid ligament are brought into tension during plantarflex-ion and contribute equally to ankle stability. In dorsiflexion, medial and lateral stretch of the middle and posterior liga-mentous fibers plays the predominant role. The differences in ankle stability may thus be related to interpersonal vari-ation in the strength of the ligaments and the orientation of the axes of rotational and translational motions of the ankle joint and tarsal mechanism.

Moreover, the tendons of the dorsiflexors, restrained in part by the inferior extensor retinaculum, have a horizontal force component preventing forward displacement of the talus. In plantarflexion, the posterior shift of the talus is limited by the lower tibial margin and the posterior talar-tibial and talofibular ligaments, as well as by possible exter-nal rotation of the fibula.

The Midtarsal Mechanism

The bones of the midtarsal area consist of the cuneiforms and the cuboid. Chopart's joint, the articular connection of these bones to the tarsal mechanism, shares a common synovial cavity that is continuous with the second and third cuneiform-metatarsal joints. The bones across these joints are connected by strong dorsal, plantar, and interosseous ligaments, making them relatively immovable with respect to each other. Forces and motions created proximal or dis-tal to this unit thus may be considered to be transferred across it, unchanged by these constrained joints.

The Tarsometatarsal Mechanism

A single line of bones proximally, the longitudinal arch sys-tems split up distally to form the most dynamic portion of the arch. In this part of the foot, the individual longitudinal tarsometatarsal chains can be moved in dorsal or plantar directions, more or less independently. Thus, the concept of the foot as a mobile weightbearing vault structure seems to be related predominantly to motion initiated at the tar-sometatarsal joints and reflected in the distal part of the foot comprising the metatarsophalangeal joints.

A striking functional anatomic feature of the tarsometa-tarsal region is the relatively immobile connection of the second metatarsal to its surrounding tarsal bones; the other metatarsal bones are far more mobile. Because the base of the second metatarsal is "locked" in a socket formed by the cuneiform bones, the distal half of the foot can be twisted around the longitudinal axis formed by the second metatarsal (Fig. 72). This possible twisting mobility, which is seated mainly in the tarsometatarsal joints with a possi-ble contribution from the talonavicular joint and calca-neocuboid joint, is known as the supination or pronation twist of the forefoot. This twisting change of shape of the metatarsal part of the foot is produced by small gliding motions with different ranges of each of the lateral 3 metatarsals and gliding and rotations of the first metatarsal in dorsal and plantar directions.

The asymmetry of the torsional tarsometatarsal mobility at both sides of the second metatarsal can be recognized in the structural relationships between the metatarsal heads. In this sense, there seems to be a principal difference between the connections between the first and second and between the second, third, fourth, and fifth metatarsals. Proximal interosseous ligaments and distal transversely running ligaments (the transverse metatarsal ligament) are found only between the heads of the second to the fifth metatarsals; they are absent between the first and second metatarsals. This is similar to the hand. Only the insertion of the transverse part of the adductor hallucis muscle pro-

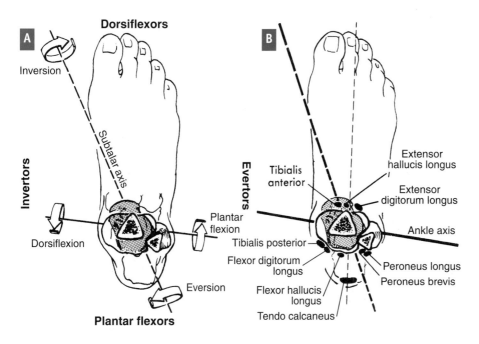

Figure 71

A, Rotation occurs about the subta-lar and ankle joint axes. **B,** The rela-tionship of the various muscles about the subtalar and ankle joint axes. (Reproduced with permission from Mann RA: Biomechanics of the foot, in *American Academy of Orthopaedic Surgeons: Atlas of Orthotics*, ed 2. St. Louis, MO, CV Mosby, 1985.)

vides an obvious anchoring of the first metatarsal to the other metatarsals distally. Moreover, the belly of the transverse adductor originates from the deep transverse metatarsal ligaments, and these origins are restricted to the spaces between the second, third, fourth, and fifth metatarsals. These features allow greater mobility of the first metatarsal ray than of the lateral three and relative immobility of the second.

The Metatarsophalangeal Mechanism

The actively stabilized phalangeal arches of the toes are of paramount importance for proper function of both the support of the arch and the mechanism of pronation-supination of the forefoot. The 5 metatarsophalangeal joints together with their phalangeal chains form 5 separate nonconstrained mechanisms.

The stabilization of the multiarticulated chain occurring in each metatarsophalangeal joint and toe against external forces appears to be similar to that described for the hand. The flexor digitorum brevis and interossei, which are major force-generating structures at the end of stance, are essential to maintain the stability of this arch. The powerful abductor, adductor, and flexor hallucis brevis are present not only for stabilization of the first metatarsal joint, but also, by virtue of their far proximal origin, have a stabilizing effect on the metatarsal cuneiform connections and even more proximal joints. The proximal origin of the interossei, unlike those in the hand, is beyond the metatarsals from the tarsal ligamentous meshwork so that the pull of the interossei is transferred across the transmetatarsal joints. This structure suggests that the interossei are stabi-

lizers of the forefoot rendering the tarsometatarsal joints rigid when weight is carried on the ball of the foot. An intrinsic minus foot, therefore, not only affects the metatarsal joints, but also deprives more proximal joints of a plantar stabilizing force.

Finally, the plantar aponeurosis bowstrings all 3 mechanisms and is connected to their bony parts as well as to the sole of the foot in an anatomically complex way. By its windlass action, it raises the longitudinal arches of the foot when the toes are dorsiflexed as well as stiffening the fibrous skeleton of the ball of the foot during push-off (Fig. 73). This effect is most evident in the medial arch and it also can be seen by dorsiflexion of the great toe. Because inversion of the tarsal mechanism leads mostly to a rise of the medial longitudinal arch, the use of this windlass mechanism is accompanied by a slight inversion of the tarsus and external rotation of the leg.

Coordinated Functions

Control of Human Movement

Human movement and CNS involvement in the control of skilled movements both have been active areas of research in recent years. Based on experimental results obtained using cats and apes, it is now accepted that commands for skilled voluntary movements are initiated from the higher centers of the CNS, descend the spinal pathways, and are decoded and executed at the muscle level. Proprioceptive

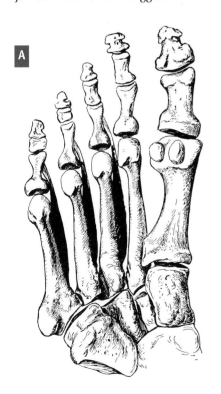
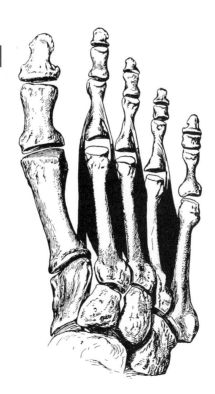

Figure 72

The interosseous muscles of the foot. **A,** Plantar. **B,** Dorsal. (Reproduced with permission from Sobotta J, Figge FHJ: *Atlas der Anatomie des Menschen*, ed 20, Vol. I. Munich, Germany, Urban & Schwarzenberg, 1993.)

feedback to the higher centers of the brain and the spinal cord is not considered essential to the performance of skilled movements. The propagation and synaptic delays involved in this process preclude the possibility of active closed-loop regulation in the course of normal movements. Such feedback is, however, useful in improving the learning proficiency of the movement or in situations in which unfamiliar movement conditions are encountered.

Spring-like behavior of the muscles plays an important role in the maintenance of posture and in the formation of movement trajectories. The muscle-joint system is dynamically similar to a mass-spring system with controllable equilibrium length. The spring-like properties of the muscle cause the joint trajectories to exhibit stable equilibrium behavior in the absence of any kind of sensory feedback; however, this spring-like behavior also exists in the presence of proprioceptive feedback.

Human movements involve active control of trajectory as well as the final position achieved by continuously varying the firing rate commands issued to the motoneurons of antagonist muscle pairs. The intrinsic muscle feedback that evolves from the spring-like behavior of the muscle provides primary movement stability during trajectory formation. This stretch reflex can be used to compensate for the asymmetries in muscle behavior away from the operating point. The spinal level controller regulates the skilled movements through the feedback servomechanism known as motor servo. The motor servo consists of the muscle spindle, the sensory pathways, and the skeletal muscle. The muscle spindle senses instantaneous changes in the spinal controller, which modulates the motoneuron firing rates. The muscle spindle receptors involved in the motor servo exhibit a nonlinear dynamic behavior characterized by low fractional power of velocity during the stretch phase.

CNS control of skilled movements involves choosing one among a number of muscle synergies available to perform the same task. A number of hypotheses have been advanced regarding the selection criteria used by the CNS. These hypotheses include energy optimal controls, quadratic cost optimization, impedance control, dynamic optimization, or, simply, the minimization of the number of muscles involved. There is little evidence that the CNS always controls any of the muscle variables in a fixed manner. Instead, there is much evidence for the flexible control of any and all variables so as to achieve the required adjustments.

Throwing

The shoulder complex is subjected to significant physical demands during the act of overhand throwing, an activity that is integral to many sports and recreational activities. Similar demands occur during stroke activities and racquet sports. Investigations involving dynamic EMG have significantly increased the level of understanding of the muscular activity of the shoulder complex as it relates to sports activities.

To throw a baseball, an athlete must generate kinetic energy and apply this energy to the ball; direct this force in order to steer the ball towards a target; and, after release of the ball, dissipate the retained energy. This is all accomplished through a complex series of coordinated muscle contractions involving both the lower and upper extremities as well as the trunk. The baseball-throwing motion has been divided into separate phases (Fig. 74). The first phase is the wind-up, which is characterized by the preparation activities performed by the athlete up until the time the ball is removed from the baseball glove. The second phase is the cocking phase, which is further divided into early cocking and late cocking. During early cocking, the arm is elevated and externally rotated. Late cocking occurs after the "lead" or "kick" leg is planted on the ground. After this foot hits the ground, late cocking continues until the maximum amount of external rotation of the arm is attained. This signals the end of the cocking phase and begins the acceleration phase. The acceleration phase of throwing is characterized by the rapid internal rotation and adduction of the arm, which results in the release of the ball. After the ball is released, the final phase of throwing is the follow-through. During the follow-through phase, the remainder of the energy in the system is dissipated.

During the wind-up, dynamic EMG of the shoulder muscles does not demonstrate a consistent pattern of activity. However, during cocking, all 3 heads of the deltoid demonstrate peak activity while holding the arm at 90°. The biceps brachii maintains appropriate elbow flexion during the cocking phase. During late cocking, amateur pitchers tend to demonstrate significantly greater activity in the supraspinatus muscle as compared to professional pitchers. The supraspinatus, infraspinatus, and teres minor all fire during cocking but begin to relax during late cocking. As the arm reaches the limit of external rotation late in cocking, the pectoralis major, latissimus dorsi, and subscapularis muscles decelerate the arm through eccentric muscle contraction.

The acceleration phase of the throw is characterized by

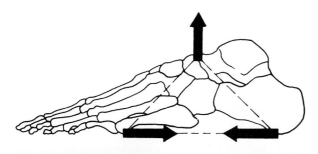

Figure 73

The intrinsic muscles of the foot, which stabilize the longitudinal arch of the foot and aid in the elevation of the arch along with the plantar aponeurosis. (Reproduced with permission from Saunders JBCM, Inman VT, Eberhart HD: The major determinants in normal and pathological gait. *J Bone Joint Surg* 1953;34A:552.)

relatively little activity in the rotator cuff and deltoid musculature. The pectoralis major, latissimus dorsi, and serratus anterior muscles contract strongly during the acceleration phase as the arm is adducted and internally rotated. Professional baseball pitchers have demonstrated significantly greater subscapularis activity during the acceleration phase when compared to amateur pitchers. Furthermore, amateur pitchers have demonstrated a tendency to use the biceps brachii more commonly during the acceleration phase.

Throughout the throwing motion, the trapezius and, especially, the serratus anterior control the scapula. This is important for the maintenance of a stable platform (glenoid) for the humeral head, as well as for the maintenance of the optimal orientation of this platform with respect to the ever-changing joint reaction forces. Fatigue of the scapular rotators jeopardizes the synchrony of the shoulder complex during throwing and may precipitate injuries to the shoulder musculature.

Once the ball is released, deceleration of the arm is required, and this is accomplished through eccentric contraction of the infraspinatus and teres minor muscles, as well as the supraspinatus, subscapularis, and posterior deltoid muscles. Protraction of the scapula is countered by eccentric contractions of the trapezius during follow-through. The entire throwing sequence usually takes less than 1 second from the start of the activity to ball release. The acceleration phase accounts for approximately 2% of the entire throwing motion. The arm internally rotates 7,000° to 8,000° per second during the acceleration phase. The ball has been calculated to accelerate from 0 mph at the onset of the acceleration phase to greater than 90 mph in approximately 80 ms. During this acceleration phase, the kinetic energy in the arm is 27,000 in-lb, which is approximately 4 times the kinetic energy in the kicking leg. This difference results from the angular velocity of the throwing arm being twice that of the kicking leg (the kinetic energy varies proportionally with the square of the angular velocity). All of this energy does not

instantly dissipate with release of the ball. The arm, still moving forward after release of the ball, must be rapidly decelerated in order that capsular ligamentous injury to the glenohumeral joint not occur. The dynamic constraints, especially the rotator cuff muscles, are the critical decelerators to prevent excessive distraction forces at the glenohumeral joint during the follow-through of each pitching motion.

Posture

Posture is the position of the total body or an individual segment relative to gravity. Posture can be thought of in static (anatomic) or dynamic (physiologic) terms. As a static term, it describes the position of the body in space or the position of the parts of the body relative to one another. Dynamically, posture denotes the precise control and neuromuscular activity that function to maintain the body's center of mass over its base of support. Even in the static-appearing condition of dual-limb stance, postural control mechanisms work constantly to maintain stability. For instance, low voltage EMG activity can be recorded intermittently in calf muscles throughout simple stance. A continuous sway mechanism is at work, with postural muscle activity in the calf counteracting and maintaining the sway. This sway and the concomitant muscle contractures are theorized to be one way in which the body in stance guards against orthostatic circulatory insufficiency.

Balance is a term that describes the control by the CNS and muscles of the inertial state of the body or any of its segments. The complex mechanism of postural control is not fully understood. Present models and thoughts concerning posture are based on experimental studies, neuromuscular theory, principles of biomechanics, and understanding of the nervous system.

Force-platform studies use the center of pressure, defined as the center of distribution of total force applied to the platform, to determine indirectly the vertical projection of

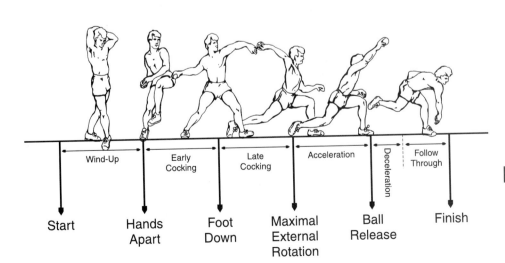

Wind-Up   Early Cocking   Late Cocking   Acceleration   Deceleration   Follow Through

Start   Hands Apart   Foot Down   Maximal External Rotation   Ball Release   Finish

Figure 74

Six phases of pitching. (Reproduced with permission from DiGiovine NM, Jobe FW, Pink M, et al: An electromyographic analysis of the upper extremity in pitching. *J Shoulder Elbow Surg* 1992;1:16.)

the location of the body's center of mass or center of gravity. In normal dual-limb stance the center of mass is in the vicinity of the sacral promontory. Technically, movement of the center of pressure depends on movement of the center of mass and the distribution of muscle forces responsible for that movement. Platform study has shown that in maintained, motionless dual-limb stance, the body's center of pressure (measured at 0.2-s intervals) fluctuates continuously around its mean center of pressure and traverses large total excursions (measured over 30 seconds of maintained stance) while remaining extremely close to the mean center of pressure.

Fluctuations of the body's center of pressure may be indicative of the sway mechanism, with total excursion indicative of total sway. With each individual sway, the center of pressure stays remarkably close to the mean center of pressure. The data show that in normal adults, the body does not deviate from its mean center of pressure, and seems to stay very close to that point automatically. Platform studies also have been used to measure differences between groups of adults. For instance, centers of pressure measured incrementally deviate farther from the mean center of pressure in elderly patients than in younger adults. Stroke victims' centers of pressure may be very poorly tuned, with very large excursions and an inability to stay close to the mean center of pressure. The center of pressure also shifts away from the weaker extremity in a hemiplegic.

Force-platform studies also allow researchers to describe an area of stability or cone of stability. The area is defined as all points from which the body can return to a point of origin without taking a step or changing the base of support. Another way of explaining this area is as the area over which weight can be safely shifted and maintained. This area is enclosed within the margin defined by the position of the center of pressure during weight shifting. Normal adults apparently are aware of the limits they can or cannot exceed to safely perform this task. Again, the elderly and stroke patients show a poorer aptitude for this task, with a resultant smaller measured area of stability.

Force-platform measurements have shown how a person can precisely maintain the center of gravity over his or her base of support during sustained weightbearing and weightshifting. Investigation, using EMG measurements, of the maintenance of posture via movement has led to the addition of synergies to postural control theory.

In experiments in which the base of support of a person in stance is moved rapidly and unexpectedly, the nervous system and body have a problem to solve. There appears to be an inordinate number of ways for the body to solve this problem, that is, potential muscle contractions or limb motions to maintain balance. The nervous system is thought to simplify this potentially complex postural problem by choosing among a set of prestructured, well-timed combinations of muscle contracture, or postural synergies. The chosen syner-

gy is the one that optimally solves the problem.

Synergies originally were theorized to simplify situations in which the body has little time (sometimes on the order of milliseconds) to react. These synergies now are thought to be important in all aspects of postural maintenance, and seem to be developed early in life. EMG studies of infants show a cephalocaudal development of synergies, with muscle timing and patterns for reliable head control developing first, followed by trunk control and then stance control. Not until an organized synergistic pattern is developed can these developmental landmarks be attained. Maturing of synergies appears to occur as the child's nervous system matures, as the body's size and muscle strength develop, and through experience. By 7 years of age, the synergistic patterns (as measured by EMG) and postural ability of the child are much like those of the normal adult.

Synergies occur around certain postural joints. The predominant synergies or joint strategies of stance occur around the ankle and hip joints. On a stable base of support in dual-limb stance, the ankle strategy predominates, with perturbations that cause the center of gravity to move forward counteracted by organized distal-to-proximal firing of the gastrocnemius-soleus and hamstrings (with turning off of the tibialis anterior). The posterior muscle firing counters the forward movement of the body and uses rotation about the ankle joint to maintain a stable center of gravity. A similar distal-to-proximal synergistic response is seen with posterior perturbation, with the tibialis anterior and rectus femoris firing sequentially to oppose the movement. The hip strategy occurs with a less stable base of support, such as a person standing on a balance beam, with trunk and hip muscles acting in a synergic proximal-to-distal sequence to maintain the center of gravity over the base of support by bending the trunk about the hip joint.

The chosen synergies appear not only to be neurologically and muscularly the optimal solution to the problem, but also work to minimize and, therefore, optimize biomechanical considerations (and perhaps energy requirements) during the adjustment. With more extreme perturbations, the hip and ankle strategies may be inadequate. The body tries to maintain its balance by lowering the center of gravity by knee bending (vertical strategy), or by changing the base of support by taking a step (step strategy).

These posture studies describe a feedback control: the body senses the perturbation and reacts via feedback using the appropriate synergy. This postural synergy feedback mechanism has been termed a postural reaction. The postural accompaniment that occurs just prior to or simultaneously with a voluntary movement might be called a "feedforward" mechanism. Feedforward involves anticipating the effect of a voluntary movement and coordinating precisely the postural adjustment (accompaniment) required to minimize the displacement of the center of gravity. Via EMG measurement, feedforward (postural accompaniment), like feedback (postural reaction), has been shown to use postural synergies.

The voluntary movement of standing up on one's toes can be used as an example of feedforward. Without the appropriate postural accompaniment, the subject will push himself or herself upward and backward, off balance. To prevent this, just prior to firing the gastrocnemius-soleus for the desired focal movement, the postural accompaniment turns off the soleus very briefly and fires a short burst of the tibialis anterior. The tibialis anterior moves the center of gravity slightly anteriorly in anticipation of the focal movement that will tend to move the center of gravity posteriorly. Postural accompaniments also occur with focal arm movements. A postural accompaniment of some sort occurs with any focal movement that alters the center of gravity, thereby keeping the center of gravity as unchanged as possible. Interestingly, the body has been shown experimentally to turn off a postural accompaniment if it senses that stability is provided from another source, such as the subject grasping a handrail.

Another mechanism of postural control occurs sequentially well before a postural accompaniment and is called a postural preparation. Examples of this are an athlete widening his or her stance or stiffening his or her postural joints prior to an anticipated collision, or an elderly or unsteady individual grabbing a handrail before arising from a chair. Postural mechanisms are thought to combine safety with efficiency. Whereas postural reactions by necessity are efficient, they may not be safe; the reaction may not be of sufficient magnitude. Postural preparations are safe, but not necessarily efficient. Postural accompaniments are both safe and efficient.

Postural maintenance through synergies is intimately integrated with all focal movements of the body. In gait, as steps are taken, the center of mass is constantly maintained safely and efficiently over the center of pressure. Postural synergies are active in undisturbed gait in the form of postural accompaniments. Evidence shows that older individuals have an altered ability to control balance and subsequent posture. For the elderly, acceleration of the head in the AP plane is significantly greater, while that noted for the hip is significantly less than in younger individuals. Acceleration of the head is only 23% of that of the hip in the AP plane in young adults, whereas it appears to be about 42% in the elderly. Furthermore, from stride to stride, variance of these numbers, as well as for lower joint moments and power, is greater for the elderly than for young adults. It is quite possible that the decrease in velocity, step length, push off, and the increase in double support seen in the elderly is a compensation to maintain balance and control during gait. EMG studies of gait show more consistent motor patterns in the elderly than in the young adult population, and kinematic observations show more consistency from stride to stride in a given individual and between individuals, with mild motion deviations, mostly at the time of double support at the hip knee, and ankle, of about 5° to 10° compared to younger adults.

Sensory input is an important contributor to postural maintenance. Visual, vestibular, and somatosensory inputs are all involved. In stance, somatosensory input depends predominantly on the body sensing its base of support. This input can influence the choice of postural strategy; for example, the sensing of a narrow base of support causes the body to choose the hip strategy over the ankle strategy. Experiments have shown that normal, healthy adults can maintain posture with vestibular input alone (while receiving altered or inhibited visual and somatosensory inputs). Elderly adults and children have problems when depending solely on vestibular input. Children also appear to choose visual cues over somatosensory cues, perhaps because the fine-tuning of sensing ankle and foot position takes longer to develop. Normal adults depend more on somatosensory input than visual input. Investigation of the effects of sensory contributions on posture control is continuing.

Experience clearly appears to be involved in postural control. The improvement of postural maintenance from childhood to adult levels, in addition to being dependent on maturity of the nervous system and the development of synergies, may best be explained by experience. Even in the normal adult, new or unusual tasks or movements may require new or unusual postural accompaniments via new synergies or novel combinations of synergies. Improvement in these new postural mechanisms develops with experience or practice. Experience may also explain why the elderly choose to maintain a smaller area of stability in platform testing. Previous experience (a fall) may prevent them from taking risks. Of course, this decreased performance in the elderly may also result from a number of factors, including deteriorating sensory input (poor vision, neuropathy), diminishing CNS control, and decreased muscle strength. Nevertheless, experience cannot be denied as an important factor, and it is an important tool used by physical therapists to help stroke victims improve their levels of postural development.

Other factors that seem to contribute to posture are muscle strength and joint range of motion. The tibialis anterior has been found to be weaker in the elderly, and this weakness may contribute to more frequent falling. Children's development of posture may depend on the development of sufficient strength for body size in addition to the aforementioned factors. Patients with neuromuscular disease (dystrophies) show deterioration of postural ability. Hemiplegics' decreased strength affects the location of the center of pressure, away from the weak extremity. Joint range of motion also plays a role. Postural synergies that might work for normal adults via an appropriate ankle strategy will not work for someone with a decreased joint range of motion (stroke victims, cerebral palsy). The ability of such patients to develop new synergies or strategies is key to their ability to maintain some level of posture.

The CNS plays a major role in postural control, as a place where sensory input is processed, experience is stored, and neuromuscular postural synergies are developed and dictated. In addition, highly abnormal postural control is found in certain CNS deficiencies. Patients who have Parkinson's disease, which affects the basal ganglia, or cerebellar disorders show decreased ability to perform simple postural tasks. Patients who have cerebellar disease have shown absent postural responses to simple focal movements, while those who have Parkinson's disease show delayed or prolonged postural synergies. The heavy network of inputs and outputs from both the cerebellum and basal ganglia to and from the cerebral cortex (the center of motor and sensory input for the body) explains why deficiencies in these areas cause postural problems. It is thought that the cerebellum and basal ganglia are involved with timing, appropriateness, and gain of postural responses. Further study is needed to better understand their respective contributions.

A published central control model summarizes currently accepted knowledge of postural control: (1) The human body can precisely and automatically maintain its center of mass over its base of support under a variety of conditions. (2) Postural control centers on the CNS, which transmits motor output and receives sensory input. Additionally, certain CNS diseases provide the most challenging questions and problems of postural maintenance. (3) Postural synergies are ways in which the CNS (with the postural muscles) derives optimal solutions for potentially complicated postural problems and combinations. (4) Sensory input plays an important role via visual, vestibular, and somatosensory inputs both in choosing postural strategies and in providing the feedback and, therefore, the experience from which a person modifies and fine-tunes the postural strategies. (5) Joint range of motion and muscle strength contribute only as much as the body is aware of any deficiencies in these areas and can thereby make postural adjustments.

The present understanding of postural control has arisen through experience, neuromuscular theory, biomechanical principles, and knowledge of the CNS. Further experimental studies continue to enhance this understanding. The orthopaedic literature has provided little input to postural control studies. Most present knowledge comes from the neurologic, biomechanical, and physical therapy literature. Nevertheless, the orthopaedist must be aware of posture as it relates to gait and to patients with neurologic and muscular diseases. The orthopaedist also should be aware of

other subsets of patients (elderly, children) who may suffer from falls or trauma because of deficiencies in postural maintenance and control.

Walking

Human gait consists of a series of multiple limb segment rotational movements that produce stable forward propulsion in an energy-conserving manner (Fig. 75). Forces produced by muscles interacting with the body's gravitational and inertial properties result in joint angular changes. The effective summation of these movements is the stride length produced and, in association with the number of steps taken per minute (cadence), the overall velocity. These latter features constitute a measure of overall performance. Timing of muscle activity, joint angular changes, and time-distance parameters (step length, phase times, cadence, velocity, and so forth) are reproducible from cycle to cycle and person to person.

The natural cadence reported in the literature varies from 101 to 122 steps per minute. Women walk faster than men, having a cadence of 122 versus 116 steps per minute. The cadence of infants and children is greater than that of adults. Children age 1 year may have a cadence as high as 180 steps per minute while 7-year-olds have been reported to have a mean cadence of about 145 steps per minute. Studies of individuals between 60 and 85 years of age seem to indicate that, in the absence of pathologic conditions, cadence does not decrease, but stride length does decrease.

Kinematic measurements of joint angles of the lower extremities also differ little between men and women and between individuals 20 and 65 years of age. From cycle to cycle for a given subject, joint angular changes vary by only approximately 2° or less at any given instant in the gait cycle. Differences between subjects may be as high as 10%. These changes, which occur at the transitions of heel strike and toe-off, are associated with differences in free walking cadence and in step length. While there is evidence that step lengths and velocities decrease for people older than 65 years of age (up to 85 years), this decrease does not appear to be related to marked changes in angular positions of the lower extremities. In the sagittal plane, angular changes show that mature gait is established by the age of 3 years. However, angular changes in the nonsagittal plane apparently take longer to achieve, and the normal degrees

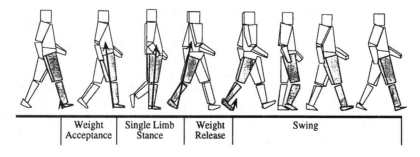

| Weight Acceptance | Single Limb Stance | Weight Release | Swing |

Figure 75

Limb movement in normal stride.

of rotation of adults seem to occur by the age of 7 years. Similarly, the walk-to-walk variability of muscle patterns seen during gait in a given subject is low although differences can be noted between the 2 sides. Patterns are apparently very similar from person to person and, at present, from 2- and 3-year-old children up to very old age.

Muscular activity and resulting limb positions and joint angular changes vary throughout the cycle (Fig. 76). The need for support and propulsion varies with the phase of the gait cycle. A normal CNS provides the control for gait to occur. Joint, ligament, bone, or muscle disease or injury produces a pattern that is different from normal, but is still controlled reproducibly by a normal CNS. Gait dysfunction from such disorders seems to be governed by a set of rules of compensation. The result, at times, may sacrifice energy efficiency, may increase joint forces and muscle effort, and may not fully compensate; but it does allow walking to be maintained. Diseases that affect the nervous system may not allow normal compensatory reactions and, in association with spasticity or weakness, may produce a walking pattern that is not readily understood by standard clinical methods.

To best understand the relationship between particular gait deviations and performance criteria, it is important to briefly review a few basic principles of gait. Whenever a person assumes an upright posture, inherent passive stability no longer exists. Unlike birds or creatures whose center of gravity lies below the pivoted hip joint, the human center of gravity is above it. A forward or backward force tends to rotate this center of gravity further away, thus making the individual susceptible to falling. Two mechanisms can prevent this. Muscles intended to reverse this trend can be activated (postural reactions), or muscles intended to extend a limb outward in the direction of movement to brace or provide a stable structure under the falling object can be activated. In normal walking, a combination of these mechanisms exists to provide stability. The leg in stance uses postural reactions. The leg in swing provides stability by reaching out a given distance at a given time. As a consequence of the latter, propulsive forces are imparted to the body to maintain forward movement. Then, this acceleration force must be decelerated when the leg hits the ground.

Thus, walking requires a greater muscular effort than quiet standing to remain stable. This dynamic stability remains only when acceleration and deceleration forces are relatively balanced. The swing of a leg may be simultane-

Muscle Sequence During Gait

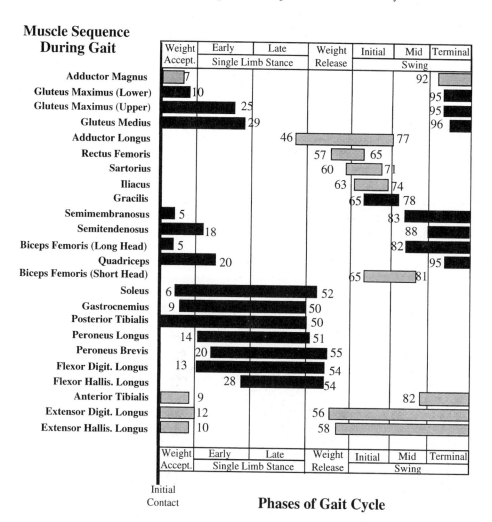

Phases of Gait Cycle

Figure 76

Muscular sequence of lower limb muscles during gait. Numbers signify percent of time in gait at which the muscle activity begins and ends.

ously balanced by the stance of the opposite leg, and acceleration of a leg similarly may be simultaneously offset by deceleration of the other. Alternatively, some balancing may be done by the same leg at a later time. In normal gait, both mechanisms operate and are confined primarily to the structures of the pelvis and below.

As cadence and velocity increase, both stance and swing times decrease. As percentages of the gait cycle, stance decreases approximately 3.5 times as rapidly as swing. In absolute time, swing time decreases little as the speed of walking changes. Cadence and stride length depend on one another; both vary as the square root of the velocity. Up to approximately 120 steps per minute, speed increases are achieved equally by increasing stride and cadence. Above 120 steps per minute, step-length levels off leaving only cadence to increase to a maximum. Additionally, in contrast to kinematic data, sagittal plane moments about the hip, knee, and ankle joints are quite variable from step to step. In particular, this variability comes between the hip and the knee, and it is present both intra- and intersubject. If the sum of these moments is examined as a reflection of the balance about the body's center of gravity, this sum remains relatively the same from step to step. Stability is controlled overall by changes in load sharing between different joints (predominantly the hip and knee).

These mechanisms are the reason for defining the phases of the gait cycle as weight acceptance, single limb stance, weight release (preswing), and swing, and are controlled by the neurologic system. The phases are relatively similar from person to person in the motions of limb segments and the active time of various muscles. The walking speed of various normal individuals is thus similar, efficient, and adaptable. For normal individuals, normal motions and normal muscular activity provide optimum results for all criteria of performance.

In neuromuscular disease, a peripheral defect alters a single or several bodily areas, thereby jeopardizing dynamic stability. Normal compensatory mechanisms that seek to correct the defect affect certain performance criteria more than others. For example, speed may be maintained close to normal at the expense of excess energy. Central defects, by attacking the control mechanisms as well as causing local abnormalities, jeopardize dynamic stability even more, thus creating an even wider discrepancy in what might be considered the normal values for various performance criteria. Because treatment does not restore normalcy, but substitutes for it, the orthopaedist must be sure that as many performance criteria as possible are improved. To best determine this, the physician must understand and analyze each gait pathology, closely examining both the primary defects and compensatory mechanisms and determining how they are related to each criterion of performance.

The process called walking is a repeated cycle of limb motions, controlled by selective muscle action, that carries the body forward while maintaining optimal upright stabili-

ty. Included are actions directed toward absorption of the shock of floor impact and conservation of energy. Except for knee flexion in swing, most joint function depends on small, but critical, 15° to 20° arcs. A 10° deviation can be obstructive.

The clearance of the foot from the ground that occurs with each of the approximately 2 million steps an individual takes each year illustrates this well. The toe is the last body segment to leave the ground at the beginning of swing and, because of the angle of the leg and foot during swing, the toe rises to no more than 2.5 cm above the ground. It then drops to 0.87 cm of clearance at midswing. This minimal toe clearance occurs at the most dangerous phase of the toe trajectory, when the horizontal velocity of the foot is at a maximum, and the body is beginning its acceleration ahead of the opposite foot in stance. As the knee extends and the foot dorsiflexes, the toe rises to a maximum of 13 cm just prior to heel strike and then lowers to the floor. Altering the subject's speed essentially does not change the overall pattern nor the maximum-minimum of the displacement of the foot from the ground. At heel contact, it has been estimated that, although the forward velocity of the body center of mass is 1.6 m/s, the velocity at the heel is 4 m/s horizontally and 0.05 m/s vertically. Thus, the heel does not strike the ground but slides and must be braked in milliseconds to zero velocity. For the elderly, heel contact velocity in the horizontal direction seems to be significantly higher (30%) despite the fact that these individuals are walking with a shorter step length and slower overall velocity.

During walking, the multiple segments of the body move at different speeds. The upper and lower extremities change their speeds and displacements to the greatest degree. Another concept of control is noted by looking at the displacement of the head, the trunk, and the pelvis. As an individual walks, vertical displacement of the head increases from 3.6 cm at slow speeds to 6.2 cm at fast speeds. Yet, during this period of change in speed, the head's lateral displacement actually decreases from 4.2 cm at slow cadences to 2.7 cm at fast cadence. The thorax and pelvis do not move in unison. When the acceleration of the head is compared to that of the pelvis, the pelvic vertical accelerations are just marginally greater than those of the head despite the greater distance from the fulcrum at which the head is located. At free speed walking, the horizontal accelerations of the head are about one half those of the pelvis, whereas in the medial lateral plane, the head's acceleration and deceleration are only about three quarters those of the pelvis. Thus, it is clear that the trunk plays an active role in reducing the translational and rotational displacements and accelerations of the head relative to the pelvis. The neurocontrol to achieve all these tasks requires extremely fine tuning.

This narrow margin between normal and abnormal function makes the diagnosis of gait deviations difficult. To overcome these limitations, objective instrumented systems for evaluating gait disorders have been developed. Their value in identifying functional problems and determining the effectiveness of treatment is becoming more and more evident. Because walking is such a complex interaction of joint motions and muscle actions, a summary of the critical events is provided as background for the literature survey.

Normal Gait

During each stride (cycle) the limb moves through 8 unique synergistic motion patterns (phases of gait) to accomplish 3 basic tasks: weight acceptance, single limb support, and limb advancement (Fig. 75). As these tasks are accomplished, the ankle and knee use 4 positions, and the hip 2 positions. A posture that is appropriate in 1 gait phase would signify dysfunction at another point in the cycle because the functional need has changed. As a result, timing often is as significant as posture. The relative significance of one joint's motion compared to the other varies among the gait phases. This factor makes observational gait analysis difficult.

Each joint has its own normal pattern of motion, moments, and joint powers as well as muscle control (Figs. 76 through 78). During stance, the stimulus is forward fall of body weight. As a result, muscle action is eccentric (that is, restraining a lengthening force). In swing, joint function is directed to clearing the floor, advancing the limb, and preparing for the next stance period. Muscle action is concentric.

Ankle The mode of foot/ankle mobility and muscular control is the most significant determinant of both limb stability and body progression.

Initial floor contact with the heel establishes the heel rocker that will be used to preserve the progression and initiate shock absorption during the limb's loading response. After heel contact, the ankle undergoes rapid plantarflexion. Vigorous deceleration of the tibialis anterior, assisted

by the extensor hallucis longus, provides a controlled heel rocker. Two purposes are served: Part of the impact shock is absorbed directly and the tibia is advanced to preserve progression and accelerate knee flexion for further shock absorption.

Controlled dorsiflexion to 10° (midstance) and subsequent heel rise (terminal stance) throughout the single limb support period are the main sources of body progression. Active deceleration of the tibial advance is a critical component of knee stability. Reversal of ankle motion toward dorsiflexion immediately follows floor contact by the forefoot. The stimulus is forward momentum of the body weight. Deceleration of this motion by soleus and gastrocnemius activity provides a controlled ankle rocker. The muscles yield as they hold to allow the tibia, and thus the body, to move forward. The restraining force, however, is sufficient to make the rate of tibial advance slower than that of the femur. This allows the knee to extend. Body weight moves across the length of the foot, reaching the metatarsal head area as the ankle attains 10° dorsiflexion. Increased (strong) gastrocnemius and soleus action stabilizes the ankle and allows the heel to rise.

The forefoot becomes the final progressional rocker. During this action, the ankle moves into slight plantar flexion (5°) just before the forwardly aligned body weight drops onto the other foot. The limb then unloads; the muscles of the gastrocnemius-soleus group promptly relax. Hence, the functions of these muscles are to decelerate tibial advance for knee stability and to stabilize the ankle for a forefoot rocker. Push-off is not their role. The large arc of plantarflexion that occurs in preswing is functionally insignificant because the limb is virtually unloaded; it contributes to clearance but not to balance. Strength demands on the gastrocnemius-soleus musculature increase as the stride is lengthened.

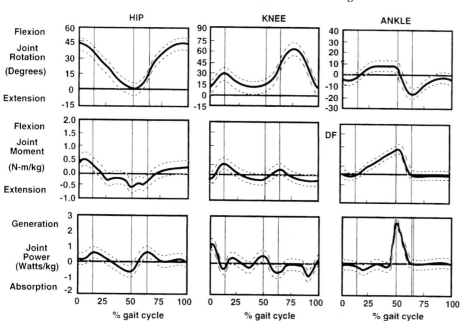

Figure 77

Joint angles, moment, and power of the hip, knee, and ankle in flexion and extension at each joint. (Adapted with permission from Gage JR: An overview of normal walking, in Greene WB (ed): *Instructional Course Lectures XXXIX*. Park Ridge, IL, American Academy of Orthopaedic Surgeons, 1990, pp 291–303.)

Dorsiflexion to neutral in swing is the final event. It is responsible for toe clearance in midswing. Three types of pathologic circumstance prevent effective ankle motion: (1) plantarflexion contracture; (2) weakness of plantarflexion muscles; and (3) weakness of dorsiflexion muscles.

Plantarflexion contracture is functionally significant when the ankle cannot attain a 5° dorsiflexed posture by the end of midstance. This angle is necessary for body weight to advance onto the forefoot. Dorsiflexion to 0° is not enough; this keeps body weight in the area of the ankle joint. A 15° plantarflexion contracture is not uncommon. Insensitivity to this posture stems from the fact that it is a natural event; it is the resting posture of the ankle and is a normal occurrence during the loading response. Contractures form as an incidental element of immobilization. Spontaneous positioning of the ankle will be in 15° of plantarflexion if specific efforts are not taken to avoid it. Inability to achieve dorsiflexion blocks the body's efforts to move forward over the supporting foot. Stride length and gait velocity are decreased. The knee may be strained into hyperextension. Forefoot pressure is prolonged and the intensity is increased, leading to pain and skin damage. Substitution of early heel-off (occurring in middle rather than terminal stance) improves progression but continues to strain the forefoot and knee.

Gastrocnemius-soleus insufficiency introduces tibial instability with a corresponding increase in quadriceps demand. If the body lacks the ability to restrain a dorsiflexion torque, body weight is kept close to the heel throughout the single limb support period. Stride length is shortened; endurance is reduced; and heel rise is delayed until the limb is unloaded. This is a very disabling situation that is difficult to recognize. The signs are persistent heel contact with excessive dorsiflexion at the end of single stance, persistent knee flexion in midstance, and lack of knee flexion during weight acceptance. All of these signs are subtle, and instrumented gait analysis may be needed to make the diagnosis. Because several motion patterns are possible, dynamic EMG also is indicated.

Clinical definition of gastrocnemius-soleus weakness is obscure. Manual testing is convenient but does not reproduce the force used in a single heel rise. Hence, this examination is woefully inadequate. Grade 5 strength supine is no better than grade 2 standing. The lesser perimalleolar plantarflexors (the peroneus group, tibialis posterior, and toe flexors) can meet the challenge of manual testing but not the standing demand. Repetitive, single limb heel rise (full range at least 20 times is normal) and instrumented force testing are the only valid measures.

Tibialis anterior weakness causes the familiar foot drop. This is the most frequently treated but least significant gait error involving the ankle. Functional significance is low because there are so many ways to adjust for it (slightly increased hip flexion, contralateral vaulting, and circumduction). Orthotic assistance at the onset of disability is indicated. Only the more severely disabled patients who lack an alternate means of lifting the foot continue to use the orthosis, however.

Knee Three essential actions occur at the knee: flexion to decrease the impact of floor contact, extension for weight-bearing stability, and flexion for toe clearance in swing.

Weight acceptance is accomplished by knee flexion of about 15°. This flexion provides valuable shock absorption, but it also introduces postural instability. Two mechanisms are involved. Body weight is behind the foot at the time of initial contact, and the heel rocker rolls the tibia forward. Both events place the body vector line behind the knee.

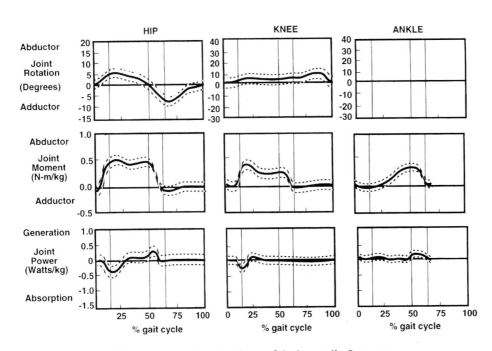

Figure 78

Joint angles, moment, and power of the hip, knee, and ankle in abduction and adduction at each joint. (Adapted with permission from Gage JR: An overview of normal walking, in Greene WB (ed): *Instructional Course Lectures XXXIX.* Park Ridge, IL, American Academy of Orthopaedic Surgeons, 1990, pp 291–303.)

Quadriceps activity preserves limb stability. When the flexion is limited to 15°, the functional demand is well tolerated. Peak stance-phase knee flexion occurs just at the onset of single limb support. Throughout midstance, the knee progressively extends over the stable tibia. As the body-weight line reaches and then moves ahead of the knee axis in late midstance, the quadriceps relax and knee extension stability depends entirely on tibial control at the ankle.

Knee flexion for swing begins in the terminal double-support period (preswing). Approximately 40° is attained passively as body weight rolls beyond the metatarsal heads, and distal stability is lost. Only if the rate of knee flexion is excessive is there any restraining muscle action. Knee flexion is increased in initial swing (60°) for toe clearance. Momentum from hip flexion and slight local knee flexion action (short head of the biceps femoris) are the sources.

The final knee action is progressive knee extension to neutral in preparation for the next weightbearing period. This begins passively in midswing and is completed by quadriceps activity in terminal swing.

Assessment of knee position is complicated by the fact that 2 bony landmarks are eccentric to the joint axes they are supposed to indicate. The greater trochanter prominence is 3 cm behind the center of the femoral head, and the apex of the lateral malleolus is 1 cm behind the ankle axis. Use of these anatomic landmarks without corrections for their eccentric alignment can indicate 15° knee flexion when that joint is seen to be fully extended on the radiograph.

There are 3 significant gait errors. Each relates to the key function listed above. (1) Inadequate knee flexion during the loading response generally is not listed, but it deprives the patient of valuable shock absorption. The primary cause is quadriceps weakness. Patients substitute by using premature ankle plantarflexion to prevent the normal heel rocker. A second substitution is increased hip extensor muscle action. Slight forward lean of the trunk provides proximal stability so the hip extensors can draw the femur back. (2) Persistent knee flexion during single-limb support increases the duration of quadriceps demand. If knee position exceeds 15°, it also increases the supporting force needed. Both situations lead to premature fatigue. A flexion contracture or persistent hamstring muscle action are well-recognized causes. Weak gastrocnemius-soleus musculature must be added to this list. Walking on a flexed knee increases energy costs because the extensor muscle must remain active. (3) Insufficient knee flexion in initial swing causes a toe drag unless the patient substitutes. Possible substitutions include lateral trunk lean, circumduction, and vaulting by the other foot. All of these alternate mechanisms increase the energy cost of walking.

Hip

Sagittal plane motion is simple. Starting from 45° of flexion, the hip progressively extends during stance. In swing there is rapid reversal into flexion for limb advancement. Demands on the extensor musculature are brief, lasting only during the weight-acceptance period. The dominant control is by the single joint muscles (gluteus maximus and adductor magnus). Relaxation of the hamstrings avoids excessive knee flexion. At the end of stance, the hip is drawn toward hyperextension, with iliacus activity being the restraining force. Limb advancement in early swing is accomplished by a mixture of low flexor muscle activities.

Hip control in the coronal plane is more demanding. Gluteus medius activity starts with the onset of stance and persists through most of the single-limb support period. The upper gluteus maximus also functions as an abductor. In addition, the hip is subjected to rotational forces as the trunk moves from behind to ahead of the supporting limb.

The significant functional errors are insufficient hip extension range and inadequacy of hip extensor, abductor, or flexion musculature. Flexion contractures commonly are accommodated by increased lumbar lordosis. In time, lumbosacral pain may be an additional complication. Patients who lack this range must lean forward. This introduces the need for a cane or crutch. Backward lean of the trunk (or lordosis) also is the postural substitution for hip extensor weakness. The 2 causes may be differentiated by timing: an extensor weakness requires accommodation at initial contact whereas demands for a flexion contracture may wait until mid or terminal stance. Hip abductor weakness leads to coronal plane instability. The immediate reaction is a drop of the contralateral side of the pelvis. Upright balance is maintained by a lateral trunk lean toward the supporting limb. Insufficiency of hip flexor strength leads to a loss of limb advancement unless the person can substitute by a contralateral lean or increased pelvic motion.

Movement Instrumentation Systems

With the dramatic improvement in types and refinements of musculoskeletal treatments, the clinician has a wide variety of options from which to select the optimal program. To best assess the proper treatment and its results, movement may now be evaluated using objective, quantifiable methods based on commercially available electronic and computer hardware and software. Recent technologic advances make clinical use of the movement laboratory feasible. Because these newer systems are becoming more available and more widely used, a summary of their characteristics and principles is provided.

The function of a movement analysis laboratory is to quantify and assess an individual patient's functional performance. At present, 5 types of instrumentation systems are applicable to clinical use: motion analysis, dynamic EMG, force plates, foot-switch stride analysis, and measurement of energy costs. Automated motion systems are replacing photography because they are more rapid and more comprehensive. Dynamic EMG provides a direct means of identifying appropriate muscle action. This is an invaluable aid in determining the appropriate surgical plan for improving the gait of persons disabled by cerebral palsy, head trauma, and stroke. Use of this technique to identify compensatory muscle action in other types of impairment also is increasing. Definition of stride characteristics by use of foot switches or other methods classifies the patient's ability to walk, and is an excellent means of measuring the functional effectiveness of treatment. Energy-cost determination identifies the physiologic strain of gait disorder. Computer equipment is required to process the data and to allow visual checks of the functioning of the system. Moments around joints and deforming forces may be calculated from the measured variables. To avoid the inconvenience of direct oxygen measurement, calculations of mechanical work and energy are being explored. However, the excessive muscular effort that may be used to minimize a limp cannot be determined by summation of segment displacement. Consequently, the ratio between the 2 sets of data is low even though the correlations are good.

Like any other laboratory test, movement analysis testing yields information; the tests themselves do not provide an interpretation of the data. This is left to the clinician.

Automated Motion Analysis

To provide an accurate measurement of human movement, motion analysis systems must (1) visualize and accurately record all movements desired; (2) identify and quantify where in space each area of interest exists at every instant in the movement cycle; and (3) calculate parameters of interest to clinicians, for example, joint angles, velocity, stance times. In current systems all 3 steps are performed using video-type cameras, specialized electronic hardware, and computers.

Movement Visualization and Recording

As every limb segment changes its position during each instant of the movement cycle, all these systems instantaneously capture all the segment positions simultaneously and perform this task multiple times during the movement (Fig. 75). For walking, such snapshots or frames of data are obtained at least 50 to 60 times per second; for faster movements, such as sports, current systems obtain these frames at least 200 times per second. Anatomic skin areas of interest are highlighted by use of markers, shapes that can be light-contrasted from the background. The marker itself can be the light source or reflective tape can be used to highlight and intensify infrared or regular light. A second camera, which simultaneously views and records the same markers, allows the 3-D position in space (X,Y,Z) of each of the markers (after further processing) to be known. If the

field of view of the camera to the marker is obscured, for example by a crutch, cane, or walker, a third camera directed at viewing the same markers often is used. Alternatively, if the view is only obscured for several snapshots or frames, computer software can later fill in the missing spots. If both sides of the body must be visualized simultaneously, careful choice of marker location is necessary to minimize the number of cameras needed.

Motion analysis systems vary as to how these visualized frames are recorded; some use VCR tape and later process and digitally record automatically or by hand off-line. In some systems, each camera is directly linked to an electronic hardware processor and the computer automatically identifies the 2-D x-y position of each marker as it is imaged on-line and computer stored. This method requires seeing and numerically recording the position of up to 25 markers from 2 to 6 cameras every fiftieth of a second. It is necessary to properly identify each marker in each frame. In all systems, this is done by identifying, via a computer software program, each marker's anatomic relationship in the first few frames of the movement. A computer program then sorts out each marker's trajectory for the cycle by automatically tracking the marker as it changes its position from frame to frame or snapshot to snapshot. From each camera's 2-D marker file, all motion analysis systems using computer software programs combine the same marker site from at least 2 camera's files to produce a 3-D file of each marker in space.

Limb Segment and Joint Position Calculations

Recorded marker positions do not represent specific joints or limb segments. They represent only a single place on or near the skin that is related to a known anatomic location, for example, distal tip of the lateral malleolus of the ankle, tibial tubercle. This positional information must then be translated into limb segment or joint positional information (Fig. 75). Where markers are placed on the skin in a given movement study is determined by how this calculation is made. Appropriate software programs have been developed to perform these calculations. A variety of different methods exist for this process. These methods vary in their degree of mathematic and biomechanical sophistication.

Calculation of Movement Parameters

A multitude of movement parameters can be calculated from these 3-D limb segment and joint positions. Certain parameters routinely are clinically useful, for example, hip flexion/extension. Other parameters may be useful in specific movement disorders, for example, toe clearance from the floor during swing. The accuracy in measurement of such parameters depends to some degree on (1) the accuracy of the camera system used, (2) the movement addressed, (3) the trueness of the 3-D motion file established, and (4) the mathematic approach used to calculate the desired parameter.

Sagittal knee movement during gait represents large angular changes (60°), marker placement on the skin does not differ significantly from patient to patient relative to the degree of the angular error that can be produced, and the mathematics used to calculate the resulting angles use a well-defined joint axis. Knee flexion-extension in almost all motion systems thus yields very similar results. However, ankle dorsiflexion-plantarflexion can be quite variable. To calculate this parameter in the simplest manner, 3 markers are used: lateral side of knee, lateral malleolus, and the dorsum or lateral side of the patient's metacarpal phalangeal joint of the foot. The angle is then calculated for each data frame of the movement cycle using simple trigonometric relationships between these points. Foot abnormalities or dynamic changes in a flexible foot during gait can cause hindfoot varus-valgus, forefoot pronation-supination, and midtarsal flexion-extension. Because the ankle angle is calculated from markers spanning these joints, the calculation program includes any combination of these motions in the sagittal ankle angle calculation and does not represent true ankle dorsiflexion-plantarflexion. To overcome such limitations, differing marker configurations and more sophisticated mathematic approaches to this angle's calculations have been developed.

The attempt for greater accuracy can lead to more markers (or cameras) being used and more difficulty in tracking individual markers during the sorting process. For different reasons, similar potential measurement inaccuracies exist in determining all the joint angles at the hip and varus-valgus and internal-external rotation of the knee. Depending on the nature of the movement, the motion system used, and the specific joint angle to be evaluated, how accurately the measurement recorded reflects and needs to reflect the real motion occurring varies with the study and the information desired.

Foot-Switch Stride Analyses

In contrast to joint angular determinations, many time-distance parameters of gait (cadence, stride length, single limb stance time) are less subject to processing variation when they are calculated from motion systems or from foot-switch stride analyses. From motion systems, such calculations are defined by selected single markers about the foot, for example, heel and frame number recording of well-defined gait events such as heel strike in frame number 5, toe-off in frame number 10. The frame in which a gait event occurs is determined by user intervention. Selecting whether a foot strike or toe-off occurs in 1 frame or in the next, a fiftieth of a second later is sometimes difficult. Distances traversed and time intervals are then calculated from the 3-D position of the marker at each of the gait events. It has been found that in addition to calculating the absolute time and distance of the gait cycle phases, normalizing each time interval to a percent of the gait cycle yields useful clinical data.

Dynamic EMG Measurement

Dynamic EMG recording represents the neurologic system's control of when a particular muscle is to be activated as well as the ability of the muscle to be activated. Investigations have established the fact that, during any functional movement, a particular muscle is activated only for a given period of time. For example, during an individual gait cycle, no muscle is activated for more than 30% to 40% of the entire cycle. Dynamic EMG does not represent the absolute force of the muscle, and the magnitude of EMG activity alone is not useful in comparing a muscle's force from one testing session to another or between subjects. However, the timing of EMG activity can be used to compare a subject's performance to normal values and to determine whether the performance is prolonged or continuously active from condition to condition and from subject to subject. Comparison in the same session of the magnitude of EMG activity during movement to that during a maximal voluntary contracture of the muscle has been found to provide useful clinical information.

The EMG signal recorded is a summation of multiple motor units and muscle fibers being activated. During the time of its activation, the magnitude and the frequency of the signal change. Sampling occurs from a given region of the muscle. The number of muscle fibers and motor units recorded varies with the method of sampling. One method obtains the signal using hair-thin electric (bipolar) wires (wire electrode) inserted into the muscle. It has been found that for most pathologic disorders, if the site of the EMG has been properly selected, the small number of motor units tested by this method accurately represents the entire muscle. The alternative to wire-electrode sampling is the use of surface electrodes. These electrodes represent a larger area of muscle motor units and muscle fibers.

The EMG signal recorded from either method represents the summation of the depolarization and repolarization of multiple muscle fibers. Because this occurs in individual muscle fibers at slightly different rates, the summation in the waveform represents negative and positive values. Wire electrodes represent the most accurate methods of recording EMG activity for such circumstances. This recording process is, however, time consuming and in certain cases, because of its invasive nature, may be a somewhat painful process. Surface-electrode recording minimizes the problem, but must be interpreted with caution. The signal picked up from surface electrodes represents transmission of the true signal through fat, fascia, and skin. Some signal is thereby reflected and/or refracted, yielding alterations in the signal's magnitude and frequency. Moreover, muscles in adjacent areas, whether laterally or deeply positioned, for example, the various components of the quadriceps (vastus intermedius, vastus lateralis, vastus medialis) represent part of the signal recorded from the muscle directly under the surface electrode, in this case the rectus femoris. In most cases, adjacent muscles are similar in activation and the signal recorded poses little problem in interpretation if surface electrode EMG is defined as measuring muscle groups, that is, quadriceps rather than rectus femoris, and is used to help understand whether regional muscle activity contributes to flexing or extending a given joint.

In addition to the electrode recorder, all dynamic EMG systems contain electrical components to ground the signal, minimize interference noise, transmit the signal, and record the signal. Both wire and surface electrodes pick up low-magnitude muscle electrical signals. The signal also contains electrical artifact noise produced by skin, muscle, wire, or electrode movement. Such noise can be equal to or larger in magnitude than that of the EMG signal. With all systems, careful placement of the electrode is essential, and an amplifier is provided as close to the origin of the signal as possible in order to minimize this noise. The signal can then be transmitted to a recording device via a cable wire system (dragged along as the patient walks) or via the airwaves (telemetry). The transmitted signals are immediately recorded and stored on tape or digitally converted and computer stored. Additional electronic hardware is necessary to synchronize the EMG signals recorded with the movement events with motion analysis systems, or with force platform systems, on-line or off-line.

The EMG data often are presented as a smoothed wave of hills and valleys; or they can be illustrated as a single horizontal bar that merely depicts the on-off activity of the muscle. Mathematic processing techniques are necessary to alter the signal for such purposes.

As the use of dynamic EMG for the evaluation of movement dysfunction has gained in popularity, its usefulness in understanding normal movement has also increased. Investigation has determined that 3 strides of EMG data per subject provide information as reliable as that obtained from 12 strides. EMG examination of 8 muscles about the ankle during manual muscle testing and 3 walking velocities (free, fast, slow) has shown that the intensity of muscle action during walking is related to the manual muscle test grades. Walking at the normal free velocity required fair (grade 3) muscle action. During slow gait, the muscle functioned at a poor (grade 2) level. Fast walking necessitated muscle action midway between fair and normal, which was interpreted as good (grade 4). Analysis of surface EMGs of 7 major muscles in adults indicates 2 general types of pattern change in lower extremity muscle activity as a function of walking speed. The fundamental phasing of muscle activity never changes, but relative amplitudes within the phases are modulated as speed increases; and different phases of activity exist for different walking speeds. The timing of most phases (expressed as percentage of the stride) decreased as speed increased. This suggests that the time base should be further normalized by stance and swing phases.

Foot-Floor Force and Pressure Recordings

The changes in direction, magnitude, and area of contact of the foot-to-ground reaction forces during the stance phase of walking are among the most relevant parameters in the assessment of human gait. Body weight and inertial forces are effective in moving the body forward and providing stability only if they are resisted by the ground. Measurement of the foot-to-ground reaction forces via platforms provides an understanding of these respective forces. These platforms, embedded in the ground, provide accurate measurements of the vertical and horizontal forces of the foot against the ground in hundredths or thousandths of seconds. The force platform must be small enough to allow only the forces on a single foot to be measured. If the platform is too small, the foot could miss the force plate. Most platforms are about 2 feet by 2 feet. To obtain information from both feet, either 2 or more force platforms must be used or the subject must walk across the force platform several times. Measurement devices within the force platform use piezoelectric or strain-gauge electronic technology and highly-insulated wire conduction systems to transmit the force measurements (after they are amplified) to a recording device. The recording devices are similar to those of EMG or motion analysis systems.

Such signals are graphically represented as absolute time during the stance phase or are normalized to the gait cycle if that cycle is synchronized to motion analysis systems.

If the external moments about the hip, knee, or ankle joints are clinically desired, further software routines are needed to calculate the resultant vector force from the vertical and fore-aft, medial-lateral forces, as well as the force's distance (moment arm) from the joint at each instant in the cycle. This calculation requires the synchronization of force platform data and motion data and further calculation of the perpendicular distance from the force vector to the joint axis. Individual software programs have been developed for this purpose; moment calculation routines therefore vary from laboratory to laboratory.

Force platforms do not provide information about the areas of contact or pressure distribution of the foot with the ground. Assessment via Harris mat provides an inexpensive qualitative snapshot of all the areas of contact of the foot with the ground during the entire stance phase. Miniature shoe devices and in-ground pedobarographs are now available to provide quantitative means of identifying the foot's vertical forces and the area of their distribution at each instant in the stance phase. These are extremely sophisticated devices; they require multiple miniature force-measuring systems and, in 1 case, highly sophisticated miniaturized amplifier and transmitting devices. The shoe-borne devices offer the advantages of not requiring the individual to walk in a confined space and of obtaining data from multiple steps and cycles. Shoe insert systems either are mats that have multiple miniature devices that come in different sizes or they use several separate small force recorders that are placed at specific locations under the foot. Based on a quantitative picture of the pressure-distribution under the human foot, a sectorial evaluation of the pressure-distribution, including an analysis of weight, area, maximum pressure, and average pressure in the different sectors, can be reported. Standardized static and dynamic pictures of the pressure-distribution of the foot can be obtained using such devices.

The normal foot-floor force pattern of a large number of normal children, young adults, and elderly people is characterized by a marked population variability, but there is a considerable step-to-step consistency and symmetry of the forces from both feet of a given subject. The force pattern in pathologic gait secondary to disorders of the foot also has shown marked repeatability.

Selected Bibliography

Shoulder

Bankart ASB: The pathology and treatment of recurrent dislocation of the shoulder joint. *Br J Surg* 1938;26:23–29.

Basmajian JV, Bazant FJ: Factors preventing downward dislocation of the adducted shoulder joint in an electromyographic and morphological study. *J Bone Joint Surg* 1959;41A:1182–1186.

Boone DC, Azen SP: Normal range of motion of joints in male subjects. *J Bone Joint Surg* 1979;61A:756–759.

Bowen MK, Warren RF: Ligamentous control of shoulder stability based on selective cutting and static translation experiments. *Clin Sports Med* 1991;10:757–782.

Bradley JP, Tibone JE: Electromyographic analysis of muscle action about the shoulder. *Clin Sports* Med 1991;10:789–805.

Colachis SC Jr, Strohm BR: Effects of suprascapular and axillary nerve blocks on muscle force in upper extremity. *Arch Phys Med Rehabil* 1971;52:22–29.

Cooper DE, O'Brien SJ, Arnoczky SP, et al: The structure and function of the coracohumeral ligament: An anatomic and microscopic study. *J Shoulder Elbow Surg* 1993;2:70–77.

Dempster WT: Mechanisms of shoulder movement. *Arch Phys Med Rehabil* 1965;46:49–70.

DiGiovine NM, Jobe FW, Pink M, et al: An electromyographic analysis of the upper extremity in pitching. *J Shoulder Elbow Surg* 1992;1:15–25.

Flatow EL: The biomechanics of the acromioclavicular, sternoclavicular, and scapulothoracic joints, in Heckman JD (ed): *Instructional Course Lectures 42.* Rosemont, IL, American Academy of Orthopaedic Surgeons, 1993, pp 237–245.

Freedman L, Munro RR: Abduction of the arm in the scapular plane: Scapular and glenohumeral movements: A roentgenographic study. *J Bone Joint Surg* 1966;48A:1503–1510.

Fukuda K, Craig EV, An KN, et al: Biomechanical study of the ligamentous system of the acromioclavicular joint. *J Bone Joint Surg* 1986;68A:434–440.

Gerber C, Ganz R: Clinical assessment of instability of the shoulder: With special reference to anterior and posterior drawer tests. *J Bone Joint Surg* 1984;66B:551–556.

Gowan ID, Jobe FW, Tibone JE, et al: A comparative electromyographic analysis of the shoulder during pitching: Professional versus amateur pitchers. *Am J Sports Med* 1987;15:586–590.

Harryman DT II, Sidles JA, Clark JM, et al: Translation of the humeral head on the glenoid with passive glenohumeral motion. *J Bone Joint Surg* 1990;72A:1334–1343.

Harryman DT II, Sidles JA, Harris SL, et al: The role of the rotator interval capsule in passive motion and stability of the shoulder. *J Bone Joint Surg* 1992;74A:53–66.

Howell SM, Galinat BJ: The glenoid-labral socket: A constrained articular surface. *Clin Orthop* 1989;243:122–125.

Howell SM, Kraft TA: The role of the supraspinatus and infraspinatus muscles in glenohumeral kinematics of anterior shoulder instability. *Clin Orthop* 1991;263:128–134.

Howell SM, Galinat BJ, Renzi AJ, et al: Normal and abnormal mechanics of the glenohumeral joint in the horizontal plane. *J Bone Joint Surg* 1988;70A:227–232.

Inman VT, Saunders JB, Abbott LC: Observations on the function of the shoulder joint. *J Bone Joint Surg* 1944;26:1–30.

Itoi E, Motzkin NE, Morrey BF, et al: Scapular inclination and inferior stability of the shoulder. *J Shoulder Elbow Surg* 1992;1:131–137.

Jobe FW, Tibone JE, Perry J, et al: An EMG analysis of the shoulder in throwing and pitching: A preliminary report. *Am J Sports Med* 1983;11:3–5.

Kronberg M, Nemeth G, Brostrom LA: Muscle activity and coordination in the normal shoulder: An electromyographic study. *Clin Orthop* 1990;257:76–85.

Kuhlman JR, Iannotti JP, Kelly MJ, et al: Isokinetic and isometric measurement of strength of external rotation and abduction of the shoulder. *J Bone Joint Surg* 1992;74A:1320–1333.

Kumar VP, Balasubramanium P: The role of atmospheric pressure in stabilizing the shoulder: An experimental study. *J Bone Joint Surg* 1985;67B:719–721.

Matsen FA III: Biomechanics of the shoulder, in Frankel VH, Nordin M (eds): *Basic Biomechanics of the Skeletal System.* Philadelphia, Lea & Febiger, 1980, pp 221–242.

Matsen FA III, Fu FH, Hawkins RJ: *The Shoulder: A Balance of Mobility and Stability.* Rosemont, IL, American Academy of Orthopaedic Surgeons, 1993.

Matsen FA, Thomas SC, Rockwood CA Jr: Anterior glenohumeral instability, in Rockwood CA Jr, Matsen FA III (eds): *The Shoulder.* Philadelphia, PA, WB Saunders, 1990, pp 526–622.

Morrey BF, An KN: Biomechanics of the shoulder, in Rockwood CA Jr, Matsen FA III (eds): *The Shoulder.* Philadelphia, PA, WB Saunders, 1990, pp 208–245.

Ovesen J, Nielsen S: Anterior and posterior shoulder instability: A cadaver study. *Acta Orthop Scand* 1986;57:324–327.

O'Brien SJ, Neves MC, Arnoczky SF, et al: The anatomy and histology of the inferior glenohumeral ligament complex of the shoulder. *Am J Sports Med* 1990;18:449–456.

Pearl ML, Harris SL, Lippitt SB, et al: A system for describing positions of the humerus relative to the thorax and its use in the presentation of several functionally important arm positions. *J Shoulder Elbow Surg* 1992;1:113–118.

Perry J: Muscle control of the shoulder, in Rowe CR (ed): *The Shoulder.* New York, Churchill Livingstone, 1988, pp 17–34.

Perry J: Anatomy and biomechanics of the shoulder in throwing, swimming, gymnastics and tennis. *Clin Sports Med* 1983;2:247–270.

Poppen NK, Walker PS: Normal and abnormal motion of the shoulder. *J Bone Joint Surg* 1976;58A:195–201.

Poppen NK, Walker PS: Forces at the glenohumeral joint in abduction. *Clin Orthop* 1978;135:167–170.

Reeves B: Experiments on the tensile strength of the anterior capsule structures of the shoulder in man. *J Bone Joint Surg* 1968;50B:858–865.

Rockwood CA Jr, Green DP (eds): *Fractures in Adults,* ed 2. Philadelphia, PA, JB Lippincott, 1984.

Schwartz R, O'Brien SJ, Warren RF, et al: Capsular restraints to anterior/posterior motion of the shoulders. *Orthop Trans* 1988;12:727.

Shevlin MG, Lehmann JF, Lucci JA: Electromyographic study of the function of some muscles crossing the glenohumeral joint. *Arch Phys Med Rehabil* 1969;50:264–270.

Soslowsky LJ, Flatow EL, Bigliani LU, et al: Articular geometry of the glenohumeral joint. *Clin Orthop* 1992;285:181–190.

Staples OS, Watkins AL: Full active abduction in traumatic paralysis of the deltoid. *J Bone Joint Surg* 1943;25:85–89.

Turkel SJ, Panio MW, Marshall JL, et al: Stabilizing mechanisms preventing anterior dislocation of the glenohumeral joint. *J Bone Joint Surg* 1981;63A:1208–1217.

Warner JJP, Caborn DNM, Berger R, et al: Dynamic capsuloligamentous anatomy of the glenohumeral joint. *J Shoulder Elbow Surg* 1993;2:115–133.

Warner JJP, Deng XH, Warren RF, et al: Superoinferior translation in the intact and vented glenohumeral joint. *J Shoulder Elbow Surg* 1993;2:99–105.

Warren RF, Kornblatt IB, Marchand R: Static factors affecting posterior shoulder stability. *Orthop Trans* 1984;8:89.

Elbow

An K-N, Morrey BF: Biomechanics of the elbow, in Mow VC, Ratcliffe A, Woo SL-Y (eds): *Biomechanics of Diarthrodial Joints.* New York, NY, Springer-Verlag, 1990, vol 2, pp 441–464.

An K-N, Morrey BF: Biomechanics, in Morrey BF, Chao EYS (eds): *Joint Replacement Arthroplasty.* New York, NY, Churchill Livingstone, 1991, pp 257–273.

Miller MD: Basic Sciences: Part I. Biomechanics, in Miller MD (ed): *Review of Orthopaedics.* Philadelphia, PA, WB Saunders, 1992, pp 37–48.

Morrey BF, Askew LJ, Chao EY, et al: A biomechanical study of normal functional elbow motion. *J Bone Joint Surg* 1981;63A:872–877.

Morrey BF, An K-N, Chao EYS: Functional evaluation of the elbow, in Morrey BF (ed): *The Elbow and Its Disorders.* Philadelphia, PA, WB Saunders, 1985, pp 73–91.

Ries MD, Hurst LC, Dee R: Biomechanics of the elbow, in Dee R, Mango E, Hurst LC (eds): *Principles of Orthopaedics Practice.* New York, McGraw-Hill, 1989, vol 1, sec B, pp 515–519.

Wrist and Hand

Anatomy and Pathophysiology of the Intrinsic Muscles and Digital Extensor Mechanism. The American Society for Hand Surgery Syllabus, 1991, chap 1.

An KN: The effect of force transmission on the carpus after procedures used to treat Kienböck's disease. *Hand Clin* 1993;9:445–454.

An KN, Chao EY, Cooney WP, et al: Forces in the normal and abnormal hand. *J Orthop Res* 1985;3:202–211.

An KN, Berger RA, Cooney WP III (eds): *Biomechanics of the Wrist Joint.* New York, NY, Springer–Verlag, 1991.

Backhouse KM, Hutchings RT: *Color Atlas of Surface Anatomy: Clinical and Applied.* Baltimore, MD, Williams & Wilkins, 1986.

Bowers WH (ed): *The Interphalangeal Joints: The Hand and Upper Limb*. Edinburgh, Scotland, Churchill-Livingstone, 1987.

Brand PW, Hollister A (eds): *Clinical Mechanics of the Hand*, ed 2. St. Louis, MO, Mosby Year-Book, 1992.

Burkhalter WE: Median nerve palsy: Intrinsic replacement in median nerve paralysis, in Green DP (ed): *Operative Hand Surgery*, ed 3. New York, NY, Churchill Livingstone, 1992, vol 2, pp 1419–1466.

Cooney WP III, Chao EYS: Biomechanical analysis of static forces in the thumb during hand function. *J Bone Joint Surg* 1977;59A:27–36.

Cooney WP III, Linscheid RL, Dobyns JH: Fractures and dislocations of the wrist, in Rockwood CA Jr, Green DP, Bucholz RW (eds): *Rockwood and Green's Fractures in Adults*, ed 3. Philadelphia, PA, JB Lippincott, 1991, pp 563–678.

Cooney WP, Garcia-Elias M, Dobyns JH, et al: Anatomy and mechanics of carpal instability. *Surg Rounds Orthop* 1989;3:15–24.

Doyle JR: Extensor tendons: Acute injuries, in Green DP (ed): *Operative Hand Surgery*, ed 3. New York, Churchill Livingstone, 1993, vol 2, pp 1925–1954.

Froimson AI: Tenosynovitis and tennis elbow: DeQuervain's disease, in Green DP (ed): *Operative Hand Surgery*, ed 3. New York, Churchill Livingstone, 1993, vol 2, pp 1989–2006.

Hall MC (ed): *Carpo-Metacarpal, Inter-metacarpal, and Interphalangeal Joints: The Locomotor System Functional Anatomy*. Springfield, IL, Charles C. Thomas, 1965, pp 272–301.

Hoppenfeld S: Physical examination of the wrist and hand, in Hoppenfeld S, Hutton R (eds): *Physical Examination of the Spine and Extremities*. New York, NY, Appleton-Century-Crofts, 1976, pp 59–104.

Imaeda T, An KN, Cooney WP III, et al: Anatomy of trapeziometacarpal ligaments. *J Hand Surg* 1993;18A:226–231.

Kauer JM: Functional anatomy of the wrist. *Clin Orthop* 1980;149:9–20.

Lampe EW: Surgical anatomy of the hand with special references to infection and trauma. *Clin Symp* 1969;21:66–109.

Lichtman DM (ed): *The Wrist and Its Disorders*. Philadelphia, PA, WB Saunders, 1988.

Littler JW: On the adaptability of man's hand with reference to the equiangular curve. *Hand* 1973;5:187–191.

Long C II, Conrad PW, Hall EA, et al: Intrinsic-extrinsic muscle control of the hand in power grip and precision handling: An electromyographic study. *J Bone Joint Surg* 1970;52A:853–867.

Miller MD: Basic sciences: Part 1, in *Biomechanics, Review of Orthopaedics*. Philadelphia, PA, WB Saunders, 1992, pp 37–48.

Norkin CC, Levangie PK (eds): *Joint Structure and Function: A Comprehensive Analysis*. Philadelphia, PA, FA Davis, 1983.

O'Driscoll SW, Horii E, Ness R, et al: The relationship between wrist position, grasp size, and grip strength. *J Hand Surg* 1992;17A:169–177.

Palmer AK, Werner FW: Biomechanics of the distal radioulnar joint. *Clin Orthop* 1984;187:26–35.

Palmer AK, Werner FW, Glisson RR, et al: Partial excision of the triangular fibrocartilage complex. *J Hand Surg* 1988;13A:391–394.

Palmer AK, Werner FW, Murhy D, et al: Functional wrist motion: A biomechanical study. *J Hand Surg* 1985;10A:39–46.

Posner MA: Ligament injuries in the wrist and hand. *Hand Clin* 1992;8:603–828.

Ries MD, Hurst L: Biomechanics of the hand and wrist, in Dee R, Mango E, Hurst LC (eds): *Principles of Orthopaedic Practice*. New York, NY, McGraw-Hill, 1989, vol 1, pp 519–529.

Ruby LK, Cooney WP III, An KN, et al: Related motion of selected carpal bones: A kinematic analysis of the normal wrist. *J Hand Surg* 1988;13A:1–10.

Ryu JY, Cooney WP III, Askew LJ, et al: Functional ranges of motion of the wrist joint. *J Hand Surg* 1991;16A:409–419.

Sarrafian SK, Melamed JL, Goshgarian GM: Study of wrist motion in flexion and extension. *Clin Orthop* 1977;126:153–159.

Spinner M (ed): *Kaplan's Functional and Surgical Anatomy of the Hand*, ed 3. Philadelphia, PA, JB Lippincott, 1984.

Steindler A (ed): *Kinesiology of the Human Body: Under Normal and Pathological Conditions*. Springfield, IL, Charles C. Thomas, 1955.

Stern P: Fractures of the metacarpals and phalanges, in Green DP (ed): *Operative Hand Surgery*, ed 3. New York, NY, Churchill Livingstone, 1993, vol 2, p 695.

Taleisnik J (ed): *The Wrist*. New York, NY, Churchill Livingstone, 1985.

Tubiana R (ed): *The Hand*. Philadelphia, PA, WB Saunders, 1981, vol 1.

Viegas SF, Tencer AF, Cantrell J, et al: Load transfer characteristics of the wrist: Part I. The normal joint. *J Hand Surg* 1987;12A:971–978.

Youm Y, Flatt AE: Kinematics of the wrist. *Clin Orthop* 1980;149:21–32.

Youm Y, McMurtry RY, Flatt AE, et al: Kinematics of the wrist: I. An experimental study of radial-ulnar deviation and flexion-extension. *J Bone Joint Surg* 1978;60A:423–431.

Spine

Adams MA, Hutton WC: The relevance of torsion to the mechanical derangement of the lumbar spine. *Spine* 1981;6:241–248.

Ahmed AM, Duncan NA, Burke DL: The effect of facet geometry on the axial torque-rotation response of lumbar motion segments. *Spine* 1990;15:391–401.

Anderson CK, Chaffin DB, Herrin GD, et al: A biomechanical model of the lumbosacral joint during lifting activities. *J Biomech* 1985;18:571–584.

Andersson GBJ: Evaluation of muscle function, in Frymoyer JW, Ducker TB, Hadler NM, et al (eds): *The Adult Spine: Principles and Practice.* New York, NY, Raven Press, 1991, vol 1, pp 241–274.

Andersson GBJ, Chaffin DB, Pope MH: Occupational biomechanics of the lumbar spine, in Pope MH, Andersson GBJ, Frymoyer JW, et al (eds): *Occupational Low Back Pain: Assessment, Treatment and Prevention.* St. Louis, MO, Mosby Year Book, 1991, pp 20–43.

Andersson GBJ, Ortengren R, Nachemson A, et al: Lumbar disc pressure and myoelectric back muscle activity during sitting: I. Studies on an experimental chair. *Scand J Rehabil Med* 1974;6:104–114.

Andersson GB, Ortengren R, Herberts P: Quantitative electromyographic studies of back muscle activity related to posture and loading. *Orthop Clin North Am* 1977;8:85–96.

Andersson GB, Ortengren R, Schultz A: Analysis and measurement of the loads on the lumbar spine during work at a table. *J Biomech* 1980;13:513–520.

Berkson MH, Nachemson A, Schultz AB: Mechanical properties of human lumbar spine motion segments: Part II. Responses in compression and shear; influence of gross morphology. *J Biomech Eng* 1979;101:53–57.

Bland JH, Boushey DR (eds): *Disorders of the Cervical Spine: Diagnosis and Medical Management.* Philadelphia, PA, WB Saunders, 1987.

Bouisset S, Zattara M: Biomechanical study of the programming of anticipatory postural adjustments associated with voluntary movement. *J Biomech* 1987;20:735–742.

Broberg KB, von Essen HO: Modeling of intervertebral discs. *Spine* 1980;5:155–167.

Crisco JJ III, Panjabi MM: The intersegmental and multisegmental muscles of the lumbar spine: A biomechanical model comparing lateral stabilizing potential. *Spine* 1991;16:793–799.

De Luca CJ: Myoelectrical manifestations of localized muscular fatigue in humans. *Crit Rev Biomed Eng* 1984;11:251–279.

Eklund JA, Corlett EN: Shrinkage as a measure of the effect of load on the spine. *Spine* 1984;9:189–194.

el Bohy AA, Yang KH, King AI: Experimental verification of facet load transmission by direct measurement of facet lamina contact pressure. *J Biomech* 1989;22:931–941.

Freivalds A, Chaffin DB, Garg A, et al: A dynamic biomechanical evaluation of lifting maximum acceptable loads. *J Biomech* 1984;17:251–262.

Frymoyer JW, Frymoyer WW, Wilder DG, et al: The mechanical and kinematic analysis of the lumbar spine in normal living human subjects in vivo. *J Biomech* 1979;12:165–172.

Goel VK, Nishiyama K, Weinstein JN, et al: Mechanical properties of lumbar spinal motion segments as affected by partial disc removal. *Spine* 1986;11:1008–1012.

Goode JD, Theodore BM: Voluntary and diurnal variation in height and associated surface contour changes in spinal curves. *Eng Med* 1983;12:99–101.

Graves JE, Pollock ML, Carpenter DM, et al: Quantitative assessment of full range-of-motion isometric lumbar extension strength. *Spine* 1990;15:289–294.

Gregersen GG, Lucas DB: An in vivo study of the axial rotation of the human thoracolumbar spine. *J Bone Joint Surg* 1967;49A:247–262.

Gunzburg R, Hutton W, Fraser R: Axial rotation of the lumbar spine and the effect of flexion: An in-vitro and in-vivo biomechanical study. *Spine* 1991;16:22–28.

Hansson TH, Keller TS, Spengler DM: Mechanical behavior of the human lumbar spine: II. Fatigue strength during dynamic compressive loading. *J Orthop Res* 1987;5:479–487.

Hirsch C, Nachemson A: New observations on the mechanical behavior of lumbar discs. *Acta Orthop Scand* 1954;23:254–283.

Horst M, Brinckmann P: 1980 Volvo award in biomechanics: Measurement of the distribution of axial stress on the end-plate of the vertebral body. *Spine* 1981;6:217–232.

Hukins DW, Kirby MC, Skoryn TA, et al: Comparison of structure, mechanical properties, and functions of lumbar spinal ligaments. *Spine* 1990;15:787–795.

Jensen KS, Mosekilde L, Mosekilde L: A model of vertebral trabecular bone architecture and its mechanical properties. *Bone* 1990;11:417–423.

Kahanovitz N, Nordin M, Verderame R, et al: Normal trunk muscle strength and endurance in women and the effect of exercises and electrical stimulation: Part 2. Comparative analysis of electrical stimulation and exercises to increase trunk muscle strength and endurance. *Spine* 1987;12:112–118.

Kazarian LE: Creep characteristics of the human spinal column. *Orthop Clin North Am* 1975;6:3–18.

Keller TS, Hansson TH, Abram AC, et al: Regional variations in the compressive properties of lumbar vertebral trabeculae: Effects of disc degeneration. *Spine* 1989;14:1012–1019.

Keller TS, Holm SH, Hansson TH, et al: 1990 Volvo Award in experimental studies: The dependence of intervertebral disc mechanical properties on physiologic conditions. *Spine* 1990;15:751–761.

Konttinen YT, Gronblad M, Antti-Poika I, et al: Neuroimmunohistochemical analysis of peridiscal nociceptive neural elements. *Spine* 1990;15:383–386.

Krag MH: Biomechanics of the cervical spine, in Frymoyer JW, Ducker TB, Hadler NM, et al (eds): *The Adult Spine: Principles and Practice*. New York, NY, Raven Press, 1991, vol 2, pp 929–965.

Krauamer J: Pressure dependent fluid shifts in the intervertebral disc. *Orthop Clin North Am* 1977;8:211–216.

Kulak RF, Belytschko TB, Schultz AB, et al: Nonlinear behavior of the human intervertebral disc under axial load. *J Biomech* 1976;9:377–386.

Lavender SA, Mirka GA, Schoenmarklin RW, et al: The effects of preview and task symmetry on trunk muscle response to sudden loading. *Hum Factors* 1989;31:101–115.

Lin HS, Liu YK, Adams KH: Mechanical response of the lumbar intervertebral joint under physiological (complex) loading. *J Bone Joint Surg* 1978;60A:41–55.

Liu YK, Goel VK, Dejong A, et al: Torsional fatigue of the lumbar intervertebral joints. *Spine* 1985;10:894–900.

Lorenz M, Patwardhan A, Vanderby R Jr: Load-bearing characteristics of lumbar facets in normal and surgically altered spinal segments. *Spine* 1983;8:122–130.

Macintosh JE, Bogduk N: 1987 Volvo award in basic science: The morphology of the lumbar erector spinae. *Spine* 1987;12:658–668.

Macintosh JE, Bogduk N: The biomechanics of the lumbar multifidus. *Clin Biomech* 1986;1:205–213.

Maroudas A, Stockwell RA, Nachemson A, et al: Factors involved in the nutrition of the human lumbar intervertebral disc: Cellularity and diffusion of glucose in vitro. *J Anat* 1975;120:113–130.

Mayer TG, Kondraske G, Mooney V, et al: Lumbar myoelectric spectral analysis for endurance assessment: A comparison of normals with deconditioned patients. *Spine* 1989;14:986–991.

Mayer TG, Tencer AF, Kristoferson S, et al: Use of noninvasive techniques for quantification of spinal range-of-motion in normal subjects and chronic low-back dysfunction patients. *Spine* 1984;9:588–595.

Moroney SP, Schultz AB, Miller JA, et al: Load-displacement properties of lower cervical spine motion segments. *J Biomech* 1988;21:769–779.

Mosekilde L, Mosekilde L: Sex differences in age-related changes in vertebral body size, density and biomechanical competence in normal individuals. *Bone* 1990;11:67–73.

Nachemson A: Lumbar intradiscal pressure, in Jayson M (ed): *The Lumbar Spine and Back Pain*. New York, NY, Grune & Stratton, 1976, pp 257–269.

National Institute for Occupational Safety and Health: *Work Practices Guide for Manual Lifting*. Cincinnati, OH, US Department of Health and Human Services, 1981, Tech Report 81–122.

Nies N, Sinnott PL: Variations in balance and body sway in middle-aged adult: Subjects with healthy backs compared with subjects with low-back dysfunction. *Spine* 1991;16:325–330.

Ogston NG, King GJ, Gertzbein SD, et al: Centrode patterns in the lumbar spine: Baseline studies in normal subjects. *Spine* 1986;11:591–595.

Panjabi M, Aburni K, Duranceau J, et al: Spinal stablity and intersegmental muscle forces: A biomechanical model. *Spine* 1989;14:194–200.

Panjabi MM, Andersson GB, Jorneus L, et al: In vivo measurements of spinal column vibrations. *J Bone Joint Surg* 1986;68A:695–702.

Panjabi MM, Brand RA Jr, White AA III: Mechanical properties of the human thoracic spine as shown by three-dimensional load-displacement curves. *J Bone Joint Surg* 1976;58A:642–652.

Panjabi M, Dvorak J, Dranceau J, et al: Three-dimensional movements of the upper cervical spine. *Spine* 1988;13:726–730.

Panjabi MM, Krag MH, Chung TQ: Effects of disc injury on mechanical behavior of the human spine. *Spine* 1984;9:707–713.

Panjabi MM, White AA III, Johnson RM: Cervical spine mechanics as a function of transection of components. *J Biomech* 1975;8:327–336.

Parnianpour M, Nordin M, Kahanovitz N, et al: The triaxial coupling of torque generation of trunk muscles during isometric exertions and the effect of fatiguing isoinertial movements on the motor output and movement patterns. *Spine* 1988;13:982–992.

Parnianpour M, Li F, Nordin M, et al: A database of isoinertal trunk strength tests against three resistance levels in sagittal, frontal, and transverse planes in normal male subjects. *Spine* 1989;14:409–411.

Pearcy MJ, Bogduk N: Instantaneous axes of rotation of the lumbar intervertebral joints. *Spine* 1988;13:1033–1041.

Penning L: Functional anatomy of joints and discs, in The Cervical Spine Research Society Editorial Committee (eds): *The Cervical Spine*, ed 2. Philadelphia, PA, JB Lippincott, 1989, pp 33–56.

Pope MH, Andersson GB, Broman H, et al: Electromyographic studies of the lumbar trunk musculature during the development of axial torques. *J Orthop Res* 1986;4:288–297.

Pope MH, Frymoyer JW, Lehmann TR: Structure and function of the lumbar spine, in Pope MH, Andersson GBJ, Frymoyer JW, et al (eds): *Occupational Low Back Pain: Assessment, Treatment and Prevention.* St. Louis, MO, Mosby Year Book, 1991, pp 3–19.

Pope MH, Svensson M, Andersson GB, et al: The role of prerotation of the trunk in axial twisting efforts. *Spine* 1987;12:1041–1045.

Pope MH, Wilder DG, Matteri RE, et al: Experimental measurements of vertebral motion under load. *Orthop Clin North Am* 1977;8: 155–167.

Posner I, White AA III, Edwards WT, et al: A biomechanical analysis of the clinical stability of the lumbar and lumbosacral spine. *Spine* 1982;7:374–389.

Reid JG, Costigan PA: Trunk muscle balance and muscle force. *Spine* 1987;12:783–786.

Ritchie JH, Fahrni WH: Age changes in lumbar intervertebral discs. *Can J Surg* 1970;13:65–71.

Roy SH, De Luca CJ, Casavant DA: Lumbar muscle fatigue and chronic lower back pain. *Spine* 1989;14:992–1001.

Schultz A, Andersson GB, Ortengren R, et al: Analysis and quantitative myoelectric measurements of loads on the lumbar spine when holding weights in standing postures. *Spine* 1982;7:390–397.

Schultz A, Cromwell R, Warwick D, et al: Lumbar trunk muscle use in standing isometric heavy exertions. *J Orthop Res* 1987;5:320–329.

Schultz AB, Warwick DN, Berkson MH, et al: Mechanical properties of human lumbar spine motion segments: Part I. Responses in flexion, extension, lateral bending and torsion. *J Biomech Eng* 1979; 101:46–52.

Seidel H, Beyer H, Brauer D: Electromyographic evaluation of back muscle fatigue with repeated sustained contractions of different strengths. *Eur J Appl Physiol* 1987;56:592–602.

Seroussi RE, Pope MH: The relationship between trunk muscle electromyography and lifting moments in the sagittal and frontal planes. *J Biomech* 1987;20:135–146.

Smidt GL, Blanpied PR, White RW: Exploration of mechanical and electromyographic responses of trunk muscles to high-intensity resistive exercise. *Spine* 1989;14:815–830.

Smith JL, Smith LA, McLaughlin TM: A biomechanical analysis of industrial manual materials handlers. *Ergonomics* 1982;25:299–308.

Snook SH: Low back pain in industry, in White AA III, Gordon SL (eds): American Academy of Orthopaedic Surgeons *Symposium on Idiopathic Low Back Pain.* St. Louis, MO, CV Mosby, 1982, pp 23–38.

Soukka A, Alaranta H, Tallroth K, et al: Leg-length inequality in people of working age: The association between mild inequality and low-back pain is questionable. *Spine* 1991;16:429–431.

Thurston AJ, Harris JD: Normal kinematics of the lumbar spine and pelvis. *Spine* 1983;8:199–205.

Urban JP, Holm S, Maroudas A, et al: Nutrition of the intervertebral disc: An in vivo study of solute transport. *Clin Orthop* 1977;129: 101–114.

White AA III, Panjabi MM: The basic kinematics of the human spine: A review of past and current knowledge. *Spine* 1978;3:12–20.

White AA III, Panjabi MM (eds): *Clinical Biomechanics of the Spine,* ed 2. Philadelphia, PA, JB Lippincott, 1991.

Wilder DG, Pope MH, Frymoyer JW: The biomechanics of lumbar disc herniation and the effect of overload and instability. *J Spinal Disord* 1988;1:16–32.

Yang JF, Winter DA, Wells RP: Postural dynamics in the standing human. *Biol Cybern* 1990;62:309–320.

Zetterberg C, Andersson GB, Schultz AB: The activity of individual trunk muscles during heavy physical loading. *Spine* 1987;12: 1035–1040.

Hip

Crowninshield RD, Johnston RC, Andrews JG, et al: A biomechanical investigation of the human hip. *J Biomech* 1978;11:75–85.

Das De S, Bose K, Balasubramaniam P, et al: Surface morphology of Asian cadaveric hips. *J Bone Joint Surg* 1985;67B:225–228.

Davy DT, Kotzar GM, Brown RH, et al: Telemetric force measurements across the hip after total arthroplasty. *J Bone Joint Surg* 1988; 70A:45–50.

Figge FHJ: *Atlas of Human Anatomy,* ed 8. New York, NY, Hafner Publishing, 1968, vol 1.

Hardt DE: Determining muscle forces in the leg during normal human walking: An application and evaluation of optimization methods. *J Biomech Eng* 1978;100:72–78.

Hodge WA, Carlson KL, Fijan RS, et al: Contact pressures from an instrumented hip endoprosthesis. *J Bone Joint Surg* 1989;71A: 1378–1386.

Patriarco AG, Mann RW, Simon SR, et al: An evaluation of the approaches of optimization models in the prediction of muscle forces during human gait. *J Biomech* 1981;14:513–525.

Paul JP, McGrouther DA: Force actions transmitted by joints in the human body. *Proc R Soc Lond [Biol]* 1976;192:163–172.

Pedotti A, Krishnan VV, Stark L: Optimization of muscle-force sequencing in human locomotion. *Math Biosci* 1978;38:57–76.

Rydell NW: Forces acting on the femoral head-prosthesis: A study on strain gauge supplied prostheses in living persons. *Acta Orthop Scand* 1966;88(suppl):1–132.

Knee

Arms S, Boyle J, Johnson R, Pope M: Strain measurement in the medial collateral ligament of the human knee: An autopsy study. *J Biomech* 1983;16:491–496.

Bartel DL, Marshall JL, Schieck RA, Wang JB: Surgical repositioning of the medial collateral ligament: An anatomical and mechanical analysis. *J Bone Joint Surg* 1977;59A:107–116.

Brantigan OC, Voshell AF: The tibial collateral ligament: Its function, its bursae, and its relation to the medial meniscus. *J Bone Joint Surg* 1943;25:121–131.

Butler DL, Noyes FR, Grood ES: Ligamentous restraints to anterior-posterior drawer in the human knee: A biomechanical study. *J Bone Joint Surg* 1980;62A:259–270.

Daniel DM, Akeson WH, O'Connor JJ (eds): *Knee Ligaments: Structure, Function, Injury, and Repair.* New York, NY, Raven Press, 1990.

Daniel DM, Malcom LL, Losse G, Stone ML, Sachs R, Burks R: Instrumented measurement of anterior laxity of the knee. *J Bone Joint Surg* 1985;67:720–726.

Feagin JA Jr: *The Crucial Ligaments: Diagnosis and Treatment of Ligamentous Injuries About the Knee.* New York, NY, Churchill Livingstone, 1988.

Frankel VH, Nordin M (eds): *Basic Biomechanics of the Skeletal System.* Philadelphia, PA, Lea & Febiger, 1980.

Fu FH, Harner CD, Johnson DL, Miller MD, Woo SL: Biomechanics of knee ligaments: Basic concepts and clinical application. *J Bone Joint Surg* 1993;75A:1716–1727.

Fukubayashi T, Torzilli PA, Sherman MF, Warren RF: An in vitro biomechanical evaluation of anterior-posterior motion of the knee: Tibial displacement, rotation, and torque. *J Bone Joint Surg* 1982;64A:258–264.

Girgis FG, Marshall JL, Monajem A: The cruciate ligaments of the knee joint: Anatomical, functional and experimental analysis. *Clin Orthop* 1975;106:216–231.

Hollinshead WH (ed): *Anatomy for Surgeons: The Back and Limbs.* New York, NY, Hoeber-Harper, 1954.

Hughston JC, Bowden JA, Andrews JR, Norwood LA: Acute tears of the posterior cruciate ligament: Results of operative treatment. *J Bone Joint Surg* 1980;62A:438–450.

Insall JN, Windsor RE, Scott WN, Kelly MA, Aglietti P (eds): *Surgery of the Knee,* ed 2. New York, NY, Churchill Livingstone, 1993.

Kaplan EB: The iliotibial tract: Clinical and morphological significance. *J Bone Joint Surg* 1958;40A:817–832.

Markolf KL, Burchfield DM, Shapiro MM, Davis BR, Finerman GA, Slauterbeck JL: Biomechanical consequences of replacement of the anterior cruciate ligament with a patellar ligament allograft. Part I: Insertion of the graft and anterior-posterior testing. *J Bone Joint Surg* 1996;78A:1720–1727.

Nicholas JA, Hershman EB (eds): *The Lower Extremity and Spine in Sports Medicine.* St. Louis, MO, CV Mosby, 1986.

Odensten M, Gillquist J: Functional anatomy of the anterior cruciate ligament and a rationale for reconstruction. *J Bone Joint Surg* 1985;67A:257–262.

Scuderi GR (ed): *The Patella.* New York, NY, Springer-Verlag, 1995.

Veltri DM, Deng XH, Torzilli PA, Maynard MJ, Warren RF: The role of the popliteofibular ligament in stability of the human knee: A biomechanical study. *Am J Sports* Med 1996;24:19–27.

Warren LF, Marshall JL: The supporting structures and layers on the medial side of the knee: An anatomical analysis. *J Bone Joint Surg* 1979;61A:56–62.

Foot and Ankle

Allard P, Thiry PS, Duhaime M: Estimation of the ligaments' role in maintaining foot stability using a kinematic model. *Med Biol Eng Comput* 1985;23:237–242.

Allard P, Eng P, Stokes IAF, et al: Modelling of the foot and ankle, in Jahss ME (ed): *Disorders of the Foot & Ankle: Medical and Surgical Management,* ed 2. Philadelphia, PA, WB Saunders, 1991.

Andrews JG: On the specification of joint configurations and motions. *J Biomech* 1984;17:155–158.

Attarian DE, McCrackin HJ, Devito DP, et al: Biomechanical characteristics of human ankle ligaments. *Foot Ankle* 1985;6:54–58.

Barnett CH, Napier JR: The axis of rotation at the ankle joint in man: Its influence upon the form of the talus and the mobility of the fibula. *J Anat* 1952;86:1–9.

Benink RJ: The constraint mechanism of the human tarsus: A roentgenological experimental study. *Acta Orthop Scand* 1985;569(suppl 215):1–135.

Bojsen-Møller F: Calcaneocuboid joint and stability of the longitudinal arch of the foot at high and low gear push off. *J Anat* 1979;129:165–176.

Cass JR, Morrey BF, Chao EYS: Three-dimensional kinematics of ankle instability following serial sectioning of lateral collateral ligaments. *Foot Ankle* 1984;5:142–149.

Castaing J, Delplace J, Le Roy JD: *La Cheville.* Paris, France, Edition Vigot, 1960.

Cavanagh PR, Rodgers MM: Pressure distribution underneath the human foot, in Perren SM, Schneider E (eds): *Biomechanics: Current Interdisciplinary Research.* Doredrecht, The Netherlands, Martinus Nijhoff Publishers, 1985.

Close JR, Inman VT, Poor PM, et al: The function of the subtalar joint. *Clin Orthop* 1967;50:159–179.

Close JR, Todd FN: The phasic activity of the muscles of the lower extremity and the effect of tendon transfer. *J Bone Joint Surg* 1959; 41A:189–208.

Duckworth T, Betts RP, Franks CI, et al: The measurement of pressures under the foot. *Foot Ankle* 1982;3:130–141.

Dul J, Townsend MA, Shiavi R, et al: Muscular synergism: I. On criteria for load sharing between synergistic muscles. *J Biomech* 1984; 17:663–673.

Dul J, Johnson GE, Shiavi R, et al: Muscular synergism: II. A minimum fatigue criterion for load sharing between synergistic muscles. *J Biomech* 1984;17:675–684.

Grundy M, Tosh BP, McLeish RD, et al: An investigation of the centres of pressure under the foot while walking. *J Bone Joint Surg* 1975;57B: 98–103.

Hicks JH: The mechanics of the foot: I. The joints. *J Anat* 1953;87:345–357.

Hicks JH: The mechanics of the foot: II. The plantar aponeurosis and the arch. *J Anat* 1954;88:25–30.

Hicks JH: The mechanics of the foot: IV. The action of muscles on the foot in standing. *Acta Anat* 1956;27:180–192.

Hicks JH: The foot as a support. *Acta Anat* 1955;25:34–45.

Huson A: Functional anatomy of the foot, in Jahss MH (ed): *Disorders of the Foot & Ankle: Medical and Surgical Management,* ed 2. Philadelphia, PA, WB Saunders, 1991.

Huson A, Van Langelaan EJ, Spoor CW: The talocrural and tarsal mechanism and tibiotalar delay. *Acta Morphol Neerl-Scand* 1986;24: 296.

Mann R, Inman VT: Phasic activity of intrinsic muscles of the foot. *J Bone Joint Surg* 1964;46A:469–481.

Mann RA, Baxter DE, Lutter LD: Running symposium. *Foot Ankle* 1981;1:190–224.

Mann R: Overview of foot and ankle biomechanics, in Jahss MH (ed): *Disorders of the Foot & Ankle: Medical and Surgical Management,* ed 2. Philadelphia, PA, WB Saunders, 1991.

Rasmussen O: Stability of the ankle joint: Analysis of the function and traumatology of the ankle ligaments. *Acta Orthop Scand* 1985; (suppl 211):1–75.

Stiehl JB (ed): *Inman's Joints of the Ankle,* ed 2. Baltimore, MD, Williams & Wilkins, 1991.

Stott JR, Hutton WC, Stokes IA: Forces under the foot. *J Bone Joint Surg* 1973;55B:335–344.

Wright DG, Desai SM, Henderson WH: Action of the subtalar and ankle-joint complex during the stance phase of walking. *J Bone Joint Surg* 1964;46A:361–382

Coordinated Functions

Frank JS, Earl M: Coordination of posture and movement. *Phys Ther* 1990;70:855–863.

Friedli WG, Cohen L, Hallett M, et al: Postural adjustments associated with rapid voluntary arm movements: I. Electromyographic data. *J Neurol Neurosurg Psychiatry* 1984;47:611–622.

Friedli WG, Hallett M, Simon SR: Postural adjustments associated with rapid voluntary arm movements. II. Biomechanical analysis. *J Neurol Neurosurg Psychiatry* 1988;51:232–241.

Horak FB: Clinical measurement of postural control in adults. *Phys Ther* 1987;67:1881–1885.

Mann RA, Hagy J: Biomechanics of walking, running and sprinting. *Am J Sports Med* 1980;8:345–350.

Mansour JM, Lesh MD, Nowak MD, et al: A three-dimensional multisegmental analysis of the energetics of normal and pathological human gait. *J Biomech* 1982;15:51–59.

Martin JP: A short essay on posture and movement. *J Neurol Neurosurg Psychiatry* 1977;40:25–29.

Morrison JB: Bioengineering analysis of force actions transmitted by the knee joint. *Biomed Eng* 1968;3:464–470.

Murray MP: Gait as a total pattern of movement. *Am J Phys Med* 1967; 46:290–333.

Murray MP, Seireg AA, Sepic SB: Normal postural stability and steadiness: Quantitative assessment. *J Bone Joint Surg* 1975;57A:510–516.

Nashner LM: Balance adjustments of humans perturbed while walking. *J Neurophysiol* 1980;44:650–664.

Nashner LM, McCollum G: The organization of human postural movement: A focal basis and experimental synthesis. *Behav Brain Sci* 1985;8:135–172.

Nashner LM: Adaptations of human movement to altered environments. *Trends Neurosci* 1982;3:358–361.

Pedotti A, Krishnan BV, Stark L: Optimization of muscle-force sequencing in human locomotion. *Math Biosci* 1978;38:57–76.

Perry J: *Gait Analysis: Normal and Pathological Function.* Thorofare, NJ, SLACK, 1992.

Pierrynowski MR, Morrison JB: Estimating the muscle forces generated in the human lower extremity when walking: A physiological solution. *Math Biosci* 1985;75:43–68.

Saunders JB, Inman VT, Eberhart HD: The major determinants in normal and pathological gait. *J Bone Joint Surg* 1953;35A:543–558.

Seireg A, Arvikar RJ: The prediction of muscular load sharing and joint forces in the lower extremities during walking. *J Biomech* 1975;8:89–102.

Sutherland DH, Olshen R, Cooper L, et al: The development of mature gait. *J Bone Joint Surg* 1980;62A:336–353.

Thorstensson A, Nilsson J, Carlson H, et al: Trunk movements in human locomotion. *Acta Physiol Scand* 1984;121:9–22.

Winter DA: *The Biomechanics and Motor Control of Human Gait: Normal, Elderly and Pathological.* Waterloo, Ontario, Canada, University of Waterloo Press, 1991.

Woollacott MH, Shumway-Cook A: Changes in posture control across the life span: A systems approach. *Phys Ther* 1990;70:799–807.

Glossary

— A —

accommodating resistance exercise A type of exercise that isolates a joint and constrains the muscle action so that the joint is moved at a constant angular velocity. The limits of this angular velocity can be set by a servocontrolled dynamometer (*also called* an isokinetic dynamometer).

accuracy The closeness of a measured reading, score, or observation to the true value.

action potential The propagating electrical potential that develops when a muscle or nerve cell is activated; the summation of nearly synchronous action potentials is referred to as a compound muscle, nerve, or sensory nerve action potential, according to the fibers activated.

active tension The amount of tension generated in muscle as a result of muscle activation (*See* passive tension).

adhesin Microbial surface structure, usually in the form of pili or fimbriae, that binds to specific receptors on epithelial cell membranes, providing for cell attachment (also to other surfaces).

adsorption Adherence of atoms, ions, or molecules to the surface of another substance.

aerobic glycolysis The metabolism of glucose to pyruvate in the presence of oxygen, with the final oxidation of its products through the mitochondrial Krebs cycle and electron transport.

afferent Toward the central nervous system.

aggrecan A large proteoglycan consisting of a protein core substituted with many glycosaminoglycan chains, and possessing the ability to form aggregates with hyaluronate and link protein.

alkaline phosphatase An enzyme that functions in skeletal mineralization as well as having numerous other biological roles.

alloantigen An antigen arising from intraspecies genetic variations (polymorphism).

allograft (*also called* homograft) A tissue or an organ transplanted between individuals of the same species, but genetically nonidentical (*See* isograft).

α (significance level) The probability of Type 1 error in an experiment involving hypothesis testing.

Amonton's law Three empirical observations regarding the nature of dry friction (1699).

amplification An increase in the amount of DNA or RNA replicated; implies a stimulated process of replication meant to produce extra DNA or RNA.

anabolic steroid Natural and synthetic sex hormones that promote protein synthesis and enhance the growth of tissue, especially muscle.

anaerobic glycolysis The metabolism of glucose in the absence of oxygen with the final oxidation to lactic acid through cytosolic glycolysis.

analysis of variance (ANOVA) The analytic method for determining whether means obtained from various samples are equivalent.

anelastic material A material without a well-defined relationship between stress and strain.

aneuploid A cell or group of cells with an abnormal amount of DNA compared with that of a normal cell, either more or less than haploid, diploid, or tetraploid.

angiogenin A factor that stimulates vessel formation.

anisotropic material A material in which the properties differ depending on direction; for example, material with oriented fibers embedded in a matrix.

annealing Heat treatment that renders metals softer and more ductile by relieving residual stresses.

anodal block Local block of nerve conduction caused by hyperpolarization of the nerve cell membrane by an electric stimulus.

anode The positive electrode and more reactive metal in a corrosion cell or battery, it is oxidized, gives up electrons, and is degraded; the positive pole of the stimulating electrode in a nerve conduction study.

anterograde From the neuronal cell body toward the axonal target.

antibody (*also called* immunoglobulin) Immune protein made by B cells in response to the presence of antigens, designed to recognize a specific antigen and lead to its elimination.

antidromic Propagation of an impulse in the direction opposite to physiologic conduction; conduction along motor nerve fibers away from the muscle and along sensory fibers away from the spinal cord.

antigen Substance capable of evoking an immune reaction.

antioncogene (*also called* recessive oncogene; tumor suppressor gene) Gene whose presence normally prevents neoplasia and whose absence or malfunction leads to the production of a neoplasm.

apophyseal growth plate Growth plate under tensile force that produces growth of nonlong bones.

apparent density The density (mass/total volume) of a porous material even though the mass occupies only a small portion of the total volume.

apoptosis Cell death induced by a series of programmed signalling events, leading to removal of cellular debris without stimulation of immune processes.

area moment of inertia (*also called* second moment of area) Resistance to bending that is solely a function of geometry, independent of material properties, and is inversely proportional to the stress caused by bending.

atactic Orientation of a polymer in which side groups are distributed on both sides of a macromolecular chain.

ATP (Adenosine 5′-triphosphate) A nucleotide whose high-energy phosphate bonds are used in metabolism to supply energy or many physiologic reactions.

attrition The wearing away of a material by friction.

autocrine A growth factor or biologically active molecule produced by a cell, it acts locally to stimulate the same cell by which it is produced.

autograft A tissue or an organ transplanted into a new position within or on the same individual.

average (x) A value, calculated from a sample, that estimates the population mean.

axon The central core of axoplasm that constitutes the conducting element of a nerve fiber; it is bounded by a surface membrane called the axolemma.

axon hillock Region of the cell body from which the axon originates, often the site of impulse initiation.

axoplasmic transport Intracellular movement of materials, both distally and centrally, within the axoplasm.

— B —

basal lamina Thin layer of extracellular matrix material, primarily collagen, laminin, and fibronectin, that surrounds muscle cells and Schwann cells; also underlies all epithelial sheets.

bending Deformation caused by transverse loading of a structure or by bending moments.

bending moment A force that tends to produce a moment to bend an object.

β (**significance level**) The probability of type 2 error in a hypothesis testing experiment.

beta-oxidation A metabolic pathway for the breakdown of long-chain fatty acids.

biglycan A small proteoglycan that consists of a short protein core and two dermatan sulfate side chains.

bioabsorbable material A material whose breakdown products are incorporated into normal physiologic and biochemical processes.

biocompatible material A material that can function in a biologic environment without known and/or significant detrimental effects on either the material or the living system.

biodegradable material A material that breaks down when placed in a biologic environment.

bioelectric potential An electric potential, generated by cellular elements and cellular metabolism, that depends on cellular viability.

biomaterial A natural biologic material or a synthetic material used to replace, treat, or augment tissue and/or organ function.

bioresorbable material A material that is broken down in vivo and removed from the implantation site.

biotribology Study of friction, lubrication, and wear of contacting biologic structures, particularly diarthrodial joints.

biphasic material A material composed of a solid phase and a fluid phase; for example, articular cartilage and meniscus.

bone densitometry General term indicating techniques for measuring bone density; the assessment of bone quantity.

bone histomorphometry Histologic quantitation of volumes, surfaces, and cell numbers involved in bone formation and resorption.

bone mass Quantity of bone in the entire skeleton.

bone modeling unit (BMU) A group of osteoblasts, osteocytes, and osteoclasts that are linked and participate in remodeling (activation, resorption, and formation) of a discrete area of bone.

bone morphogenic proteins (BMP) A family of growth and differentiation factors belonging to the TGF-β super family, which stimulates bone and cartilage differentiation and bone growth.

boundary lubrication Separation of the sliding contacts of two bodies by a layer of adsorbed molecules on each surface.

brittle Sustaining little or no permanent deformation prior to failure.

bulk modulus Proportionality constant between change of volume per unit volume and the applied pressure, analogous to Young's modulus.

— C —

calcitonin A protein produced by parafollicular cells of the thyroid that decreases serum calcium by inhibiting osteoclast activity and accelerates growth plate calcification.

cambium The inner cellular layer of the periosteum that interfaces with bone.

capacitance (C) The property that permits storage of electrical energy as a result of electric displacement when opposite surfaces of conducting plates separated by an insulator carry opposite electrical charges; it is determined by the area of the two plates and the distance between them and is measured in farads (F); increasing or decreasing the distance between plates will increase the capacitance.

carbohydrate A compound of carbon, hydrogen, and oxygen: $(CH_2O)_n$; the most important dietary carbohydrates are starches, sugars, and celluloses.

carbohydrate loading An exercise and diet regimen that elevates muscle glycogen by regulating exercise level and emphasizing dietary carbohydrate.

carcinogen Agent associated with an increase in cancer production.

casting Fabrication of parts by pouring molten material (such as metal) into molds.

cathode The negative electrode and less reactive metal in a corrosion cell, it is reduced and does not corrode; the negative pole of the stimulating electrode in nerve conduction studies.

centroid The point at which an object's geometry may be considered to be concentrated; for an object with uniform density, the centroid is located at the center of mass.

ceramic Inorganic, ionically bonded materials often have a metallic oxide component.

channel Pathway through a membrane allowing passage of ions or molecules.

chemokine A polypeptide factor with a chemotactic activity, usually for cells of the immune system (monocytes, neutrophils, T or B cells).

chemotaxis The movement of a cell up or down a concentration gradient of a chemical agent.

χ^2-statistic The statistic used in frequency analysis to compare expected proportions.

chondrocalcinosis The excessive presence of calcium salts in cartilaginous structures of joints.

chondron The region within articular cartilage that contains the chondrocyte or a group of chondrocytes and its pericellular and territorial matrices.

chromosome A nuclear structure containing a linear strand of DNA; humans have 46 chromosomes (23 pairs).

coefficient of determination (r^2) The "goodness of fit" statistic that represents the total fraction of the data explained by a linear relationship.

coefficient of friction The resistance of relative motion of two objects in contact measured by dividing the frictional force by the compressive load (*See* Amonton's law).

cold flow Plastic deformation during creep.

collagen A large family of genetically distinct proteins, each of which has a triple helix fibrillar component, and which form a major proportion of the organic matrix of bone, cartilage, tendon, ligament, and skin.

collagenase Metalloprotease that cleaves native collagen in the triple helical region.

component of a force The magnitude of force in a specific direction; in three dimensions, a force has three components.

compliance The inverse stiffness (m/N); the motion caused by a load divided by that load.

compression A force tending to squeeze or crush an object.

concentration cell An electrochemical cell arising from unequal electrolyte concentrations between compartments.

concentric activation (*also called* concentric action) The shortening of a muscle during activation (*See* eccentric activation).

conduction (g) The readiness with which an electric current is conducted; the reciprocal of resistance: g = 1/R.

conduction velocity Speed of propagation of an action potential along a nerve or muscle fiber.

contact guidance Notion that axon outgrowth is directed by mechanical features of the local environment.

contact healing (*also called* primary bone healing) A term previously used to indicate healing of a fracture without callus formation when bone fragments are touching.

copolymer Macromolecules composed of more than one type of monomer.

correlation coefficient (r) The "goodness of fit" statistic that represents the degree to which the experimental data fit a line; the square root of the coefficient of determination; positive for positive slopes and negative for negative slopes.

corrosion Electrochemical destruction of a metal.

couple The moment formed by two parallel forces of equal magnitude and opposite direction; a pure moment with a resultant force of zero.

coupling Motion in which rotation or translation of a rigid body about one axis is associated with rotation or translation of that same rigid body about another axis.

covalent bond Atomic bonding produced by the sharing of a pair of electrons between two adjacent atoms.

crack A flaw or hole inside or on the surface of an object.

cramp An involuntary (painful) condition of muscle characterized by a powerful activation of the muscle.

creep A viscoelastic property of materials whereby the deformation continues to increase, without the loss of material, when subjected to a constant force.

cross-linking Association of adjacent polymers through covalent bonds.

current (I) The amount of charge moved per unit of time; in biologic systems it is carried by ions and flows in the direction of the positive ions; measured in amperes (A).

cytokine Generic term for proteins that mediate cell function by binding to specific cell-surface receptors; a group of growth factors; this term replaces the earlier used terms lymphokine and monokine (See interleukin).

— D —

dalton (d) Measurement of molecular mass in which 1 dalton = 0.9997 mass unit or one sixteenth of the mass of oxygen 16.

Darcy's law Linear relationship between fluid flux and pressure gradient.

decorin A small proteoglycan that contains a short protein core and one dermatan sulfate side chain; it coats the surfaces of collagen fibers.

degree of freedom The number of independent quantities needed to describe the position of an object; for example, six degrees of freedom describe the position of any segment of the body in three dimensions (three angles and three coordinates of a point on the body). When there are constraints, the degrees of freedom will be reduced accordingly; in one degree of freedom a rigid body either translates back and forth along a straight line or rotates clockwise and counterclockwise.

depolarization Reduction in the magnitude of the resting membrane potential toward zero.

descriptive statistics Numeric expressions that serve to describe a sample; for example, mean (x).

desmosome A small, discrete, circular, dense body that forms the site of attachment between certain epithelial cells.

differential melting Surface melting results from the brief application of heat from an external source.

diffusion bonding Adhesion of two materials in contact by the movement of surface atoms between them.

dilatation An increase or decrease in volume per unit volume.

diploid Twice haploid; the amount of DNA in a normal resting human cell (the G_0/G_1 phase of the cell cycle).

DNA (deoxyribonucleic acid) A nucleic acid that constitutes the genetic material of all cellular organisms and the DNA viruses; it is the autoreproducing component of chromosomes and of many viruses.

dominant oncogene A proto-oncogene that when mutated (altered) transforms the cell to a malignant phenotype by a variety of mechanisms; for example, by acting as a growth factor.

Donnan ion distribution Concentration of counter-ions in the interstitium resulting from charges fixed on the porous-permeable solid matrix.

Donnan osmotic pressure Component of swelling pressure resulting from excess ionic particles due to Donnan ion distribution within the interstitium.

drag coefficient Proportionality factor between drag force and flow speed.

dual-energy x-ray absorptiometry (DEXA) Radiographic technique that measures bone density and cross-sectional geometry.

ductile Capacity to sustain large amounts of permanent deformation without failing.

dynamic shear modulus Response of a viscoelastic material resulting from sinusoidal excitation.

dynamics Study of relationships between forces, moments, and motions of objects.

— E —

eccentric activation (also called eccentric action) Muscle activation with simultaneous muscle lengthening.

efferent Away from the central nervous system.

eicosanoids Biologically active substances derived from arachidonic acid, including the prostaglandins and leukotrienes.

elastic deformation Deformation that disappears when the stress is removed.

elastic limit Strain beyond which permanent deformation occurs.

elastic modulus Measure of material stiffness defined by dividing stress (measured in pascals) by strain; for linear materials, it is the slope of the stress-strain curve.

elastohydrodynamic lubrication Condition that occurs when the deformation of bearing surfaces becomes important in hydrodynamic lubrication.

electrodiagnosis Recording and analysis of responses from nerves and muscle to electric stimulation, and identification of patterns of insertion, spontaneous, involuntary, and voluntary action potentials.

electromyography Recording and study of insertion, spontaneous, and voluntary electric activity of muscle.

endochondral ossification Bone development through the formation of a cartilage model.

endomysium Connective tissue surrounding the muscle cell.

endoneurial tube Term describing the endoneurial sheath and the column of tissue it encloses.

endoneurium Connective tissue that forms the supporting framework for the nerve fibers and capillaries inside a fascicle.

endotenon A loose connective tissue that surrounds individual fascicles of a tendon.

endurance limit Repetitive stress that can be endured indefinitely by a material; for stresses below the endurance limit, fatigue life is theoretically infinite.

engineering stress Applied force divided by unstressed (original) area.

enhancer Portion of DNA that assists in initiating transcription (constructing mRNA from DNA), but is not necessary for the process.

enzyme A protein molecule that catalyzes a chemical reaction of other substances without itself being destroyed or altered during the reaction; the six main groups are oxidoreductases, transferases, hydrolases, lyases, isomerases, and ligases.

epigenesis Production of a neoplasm due to the expression of genes present in the genome, but not normally activated or expressed.

epimysium Connective tissue surrounding the entire muscle.

epineurium Connective tissue that envelops the nerve and extends internally to separate and enclose individual fascicles so that they are embedded in it.

epiphysis The end of a long bone formed by the secondary center of ossification and covered by articular cartilage.

equilibrium Point at which the sum of all forces and moments acting on an object equals zero; such that $\Sigma F = 0$ and $\Sigma M = 0$.

equilibrium potential Membrane potential at which there is no net passive movement of a permanent ion species into or out of a cell.

equipollent force system System in which the action of a force about a point p is equivalent to the force acting at that point plus a couple that is equal to the moment of the force about the point p.

ergotism Poisoning from excessive or misdirected use of ergot as a medicine or from eating ergotized grain containing the fungus *Claviceps purpura*; characterized by necrosis of the extremities caused by contractions of the peripheral vascular bed.

exon Portion of a gene that codes for mRNA.

— F —

F-statistic The statistic created by the ratio of two variances, it can be used in ANOVA to compare whether a number of means are equivalent.

facultative Ability to live under more than one set of environmental conditions.

fascicle Bundle of nerve fibers and their related endoneurial tissue.

fasciculation Random spontaneous twitching of a group of muscle fibers or a motor unit.

fast-glycolytic (FG) fiber A fast-twitch muscle fiber characterized by low aerobic and high anaerobic capacities.

fast-oxidative glycolytic (FOG) fiber A fast-twitch muscle fiber characterized by high aerobic activity and moderate anaerobic activity.

fast-twitch (FT) muscle fiber A muscle fiber characterized by fast contraction time in response to electrical stimulation of the nerve and muscle.

fatigue Structural failure caused by repetitive stresses below the ultimate strength.

fibrillation A small, local, involuntary muscle contraction resulting from spontaneous activation of single muscle fibers.

fibroblast growth factor (FGF) Peptide hormone derived from the pituitary and from cartilage; it is a potent stimulator of proliferation.

fibronectin A glycoprotein found in connective tissue matrices, including bone, fibrous tissue, and cartilage, that is also a major component of serum. Fibronectin is synthesized by many connective tissue cells, including osteoblasts, and may play a role in cell-matrix interactions during osteoblast maturation.

flow-dependent viscoelasticity Creep and stress-relaxation phenomena resulting from interstitial fluid flow through porous-permeable material, for example, articular cartilage.

flow-independent viscoelasticity (*also called* intrinsic viscoelasticity) Creep and stress-relaxation phenomena resulting from molecular rearrangement within the solid matrix of a porous-permeable material.

fluorocytometry A technique used to measure cells, nuclei, or other cellular components that are prelabeled with a fluorochrome and passed single-file through an exciting wavelength of light; the amount of fluorescence emitted from each cell is directly proportional to the cellular content of the component (DNA, proteins, etc.) under investigation.

force A type of vector that describes a push or pull; for example, a push with a magnitude of 10 pounds, acting from left to right.

forging Fabrication by plastic deformation.

fracture Failure resulting from the unbounded growth of a crack.

fracture toughness A material property that is measured by the energy required to cause crack propagation in the material.

free-body diagram Partial model of an object that is used to isolate it from the environment to explore all the forces that act on it.

frequency analysis The analytic technique that determines the probability that certain numbers of frequencies of observations are independent.

friction Resistance to relative sliding motion between two surfaces in contact.

F wave Long-latency motor response resulting from antidromic activation of α motoneurons in the spinal cord.

— G —

gap healing Healing by bone formation across a reduced fracture where gap exists.

gene A segment of a DNA molecule that contains all the information required for synthesis of a product (polypeptide chain of RNA molecule), including both coding and noncoding sequences.

gene enhancer Regions of a gene that regulate rates of transcription.

gene promotor Regulatory portion of DNA that is found adjacent to the transcription start site of a gene and that controls initiation of transcription.

genome The complete complement of genetic information of an organism.

germ line defect An inherited DNA mutation that is present in the DNA of all cells in the organism; the resulting alteration is usually subtle and not recognized at birth.

glass An amorphous, undercooled liquid of extremely high viscosity that has all the appearance of a solid.

glass transition temperature (T_g) The temperature at which the behavior of an amorphous material changes from brittle to viscous.

glia Neuroglia; supporting structure of nerve tissue composed of astrocytes and oligodendrocytes in the central nervous system, Schwann cells in the peripheral nervous system, and satellite cells in ganglia.

glycosaminoglycan (GAG) Repeating units of sulfated disaccharides, including keratan sulfate, dermatan sulfate, heparan sulfate, chondroitin 4-sulfate and chondroitin 6-sulfate; varying numbers of GAGs are covalently bound to serine residues of core proteins unique to each proteoglycan (eg, aggrecan).

graded potential Local change in the membrane potential of a neuron.

groove of Ranvier Cells that surround the cartilaginous component of the growth plate at the junction between the reserve and proliferative zones and function in the circumferential enlargement of the growth plate.

ground electrode Electrode placed between the stimulating and recording electrodes in nerve conduction studies.

growth cone Specialized end of a growing axon (or dendrite) that generates the motive force for elongation.

growth factor Polypeptides that are released by certain cells and bind to specific cell membrane receptors to stimulate cell division.

growth plate (*also called* physis; epiphyseal plate) A cartilaginous structure composed of a proliferative and a hypertrophic zone that produces a large extracellular matrix, which serves as a template for bone formation (*See* endochondral ossification).

— H —

haploid The amount of DNA in a normal human egg or sperm cell, or half that found in a normal cell.

hardness A surface property of a material that impacts resistance to penetration or scratching.

haversian bone Mature bone formed by whole or fractured osteons usually arranged longitudinally.

haversian canal Freely anastomosing channels within cortical bone containing blood vessels, lymph vessels, and nerves.

helical axis *See* screw axis.

Hertz (Hz) Unit of frequency equivalent to one cycle per second.

heterogenous Nonuniform.

heterograft *See* xenograft.

histocompatibility complex *See* human leukocyte antigen.

homograft *See* allograft.

Hooke's laws A linear relationship, $F = kx$, defining the response of an elastic material between load (F) and deformation (x), where k is a constant that defines the stiffness of the material.

hot isostatic pressing Consolidation under high temperature and pressure of metal powder into a fine-grained material.

H reflex Electrically-evoked spinal monosynaptic reflex involving the Ia afferent fibers from the muscle spindles and motor axons.

human leukocyte antigen (HLA) The human major histocompatibility complex, which lies on chromosome 6 and is divided into four main regions, A, B, C, and D, each encoding for different types of cell surface molecules.

hyaline cartilage A cartilage composed of a smooth, glasslike extracellular matrix in which the predominant type of cartilage is type II collagen. Articular cartilage is a hyaline cartilage.

hyaluronic acid (or hyaluronan) A linear polymer of repeating disaccharide units consisting of N-acetyl glucosamine and glucuronic acid, molecular weights in excess of 10^6 daltons. Serves as backbone for the formation of proteoglycan aggregates in the extracellular matrix.

hybridoma Activated B-lymphocyte (plasma cell) combined with myeloma cell to produce an immortal population of cells capable of producing a single specific antibody.

hydrodynamic lubrication Separation of sliding contacts between two bodies by a layer of lubricant in the form of a liquid or gas.

hydrogen bond Secondary noncovalent bond in which a hydrogen atom is attracted to electrons of neighboring atoms.

hydroxyapatite (*also called* apatite) Naturally occurring mineral $[Ca_{10}(PO_4)_6(OH)_2]$ found as the major inorganic constituent of bone matrix.

hyperplasia An abnormal increase in the number of cells in a tissue or organ.

hypertrophic zone That portion of the growth plate in which the chondrocytes enlarge and matrix calcification occurs.

hypertrophy An abnormal increase in the size of a cell or organ.

hypophosphatasia A genetic deficiency in alkaline phosphatase resulting in deficient cartilage mineralization and a clinical picture similar to rickets.

hysteresis Conversion of strain energy to heat during cyclic loading; that is, mechanical energy is lost during each cycle.

— I —

immunity In materials, resistance to corrosion.

indirect calorimetry A method of estimating metabolic rate and energy sources by measuring the amount of oxygen used by the body.

instant center of rotation (ICR) The point about which an object appears to be rotating; this concept is valid only for two-dimensional motion.

insulin-like growth factors (IGF) Peptides that are structurally similar to insulin and stimulate cell proliferation.

integrins Transmembrane proteins that function in the attachment of cells to the extracellular matrix and in the transduction of mechanical stimuli in cellular metabolism.

interleukin Polypeptide mediator in the class designated as cytokines; most interleukins are regulators of the immune response, including inflammatory mechanisms.

intramembranous ossification Bone formation directly within a fibrous mesenchymal connective tissue.

interneuron Neuron that intervenes between sensory and effector neurons.

intron Portion of a gene that does not code for mRNA.

ionic bond Atomic bonding through coulombic attraction of oppositely charged ions.

isograft A tissue or an organ transplanted between genetically identical individuals.

isokinetic A term used to describe the conditions of muscle activation; when applied to isolated muscles, it implies a constant velocity of shortening or lengthening, and when applied to the action of muscles moving joints, it implies a constant angular velocity of joint rotation.

isometric A term used to describe the conditions of muscle activation; when applied to isolated muscle, it implies that the muscle length is held constant, and when applied to the action of muscles moving joints, it implies that the angular position is set at a given position and not allowed to rotate.

isotactic Orientation of a polymer in which all side groups are on one side of the carbon chain.

isotonic A term used to describe the conditions of muscle activation; when applied to isolated muscles, it implies that the load on the muscle is constant, and when applied to the action of muscles moving joints, it implies that the load-resisting angular rotation of the joint is constant.

isotropy Having the same material properties independent of direction.

— J —

jitter Variability with consecutive discharges of the interpotential interval between two muscle fiber action potentials belonging to the same motor unit.

— K —

k-space Frequency domain as opposed to spatial domain.

kinematics Description of motion, regardless of how the motion came about.

kinesiology Study of motion in the human body.

kinetics Study of the forces that bring about motion.

Krebs cycle (*also called* tricarboxylic acid cycle; citric acid cycle) A sequence of chemical reactions in the metabolic pathways degrading glucose to carbon dioxide and water.

kurtosis The degree to which the variability of a distribution matches the variability of a normal distribution.

— L —

lamellar bone Organized bone so named because of its laminar appearance.

latency Interval between the onset of a stimulus and the onset of a response.

leptokurtotic Kurtosis of a distribution in which a greater number of observations are obtained near the tails of the distribution than near the mean.

lineal strain (ε) Change of length (Δl) divided by original length (l_o), such that $\varepsilon = \Delta l / l_o$; in three dimensions, there are three lineal strains.

linear regression The analytic technique whereby a line is fit through a data set yielding a correlation coefficient and a *p* value.

link protein Small globular protein that associates with the core protein of an aggrecan molecule and hyaluronate to form a stable proteoglycan aggregate.

linkage analysis The use of marker genes associated with a restriction fragment length polymorphism to locate an abnormal gene in the same chromosome; the inheritance pattern of the clinical features of the disorder must be known.

loss modulus Amount of energy lost per unit volume in a viscoelastic material as a result of sinusoidal excitation over one cycle.

lubrication Reduction of frictional resistance by an interposed material (lubricant).

lyophilization (*also called* freeze drying) The process of drying a sample by freezing the solution and evaporating the ice under a vacuum.

— M —

major histocompatibility complex (MHC) A cluster of genes important in immune recognition and signaling between cells of the immune system; originally identified as a locus encoding molecules present on cell surfaces, such that animals that differed at this locus would rapidly reject each other's tissue grafts.

material property Any physical characteristic of an object's substance, for example, heat conduction, diffusivity, thermal expansion, and melting point, that is independent of the object's structure and geometry.

matrix vesicle Small membrane-bound vesicles found in the extracellular matrix of the hypertrophic zone of the growth plate. They are derived from the plasma membrane of bone cells and chondrocytes; they sequester calcium and have a role in matrix mineralization.

maximal oxygen consumption The maximal rate at which oxygen can be consumed by an exercising individual, indicative of the aerobic system of that individual.

mean (μ) A number that typifies a set of numbers, such as an arithmetic mean or average.

mechanical property A subset of material properties that relates stresses to strains; for linear elastic materials, the proportionality constants are Young's modulus, shear modulus, Poisson's ratio, etc.

membranous bone formation Bone formation without a cartilaginous template (*See* intramembranous ossification).

mesenchyme Embryonic mesodermal tissue forming a network of cells. In the adult, mesenchymal stem cells reside in the bone marrow and give rise to osteocytes, chondrocytes, adipocytes, fibrocytes, and myocytes.

mesotenon (*also called* mesotendineum) The synovial layer that passes from the tendon to the wall of the tendon sheath.

messenger RNA (mRNA) An RNA molecule that transmits information from DNA to the protein synthesis machinery of the cell.

metallic bond Interatomic bond in metals characterized by delocalized electrons shared by many atoms.

metalloproteinase Class of degradative enzymes (collagenases, stromelysin, and gelatinases) that depend on zinc for enzyme activity and are important for normal matrix turnover as well as for the pathologic degradation of the cartilage matrix in both articular and growth plate tissue.

mineralization The addition of mineral deposits on already deposited mineral nuclei.

mitogen An agent that stimulates DNA synthesis and cell division.

modulus Proportional constant between stresses and strains; for example, Young's modulus, shear modulus, bulk modulus.

molecular weight Mass, in grams, of 6.02×10^{23} (Avogadro's number) molecules; for polymers, the average molecular size; M_n is the number-average molecular weight and M_2 is the weight-average molecular weight.

moment (*also called* torque) The tendency of a force, measured in N•m or ft-lb, to cause rotations about an axis; a vector having a magnitude defined by the product of the magnitude of the force and the perpendicular distance between the axis and the line of application of the force.

moment of inertia Resistance of a geometric shape to deformation; solely a function of geometry, independent of material properties (*See* area moment of inertia).

monomer The smallest repeating unit in a polymer.

motion segment The basic anatomic unit of the spine, it comprises two vertebrae and their intercalated soft tissue; the functional spinal unit.

motoneuron Nerve cell that innervates skeletal muscle.

motor end plate The synapse between a motoneuron and a muscle fiber.

motor point The anatomic site at which the motor nerve enters the muscle; the point over a muscle at which a contraction may be elicited by a minimal-intensity, short-duration electric stimulus.

motor unit An alpha motoneuron and the muscle fibers innervated by it.

motor unit territory Muscle area over which muscle fibers belonging to an individual motor unit are distributed.

mucopolysaccharidoses A group of genetically inherited diseases that are characterized by a deficiency of enzymes responsible for the degradation of polysaccharides, resulting in the accumulation of undegraded glycosaminoglycans in the lysosome.

multivariate analysis An analytic technique that operates on a number of variables simultaneously; for example, stepwise linear regression.

muscle activation The process by which muscle shortens or resists lengthening by mechanisms involving contractile protein interactions and metabolic energy.

muscle contraction The attempt of muscle to shorten and generate tension in response to activation, although the muscle may actually remain the same length or lengthen if the opposing load is large enough.

muscle fatigue Inability of muscle to maintain a given force or exercise intensity due to factors in the muscle itself or in the peripheral or central nervous systems.

muscle twitch A brief period of contraction followed by relaxation in the response of a motor unit to a stimulus (nerve impulse).

mutagen An agent that causes an alteration (mutation) in the DNA, which can lead to neoplasia.

mutagenesis The introduction of an alteration into an organism's genome, resulting in a structural and functional change of the encoded protein.

M wave Short latency orthodromic response resulting from antidromic activation of alpha motoneurons in the spinal cord; compound action potential evoked from a muscle by a single electric stimulus to its motor nerve.

myositis ossificans Development of heterotopic bone in muscle.

— N —

nerve fiber The connecting unit of a nerve composed of a central core, the axon, enveloped in a complex covering comprised of a single layer of Schwann cells, a basement membrane, and a sheath of endoneurial tissue.

neuropathy Nerve lesions not caused by physical injury; may be a consequence of toxic and metabolic disturbances and primary vascular disease.

neurapraxia Failure of nerve conduction, usually reversible, caused by metabolic or microstructural abnormalities without disruption of the axon.

neurotmesis Partial or complete severance of a nerve, with disruption of the axons, their myelin sheaths, and the supporting connective tissue; results in degeneration of the axons distal to the injury site.

neutral axis The line of intersection between the plane of loading on a beam and the neutral plane.

neutral plane The plane within a bent beam on which the stress is zero; this plane divides the compressive and tensile regions within the beam.

newton A unit of force named after Sir Isaac Newton in which 1 N = 0.225 lb.

newtonian fluid A fluid in which the shear stress (τ) is linearly proportional to the rate of shear (γ), and the viscosity (η) may depend on temperature: $\tau = \eta\gamma$.

node of Ranvier Localized area devoid of myelin that occurs at intervals along a myelinated axon.

normal distribution The probability distribution described by the function:

$$y = \frac{e^{\frac{-(x-\mu)^2}{2\sigma^2}}}{\sigma\sqrt{2\pi}}$$

which represents the probability of obtaining an observation a certain distance away from the mean within a standard sample.

normal stress A force acting perpendicular to the area of interest divided by that area.

Northern hybridization A method to quantitate the levels of specific mRNA species in a tissue or cell population, while using chemically or radiologically labeled rDNA fragments complementary to the target.

nucleation The first deposition of mineral crystal in cartilage or bone matrix.

nucleotide A compound composed of a base (purine or pyrimidine), a sugar (ribose or deoxyribose), and a phosphate group.

— O —

Ohm's law Relates current (I) to voltage (V) and resistance (R); V = IR.

oncogene Either of two types of abnormal genes (proto-oncogenes and antioncogenes) associated with the production of a neoplasm.

orthodromic Propagation of an impulse in the direction of physiologic conduction; conduction along motor nerve fibers towards the muscle and along sensory nerve fibers toward the spinal cord.

osteoblast An active bone-forming cell that produces type I collagen, responds to parathyroid hormone, and releases osteocalcin when stimulated by 1,25-dihydroxyvitamin D_3.

osteocalcin (bone gla protein) A bone matrix protein synthesized by osteoblasts, characterized by vitamin K dependent gamma-carboxylated glutamic residues that give this protein mineral-binding properties. This protein is thought to be important in mineralization.

osteoclast A multinucleated bone cell that resorbs bone matrix when activated.

osteocyte A mature bone cell surrounded by bone matrix and active in bone mineral homeostasis.

osteogenesis imperfecta A genetic defect in type I collagen metabolism that results in bone fragility.

osteoid Unmineralized bone matrix.

osteomalacia Condition characterized by insufficiently mineralized bone matrix, although the mass of bone can be normal, decreased, or increased (*See* rickets).

osteon A haversian canal with its concentrically arranged lamellae.

osteopenia Generic term that describes neither a specific disease state nor a diagnosis, but a radiographic appearance of decreased bone density.

osteopontin A bone matrix glycoprotein that is synthesized by cells in the osteoblast lineage and is expressed strongly just prior to mineralization and may regulate this process. It may also be important in osteoblast and osteoclast attachment to the matrix.

osteoporosis A decrease in bone mass per unit volume of normally mineralized bone.

outcomes research A type of clinical research in which specific outcomes (such as range of motion, patient satisfaction, or subjective pain) are used as measures of the success of a particular clinical treatment.

— P —

paracrine Local action of molecules (such as growth factors) that are produced by one cell on another cell within the same tissue.

paramagnetic agent An atom or molecule with unpaired electrons that, when placed in a magnetic field, generates its own small magnetic field that adds and/or subtracts from the main magnetic field.

paratenon The material that separates the tendon from the sheath.

parathyroid hormone (PTH) A protein produced by the parathyroid gland, it is important in calcium metabolism and bone homeostasis.

pascal A measure of pressure or stress in the formula $Pa = N/m^2$; $MPa = 10^6 Pa = N/mm^2 = 145$ psi, $GPa = 10^9 Pa$.

passive tension The tension generated in stretched muscle due to the inherent properties of the tissue and not to muscle activation.

pennation angle The angle of muscle fibers with respect to the direction of the resultant force of the muscle-tendon unit.

perichondral ring of LaCroix The fibrous structure that surrounds the cartilaginous portion of the growth plate, is contiguous with the periosteum of the metaphysis, and lends mechanical support to the growth plate.

perimysium Connective tissue surrounding a fascicle.

perineural Around the nerve trunk.

perineurium Thin sheath of specialized perineurial or lamellar cells, arranged in concentric layers, that encircle a bundle of nerve fibers.

permeability coefficient The proportionality constant (k) between volume fluid per unit area and pressure gradient, it determines the ease of fluid flow through a porous material; it is inversely related to diffusive drag coefficient (K) by: $k = \phi^2/K$, where ϕ is porosity.

p-glycoprotein A molecule embedded in the cell membrane encoded by the MOR-1 gene, it actively pumps certain classes of molecules, drugs, or toxins from the cell's cytoplasm.

phenotype Physical characteristics expressed by an individual.

phosphocreatine (PC) A chemical compound stored in muscle. It serves to store energy in the form of high-energy phosphate bonds. Hydrolysis of these bonds allows use of this energy for the formation of ATP and thus for use in muscle contraction.

physeal growth plate Growth plate that produces long bone growth under compressive force (*See* growth plate).

physiochemical forces Forces derived from the charged nature of constituents within a material; for example, charged proteoglycan gives rise to Donnan osmotic pressure and charge-to-charge repulsion.

physiologic cross-sectional area (PCSA) The sum of the cross-sectional areas of all the muscle fibers in the muscle; it is calculated by dividing the muscle's volume by the length of individual muscle fibers.

piezoelectric potential An electric potential generated by the deformation of a solid material that contains fixed charges but is neutral because of the presence of counterions or electrons.

plasmid An extrachromosomal element that replicates and is transferred independently of the host (bacterial) chromosome and usually is not essential to the host's basic functioning; independent piece of DNA (usually nonhuman) that can replicate.

plastic deformation Permanent change in shape of an object even after the load has been removed.

platelet-derived growth factor (PDGF) Glycoprotein growth factor produced by mesenchymal cells or released by platelets during clotting. It stimulates cell proliferation and chemotaxis in cartilage, bone, and many other cell types.

platykurtotic A distribution property in which a greater number of observations are obtained near the mean than near the tails of the distribution.

point mutation An alteration in the genomic DNA at a single nucleotide; depending on the base change (A to T or G to C), it may or may not alter the genetic code and resulting protein product.

Poisson's ratio A material property defining the lateral expansion (or contraction) of a deformable object transverse (at 90°) to the direction of loading; when an object is stretched, it also will contract in the transverse direction, and vice versa.

polar moment of inertia Resistance to twisting; it is solely a function of geometry, independent of material properties; the stress caused by torsion is proportional to the applied torque and inversely proportional to the polar moment of inertia.

polygeneic inheritance Effects of multiple genes and alleles interacting with environmental factors to influence form, function, and incidence of any trait.

polymer Molecule composed of many repeating units (mers).

polymerase chain reaction (PCR) A method for the repetitive synthesis of specific DNA sequences in vitro.

polymorphism The variability of nucleic acid sequences among different individuals. Polymorphisms are usually silent, ie, they do not lead to structural or functional abnormalities.

population In statistics, the entire collection of elements about which information is desired.

porosity Ratio of void (or fluid) volume to apparent (total) volume of a porous material (*See* solidity).

power grip The forceful finger flexion used to maintain an object against the palm of the hand.

precess The motion of the rotation axis of a rigid body, as a spinning top, when a disturbing force is applied while the body is rotating; the rotation axis, moving in a cone with one end of the rotating body at its vertex.

precision The closeness of repeated measurements of the same quantity; the repeatability of a particular measurement.

precision grip Grip associated with fine tactile sensibility at the fingertips; requires fine kinesthetic control; does not involve the palm.

prehension The grasping or taking hold of an object between any two surfaces of the hand.

primary bone healing *See* contact healing.

primary ossification center Site of initial bone formation in the cartilaginous template of a bone.

primary spongiosa Woven bone formed on calcified cartilage during endochondral ossification.

proliferative zone A region of the growth plate primarily responsible for longitudinal growth through chondrocyte proliferation.

promotor DNA sequences upstream of the coding sequences that are necessary for binding of RNA polymerase, and thus initiation of transcription.

proportional limit The end of the linear range of the stress-strain curve.

prospective study An experimental study in which the data are acquired after the experimental design is proposed.

protein A macromolecule linked in a linear array.

proteoglycan Major constituent of the organic matrix of all connective tissues; plays a major role in the structural and biologic properties of the tissue. Member of a family of macromolecules consisting of a core protein and covalently linked glycosaminoglycan side chains.

proteoglycan aggregate A complex composed of proteoglycans, hyaluronate, and link proteins.

proto-oncogene A normal gene that when initiated becomes an oncogene; a dominant oncogene.

p **value** The probability obtained from a statistical analysis that a type 1 error will occur.

— Q —

quantitative computed tomography (QCT) Quantitative measurement of bone density at various sites using CT images.

quantitative ultrasound Ultrasound technique dedicated to measure ultrasound attenuation or speed of sound in bone. This technique provides an assessment of bone density and strength.

— R —

rad (radiation absorbed dose) Unit of absorbed dose of ionizing radiation equal to an energy of 100 ergs per gram of irradiated material; 100 rads = 1 joule/kg = 1 Gy.

radiogrammetry Technique used to measure bone dimensions on radiographs.

radiographic absorptiometry Technique used to measure bone density on conventional or digital radiographs.

Rb gene (retinoblastoma gene) The oncogene (recessive) associated with retinoblastoma and an oncogene associated with some cases of osteosarcoma.

recessive oncogene An antioncogene.

reciprocal inhibition Simultaneous inhibition of antagonists and excitation of homonymous and synergistic motoneurons.

recombinant DNA A DNA fragment that is removed from its original source and ligated with DNA from another source.

recruitment An increase in muscular force by adding (recruiting) the activities of more motoneurons and motor units of the central nervous system in response to a prolonged stimulus.

recrystallization The formation of new annealed grains in metals from strain-hardened grains.

recrystallization temperature Temperature above which recrystallization is spontaneous, and which depends on the specific material and the strain state.

reference electrode Electrode placed distal to the active recording electrode on the tendon during motor nerve conduction studies and over the nerve during sensory studies.

rem Dosage of ionizing radiation that will cause the same biologic effect as one roentgen of x-ray or gamma radiation dosage; for clinical diagnostic radiographic procedures, 1 rem = 1 rad.

repeated measures Measurements that are taken from a population from the same sampling element; for example, measuring blood pressure in the same individuals over time.

reserve zone Portion of the growth plate consisting of sparse regularly shaped chondrocytes in an abundant matrix; its functions are storage and matrix production.

resilience The capacity of strained material to recover its size and shape after the deforming load is removed.

resistance (R) The hindrance to movement of electrical charges measured in ohms (Ω); its strength depends on the material through which the particles are moving. Current flowing through a resistance will produce a voltage: V = IR.

resting membrane potential Voltage across the membrane of an excitable cell at rest.

restriction enzyme Endonuclease that cleaves DNA at specific sites, producing restriction fragments.

restriction fragment length polymorphism (RFLP) Variation in the lengths of DNA restriction fragments because of differences in the nucleic acid sequence.

retrograde From the axon terminal toward the cell body.

retrospective study An experiment in which the data are already acquired by the time the specific experiment is designed.

rickets Condition characterized by insufficient mineralization of growth plate in the immature skeleton (*See* osteomalacia).

RNA (ribonucleic acid) Nucleic acid composed of ribonucleotide monomers, each containing ribose, a phosphate group, and a purine or pyrimidine; found in all cells (in the nucleus and cytoplasm) in particulate and nonparticulate form, and also in many viruses.

roentgen (R) Unit of radiation exposure equal to 2.58×10^{-4} coulombs/kg of air; applies only to X and gamma irradiation below 3 meV.

rotation Revolving motion of an object about a point or an axis.

— S —

sample A collection of individual observations selected in accordance with a specified procedure.

sample size (n) The number of independent observations that make up a sample; sample size is related to statistical power in hypothesis testing.

sarcolemma Muscle-cell membrane and its associated basement membrane.

screw axis (*also called* helical axis) Any motion can be resolved into a rotation and a translation. In three dimensions, an object's motion may be described as a combination of rotation about an axis and translation parallel to the same axis. This unique axis is called the screw axis.

scurvy A nutritional disorder caused by a deficiency of vitamin C.

secondary ossification center Located usually at the ends of bones, a site of bone formation in the cartilaginous template of a bone, which occurs after primary ossification.

secondary spongiosa Trabecular lamellar bone formed after the resorption of the primary spongiosa.

selectivity Ability of an axon to chose appropriately among potential synaptic partners.

semicrystalline A polymer conformation consisting of ordered regions in a matrix of randomly oriented chains; the degree of crystallinity has a strong effect on the mechanical properties.

shear modulus (G or μ) The proportionality constant between shear stress and shear strain.

shear strain Change of angle between two lines inscribed in a material, which were originally at 90°; in three dimensions, there are three shear strains.

shear stress A force acting parallel to the area of interest divided by that area.

shear thinning Decrease in viscosity with increasing shear rate.

SI units (*also called* System International units) Units of physical quantities; commonly force, Newton (N) = 0.225 lb; length, meter (m) = 39.37 in; time, seconds (s); and stress, pascal (Pa) = N/m^2 = 1.45×10^{-4} psi.

significance level (α) The probability of type 1 error in an experiment involving hypothesis testing.

single x-ray absorptiometry (SXA) X-ray technique dedicated to measuring bone density in the peripheral skeleton.

sintering A method by which high pressure produces the temperatures used to bond particulate matter into a solid.

sinusoidal excitation A periodic (sine function) deformation or stress imposed on a material.

size principle The principle governing an increase in muscle activation by central nervous system recruitment of motor nerves and motor units in order of size from smallest to largest.

skew The property of a distribution that "leans" either to the right or to the left; skewed distributions are, by definition, not normally distributed.

slow-oxidative (SO) muscle fiber A slow-twitch muscle fiber characterized by fatigue resistance and high aerobic capacity.

slow-twitch (ST) muscle fiber A muscle fiber characterized by high aerobic capacity and low anaerobic capacity.

s-n curve Plot of fatigue stress (s) versus number (n) of cycles to failure.

solidity Ratio of solid volume to apparent (total) volume of a porous material (*See* porosity).

somatic defect An abnormality that is present only in the cells of the abnormal tissue of the organism with the neoplasia, not in the normal cells.

Southern hybridization (*also called* Southern blot) Detection of a specific DNA sequence (target sequence) using a fragment of radioactively labeled single-stranded DNA (a probe), which binds to the complementary target sequence, creating a DNA-DNA hybrid (*See* Northern hybridization).

splicing Removal of intronic sequences from newly transcribed RNA, resulting in the production of mRNA.

spring A linear elastic structure in which the force-deformation relationship is defined by F = kx, where k is the stiffness.

squeeze-film lubrication Type of lubrication in which two bearing surfaces are loaded perpendicular to each other, causing the lubricant to be squeezed from the gap.

standard deviation (s) The square root of the sample variance; a measure of population variability that is expressed in terms of the original measurement units.

standard error of the mean (SEM) The error associated with estimating the mean value of a sample.

statics Study of structures in mechanical equilibrium.

statistical power (1-β) The probability that, if a negative result is obtained, it truly represents a negative result and not simply inadequate sample size.

stem cell A cell type that when it divides creates a daughter cell with a variety of differentiation potentials and another stem cell. These cells have the ability of self-renewal and regeneration.

stiffness Resistance of a structure to a deformation.

stimulus artifact In nerve conduction studies, deflection from the baseline resulting from direct conduction of the stimulus.

storage modulus Amount of energy stored per unit volume in a viscoelastic material as a result of sinusoidal excitation over one cycle.

strain Measure of deformation having six components (three lineal strain and three shear strain).

strain energy The amount of energy stored in a loaded material associated with the deformation of the material from its undeformed state.

strain energy density Work required to produce a given strain in a unit volume of a material under load, expressed in $Joules/meter^3 = Newtons/meter^2$.

strain rate Speed at which a material is deformed.

streaming potentials Electrical potentials produced by the flow of an electrolyte fluid through a porous charged matrix; the material itself is neutral because of the presence of counterions and electrons.

strength Maximum resistance to strain before mechanical failure begins.

stress A physical quantity defined as force per unit area (F/A) and consisting of six components: three normal stresses and three shear stresses (*See* tensor).

stress concentration Increased level of stress around a flaw caused by the presence of that flaw, such as a crack, hole, or discontinuity (*See* stress riser).

stress relaxation Decrease in stress at constant strain by internal molecular rearrangement.

stress riser A flaw (crack, hole, or discontinuity) in a material that increases local stress (*See* stress concentration).

stress shielding A decrease in physiologic stress in a biologic material caused when a stiffer structure (such as a rod, plate, or implant) acts in parallel with the biological material (such as bone tissue).

stress-strain plot The experimental data relating stress (F/A) to strain ($\Delta l/l$).

stromelysin (MMP-3) Member of the metalloprotease family with broad substrate specificity. It degrades many components of the extracellular matrix, including aggrecans but not collagen fibrils.

structure Any object of finite size and consisting of geometrically shaped materials; for example, a bridge, airplane, femur, tibia, or humerus.

subchondral bone The bone of the epiphysis underlying and supporting articular cartilage.

swelling An increase (or decrease) of size, weight, or water content of an object as a result of changing environmental conditions; for example, changes in ion concentration.

swelling pressure of cartilage Sum of Donnan osmotic pressure and charge-to-charge repulsive forces in cartilage.

synapse A specialized apposition between a neuron and its target cell for transmission of information by release and reception of chemical transmitter agent.

syndiotactic Orientation of a polymer in which the side groups are on alternate sides of the macromolecular chain.

— T —

tan δ A property of viscoelastic materials that measures the ratio of loss modulus to the storage modulus; δ = phase angle.

temporal dispersion Relative desynchronization resulting from different rates of conduction of two or more synchronously evoked components of a compound action potential from the stimulation point to the record electrode.

tensile strength The maximum stress reached before a specimen in a uniaxial tensile test begins to fail.

tension A force tending to elongate an object; a pull.

tensor A mathematical quantity representing stresses and strains; in three dimensions it has six independent components.

tetanus The contractile condition of muscle in which a higher frequency of stimulation produces no increase in the muscle force.

tetraploid Four times haploid, or twice the amount of DNA in a normal resting human cell; the amount of DNA in a normal human cell in G_2 phase of the cell cycle.

threshold Term generally used to refer to the voltage level at which an action potential is initiated in a single axon or a group of axons; operationally defined as the intensity that produces a response in about 50% of equivalent trials.

tidemark Demarcation between the deep uncalcified and calcified zones of articular cartilage; it appears as one or more wavy lines on histologically stained tissues.

tissue inhibitor of metalloproteinase (TIMP) A family of naturally occurring inhibitors of metalloproteases.

torque Synonym to moment of a force (*See* moment *and* couple).

torsion Deformation caused by twisting (torquing) of a shaft.

toughness Qualitative term for the ability of a material to absorb energy before failure; usually associated with large deformations; for example, rubber or plastic.

transcription The production of a complementary RNA molecule from a DNA template, which occurs in the nucleus of eukaryotic cells and is mediated by the enzyme RNA polymerase.

transformation Inserting into a bacterium a plasmid (independent self-replicating DNA) with added recombinant DNA.

transforming growth factors A group of growth factors originally discovered because of their ability to stimulate independent growth. It is now known that their major role is that of growth and differentiation factors. The TGF-β family constitutes a large family of structurally and functionally related growth factors. A major subgroup are the bone morphogenic proteins (BMPs).

transgene A gene that is not normally found in an organism, but was artifically placed into the single-celled embryo and therefore is present in all cells of that organism.

transgenic animal An animal that develops from a fertilized egg into which a foreign gene (transgene) has been inserted.

translation (biologic) The process of protein synthesis using the sequence information specified in mRNA. This process is mediated by a complex machinery assembled on ribosomes.

translation (mechanical) Linear motion of an object without rotation.

transverse isotropy Isotropy in a plane, with material properties distinctly different along the axis perpendicular to this plane; for example, laminated structures such as mica or cortical bone.

trophic Ability of one tissue or cell to support another; usually applied to long-term interactions between pre- and postsynaptic cells.

tropic An influence of one cell or tissue on the direction of movement or outgrowth of another.

tropism Orientation of growth in response to an external stimulus.

tropocollagen A word previously used to describe a single collagen molecule that results from the winding of three alpha chains.

t-**statistic** The statistic used to compare two means obtained from two different samples.

tumor suppressor gene A gene coding for a protein that inhibits (suppresses) the growth of transformed cells. These proteins are often involved in the control of cell division in normal cells.

twitch A brief contractile response of a skeletal muscle elicited by a single volley of impulses in the neurons supplying it.

type I fiber A slow-oxidative (SO) muscle fiber.

type II fiber A fast-oxidative glycolytic (FOG) or fast-glycolytic (FG) muscle fiber.

— U —

ultimate strain Maximum strain sustained by the specimen prior to failure of the material.

ultimate stress Maximum stress (resistance divided by the original area) sustained by a specimen prior to failure of the material.

unit cell The smallest repetitive volume that possesses the symmetry of a crystal lattice.

univariate analysis Any statistical analytic technique that operates on a single variable at a time; for example, one-way analysis of variance.

— V —

van der Waals forces Weak secondary forces that attract neutral atoms and molecules.

variable The actual property measured by means of individual observations.

variance (s^2) The variance measure of the spread of data about the sample mean.

variate A single reading, score, or observation of a given variable.

vector A plasmid designed to transfer specific fragments of DNA into a bacterial or prokaryotic host.

viscoelastic In biology, a property of a tissue that exhibits both viscous and elastic behavior (creep and stress relaxation); the material's stress-strain behavior depends on strain rate.

viscosity (η) Resistance (τ) offered by a fluid to shearing (γ), given by Newton's law for viscous fluids: $\tau = \eta\gamma$.

viscous A property of the fluid that offers resistance to flow; for example, frictional drag.

vitreous Glassy or amorphous.

vitrification Solidification by cooling to produce an amorphous, glassy material.

voltage The potential for separated charges to do work; the amount of work done by an electric charge when moving from one point to another measured in volts (V).

voxel Volume element of an image (ie, pixel $\times$ slide thickness).

— W —

wear Unintended removal of surface material during normal functional use.

wear debris Particles produced by wear.

Wolff's law A law that states that the remodeling of bone or soft tissue is influenced and modulated by mechanical stresses.

work hardening Increased hardness (and strength) from plastic deformation at ambient temperature.

woven bone Immature bone without laminar or osteonal organization.

— X —

xenograft (*also called* heterograft) Material transplantation between individuals of different species.

yield strength (*also called* yield stress) Stress necessary to cause plastic flow.

— Y —

Young's modulus (E) The intrinsic stiffness of a linear material in tension or compression expressed as the ratio of stress to strain: E = stress/strain.

Index

Page references followed by t or f indicate
tables or figures, respectively.

— A —